Oxford Textbook of
Osteoarthritis and Crystal Arthropathy

THIRD EDITION

Edited by

Michael Doherty

Johannes Bijlsma

Nigel Arden

David J. Hunter

Nicola Dalbeth

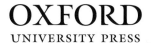

OXFORD
UNIVERSITY PRESS

Great Clarendon Street, Oxford, OX2 6DP,
United Kingdom

Oxford University Press is a department of the University of Oxford.
It furthers the University's objective of excellence in research, scholarship,
and education by publishing worldwide. Oxford is a registered trade mark of
Oxford University Press in the UK and in certain other countries

First Edition published in 1998
Second Edition published in 2003

Impression: 1

Published in the United States of America by Oxford University Press
198 Madison Avenue, New York, NY 10016, United States of America

British Library Cataloguing in Publication Data
Data available

Library of Congress Control Number: 2016939454

ISBN 978–0–19–966884–7

Printed in Great Britain by
Bell & Bain Ltd., Glasgow

Contents

Abbreviations

AAOS	American Academy of Orthopaedic Surgeons		EOA	erosive osteoarthritis
ACE	angiotensin-converting enzyme		ePi	extracellular inorganic phosphate
ACL	anterior cruciate ligament		ePPi	extracellular inorganic pyrophosphate
ACR	American College of Rheumatology		ES	effect size
ACTH	adrenocorticotropic hormone		ESR	erythrocyte sedimentation rate
ADAMTS	a disintegrin and metalloproteinase with thrombospondin-like motifs		ESWT	extracorporeal shock wave therapy
ADL	activity of daily living		EU	European Union
ADR	adverse drug reaction		EULAR	European League Against Rheumatism
AGE	advanced glycation end product		FAI	femoroacetabular impingement
AMP	adenosine monophosphate		FDA	Food and Drug Administration
BCP	basic calcium phosphate		FEUA	fractional excretion of uric acid
BGA	behavioural graded activity		FGF	fibroblast growth factor
BLOKS	Boston–Leeds Osteoarthritis Knee Score		FLASH	fast low-angle shot
BME	bone marrow oedema		FM	fibromyalgia
BMI	body mass index		FSE	fast spin-echo
BML	bone marrow lesion		GDF	growth differentiation factor
BMP	bone morphogenetic protein		GFR	glomerular filtration rate
BSR	British Society of Rheumatology		GI	gastrointestinal
CAD	coronary artery disease		GMP	guanosine monophosphate
CC	chondrocalcinosis		GRE	gradient-recalled echo
CCI	central credible interval		GWAS	genome-wide association study
CI	confidence interval		HA	hyaluronic acid
CKD	chronic kidney disease		HaOA	hand osteoarthritis
CMC	carpometacarpal		HR	hazard ratio
CNS	central nervous system		ICF	International Classification of Functioning, Disability and Health
COMT	catechol-O-methyltransferase			
COX	cyclooxygenase		IGF	insulin-like growth factor
CPP	calcium pyrophosphate		IL	interleukin
CPPD	calcium pyrophosphate crystal deposition		JSN	joint space narrowing
CRP	C-reactive protein		JSW	joint space width
CS	corticosteroid or chondroitin sulphate		KL	Kellgren and Lawrence
CT	computed tomography		LD	linkage disequilibrium
DESS	dual-echo steady-state		mAb	monoclonal antibody
dGEMRIC	delayed gadolinium-enhanced magnetic resonance imaging of cartilage		MAPK	mitogen-activated protein kinase
			MCID	minimal clinically important difference
			MCP	metacarpophalangeal
DIP	distal interphalangeal		MMP	matrix metalloproteinase
DMOAD	disease-modifying osteoarthritis drug		MOAKS	MRI Osteoarthritis Knee Score
EAI	episode of acute inflammation		MOC	model(s) of care
ECM	extracellular matrix		MRI	magnetic resonance imaging
eGFR	estimated glomerular filtration rate		MSU	monosodium urate
EMA	European Medicines Agency		MTP	metatarsophalangeal

NGF	nerve growth factor		SF	synovial fluid
NGOA	nodal generalized osteoarthritis		SLRP	small leucine-rich proteoglycan
NHS	National Health Service		SMD	standardized mean difference
NHANES	National Health and Nutrition Examination Survey		SMOAD	structure-modifying osteoarthritis drug
NO	nitric oxide		SNP	single nucleotide polymorphism
NSAID	non-steroidal anti-inflammatory drug		SNR	signal-to-noise ratio
OA	osteoarthritis		SPGR	spoiled gradient-echo
OAI	Osteoarthritis Initiative		SSM	statistical shape modelling
OARSI	Osteoarthritis Research Society International		SUA	serum urate
OMERACT	Outcome Measures in Rheumatology		sxHaOA	symptomatic hand osteoarthritis
OR	odds ratio		sxHOA	symptomatic hip osteoarthritis
PAR	protease-activated receptor		sxKOA	symptomatic knee osteoarthritis
PDGF	platelet-derived growth factor		sxOA	symptomatic osteoarthritis
PEDro	Physiotherapy Evidence Database		TENS	transcutaneous electrical nerve stimulation
PIP	proximal interphalangeal		THR	total hip replacement
PPi	inorganic pyrophosphate		TJR	total joint replacement
PPT	pressure pain threshold		TKA	total knee arthroplasty
PTHrP	parathyroid hormone-related protein		TKR	total knee replacement
RA	rheumatoid arthritis		TNF	tumour necrosis factor
RCT	randomized controlled trial		ULD	urate-lowering drug
rHaOA	radiographic hand osteoarthritis		ULT	urate-lowering therapy
rHOA	radiographic hip osteoarthritis		US	ultrasound
rKOA	radiographic knee osteoarthritis		VAS	visual analogue scale
rOA	radiographic osteoarthritis		VEGF	vascular endothelial growth factor
ROS	reactive oxygen species		WHO	World Health Organization
RR	relative risk		WOMAC	Western Ontario and McMaster Universities Osteoarthritis Index
SAMe	S-adenosylmethionine			
SE	spin-echo		WORMS	Whole-Organ Magnetic Resonance Imaging Score
SES	socioeconomic status		XO	xanthine oxidase

Contributors

Associate Professor Abhishek Abhishek, Academic Rheumatology, School of Medicine, University of Nottingham, Nottingham, UK

Associate Professor Ilana N. Ackerman, Department of Epidemiology and Preventive Medicine, Monash University, Melbourne; Department of Medicine (Royal Melbourne Hospital), The University of Melbourne, Melbourne, Australia

Professor Kelli D. Allen, Thurston Arthritis Research Center, University of North Carolina, Chapel Hill, NC, USA

Professor Nigel Arden, Botnar Research Centre, University of Oxford, Oxford; University of Southampton, Southampton General Hospital, Southampton, UK

Professor Richard Aspden, Arthritis and Musculoskeletal Medicine, University of Aberdeen, Institute of Medical Sciences, School of Medicine, Medical Sciences and Nutrition, Aberdeen, UK

Professor Bernard Bannwarth, Groupe Hospitalier Pellegrin and Division of Therapeutics, University of Bordeaux, Bordeaux, France

Professor Thomas Bardin, Hôpital Lariboisière and Université Paris Diderot Paris Cité Sorbonne, Paris, France

Professor David Beard, Nuffield Department of Orthopaedics, Rheumatology and Musculoskeletal Sciences, University of Oxford, Oxford, UK

Professor Kim L. Bennell, Centre for Health, Exercise and Sports Medicine, University of Melbourne, Melbourne, Australia

Professor Francis Berenbaum, Rheumatology Department, Sorbonnes Universités UPMC Univ Paris 06, INSERM UMRS_938, DHU i2B, Assistance Publique-Hopitaux de Paris, Hôpital Saint-Antoine, Paris, France

Dr Nick J. Besselink, University Medical Centre Utrecht, Utrecht, The Netherlands

Professor Sita M. A. Bierma-Zeinstra, Erasmus University Medical Center, Rotterdam; Department of General Practice, Rotterdam, The Netherlands

Professor Johannes Bijlsma, University of Utrecht, Utrecht; University of Amsterdam and Free University at Amsterdam, Amsterdam, The Netherlands

Dr Esmeralda N. Blaney Davidson, Radboud University Medical Centre, Nijmegen, The Netherlands

Professor Henning Bliddal, The Parker Institute, Copenhagen University Hospital Bispebjerg-Frederiksberg, Denmark

Dr Daniel Bossen, ACHIEVE – Centre of Applied Research, Faculty of Health, Amsterdam University of Applied Sciences, Amsterdam, The Netherlands

Adjunct Associate Professor Caroline A. Brand, Department of Epidemiology and Preventive Medicine, Monash University, Melbourne; Melbourne EpiCentre, The University of Melbourne and Melbourne Health, Melbourne, Australia

Dr Leigh F. Callahan, Thurston Arthritis Research Center, University of North Carolina, Chapel Hill, NC, USA

Dr Sandra P. Chinchilla, Rheumatology Division, Hospital Universitario Cruces, Barakaldo, Spain

Professor Robin Christensen, The Parker Institute, Copenhagen University Hospital Bispebjerg-Frederiksberg, Denmark

Professor Daniel O. Clegg, Department of Veterans Affair Medical Centre and University of Utah, Salt Lake City, UT, USA

Professor Nicola Dalbeth, University of Auckland and Auckland District Health Board, Auckland, New Zealand

Dr Mariëtte de Rooij, Amsterdam Rehabilitation Research Center, Reade, Amsterdam, The Netherlands

Professor Joost Dekker, Department of Rehabilitation Medicine, and Department of Psychiatry, VU University Medical Center, Amsterdam, The Netherlands

Dr Leticia A. Deveza, Department of Rheumatology, Royal North Shore Hospital and Institute of Bone and Joint Research, Kolling Institute of Medical Research, University of Sydney, Sydney, Australia

Professor Paul Dieppe, University of Exeter Medical School, Exeter, UK

Professor Michael Doherty, Academic Rheumatology, School of Medicine, University of Nottingham, Nottingham, UK

Professor Changhai Ding, Menzies Institute for Medical Research, University of Tasmania, Hobart, Tasmania; Institute of Bone & Joint Research, University of Sydney, Sydney, Australia

Dr Fiona Dobson, Department of Physiotherapy, University of Melbourne, Melbourne, Australia

Professor Krysia S. Dziedzic, Arthritis Research UK Primary Care Centre, Research Institute for Primary Care and Health Sciences, Keele University, Keele, UK

Dr Emilio Filippucci, Clinica Reumatologica, Università Politecnica delle Marche, Ospedale 'C. Urbani', Jesi, Ancona, Italy

Dr Steven R. Goldring, Weill Cornell Medical College, Hospital for Special Surgery, New York, NY, USA

Professor Walter Grassi, Department of Rheumatology, Università Politecnica delle Marche, Ospedale 'C. Urbani', Jesi, Ancona, Italy

Dr Jenny Gregory, Arthritis and Musculoskeletal Medicine, University of Aberdeen, Institute of Medical Sciences, School of Medicine, Medical Sciences and Nutrition, Aberdeen, UK

Professor Ali Guermazi, Department of Radiology, Boston University School of Medicine, Boston, MA, USA

Dr Gillian Hawker, Sir John and Lady Eaton Professor and Chair, University of Toronto, Women's College Hospital, Toronto, Canada

Dr Daichi Hayashi, Department of Radiology, Boston University School of Medicine, Boston, MA, USA

Professor Berit L. Heitmann, The Parker Institute, Copenhagen University Hospital Bispebjerg-Frederiksberg, Denmark

Professor Marius Henriksen, The Parker Institute, Copenhagen University Hospital Bispebjerg-Frederiksberg, Denmark

Dr Samantha Hider, Arthritis Research UK Primary Care Centre, Research Institute for Primary Care and Health Sciences, Keele University, Keele, UK

Professor Rana S. Hinman, Centre for Health, Exercise and Sports Medicine, University of Melbourne, Melbourne, Australia

Professor Marc C. Hochberg, University of Maryland School of Medicine, Baltimore, MD, USA

Dr Melanie A. Holden, Arthritis Research UK Primary Care Centre, Research Institute for Primary Care and Health Sciences, Keele University, Keele, UK

Dr Jasmijn Holla, Amsterdam Rehabilitation Research Center, Reade, Amsterdam, The Netherlands

Professor David J. Hunter, Department of Rheumatology, Royal North Shore Hospital and Institute of Bone and Joint Research, Kolling Institute of Medical Research, University of Sydney, Sydney, Australia

Professor Susan Jaglal, Department of Physical Therapy, and Toronto Rehabilitation Institute, Toronto; University Health Network Chair at the University of Toronto, Toronto, Canada

Dr Tim L. Jansen, Radboud University Nijmegen Medical Centre, Nijmegen; Department of Rheumatology, VieCuri Medical Centre, Venlo and Scientific Institute IQ HealthCare, RadboudUMC, Nijmegen, The Netherlands

Dr Xingzhong Jin, Menzies Institute for Medical Research, University of Tasmania, Hobart, Tasmania; Australian Institute of Health Innovation, Macquarie University, Sydney, Australia

Dr Adrian Jones, Department of Rheumatology, Nottingham University Hospitals NHS Trust, Nottingham, UK

Dr Joanne M. Jordan, Thurston Arthritis Research Center, University of North Carolina, Chapel Hill, NC, USA

Dr Robert T. Keenan, Division of Rheumatology, Duke University School of Medicine, Durham, NC, USA

Assistant Professor Puja Khanna, Division of Rheumatology, Department of Internal Medicine, University of Michigan, Ann Arbor, MI, USA

Professor Margreet Kloppenburg, Departments of Rheumatology and Clinical Epidemiology, Leiden University Medical Center, Leiden, The Netherlands

Professor Floris P. J. G. Lafeber, University Medical Centre Utrecht, Utrecht, The Netherlands

Associate Professor Linda Li, Department of Physical Therapy, University of British Columbia, Vancouver, Canada

Professor L. Stefan Lohmander, Lund University, Department of Clinical Sciences Lund, Orthopedics, Lund, Sweden

Ms Anne Lyddiatt, Patient Partners in Arthritis Program, Ingersoll, Ontario, Canada

Associate Professor Simon C. Mastbergen, University Medical Centre Utrecht, Utrecht, The Netherlands

Professor Jason J. McDougall, Departments of Pharmacology and Anaesthesia, Pain Management & Perioperative Medicine, Dalhousie University, Halifax, Nova Scotia, Canada

Professor Philip Mease, Division of Rheumatology Research, Swedish Medical Center, Seattle; University of Washington School of Medicine, Seattle, WA, USA

Professor Tony R. Merriman, University of Otago, Dunedin, New Zealand

Dr Paul Monk, Nuffield Department of Orthopaedics, Rheumatology and Musculoskeletal Sciences, University of Oxford, Oxford, UK

Dr Sarah Munce, Toronto Rehabilitation Institute, University Health Network, Toronto, Canada

Professor Michael C. Nevitt, Department of Epidemiology and Biostatistics, University of California, San Francisco, CA, USA

Dr Christelle Nguyen, Université Paris Descartes, Service de Rééducation et de Réadaptation de l'Appareil Locomoteur et des Pathologies du Rachis, Hôpital Cochin, Paris; Laboratoire de Pharmacologie, Toxicologie et Signalisation Cellulaire, INSERM UMR-S 1124, UFR Biomédicale des Saints Pères, Paris, France

Dr Tadashi Okano, Department of Orthopedic Surgery, Osaka City University Graduate School of Medicine, Osaka, Japan

Dr Professor Terence W O'Neill, Arthritis Research UK Centre for Epidemiology, University of Manchester, Manchester, UK

Dr Sneha Pai, Division of Rheumatology, Rutgers Robert Wood Johnson Medical School, New Brunswick, NJ, USA

Professor Eliseo Pascual, Universidad Miguel Hernández and Hospital General Universitario de Alicante, Alicante, Spain

Associate Professor Fernando Perez-Ruiz, Rheumatology Division, Hospital Universitario Cruces, Department of Medicine of the Medicine and Nursery School, Basque Country University, and BioCruces Health Research Institute, Spain

Professor Andrew Price, Nuffield Department of Orthopaedics, Rheumatology and Musculoskeletal Sciences, University of Oxford, Oxford, UK

Professor François Rannou, Université Paris Descartes, Service de Rééducation et de Réadaptation de l'Appareil Locomoteur et des

Pathologies du Rachis, Hôpital Cochin, Paris; Laboratoire de Pharmacologie, Toxicologie et Signalisation Cellulaire, INSERM UMR-S 1124, UFR Biomédicale des Saints Pères, Paris, France

Professor Pascal Richette, Université Paris Diderot, UFR médicale, Paris; Assistance Publique-Hôpitaux de Paris, Hôpital Lariboisiére, Fédération de Rhumatologie, Paris; INSERM 1132, Université Paris-Diderot, Hôpital Lariboisière, Paris, France

Dr Edward Roddy, Arthritis Research UK Primary Care Centre, Research Institute for Primary Care and Health Sciences, Keele University, Keele, UK

Associate Professor Frank W. Roemer, Department of Radiology, University of Erlangen-Nuremberg, Erlangen, Germany; Department of Radiology, Boston University School of Medicine, Boston, MA, USA

Dr Juliet Rogers, Bristol Royal Infirmary, Bristol, UK

Dr Jos Runhaar, Erasmus University Medical Center Rotterdam; Department of General Practice, Rotterdam, the Netherlands

Associate Professor Allen D. Sawitzke, University of Utah, Salt Lake City, UT, USA

Dr Naomi Schlesinger, Division of Rheumatology, Rutgers Robert Wood Johnson Medical School, New Brunswick, NJ, USA

Dr Lee S. Simon, SDG LLC, Cambridge, MA, USA

Dr Francisca Sivera, Department of Rheumatology, Hospital General Universitario de Elda, Alicante, Spain

Professor Dawn Stacey, School of Nursing, Faculty of Health Sciences, University of Ottawa; Patient Decision Aids Research Group, Ottawa Hospital Research Institute, Ottawa, Canada

Dr Martin J. Thomas, Arthritis Research UK Primary Care Centre, Research Institute for Primary Care and Health Sciences, Keele University, Keele, UK

Associate Professor Jonas Bloch Thorlund, Department of Sports Science and Clinical Biomechanics, University of Southern Denmark, Odense, Denmark

Dr Irati Urionagüena, Rheumatology Division, Hospital Universitario Cruces, Barakaldo, Spain

Associate Professor Ana M. Valdes, Academic Rheumatology, School of Medicine, University of Nottingham, Nottingham, UK

Associate Professor Peter M. van der Kraan, Radboud University Medical Centre, Nijmegen, The Netherlands

Dr Marike van der Leeden, Department of Rehabilitation Medicine, VU University Medical Center, Amsterdam; Amsterdam Rehabilitation Research Center, Reade, Amsterdam, The Netherlands

Dr Ans Van Ginckel, Centre for Health, Exercise and Sports Medicine, University of Melbourne, Melbourne, Australia

Professor Cindy Veenhof, Department of Rehabilitation, Nursing Science & Sports, Brain Center Rudolf Magnus, University Medical Center Utrecht, Utrecht, The Netherlands

Professor Joel A. Vilensky, Indiana University School of Medicine-Fort Wayne, Fort Wayne, IN, USA

Professor David A. Walsh, Arthritis Research UK Pain Centre, University of Nottingham, Nottingham, UK

Dr Xia Wang, Menzies Institute for Medical Research, University of Tasmania, Hobart, Tasmania

Professor Esther Waugh, Department of Physical Therapy, University of Toronto, Toronto; Women's College Hospital, Toronto, Canada

Dr Laura A. Wyatt, Arthritis Research UK Pain Centre, University of Nottingham, Nottingham, UK

Dr Shirley P. Yu, Department of Rheumatology, Royal North Shore Hospital, Sydney, Australia

Professor Weiya Zhang, Academic Rheumatology, School of Medicine, University of Nottingham, Nottingham, UK

Dr Zhaohua Zhu, Menzies Institute for Medical Research, University of Tasmania, Hobart, Tasmania, Australia

SECTION 1

What is osteoarthritis?

CHAPTER 1

Introduction: what is osteoarthritis?

Michael Doherty, Johannes Bijlsma,
Nigel Arden, David J. Hunter, and Nicola Dalbeth

Definition

Osteoarthritis (OA) is by far the most common form of arthritis worldwide and symptomatic OA is recognized as an important cause of disability and participation restriction in middle-aged and older adults [1]. It can be defined and diagnosed in several ways:

1. *Pathological changes.* OA is a condition confined to synovial (diarthrodial) joints that results in (a) focal narrowing of articular hyaline cartilage together with (b) bone remodelling and marginal new bone (osteophyte) formation (Figure 1.1) [2]. Although historically cartilage and subsequently bone have been the main focus of research interest, increasingly it is recognized that all joint tissues that comprise the joint (articular hyaline cartilage, fibrocartilage, bone, synovium/capsule, and muscle) are involved in OA.

2. *Changes on imaging.* Plain radiographic features reflect underlying cartilage and bone pathology and include focal joint space narrowing and marginal osteophyte, with varying degrees of subchondral bone sclerosis, bone 'cysts', osteochondral 'loose'

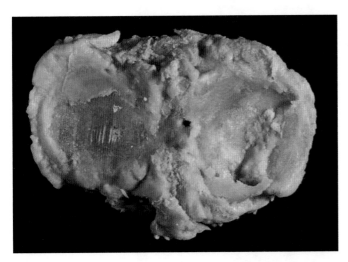

Figure 1.1 Gross pathology of human tibial plateaux affected by osteoarthritis, showing marked focal cartilage loss, eburnation ('polishing') and furrowing due to wear of the exposed bone, and marginal irregularity caused by osteophytes.

bodies, and eventual bone attrition and deformity (Figure 1.2). Magnetic resonance imaging is much more sensitive than radiographs and may show additional physiological and structural changes including bone marrow lesions, synovial hypertrophy and effusion, initial mild expansion of cartilage thickness (due to increased water content), and eventual focal hyaline cartilage loss (often with meniscal pathology/extrusion in knee OA).

3. *Physical signs.* These vary according to the joint involved, but typical features include reduced range of movement, bony swelling, and coarse crepitus (Figure 1.3) [3]. There may also be modest soft tissue swelling and effusion, and eventual muscle weakness and wasting, joint deformity (Figures 1.4 and 1.5), and occasional instability. Joint line and/or peri-articular tenderness may be present in symptomatic joints.

4. *Associated symptoms.* OA pain is typically worse with joint use and relieved by rest ('usage' or 'mechanical' pain), associates with only short-lived early morning and inactivity stiffness, affects one or a few joints at any one time, and predominately affects people over the age of 40 [3]. More persistent pain, especially at night, may also occur with large joint, especially hip, OA. Symptoms may fluctuate in severity from day to day but, in general, change only slowly with time. Apart from pain, functional impairment is an important problem that may result in participation restriction and reduced quality of life.

There are a number of diagnostic and classification criteria for OA, primarily at the knee, hip, and hand, which are used for inclusion criteria for clinical trials and for case definition for epidemiological and genetic studies. These often use algorithms to allow classification based on different combinations of features which may include simple demographics (e.g. over age 38), clinical features such as crepitus or bony swelling, presence of symptoms (e.g. pain for most days of the past month, morning stiffness of less than half an hour), plain radiographic changes of OA, and sometimes other investigations (e.g. synovial fluid characteristics, negative serum rheumatoid factor). However, for everyday clinical purposes the diagnosis of OA is made on the basis of a full history and clinical examination, and takes into account the presence of typical symptoms and/or signs and absence of features to suggest an alternative cause in the context of a specific individual.

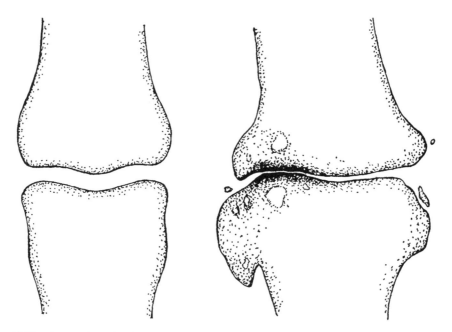

Figure 1.2 Diagram of normal (left) and osteoarthritic (right) joint, showing focal joint-space narrowing, adjacent subchondral sclerosis, marginal osteophyte, cysts, and osteochondral bodies typical of OA.

The weighting of various aspects within an individual is variable, and use of imaging and other investigations are not usually required (see Chapter 15).

Observations on the nature of osteoarthritis

Our views of OA and its pathogenesis continue to change. OA was previously considered a 'degenerative' disease, the inevitable accompaniment of ageing, with 'wear and tear' the principal driving pathogenic mechanism. However, now OA is increasingly viewed as a metabolically active, dynamic process including tissue repair as well as damage which may be triggered not just by mechanical, but also by a variety of metabolic and inflammatory insults.

Any view of OA needs to take into account the following general observations:

1. *The phylogenetic and evolutionary preservation of OA.* The study of ancient skeletal remains suggests that OA has accompanied

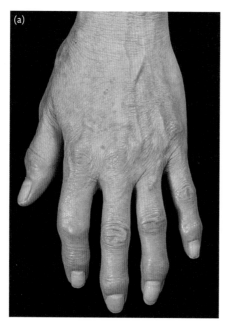
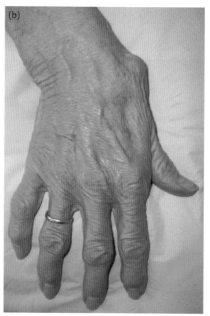

Figure 1.3 Two women with hand OA: (a) the younger on the left, showing thumb and finger interphalangeal bony swelling, some fingers with radial/ulnar deviation (very characteristic of osteoarthritis); and (b) the older women on the right, showing similar but less pronounced interphalangeal changes, but marked bony swelling and proximal/radial subluxation of the thumb-base (first carpometacarpal joint).

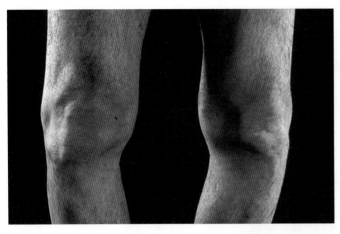

Figure 1.4 Typical varus deformity, with bony swelling and small effusions, in a 65-year-old man with knee osteoarthritis.

mankind throughout our evolutionary history (see Chapter 2) [4–7]. Structural changes equivalent to OA are also found in other animals with diarthrodial (synovial) joints that fuse their epiphyses in the adult [8–10]. Indeed, archaeological evidence supports the evolutionary antiquity of the condition in many species [6,7] including dinosaurs [11], which suggests that OA is not necessarily 'all bad' and may have been conserved throughout animal evolution for a reason, for example, as an adaptive response to joint injury.

2. *The dynamic nature of the OA process.* OA is a metabolically active process that involves all tissues that comprise the joint. Pathologically it is usually characterized by exuberant new bone formation (most evident as osteophyte) and bone remodelling, synovial hyperplasia, and capsular thickening (see Chapter 3). Although focal loss of hyaline cartilage is a cardinal feature, articular chondrocytes in an OA joint, at least initially, multiply in number and increase their activity, producing more matrix components and assuming a hypertrophic phenotype [12]. Formation of new fibrocartilage is evident at the joint margins and this undergoes endochondral ossification to form osteophytes (Figure 1.6). In the synovium, synoviocytes may

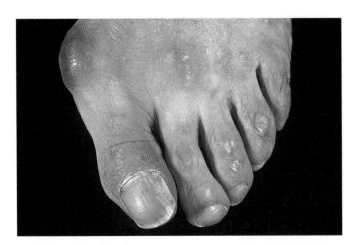

Figure 1.5 Hallux valgus, with accompanying longitudinal rotation of the big toe, due to OA of the first metatarsophalangeal joint.

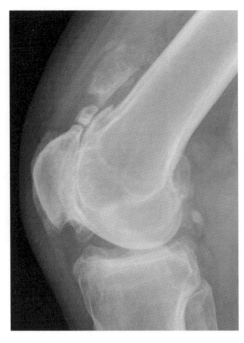

Figure 1.6 Lateral knee radiograph showing marked patello-femoral narrowing, florid osteophyte formation, and multiple, variably sized osteochondral bodies anteriorly in the suprapatellar pouch and posteriorly.

undergo chondroid metaplasia to produce fibrocartilage which again may ossify and produce slowly enlarging osteochondral bodies (Figure 1.6) (see Chapter 3). The biochemical changes in OA cartilage differ from those of ageing alone and include an increased turnover of many matrix components [13], and expression of chondroitin epitopes that are normally evident in young (growth) cartilage [14]. Similar dynamic processes to those occurring in cartilage also occur within the other tissues involved in OA including bone and synovium. These features alone negate the use of the term 'degenerative joint disease' and suggest a generalized attempt by all joint components to product new tissue in response to joint insults.

3. *The discordance between structural change, symptoms, and disability.* It is striking that clinical and radiographic evidence of OA may often be present without symptoms or compromised function [15–17]. Asymptomatic OA is particularly prevalent at certain sites, such as finger joints and lower cervical and lumbar apophyseal joints, but is not uncommon even in large weight-bearing joints. Probably all of us develop OA somewhere in our skeleton as we mature and age, but in the vast majority of joints this does not associate with evident problems. Thus there is a marked difference between the *disease* OA (structural change identified by imaging or clinical examination) and the *illness* OA (patient-reported symptoms) [18].

4. *The good outcome in many cases of symptomatic OA.* Although the effects of OA on an individual may be dramatic [19], OA is not inevitably progressive. Many OA patients have phases or 'flares' of symptoms, and eventual slow resolution of pain and stiffness. This is particularly likely for finger joints affected by nodal OA [20], but may also occur at hips and knees [21,22]. Although symptoms may resolve, the structural changes of OA persist and stabilize. Replacement of lost hyaline cartilage does

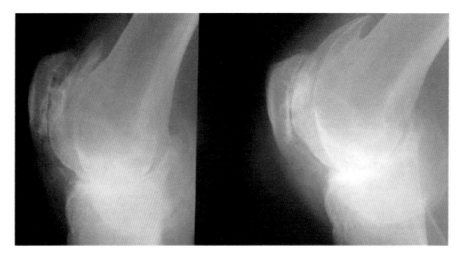

Figure 1.7 Lateral knee radiographs of a 68-year-old lady taken 3 years apart showing remodelling. During this time she has lost weight and her symptoms were improved.

not occur, but in rare cases radiographs may show 'improvement' with remodelling of bony contours with limited fibrocartilage replacement, which may show as an increase in inter-bone distance (Figure 1.7) [23].

The perspective of osteoarthritis as the inherent repair process of synovial joints

All the above observations are readily accommodated by the perspective of OA as a potential repair process in response to joint insult and cartilage destruction (Figure 1.8) [12,24]. In this perspective, a wide variety of insults may trigger the need to repair. Once the process is initiated, all the tissues in the joint are involved in what may be considered an adaptive response [12,24,25].

The increased metabolic activity by cartilage, new bone formation, and remodelling of the joint may help keep pace with tissue loss and redistribute mechanical forces across the compromised

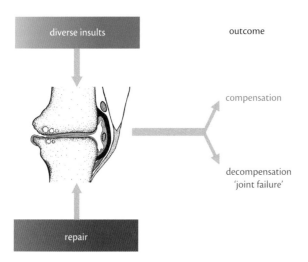

Figure 1.8 Schematic representation of OA as a repair process triggered by a variety of joint insults, involving response by all the joint tissues, and showing variable outcome.

joint. Marginal osteophyte and capsular thickening may help to sustain joint stability. The outcome of an OA joint depends on the balance between the severity and chronicity of the insult, and the effectiveness of the repair response. In many instances the repair and remodelling successfully counter and rectify the adverse effects of the insult ('compensated OA') with little in the way of any perceived symptoms or functional restriction. However, in some cases overwhelming insult or poor tissue response lead to 'decompensated' OA, with the need for continuing attempted repair and remodelling and an increased likelihood of associating with symptoms, disability, and progression of structural damage. This equates to '*joint failure*' of the diarthrodial joint, analogous to renal or cardiac failure, in which a similar end-stage may result from diverse individual triggers. Such a scenario could readily explain the *marked heterogeneity* of OA with different sites of involvement, different numbers of joints affected, and marked variability of outcome.

If OA is, in general, a slow but often successful repair process, this also explains its frequent presence in the absence of symptoms or impaired function, its generally benign natural history, and its widespread presence in humans and other animals. If such a perspective is correct, the concept of OA as a single 'disease' should be replaced by the concept of OA as a 'process', with diverse triggers and outcomes. A number of consequences of such a perspective require emphasis:

1. Although these triggers share a common phenotypic expression as 'OA', the way in which they insult the joint may vary greatly and involve hereditary, constitutional, metabolic, endocrine, environmental, or biomechanical mechanisms (Figure 1.9).

2. The site of primary insult may be any tissue in the joint (bone, cartilage, synovium, capsule, ligament, muscle), because all are essential to its health and integrity.

3. Risk factors and mechanisms involved in the development of OA need not be the same as those that determine progression or non-progression.

4. Risk factors for structural OA are not synonymous for risk factors for pain and disability—these need examination in their own right (see Chapter 15).

Osteoarthritis—a common complex disorder

genetic and racial factors
gender, hormonal status
age
obesity
bone density
muscle strength
nutrition

joint shape
joint alignment
joint laxity

trauma
joint usage
- occupational
- recreational

constitutional susceptibility

biomechanical factors

Figure 1.9 Recognized risk factors for development of OA.

5. Caution must be exercised in extrapolating knowledge of the pathogenesis of OA from one joint site to another, or from one clinical form or model of OA, to OA in general.

A variety of biochemical and biomechanical triggers and mechanisms have been studied in OA, particularly with respect to cartilage. It is often difficult, however, to disentangle deleterious initiating factors from events linked to tissue response, especially when studying established, particularly end-stage, disease. Physical and biomechanical factors, though usefully separated in test systems, are likely to be inexorably linked and interdependent *in vivo*. Sharp polarization between them is likely to be artificial. Furthermore, we should not assume an 'all-or-none' or linear response, for initiating or perpetuating triggers. For example, we know that a certain amount of regular loading is required for the health of both cartilage and bone, and that either too little or too much loading may result in cartilage fibrillation and thinning [26]. Such U-shaped response curves may cause problems for the unwary.

Subsets of osteoarthritis

The rationale for attempting to divide the heterogeneous group of people with OA into more homogeneous subsets or phenotypes is to better identify individual triggers and mechanisms, and to potentially consider stratified care in which certain treatments are selected according to the presence of individual phenotypic characteristics (see Chapter 21 for an overview discussion of management). Although subsets have been defined in various ways, for example, by radiographic appearance (*atrophic* versus *hypertrophic*) [27] (Figure 1.10), by the presence of florid inflammation ('*inflammatory OA*' [28]) or calcium crystals (e.g. '*pyrophosphate arthropathy*' [29], *apatite associated destructive arthritis* [30,31]) separation at least according to the *site* and *number* of joints affected appears important [32] and justified in terms of different profiles of risk factors for development and progression and for the targeted management of OA. Probably the best accepted 'subset' is nodal generalized OA (NGOA) [32] (Figure 1.3) characterized by polyarticular involvement of finger interphalangeal joints (with nodes, radial/ulnar deviation, and retained stability), strong heritability and female predominance, onset in middle age ('menopausal arthritis'), generally good prognosis for hand outcomes, and subsequent increased risk of OA at other sites, especially the knee.

Caveats to defining subsets, however, include the lack of clear distinction between many subsets. For example, 'inflammatory' [28] or 'erosive' [33] hand OA (EOA) predominantly targets finger interphalangeal joints and is characterized clinically by more marked pain, early morning stiffness, soft tissue swelling, and disability than common hand OA [20,28] and structurally by subchondral bone erosion and marked cartilage and bone attrition [33] (Figure 1.11) sometimes resulting in instability or spontaneous fusion which do not occur in NGOA. Unlike NGOA there is no increased predisposition to OA at other joint sites. However, radiographic features of EOA are reported to occur commonly in just one or a few finger joints of people with NGOA in both hospital [34] and population-based settings [35], suggesting more of a spectrum of severity than two distinct entities [34,35]. Other caveats include the occurrence of different subsets at different sites within the same individual and evolution from one subset to another within the

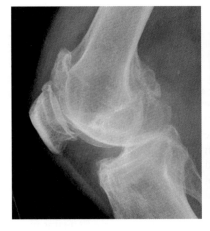 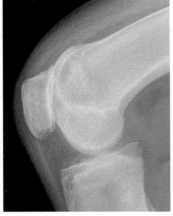

Figure 1.10 Contrasting examples of atrophic and hypertrophic OA at the knee. The lateral radiograph on the left shows florid femoral osteophyte formation anteriorly and posteriorly as well as superior and inferior patellar and tibial osteophyte, whereas the only definite osteophyte seen in the knee on the right is a small superior patellar osteophyte.

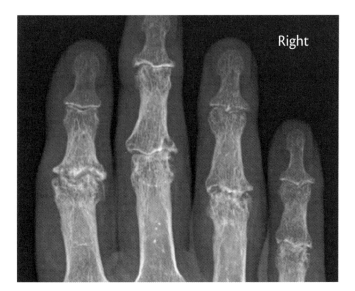

Figure 1.11 Changes of erosive hand OA. Subchondral erosion at different stages in multiple interphalangeal joints, with 'gull-wing' appearance apparent particularly in the middle finger distal interphalangeal joint, and the 'saw-tooth' pattern particularly seen in the ring finger proximal interphalangeal joint.

same joint. Furthermore, it is now apparent that there is interaction between what traditionally has been considered *primary* (hereditary, constitutional) and *secondary* (mechanical, traumatic) forms of OA based on presumed aetiology. For example, young adults who undergo meniscectomy for meniscal injury are more likely to develop subsequent post-meniscectomy knee OA in middle and older age, and for it to be more severe, if they also have hand OA [36,37]. Furthermore, examining combined genetic variants associated with knee OA it appears that people with 'post-traumatic secondary' knee OA severe enough to come to joint replacement have at least as high a genetic contribution as people coming to arthroplasty for non-traumatic 'primary' knee OA [38]. Therefore the descriptors 'primary' and 'secondary' are no longer used.

An alternative to subgroup characterization is to recognize OA as a common complex disorder with multiple risk factors and a wide spectrum of phenotypic presentations, and to identify the risk profile for each individual. Addressing any modifiable risk factors (e.g. overweight, muscle weakness, and certain adverse mechanical factors) may then be incorporated within the management plan.

Why does osteoarthritis target certain joints more than others?

An intriguing aspect of OA that remains unexplained is its site specificity. Only certain synovial joints show a high prevalence of OA, with others being relatively spared (Figure 1.12). One hypothesis to explain this distribution relates to human evolution [39]. Joints that have undergone major changes in orientation and function, to permit our bipedal gait and associated liberation of the upper limb, may not yet have adapted to their new functional requirements: they may be under-designed (that is, have poor functional reserve), and, therefore, more frequently require a reparative response in the face of insult. The distribution of OA in humans and other animals is largely consistent with this theory, though further testing of the hypothesis is clearly problematic. Within individual

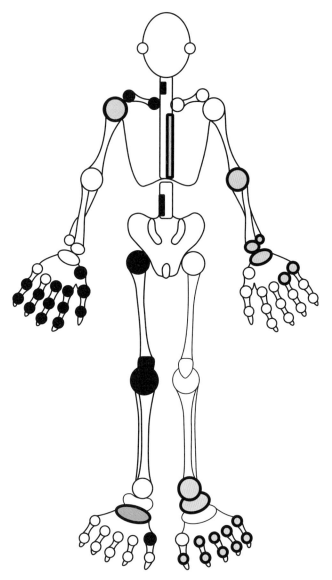

Figure 1.12 Targeted distribution of OA in human beings. Common target sites are shown on the left in black (moderately common sites in older age shown in grey), whereas relatively spared sites of involvement are shown on the right in blue.

joints, there is additional specificity with respect to sites of maximal cartilage loss. For large joints, this most commonly occurs at sites of maximum load bearing, supporting the importance of physical factors. Although this biomechanical explanation fits the majority of cases of large joint OA, topographical variation certainly occurs and has been used as a basis for subset classification. For example, at the hip, superior (lateral, intermediate, medial), axial, and medial patterns of femoral head migration are recognized and have different associations (Figure 1.13) [40].

The strong association with ageing

The strong association between *ageing* and OA prevalence for all sites of involvement remains unexplained. Certain aspects of OA are particularly common in the elderly, for example, marked calcium crystal deposition (basic calcium phosphate (BCP—mainly apatite) and calcium pyrophosphate (CPP) crystals), involvement

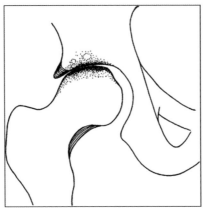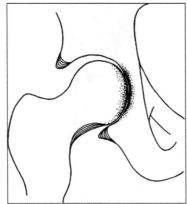

Figure 1.13 Two examples of patterns of hip OA defined radiographically by site of maximum joint space narrowing: supero-lateral hip OA (left) and medial hip OA (right).

of atypical sites (e.g. glenohumeral, radiocarpal, and mid-foot joints), and rapidly destructive OA of large joints (hip, knee, and glenohumeral joints). The mechanism underlying these striking age associations may relate to age-related decline in muscle function, impaired joint proprioception, reduction of vascular supply and nutrition of joint tissues, or reduced regenerative potential of connective tissue. All of these might lower resistance to insult, tip a compensated OA joint toward decompensation, and favour more rapid progression and poor outcome. There is a dramatic decline with ageing in the biomechanical properties of cartilage matrix [41], probably caused by subtle but cumulative changes in the structure of collagens, proteoglycans, and matrix proteins. Certainly the effect of ageing on both normal and OA tissues deserves further study.

The association between crystals and osteoarthritis

In contrast to immature cartilage involved in endochondral ossification during growth, normal mature cartilage does not readily form calcium crystals within its matrix. However, with increasing age and especially with development of OA, calcium crystal formation within articular hyaline and fibrocartilage again becomes common. Indeed, examination of OA articular cartilage removed at the time of total knee or hip replacement (i.e. 'end-stage' OA) reveals BCP crystal deposition in 100% of cases and CPP crystal deposition in 20% of cases, suggesting that cartilage mineralization is an integral part of the OA process rather than a marker of a subset of OA [42,43].

Certain physicochemical conditions are required for crystal formation [44]. Firstly there must be sufficient concentration of the constituents (the 'seed') that form the crystal (i.e. the ionic product needs to be above the saturation point at which crystals can form). Secondly, physical factors such as pH, temperature, and the physical matrix in which the solution occurs (the 'soil') need to be conducive to crystal nucleation and growth. In many tissues, including cartilage, the normal balance between tissue inhibitors and promotors of crystallization favours inhibition and this prevents inappropriate crystal formation despite the tissue having many components in solution at a concentration above their saturation point. However, changes related to ageing, such as reduction in cartilage proteoglycan (an inhibitor [45]) and increase in lipid (a promotor) may tip the balance in favour of crystal formation, but in OA this shift in

balance is far greater and involves additional factors such as reduction in type II collagen (an inhibitor) [44] and an increase in type I collagen (a promotor) [46]. In addition to changes in 'soil' factors, hypertrophic chondrocytes in OA associate with increased levels of extracellular pyrophosphate and this increase stimulates formation of BCP, and at higher levels CPP, crystals [47] (see Chapters 50 and 54).

Comparison between OA and growth cartilage is of interest with respect to cartilage mineralization in OA. Metabolically active hypertrophic chondrocytes, adjacent vascularity, and tendency to readily calcify cartilage are all features of endochondral ossification which is required as our skeleton is growing. In normal adult articular cartilage, chondrocytes become less active and lose the hypertrophic phenotype, vascularity recedes, matrix epitopes take on adult characteristics, and cartilage becomes resistant to crystal formation. However, if OA develops, chondrocytes again multiply and assume the hypertrophic phenotype, there is angiogenesis and increased vascularity, matrix neo-epitopes re-appear [14], and the cartilage again is prone to calcification. It is as if the OA joint is reverting to the immature form, which of course is well designed to produce new tissue. This view again is consistent with the perspective of OA as an inherent repair process.

The hardness and stability of crystals confer a clear biological advantage when they occur in the correct tissue, for example, BCP mineralization of our bones and teeth. However, when such hard particles form in adult cartilage they can cause adverse mechanical effects and trigger both acute and chronic inflammation through interaction between their negatively charged, irregular surface and the body's defence mechanisms (e.g. triggering of the innate immune response and complement activation). Whether BCP and CPP crystals are deleterious (through 'microcrystal-induced stress') or potentially beneficial to OA cartilage, or are just incidental 'innocent bystanders' remains unclear [44] (see Chapters 50 and 54).

Apart from the association with calcium crystals OA also shows a positive association with urate crystal deposition and gout [48]. This occurs at the disease level in that people presenting with incident gout are more likely than matched controls to have a prior diagnosis of OA (adjusted odds ratio for the preceding 10 years 1.20, 95% confidence interval (CI) 1.13–1.27) and more likely to develop OA in subsequent years (adjusted hazard ratio 1.45,

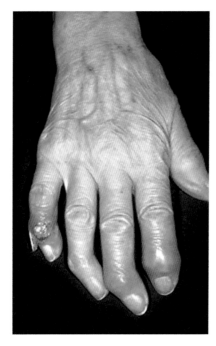

Figure 1.14 Tophi targeting distal interphalangeal joints in an older lady with pre-existing nodal OA. The discharging tophus in her little finger led to her presentation and diagnosis of gout.

95% CI 1.35–1.54) [49]. It also occurs at the local level in that peripheral joints affected by OA appear more prone than normal joints to develop gout (Figure 1.14) [48]. Possible reasons for this include the altered balance of matrix inhibitors and promotors of crystal formation in OA cartilage [48], possible epitaxial growth of urate crystals on calcium crystals [48], and encouragement of ordered urate crystal nucleation and growth by exposed collagen fibres in OA [50]. However, the finding that higher synovial fluid uric acid levels associates with greater OA severity [51] suggests the possibility of other pathogenic mechanisms to link the two conditions related to hyperuricaemia rather than crystal formation per se.

There are a number of ways in which OA and gout may associate and interact (Figure 1.15). They may co-associate because (1) they share certain risk factors in common (e.g. ageing, overweight, and metabolic syndrome); (2) OA tissues encourage urate crystal

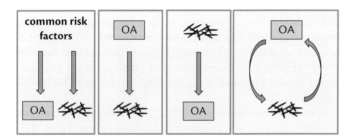

Figure 1.15 Possible explanations for the association between OA and gout: both may develop in parallel through sharing of common risk factors; OA may predispose to urate crystal formation; urate crystal may damage the joint and lead to OA; or OA may encourage crystal deposition which in turn leads to further joint damage (i.e. an 'amplification loop' interaction).

deposition; (3) gout causes joint damage via crystals or elevated urate, or both; or (4) urate crystals deposit more readily in OA cartilage where they then initiate and progress further joint damage—this more unifying interpretation is equivalent to the 'amplification loop' hypothesis suggested for the association between OA and calcium crystal deposition [52].

Conclusion

OA is a common complex disorder with multiple risk factors and varied phenotypic expression. Various observations, including the fact that most OA is clinically occult, support the perspective of OA as a potential repair process that involves all joint tissues in the adaptive response to joint insult. Although a number of subsets of OA have been proposed, probably the best differentiating factors are the site and number of joints affected. Ageing is a striking risk factor at all sites. There is also a strong association between OA and calcium crystals, with deposition of BCP in cartilage appearing to be an integral part of the OA process, at least in large joints. OA also associates with gout, the second most common form of arthritis after OA. It is for these reasons that crystal arthropathies are given greater prominence in this third edition of the textbook which previously was entitled *Osteoarthritis*.

References

1. Song J, Chang RW, Dunlop D. Population impact of arthritis on disability in older adults. *Arthritis Rheum* 2006; 55:248–55.
2. Loeser RF, Goldring SR, Scanzello CR, Goldring MB. Osteoarthritis: a disease of the joint as an organ. *Arthritis Rheum* 2012; 64(6):1697–707.
3. Abhishek A, Doherty M. Diagnosis and clinical presentations of osteoarthritis. *Rheum Dis Clin North Am* 2010; 39(1):45–66.
4. Ruffer MA, Rietti A. On osseous lesions in ancient Egyptians. *J Pathol Bacteriol* 1911; 16:439–65.
5. Rogers J, Watt I, Dieppe P. Arthritis in Saxon and medieval skeletons. *Br Med J* 1981; 283:1668–70.
6. Jurmain RD, Kilgore L. Skeletal evidence of osteoarthritis: a palaeo-pathological perspective. *Ann Rheum Dis* 1995; 54:443–50.
7. Hutton C. Generalised osteoarthritis: an evolutionary problem. *Lancet* 1987; 1:1463–5.
8. Fox H. Chronic arthritis in wild mammals. *Trans Am Phil Soc* 1939; 31:71–148.
9. Bennett GA, Bauer W. A systematic study of the degeneration of articular cartilage in bovine joints. *Am J Pathol* 1931; 7:399–414.
10. Sokoloff L. Natural history of degenerative joint disease in small laboratory animals. *AMA Arch Pathol* 1956; 62:118–28.
11. Rothschild B. Radiological assessment of osteoarthritis in dinosaurs. *Ann Carnegie Mus* 1990; 59:295–301.
12. Bland JH, Cooper, SM. Osteoarthritis: a review of the cell biology involved and evidence for reversibility. Management rationally related to known genesis and pathophysiology. *Semin Arthritis Rheum* 1984; 14:106–33.
13. Hammerman D. The biology of osteoarthritis. *N Engl J Med* 1989; 320:1322–30.
14. Caterson B, Mahmoodian F, Sorrell JM, et al. Modulation of native chondroitin sulphate structure in tissue development and in disease. *J Cell Sci* 1990; 97:411–17.
15. Lawrence JS, Bremner JM, Bier F. Osteoarthrosis: prevalence in the population and relationship between symptoms and X-ray changes. *Ann Rheum Dis* 1966; 25:1–23.
16. Davis MA, Ettinger WH, Neuhaus JM, Barclay JD, Segal MR. Correlates of knee pain among US adults with and without radiographic knee osteoarthritis. *J Rheumatol* 1992; 19:1943–9.
17. Hadler NM. Knee pain is the malady—not osteoarthritis. *Ann Intern Med* 1992; 116:598–9.

18. Lane NE, Brandt K, Hawker G, et al. OARSI-FDA initiative: defining the disease state of osteoarthritis. *Osteoarthritis Cartilage* 2011; 19(5):478–82.

19. Atkinson JP. A remembrance of Fred, the lowland gorilla. *Arthritis Rheum* 1996; 39:891–3.

20. Patrick M, Aldridge S, Hamilton E, Manhire A, Doherty M. A controlled study of hand function in nodal and erosive osteoarthritis. *Ann Rheum Dis* 1989; 48:978–82.

21. Danielsson LG. Incidence and prognosis of coxarthrosis. *Acta Orthop Scand* 1964; 64(Suppl.):1–114.

22. Hernborg JS, Nilsson BE. The natural course of untreated osteoarthritis of the knee. *Clin Orthop Rel Res* 1977; 123:130–7.

23. Perry GH, Smith MJG, Whiteside CG. Spontaneous recovery of the joint space in degenerative hip disease. *Ann Rheum Dis* 1972; 31:440–8.

24. Radin EL, Burr DB. Hypothesis: joints can heal. *Semin Arthritis Rheum* 1984; 13:293–302.

25. Mankin HJ. The reaction of cartilage to injury and osteoarthritis. *N Engl J Med* 1974; 291:1285–92.

26. Buckwalter JA. Osteoarthritis and articular cartilage use, disuse and abuse: experimental studies. *J Rheumatol* 1995; 22:13–15.

27. Solomon L. Osteoarthritis, local and generalised: a uniform disease? *J Rheumatol* 1983; 10(Suppl. 9):13–15.

28. Ehrlich G. Inflammatory osteoarthritis: I. The clinical syndrome. *J Chron Dis* 1972; 25:317–28.

29. Doherty M, Dieppe PA. Clinical aspects of calcium pyrophosphate dehydrate crystal deposition. *Rheum Dis Clin NA* 1988; 14:395–414.

30. Dieppe PA, Doherty M, MacFarlane DG, et al. *Br J Rheumatol* 1984; 23:84–91.

31. Halverson PB, McCarty DJ, Cheung H, Ryan LM. Milwaukee shoulder syndrome: eleven additional cases with involvement of the knee in seven basic calcium phosphate deposition. *Sem Arthritis Rheum* 1984; 14:36–44.

32. Kellgren JH, Moore R. Generalised osteoarthritis and Heberden's nodes. *Br Med J* 1952; 1:181–7.

33. Kidd KL, Peter JB. Erosive osteoarthritis. *Radiology* 1966; 86:640–7.

34. Addimanda O, Mancarella L, Dolzani P, et al. Clinical and radiographic distribution of structural damage in erosive and nonerosive hand osteoarthritis. *Arthritis Care Res* 2012; 64:1046–53.

35. Marshall M, Nicholls E, Kwok W-Y, et al. Erosive osteoarthritis: a more severe form of radiographic hand osteoarthritis rather than a distinct entity? *Ann Rheum Dis* 2015; 74:136–41.

36. Doherty M, Watt I, Dieppe PA. Influence of primary generalised osteoarthritis on development of secondary osteoarthritis. *Lancet* 1983; 2:8–11.

37. Englund M, Paradowski PT, Lohmander LS. Association of radiographic hand osteoarthritis with radiographic knee osteoarthritis after meniscectomy. *Arthritis Rheum* 2004; 50(2):469–75.

38. Valdes AM, Doherty SA, Muir KR, et al. The genetic contribution to severe post-traumatic osteoarthrtitis. *Ann Rheum Dis* 2013; 72:1687–90.

39. Hutton, C. Generalised osteoarthritis: an evolutionary problem. *Lancet* 1987; 2:1463–5.

40. Ledingham J, Dawson S, Preston B, Milligan G, Doherty M. Radiographic patterns and associations of osteoarthritis of the hip. *Ann Rheum Dis* 1992; 51:1111–16.

41. Kempson GE. Age-related changes in the tensile properties of human articular cartilage: a comparative study between the femoral head of the hip joint and the talus of the ankle joint. *Biochim Biophys Acta* 1991; 1075:223–30.

42. Fuerst M, Bertrand J, Lammers L, et al. Calcification of articular cartilage in human osteoarthritis. *Arthritis Rheum* 2009; 60:2694–703.

43. Fuerst M, Niggemeyer O, Lammers L, et al. Articular cartilage mineralization in osteoarthritis of the hip. *BMC Musculoskelet Disord* 2009; 10:166.

44. Ea H-K, Nguyen C, Bazin D, et al. Articular cartilage calcification in osteoarthritis—insights into crystal-induced stress. *Arthritis Rheum* 2011; 63:10–18.

45. Chen CC, Boskey AL, Rosenberg LC. The inhibitory effect of cartilage proteoglycans on hydroxyapatite growth. *Calcif Tissue Int* 1984; 36:285–90.

46. Jubeck B, Gohr C, Fahey M, et al. Promotion of articular cartilage matrix vesicle mineralization by type I collagen. *Arthritis Rheum* 2008; 58:2809–17.

47. Thouverey C, Bechkoff G, Pikula S, Buchet R. Inorganic pyrophosphate as a regulator of hydroxyapatite or calcium pyrophosphate dihydrate mineral deposition by matrix vesicles. *Osteoarthritis Cartilage* 2009; 17:64–72.

48. Roddy E, Doherty M. Gout and osteoarthritis: a pathogenetic link? *Joint Bone Spine* 2012; 79:425–7.

49. Kuo C-F, Grainge MJ, Mallen C, Zhang W, Doherty M. Comorbidities in patients with gout prior to and following diagnosis: case control study. *Ann Rheum Dis* 2016; 75(1):210–17.

50. Pascual E, Martínez A, Ordónez S. Gout: the mechanism of urate crystal nucleation and growth. A hypothesis based in facts. *Joint Bone Spine* 2013; 80:1–4.

51. Denoble AE, Huffman KM, Stabler TV, et al. Uric acid is a danger signal of increasing risk for osteoarthritis through inflammasome activation. *Proc Natl Acad Sci U S A* 2011; 108:2088–93.

52. Doherty M, Watt I, Dieppe PA. Localised chondrocalcinosis in post-meniscectomy knees. *Lancet* 1982; 1:1207–10.

CHAPTER 2

Palaeopathology of osteoarthritis

Juliet Rogers and Paul Dieppe

Palaeopathology and osteoarthritis: an introduction

Palaeopathology is a term first used by Schufeldt [1] and subsequently popularized by Sir Marc Armand Ruffer [2] at the beginning of the twentieth century as 'the study of disease in the past'. Ruffer was a pathologist in Cairo whose interest was aroused by the study of the extensive collection of mummies and other human remains which were being discovered with great frequency during this period. Palaeopathological evidence is, of course, not restricted to the study of mummified human remains although, because of soft tissue preservation, they are ideal. Paintings, drawings, sculpture, literature, and early medical texts can all be used as evidence for the presence and identification of early disease. The most widespread, common, and direct type of evidence however, particularly for disorders that affect the skeleton, is that derived from the study of human skeletal remains from archaeological sites. Apart from the interest in the occurrence of particular diseases at different time periods, palaeopathology can provide invaluable evidence for the frequency, distribution, and variation of expression of individual pathologies through time [3].

From the earliest organized studies of human skeletal remains, it has been evident that joint disease is the most frequent type of postcranial pathology to be seen. Despite diagnostic confusion and variation in terminology, what is now recognized as osteoarthritis (OA) is, by far, the most common form of these joint diseases: it is reported in hominid fossils [4], from Neolithic sites [5], and from Egyptian mummies [6]. The presence of OA is ubiquitous in all the other skeletal sites from earliest times to the post-medieval period [7], in the United Kingdom, Europe [8], the United States [9], and other areas of the world [10].

Recognition of osteoarthritis

OA is customarily recognized in skeletal material by a combination of morphological changes. As in other palaeopathological conditions these are generally very easy to see, although postmortem damage may mask some changes. The advantage of skeletal material over clinical observation is the opportunity for direct viewing of every joint in the body from every angle. This allows the recording of OA in unreported or underreported situations and of skeletal changes that are not apparent clinically or radiographically. Conversely, there is the disadvantage that all joints may not be present in every skeleton, thus reducing the quantity and completeness of information for analysis.

The most frequent change is the presence of a rim of osteophyte at the margin of the joint surfaces. Osteophytes are also frequently observed along the upper or lower margins of the vertebral bodies. Around the articular margins, the osteophyte may take the form of a thin, sharp rim, a flat ribbon, or a large florid and irregular fringe of bone (Figure 2.1). They may circle the entire joint margin or only a part. The joint surface itself may exhibit several different abnormalities, either alone or in combination. There may be small areas of new bone formation, 1–2 cm in diameter, in the form of 'buttons' or 'pancakes' of osteophyte on the articular surface itself (Figure 2.2). Frequently there are areas of pitting, with the openings occasionally visibly connecting with subchondral cysts (Figure 2.3). The pits can also be very small in diameter and they may be widely spaced or crowded together. The alteration of the shape or contour of the affected bones may also be seen and can now be measured [11]. The most striking abnormalities, however, are the clearly delineated areas of eburnation or polishing of the joint surface (Figure 2.4). On some joints the eburnated areas are grooved or scored [12] (Figure 2.5). This polishing is, presumably, caused by the total degradation of the cartilage, and the friction of the two opposing bone surfaces rubbing together.

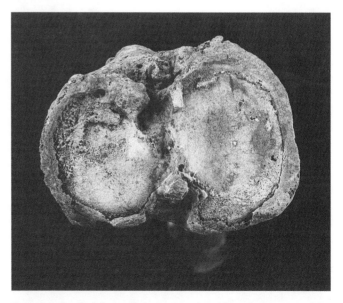

Figure 2.1 The tibial plateau of a knee joint with prolific osteophytes around the entire joint margin.

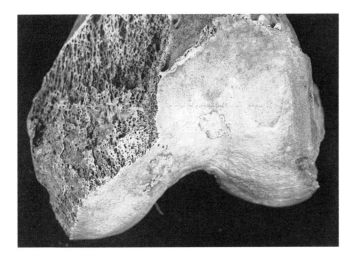

Figure 2.2 The anterior surface of a distal femoral condyle. There is extensive postmortem damage to the medial condyle but it is still possible to see the surface osteophyte both on the medial condyle and the patellofemoral joint.

Disease definition and assessment

There are, then, several different morphological changes that may be indicative of OA. The relationship between them is often assumed to be linear, as in the radiological stages developed by Kellgren and Lawrence [13]. In this model, osteophyte on its own is scored as being the mildest and earliest sign of OA, developing

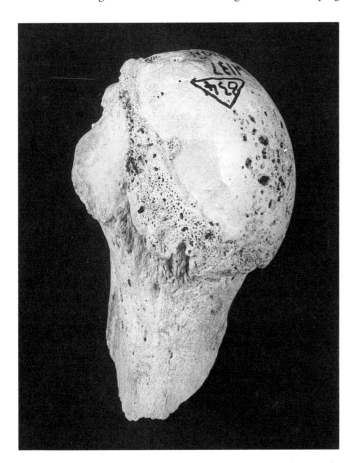

Figure 2.3 Humeral head with marginal osteophytes, eburnation, and pitting of the articular surface. In this example, the pits are restricted to the eburnated area.

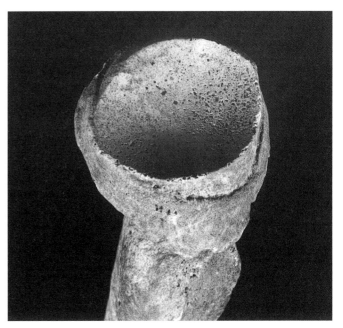

Figure 2.4 Proximal radial joint with marked bony contour change and eburnation.

to the most severe and latest stage marked by the presence of eburnation with grooves. However, osteophytes are an extremely common phenomenon and there is clinical evidence to suggest that they may be a marker of activity or age, rather than OA [14]. Particularly in skeletal material, they are easily seen by the direct observation of joints. If, therefore, a positive score for OA is recorded whenever osteophyte is present on its own, OA will be reported with an unexpectedly and erroneously high frequency in many joints. In many reports considering OA in skeletal populations, it is not always clear which diagnostic criteria have been used to score OA as present or absent. Furthermore, a study on the interobserver variation in coding OA in skeletal material [15] found that frequently there was incomplete agreement as to

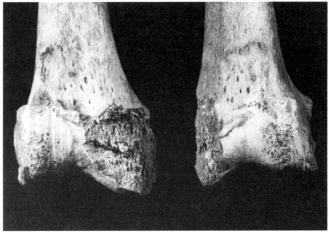

Figure 2.5 Patellofemoral joints in medieval knees, from the site at Barton-on-Humber. Despite postmortem damage, the grooves can clearly be seen on the eburnated lateral facet of the patellofemoral joint.

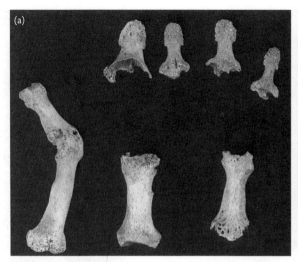
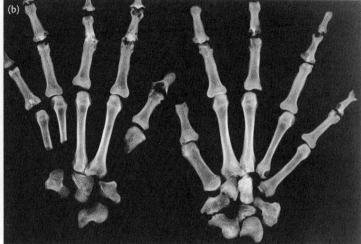

Figure 2.6 (a) Selected medial and distal phalanges of a skeleton, showing areas of erosion and fusion of one proximal and medial phalanx. (b) X-ray of hand bones from the same skeleton: a possible diagnosis of erosive OA was made for this specimen.

whether particular pathological changes were present, and only half the observers agreed on the severity of the changes. It is the case that many different scoring systems can and have been used [16]. These often bear no relationship to the clinical scoring systems, which can add to the confusion and may impair the comparison of skeletal data both between archaeological populations and with clinical data.

Examination of the relationship between visual, radiographic, and pathological changes can be used to help standardize the diagnostic criteria for OA in a palaeopathological context. Inspection of a series of cadaveric knees with OA demonstrates that the region of cartilage degradation has a sharply delineated margin enclosing an area of eburnation. Because of this good correlation between eburnation and cartilage degradation, the presence of eburnation is taken as a pathognomonic sign of the presence of OA. Osteophyte is more problematic, as outlined earlier. The relationship of pitting and bony contour change to the soft tissue pathology and how this relates in dry bone to the X-ray changes is also unclear. So again it is seen that the presence of osteophytes, pitting, or contour change on its own should not be used as a marker for OA. Only if two of the group (pitting of joint surface, osteophyte, bony contour change) are found together [17] should OA be considered as present.

There are, of course, many other bony changes that can be recognized in joints, such as erosion, periosteal reactions, and fractures. Some of these, such as erosions, may be due to other forms of arthropathy, which may give rise to secondary OA change. A diagnosis of erosive OA (EOA) has been suggested in one skeleton, a female recovered from a site in London [18]. The distribution of the erosions on the articular surfaces of the interphalangeal joints and in the carpal bones, with proliferative new bone around the joint margins, is characteristic of EOA (Figure 2.6). The radiological appearance confirmed the main involvement of the proximal and distal interphalangeal joints. The predominant abnormality was ill-defined bone destruction at the articular surfaces, producing in some fingers a 'gull-wing' abnormality and one proximal interphalangeal joint was ankylosed.

The prevalence of osteoarthritis

The aim of most research on the occurrence of OA in the past is to compare the frequency, distribution, or characteristics between various ancient populations and how and why they might differ from those seen now. For this one needs agreed and comparable data and work has begun to address this problem [16,19,20]. Even with agreed operational definitions for OA in palaeopathological material, as discussed earlier, there are still problems. In order that data collected from ancient skeletal populations can be related to modern information, it must be comparable. Clinical data are frequently obtained on the basis of radiographic assessments [13,21]. The visual inspection of skeletal material enables morphological alterations to be observed very easily, but it is not always clear that the visual and radiographic assessments of an osteoarthritic joint are comparable. A study by Rogers et al. [22] demonstrated a frequency of OA in a series of 24 skeletal knees ranging from 21% by visual assessment to 8% in the same knees radiologically assessed (Table 2.1). There is also considerable variation between authors in the way that individual joints are classified. The shoulder joint, for instance, may be defined as the glenohumeral joint or as the glenohumeral joint and acromioclavicular joint [7,9]. Clearly, differences in the definition of what constitutes a particular joint can also produce widely varying values. The knee is another joint that can suffer from confusion over definition between different researchers, some collecting data on the joint as a whole and others recording compartmental changes as separate joints.

Table 2.1 Frequency of OA in a series of 24 skeletal knees

Normal	Visual appearance		Radiological appearance
	Osteophyte only (eburnation)	OA	
8 knees	11 knees	5 knees	2 knees
(33.3%)	(41%)	(21%)	(8%)

Source data: [24].

A further major problem arises from the paucity of data available on skeletons collected for examination, and the absence of information about the extent to which they are representative of the population from which they come. For example, some burial sites may have a high concentration of clergy, or of some other unrepresentative section of society. It is also difficult to age skeletons accurately, the methods [20] used by biological anthropologists are generally imprecise, only allowing for ageing within a decade after skeletal maturation has been achieved, and with no differentiation after the age of 50, in most cases. For all of these reasons we cannot make accurate comparisons of the prevalence of OA in the modern and ancient populations.

Despite this, much interesting and valuable information on the overall prevalence of OA in different populations has been obtained.

Most authors reporting on many different skeletal groups from a wide and varying time span agree that OA is the most commonly reported pathological change and the most frequently occurring joint disease [23]. In a group of Roman British skeletons from Cirencester, for example, Wells [24] reported that 44.8% of the adult population had OA somewhere in the skeleton. When these figures were examined by sex, 51.5% of males and 32.9% of females were affected. In a medieval site in York [25], at Fishergate, 46.9% of adults had OA in at least one joint—48% of males and 43.8% of females. Rogers [26] found that only 15% of adult Roman British skeletons had OA—but there were only 15 Roman British skeletons recovered from the site (St Oswald's Priory, Gloucestershire). Larger numbers were recovered for the periods dating, respectively, 900–1120, 1120–1230, and 1600–1850. For the first of these periods, 22% of adults were reported as having OA—28.5% of males and 26.6% of females. The second, later medieval period had 24% of adults with OA—37.5% of males and 25% of females; and, in the post-medieval period dating 1600–1850, the frequency of OA in all adults was 34%—33.3% of males and 39.4% of females. Another site that yielded contemporary skeletal material to support the findings of the last phase of St Oswald's Priory was Christ Church, Spitalfields, in London. Three hundred and eighty-seven named skeletons were recovered from among a larger assemblage from the crypt of this church. Waldron [27] reported a prevalence of 30.9% of adults with OA, with 34.5% of males and 24.3% of females showing signs of OA change.

Site-specific prevalence

Many reports do not present an overall prevalence of OA for their skeletons but concentrate on the frequency of occurrence at particular joints. The majority of authors agree that OA most commonly affects the spinal facet joints. The prominence of spinal OA is a reasonably constant finding. When more detailed analysis of the peak level of affected vertebrae is undertaken there is also uniformity. Waldron [27] reports that the Spitalfields skeletons have a peak occurrence at cervical 4/5, thoracic 4/5, and lumbar 5 joints. Jurmain and Kilgore [28] find an almost identical picture in a medieval Nubian sample. Merbs [29], in a detailed and extensive study of Inuit skeletons, found a very similar distribution with peaks of OA frequency at cervical 2/4, thoracic 4/5, and lumbar 5 joints. As well as facet joint involvement of the cervical spine, OA of the odontoid component of atlanto-axial joints is also frequently observed (Figure 2.7).

The frequency of OA at peripheral joints varies more widely between populations, with Jurmain and Kilgore [28], for instance,

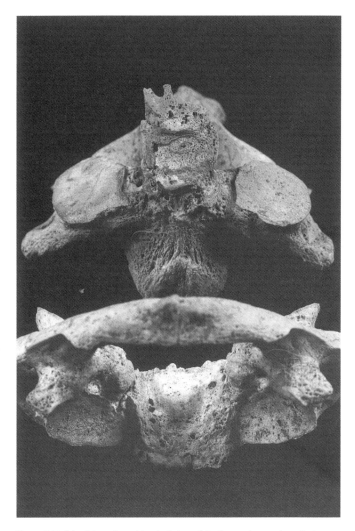

Figure 2.7 OA of the odontoid articulation of the first and second cervical vertebra with osteophyte and eburnation.

stating that the shoulder and hip are less involved than the knee or elbow, whereas Waldron [7] found the converse. Table 2.2 displays the frequency of OA at different joint sites reported by seven authors for seven different skeletal assemblages. It will be seen that there is a wide variation, some of which can be explained by the inclusion of the acromioclavicular joint within the scoring of the shoulder [7,9]. Other variations are likely to be due to the inclusion of too wide a range of bony change within the definition of OA [8,9,25]. The variations seen from the skeletons from the other sites are likely to be real, as the data was collected using the same operational definition of OA.

It can be seen from Table 2.2 that the ankle is very rarely involved in OA, which is similar to the pattern seen today [30]. Other differences are apparent, however, and the findings reported for knee and elbow joint OA raise particularly interesting issues. Rogers and Dieppe [31] reported that in the earlier historical period, hip OA was more frequent than knee OA, but that this ratio changed in the post-medieval period with knee OA becoming more frequent than hip OA. This differs from the pattern most frequently seen in archaeological skeletons in the United States [9,28], where hip OA is less common than knee OA. Not many skeletal reports have covered the precise distribution of knee OA into its component

Table 2.2 OA of different joints in various skeletal populations

Archaeological site	Joints (% skeletons affected)						
	Spine	Shoulder	Elbow	Wrist	Hip	Knee	Ankle
SE USA [8]	—	35.0	40.0	15.0	3.0	27.0	8.0
Fishergate, York [24]	—	12.5	17.0	15.0	18.2	15.2	4.0
Dordrecht, Holland [7]	36.8	14.3	5.6	—	12.0	5.2	—
Trowbridge, Wilts [27]	—	2.9	1.9	1.4	3.4	1.4	0.4
Castledyke, N. Lincs. [37]	—	7.6	1.8	5.2	2.3	3.8	0.0
England							
Premedieval	31.9	31.9	2.1	8.5	12.8	2.1	0.0
Medieval	31.7	33.5	2.1	3.6	5.7	5.0	0.0
Postmedieval	24.0	27.7	2.6	1.9	2.9	4.4	0.0
St Oswald's Priory, Glos [25]							
Early medieval	18.6	0.0	0.9	5.7	1.9	0.0	0.0
Medieval	22.5	0.9	0.0	2.7	4.6	0.9	0.0
Postmedieval	25.9	0.0	4.6	8.0	3.4	5.7	0.0

subjoints of patellofemoral and tibiofemoral compartments. In the same study of over 785 skeletons [31], despite the changing frequency of knee OA, the majority of affected compartments were patellofemoral. This finding has been confirmed by Waldron [7], but again skeletal populations from the United States seem to differ. Merbs [29] reported that the lateral compartment was more frequently involved than the other compartments. In some United States populations the medial and patellofemoral compartments are equally involved. There has been one study of large-joint osteoarthritis in an Asian (Japanese) population which again suggests change over time, as well as some differences between Asian and Caucasian skeletal populations, as might be expected [32]. One of the most important risk factors for tibiofemoral knee OA is obesity, so it is possible that the relative infrequency of tibiofemoral knee OA in old European populations is explained by a lower prevalence of severe obesity in the past. The elbow joint is interesting for different reasons. It has been found, in several different populations, that skeletal evidence of OA is extremely common in the elbow joint. However, it is rarely reported in contemporary clinical descriptions of OA [33]. This raises the intriguing possibility that elbow OA is relatively asymptomatic, which would result in us not looking for it and therefore not finding it, in the modern clinical setting [33–35]. Further investigation is needed to find the true prevalence of different joint involvement in different groups and their implications.

Generalized osteoarthritis and generalized bone formation

The examination of skeletons affords us a unique opportunity to investigate the association of OA between different joints, and thus that of the existence and patterns of 'generalized' forms of OA, and to look for associations between OA and other skeletal changes. However, this has not been possible for most investigators because the requirements include relatively large numbers of

skeletons with most joints preserved, in addition to sophisticated statistical analyses. The authors have been able to do such work, in conjunction with statistician Lee Shepstone, using a group of 563 well-preserved skeletons from Barton-on-Humber in the United Kingdom. We have obtained good evidence for the existence of at least two forms of generalized OA (i.e. clusters of joints with OA at a much higher association between them than would be expected by chance) [36]. We have also found that osteophyte formation as well as eburnation have a higher than expected association with the ossification of entheses, resulting in the concept of a subsection of bone formers in the population (i.e. people whose skeletons react to insult with more bone formation than is generally the case) [37,38]. Interestingly, Hardcastle and colleagues have recently shown that in people with abnormally high bone mass there is an association between osteoarthritis, osteophyte formation, and enthesophytes, supporting the concept of there being a subset of OA characterized by a generalized increase in bone formation [39].

The interpretation of osteoarthritis in osteoarchaeology

In most osteoarchaeological and palaeopathological investigations, a special interest is taken in the precise pattern and distribution of OA in different populations. This is because the perception is that OA results from biomechanical stress and that, thus, the pattern of involvement is an imprint of the activity or occupations of the early populations under investigation. A quotation by Calvin Wells [24] regarding OA perhaps best exemplifies this approach: 'It is the most useful of all diseases for reconstructing the lifestyle of early populations. Its anatomical localization reflects very closely their occupation and activities …'.

This concept has helped the widespread dissemination of a preconceived idea of OA as only being caused by activities and occupation. For instance, in a report [38] on the examination of over a thousand skeletons from the Romano–British site at Poundbury, the discussion of OA and other joint disease is placed in a chapter entitled 'Lifestyle and occupation'.

But this approach has also led to some extremely thorough and detailed examinations of the patterns and distributions of the series of bony changes seen in OA. Some of the variations of distribution are, in fact, very likely to be influenced by biomechanical and activity-related changes. However, this somewhat simplistic approach of equating a particular pattern with a particular activity has been questioned [40]. It is very difficult, if not impossible, to test the connection between activity and OA pattern and distribution in an archaeological sample. This is because it is not usually known how representative of the whole historic population the excavated skeletons are. Furthermore, there is rarely, if ever, documentation to link skeletons with particular activities.

The excavation of the 387 named skeletons from Christ Church, Spitalfields, provided a unique opportunity to investigate this further, as there was evidence for the occupation actually followed by these populations. Many of them had been weavers. Waldron and Cox [41], in a case–control study, found no relationship between occupation and OA of the hands or any other joint site.

Comparative animal data

Investigation of the variance of distribution between human populations and primate skeletons is also proving to be a useful area of investigation, providing more insight into the potential contribution of mechanical factors in the pathogenesis of OA at particular joint sites. Jurmain and Kilgore [28] and Lim et al. [42] have shown that there is a similar distribution of OA of the interphalangeal joints between an age-matched group of macaque and human skeletons, but that there was a much lower frequency of thumb-base OA in the macaque group. Investigation of knee OA in the same group of subjects also showed differences, with the humans having a high prevalence of patellofemoral OA. The converse is true of the macaques [43].

Rothschild has reviewed the reasons for skeletal 'palaeorheumatology' being able to make valuable contributions to our understanding of OA and other rheumatic diseases, which include the new ability to extract and analyse DNA from animal and human skeletal remains [44].

Conclusion

It is clear from the brief discussion of the palaeopathology of OA that there are many limitations both in the material and in the methodology and interpretation of findings. Nevertheless, it is also clear that the investigation of the nature and epidemiology of a disease such as OA in earlier populations can provide a valuable type of information to enhance and complement the current research into OA [29,45]. Furthermore, the access to skeletal material provides a unique resource for the investigation of specific questions such as the relationship between the visual, radiological, and pathological appearance of particular pathological changes. Skeletal material can also provide a source of information about the relationship of changes [37,45] throughout the entire skeleton, rather than being restricted to a few symptomatic joints, thus enhancing the possibility of learning something about a systemic bony response.

Acknowledgement

Tragically, Juliet Rogers died in November 2001 during the production of the Second Edition of *Osteoarthritis*. Her contribution to the palaeopathology of joint and bone disease was truly outstanding. In addition, she will be remembered by all who knew her as an exceptionally warm and generous individual. She is sadly missed.

Recommended reading

Lim K, Rogers J, Shepstone L, Dieppe P. The evolutionary origins of OA: a comparative skeletal study of hand disease in two primates. *J Rheumatol* 1995; 22(11):2132–4.

This evolutionary hypothesis of OA was first proposed by Charles Hutton in 1987. This paper describes one of the few studies that has tested and extended the hypothesis, using skeletal material from a variety of different primates and relating the distribution of OA to their morphology and joint usage. An example of a palaeopathological study that provides data of relevance to the pathogenesis of OA.

Rogers J, Shepstone L, Dieppe P. Bone formers: osteophyte and enthesophyte formation are positively associated. *Ann Rheum Dis* 1997; 56:85–90.

This paper reports an association between the formation of enthesophytes and osteophytes, the data being derived from a large collection of skeletons from Barton-on-Humber in the United Kingdom. It suggests that the generalized tendency for the skeleton to produce bone in response to stress is more pronounced in some individuals ('bone formers') than others, and that this goes some way to explaining the heterogeneity of the OA phenotype.

Rogers J, Waldron T. *A Field Guide to Joint Disease in Archaeology.* London: Wiley; 1995.

This excellent book is the current definitive guide to the examination and interpretation of findings on old skeletons. If you want a more readily available journal article, and to confine your attention to arthropathies, then the related reference (J Archaeol Sci 1987; 16:611–25) is an alternative, but the book is a fascinating read and highly recommended.

Ruffer MA. Studies in palaeopathology in Egypt. *J Pathol Bacteriol* 1913; 18:149–62.

This is the first significant publication on the use of ancient human remains as a means of exploring disease. Ruffer used mummies as they were more readily available to him than skeletons, which are now the main source of material.

Waldron T. Prevalence and distribution of OA in a population from Georgian and early Victorian London. *Ann Rheum Dis* 1991; 50:301–7.

A large, well-conducted study of osteoarthritis in skeletons. This collection is unique, because complete information on age at death and occupation are available, allowing much more informative comparisons with contemporary data to be made. (See also Waldren and Cox, Brit J Ind Med 1989; 46:420–2).

References

1. Schufeldt RW. Notes on paleopathology. *Pop Sci Monthly* 1893; 42:679–84.
2. Ruffer MA. Studies in palaeopathology in Egypt. *J Pathol Bacteriol* 1913; 18:149–62.
3. Rogers J, Dieppe P. Skeletal palaeopathology of the rheumatic diseases. Where are we now? *Ann Rheum Dis* 1990; 49:885–6.
4. Strauss WL, Cave AJ. Pathology and posture of Neanderthal man. *Quart Rev Biol* 1957; 32:348–63.
5. Rogers JM. The skeletal remains. In Saville A (ed) *Hazelton Long Barrow*. London: English Heritage; 1990:182–97.
6. Ruffer MA. Arthritis deformans and spondylitis in ancient Egypt. *J Pathol Bacteriol* 1918; 22:152–96.
7. Waldron T. Changes in the distribution of OA over historical time. *Int J Osteoarchaeol* 1995; 5:385–9.

8. Maat G, Mastwijk RW, van der Velde EA. Skeletal distribution of degenerative changes in vertebral osteophytosis, vertebral OA and DISH. *Int J Osteoarchaeol* 1995; 5(3):289–98.

9. Bridges P. Degenerative joint disease in hunter gatherers and agriculturalists from the South Eastern United States. *Am J Phys Anthropol* 1991; 85:379–91.

10. Kricum ME. Paleoradiology of the prehistoric Australian aboriginies. *Am J Roentgenol* 1994; 163:241–7.

11. Shepstone L, Rogers J, Kirwan J, Silverman B. The shape of the distal femur: a palaeopathological comparison of eburnated and non-eburnated femora. *Ann Rheum Dis* 1999; 58:72–8.

12. Rogers J, Dieppe P. Ridges and grooves on the bony surfaces of osteoarthritic joints. *Osteoarthritis Cartilage* 1993; 1:167–70.

13. Kellgren JH, Lawrence JS. Radiological assessment of OA. *Ann Rheum Dis* 1957; 16:494–501.

14. Hernborg J, Nilsson BE. The relationship between osteophytes in the knee joint, OA and ageing. *Acta Orthop Scand* 1973; 44:69.

15. Waldron T, Rogers J. Inter-observer variation in coding OA in human skeletal remains. *Int J Osteoarchaeol* 1991; 1:49–56.

16. Bridges P. The effect of variation in methodology on the outcome of osteoarthritic studies. *Int J Osteoarchaeol* 1993; 3:289–95.

17. Rogers J, Waldron T. *A Field Guide to Joint Disease in Archaeology.* London: Wiley; 1995:32–46.

18. Rogers J, Waldron T, Watt I. Erosive osteoarthritis in a mediaeval skeleton. *Int J Osteoarchaeol* 1991; 1:151–3.

19. Rogers J, Waldron T, Dieppe P, Watt I. Arthropathies in palaeopathology: the basis of classification according to most probable cause. *J Archaeol Sci* 1987; 16:611–25.

20. Buikstra JE, Ubelaker DH (eds). *Standards for Data Collection from Human Skeletal Remains.* Arkansas Arch Survey Research Series No. 44. Fayetteville, AR: Arkansas Archeological Survey; 1994.

21. van Saase J, van Romande IK, Cars A, Vandenbrouke J, Valkenberg H. Epidemiology of OA: the Zoctermeer survey. Comparison of radiological arthritis in a Dutch population with that in 10 other populations. *Ann Rheum Dis* 1989; 48:271–80.

22. Rogers J, Watt I, Dieppe P. Comparison of visual and radiographic detection of bony changes at the knee joint. *Br Med J* 1990; 300:367–8.

23. Ortner DJ, Putschar W. Identification of pathological conditions in human skeletal remains. *Smithson Contr Anthropol* 1985; 28:419.

24. Wells C. The human burials. In McWhirr A, Viner L, Wells C (eds) *Romano-British Cemeteries at Cirencester.* Cirencester: Excavation Committee; 1982:135–202.

25. Stroud G. The human bones. In Stroud G, Kemp RL (eds) *Cemeteries of St Andrew Fishergate.* York: York Archaeological Trust; 1993:160–241.

26. Rogers J. The human skeletons. In Heighway C (ed) *St Oswald's Priory.* Research Report for the Council for British Archaeology. London: Council for British Archaeology; 2001.

27. Waldron T. Prevalence and distribution of OA in a population from Georgian and early Victorian London. *Ann Rheum Dis* 1991; 50:301–7.

28. Jurmain RD, Kilgore L. Skeletal evidence of osteoarthritis, a palaeopathological perspective. *Ann Rheum Dis* 1995; 54:443–50.

29. Merbs CF. *Patterns of Activity-Induced Pathology in a Canadian Inuit Population.* Ottawa: National Museums of Canada; 1983.

30. Huch K, Kuettner KE, Dieppe P. Osteoarthritis in ankle and knee joints. *Sem Arthritis Rheum* 1997; 26:667–74.

31. Rogers J, Dieppe P. Is tibio-femoral osteoarthritis in the knee joint a new disease? *Ann Rheum Dis* 1994; 53:612–13.

32. Inoue K, Hakuda S, Fardellon P, et al. Prevalence of large joint osteoarthritis in Asian and Caucasian skeletal populations. *Rheumatology* 2001; 40:70–3.

33. Cushingham J, Dieppe P. Study of 500 patients with limb joint osteoarthritis. I. Analysis by age, sex, and distribution of symptomatic joint sites. *Ann Rheum Dis* 1991; 50:8–13.

34. Debono L, Mafart B, Jeusel E, Gulpert G. Is the incidence of elbow osteoarthritis underestimated? Insights from paleopathology. *Joint Bone Spine* 2004; 71: 397–400.

35. Doherty M, Preston B. Primary osteoarthritis of the elbow. *Ann Rheum Dis* 1989; 48:743–7.

36. Rogers J, Shepstone L, Dieppe P. Osteoarthritis—a system disorder of bone. *Arthritis Rheum* 2004; 50:452–7

37. Rogers J, Shepstone L, Dieppe P. Bone formers: osteophyte and enthesophyte formation are positively associated. *Ann Rheum Dis* 1997; 56:85–90.

38. Molleson T. The human remains. In Farewell DE, Molleson T (eds) *Poundbury, Vol. 2.* Monograph Series, No. 11, Dorchester: Dorset Natural History and Archaeological Society; 1993:142–214.

39. Hardcastle S, Dieppe P, Gregson CL, et al. Osteophytes, enthesophytes and high bone mass: a bone forming triad with potential relevance to osteoarthritis. *Arthritis Rheum* 2014; 66:2429–39.

40. Jurmain RD. Degenerative changes in peripheral joints as indicators of mechanical stress: opportunities and limitations. *Int J Osteoarchaeol* 1991; 3–4:247–52.

41. Waldron HA, Cox M. Occupational arthropathy evidence from the past. *Brit J Ind Med* 1989; 46:420–2.

42. Lim K, Rogers J, Shepstone L, Dieppe P. The evolutionary origins of OA: a comparative skeletal study of hand disease in two primates. *J Rheumatol* 1995; 22(11):2132–4.

43. Rogers J, Lim K, Shepstone L, Turnquist J. Distribution of knee OA in human and macaque skeletons. *Am J Phys Anthropol* 1996; 22(Suppl):202.

44. Rothschild B. Contributions of paleorheumatology to understanding contemporary disease. *Rheumatismo* 2002; 54:272–84.

45. Dieppe PA, Rogers J. Two dimensional epidemiology. *Brit J Rheumatol* 1985; 24:310–12.

CHAPTER 3

Morphological aspects of pathology

Laura A. Wyatt and Michael Doherty

Introduction

Osteoarthritis (OA) is the commonest condition to affect the synovial joints. Any synovial joint can be affected by OA, however most research on the pathology of human OA relates to large joints, specifically knees and hips. Established OA is characterized by a mixture of tissue loss and new tissue production resulting in the classic combination of focal loss of articular hyaline cartilage together with bone remodelling and osteophyte formation. It is this combination of focal hyaline cartilage loss, bone remodelling, and osteophyte formation that defines OA pathologically. However, pathological alterations characteristically occur in all joint tissues in OA making it a disease of the whole joint [1]. Indeed, in recent years there has been growing interest in the synovial changes that are observed in OA and their contribution to the changes in cartilage and overall progression of OA pathogenesis [2]. Clearly, understanding specific pathological alterations in OA and how these relate to patient-centred outcomes is crucial for logical development of targeted treatments. This chapter aims to summarize the overall gross morphological aspects of OA pathology. More detailed coverage of pathophysiology in the individual tissues will be covered in Chapters 4–7.

Normal articular cartilage

Pathological modifications in the articular cartilage are a key feature in OA pathogenesis. However, before discussing the morphological changes OA the normal histological and macroscopic features of the articular cartilage must first be considered.

Articular cartilage is a highly specialized and unique tissue lining the articulating surfaces of the joint. In the healthy joint the cartilage is a firm material with a white to off-white colour and a smooth unbroken surface with no limiting boundary membrane [3]. With lubrication from the viscous synovial fluid, this smooth surface facilitates a low-friction motion during movement. It also acts as a protective connective tissue to bear and distribute mechanical loads across the joint and to protect the underlying subchondral bone. Articular cartilage has a very limited capacity to repair [4]. The functional capabilities of the articular cartilage are dependent upon the highly specialized structure and composition of the tissue.

Healthy mature articular cartilage is aneural, avascular, and alymphatic. This is advantageous for load-bearing tissue since otherwise these structures would be compressed and activated under load. Oxygen and nutrients are supplied in part through diffusion from the synovial fluid which is in direct contact with the articular surface, but also from diffusion from the subchondral blood vessels which supply nutrients to the calcified cartilage.

Cartilage is comprised of just a single cell type, the chondrocyte. Chondrocytes are specialized cells embedded in lacunae within the highly organized extracellular matrix (ECM). Chondrocytes are relatively sparse and comprise only around 1% of total tissue volume [5]. The ECM is produced by the chondrocytes and consists mainly of water (75–80%) and structural macromolecules (predominantly collagen type II and proteoglycan), in addition to non-collagenous molecules and glycoproteins [6].

The shape and volume of cartilage is maintained by the collagenous framework. This provides a scaffold of fibrils, each a triple helix linked by disulphide bonds, analogous to a spring mattress, being readily bent when compressed but having very high tensile strength if stretched lengthways. The collagen framework entraps macromolecules including proteoglycans and highly charged hydrophilic sugar and protein molecules. Proteoglycans have a high affinity for water but rarely if ever become saturated and are essential for maintaining the high osmotic potential of the cartilage. The ability of cartilage to retain water is critical for its highly specialized function. When proteoglycan macromolecules draw in water they expand within the surrounding collagen framework and push it out to its full volume, maintaining the shape of the cartilage and limiting further expansion of the proteoglycans. However, when cartilage undergoes loading, water is squeezed laterally allowing the cartilage thickness to diminish and to absorb some of the load. When loading is removed the water rapidly returns under osmotic pressure to allow the cartilage to resume its normal volume again. The compressive and tensile resilience of the articular cartilage is facilitated by the proteoglycans and collagenous network, respectively [7].

The major proteoglycan present in cartilage is aggrecan. It is constructed of a protein core with many sulphated, highly negatively charged glycosaminoglycan (GAG) side chains (chondroitin sulphate and keratan sulphate) attached [5,8]. Hyaluronic acid together with link proteins forms a large supramolecular complex with the aggrecan protein core.

Histologically the articular cartilage is an elaborate, organized tissue. Morphological differences in the chondrocytes, collagen fibrils, and proteoglycan content allow for identification of four distinct anatomical layers. Adjacent to the subchondral bone is the calcified cartilage, followed by the deep (radial), middle (transitional), and superficial (tangential) layers. The latter three are non-calcified tissue [9]. The tidemark is a 2–5 μm thick mineralizing front marking the boundary between the deep and calcified layer [10].

Of all four zones the superficial is the thinnest (10–20% of articular cartilage thickness). Chondrocytes in this zone are of a flattened appearance. Collagen bundles (20 nm diameter) are tightly packed and orientated parallel to the superficial surface and aggrecan content is low. About half of the cartilage volume (40–60%) is occupied by the middle zone [4]. Here chondrocytes are more sparsely distributed, and are more spherical in shape. Collagen fibrils have a larger diameter (70–120 nm) and are arranged in radial bundles [8]. In the deep zone (approximately 30% of cartilage volume), collagen fibrils have the largest diameter and are arranged perpendicular to the articular surface. Proteoglycan is abundant and chondrocytes are arranged in columns perpendicular to the articular surface.

Morphological changes in the articular cartilage

OA is a metabolically dynamic process, characterized both by tissue attrition and synthesis. A variety of joint insults may mediate the onset of OA and in general OA development and progression is very slow. The early phase of OA is characterized by increased synthesis of collagen type II and aggrecan by the articular chondrocytes in medial and deep layers [11]. As OA progresses, the balance may shift in favour of joint degradation promoting release of proteolytic enzymes, matrix metalloproteinases (MMPs) from chondrocytes

[12], possibly mediated by proinflammatory cytokines such as interleukin 1 (IL1) and tumour necrosis factor alpha (TNFA) [13].

The appearance and extent of articular cartilage loss can be determined macroscopically (Figures 3.1 and 3.2). Normal cartilage is a white homogenous colour and firm in nature (Figure 3.1a, b). Although cartilage loss is a characteristic feature of established OA, an initial increase in cartilage thickness due to increased water content may be detected in the earliest stages [14]. Alterations are typified by initial softening and swelling of the articular surface which is of a light brown colouration (Figure 3.1c, d). In OA, various collagenases and MMPs break down macromolecules in the cartilage into smaller pieces, increasing the ability to draw more water into the cartilage, thus increasing thickness and turgor pressure. Eventually the collagen framework is compromised by the increased turgor pressure which mediates cartilage loss.

With OA progression, fibrillation of the superficial layer can be observed. In advanced cases the cartilage may be grey, red, or dark brown in appearance. In cases with severe macroscopic appearances, focal cartilage loss may expose the subchondral bone (Figure 3.1d) [3].

Histological features of osteoarthritic articular cartilage include fibrillation of the articular surface and phenotypic modifications in chondrocyte morphology, which include a variable mixture of hypercellularity, cloning and hypocellularity (Figures 3.3 and 3.4) [15].

Cartilage fibrillation is a key feature of OA, and can be assessed microscopically. The early phases of OA are characterized by the appearance of vertical clefts in the articular surface (Figure 3.3a). As the disease progresses, fibrillations extend deeper through the

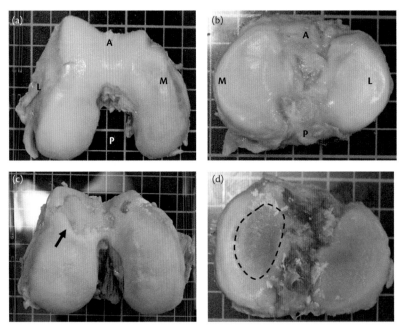

Figure 3.1 Macroscopic appearance of femoral condyle (a, c) and tibial plateau (b, d) articular surfaces obtained from cadaver donors. (a) Normal cartilage appearance in lateral aspect of the femoral condyle typified by a smooth unbroken surface. Mild swelling and softening is observed on the medial surface. (b) Normal white homogenous colouration of the medial and lateral surface of the tibial plateaux. (c) Cartilage defects observed in a femoral condyle. Coarsely broken surface indicated by arrow. (d) Cartilage defects in the medial and lateral aspect of the tibial plateaux. An area of subchondral bone exposure in the medial compartment is indicated by the dotted circle. A, anterior; L, lateral; M, medial; P, posterior.
Courtesy of Prof. David Walsh.

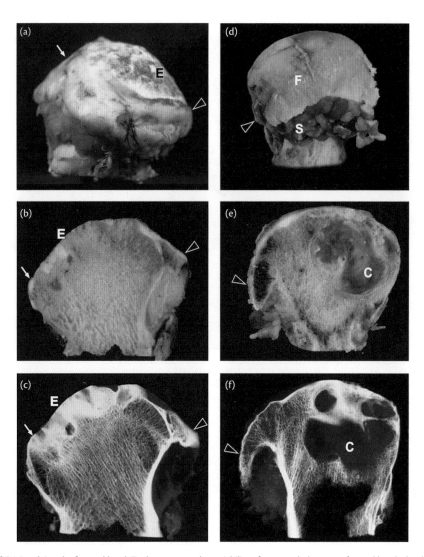

Figure 3.2 Gross pathology of OA involving the femoral head. To demonstrate the variability of gross pathology, two femoral heads that have been removed surgically because of OA are illustrated. Both specimens show extensive remodelling. The femoral head is shown in (a), (b), and (c), with extensive eburnation of the surface and articular plate bone sclerosis: (a) surface; (b) cut surface; (c) specimen X-ray of (b). Prominent features of OA include cartilage erosion, closed arrow; bone eburnation, E; osteophyte formation, arrow head. The femoral head with a relative preservation of cartilage, extreme subchondral bone cyst formation, and extreme osteophyte formation is shown in (d), (e), and (f): (d) surface; (e) cut surface; (f) specimen X-ray of (e). Prominent OA features include cartilage fibrillation, F; synovial hypertrophy, S; osteophyte formation, open arrow head; cyst formation, C.

cartilage; in advanced OA, large clefts may penetrate the tidemark to enter the calcified cartilage (Figure 3.4).

During OA, there is alteration in proteoglycan content. In the early phases of OA, proteoglycan loss from the superficial layer is observed [15]. Furthermore there are changes in the molecular structure of proteoglycans, from the normal aggregated form to non-aggregated form. The elevated non-aggregated proteoglycan content may lead to chondromalacia (cartilage softening), which may be detected by mechanical probing at arthroscopy. Normally, the low permeability of the matrix membrane and hydraulic pressure maintains the stiffness of the cartilage which is essential for distributing compressive and tensile stresses over the bone. Subsequently, aberrant breakdown of the non-aggregated form of proteoglycan increases hydraulic permeability, reducing the fluid pressure thus resulting in loss of stiffness and chondromalacia [16].

Fibrillation is a consequence of impaired integrity of the collagen network and reduced fluid pressure as described above. In addition, fibrillation may in part result from the reduced adhesion of chondrocytes to fibronectin, a high-molecular-weight glycoprotein [17]. In relation to fibrillation, water content in the cartilage is significantly increased in early OA [18]. These features, along with the altered proteoglycan composition all contribute to increased permeability and decreased stiffness of the ECM.

Osteoarthritic tissue can lose its ability to remain avascular and aneural, which may be attributed to loss of tidemark integrity. Breaching of the tidemark by channels originating in the subchondral bone and entering the non-calcified cartilage has been observed in OA (Figure 3.3b) [19,20]. Tidemark integrity is physiologically important in preventing macromolecular diffusion and maintaining the chondro-osseous barrier. Loss of tidemark integrity may permit growth factors such as vascular endothelial growth

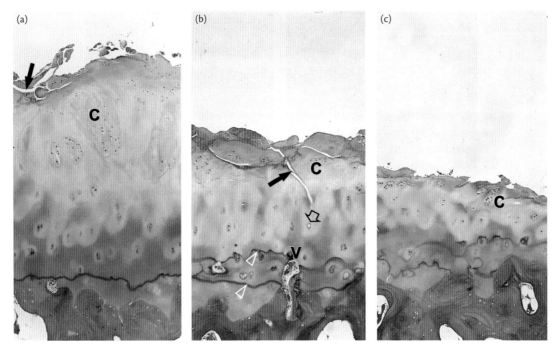

Figure 3.3 Microscopic pathology of OA articular cartilage. The photomicrographs are taken from different areas of the same specimen: (a) early OA; horizontal fibrillation (closed arrow), chondrocyte clusters, C. (b) moderate OA, vertical fissure (closed arrow), chondrocyte death (open arrow), tidemark undulation and duplication (open arrow head), vascular penetration into cartilage, V, chondrocyte clusters, C. (c) Advanced OA, with cartilage erosion, cartilage matrix disorganization and chondrocyte clusters, C. Haematoxylin and eosin stain, magnification ×40.

factor to enter the subchondral bone from the non-calcified cartilage matrix to induce osteochondral angiogenesis [21]. The tidemark may be duplicated in OA [19], but it may also be a feature of normal ageing [22].

Calcium crystals in osteoarthritis

Mineralization of the cartilage and deposition of basic calcium phosphate (BCP—predominantly carbonate-substituted hydroxyapatite but also octacalcium phosphate and tricalcium phosphate) and calcium pyrophosphate (CPP) dihydrate crystals are a common finding in late established OA, certainly at the knee [23].

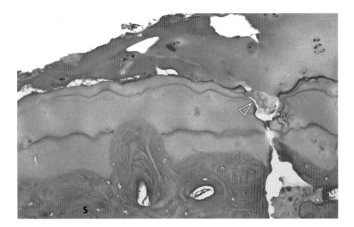

Figure 3.4 The articular plate in advanced OA. The cartilage is eroded. The tidemark shows undulation and duplication. The subchondral bone (S) is thickened and a fracture through the subchondral bone and calcified cartilage is present (open arrow head). Haematoxylin and eosin stain, magnification ×100.

Mineralization of the cartilage is a key feature of endochondral ossification. Endochondral ossification describes the process of embryonic and juvenile bone formation from cartilaginous tissue. During development, chondrocytes divide rapidly and are very active in secreting components of the ECM including aggrecan and type II collagen. Calcification and ossification of the cartilage bone ends is required to allow bone growth and this is promoted in part through secretion of type X collagen, which can encourage crystal nucleation, from the hypertrophic chondrocytes [23]. Furthermore, during growth the cartilage has a rich blood supply and displays immature antigenic epitopes.

In the healthy mature joint the cartilage is avascular, aneural, and displays mature antigenic epitopes. Furthermore the normal adult chondrocyte phenotype is stabilized and shows lower synthetic activity than during growth. However, when OA develops, the cartilage reverts back to an immature state which is ideally suited to producing new tissue. Immature epitopes reappear ('neo-epitopes'), and the usually avascular and aneural cartilage may be invaded by blood and nerve vessels from the underlying subchondral bone [20]. Furthermore the chondrocyte phenotype reverts to the hypertrophic form (Figure 3.5b) and increases its production of ECM components.

Hypertrophic chondrocyte differentiation is closely associated with BCP and CPP production, and calcium crystals are located close to areas of chondrocyte hypercellularity. BCPs are found in cartilage in all cases of severe knee OA [23] making BCP crystal deposition an integral aspect of OA rather than a marker for a particular subset. CPP crystals also occur in cartilage in around 20% of knees with end-stage knee OA [23]. Interestingly peripheral joints with OA are particularly prone to urate crystal deposition in people with gout [24] so the association between OA and crystal deposition is not restricted to calcium crystals.

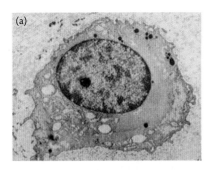
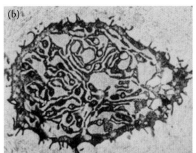

Figure 3.5 Chondrocyte appearance visualized using electron microscopy. (a) Chondrocyte in lacuna from normal hyaline cartilage. (b) Chondrocyte from osteoarthritic cartilage showing great increase in endoplasmic reticulum associated with increased production of matrix components (hypertrophic chondrocyte phenotype).

In normal adult cartilage, inhibitors of crystal nucleation and growth (e.g. proteoglycan) usually prevent cartilage calcification. During ageing there is reduction in proteoglycan and increase in crystal promotors (e.g. lipid), but in OA there is an even greater reduction in inhibitors such as proteoglycan and an increase in other promotors such as osteopontin, cartilage intermediate layer protein (CILP), chondrocyte matrix vesicles, and upregulation of expression of various transglutaminases. Furthermore, extracellular concentration of inorganic pyrophosphate increases around hypertrophic OA chondrocytes and this can influence formation of both BCP and CPP crystals.

Morphological alterations in the subchondral bone

Subchondral bone is a highly dynamic and adaptive tissue, which is capable of remodelling in response to local mechanical stress. The subchondral bone plays an important role in OA pathogenesis. Osteoarthritic morphological alterations in the subchondral bone include bone remodelling, microfractures, and localized areas of osteonecrosis, trabecular thickening, and osteophyte formation. The crucial involvement of the subchondral bone in OA pathology was first proposed by Radin and colleagues [25] who suggested that subchondral bone pathology precedes articular cartilage pathology. Conversely stress in the articular cartilage may over time induce microfractures in the trabecular bone. Subsequent repair of these microfractures may increase subchondral bone stiffness, impairing the ability for the bone to act as a shock absorber which increases forces in overlying articular cartilage inducing secondary damage.

Bone marrow pathology

Radiographs and magnetic resonance imaging (MRI) are valuable, non-invasive investigative techniques which have been pivotal in characterizing osteoarthritic modifications in the subchondral bone. Morphological alterations in the subchondral bone marrow exist in OA. Typically subchondral bone marrow spaces occupy fatty marrow tissue, but during OA focal areas of fatty marrow may be replaced with fibrovascular tissue [20,26]. The histological appearances of bone marrow lesions (BMLs) on MRI have been characterized as manifestations of bone marrow necrosis, fibrosis, and oedema in addition to bone marrow bleeding [27]. Fibrovascular bone marrow replacement may be associated with bone marrow lesions on MRI [27], in addition to osteochondral angiogenesis [20].

BML development may be associated with other pathological changes within the osteoarthritic joint such as cartilage degeneration [28], subchondral cysts [29], and subchondral attrition [30]. Nevertheless, different pathological characteristics typically coincide and it is therefore difficult to prove causality.

Osteophytes

Osteophytes are cartilaginous and osseous spurs which develop predominantly along the joint margin, but also can be located centrally (e.g. the inter-condylar site and tibial 'spiking' at the knee, and bone 'buttons' rising into the cartilage from subchondral bone (see Chapter 2, Figure 2.2). Osteophytes are a hallmark feature of OA which can be assessed radiographically [31,32] and form part of the diagnostic criteria for OA [33]. Periosteal and synovial mesenchymal stem cells are thought to be osteophyte precursors [34]. Osteophytosis occurs primarily through the process of endochondral ossification with an initial fibrocartilaginous outgrowth at the joint margin that then undergoes calcification and ossification (Figure 3.6). At the inferior aspect of the femoral neck osteophyte derives from periosteum and such periosteal osteophyte ('buttressing') may appear as a separate distinct layer from the underlying bone. Bone morphogenetic proteins, in addition to transforming growth factor beta (TGFβ) and basic fibroblast growth factor (bFGF) [35] may play a key role in the development of osteophytes. Osteophytes tend to occur at characteristic places within a joint and

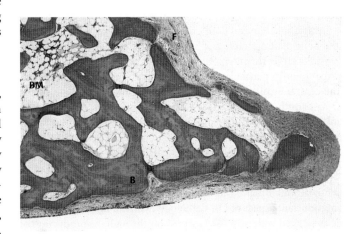

Figure 3.6 An osteophyte at the articular margin; fibrocartilage, F, bone, B, haematopoietic bone marrow, BM. Haematoxylin and eosin stain, magnification ×2.5.

may act as a protective mechanism to stabilize the osteoarthritic joint [36].

Bone remodelling

Bone is a dynamic tissue; homeostasis is maintained by continuous resorption (destruction) and formation by osteoclasts and osteoblasts, respectively. Homeostatic activity is disrupted during OA in favour of increased bone formation, leading to osteophyte formation, sclerosis and bone remodelling. Bone remodelling is considered to be largely a consequence of mechanical loading in addition to other pathological changes. Wolff's law of bone describes the ability of bone to adapt to mechanical loading by remodelling itself in terms of shape, trabecular alignment, and thickening to be better able to accommodate the loading. Remodelling of the subchondral bone leads to narrowing of the joint space which can be assessed radiographically [31,32].

As OA progresses, the shape of the bone ends may change considerably due to remodelling but also to attrition. An example of this is increasing non-sphericity of the femoral head and reduction in the neck-shaft-angle as hip OA progresses. Conversely, non-sphericity of the femoral head ('pistol grip' deformity) may associate with femoroacetabular impingement and be a risk factor for hip OA, leading some to suggest that slow bone remodelling may be a very early, or even the first abnormality, relating to OA. Because some morphological changes may be both a cause and a consequence of OA there is considerable interest in studying morphological variation prospectively in community cohorts.

In end-stage OA, full-thickness cartilage loss can expose the subchondral bone, which in turn, is more vulnerable to sclerosis. Mechanical grinding of the two adjacent bone ends may lead to a very polished-looking appearance ('eburnation') sometimes with deep grooves which reflect the wear pattern but which may help stability (see Chapter 2, Figure 2.5). Subchondral bone 'cysts' form beneath remodelled joint surfaces, often under areas where the cartilage is absent, and are commonly seen in OA joints. Subchondral bone cysts may originate from localized microfractures and osteonecrotic lesions in the bone mediated by increased mechanical pressure (the bone contusion theory) [29,37]. Alternatively synovial fluid may enter the subchondral bone through microfissures in the calcified cartilage (synovial fluid intrusion theory) [38,39]. Bone necrosis in the superficial layers of bone is thought to result from increased local biomechanical stress on the bone surface.

Central subchondral bone erosions and collapse of the subchondral bone plate are radiographic features of 'erosive hand OA' [40]. Erosions target the interphalangeal joints and the first carpometacarpal joint in particular, and lead to cartilage and bone attrition. The central erosions are depicted radiographically as a 'gull-wing' or 'saw-tooth' appearance (see Chapter 2, Figure 2.6). Furthermore, ankylosis of affected interphalangeal joints may occur and this is not a feature of other forms of OA.

Synovium

Synovial inflammation in OA is increasingly being recognized as an important aspect of OA pathology. Synovial inflammation may be associated with pain [41,42], possibly through the production of proinflammatory cytokines which can sensitize nerves and through increase in intracapsular pressure. The synovium has a rich blood and nerve supply [43]. The functions of the normal synovium include production of synovial fluid to lubricate the articular cartilage surfaces [44], facilitating nutrient and oxygen delivery to the chondrocytes and removing waste products of matrix degradation from the synovial cavity [2].

Histologically three synovial subtypes have been identified; fibrous, areola, and adipose [45].

Two morphologically distinct synovial layers exist: the lining (intima) and sublining (subintima). The synovium is composed of two major types of synovial cells (synoviocytes): type A cells are resident macrophages, whereas type B are fibroblast-like synoviocytes [45,46].

The normal synovium consists of a one- to four-cell thick synovial lining [45,47]. The synovial sublining is typified by a sparse cellular distribution, in addition to adipocytes and a dispersed distribution of blood and lymphatic vessels. Furthermore there are very few inflammatory cells present [45,47]. Synovial inflammation may be a feature of both early [48] and end-stage OA [47]. The degree and extent of synovial change can be characterized either histologically [47,49] or through imaging.

The OA synovium may show variable, but sometimes marked proliferation of the synoviocytes in the lining layer (hyperplasia), which may be more than seven cells deep [47], in addition to synoviocyte hypertrophy. Moreover, there may be infiltration of inflammatory cells such as macrophages (Figure 3.7), and in severe inflammation, localized perivascular lymphoid aggregates containing T and B lymphocytes and macrophages also may be observed [47]. Synovial villus formation and increased vascularity [50] may also occur. Increased synovial cytokine and chemokine synthesis is suggested to be a feature of early OA [48]. However, reduced synovial lymphatic vessels have been observed recently in OA and reduced lymphatic clearance may contribute to some of the synovial hypertrophy and increase in synovial fluid volume seen in OA [51].

Cartilage fragments may be incorporated in the synovial lining, exacerbating inflammation ('debris synovitis') which in turn, through the release of proinflammatory cytokines such as IL1B and TNFA mediates further damage to the surrounding joint tissues. Furthermore, BCP and CPP crystals within the joint may contribute to low-grade synovial inflammation and cartilage degradation through the production of proinflammatory mediators such as nitric oxide, MMP13, and prostaglandin E2 [52].

The synovial reaction in OA generally is far less marked than that observed in rheumatoid arthritis (RA). In RA, synovial

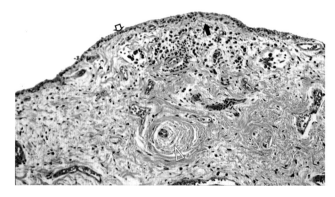

Figure 3.7 OA synovium synovial lining cells (open arrow), subintimal fibrosis (closed arrow head); perivascular fibrosis (closed arrow); infiltrate of plasma cells and lymphocytes, P. Haematoxylin and eosin stain, magnification ×20.

inflammation is chronic and widespread whereas in OA, it is usually more focal. Furthermore marginal erosions commencing at the 'bare areas' of the joint where synovium is directly opposed to the bone cortex are a hallmark feature of RA but are not observed in patients with OA.

Osteochondral 'loose bodies' are a not infrequent feature in OA. These are composed of fragments of bone and/or cartilage and although they may exist loose within the joint they predominantly are incorporated within the synovial lining. Cartilaginous loose bodies containing chondrocytes can increase in size and eventual calcify and ossify into bony tissue. Apart from synovial uptake of cartilage and bone shards, some osteochondral bodies may arise locally through chondroid metaplasia of synoviocytes.

Synovial fluid

Normal synovial fluid is an ultrafiltrate of plasma to which is added hyaluronic acid and other synovium-produced molecules to make it highly viscous. The cell content is almost zero and limited to mononuclear cells and macroscopically it is viscous, pale, yellow to colourless in appearance. In OA, there is an increase in volume of the synovial fluid and an accompanying decrease in viscosity due to a decrease in hyaluronic acid and other macromolecules. The cell count may increase but remains predominantly mononuclear cells. The fluid may contain cartilage debris and calcium crystals. CPP crystals may be seen and identified using ordinary light or phase contrast microscopy, but under polarized light microscopy 60% are non-birefringent while others exert weak positive birefringence. They are small (<15 μm) and polymorphic, varying in shape from a rhombus to thin needles; rods or thick needles and parallelepipeds are intermediate forms. BCP crystals are too small to be visualized by ordinary microscopy but aggregates of BCP crystals may be seen under light microscopy if stained with Alizarin red S at acidic pH. Fibroblast-like synoviocytes play an active role in BCP formation [53]. An increase in proinflammatory cytokines in the synovial fluid is a reported feature of OA [54].

Meniscal pathology

Fibrocartilage menisci and discs occur in the knee, temporomandibular and sternoclavicular joints, and there is also a triangular fibrocartilage disc at the wrist. The large knee menisci are responsible for proprioception, reducing friction and shock absorption by dissipating weight throughout the joint. Menisci are comprised of chondrocytes set within a collagenous matrix (mainly type I collagen), with glycoproteins, proteoglycans, and elastin [55]. Two distinct regions of the knee menisci have been identified histologically: the inner and outer region. Normally, the inner two-thirds of the menisci are avascular. In knee OA, there is an increase in meniscal vascular densities in addition to CGRP-immunoreactive nerves at the fibrocartilage junction. Angiogenesis and neuronal growth in the meniscus in OA may contribute to symptomatic OA [56]. Furthermore, in OA, mild meniscal pathology is characterized histologically by mild clefts to the collagen bundles, in addition to slight hypocellularity of the chondrocytes. Severe knee meniscal changes are identified by severe cleft and cyst formation, more pronounced regions of chondrocyte hypocellularity [56–58] and herniation and extrusion from the tibiofemoral compartment.

Fibrous tissues and other joint structures

Other tissues that comprise the joint are also affected by OA. The intra-articular ligaments and capsule provide essential support and stability to the joint. Both structures are composed of highly orientated type I collagen fibres. During OA there are pathological changes that include thickening of the joint capsule and intra-articular ligaments, such changes possibly helping to stabilize the compromised OA joint as part of the repair process. Lacerations and scar tissue are evident microscopically in the ligaments and capsular tissue in OA. Although thickening and contracture are usual, the ligaments and capsule may lose some of their stabilizing potential and resulting instability may further facilitate joint pathology. Distortion of the capsule may be precipitated by increased synovial effusion in the joint and equally alterations in the capsule impair fluid diffusion in the joint cavity. Enthesophytes at the insertions of the capsule, ligaments, and tendons may also occur more commonly in OA and be a marker of a bone-forming phenotype [59].

As in any arthropathy, the muscles that act over the OA joint may show generalized atrophy of type II muscle fibres, which clinically may associate with muscle weakness, wasting, and reduced proprioception [60,61]. Such muscle alterations may have multiple causes such as reduced activity, inhibition due to pain, and local spinal reflex inhibition.

Is osteoarthritis a disease of mechanics or inflammation?

The precipitating mechanism driving the onset of OA has been widely debated. Evidence for OA as a disease of mechanics has been proposed and is most widely accepted [62]. The mechanical theory suggests that increased mechanical loading across a joint can induce OA. Furthermore this theory suggests that inflammation in OA is a secondary feature of the disease caused by incorporation of joint products into the synovial lining initiating an inflammatory response.

In contrast, various researchers have argued for a more central role of low-grade synovial inflammation in mediating OA pathogenesis [2]. Synovial inflammation has been well characterized in OA, although the changes are far less severe than that seen in RA and marginal erosions, osteopenia, and marked clinical inflammation are not features of OA. Furthermore, cartilage loss is characteristically focal in OA but more generalized in conditions with synovitis as a key driver of disease. Nevertheless, different levels of inflammation have been reported in OA, and imaging and histological studies have associated synovial changes with pain [41,42,63].

There is a wide spectrum of severity of OA, with variable involvement of the various joint tissues, and based on the perspective of OA as the inherent repair process of synovial joints it may be that some joint insults that initiate OA have a synovitis element (e.g. 'secondary' OA following recognized RA, infection, seronegative spondyloarthropathy, etc.) whereas more commonly it is single or repetitive biomechanical trauma/injury to one or more tissue components that triggers the joint-wide OA process.

Joint pathology in osteoarthritis and normal ageing

Age is a major risk factor for OA. However OA is not an inevitable consequence of ageing. The differences between OA and normal

Table 3.1 Comparison of OA and normal age-related changes in the joint

Feature	OA	Ageing
Cartilage loss sites	Focal	General, all layers
Cartilage water content	Initial increase (oedema)	Dehydration
Proteoglycan content	Irreversible proteoglycan depletion	Decreased proteoglycan synthesis
Cartilage collagen	Degradation	Increased advanced glycation end products
Cartilage texture	Chondromalacia	Stiffness
Chondrocyte activity	Increased proliferation and death	Decreased activity
Bone	Subchondral remodelling	Osteopenia
Synovium	Mild, focal inflammation	Atrophy
Muscle	Atrophy	Atrophy

age-related changes are summarized in Table 3.1. In OA, cartilage loss is focal, whereas in ageing, cartilage loss occurs from all layers. In OA, water content in the cartilage ECM is initially increased as the breakdown of macromolecules draw water into the tissue. Such changes are not apparent in normal ageing in which progressive dehydration occurs.

In normal ageing, there is a decrease in proteoglycan synthesis [64] which contrasts with the progressive degradation of proteoglycan in OA [4] and accumulation of non-aggregated proteoglycan content which may lead to chondromalacia. The progressive destruction of articular cartilage in OA is attributed partly to the breakdown of type II collagen fibres by various collagenases and MMPs. The tensile strength of the cartilage decreases from around 30 years of age [65] and during ageing the collagen framework increases in stiffness. Increased stiffness may be attributed to both the accumulation [66] and crosslinking [67] of non-enzymatic advanced glycation end products in the collagen framework. Cartilage stiffness may contribute to the propensity of the joint to develop OA.

Chondrocytic phenotypes in OA are characterized by increased proliferation, which are evident microscopically as chondrocyte clusters located towards the superficial surface of the articular cartilage. Furthermore chondrocyte death (or hypocellularity) is mediated by apoptosis in OA. During ageing, articular chondrocytes display a decline in activity, impairing their ability to maintain homeostasis of the ECM [68]. This contrasts with the active hypertrophic chondrocyte phenotype which is characteristic of OA. Similarly the subchondral bone remodelling and formation of marginal and central tissue which is a typical feature of OA is not associated with normal ageing. Rather, ageing associates more with diminution in bone mineral density and osteopenia.

The synovial response in OA is typified by low-grade localized inflammation, whereas synovial atrophy is a feature of ageing.

However, muscle atrophy is a feature that is common to both OA and ageing, though in normal ageing sarcopenia and malnutrition may play important roles in addition to other factors [69].

In conclusion, in OA characteristic pathological changes occur in all the joint tissues which are different from those due to ageing alone. These vary in severity and emphasis and usually change only slowly with time. Overall OA is characterized by the combination of both new tissue production and tissue attrition, manifesting typically as focal loss of articular cartilage, bone remodelling, and marginal osteophyte formation. Varying degrees of synovial hyperplasia and inflammation, increased synovial fluid volume, and capsular thickening are also recognized features. OA cartilage encourages calcium crystal deposition and also associates with periarticular type II muscle atrophy and enthesophytes.

References

1. Loeser RF, Goldring SR, Scanzello CR, Goldring MB. Osteoarthritis: a disease of the joint as an organ. *Arthritis Rheum* 2012; 64(6):1697–707.
2. Sellam J, Berenbaum F. The role of synovitis in pathophysiology and clinical symptoms of osteoarthritis. *Nat Rev Rheumatol* 2010; 6(11):625–35.
3. Walsh DA, Yousef A, McWilliams DF, et al. Evaluation of a Photographic Chondropathy Score (PCS) for pathological samples in a study of inflammation in tibiofemoral osteoarthritis. *Osteoarthritis Cartilage* 2009; 17(3):304–12.
4. Pearle AD, Warren RF, Rodeo SA. Basic science of articular cartilage and osteoarthritis. *Clin Sports Med* 2005; 24(1):1–12.
5. Buckwalter JA, Mankin HJ, Grodzinsky AJ. Articular cartilage and osteoarthritis. *Instr Course Lect* 2005; 54:465–80.
6. Heijink A, Gomoll AH, Madry H, et al. Biomechanical considerations in the pathogenesis of osteoarthritis of the knee. *Knee Surg Sports Traumatol Arthrosc* 2012; 20(3):423–35.
7. Goldring MB, Marcu KB. Cartilage homeostasis in health and rheumatic diseases. *Arthritis Res Ther* 2009; 11(3):224.
8. Madry H, Luyten FP, Facchini A. Biological aspects of early osteoarthritis. *Knee Surg Sports Traumatol Arthrosc* 2012; 20(3):407–22.
9. Poole CA. Articular cartilage chondrons: form, function and failure. *J Anat* 1997; 191(Pt 1):1–13.
10. Pesesse L, Sanchez C, Henrotin Y. Osteochondral plate angiogenesis: a new treatment target in osteoarthritis. *Joint Bone Spine* 2011; 78(2):144–9.
11. Aigner T, Vornehm SI, Zeiler G, et al. Suppression of cartilage matrix gene expression in upper zone chondrocytes of osteoarthritic cartilage. *Arthritis Rheum* 1997; 40(3):562–9.
12. Reboul P, Pelletier JP, Tardif G, et al. The new collagenase, collagenase-3, is expressed and synthesized by human chondrocytes but not by synoviocytes. A role in osteoarthritis. *J Clin Invest* 1996; 97(9):2011–9.
13. Fernandes JC, Martel-Pelletier J, Pelletier JP. The role of cytokines in osteoarthritis pathophysiology. *Biorheology* 2002; 39(1–2):237–46.
14. Cotofana S, Buck R, Wirth W, et al. Cartilage thickening in early radiographic knee osteoarthritis: a within-person, between-knee comparison. *Arthritis Care Res* 2012; 64(11):1681–90.
15. Mankin HJ, Dorfman H, Lippiello L, Zarins A. Biochemical and metabolic abnormalities in articular cartilage from osteo-arthritic human hips. II. Correlation of morphology with biochemical and metabolic data. *J Bone Joint Surg Am* 1971; 53(3):523–37.
16. Setton LA, Mow VC, Müller FJ, et al. Mechanical properties of canine articular cartilage are significantly altered following transection of the anterior cruciate ligament. *J Orthop Res* 1994; 12(4):451–63.
17. Piperno M, Reboul P, Hellio le Graverand MP, et al. Osteoarthritic cartilage fibrillation is associated with a decrease in chondrocyte adhesion to fibronectin. *Osteoarthritis Cartilage* 1998; 6(6):393–9.

18. Berberat JE, Nissi MJ, Jurvelin JS, Nieminen MT. Assessment of interstitial water content of articular cartilage with T1 relaxation. *Magn Reson Imaging* 2009; 27(5):727–32.
19. Suri S, Gill SE, Massena de Camin S, et al. Neurovascular invasion at the osteochondral junction and in osteophytes in osteoarthritis. *Ann Rheum Dis* 2007; 66(11):1423–8.
20. Walsh DA, McWilliams DF, Turley MJ, et al. Angiogenesis and nerve growth factor at the osteochondral junction in rheumatoid arthritis and osteoarthritis. *Rheumatology (Oxford)* 2010; 49(10):1852–61.
21. Franses RE, McWilliams DF, Mapp PI, Walsh DA. Osteochondral angiogenesis and increased protease inhibitor expression in OA. *Osteoarthritis Cartilage* 2010; 18(4):563–71.
22. Lane LB, Bullough PG. Age-related changes in the thickness of the calcified zone and the number of tidemarks in adult human articular cartilage. *J Bone Joint Surg Br* 1980; 62(3):372–5.
23. Fuerst M, Bertrand J, Lammers L, et al. Calcification of articular cartilage in human osteoarthritis. *Arthritis Rheum* 2009; 60(9):2694–703.
24. Roddy E, Doherty M. Gout and osteoarthritis: a pathogenetic link? *Joint Bone Spine* 2012; 79(5):425–7.
25. Radin EL, Rose RM. Role of subchondral bone in the initiation and progression of cartilage damage. *Clin Orthop Relat Res* 1986; 213:34–40.
26. Milgram JW. Morphologic alterations of the subchondral bone in advanced degenerative arthritis. *Clin Orthop Relat Res* 1983; 173:293–312.
27. Zanetti M, Bruder E, Romero J, Hodler J. Bone marrow edema pattern in osteoarthritic knees: correlation between MR imaging and histologic findings. *Radiology* 2000; 215(3):835–40.
28. Hunter DJ, Zhang Y, Niu J, et al. Increase in bone marrow lesions associated with cartilage loss: a longitudinal magnetic resonance imaging study of knee osteoarthritis. *Arthritis Rheum* 2006; 54(5):1529–35.
29. Crema MD, Roemer FW, Zhu Y, et al. Subchondral cystlike lesions develop longitudinally in areas of bone marrow edema-like lesions in patients with or at risk for knee osteoarthritis: detection with MR imaging—the MOST study. *Radiology* 2010; 256(3):855–62.
30. Roemer FW, Neogi T, Nevitt MC, et al. Subchondral bone marrow lesions are highly associated with, and predict subchondral bone attrition longitudinally: the MOST study. *Osteoarthritis Cartilage* 2010; 18(1):47–53.
31. Kellgren JH, Lawrence JS. Radiological assessment of osteo-arthrosis. *Ann Rheum Dis* 1957; 16(4):494–502.
32. Nagaosa Y, Mateus M, Hassan B, Lanyon P, Doherty M. Development of a logically devised line drawing atlas for grading of knee osteoarthritis. *Ann Rheum Dis* 2000; 59(8):587–95.
33. Altman R, Asch E, Bloch D, et al. The American College of Rheumatology criteria for the classification and reporting of osteoarthritis of the knee. *Arthritis Rheum* 1986; 29:1039–49.
34. van der Kraan, PM, van den Berg WB. Osteophytes: relevance and biology. *Osteoarthritis Cartilage* 2007; 15(3):237–44.
35. Uchino M, Izumi T, Tominaga T, et al. Growth factor expression in the osteophytes of the human femoral head in osteoarthritis. *Clin Orthop Relat Res* 2000; 377:119–25.
36. Pottenger LA, Phillips FM, Draganich LF. The effect of marginal osteophytes on reduction of varus-valgus instability in osteoarthritic knees. *Arthritis Rheum* 1990; 33(6):853–8.
37. Li G, Yin J, Gao J, et al. Subchondral bone in osteoarthritis: insight into risk factors and microstructural changes. *Arthritis Res Ther* 2013; 15(6):223.
38. Landells JW. The bone cysts of osteoarthritis. *J Bone Joint Surg Br* 1953; 35-B(4):643–9.
39. Pallante-Kichura AL, Cory E, Bugbee WD, Sah RL. Bone cysts after osteochondral allograft repair of cartilage defects in goats suggest abnormal interaction between subchondral bone and overlying synovial joint tissues. *Bone* 2013; 57(1):259–68.
40. Punzi L, Ramonda R, Sfriso P. Erosive osteoarthritis. *Best Pract Res Clin Rheumatol* 2004; 18(5):739–58.
41. Hill CL, Hunter DJ, Niu J, et al. Synovitis detected on magnetic resonance imaging and its relation to pain and cartilage loss in knee osteoarthritis. *Ann Rheum Dis* 2007; 66(12):1599–603.
42. Baker K, Grainger A, Niu J, et al. Relation of synovitis to knee pain using contrast-enhanced MRIs. *Ann Rheum Dis* 2010; 69(10):1779–83.
43. Mapp PI. Innervation of the synovium. *Ann Rheum Dis* 1995; 54(5):398–403.
44. Swann DA, Bloch KJ, Swindell D, Shore E. The lubricating activity of human synovial fluids. *Arthritis Rheum* 1984; 27(5):552–6.
45. Smith MD. The normal synovium. *Open Rheumatol J* 2011; 5:100–6.
46. Iwanaga T, Shikichi M, Kitamura H, et al. Morphology and functional roles of synoviocytes in the joint. *Arch Histol Cytol* 2000; 63(1):17–31.
47. Haywood L, McWilliams DF, Pearson CI, et al. Inflammation and angiogenesis in osteoarthritis. *Arthritis Rheum* 2003; 48(8):2173–7.
48. Benito MJ, Veale DJ, FitzGerald O, van den Berg WB, Bresnihan B. Synovial tissue inflammation in early and late osteoarthritis. *Ann Rheum Dis* 2005; 64(9):1263–7.
49. Krenn V, Morawietz L, Burmester GR, et al. Synovitis score: discrimination between chronic low-grade and high-grade synovitis. *Histopathology* 2006; 49(4):358–64.
50. Walsh DA, Bonnet CS, Turner EL, et al. Angiogenesis in the synovium and at the osteochondral junction in osteoarthritis. *Osteoarthritis Cartilage* 2007; 15(7):743–51.
51. Walsh DA, Verghese P, Cook GJ, et al. Lymphatic vessels in osteoarthritic human knees. *Osteoarthritis Cartilage* 2012; 20(5):405–12.
52. Liu YZ, Jackson AP, Cosgrove SD. Contribution of calcium-containing crystals to cartilage degradation and synovial inflammation in osteoarthritis. *Osteoarthritis Cartilage* 2009; 17(10):1333–40.
53. Sun Y, Mauerhan DR, Franklin AM, et al. Fibroblast-like synoviocytes induce calcium mineral formation and deposition. *Arthritis* 2014; 2014:812678.
54. Hoff P, Buttgereit F, Burmester GR, et al. Osteoarthritis synovial fluid activates pro-inflammatory cytokines in primary human chondrocytes. *Int Orthop* 2013; 37(1):145–51.
55. McDevitt CA, Webber RJ. The ultrastructure and biochemistry of meniscal cartilage. *Clin Orthop Relat Res* 1990; 252:8–18.
56. Ashraf S, Wibberley H, Mapp PI, et al. Increased vascular penetration and nerve growth in the meniscus: a potential source of pain in osteoarthritis. *Ann Rheum Dis* 2011; 70(3):523–9.
57. Ishihara G, Kojima T, Saito Y, Ishiguro N. Roles of metalloproteinase-3 and aggrecanase 1 and 2 in aggrecan cleavage during human meniscus degeneration. *Orthop Rev (Pavia)* 2009; 1(2):e14.
58. Copenhaver W, Kelly DR, Wood RL. The connective tissues: cartilage and bone. In Wilfred M, Douglas EK, Richard LW (eds) *Bailey's Textbook of Histology*, 17th ed. Philadelphia, PA: Williams & Wilkins; 1978:170–8.
59. Hardcastle SA, Dieppe P, Gregson CL, et al. Osteophytes, enthesophytes, and high bone mass: a bone-forming triad with potential relevance in osteoarthritis. *Arthritis Rheumatol* 2014; 66(9):2429–39.
60. Loureiro A, Mills PM, Barrett RS. Muscle weakness in hip osteoarthritis: a systematic review. *Arthritis Care Res (Hoboken)* 2013; 65(3):340–52.
61. Valderrabano V, von Tscharner V, Nigg BM, et al. Lower leg muscle atrophy in ankle osteoarthritis. *J Orthop Res* 2006; 24(12):2159–69.
62. Felson DT. Osteoarthritis as a disease of mechanics. *Osteoarthritis Cartilage* 2013; 21(1):10–5.
63. Stoppiello LA, Mapp PI, Wilson D, et al. Structural associations of symptomatic knee osteoarthritis. *Arthritis Rheumatol* 2014; 66(11):3018–27.
64. DeGroot J, Verzijl N, Bank RA, et al. Age-related decrease in proteoglycan synthesis of human articular chondrocytes: the role of nonenzymatic glycation. *Arthritis Rheum* 1999; 42(5):1003–9.
65. Kempson GE. Relationship between the tensile properties of articular cartilage from the human knee and age. *Ann Rheum Dis* 1982; 41(5):508–11.

66. Verzijl N, DeGroot J, Oldehinkel E, et al. Age-related accumulation of Maillard reaction products in human articular cartilage collagen. *Biochem J* 2000; 350(Pt 2):381–7.

67. Verzijl N, DeGroot J, Ben ZC, et al. Crosslinking by advanced glycation end products increases the stiffness of the collagen network in human articular cartilage: a possible mechanism through which age is a risk factor for osteoarthritis. *Arthritis Rheum* 2002; 46(1):114–23.

68. Loeser RF. Aging and osteoarthritis: the role of chondrocyte senescence and aging changes in the cartilage matrix. *Osteoarthritis Cartilage* 2009; 17(8):971–9.

69. Hügle T, Geurts J, Nüesch C, Müller-Gerbl M, Valderrabano V. Aging and osteoarthritis: an inevitable encounter? *J Aging Res* 2012; 2012:950192.

SECTION 2

Tissues

CHAPTER 4

Cartilage (including meniscus)

Peter M. van der Kraan and
Esmeralda N. Blaney Davidson

Introduction

This chapter will give an overview of tissues unique to synovial joints, articular cartilage, and meniscus. Their development and cellular and (bio)chemical composition will be described along with the most profound changes that occur during osteoarthritis (OA). In addition, the role of growth factors and loading in maintenance and loss of cartilage homeostasis is discussed.

Development of articular cartilage and meniscus

Synovial joints consist of bone, ligament, synovium, capsule, and articular cartilage and are characterized by being highly movable. This tissue is unique in being both aneural and avascular, having a low cell density and an almost frictionless surface. During embryogenesis, articular cartilage is either formed at the interzone that arises in the anlagen of long bones, such as the humerus, radius, and ulnus, or is formed at the ends of bony structures that develop as discrete entities, like the carpals [1]. Articular cartilage is not just a remnant of the embryonic epiphyses but arises from a distinct cell population called interzone cells [2]. This interzone is a zone of flat cells interrupting the adjacent cartilaginous elements, which are thought to be derived from dedifferentiated chondrocytes [3]. The cells of the interzone are considered to generate several joint tissues, including articular cartilage and menisci [2]. However, invading cells, without a cartilage history, also contribute to the formation of these tissues [4].

When a joint is formed its size increases until adolescence. The growth of articular cartilage appears to be appositional and to be based on a population of progenitor cells in the articular cartilage surface [5]. During late embryogenesis and shortly after birth, synovial joints undergo cavitation, creating a fluid-filled cavity. Joint movement is important in the formation of the cavity and the generation of a population of surface zone cartilage cells that produce the lubricating protein lubricin [6]. Nevertheless, it has to be noted that fundamentally different mechanisms can contribute to the development of different joints, as has been shown for elbow and knee formation in mice [7].

The chondrocyte and the building blocks of articular cartilage and meniscus

Articular cartilage

Articular cartilage is aneural, avascular, and alymphatic and is considered to contain only one cell type, the chondrocyte. In adult human articular cartilage, these cells only represent a small portion of the tissue volume (maximally 5%), have a modest need for oxygen and nutrients, and do not divide. These attributes make it possible that articular chondrocytes survive in the body after death for days or even weeks at a low temperature [8].

Articular cartilage can largely be divided in four zones from top to bottom (see Figure 4.1). The superficial zone, the middle (transitional) zone, the deep (radial) zone, and the calcified zone. The calcified cartilage is separated from the remainder by the tidemark, while on the surface a not well-defined layer of glycoproteins

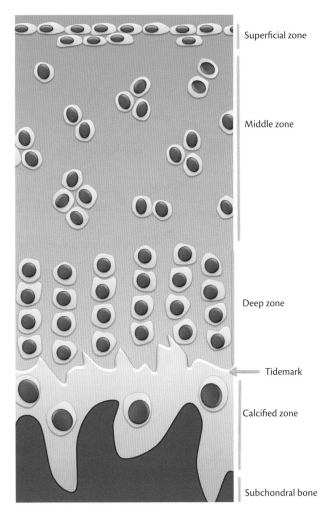

Figure 4.1 Schematic structure of articular cartilage. The difference in cellular distribution in the different layers is depicted.

is found, the lamina splendens. Although articular chondrocytes are considered a single cell type, morphological differences can be observed within the matrix. The form and size of the chondrocytes and the orientation of collagen fibrils varies from layer to layer. Surface zone cells are flattened and stretched parallel to the cartilage surface. These surface zone cells express stem cell markers and most likely represent a progenitor cell population of articular cartilage [9]. Middle and deep zone cells are round. In the middle zone the cells are solitary or in small groups up to four cells while in the deep zone the cells are aligned in columns. In the calcified zone the cells are enlarged and hypertrophic. Collagen fibrils in the surface zone run parallel to the articular surface, aligned in the direction of stress caused by motion, while in the deep layer, collagen fibrils penetrate the calcified zone perpendicular to the surface plane. The middle and deep layers show a change of the collagen fibril orientation from parallel to perpendicular. In the meniscus, collagen fibrils demonstrate a radial orientation in the surface zone and are circumferential in the remainder of the tissue, a pattern consistent with transmission of compressive loads in the joint [10].

The extracellular matrix (ECM) of articular cartilage can be divided into the interterritorial matrix and the pericellular matrix, surrounding the chondrocytes. The pericellular matrix, together with the embedded chondrocytes (one to four cells), make up a specific structure that is called a chondron [11]. The main structural component of articular cartilage is water. Besides water, all structural components of articular cartilage are synthesized by the chondrocytes (see Figure 4.2 and Table 4.1). Collagen type II is the most abundant protein on a weight base [12]. Collagen type II forms a supramolecular complex in the ECM in combination with collagen IX and XI [13]. These collagens build a heteropolymer in which collagen type IX decorates the collagen type II fibrils while collagen type XI is embedded in the collagen type II fibrils. The terminal NC4 globular domain of α1(IX) projects from the fibril surfaces and interacts with other matrix molecules [14]. Collagen type III is also present in articular cartilage and linked to collagen type II as a minor, but general component [15]. A filamentous network is formed in the pericellular matrix of the chondron by collagen type VI [16]. Collagen type X is only found in the calcified zone of articular cartilage and a marker for chondrocyte hypertrophy.

On a weight base, collagen is the dominant protein in articular cartilage but on a molar base this is challenged by other matrix molecules. The major aggregating proteoglycan of cartilage, aggrecan, consists of a central linear core protein with three globular domains (G1, G2, and G3). The G1 domain binds to the glycosaminoglycan hyaluronan, a bond that is strengthened by link protein. The aggrecan core protein has covalently bound, between G2 and G3, about a hundred chondroitin sulphate chains, and a smaller number of keratan sulphate chains [17]. The glycosaminoglycan chains are heterogeneous in length and sulphation, which changes during development and ageing [18]. The glycosaminoglycan chains are highly negatively charged, mainly due to the sulphate groups, and thereby provide a very high fixed charge density to the cartilage. This results in high osmotic strength that retains water in the

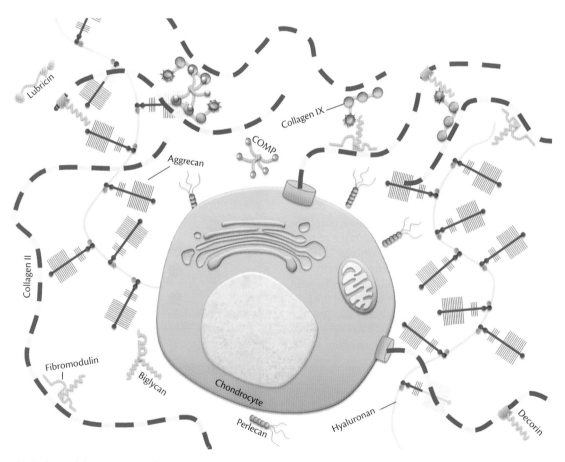

Figure 4.2 Simplified scheme of the components of the articular cartilage matrix. Note that the components do not show actual relative differences in size.

Table 4.1 Major matrix constituents of articular cartilage

Name	Characteristics	Location	References
Collagen II	Cartilage specific, α1(II)	Extracellular matrix	[128]
Collagen III	α1(III)	Extracellular matrix	[15]
Collagen VI	α1(VI), α2(VI), α3(VI), α4(VI), α5(VI), α6(VI)	Pericellular matrix	[129]
Collagen IX	α1(IX), α2(IX), α3(IX)	On the surface of collagen II	[130]
Collagen X	α1(X)	Calcified cartilage	[131]
Collagen XI	Cartilage specific, α1(XI), α2(XI), α3(XI), (α1(V))	Inside collagen II fibres	[132]
Aggrecan	Large aggregating proteoglycan	Extracellular matrix	[133]
Link protein	Binds aggrecan and hyaluronan	Extracellular matrix	[134]
Hyaluronan	Glycosaminoglycan, binds aggrecan	Extracellular matrix	[135]
Perlecan	Large proteoglycan,	Pericellular matrix	[136]
Small leucine-rich repeat proteoglycans (SLRPs)	Small proteoglycans, bind to collagens, regulate fibrillogenesis	Extracellular matrix	[137]
COMP	Regulates fibrillogenesis	Extracellular matrix	[138]
Matrilins	Binds collagen, SLRPs, and COMP	Extracellular matrix	[25]
Lubricin	Lubricates cartilage surface	Superficial zone	[139]

cartilage and plays a major role in the strain resilient properties of articular cartilage. The fixed charge density is mainly a function of chondroitin sulphate. Keratan sulphate binds with high affinity to collagen and in this way has an important function in the network formation in articular cartilage [19].

Besides aggrecan, the proteoglycan perlecan has a crucial function in articular cartilage. Mice deficient in perlecan have defective cartilage formation while functional mutations in humans result in Schwartz–Jampel syndrome, characterized by chondrodysplasia [20]. Perlecan is a so-called heparan sulphate proteoglycan that is localized in the pericellular matrix and has an essential function in sequestering growth factors, such as fibroblast growth factor, in this way promoting specific cellular functions [21]. Cartilage not only contains large proteoglycans, such as aggrecan and perlecan, but also a number of small proteoglycans, small leucine-rich proteoglycans (SLRPs). To this family of SLRPs belong, amongst others, decorin, lumican, biglycan, fibromodulin, asporin, and chondroadherin. The SLRPs have specific functions in fibrillogenesis and matrix assembly [22]. Another molecule important in collagen fibrillogenesis is cartilage oligomeric protein (COMP) that is found in tissues under load, such as articular cartilage. COMP consist of five identical subunits which extent as five arms ending in a globular domain [23]. This globular domain at the end of the arms binds to a number of matrix molecules. One COMP molecule can bind five collagen molecules, bringing these together and facilitating fibril formation [24]. The articular cartilage-specific molecule matrilin-3 forms heterotetramers and can bind to various other matrix molecules [25]. In cartilage, matrilin is positioned between collagen type VI and decorin or biglycan but can also bind to aggrecan [26]. The SLRPs, COMP, and matrilins all have a function in fibrillogenesis and organization of the extracellular, and pericellular, matrix. Therefore these molecules play an essential role in the assembly and maintains of the cartilage matrix.

Another molecule essential for proper articular cartilage functioning is lubricin, also called proteoglycan 4. Mutations in lubricin cause camptodactyly-arthropathy-coxa vara-pericarditis syndrome which is amongst others characterized by joint pathology [27]. Lubricin is produced by surface zone chondrocytes and has a major function in reduction of friction between opposing cartilage surfaces [28]. Although not all functions of the cartilage matrix molecules are fully elucidated it is clear that articular cartilage is a highly specialized tissue with a unique composition and function.

Meniscus

Menisci are fibrocartilaginous wedge-shaped structures that in the knee joint are positioned between the tibial plateau and the femoral condyle. Similar formations can be found in other joints. In adults only the outer rim of the menisci is vascularized. The outer part contains fibroblast-like cells while in the inner part chondrocyte-like cells are embedded. Like in articular cartilage, the meniscal surface contains flattened cells that might have progenitor attributes.

Collagen fibrils of meniscus are oriented circumferentially in the central part and radially in the surface region, adapted to its mechanical role [10]. The main collagen in menisci is type I, which is a major difference with articular cartilage, but also collagens type II, III, V, VI, and X are present [29]. Besides the collagens, aggrecan and link protein are structural components with comparable functions as in articular cartilage. Less is known about the matrix composition and molecular function of meniscus than those of articular cartilage, but it has been shown that SLRPs, fibronectin, and thrombospondin can be found in this tissue (see Table 4.2) [30–32]. The presence of elastin in menisci can be related to the mechanical function of the menisci, being distribution of load by its strain- and compressive-resistant properties [33].

Table 4.2 Major matrix constituents of the meniscus

Name	Type	Location	References
Collagen I	α1(I), α2(II)	Extracellular matrix	[29]
Collagen II	α1(II)	Loaded areas	[29]
Collagen type III	α1(III)	Extracellular matrix	[29]
Collagen type V	α1(V), α2(V), α3(V)	Extracellular matrix	[29]
Collagen type VI	α1(VI), α2(VI), α3(VI), α4(VI), α5(VI), α6(VI)	Pericellular matrix	[140]
Collagen type X	α1(X)	Calcified zones	[141]
Aggrecan	Large aggregating proteoglycan	Extracellular matrix	[142]
Link protein	Binds aggrecan and hyaluronan	Extracellular matrix	[143]
Small leucine-rich repeat proteoglycans (SLRPs)	Small proteoglycans, bind to collagens, regulate fibrillogenesis	Extracellular matrix	[30]
Fibronectin	Glycoprotein	Extra/ pericellular matrix	[31]
Thrombospondin	Glycoprotein	Extracellular matrix	[32]
Elastin	Forms elastic fibres	Extracellular matrix	[33]

Mechanical function of cartilage and the meniscus

Synovial joints are mechanical organs and the main function of articular cartilage and menisci is to deal with mechanics and to make smooth movement possible. This is made possible by the structural and biochemical make-up of articular cartilage and menisci. Articular cartilage minimizes contract stresses and provides lubrication. The tissue deforms when load is applied and in this way distributes the load over an increased contact area. The tissue deformation results in compressive, tensile, and shear stresses.

The mechanical function of cartilage is mainly determined by the entrapped water, the collagen network, and hyaluronan/aggrecan complexes [34]. The aggrecan molecules have, due to their sulphate groups, a very high fixed charge density. The cation concentration in the tissue is much higher than in the surrounding synovial fluid. This leads to an osmotic pressure difference which causes swelling of the tissue [35]. Unloaded cartilage is pre-stressed, due to the fact that the collagen network limits the expansion of the aggrecan molecules to about 10% of their maximum volume. During compressive load, water is pressed through the ECM which causes a redistribution of fluid in the tissue. Only when fluid flow within the tissue has come to an end, will the applied load be countered by the solid matrix. Unloading will again initiate movement of fluid until the original unloaded state has been reached [36]. However, in conditions of rapid loading and unloading a state of equilibrium will be hardly ever acquired. Loading of cartilage leads not only to compression but also to tensile and shearing forces within the tissue. The cartilage pre-stress generated by the aggrecan complexes within the collagen network contributes to the shear stiffness of cartilage [37].

The friction coefficient of articular cartilage is extremely low. The low friction is not only caused by lubricating molecules, like lubricin, but is also dependent on fluid film lubrication [38]. Fluid film lubrication is supported by interstitial pressurized fluid flow that is a result of applied compression.

Articular cartilage is tissue that not only enables 'mechanics' but also relies highly on these mechanical stimuli for its homeostasis. Non-loaded articular cartilage rapidly deteriorates, and therefore also for this tissue the motto 'use it or lose it' is true [39]. Chondrocytes react to mechanical stimuli and an important role is attributed to the pericellular matrix to transduce mechanical signals from the environment to the cells [40]. How chondrocytes react to mechanical forces is not fully clear. Loading induces chondrocyte deformation and this affects chondrocyte metabolism [41]. On the other hand, loading might activate growth factor signalling and in this way activate chondrocytes in an indirect manner [42].

Like articular cartilage, the meniscus has to endure different forces such as compression, tension, and shear. Menisci are wedge-shaped and adapted to stabilization of the arched femoral condyle with the flat tibial plateau. During movement, the meniscus is deformed radially that results in shear forces in the collagen fibres within the meniscus. Axial forces in the knee joint result in compression of the menisci. The orientation of the collagen fibres and aggrecan within the menisci are fine-tuned to these functional demands. Intact menisci cover about 60% of the contact areas between the tibial plateau and the femoral condyles and transmit approximately half of the load in the joint but the contact area is greatly dependent on the degree of flexion of the knee [43].

Role of growth factors in the homeostasis of articular cartilage and meniscus

For cartilage to remain intact it relies on local signals by growth factors, most of which are produced and stored in cartilage itself or produced by synovial tissue. They stimulate production of proteoglycans and/or collagens to keep the cartilage intact. But they also prevent MMP (matrix metalloproteinase) and ADAMTS (a disintegrin and metalloproteinase with thrombospondin-like motifs) production and/or activation thereby protecting cartilage from enzymatic degradation. In some cases they can even induce enzyme production and by delicately balancing production and breakdown of the ECM play a role in cartilage remodelling. The factors discussed here are insulin-like growth factor 1 (IGF1), transforming growth factor beta (TGFβ), bone morphogenetic proteins (BMPs), growth differentiation factors (GDFs), fibroblast growth factor (FGF), wingless-type MMTV integration site family (WNT), platelet-derived growth factor (PDGF), Indian hedgehog (IHH), and vascular endothelial growth factor (VEGF).

Insulin-like growth factor 1

IGF1 is produced in bone and cartilage. It is even considered by some investigators to be the main anabolic growth factor for articular cartilage. It is a major chondrocyte stimulator of proteoglycan and collagen synthesis in cartilage and inhibits matrix degradation in a dose-dependent manner [44]. Not only does it stimulate cartilage ECM synthesis, but it also protects cartilage by counteracting catabolic effects of the cytokine interleukin 1 (IL1) [45]. Strikingly, with age and OA, chondrocytes become unresponsive to IGF1 [44], which might make it prone to damage. This lower responsiveness is considered, at least in part, to be dependent on the high expression of IGF-binding proteins which prevent its signalling [44].

Transforming growth factor β

TGFβ and its family members are pivotal in cartilage homeostasis. TGFβ stimulates the production of cartilage ECM molecules, like collagens and aggrecan, both in chondrocytes and meniscal fibrochondrocytes. Even though both articular chondrocytes and meniscal fibrochondrocytes respond to TGFβ by increasing proteoglycan synthesis, the aggrecan fragments that are found when exposed to TGFβ are slightly different. There are more fragments in explants of articular chondrocytes, which seems to point to higher remodelling in articular cartilage. Besides enhancing ECM production, TGFβ also prevents degradation of ECM by increasing levels of protease inhibitors like TIMP. In addition, TGFβ can counteract catabolic factors such as IL1 and tumour necrosis factor alpha (TNFα) preventing cartilage degradation [46]. Disruption of TGFβ signalling results in cartilage degeneration [47]. Even though TGFβ generally seems to have protective effects on cartilage, there is some debate whether or not TGF-β is protective for cartilage, as it has also been found and suggested to lead to cartilage damage [48]. These different findings might be due to the different signalling pathways that can be activated by TGFβ which have been shown to have different downstream effects in chondrocytes [49]. Therefore, whether TGFβ is beneficial or deleterious is most likely context and dose dependent.

Bone morphogenetic proteins

Bone morphogenetic proteins (BMPs) belong to the TGFβ superfamily and are extensively studied in chondrogenesis and expressed by chondrocytes of both articular and meniscal origin. Of the vast number of BMPs, BMP2, -4, and -7 have been studied the most. BMP2 stimulates ECM production in chondrocytes and reverses IL-1-induced proteoglycan inhibition. BMP7 is predominantly found in the superficial and middle layers of cartilage [50]. It has been found to have chondroprotective effects in in vivo OA models [51] and stimulates collagen type II and aggrecan expression while inhibiting MMP expression in meniscus repair [52]. Its expression is found to be reduced with age [53]. BMP4 also shows anabolic effects, but whether or not it is chondroprotective is unclear. For BMP4, an age-dependent difference in response is found [54]. Besides having a stimulating effect on cartilage ECM production, BMPs are not solely beneficial for cartilage maintenance. On the one hand, BMPs promote ECM production, but on the other hand, BMPs are involved in chondrocyte terminal differentiation. The latter is considered a deleterious quality when it comes to articular cartilage, as induction of terminal differentiation implies loss of the articular cartilage state. Given the age-dependent alterations, it might be age-dependent whether or not BMPs protect cartilage or induce deleterious effects.

Growth differentiation factors

GDFs are a subfamily of the BMPs that are important in skeletal development. For articular cartilage in particular, GDF5 is researched, due to its importance in the formation of articular cartilage during joint development. It is very popular in cartilage tissue engineering where GDF5 inhibits expression of MMP13 and ADAMTS4, while stimulating aggrecan and SOX9 expression [55]. In the same study, this function is suggested to operate via inhibition of WNT signalling, which is discussed later. In another study, GDF5 promoted chondrogenesis, but also chondrocyte hypertrophy, an attribute that would not be beneficial for articular cartilage maintenance [56]. Mutations in GDF5 lead to joint abnormalities [57]. This seems to indicate a role in homeostasis, but could also merely reflect alterations in joint formation. Polymorphisms in humans that result in reduced transcriptional activity of GDF5 are associated with OA susceptibility suggesting a role in homeostasis. But whether or not this is really due to a function in cartilage maintenance is unknown.

Fibroblast growth factors

Three members of the FGF family have been implicated in cartilage homeostasis: FGF2, -8, and -18. The role of FGF2 is not clear as both anabolic and catabolic effects have been described. The majority of FGF2 studies find an anabolic role in cartilage repair in vivo, which seems predominantly dependent on increased cell proliferation rather than enhanced ECM production. The same holds true for meniscal cells. This enhanced proliferation is associated with loss of a chondrocyte phenotype. Also, FGF2 is found to counteract IGF1 and BMP7 and to stimulate expression of MMPs. On the other hand, FGF2 is found to be chondroprotective in vivo as FGF2-null mice show accelerated spontaneous and surgically-induced OA [58]. This effect is said to be associated with an increase in ADAMTS5 expression in mice lacking FGF2. The controversy in FGF2 effects lies in the type of receptor that is used. Human adult chondrocytes express all four subtypes of the FGF receptor, with significantly higher concentrations of FGFR1 and FGFR3. FGF2 can signal via both these receptors, but its catabolic effects run primarily via FGFR1, whereas beneficial effects are dependent on FGFR3. FGF8 has catabolic effects in rat articular cartilage, but whether or not this translates to human adult cartilage has not yet been established [59]. FGF18 has anabolic effects in human articular chondrocytes, by activation of the FGFR3 pathway [60]. FGF18 induces ECM production, cartilage formation, and reduces cartilage degeneration in an OA model. Also in a rat meniscal tear model, FGF18 is shown to be beneficial [61]. One proposed major difference between FGF2 and FGF18 is that FGF2 induces BMP-inhibitor noggin, whereas FGF18 suppresses its expression [62].

Wingless-type MMTV integration site family

WNT signalling is implicated in cartilage homeostasis. The WNT family consists of many members and different downstream signalling pathways, which can be separated into canonical WNT signalling via β-catenin and non-canonical signalling. In general, WNTs seem to have beneficial effects on chondrogenesis, but when it comes to cartilage maintenance it seems like WNTs predominantly have deleterious effects. Many WNTs activate chondrocyte dedifferentiation—WNT3A, WNT5A, WNT7A [63–66]—but where some suppress MMP expression and/or activity (WNT7B) others promote this (WNT1, WNT5A) [67–69]. WNT3A and WNT7A cause loss of collagen type II synthesis [66]. In addition, WNT3A promoted cell proliferation and loss of expression of collagen type II, aggrecan, and SOX9 in human articular chondrocytes [70]. The canonical WNT signalling mediator β-catenin has even been found to be implicated in opposing effects, where it induces an OA phenotype in a mouse model, whereas it inhibits deleterious nuclear factor kappa B activity and MMP expression in human chondrocytes [71,72]. From joint formation we can learn that the level of WNT signalling is crucial in determining chondrocyte fate. Having too much or too little WNT signalling can alter chondrocyte fate into becoming a chondrocyte, or even losing articular chondrocyte state and undergoing hypertrophy (discussed in more detail in Chapter 9). Overall this shows that WNT signalling has to be delicately balanced to maintain chondrocytes in their articular chondrocyte state, and their effects can even be species and tissue dependent. Until now, it is still unclear what the exact function in human cartilage is.

Platelet-derived growth factor

PDGF is important in wound healing and is produced by chondrocytes. It is believed to be capable of enhancing tissue regeneration and repair [44]. *In vitro*, PDGF stimulates proliferation and GAG production in meniscal cells from all areas of the meniscus, and enhances cellularity in meniscal explants [73]. In chondrocytes, PDGF induces proliferation and proteoglycan production, but does not alter collagen production [74]. In addition, besides stimulating GAG content in cartilage explants, it also inhibits catabolic degradation of proteoglycans in this system, indicating an impact on cartilage homeostasis [75]. In contrast, exposure to IL1 results in upregulation of PDGF receptors in chondrocytes and in this same experiment adding PDGF augments IL1-induced MMP expression [44]. This MMP expression is considered deleterious, but could also reflect a function of PDGF in cartilage remodelling. Whether or not PDGF truly contributes in a beneficial way to cartilage homeostasis is not clear, but it does seem to promote cartilage repair.

Indian hedgehog

IHH is a well-known regulator of cartilage differentiation, where it together with PTHrP regulates the speed of chondrocyte differentiation in cartilage development [76]. IHH is primarily secreted by prehypertrophic chondrocytes and regulates chondrocyte hypertrophy by inhibition of PTHrP. Transgenic mice with elevated IHH levels show increased chondrocyte hypertrophy and cartilage damage which resembles human OA [77], which would indicate IHH is deleterious for cartilage homeostasis. In human OA articular cartilage, IHH expression was found upregulated and correlated with damage [78]. Conditional deletion of IHH attenuated OA progression, which would suggest one should inhibit IHH to maintain cartilage in its healthy state [77].

Vascular endothelial growth factor

VEGF is an angiogenic factor and is not expressed in human articular cartilage under physiological conditions. In contrast, in diseased cartilage, like during OA, VEGF and its receptors are expressed, which is suggested to stimulate blood vessel penetration from subchondral bone into articular cartilage, thereby contributing to disease progression [79]. Thus VEGF does not seem to function in normal cartilage homeostasis, but does seem to play a role in OA conditions. However, the exact mechanism thereof is not clear yet.

Overall it has become clear that there are many growth factors that influence cartilage homeostasis, even more than discussed in this chapter. Most of these growth factors have divergent effects, either good or bad, depending on the state of the chondrocyte/cartilage and are influenced by other factors, like IL1 or other growth factors. Therefore, to maintain healthy cartilage these factors have to be delicately balanced out. Altering this delicate balance will result in changes in chondrocyte differentiation, and altered production of ECM molecules and cartilage degrading enzymes.

Growth factors in chondrocyte differentiation and hypertrophy

In the past, OA was considered a 'wear and tear' disease, in which cartilage degenerates due to (over)use. This is still the view of the general public, but research has identified that there are changes in the articular cartilage that are not due to (over)use and occur prior to mechanical damage. One of the hallmarks in cartilage degeneration is expression of collagen type X and MMP13. These are markers of chondrocyte hypertrophy. Chondrocytes normally undergo hypertrophy during endochondral bone formation. During this process, precursor cells differentiate into chondrocytes, but thereafter differentiate further into hypertrophic chondrocytes and eventually cartilage is replaced by bone. Currently many researchers believe that chondrocytes in OA lose their articular chondrocyte state by undergoing a process that highly resembles this chondrocyte differentiation into hypertrophy. Growth factors play a major role in the maintenance of articular chondrocytes and/or transition into hypertrophic chondrocytes. Some growth factors actively block chondrocyte hypertrophy and are therefore considered protective for the articular chondrocyte phenotype, whereas others promote chondrocyte hypertrophy. A delicate balance between all players will ultimately determine whether the articular chondrocyte phenotype is maintained or lost. Here, the role of the growth factors known to be involved in cartilage homeostasis will be further discussed in light of chondrocyte differentiation.

Transforming growth factor β

TGFβ signals via two classes of receptors: the type I and the type II receptors. The type II receptor (TGFβ type II receptor) is a common receptor that drives all different types of TGFβ signalling downstream, and therefore the type I receptor is considered dominant in determining whether either SMAD2/3 is activated (by type I receptor ALK5) or SMAD1/5/8 (by type I receptor ALK1). In addition, TGFβ signals via MAPK pathways using the same receptors. From developmental studies in mice it became clear that Smad2/3 inhibits hypertrophic differentiation [80], whereas Smad1/5/8 promotes hypertrophy [81]. Therefore, TGFβ signalling can have a dual role in both inhibiting and promoting chondrocyte hypertrophy depending on the active signalling pathway. SMAD2/3 is a dominant pathway in healthy articular cartilage, and via that pathway TGFβ actively represses chondrocyte hypertrophy [49]. Also in *in vitro* models of chondrogenesis, the addition of TGFβ arrests hypertrophic differentiation. However, with ageing and OA, there is a shift towards more dominant ALK1 signalling, which has been found to promote MMP13 expression in chondrocytes [49]. In contrast, other researchers propose that the ALK1 signalling via SMAD1/5/8 is a reparative phenotype, whereas ALK5 SMAD2/3 signalling is a fibrotic phenotype [48]. The jury is still out regarding whether TGFβ is beneficial or deleterious and via which signalling pathway in articular cartilage. At least *in vitro*, TGFβ is crucial for the transition from stem cell into chondrocyte, but whether or not this holds true *in vivo* remains to be determined.

Bone morphogenetic proteins

BMPs signal via the SMAD1/5/8 pathway, using similar classes, but different types of receptors compared to TGFβ. For BMPs, the type II receptor is a specific BMP receptor, and type I receptors are ALK1, -2, -3, and -6. Like TGFβ, BMPs are crucial in embryonic development and promote chondrogenesis. BMPs are involved in all phases of chondrogenesis. But unlike TGFβ, most BMPs are not considered to actively block terminal differentiation, but even promote this process. It is thought that BMPs act together with transcription factor RUNX2 to control chondrocyte terminal differentiation [82]. BMP7 however, is different than the other BMPs as it can actively suppress chondrocyte hypertrophy and therefore could be protective for articular cartilage [83]. Exposure of articular chondrocytes or stem cells to BMPs does not automatically lead to chondrocyte hypertrophy [84]. Most likely it depends on whether or not there are abundant other factors, like other growth factors such as TGFβ or FGF or BMP inhibitors like noggin, gremlin, and chordin, are present to suppress this process.

Growth differentiation factors

Much like the other members of the bone morphogenetic proteins, GDF5 also promotes both chondrogenesis as well as chondrocyte hypertrophy. It is crucial in regulating joint morphogenesis as without it, no joint is formed [57]. GDF5 is expressed in the early cartilage condensations and can increase the size of a condensating chondrogenic nodule *in vitro* [85]. Besides enhancing the condensation phase of chondrogenesis, some studies show increased proliferation of chondrocytes in response to GDF5 [86]. Not all studies show this, which might be due to a difference in experimental setup and the effect being very transient. In addition, GDF5 can accelerate chondrocyte differentiation in limb mesenchymal cell cultures, but this does not seem to reflect a physiological function of GDF5 as it is normally not expressed in or near the hypertrophic zone [85]. In humans, the closely related protein GDF6 is expressed in these areas and might promote terminal differentiation of chondrocytes there [87].

Insulin-like growth factor 1

IGF1 signals via the IGF1R, which is a type II tyrosine kinase receptor, activating PI3K and the MAPK pathways. IGF1 increases chondrocyte proliferation [88], and synergizes with TGFβ to promote chondrogenesis [89]. In later phases of chondrogenic differentiation the role of IGF1 is less clear. In *Igf1* null mice, Wang et al. identified that Igf1 is involved in chondrocyte hypertrophy to at least some extent [90]. *Igf1* null mice still differentiate towards hypertrophy, with expression of collagen type X and ALP, but hypertrophy is reduced compared to normal and the hypertrophic cells are smaller. Another group shows that IGF1 promotes chondrocyte differentiation, but only in low concentrations and that this is dependent on the state of the cell [91]. In proliferating chondrocytes, IGF1 is capable of inducing ERK activation (active signal through the MAPK pathway), but in hypertrophic chondrocytes, IGF can no longer do this. Hence, the cellular state might define the responsiveness to IGF-1. Mushtaq et al. concludes, similar to Wang et al. that murine *Igf1* is predominantly expressed in the hypertrophic zone and that it augments chondrocyte hypertrophy [92]. Since *Igf1* null mice do still show chondrocyte hypertrophy, it might very well be the case that IGF1 cannot induce hypertrophy itself, but can contribute once hypertrophy has already set in.

Fibroblast growth factors

FRF2 has been researched quite extensively in chondrogenic differentiation. Not only does it play a role in chondrogenic differentiation itself, it enhances chondrogenic potential of stem cells prior to being triggered to become chondrocytes [93]. This is perceived as a 'priming' of stem cells for enhanced chondrogenesis. This priming with FGF2 results in generation of larger cartilage constructs *in vitro*, with more proteoglycan production [93]. Once chondrogenesis sets in, FGF2 inhibits hypertrophy, as measured by reduced chondrocyte hypertrophy markers [94]. This is supported by *in vivo* studies that show FGF2 has an inhibitory effect on chondrocyte hypertrophy [95]. In addition, a combination of FGF2 with SOX9 can even decrease collagen type X expression in OA chondrocytes *in vitro* [96]. The effects of FGF2 as well as FGF8 in chondrogenesis, either promoting or inhibiting, are shown highly dependent on the stage of chondrogenesis.

From mouse knock-out studies it is clear that FGF18 is required for chondrogenesis, and does this by signalling via the FGFR3 receptor [97]. It regulates chondrocyte proliferation as well as differentiation, but it also plays a role in chondrocyte hypertrophy: *Fgf18* knockout mice show delayed initiation of chondrocyte hypertrophy as well as decreased proliferation in early stages of chondrogenesis [98].

Wingless-type MMTV integration site family

As stated in Chapter 9, the balance in WNT signalling is crucial in determining chondrocyte fate. WNTs are important in limb development and have a major impact on chondrogenesis. During joint development, several WNTs are expressed in the presumptive joint region, such as WNT9A, -4, and -16 [99]. WNT3A and WNT5A keep progenitor cells in a proliferative state and thereby prevent chondrogenesis [63,64]. Thereafter, by having a slightly lower WNT signal via β-catenin, cells are allowed to express chondrogenic marker SOX9 [63]. Where WNT4 blocks the initiation of chondrogenesis, it accelerates terminal differentiation of chondrocytes [100]. Wnt1 and Wnt7a block chondrogenesis in a chick limb model [63]. In pre-hypertrophic chondrocytes WNT5A, WNT5B, and WNT11 are expressed [63,101]. Of these WNTs, WNT5A and -5B promote early chondrogenesis and inhibit the progression into chondrocyte hypertrophy and as such block terminal differentiation [63]. In contrast, WNT7B, -8C, -9A and -16 are found to enhance chondrocyte hypertrophic maturation [63,102]. WNT signalling has been proposed to stimulate chondrocyte hypertrophy through inhibition of parathyroid hormone-related protein (PTHrP) [103]. In general, activation of canonical WNTs inhibit early stages of chondrogenesis whereas WNT5A and WNT5B promote early chondrogenesis by activating non-canonical signalling [63]. WNT signalling is in general implicated in inducing chondrocyte hypertrophy, but exceptions are to be found [63].

Platelet-derived growth factor

PDGF is less popular in chondrogenesis research, but it has been found to promote chondrocyte proliferation, promote matrix production which is typical to resting zone chondrocytes, and maintain chondrocytes in a less mature phenotype, indicating a blockage of hypertrophy [74]. PDGF-AA effects on chondrogenesis are stage-dependent as it can both increase and inhibit chondrogenesis in similar culturing conditions in different stages of development. PDGF-BB initially decreases cartilage formation in tissue engineered constructs, but eventually increases cartilage formation and decreases the formation of hypertrophic cells [104]. PDGF is one component of PRP (platelet-rich plasma), together with TGFβ, IGF, FGF2, and VEGF. It has received attention due to the high growth factor content and is used as a patient's own substance to promote chondrogenesis in cartilage tissue engineering. The knowledge about PDGF in chondrogenesis is scattered and often PDGF is combined with other growth factors to improve their function. It seems that pre-treatment of stem cells with PDGF results in better cartilage constructs [104].

Indian hedgehog

IHH is produced by prehypertrophic and hypertrophic chondrocytes and stimulates the production of PTHrP by early chondrocytic cells. The balance between IHH and PTHrP determines the differentiation state of chondrocyte differentiation as well as the speed of differentiation in the growth plate [76]. However, IHH also has PTHrP-independent functions, where it promotes chondrocyte hypertrophy on its own [105]. It has even been shown in stem cell differentiation that IHH is pivotal in TGFβ-induced chondrogenesis and can drive chondrogenic differentiation when TGFβ signalling is inhibited [106]. It is also found that IHH plays a role in early chondrogenesis by interacting with RUNX2 and RUNX3 [107]. IHH alone is sufficient to induce chondrogenesis without addition of growth factors like TGFβ or BMP2, but eventually, IHH-treated samples show higher degrees of hypertrophy [108]. Since IHH can induce chondrogenesis on its own, this clearly shows that IHH function goes beyond stimulation of hypertrophy alone.

Vascular endothelial growth factor

During chondrogenesis *in vitro*, VEGF as well as its receptor are expressed, but its function is still not entirely clear. *In vivo*, VEGF is found in hypertrophic chondrocytes of the growth plate, not in quiescent and proliferating chondrocytes [109]. Early in development, the presence of exogenous high levels of VEGF stimulates angiogenesis while chondrogenesis is prevented. The authors suggest that vascular regression is required to enable mesenchymal condensation and chondrogenesis [110]. Without VEGF, chondrocytes die in epiphyseal regions during endochondral bone formation, which makes VEGF a crucial survival factor [111]. A major function of VEGF seems to lie in the vascularization during endochondral bone formation and blocking VEGF results in delayed removal of terminal hypertrophic chondrocytes [111]. In adult tissue, VEGF can induce new chondrocyte differentiation in articular cartilage repair [112]. On the other hand, blocking of VEGF improved chondrogenic potential of mouse stem cells treated with BMP4 and TGFβ and improved cartilage repair *in vivo*, and did this even in osteoarthritic conditions [113].

For each growth factor discussed here, it has become clear that the effects on chondrogenesis depend on the differentiation state of the chondrocyte, culture conditions, *in vitro* or *vivo*, and the presence of other factors. In this whirlpool of options different researchers often find opposite effects of growth factors depending on the research conditions. Therefore it is crucial to discern which state the chondrocytes are in, which phase of chondrogenesis is researched, and which other factors might manipulate the outcome. For some growth factors, roles in specific phases of chondrogenesis (i.e. condensation, early chondrogenesis, hypertrophy, etc.) are clearer than others, but much is still under debate. In order to steer chondrogenesis in a desired direction, it might take more than just interfering with one particular factor, but rather a complicated but well-balanced pool of factors might do the trick. A trick that Mother Nature knows best.

In terms of articular cartilage maintenance, changes in growth factors levels can have a major impact. They can trigger articular chondrocytes to leave their frozen, healthy, articular chondrocyte state and differentiate towards hypertrophy. A small change in one particular growth factor in most cases will likely be buffered by others, but when multiple levels start to change, this might very well be a deleterious trigger. The growth plate is a perfect example of how gradients manipulate chondrocyte differentiation, and shows how slight alterations can have a major impact.

With age, but also by triggers like mechanical injury or inflammation, not only the environment, but the chondrocytes themselves also start to change. They start expressing different receptor levels for particular growth factors (for instance, TGFβ or FGF), or different co-factors which manipulate growth factor signalling (for instance, IGF1). In this case, the levels of growth factors may remain unaltered, but how the chondrocytes deal with growth factors may become very different. One can imagine that once cartilage becomes osteoarthritic, with all of these changes it is almost impossible to restore the balance.

Aggrecanases and matrix metalloproteinases in cartilage matrix degradation in osteoarthritis

The main structural characteristic of OA is (focal) degradation of articular cartilage, but menisci are also damaged in the OA process. During OA, proteolytic enzymes produced by deranged chondrocytes are thought to play a crucial role in the degradation of articular cartilage. The cells that in healthy cartilage are in charge of maintaining homeostasis, degrade their own matrix in the OA situation. While limited degradation of aggrecan is shown to be reversible, loss of collagen type II is thought to be a process of no return. However, loss of aggrecan from the matrix will render the matrix more vulnerable to further proteolytic degradation and mice with an aggrecanase degradation-resistant mutation show diminished cartilage damage during experimental OA [114].

It is widely accepted that the major aggrecanase involved in cartilage breakdown in OA belongs to the ADAMTS family. Although for a long time MMP activity was suspected as the main degrader of aggrecan it has become clear that the key cleavage site in aggrecan in OA cartilage is MMP insensitive, but can be cleaved by ADAMTS activity. The major candidate involved in aggrecan break down in OA cartilage appeared to be either ADAMTS4 or -5 [115]. Studies in mice indicate that ADAMTS5 is the major aggrecanase in cartilage *in vivo* but the jury is still out whether it is either ADAMTS4 or -5 in human cartilage [116]. However, the aggrecan-degrading activity under physiological conditions of ADAMTS5 is about 1000-fold higher than ADAMTS4, suggesting that ADAMTS5 should be the major destructive enzyme of aggrecan [117]. These findings have pushed a lot of effort in the development of ADAMTS5 inhibitors to block cartilage degradation in OA [118]. In an experimental model of OA in rats, application of an ADAMTS5 inhibitor resulted in reduction of progressive cartilage damage [119]. It has to be kept in mind that inhibition of cartilage damage in slowly developing human OA might not be as effective as in acute post-traumatic experimental OA.

Although all typical collagenases (MMP1, -8, -13, and -14) can cleave collagen type II, resulting in the generation of the characteristic three-quarter and one-quarter collagen fragments, it is now widely accepted that in human articular cartilage MMP13 is the major degrader of collagen type II [120]. It has been established that MMP13 expression is strikingly increased in osteoarthritic cartilage, both on mRNA and protein level and both in animal models and human OA [121,122]. Moreover, *Mmp13* knockout mice are partly protected against cartilage damage in experimental OA [123]. These data indicate that inhibition of MMP13 is an attractive option for OA therapy. However, application of MMP inhibitors in patients has resulted in a painful, joint-stiffening tendonitis-like side effect, termed 'musculoskeletal syndrome' or fibroplasia [124]. To overcome these problems research has been directed at the development of specific MMP13 blockers that do not show these side effects.

The biochemical pathways in meniscus degradation in OA are less well studied than cartilage degradation but it can be anticipated that similar mechanisms are involved. Pro-inflammatory stimulation of human meniscus cells resulted in increased MMP production and catabolic gene expression [125]. Damaged menisci showed increased expression of ADAMTS5 and MMP3 in the chondrocyte-like cells of menisci, indicating that these enzymes could be involved in meniscal degradation [126]. Moreover, in addition to enzymatic degradation, mechanical disruption of the tissue will occur in a damaged joint. Displacement of menisci, meniscal extrusion, has been shown to be associated with OA severity, so in knee OA not only degradation of articular cartilage is characteristic but also meniscal damage [127].

Repair of articular cartilage and meniscus

Damaged articular cartilage has very little capacity to regenerate, although some repair capability seems to be present under the right conditions. However, the limited self-renewal has inspired researchers to develop biology-based methods to repair cartilage to prevent total joint replacement by non-biological materials. Most efforts until now are focused on the repair of focal cartilage defects, not on damaged cartilages in OA joints, to prevent further damage and OA development. The main technique to stimulate the formation of fibrocartilage at the defect site, by contacting the bone marrow, is by microfracture of the subchondral plate or Pridie drilling. A newer, now commonly used technique is (matrix-induced) autologous chondrocyte implantation in which chondrocytes are harvested in the joint from a relatively unloaded location, cultured, and transferred, most times within a scaffold, to the cartilage defect. Since this method has the drawback that a new defect has to be created within the joint to obtain chondrocytes, alternative cell sources have been explored, most commonly mesenchymal stromal cells from bone marrow or fat tissue. Challenges to acquire stable articular cartilage from these cells is the control of cellular differentiation into articular chondrocytes and the maintenance of this phenotype by prevention of hypertrophy and terminal differentiation of these cells. Although *in vitro* these goals are not easily

reached, it can be expected that the joint environment will facilitate better maintenance of the differentiated chondrocyte phenotype. On the other hand, the conditions in an OA joint, both mechanically and biochemically, might even accelerate unwanted changes in chondrocyte phenotype. An attractive option, needing only one operation and no cell harvesting, is the development of smart cell-free scaffolds that induce and guide the formation of stable articular cartilage in the cartilage defect.

In earlier times, damaged menisci were not repaired but removed from the knee joint. Since this appeared to be associated with a higher incidence of OA development this procedure has been abandoned and nowadays only partial meniscectomy is carried out, or meniscal tears are sutured if possible. To replace damaged meniscus similar routes have been followed as for articular cartilage lesions but in addition fully artificial menisci are being developed to replace damaged menisci. What will be the optimal solution to repair damaged menisci will hopefully become clear within the next decade.

It is clear that both articular cartilage and meniscus are unique tissues that primarily have a mechanical function. Loss of tissue integrity leads to progressive loss of this function. It is of utmost importance to understand and to adequately diagnose age- and disease-related degradation of these tissues to be able to interfere with disease development at an early stage. Alternatively, technology should be developed to make it possible to repair damaged tissue to restore long-lasting joint function.

References

1. Craig FM, Bentley G, Archer CW. The spatial and temporal pattern of collagens I and II and keratan sulphate in the developing chick metatarsophalangeal joint. *Development* 1987; 99(3):383–91.
2. Archer CW, Morrison H, Pitsillides AA. Cellular aspects of the development of diarthrodial joints and articular cartilage. *J Anat* 1994; 184(Pt 3):447–56.
3. Mitrovic D. Development of the diarthrodial joints in the rat embryo. *Am J Anat* 1978; 151(4):475–85.
4. Koyama E, Shibukawa Y, Nagayama M, et al. A distinct cohort of progenitor cells participates in synovial joint and articular cartilage formation during mouse limb skeletogenesis. *Dev Biol* 2008; 316(1):62–73.
5. Hayes AJ, MacPherson S, Morrison H, Dowthwaite G, Archer CW. The development of articular cartilage: evidence for an appositional growth mechanism. *Anat Embryol* 2001; 203(6):469–79.
6. Osborne AC, Lamb KJ, Lewthwaite JC, Dowthwaite GP, Pitsillides AA. Short-term rigid and flaccid paralyses diminish growth of embryonic chick limbs and abrogate joint cavity formation but differentially preserve pre-cavitated joints. *J Musculoskelet Neuronal Interact* 2002; 2(5):448–56.
7. Kahn J, Shwartz Y, Blitz E, et al. Muscle contraction is necessary to maintain joint progenitor cell fate. *Dev Cell* 2009; 16(5):734–43.
8. Lasczkowski GE, Aigner T, Gamerdinger U, Weiler G, Bratzke H. Visualization of postmortem chondrocyte damage by vital staining and confocal laser scanning 3D microscopy. *J Forensic Sci* 2002; 47(3):663–6.
9. Dowthwaite GP, Bishop JC, Redman SN, et al. The surface of articular cartilage contains a progenitor cell population. *J Cell Sci* 2004; 117(Pt 6):889–97.
10. Aspden RM, Yarker YE, Hukins DW. Collagen orientations in the meniscus of the knee joint. *J Anat* 1985; 140(Pt 3):371–80.
11. Poole CA, Flint MH, Beaumont BW. Chondrons in cartilage: ultrastructural analysis of the pericellular microenvironment in adult human articular cartilages. *J Orthop Res* 1987; 5(4):509–22.

12. Eyre DR, Weis MA, Wu JJ. Articular cartilage collagen: an irreplaceable framework? *Eur Cell Mater* 2006; 12:57–63.

13. Eyre DR, Wu JJ, Fernandes RJ, Pietka TA, Weis MA. Recent developments in cartilage research: matrix biology of the collagen II/IX/XI heterofibril network. *Biochem Society Trans* 2002; 30(Pt 6):893–9.

14. Eyre D. Collagen of articular cartilage. *Arthritis Res* 2002; 4(1):30–5.

15. Wu JJ, Weis MA, Kim LS, Eyre DR. Type III collagen, a fibril network modifier in articular cartilage. *J Biol Chem* 2010; 285(24):18537–44.

16. Poole CA, Ayad S, Gilbert RT. Chondrons from articular cartilage. V. Immunohistochemical evaluation of type VI collagen organisation in isolated chondrons by light, confocal and electron microscopy. *J Cell Sci* 1992; 103(Pt 4):1101–10.

17. Heinegard D, Wieslander J, Sheehan J, Paulsson M, Sommarin Y. Separation and characterization of two populations of aggregating proteoglycans from cartilage. *Biochem J* 1985; 225(1):95–106.

18. Bayliss MT, Osborne D, Woodhouse S, Davidson C. Sulfation of chondroitin sulfate in human articular cartilage. The effect of age, topographical position, and zone of cartilage on tissue composition. *J Biol Chem* 1999; 274(22):15892–900.

19. Hedlund H, Hedbom E, Heinegård D, et al. Association of the aggrecan keratan sulfate-rich region with collagen in bovine articular cartilage. *J Biol Chem* 1999; 274(9):5777–81.

20. Nicole S, Davoine CS, Topaloglu H, et al. Perlecan, the major proteoglycan of basement membranes, is altered in patients with Schwartz-Jampel syndrome (chondrodystrophic myotonia). *Nat Genet* 2000; 26(4):480–3.

21. Melrose J, Hayes AJ, Whitelock JM, Little CB. Perlecan, the 'jack of all trades' proteoglycan of cartilaginous weight-bearing connective tissues. *BioEssays* 2008; 30(5):457–69.

22. Heinegard D. Proteoglycans and more—from molecules to biology. *Int J Exp Pathol* 2009; 90(6):575–86.

23. Oldberg A, Antonsson P, Lindblom K, Heinegard D. COMP (cartilage oligomeric matrix protein) is structurally related to the thrombospondins. *J Biol Chem* 1992; 267(31):22346–50.

24. Halasz K, Kassner A, Morgelin M, Heinegard D. COMP acts as a catalyst in collagen fibrillogenesis. *J Biol Chem* 2007; 282(43):31166–73.

25. Klatt AR, Nitsche DP, Kobbe B, et al. Molecular structure and tissue distribution of matrilin-3, a filament-forming extracellular matrix protein expressed during skeletal development. *J Biol Chem* 2000; 275(6):3999–4006.

26. Wiberg C, Klatt AR, Wagener R, et al. Complexes of matrilin-1 and biglycan or decorin connect collagen VI microfibrils to both collagen II and aggrecan. *J Biol Chem* 2003; 278(39):37698–704.

27. Marcelino J, Carpten JD, Suwairi WM, et al. CACP, encoding a secreted proteoglycan, is mutated in camptodactyly-arthropathy-coxa vara-pericarditis syndrome. *Nat Genet* 1999; 23(3):319–22.

28. Jay GD, Torres JR, Rhee DK, Helminen HJ, Hytinnen MM, Cha CJ, et al. Association between friction and wear in diarthrodial joints lacking lubricin. *Arthritis Rheum* 2007; 56(11):3662–9.

29. Eyre DR, Wu JJ. Collagen of fibrocartilage: a distinctive molecular phenotype in bovine meniscus. *FEBS Lett* 1983; 158(2):265–70.

30. Melrose J, Fuller ES, Roughley PJ, et al. Fragmentation of decorin, biglycan, lumican and keratocan is elevated in degenerate human meniscus, knee and hip articular cartilages compared with age-matched macroscopically normal and control tissues. *Arthritis Res Ther* 2008; 10(4):R79.

31. Scanzello CR, Markova DZ, Chee A, et al. Fibronectin splice variation in human knee cartilage, meniscus and synovial membrane: observations in osteoarthritic knee. *J Orthop Res* 2015; 33(4):556–62.

32. Miller RR, McDevitt CA. Thrombospondin in ligament, meniscus and intervertebral disc. *Biochim Biophys Acta* 1991; 1115(1):85–8.

33. Hopker WW, Angres G, Klingel K, Komitowski D, Schuchardt E. Changes of the elastin compartment in the human meniscus. *Virchows Archiv A Pathol Anat Histopathol* 1986; 408(6):575–92.

34. Mow VC, Guo XE. Mechano-electrochemical properties of articular cartilage: their inhomogeneities and anisotropies. *Annu Rev Biomed Eng* 2002; 4:175–209.

35. Wilson W, van Donkelaar CC, van Rietbergen B, Huiskes R. A fibril-reinforced poroviscoelastic swelling model for articular cartilage. *J Biomech* 2005; 38(6):1195–204.

36. Likhitpanichkul M, Guo XE, Mow VC. The effect of matrix tension-compression nonlinearity and fixed negative charges on chondrocyte responses in cartilage. *Mol Cell Biomech MCB* 2005; 2(4):191–204.

37. Maroudas AI. Balance between swelling pressure and collagen tension in normal and degenerate cartilage. *Nature* 1976; 260(5554):808–9.

38. Ateshian GA. The role of interstitial fluid pressurization in articular cartilage lubrication. *J Biomech* 2009; 42(9):1163–76.

39. Hinterwimmer S, Krammer M, Krotz M, et al. Cartilage atrophy in the knees of patients after seven weeks of partial load bearing. *Arthritis Rheum* 2004; 50(8):2516–20.

40. Wilusz RE, Sanchez-Adams J, Guilak F. The structure and function of the pericellular matrix of articular cartilage. *Matrix Biol* 2014; 39:25–32.

41. Szafranski JD, Grodzinsky AJ, Burger E, et al. Chondrocyte mechanotransduction: effects of compression on deformation of intracellular organelles and relevance to cellular biosynthesis. *Osteoarthritis Cartilage* 2004; 12(12):937–46.

42. Madej W, van Caam A, Blaney Davidson EN, van der Kraan PM, Buma P. Physiological and excessive mechanical compression of articular cartilage activates Smad2/3P signaling. *Osteoarthritis Cartilage* 2014; 22(7):1018–25.

43. Fukubayashi T, Kurosawa H. The contact area and pressure distribution pattern of the knee. A study of normal and osteoarthrotic knee joints. *Acta Orthopaed Scand* 1980; 51(6):871–9.

44. Schmidt MB, Chen EH, Lynch SE. A review of the effects of insulin-like growth factor and platelet derived growth factor on in vivo cartilage healing and repair. *Osteoarthritis Cartilage* 2006; 14(5):403–12.

45. Montaseri A, Busch F, Mobasheri A, et al. IGF-1 and PDGF-bb suppress IL-1beta-induced cartilage degradation through down-regulation of NF-kappaB signaling: involvement of Src/PI-3K/AKT pathway. *PLoS ONE* 2011; 6(12):e28663.

46. Blaney Davidson EN, van der Kraan PM, van den Berg WB. TGF-beta and osteoarthritis 1. *Osteoarthritis Cartilage* 2007; 15(6):597–604.

47. Serra R, Johnson M, Filvaroff EH, et al. Expression of a truncated, kinase defective TGF-beta type II receptor in mouse skeletal tissue promotes terminal chondrocyte differentiation and osteoarthritis. *J Cell Biol* 1997; 139(2):541–52.

48. Plaas A, Velasco J, Gorski DJ, et al. The relationship between fibrogenic TGFbeta1 signaling in the joint and cartilage degradation in post-injury osteoarthritis. *Osteoarthritis Cartilage* 2011; 19(9):1081–90.

49. Blaney Davidson EN, Remst DF, Vitters EL, et al. Increase in ALK1/ALK5 ratio as a cause for elevated MMP-13 expression in osteoarthritis in humans and mice. *J Immunol* 2009; 182(12):7937–45.

50. Erlacher L, Ng CK, Ullrich R, Krieger S, Luyten FP. Presence of cartilage-derived morphogenetic proteins in articular cartilage and enhancement of matrix replacement in vitro. *Arthritis Rheum* 1998; 41(2):263–73.

51. Hurtig M, Chubinskaya S, Dickey J, Rueger D. BMP-7 protects against progression of cartilage degeneration after impact injury. *J Orthop Res* 2009; 27(5):602–11.

52. Forriol F, Ripalda P, Duart J, Esparza R, Gortazar AR. Meniscal repair possibilities using bone morphogenetic protein-7. *Injury* 2014; 45 Suppl 4:S15–21.

53. Chubinskaya S, Kumar B, Merrihew C, et al. Age-related changes in cartilage endogenous osteogenic protein-1 (OP-1). *Biochim Biophys Acta* 2002; 1588(2):126–34.

54. Luyten FP, Chen P, Paralkar V, Reddi AH. Recombinant bone morphogenetic protein-4, transforming growth factor-beta 1, and activin A enhance the cartilage phenotype of articular chondrocytes in vitro. *Exp Cell Res* 1994; 210(2):224–9.

55. Enochson L, Stenberg J, Brittberg M, Lindahl A. GDF5 reduces MMP13 expression in human chondrocytes via DKK1 mediated canonical Wnt signaling inhibition. *Osteoarthritis Cartilage* 2014; 22(4):566–77.

56. Coleman CM, Vaughan EE, Browe DC, et al. Growth differentiation factor-5 enhances in vitro mesenchymal stromal cell chondrogenesis and hypertrophy. *Stem cells and development* 2013; 22(13):1968–76.

57. Masuya H, Nishida K, Furuichi T, et al. A novel dominant-negative mutation in Gdf5 generated by ENU mutagenesis impairs joint formation and causes osteoarthritis in mice. *Hum Mol Genet* 2007; 16(19):2366–75.

58. Chia SL, Sawaji Y, Burleigh A, et al. Fibroblast growth factor 2 is an intrinsic chondroprotective agent that suppresses ADAMTS-5 and delays cartilage degradation in murine osteoarthritis. *Arthritis Rheum* 2009; 60(7):2019–27.

59. Uchii M, Tamura T, Suda T, et al. Role of fibroblast growth factor 8 (FGF8) in animal models of osteoarthritis. *Arthritis Res Ther* 2008; 10(4):R90.

60. Ellsworth JL, Berry J, Bukowski T, et al. Fibroblast growth factor-18 is a trophic factor for mature chondrocytes and their progenitors. *Osteoarthritis Cartilage* 2002; 10(4):308–20.

61. Moore EE, Bendele AM, Thompson DL, et al. Fibroblast growth factor-18 stimulates chondrogenesis and cartilage repair in a rat model of injury-induced osteoarthritis. *Osteoarthritis Cartilage* 2005; 13(7):623–31.

62. Reinhold MI, Abe M, Kapadia RM, Liao Z, Naski MC. FGF18 represses noggin expression and is induced by calcineurin. *J Biol Chem* 2004; 279(37):38209–19.

63. Lories RJ, Corr M, Lane NE. To Wnt or not to Wnt: the bone and joint health dilemma. *Nature reviews. Rheumatology* 2013; 9(6):328–39.

64. Leucht P, Minear S, Ten Berge D, Nusse R, Helms JA. Translating insights from development into regenerative medicine: the function of Wnts in bone biology. *Seminars in cell & developmental biology* 2008; 19(5):434–43.

65. Hwang SG, Yu SS, Lee SW, Chun JS. Wnt-3a regulates chondrocyte differentiation via c-Jun/AP-1 pathway. *FEBS Lett* 2005; 579(21):4837–42.

66. Ma B, Landman EB, Miclea RL, et al. WNT signaling and cartilage: of mice and men. *Calcif Tissue Int* 2013; 92(5):399–411.

67. Ma B, van Blitterswijk CA, Karperien M. A Wnt/beta-catenin negative feedback loop inhibits interleukin-1-induced matrix metalloproteinase expression in human articular chondrocytes. *Arthritis Rheum* 2012; 64(8):2589–600.

68. Blavier L, Lazaryev A, Shi XH, et al. Stromelysin-1 (MMP-3) is a target and a regulator of Wnt1-induced epithelial-mesenchymal transition (EMT). *Cancer biology & therapy* 2010; 10(2):198–208.

69. Yamagata K, Li X, Ikegaki S, et al. Dissection of Wnt5a-Ror2 signaling leading to matrix metalloproteinase (MMP-13) expression. *J Biol Chem* 2012; 287(2):1588–99.

70. Nalesso G, Sherwood J, Bertrand J, et al. WNT-3A modulates articular chondrocyte phenotype by activating both canonical and noncanonical pathways. *J Cell Biol* 2011; 193(3):551–64.

71. Harada N, Tamai Y, Ishikawa T, et al. Intestinal polyposis in mice with a dominant stable mutation of the beta-catenin gene. *EMBO J* 1999; 18(21):5931–42.

72. Zhong L, Ma B, Post JN, Karperien M. Role of TCF4 in signaling crosstalk with NFκB in human chondrocytes. *Osteoarthritis Cartilage*; 21:S122–23.

73. Tumia NS, Johnstone AJ. Platelet derived growth factor-AB enhances knee meniscal cell activity in vitro. *Knee* 2009; 16(1):73–6.

74. Kieswetter K, Schwartz Z, Alderete M, Dean DD, Boyan BD. Platelet derived growth factor stimulates chondrocyte proliferation but prevents endochondral maturation. *Endocrine* 1997; 6(3):257–64.

75. Schafer SJ, Luyten FP, Yanagishita M, Reddi AH. Proteoglycan metabolism is age related and modulated by isoforms of platelet-derived growth factor in bovine articular cartilage explant cultures. *Arch Biochem Biophys* 1993; 302(2):431–8.

76. Kronenberg HM, Lee K, Lanske B, Segre GV. Parathyroid hormone-related protein and Indian hedgehog control the pace of cartilage differentiation. *J Endocrinol* 1997; 154 Suppl:S39–45.

77. Zhou J, Wei X, Wei L. Indian Hedgehog, a critical modulator in osteoarthritis, could be a potential therapeutic target for attenuating cartilage degeneration disease. *Connect Tissue Res* 2014; 55(4):257–61.

78. Wei F, Zhou J, Wei X, et al. Activation of Indian hedgehog promotes chondrocyte hypertrophy and upregulation of MMP-13 in human osteoarthritic cartilage. *Osteoarthritis Cartilage* 2012; 20(7):755–63.

79. Enomoto H, Inoki I, Komiya K, et al. Vascular endothelial growth factor isoforms and their receptors are expressed in human osteoarthritic cartilage. *Am J Pathol* 2003; 162(1):171–81.

80. Yang X, Chen L, Xu XL, et al. TGF-beta/Smad3 signals repress chondrocyte hypertrophic differentiation and are required for maintaining articular cartilage. *J Cell Biol* 2001; 153(1):35–46.

81. Retting KN, Song B, Yoon BS, Lyons KM. BMP canonical Smad signaling through Smad1 and Smad5 is required for endochondral bone formation. *Development* 2009; 136(7):1093–104.

82. van der Kraan PM, Blaney Davidson EN, van den Berg WB. Bone morphogenetic proteins and articular cartilage: to serve and protect or a wolf in sheep clothing's? *Osteoarthritis Cartilage* 2010; 18(6):735–41.

83. Caron MM, Emans PJ, Cremers A, et al. Hypertrophic differentiation during chondrogenic differentiation of progenitor cells is stimulated by BMP-2 but suppressed by BMP-7. *Osteoarthritis Cartilage* 2013; 21(4):604–13.

84. Blaney Davidson EN, Vitters EL, van Lent PL, et al. Elevated extracellular matrix production and degradation upon bone morphogenetic protein-2 (BMP-2) stimulation point toward a role for BMP-2 in cartilage repair and remodeling. *Arthritis Res Ther* 2007; 9(5):R102.

85. Buxton P, Edwards C, Archer CW, Francis-West P. Growth/differentiation factor-5 (GDF-5) and skeletal development. *J Bone Joint Surg Am* 2001; 83-A Suppl 1(Pt 1):S23–30.

86. Francis-West PH, Abdelfattah A, Chen P, et al. Mechanisms of GDF-5 action during skeletal development. *Development* 1999; 126(6):1305–15.

87. Chang SC, Hoang B, Thomas JT, et al. Cartilage-derived morphogenetic proteins. New members of the transforming growth factor-beta superfamily predominantly expressed in long bones during human embryonic development. *J Biol Chem* 1994; 269(45):28227–34.

88. Trippel SB, Corvol MT, Dumontier MF, et al. Effect of somatomedin-C/insulin-like growth factor I and growth hormone on cultured growth plate and articular chondrocytes. *Pediatr Res* 1989; 25(1):76–82.

89. Elder BD, Athanasiou KA. Systematic assessment of growth factor treatment on biochemical and biomechanical properties of engineered articular cartilage constructs. *Osteoarthritis Cartilage* 2009; 17(1):114–23.

90. Wang J, Zhou J, Cheng CM, Kopchick JJ, Bondy CA. Evidence supporting dual, IGF-I-independent and IGF-I-dependent, roles for GH in promoting longitudinal bone growth. *J Endocrinol* 2004; 180(2):247–55.

91. Phornphutkul C, Wu KY, Yang X, Chen Q, Gruppuso PA. Insulin-like growth factor-I signaling is modified during chondrocyte differentiation. *J Endocrinol* 2004; 183(3):477–86.

92. Mushtaq T, Bijman P, Ahmed SF, Farquharson C. Insulin-like growth factor-I augments chondrocyte hypertrophy and reverses glucocorticoid-mediated growth retardation in fetal mice metatarsal cultures. *Endocrinology* 2004; 145(5):2478–86.

93. Solchaga LA, Penick K, Goldberg VM, Caplan AI, Welter JF. Fibroblast growth factor-2 enhances proliferation and delays loss of chondrogenic potential in human adult bone-marrow-derived mesenchymal stem cells. *Tissue Eng Part A* 2010; 16(3):1009–19.

94. Richter W, Bock R, Hennig T, Weiss S. Influence of FGF-2 and PTHrP on chondrogenic differentiation of human mesenchymal stem cells. *J Bone Joint Surg Br* 2009; 91-B(Supp III):444.

95. Mancilla EE, De Luca F, Uyeda JA, Czerwiec FS, Baron J. Effects of fibroblast growth factor-2 on longitudinal bone growth. *Endocrinology* 1998; 139(6):2900–4.

96. Cucchiarini M, Ekici M, Schetting S, Kohn D, Madry H. Metabolic activities and chondrogenic differentiation of human mesenchymal stem cells following recombinant adeno-associated virus-mediated gene transfer and overexpression of fibroblast growth factor 2. *Tissue Eng Part A* 2011; 17(15–16):1921–33.

97. Davidson D, Blanc A, Filion D, et al. Fibroblast growth factor (FGF) 18 signals through FGF receptor 3 to promote chondrogenesis. *J Biol Chem* 2005; 280(21):20509–15.

98. Liu Z, Lavine KJ, Hung IH, Ornitz DM. FGF18 is required for early chondrocyte proliferation, hypertrophy and vascular invasion of the growth plate. *Dev Biol* 2007; 302(1):80–91.

99. Guo X, Day TF, Jiang X, et al. Wnt/beta-catenin signaling is sufficient and necessary for synovial joint formation. *Genes Dev* 2004; 18(19):2404–17.

100. Church V, Nohno T, Linker C, Marcelle C, Francis-West P. Wnt regulation of chondrocyte differentiation. *J Cell Sci* 2002; 115(Pt 24):4809–18.

101. Witte F, Dokas J, Neuendorf F, Mundlos S, Stricker S. Comprehensive expression analysis of all Wnt genes and their major secreted antagonists during mouse limb development and cartilage differentiation. *Gene Expr Patterns* 2009; 9(4):215–23.

102. Dong YF, Soung do Y, Schwarz EM, O'Keefe RJ, Drissi H. Wnt induction of chondrocyte hypertrophy through the Runx2 transcription factor. *J Cell Physiol* 2006; 208(1):77–86.

103. Guo X, Mak KK, Taketo MM, Yang Y. The Wnt/beta-catenin pathway interacts differentially with PTHrP signaling to control chondrocyte hypertrophy and final maturation. *PLoS ONE* 2009; 4(6):e6067.

104. Lohmann CH, Schwartz Z, Niederauer GG, et al. Pretreatment with platelet derived growth factor-BB modulates the ability of costochondral resting zone chondrocytes incorporated into PLA/PGA scaffolds to form new cartilage in vivo. *Biomaterials* 2000; 21(1):49–61.

105. Mak KK, Kronenberg HM, Chuang PT, Mackem S, Yang Y. Indian hedgehog signals independently of PTHrP to promote chondrocyte hypertrophy. *Development* 2008; 135(11):1947–56.

106. Handorf A, Chamberlain CS, Li WJ. Endogenously-produced Indian Hedgehog regulates TGFbeta-driven chondrogenesis of human bone marrow stromal/stem cells. *Stem Cells Dev* 2014; 24(8):995–1007.

107. Kim EJ, Cho SW, Shin JO, et al. Ihh and Runx2/Runx3 signaling interact to coordinate early chondrogenesis: a mouse model. *PLoS ONE* 2013; 8(2):e55296.

108. Steinert AF, Weissenberger M, Kunz M, et al. Indian hedgehog gene transfer is a chondrogenic inducer of human mesenchymal stem cells. *Arthritis Res Ther* 2012; 14(4):R168.

109. Carlevaro MF, Cermelli S, Cancedda R, Descalzi Cancedda F. Vascular endothelial growth factor (VEGF) in cartilage neovascularization and chondrocyte differentiation: auto-paracrine role during endochondral bone formation. *J Cell Sci* 2000; 113(Pt 1):59–69.

110. Yin M, Pacifici M. Vascular regression is required for mesenchymal condensation and chondrogenesis in the developing limb. *Dev Dyn* 2001; 222(3):522–33.

111. Zelzer E, Mamluk R, Ferrara N, et al. VEGFA is necessary for chondrocyte survival during bone development. *Development* 2004; 131(9):2161–71.

112. Kolostova K, Taltynov O, Pinterova D, et al. Wound healing gene therapy: cartilage regeneration induced by vascular endothelial growth factor plasmid. *Am J Otolaryngol* 2012; 33(1):68–74.

113. Kubo S, Cooper GM, Matsumoto T, et al. Blocking vascular endothelial growth factor with soluble Flt-1 improves the chondrogenic potential of mouse skeletal muscle-derived stem cells. *Arthritis Rheum* 2009; 60(1):155–65.

114. Little CB, Meeker CT, Golub SB, et al. Blocking aggrecanase cleavage in the aggrecan interglobular domain abrogates cartilage erosion and promotes cartilage repair. *J Clin Invest* 2007; 117(6):1627–36.

115. Sandy JD, Flannery CR, Neame PJ, Lohmander LS. The structure of aggrecan fragments in human synovial fluid. Evidence for the involvement in osteoarthritis of a novel proteinase which cleaves the Glu 373-Ala 374 bond of the interglobular domain. *J Clin Invest* 1992; 89(5):1512–6.

116. Stanton H, Rogerson FM, East CJ, et al. ADAMTS5 is the major aggrecanase in mouse cartilage in vivo and in vitro. *Nature* 2005; 434(7033):648–52.

117. Gendron C, Kashiwagi M, Lim NH, et al. Proteolytic activities of human ADAMTS-5: comparative studies with ADAMTS-4. *J Biol Chem* 2007; 282(25):18294–306.

118. Maingot L, Leroux F, Landry V, Dumont J, Nagase H, Villoutreix B, et al. New non-hydroxamic ADAMTS-5 inhibitors based on the 1,2,4-triazole-3-thiol scaffold. *Bioorg Med Chem Lett* 2010; 20(21):6213–6.

119. Chen P, Zhu S, Wang Y, et al. The amelioration of cartilage degeneration by ADAMTS-5 inhibitor delivered in a hyaluronic acid hydrogel. *Biomaterials* 2014; 35(9):2827–36.

120. Billinghurst RC, Dahlberg L, Ionescu M, et al. Enhanced cleavage of type II collagen by collagenases in osteoarthritic articular cartilage. *J Clin Invest* 1997; 99(7):1534–45.

121. Huebner JL, Otterness IG, Freund EM, Caterson B, Kraus VB. Collagenase 1 and collagenase 3 expression in a guinea pig model of osteoarthritis. *Arthritis Rheum* 1998; 41(5):877–90.

122. Moldovan F, Pelletier JP, Hambor J, Cloutier JM, Martel-Pelletier J. Collagenase-3 (matrix metalloprotease 13) is preferentially localized in the deep layer of human arthritic cartilage in situ: in vitro mimicking effect by transforming growth factor beta. *Arthritis Rheum* 1997; 40(9):1653–61.

123. Little CB, Barai A, Burkhardt D, et al. Matrix metalloproteinase 13-deficient mice are resistant to osteoarthritic cartilage erosion but not chondrocyte hypertrophy or osteophyte development. *Arthritis Rheum* 2009; 60(12):3723–33.

124. Clark IM, Parker AE. Metalloproteinases: their role in arthritis and potential as therapeutic targets. *Expert Opin Ther Targets* 2003; 7(1):19–34.

125. Stone AV, Loeser RF, Vanderman KS, et al. Pro-inflammatory stimulation of meniscus cells increases production of matrix metalloproteinases and additional catabolic factors involved in osteoarthritis pathogenesis. *Osteoarthritis Cartilage* 2014; 22(2):264–74.

126. Ishihara G, Kojima T, Saito Y, Ishiguro N. Roles of metalloproteinase-3 and aggrecanase 1 and 2 in aggrecan cleavage during human meniscus degeneration. *Orthop Rev* 2009; 1(2):e14.

127. Englund M, Guermazi A, Lohmander LS. The meniscus in knee osteoarthritis. *Rheum Dis Clin North Am* 2009; 35(3):579–90.

128. Eyre DR, Muir H. The distribution of different molecular species of collagen in fibrous, elastic and hyaline cartilages of the pig. *Biochem J* 1975; 151(3):595–602.

129. Poole CA, Ayad S, Schofield JR. Chondrons from articular cartilage: I. Immunolocalization of type VI collagen in the pericellular capsule of isolated canine tibial chondrons. *J Cell Sci* 1988; 90(Pt 4):635–43.

130. Wu JJ, Eyre DR. Cartilage type IX collagen is cross-linked by hydroxypyridinium residues. *Biochem Biophys Res Comm* 1984; 123(3):1033–9.

131. Kielty CM, Kwan AP, Holmes DF, Schor SL, Grant ME. Type X collagen, a product of hypertrophic chondrocytes. *Biochem J* 1985; 227(2):545–54.

132. Morris NP, Bachinger HP. Type XI collagen is a heterotrimer with the composition (1 alpha, 2 alpha, 3 alpha) retaining non-triple-helical domains. *J Biol Chem* 1987; 262(23):11345–50.

133. Heinegard D, Hascall VC. Aggregation of cartilage proteoglycans. 3. Characteristics of the proteins isolated from trypsin digests of aggregates. *J Biol Chem* 1974; 249(13):4250–6.

134. Doege K, Hassell JR, Caterson B, Yamada Y. Link protein cDNA sequence reveals a tandemly repeated protein structure. *Proc Natl Acad Sci U S A* 1986; 83(11):3761–5.

135. Hardingham TE, Muir H. Hyaluronic acid in cartilage and proteoglycan aggregation. *Biochem J* 1974; 139(3):565–81.

136. Arikawa-Hirasawa E, Watanabe H, Takami H, Hassell JR, Yamada Y. Perlecan is essential for cartilage and cephalic development. *Nat Genet* 1999; 23(3):354–8.

137. Archer CW, Morrison EH, Bayliss MT, Ferguson MW. The development of articular cartilage: II. The spatial and temporal patterns of glycosaminoglycans and small leucine-rich proteoglycans. *J Anat* 1996; 189(Pt 1):23–35.

138. Shen Z, Heinegard D, Sommarin Y. Distribution and expression of cartilage oligomeric matrix protein and bone sialoprotein show marked changes during rat femoral head development. *Matrix Bioll* 1995; 14(9):773–81.

139. Flannery CR, Hughes CE, Schumacher BL, et al. Articular cartilage superficial zone protein (SZP) is homologous to megakaryocyte stimulating factor precursor and is a multifunctional proteoglycan with potential growth-promoting, cytoprotective, and lubricating properties in cartilage metabolism. *Biochem Biophys Res Commun* 1999; 254(3):535–41.

140. McDevitt CA, Webber RJ. The ultrastructure and biochemistry of meniscal cartilage. *Clin Orthop Relat Res* 1990(252):8–18.

141. Bluteau G, Labourdette L, Ronziere M, et al. Type X collagen in rabbit and human meniscus. *Osteoarthritis Cartilage* 1999; 7(5):498–501.

142. McNicol D, Roughley PJ. Extraction and characterization of proteoglycan from human meniscus. *Biochem J* 1980; 185(3):705–13.

143. Fife RS. Identification of link proteins and a 116,000-Dalton matrix protein in canine meniscus. *Arch Biochem Biophys* 1985; 240(2):682–8.

CHAPTER 5

Pathophysiology of periarticular bone changes in osteoarthritis

Steven R. Goldring

Periarticular bone structure and physiology

Joint structures are divided into three categories based on their anatomy and functional properties. They include diarthrodial joints (e.g. the knee or hip joints), which are highly mobile and have a synovial lining; amphiarthroses (e.g. intervertebral discs), in which the adjacent bones are separated by articular cartilage or fibrocartilage and for which there is limited motion; and synarthroses, in which fibrous tissue separates adjoining bones [1–3]. The diarthrodial joints and amphiarthroses are the principal joints affected by the osteoarthritic (OA) process. This chapter will focus on the anatomy, pathology, and pathophysiology of OA changes in periarticular bone in diarthrodial joints.

Under physiological conditions periarticular bone in diarthrodial joints forms a biocomposite with the overlying calcified and hyaline articular cartilage. The composition and structure of these tissues are optimally adapted to provide structural stability and transfer mechanical loads across the joint. During the evolution of the OA process, the periarticular bone undergoes striking alterations in its composition and structural organization and importantly the physiological equilibrium and interaction with the overlying cartilage is disrupted [3,4].

The subchondral bone is organized into two distinct anatomical components consisting of a zone of plate-like compact cortical bone that overlies a network of trabecular bone that encloses the bone marrow and bone marrow space (Figure 5.1). The bone at the joint margins is comprised of cortical bone lined by periosteum. It is the site of attachment of the synovium and entheseal structures where tendons and ligaments insert [2,3]. Throughout postnatal life, periarticular bone retains the capacity to adapt its structural and functional properties in response to local biomechanical influences and systemic factors such as endocrine hormones, as well as the effects of soluble products generated in the adjacent joint tissues. These adaptive changes are mediated by the coordinated cellular activities of osteoclasts and osteoblasts that remodel the cortical and trabecular bone through a process of osteoclast-mediated bone resorption, followed by a phase of bone formation mediated by osteoblasts [5]. Bone remodelling provides a mechanism for adapting the skeleton to local biomechanical and physiological mediators and for responding to systemic hormonal influences. Importantly, it also provides a cellular mechanism

for replacing bone that has undergone damage from repetitive or excessive mechanical loading [6–8].

Although the activities of osteoclasts and osteoblasts are the ultimate determinants of the composition and structural organization of the bone tissue, there is a third cell type in bone, the osteocyte, that plays an essential role in regulating the remodelling and adaptive changes in the skeleton [9–11]. Osteocytes form an interconnected network within the bone matrix and with the cells on the bone surface, including osteoclasts and osteoblasts. They are optimally positioned within the bone matrix to act as a mechanosensor that responds to local biomechanical influences as well as recognizing structural damage to the bone matrix [6–8]. Osteocytes also have the capacity to respond to systemic hormones and local soluble mediators and to signal to osteoclasts and osteoblasts to control the bone remodelling machinery.

The capacity of bone to adapt to its local mechanical influences is embodied in *Wolff's law* that states that the structural organization and material properties of bone are determined by the magnitude and characteristics of applied load [12]. In this paradigm, at a given anatomical site, exposure of the bone tissue to increased loads results in a cell-mediated adaptive increase in bone mass, and a decrease in loading is translated into a decrease in bone mass. As will be discussed in the following section, alterations in

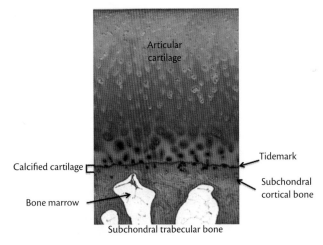

Figure 5.1 Histological cross-section of a normal knee joint.
Courtesy of Edward DiCarlo, MD, Hospital for Special Surgery, New York, NY.

the organization and structural properties of periarticular bone in part are a reflection of an adaptation to the local biomechanical environment and as such are a reflection of the past loading history.

Bone pathology in osteoarthritis

As described in the preceding section, the periarticular bone in diarthrodial joints can be segregated into distinct anatomical and functional compartments. As the OA process evolves, each of these anatomical sites, including the subchondral cortical bone plate, the subchondral trabecular bone and the bone at the joint margins exhibit distinct structural and functional properties reflecting the unique biological and biomechanical influences at these locations. A hallmark of osteoarthritis (OA) in human subjects is the development of increased thickness of the subchondral cortical bone plate that is demonstrated radiographically as bone sclerosis [2,4,13–16] (Figure 5.2). In addition, there is development of so-called bone attrition at this site, which manifests as progressive flattening and deformation of the subchondral articular contour [17–19].

The alterations in the subchondral cortical bone are mediated via the activities of osteoclasts and osteoblasts that respond to local biomechanical forces and through a process of remodelling and modelling (direct apposition of bone to existing bone surfaces) increase the volumetric bone mass, resulting in thickening of the subchondral bone plate. The effect of the increase in bone remodelling affects not only the bone volume in this compartment but can modify the material properties of the newly formed bone matrix [20–22]. This is related to the observation that in states of high bone turnover, there is attenuation of mineral accretion by the rapid remodelling process, which leads to a state of relative hypomineralization. These changes in the state of mineralization reduce the elastic modulus of the bone, which increases its tendency to deform under load, thereby enhancing its susceptibility to both micro- as well as macrodamage. The relationship between these changes and the development of bone marrow lesions (BMLs) and bone cysts in subchondral bone will be discussed later in this section. These material property changes not only adversely affect the integrity of the subchondral bone, but also disrupt the physiological relationship between the subchondral bone and overlying calcified and articular cartilage potentially contributing to accelerating deterioration in the integrity of joint cartilage [13,20,23].

As shown in Figure 5.1, under physiological conditions the subchondral bone is separated from hyaline articular cartilage by a thin zone of calcified cartilage. The region between the articular and calcified cartilage is marked by the so-called *tidemark* that can be identified by its enhanced metachromatic staining pattern. During the evolution of the OA process, the zone of calcified cartilage is penetrated by blood vessels that extend from the subchondral bone and adjacent marrow spaces. This is accompanied by expansion and advancement of the zone of calcified cartilage into the overlying articular cartilage associated with duplication of the tidemark [4,13,24]. Within the deeper zones of the calcified cartilage the matrix undergoes mineralization and is remodelled to form new bone tissues (Figure 5.3). These events, including vascular invasion and new bone formation, recapitulate many of the features of the growth plate during the development and growth of long bones [25–28].

In contrast to the progressive increases in bone mass in the subchondral bone plate in OA, a variety of techniques, including computed tomography (CT), magnetic resonance imaging (MRI), and radiographic techniques indicate that the OA process is accompanied by a progressive loss of subchondral trabecular bone [13,29–31]. Particularly informative have been the studies using a computerized method of bone textural image analysis (fractal signature analysis), which demonstrates that OA progression is associated with thinning and fenestration of vertical trabeculae consistent with the development of osteoporotic bone loss. Recently, Kraus and co-workers using the radiographic fractal signature analysis technology confirmed the previous observations indicating the presence of osteoporotic changes in subchondral trabecular bone

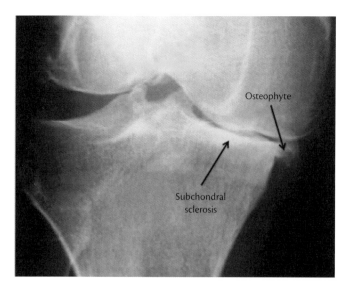

Figure 5.2 Knee radiograph demonstrating subchondral sclerosis and osteophyte formation at the joint margin.

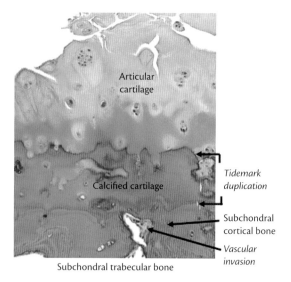

Figure 5.3 Subchondral bone changes associated with advanced osteoarthritis. There is advancement of the calcified cartilage into the lower zones of the articular cartilage with duplication of the tidemark and vascular invasion of the subchondral cortical bone.

Courtesy of Edward DiCarlo, MD, Hospital for Special Surgery, New York, NY.

and further demonstrated that this technique could be used as an outcomes measure in OA studies and as a tool to predict patients at increased risk for OA progression [32].

The mechanisms underlying the reduced bone mass in the subchondral trabecular bone reflect the adaptation of the bone at this site to the local biomechanical and biological environment. The progressive increase in bone volume and sclerosis that characterizes the subchondral cortical bone results in shielding of the underlying trabecular bone from load transfer. The relative reduction in load transfer is sensed by the osteocytes in the trabecular bone compartment resulting in activation of bone resorption and progressive bone loss via the bone remodelling process. In our own studies, we have used an *in vivo* tibial loading model to investigate the adaptive responses of subchondral bone (and cartilage) to mechanical loading and to define the role of mechanical loading on the development of OA bone pathology [33]. We observed increased subchondral cortical thickness in regions exposed to loading with associated decrease in bone mass in the underlying trabecular bone, thus recapitulating the effects of loading on bone remodelling observed in human OA. As discussed below, recent studies have provided insights into the cellular and molecular mechanisms by which mechanical loading regulates bone remodelling and how the phenomenon of stress shielding contributes to bone loss.

Osteophytes are an additional hallmark of OA. They represent fibrocartilaginous and skeletal outgrowths that are localized to the joint margins. Animal models of OA have shown that osteophyte formation is initiated by proliferation of periosteal cells at the joint margins. This is followed by differentiation of these cells into chondrocytes, which hypertrophy and through a process of endochondral ossification create a bony outgrowth at the joint margin [34]. The localization of osteophytes to sites of tensile and compressive loading strongly implicates a role for local biomechanical factors in the formation of osteophytes. Importantly, several lines of evidence support the concept that osteophytes represent a skeletal adaptation to local mechanical factors that in fact contribute to maintenance of joint function and stability [34–36].

As described above, BMLs are a characteristic feature of OA. BMLs were originally identified as regions of so-called bone marrow oedema detectible by increased signal intensity using fluid-sensitive magnetic resonance sequences [37,38] (Figure 5.4). BMLs characteristically are localized to regions of the subchondral bone that are associated with sites of OA pathology in the adjacent overlying cartilage, suggesting that a common mechanism related to the adverse effects of loading are involved in the pathogenesis of both the bone and cartilage changes. Histological examination of the bone tissue corresponding to the sites of BMLs reveals the presence of osteoclasts and osteoblasts associated with marrow fibrosis and fat necrosis and microfractures of the trabecular bone. These findings indicate that the MRI signals are not generated by actual 'oedema' but rather by the replacement of the haematopoietic marrow with the reactive bone remodelling and repair process associated with the local bone microdamage [39,40]. The presence of microfractures and localized bone remodelling is consistent with activation of bone repair via a mechanism of targeted bone remodelling initiated by bone damage [4,8,41]. Of interest, bone cysts, another characteristic feature of OA, frequently develop in the focal areas of bone damage and necrosis, suggesting a common mechanism by which excessive mechanical loading and resultant bone

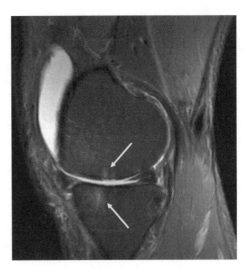

Figure 5.4 MRI using fat-suppressed T2-weighted; fast spin-echo (STIR) sequence demonstrating the presence of bone marrow lesions in the distal femur and proximal tibia in a patient with OA.
Courtesy of Hollis Potter, MD, Hospital for Special Surgery, New York, NY.

damage lead to the development of BMLs and bone cysts [42,43]. Importantly, the presence of BMLs correlate with pain and also are predictive of OA disease progression [38,44–49].

Mechanisms of deregulated bone remodelling in osteoarthritis

Insights into the mechanisms that contribute to the bone pathology in OA have come from the recognition of the key role of osteocytes in regulating bone remodelling [7,50]. As described previously, osteocytes are distributed throughout the mineralized bone matrix where they are ideally positioned to sense local biomechanical and biological signals to regulate bone remodelling and adaptation. They mediate their effects via both cell–cell contact with osteoclasts and osteoblasts but also via paracrine signalling through the release of soluble mediators, including prostanoids, nitric oxide, and nucleotides, as well as the release of cytokines and growth factors, including insulin like growth factor 1 (IGF1), vascular endothelial growth factor (VEGF), interleukin 6 (IL6), and transforming growth factor beta (TGFβ) [51–56].

Recent studies have helped to further define the essential role of osteocytes in regulating the effects of mechanical factors on bone remodelling [9,10,57,58,59]. In initial studies, Robling and co-workers [57–59] showed that osteocytes are a major source of dickkopf-related protein 1 (DKK1) and sclerostin (a product of the *SOST* gene), two inhibitors of the WNT/beta-catenin signalling pathway that plays a key role in regulating osteoblast differentiation and activity. They demonstrated that mechanical loading decreased the expression of sclerostin and DKK1 in osteocytes, resulting in up-regulation of WNT/beta-catenin signalling and enhanced bone formation. In contrast, they showed that unloading resulted in increased expression of sclerostin and DKK1 resulting in reduced bone formation.

More recent studies by Xiong and Nakashima have demonstrated an additional mechanism by which osteocytes regulate bone remodelling [9,10]. They showed that osteocytes produce two molecules that are the key regulators of osteoclast differentiation and activity, receptor activator of nuclear factor kappa B ligand (RANKL), which induces osteoclast differentiation and activity and osteoprotegerin (OPG) that inhibits RANKL-induced osteo-clastogenesis. The studies demonstrated that mice lacking RANKL in osteocytes were resistant to bone loss induced by mechanical unloading confirming the results of previous studies by Tatsumi et al. [60].

Direct evidence supporting a role of the WNT/beta-catenin pathway and its inhibitors in the development of OA joint pathology has been provided by several recent studies [61–64]. For example, Chan et al. [62] studied osteochondral samples from human OA joint tissue and osteochondral sections from sheep and mice with surgically induced OA and found that osteocyte sclerostin was decreased in regions of subchondral bone with increased bone formation. These sites conformed to regions of increased mechanical loading. Appel et al. observed similar decreases in sclerostin expression in regions of subchondral bone sclerosis in osteochondral samples from patients with OA [61]. Chan et al. [62] also noted increased sclerostin in chondrocytes in regions of focal cartilage damage and chondrocyte clusters. They also showed that sclerostin inhibited WNT/beta-catenin signalling and blocked IL1-induced increases in metalloproteinase and aggrecanase production in chondrocytes, implicating a role for sclerostin in the cartilage pathology associated with OA.

In addition to sclerostin and the RANKL/OPG system, other factors have been implicated in the pathogenesis of bone pathology in OA. Zhen et al. [65] demonstrated that TGFβ levels were elevated in subchondral bone from patients with OA and that overexpression of TGFβ in osteoblasts in transgenic mice resulted in induction of OA bone and cartilage pathology. In contrast, inhibition of TGFβ activity in the subchondral bone attenuated the development of OA in a murine model. In addition to TGFβ, other soluble mediators have been shown to regulate bone remodelling in response to mechanical loading. For example, Galea et al. showed that prostaglandin E2 (PGE2) is induced in osteocytes in response to mechanical loading, and signalling through its EP4 receptor results in rapid suppression of sclerostin [66].

As described above, in addition to alterations in the architecture and properties of subchondral bone in OA, there also are striking changes in the zone of calcified cartilage that separates the subchondral bone from the overlying articular cartilage. In a series of studies, Walsh and co-workers [25–27,67–70] examined sites of vascular invasion into the calcified cartilage in tissue retrieved from patients undergoing total joint replacement for end-stage OA. They found that the bone marrow adjacent to sites of vascular invasion was replaced by a fibrovascular stroma with cells expressing VEGF, platelet-derived growth factor, and hepatocyte growth factor that likely were responsible for the angiogenic activity. In addition, they detected VEGF expression in chondrocytes with morphological features of hypertrophic chondrocytes in the deep layers of the articular cartilage in regions associated with the new vessel formation recapitulating the functional role of these cells in the physiologic growth plate. They also noted the presence of sensory nerve fibres expressing nerve growth factor in the vascular channels and speculated that the sensory fibres could be a potential source of symptomatic pain.

Role of bone and cartilage in osteoarthritis pathogenesis

Multiple risk factors contribute to the pathogenesis of OA, including the effects of ageing, sex, genetic factors, joint injury, metabolic influences, synovial inflammation, and biomechanical factors including joint loading, alignment, and shape [16]. Importantly, OA should be considered a 'whole-joint disease' and not just a disease of cartilage or bone since all of the joint tissues are affected. Nevertheless, there remains controversy regarding the initial structural and composition changes in OA and whether these alterations occur first in the cartilage or the bone and the causal relationship between the pathology in each of these tissues. In considering this issue, it is important to recognize that the subchondral bone and articular cartilage form a functional biocomposite and under physiological conditions the individual components of this structural entity interact cooperatively and synergistically with each other to transfer and distribute load during weight bearing and locomotion. Pathological processes such as joint injury may initially target the bone or cartilage or in certain genetic disorders the pathological process may primarily affect either the bone or the cartilage. However, because of their intimate structural and functional relationship, any process that affects the bone or cartilage will inevitably affect the physiological relationship between these two tissues and affect the other tissue. A relevant question with respect to treatment of OA is whether independently targeting either the bone or cartilage to restore a physiological state can alter the natural history of OA. This section will focus primarily on the role of biomechanical factors in OA pathogenesis to address the question of the role of cartilage or bone in initiating the OA process.

The early studies of Radin and Rose focused attention on the skeletal changes as the principal effector of the OA process [71]. They hypothesized that the initial event in OA was an increase in the thickness and volume of the subchondral bone resulting in increased subchondral bone stiffness. They speculated that this would result in increased load transfer to the chondrocytes in the overlying cartilage matrix deregulating chondrocyte function and producing cartilage matrix loss. This theory can be challenged by the studies of Day et al, as well as others, that indicate that despite the volumetric increase in subchondral cortical bone in OA, the modulus is decreased and that the bone is less stiff [20,23,41,72]. It is likely that the material properties of the subchondral bone in fact are not fixed during the evolution of OA and that at various stages the modulus may transition to a different state. This is also accompanied by a change in the contour (identified as 'attrition') of the subchondral bone, which may have a more significant adverse effect on the overlying articular cartilage [17–19]. As discussed above, in our own studies using an *in vivo* tibial loading model, we observed synchronous alterations in the articular cartilage and bone using histopathological analysis and radiological imaging, indicating that both tissues were responding to the load transfer [33]. It is most likely that in an adverse loading environment that both tissues respond with an adaptive alteration in their structural and functional properties. The initial detection of alterations in the bone tissue in human studies may reflect the more rapid capacity of bone cells to modulate their function and alter their extracellular matrix compared to chondrocytes [73–77]. An additional factor may be the sensitivity of the analytic techniques to assess the composition and structural properties of bone and cartilage.

Therapeutic approaches to modulate bone pathology

The extensive alterations in periarticular bone that characterize the OA process have identified bone remodelling as an attractive target for therapeutic intervention. Principal attention has focused on targeting the osteoclast and osteoclast-mediated resorption since this would be expected to slow the rate of bone remodelling and potentially avert the pathological alterations in bone structure and thereby indirectly reduce the adverse effects of these bone changes on cartilage homeostasis. Multiple studies in animal models of OA have confirmed the efficacy of bisphosphonates in attenuating the periarticular bone changes and providing a chondroprotective effect [78–86]. Based on the favourable effects of bisphosphonate therapy in animal models of OA, phase II and III studies with oral risedronate were initiated in human subjects with OA. Although results from the initial phase II studies indicated a potential beneficial effect, the subsequent phase III trial did not demonstrate clinical efficacy [14,87–89]. Analysis of biochemical markers of bone and cartilage degradation were reduced by the treatments, but the X-rays failed to show attenuation of structural cartilage loss as assessed by joint space narrowing. Of interest, in a secondary analysis using fractal signature analysis, the treatment did attenuate subchondral trabecular bone loss in a subset of patients with more rapid cartilage loss demonstrating that the bisphosphonate could modify the periarticular bone changes [14].

Epidemiological studies in patients with OA suggest that bisphosphonates may affect the natural history of BMLs [90,91]. Support for this concept is provided by a recent proof-of-concept study in which the authors investigated the effects of zoledronic acid on the natural history of BMLs detected by MRI and associated pain and function [92]. They showed that pain scores and the size of BMLs were reduced in patients receiving zoledronic acid compared to a matched control population. Based on these observations, as well as the results from animal models, there remains interest in pursuing further evaluation of the benefit of bisphosphonates for OA therapy but challenges remain in study design and the need for more sensitive and specific methods such as MRI for assessing cartilage changes.

Calcitonin is an additional antiresorptive therapy that has been evaluated for the treatment of OA. Several studies in animal models have demonstrated a beneficial effect of calcitonin on periarticular bone remodelling and chondroprotection. The chondroprotective effect has been in part attributed to a direct effect of calcitonin on chondrocyte function [93–98]. In our own studies, we evaluated the effects of an intra-articular injection of a hyaluronic acid calcitonin conjugate in a rabbit OA model and demonstrated a chondroprotective effect [99]. Preliminary studies exploring a biologically active oral formulation of calcitonin for the treatment of human subjects with OA have reported beneficial effects on joint pain and biochemical markers of bone and cartilage degradation [100–102]. Further studies are needed to establish the potential efficacy of calcitonin in human subjects with OA.

Strontium ranelate is an additional agent that has been evaluated for the treatment of OA. It was originally developed for the treatment of osteoporosis based on its ability to favourably modulate the relationship between bone resorption and formation. Although there remains uncertainty regarding its mechanism of action, there is evidence that it exerts its effects via modulation of the RANKL/OPG ratio favouring a reduction in bone resorption [103]. A recent randomized clinical trial in patients with radiographic and clinical evidence of knee OA demonstrated that treatment with strontium ranelate attenuated radiographic progression compared to a placebo-treated control population [104]. *In vitro* studies suggest that strontium ranelate also has a beneficial effect on chondrocyte-mediated cartilage remodelling [105]. These *in vitro* observations are supported by studies in a canine anterior cruciate ligament injury model, which showed a reduction in cartilage damage in animals treated with strontium ranelate [106].

Given the evidence that antiresorptive therapies targeting osteoclast-mediated bone resorption exhibit beneficial effects in animal models of OA and also show promising results in clinical trials in human subjects with OA, there is interest in exploring the potential beneficial effects of additional antiresorptive therapies that have been developed for the treatment of osteoporosis. These include agents that inhibit cathepsin K activity or block the pro-osteoclastogenic effects of RANKL.

Conclusion

During the evolution of the OA process, the periarticular bone undergoes marked changes in its composition, structure, and functional properties. These changes are mediated by the cells that remodel and adapt the skeleton under physiological conditions. Ageing, sex, and metabolic factors increase the risk for the development of OA, but in general the structural alterations in the periarticular bone reflect the adverse effects of altered biomechanical forces on the cells that remodel the periarticular bone. Studies in animal models of OA provide evidence that therapeutically targeting the bone remodelling machinery can attenuate the progression of OA bone pathology and provide a 'chondroprotective effect' by reducing cartilage breakdown and loss. These findings in animal studies, as well as the observed beneficial effects of bisphosphonate therapy on BMLs in human subjects [92], provide support for the concept that targeting bone remodelling represents a rational approach for preventative OA therapy. The availability of additional bone active agents such as cathepsin K or RANKL inhibitors that regulate bone remodelling via differential mechanisms represent new opportunities that warrant further exploration. The heterogeneity of the human OA population and the lack of widely accepted sensitive and specific tools for assessing bone pathology and disease progression present challenges to extending the favourable results of the animal studies to human subjects with OA. Advances in the development and implementation of these diagnostic tools will enable more rigorous evaluation of therapies that target bone and cartilage pathology in OA.

References

1. Goldring SR, Goldring MB. Biology of the normal joint. In Firestein GS, Budd RC, Gabriel SE, McInnes IB, O'Dell JR (eds) *Kelly's Textbook of Rheumatology*, 9th ed. Philadelphia, PA: Saunders; 2013:1–19.
2. Goldring MB, Goldring SR. Osteoarthritis. *J Cell Physiol* 2007; 213(3):626–34.
3. Goldring SR. Role of bone in osteoarthritis pathogenesis. *Med Clin North Am* 2009; 93(1):25–35, xv.
4. Burr DB. Anatomy and physiology of the mineralized tissues: role in the pathogenesis of osteoarthrosis. *Osteoarthritis Cartilage* 2004; 12(Suppl A):S20–30.
5. Eriksen EF. Cellular mechanisms of bone remodeling. *Rev Endocr Metab Disord* 2010; 11(4):219–27.
6. Kennedy OD, Schaffler MB. The roles of osteocyte signaling in bone. *J Am Acad Orthop Surg* 2012; 20(10):670–1.
7. Schaffler MB, Kennedy OD. Osteocyte signaling in bone. *Curr Osteoporos Rep* 2012; 10(2):118–25.

8. Martin RB. Targeted bone remodeling involves BMU steering as well as activation. *Bone* 2007; 40(6):1574–80.
9. Nakashima T, Hayashi M, Fukunaga T, et al. Evidence for osteocyte regulation of bone homeostasis through RANKL expression. *Nat Med* 2011; 17(10):1231–4.
10. Xiong J, Onal M, Jilka RL, et al. Matrix-embedded cells control osteoclast formation. *Nat Med* 2011; 17(10):1235–41.
11. Dallas SL, Prideaux M, Bonewald LF. The osteocyte: an endocrine cell … and more. *Endocr Rev* 2013; 34(5):658–90.
12. Frost HM. Bone's mechanostat: a 2003 update. *Anat Rec A Discov Mol Cell Evol Biol* 2003; 275(2):1081–101.
13. Buckland-Wright C. Subchondral bone changes in hand and knee osteoarthritis detected by radiography. *Osteoarthritis Cartilage* 2004; 12(Suppl A):S10–9.
14. Buckland-Wright JC, Messent EA, Bingham CO, 3rd, Ward RJ, Tonkin C. A 2 yr longitudinal radiographic study examining the effect of a bisphosphonate (risedronate) upon subchondral bone loss in osteoarthritic knee patients. *Rheumatology (Oxford)* 2007; 46(2):257–64.
15. Goldring MB, Goldring SR. Articular cartilage and subchondral bone in the pathogenesis of osteoarthritis. *Ann N Y Acad Sci* 2010; 1192:230–7.
16. Loeser RF, Goldring SR, Scanzello CR, Goldring MB. Osteoarthritis: a disease of the joint as an organ. *Arthritis Rheum* 2012; 64(6):1697–707.
17. Reichenbach S, Guermazi A, Niu J, et al. Prevalence of bone attrition on knee radiographs and MRI in a community-based cohort. *Osteoarthritis Cartilage* 2008; 16(9):1005–10.
18. Neogi T, Felson D, Niu J, et al. Cartilage loss occurs in the same subregions as subchondral bone attrition: a within-knee subregion-matched approach from the Multicenter Osteoarthritis Study. *Arthritis Rheum* 2009; 61(11):1539–44.
19. Neogi T, Nevitt M, Niu J, et al. Subchondral bone attrition may be a reflection of compartment-specific mechanical load: the MOST Study. *Ann Rheum Dis* 2010; 69(5):841–4.
20. Day JS, Ding M, van der Linden JC, et al. A decreased subchondral trabecular bone tissue elastic modulus is associated with pre-arthritic cartilage damage. *J Orthop Res* 2001; 19(5):914–8.
21. Faibish D, Ott SM, Boskey AL. Mineral changes in osteoporosis: a review. *Clin Orthop Relat Res* 2006; 443:28–38.
22. Meunier PJ, Boivin G. Bone mineral density reflects bone mass but also the degree of mineralization of bone: therapeutic implications. *Bone* 1997; 21(5):373–7.
23. Day JS, Van Der Linden JC, Bank RA, et al. Adaptation of subchondral bone in osteoarthritis. *Biorheology* 2004; 41(3–4):359–68.
24. Bullough PG. The role of joint architecture in the etiology of arthritis. *Osteoarthritis Cartilage* 2004; 12(Suppl A):S2–9.
25. Ashraf S, Walsh DA. Angiogenesis in osteoarthritis. *Curr Opin Rheumatol* 2008; 20(5):573–80.
26. Suri S, Gill SE, Massena de Camin S, et al. Neurovascular invasion at the osteochondral junction and in osteophytes in osteoarthritis. *Ann Rheumat Dis* 2007; 66(11):1423–8.
27. Suri S, Walsh DA. Osteochondral alterations in osteoarthritis. *Bone* 2012; 51(2):204–11.
28. Walsh DA, McWilliams DF, Turley MJ, et al. Angiogenesis and nerve growth factor at the osteochondral junction in rheumatoid arthritis and osteoarthritis. *Rheumatology (Oxford)* 2010; 49(10):1852–61.
29. Messent EA, Ward RJ, Tonkin CJ, Buckland-Wright C. Differences in trabecular structure between knees with and without osteoarthritis quantified by macro and standard radiography, respectively. *Osteoarthritis Cartilage* 2006; 14(12):1302–5.
30. Chiba K, Ito M, Osaki M, Uetani M, Shindo H. In vivo structural analysis of subchondral trabecular bone in osteoarthritis of the hip using multi-detector row CT. *Osteoarthritis Cartilage* 2011; 19(2):180–5.
31. Carballido-Gamio J, Joseph GB, Lynch JA, Link TM, Majumdar S. Longitudinal analysis of MRI T2 knee cartilage laminar organization in a subset of patients from the osteoarthritis initiative: a texture approach. *Magn Reson Med* 2011; 65(4):1184–94.
32. Kraus VB, Feng S, Wang S, et al. Subchondral bone trabecular integrity predicts and changes concurrently with radiographic and magnetic resonance imaging-determined knee osteoarthritis progression. *Arthritis Rheum* 2013; 65(7):1812–21.
33. Ko FC, Dragomir C, Plumb DA, et al. In vivo cyclic compression causes cartilage degeneration and subchondral bone changes in mouse tibiae. *Arthritis Rheum* 2013; 65(6):1569–78.
34. van der Kraan PM, van den Berg WB. Osteophytes: relevance and biology. *Osteoarthritis Cartilage* 2007; 15(3):237–44.
35. Pottenger LA, Phillips FM, Draganich LF. The effect of marginal osteophytes on reduction of varus-valgus instability in osteoarthritic knees. *Arthritis Rheum* 1990; 33(6):853–8.
36. Messent EA, Ward RJ, Tonkin CJ, Buckland-Wright C. Osteophytes, juxta-articular radiolucencies and cancellous bone changes in the proximal tibia of patients with knee osteoarthritis. *Osteoarthritis Cartilage* 2007; 15(2):179–86.
37. Wilson AJ, Murphy WA, Hardy DC, Totty WG. Transient osteoporosis: transient bone marrow edema? *Radiology* 1988; 167(3):757–60.
38. Xu L, Hayashi D, Roemer FW, Felson DT, Guermazi A. Magnetic resonance imaging of subchondral bone marrow lesions in association with osteoarthritis. *Semin Arthritis Rheum* 2012; 42(2):105–18.
39. Leydet-Quilici H, Le Corroller T, Bouvier C, et al. Advanced hip osteoarthritis: magnetic resonance imaging aspects and histopathology correlations. *Osteoarthritis Cartilage* 2010; 18(11):1429–35.
40. Taljanovic MS, Graham AR, Benjamin JB, et al. Bone marrow edema pattern in advanced hip osteoarthritis: quantitative assessment with magnetic resonance imaging and correlation with clinical examination, radiographic findings, and histopathology. *Skeletal Radiol* 2008; 37(5):423–31.
41. Burr DB, Schaffler MB. The involvement of subchondral mineralized tissues in osteoarthrosis: quantitative microscopic evidence. *Microsc Res Tech* 1997; 37(4):343–57.
42. Carrino JA, Blum J, Parellada JA, Schweitzer ME, Morrison WB. MRI of bone marrow edema-like signal in the pathogenesis of subchondral cysts. *Osteoarthritis Cartilage* 2006; 14(10):1081–5.
43. Bancroft LW, Peterson JJ, Kransdorf MJ. Cysts, geodes, and erosions. *Radiol Clin N Am* 2004; 42(1):73–87.
44. Crema MD, Roemer FW, Zhu Y, et al. Subchondral cystlike lesions develop longitudinally in areas of bone marrow edema-like lesions in patients with or at risk for knee osteoarthritis: detection with MR imaging—the MOST study. *Radiology* 2010; 256(3):855–62.
45. Felson DT, McLaughlin S, Goggins J, et al. Bone marrow edema and its relation to progression of knee osteoarthritis. *Ann Internal Med* 2003; 139(5 Pt 1):330–6.
46. Hernandez-Molina G, Neogi T, Hunter DJ, et al. The association of bone attrition with knee pain and other MRI features of osteoarthritis. *Ann Rheumat Dis* 2008; 67(1):43–7.
47. Roemer FW, Frobell R, Hunter DJ, et al. MRI-detected subchondral bone marrow signal alterations of the knee joint: terminology, imaging appearance, relevance and radiological differential diagnosis. *Osteoarthritis Cartilage* 2009; 17(9):1115–31.
48. Roemer FW, Hunter DJ, Guermazi A. MRI-based semiquantitative assessment of subchondral bone marrow lesions in osteoarthritis research. *Osteoarthritis Cartilage* 2009; 17(3):414–5.
49. Hunter DJ, Zhang Y, Niu J, et al. Increase in bone marrow lesions associated with cartilage loss: a longitudinal magnetic resonance imaging study of knee osteoarthritis. *Arthritis Rheum* 2006; 54(5):1529–35.
50. Bonewald LF. The amazing osteocyte. *J Bone Miner Res* 2011; 26(2):229–38.
51. Caballero-Alias AM, Loveridge N, Pitsillides A, et al. Osteocytic expression of constitutive NO synthase isoforms in the femoral neck cortex: a case-control study of intracapsular hip fracture. *J Bone Miner Res* 2005; 20(2):268–73.
52. Cheng B, Kato Y, Zhao S, et al. PGE$_2$ is essential for gap junction-mediated intercellular communication between osteocyte-like MLO-Y4 cells in response to mechanical strain. *Endocrinology* 2001; 142(8):3464–73.

53. Schaffler MB, Cheung WY, Majeska R, Kennedy O. Osteocytes: master orchestrators of bone. *Calcif Tissue Int* 2014; 94(1):5–24.

54. Kennedy OD, Laudier DM, Majeska RJ, Sun HB, Schaffler MB. Osteocyte apoptosis is required for production of osteoclastogenic signals following bone fatigue in vivo. *Bone* 2014; 64:132–7.

55. Lau KH, Baylink DJ, Zhou XD, et al. Osteocyte-derived insulin-like growth factor I is essential for determining bone mechanosensitivity. *Am J Physiol Endocrinol Metab* 2013; 305(2):E271–81.

56. Kennedy OD, Herman BC, Laudier DM, et al. Activation of resorption in fatigue-loaded bone involves both apoptosis and active pro-osteoclastogenic signaling by distinct osteocyte populations. *Bone* 2012; 50(5):1115–22.

57. Robling AG, Bellido T, Turner CH. Mechanical stimulation in vivo reduces osteocyte expression of sclerostin. *J Musculoskelet Neuronal Interact* 2006; 6(4):354.

58. Robling AG, Niziolek PJ, Baldridge LA, et al. Mechanical stimulation of bone in vivo reduces osteocyte expression of Sost/sclerostin. *J Biol Chem* 2008; 283(9):5866–75.

59. Tu X, Rhee Y, Condon KW, et al. Sost downregulation and local Wnt signaling are required for the osteogenic response to mechanical loading. *Bone* 2012; 50(1):209–17.

60. Tatsumi S, Ishii K, Amizuka N, et al. Targeted ablation of osteocytes induces osteoporosis with defective mechanotransduction. *Cell Metab* 2007; 5(6):464–75.

61. Appel H, Ruiz-Heiland G, Listing J, et al. Altered skeletal expression of sclerostin and its link to radiographic progression in ankylosing spondylitis. *Arthritis Rheum* 2009; 60(11):3257–62.

62. Chan BY, Fuller ES, Russell AK, et al. Increased chondrocyte sclerostin may protect against cartilage degradation in osteoarthritis. *Osteoarthritis Cartilage* 2011; 19(7):874–85.

63. Funck-Brentano T, Bouaziz W, Marty C, et al. Dkk1-mediated inhibition of Wnt signaling in bone ameliorates osteoarthritis. *Arthritis Rheumatol* 2014; 66(11):3028–39.

64. Roudier M, Li X, Niu QT, et al. Sclerostin is expressed in articular cartilage but loss or inhibition does not affect cartilage remodeling during aging or following mechanical injury. *Arthritis Rheum* 2013; 65(3):721–31.

65. Zhen G, Wen C, Jia X, et al. Inhibition of TGF-beta signaling in mesenchymal stem cells of subchondral bone attenuates osteoarthritis. *Nat Med* 2013; 19(6):704–12.

66. Galea GL, Sunters A, Meakin LB, et al. Sost down-regulation by mechanical strain in human osteoblastic cells involves PGE2 signaling via EP4. *FEBS Lett* 2011; 585(15):2450–4.

67. Ashraf S, Mapp PI, Walsh DA. Contributions of angiogenesis to inflammation, joint damage, and pain in a rat model of osteoarthritis. *Arthritis Rheum* 2011; 63(9):2700–10.

68. Ashraf S, Wibberley H, Mapp PI, et al. Increased vascular penetration and nerve growth in the meniscus: a potential source of pain in osteoarthritis. *Ann Rheumat Dis* 2011; 70(3):523–9.

69. Walsh NC, Gravallese EM. Bone loss in inflammatory arthritis: mechanisms and treatment strategies. *Curr Opin Rheumatol* 2004; 16(4):419–27.

70. Walsh NC, Reinwald S, Manning CA, et al. Osteoblast function is compromised at sites of focal bone erosion in inflammatory arthritis. *J Bone Miner Res* 2009; 24(9):1572–85.

71. Radin EL, Rose RM. Role of subchondral bone in the initiation and progression of cartilage damage. *Clin Orthop Relat Res* 1986(213):34–40.

72. Burr DB, Gallant MA. Bone remodelling in osteoarthritis. *Nat Rev Rheumatol* 2012; 8(11):665–73.

73. Goldring MB, Berenbaum F. The regulation of chondrocyte function by proinflammatory mediators: prostaglandins and nitric oxide. *Clin Orthop* 2004; 427(Suppl):S37–46.

74. Goldring SR, Goldring MB. The role of cytokines in cartilage matrix degeneration in osteoarthritis. *Clin Orthop* 2004; 427(Suppl):S27–36.

75. Maroudas A, Bayliss MT, Uchitel-Kaushansky N, Schneiderman R, Gilav E. Aggrecan turnover in human articular cartilage: use of aspartic acid racemization as a marker of molecular age. *Arch Biochem Biophys* 1998; 350(1):61–71.

76. Plaas A, Osborn B, Yoshihara Y, et al. Aggrecanolysis in human osteoarthritis: confocal localization and biochemical characterization of ADAMTS5-hyaluronan complexes in articular cartilages. *Osteoarthritis Cartilage* 2007; 15(7):719–34.

77. Sandell LJ, Aigner T. Articular cartilage and changes in arthritis. An introduction: cell biology of osteoarthritis. *Arthritis Res* 2001; 3(2):107–13.

78. Hayami T, Pickarski M, Wesolowski GA, et al. The role of subchondral bone remodeling in osteoarthritis: reduction of cartilage degeneration and prevention of osteophyte formation by alendronate in the rat anterior cruciate ligament transection model. *Arthritis Rheum* 2004; 50(4):1193–206.

79. Hayami T, Pickarski M, Zhuo Y, et al. Characterization of articular cartilage and subchondral bone changes in the rat anterior cruciate ligament transection and meniscectomized models of osteoarthritis. *Bone* 2006; 38(2):234–43.

80. Karsdal MA, Bay-Jensen AC, Lories RJ, et al. The coupling of bone and cartilage turnover in osteoarthritis: opportunities for bone antiresorptives and anabolics as potential treatments? *Ann Rheumat Dis* 2014; 73(2):336–48.

81. Moreau M, Rialland P, Pelletier JP, et al. Tiludronate treatment improves structural changes and symptoms of osteoarthritis in the canine anterior cruciate ligament model. *Arthritis Res Ther* 2011; 13(3):R98.

82. Pelletier JP, Troncy E, Bertaim T, et al. Treatment with tiludronic acid helps reduce the development of experimental osteoarthritis lesions in dogs with anterior cruciate ligament transection followed by reconstructive surgery: a 1-year study with quantitative magnetic resonance imaging. *J Rheumatol* 2011; 38(1):118–28.

83. Shirai T, Kobayashi M, Nishitani K, et al. Chondroprotective effect of alendronate in a rabbit model of osteoarthritis. *J Orthop Res* 2011; 29(10):1572–7.

84. Strassle BW, Mark L, Leventhal L, et al. Inhibition of osteoclasts prevents cartilage loss and pain in a rat model of degenerative joint disease. *Osteoarthritis Cartilage* 2010; 18(10):1319–28.

85. Zhu S, Chen K, Lan Y, et al. Alendronate protects against articular cartilage erosion by inhibiting subchondral bone loss in ovariectomized rats. *Bone* 2013; 53(2):340–9.

86. Lampropoulou-Adamidou K, Dontas I, Stathopoulos IP, et al. Chondroprotective effect of high-dose zoledronic acid: an experimental study in a rabbit model of osteoarthritis. *J Orthop Res* 2014; 32(12):1646–51.

87. Spector TD, Conaghan PG, Buckland-Wright JC, et al. Effect of risedronate on joint structure and symptoms of knee osteoarthritis: results of the BRISK randomized, controlled trial [ISRCTN01928173]. *Arthritis Res Ther* 2005; 7(3):R625–33.

88. Garnero P, Aronstein WS, Cohen SB, et al. Relationships between biochemical markers of bone and cartilage degradation with radiological progression in patients with knee osteoarthritis receiving risedronate: the Knee Osteoarthritis Structural Arthritis randomized clinical trial. *Osteoarthritis Cartilage* 2008; 16(6):660–6.

89. Bingham CO, 3rd, Buckland-Wright JC, Garnero P, et al. Risedronate decreases biochemical markers of cartilage degradation but does not decrease symptoms or slow radiographic progression in patients with medial compartment osteoarthritis of the knee: results of the two-year multinational knee osteoarthritis structural arthritis study. *Arthritis Rheum* 2006; 54(11):3494–507.

90. Carbone LD, Nevitt MC, Wildy K, et al. The relationship of antiresorptive drug use to structural findings and symptoms of knee osteoarthritis. *Arthritis Rheum* 2004; 50(11):3516–25.

91. Raynauld JP, Martel-Pelletier J, Berthiaume MJ, et al. Correlation between bone lesion changes and cartilage volume loss in patients with osteoarthritis of the knee as assessed by quantitative magnetic resonance imaging over a 24-month period. *Ann Rheumat Dis* 2008; 67(5):683–8.

92. Laslett LL, Dore DA, Quinn SJ, et al. Zoledronic acid reduces knee pain and bone marrow lesions over 1 year: a randomised controlled trial. *Ann Rheumat Dis* 2012; 71(8):1322–8.

93. Behets C, Williams JM, Chappard D, Devogelaer JP, Manicourt DH. Effects of calcitonin on subchondral trabecular bone changes and on osteoarthritic cartilage lesions after acute anterior cruciate ligament deficiency. *J Bone Miner Res* 2004; 19(11):1821–6.

94. Manicourt DH, Altman RD, Williams JM, et al. Treatment with calcitonin suppresses the responses of bone, cartilage, and synovium in the early stages of canine experimental osteoarthritis and significantly reduces the severity of the cartilage lesions. *Arthritis Rheum* 1999; 42(6):1159–67.

95. Sondergaard BC, Catala-Lehnen P, Huebner AK, et al. Mice overexpressing salmon calcitonin have strongly attenuated osteoarthritic histopathological changes after destabilization of the medial meniscus. *Osteoarthritis Cartilage* 2012; 20(2):136–43.

96. Sondergaard BC, Madsen SH, Segovia-Silvestre T, et al. Investigation of the direct effects of salmon calcitonin on human osteoarthritic chondrocytes. *BMC Musculoskelet Disord* 2010; 11:62.

97. Karsdal MA, Sondergaard BC, Arnold M, Christiansen C. Calcitonin affects both bone and cartilage: a dual action treatment for osteoarthritis? *Ann N Y Acad Sci* 2007; 1117:181–95.

98. Sondergaard BC, Oestergaard S, Christiansen C, Tanko LB, Karsdal MA. The effect of oral calcitonin on cartilage turnover and surface erosion in an ovariectomized rat model. *Arthritis Rheum* 2007; 56(8):2674–8.

99. Mero A, Campisi M, Favero M, et al. A hyaluronic acid-salmon calcitonin conjugate for the local treatment of osteoarthritis: chondro-protective effect in a rabbit model of early OA. *J Control Release* 2014; 187:30–8.

100. Manicourt DH, Azria M, Mindeholm L, Thonar EJ, Devogelaer JP. Oral salmon calcitonin reduces Lequesne's algofunctional index scores and decreases urinary and serum levels of biomarkers of joint metabolism in knee osteoarthritis. *Arthritis Rheum* 2006; 54(10):3205–11.

101. Manicourt DH, Devogelaer JP, Azria M, Silverman S. Rationale for the potential use of calcitonin in osteoarthritis. *J Musculoskelet Neuronal Interact* 2005; 5(3):285–93.

102. Karsdal MA, Byrjalsen I, Alexandersen P, et al. Treatment of symptomatic knee osteoarthritis with oral salmon calcitonin: results from two phase 3 trials. *Osteoarthritis Cartilage* 2015; 23(4):532–43.

103. Atkins GJ, Welldon KJ, Halbout P, Findlay DM. Strontium ranelate treatment of human primary osteoblasts promotes an osteocyte-like phenotype while eliciting an osteoprotegerin response. *Osteoporos Int* 2009; 20(4):653–64.

104. Reginster Y, Badurski J, Bellamy N, et al. Efficacy and safety of strontium ranelate in the treatment of knee osteoarthritis: results of a double-blind, randomised placebo-controlled trial. *Ann Rheum Dis* 2013; 72(2):179–86.

105. Henrotin Y, Labasse A, Zheng SX, Galais P, Tsouderos Y. Crielaard JM, Reginster,JY. Strontium ranelate increases cartilage matrix formation. *J Bone Miner Res* 2001; 16(2):299–308.

106. Pelletier JP, Kapoor M, Fahmi H, et al. Strontium ranelate reduces the progression of experimental dog osteoarthritis by inhibiting the expression of key proteases in cartilage and of IL-1beta in the synovium. *Ann Rheum Dis* 2013; 72(2):250–7.

CHAPTER 6

Synovium and capsule

Floris P. J. G. Lafeber, Nick J. Besselink, and Simon C. Mastbergen

The synovial membrane

The most common and movable type of joint is the diarthrodial joint, consisting of (at least two) articulating bones, covered by articular cartilage, and a closed joint cavity, formed by the surrounding joint capsule (Figure 6.1). The combination of these components provides support and mobility. The low-friction cartilage surfaces allow for smooth flexible motion under high weight-bearing conditions. The joint capsule consists of an outer fibrous layer and an inner more cellular layer, the synovial membrane. The latter supports smooth motion by lubricating the cartilage joint surfaces.

The outer fibrous layer, the articular capsule, is made up of dense connective tissue, and attaches to the end of each bone. It is continuous with the periosteum, and thus surrounds the entire synovial joint. The dense fibrous collagen tissue of the capsule is firmly attached to the bone with so-called Sharpey's fibres. The capsule is densely innervated and is, together with tendons and muscles, responsible for joint stability and proprioception. These in turn are,

in addition to smooth movement, responsible for optimal function of the synovial joint.

The synovial membrane consists of two distinct layers: the intimal lining and the supportive sublining layer. The intimal lining is in direct contact with the intra-articular cavity and is the source of lubricious synovial fluid. The two major lubricating components that are important in reducing friction are lubricin (also called proteoglycan 4; PRG4) and hyaluronic acid (HA) [1]. These lubricants not only have a lubricating effect but are also reported to have joint protective effects by, for example, inhibiting inflammatory activities and adherence of cells and proteins to the articular surface [2–7].

The articular cartilage, unlike the synovial membrane, is not vascularized or provided with lymphatic drainage and therefore depends on the synovium for providing all the essential nutrients. The semipermeable membrane does this by controlling molecular traffic in and out of the joint space. High-molecular-weight molecules like HA and PRG4 do not cross the membrane, whilst small molecules like cytokines and chemokines can. This leads to retention of lubrication molecules in the synovial fluid, and keeps other high-molecular-weight molecules, like plasma proteins, out [2,8–10]. In this way the synovial membrane is essential for nutrition and lubrication of cartilage (Figure 6.1).

The synovial surface is an integration of lining cells, vessels, and nerve endings [11]. The synovial lining lacks epithelial cells, tight junctions, and desmosomes and the synovial cells (synoviocytes) are not fixed on a basement membrane, but are loosely organized over three or four layers [12]. Synoviocytes are classically subdivided into two types, macrophage and fibroblast-like synoviocytes, also referred to as 'type A' and 'type B' synoviocytes, respectively.

Type A synoviocytes express markers of haematopoietic origin, most similar to the monocyte/macrophage lineage [13]. Being mainly phagocytic, these cells have lysosomes and a large Golgi complex. They are involved in removal of waste products from the synovial cavity as a result of tissue turnover. Type B synoviocytes are mesenchymal cells that display many characteristics of fibroblasts. They are involved in the production of molecules such as collagens, PGR4, and HA [14]. Note that production and intra-articular release of such molecules is not unique for the synovial membrane but that these molecules are also produced by the (superficial) cartilage chondrocytes [3].

The synovial membrane is additionally a source of mesenchymal stem cells that are potentially able to differentiate into cartilage,

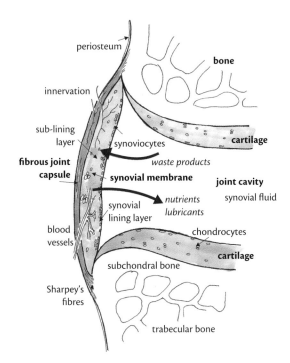

Figure 6.1 Synovial joint.

bone, and adipose tissue. Therefore, the synovium is considered to contribute to the regeneration and repair of degenerated tissue in the joint although to what extent and how, still remains elusive [15,16].

Synovial changes (synovitis) in osteoarthritis

Data on synovial changes in osteoarthritis have been obtained over the past decades from numerous *ex vivo* and *in vitro* human studies as well as *in vivo* animal disease models. It should be recognized that data from animal models in general and also data from synovial changes in animal models of osteoarthritis are not always translatable, or at least were not confirmed to be translatable, to human disease [17–19].

Most of the literature on synovitis in human osteoarthritis originates from studies of the larger joints such as the knee. This is not only simply because this joint is more accessible for obtaining synovial tissue biopsies and synovial fluid, but of course also because of the high incidence of osteoarthritis in this joint. Additionally, the involvement of structures like cruciate ligaments, menisci, and (patellar) fat pads, of relevance to joint degeneration, can easily be studied in the knee joint.

However, synovial changes may differ between joint types, as there are clear differences between synovial joints. Specifically the large fat pad might be of relevance. This is an important source of inflammation [20], and differs in the knee compared to, for example, the hip, with less surrounding adipose tissue [21]. Another example is the characteristic erosive hand osteoarthritis which is explicitly synovitis driven, not often as explicitly seen in other joints [22,23].

Even within the same joint, synovial changes are not always equally distributed and can vary in location within the affected joint, being patchy in character and confined to areas near sites of cartilage damage [24,25]. Cartilage destructive properties and angiogenesis can be strikingly different in inflamed and non-inflamed areas of synovial tissue in individual patients with osteoarthritis [26]. The synovial tissue inflammatory cell infiltrate and synovial fluid proinflammatory cytokines can differ significantly between different forms of knee osteoarthritis [27]. Correlations have been reported between the region of inflammation and the severity of cartilage damage [28], supporting this.

The location of inflammation can also determine the severity of symptoms; for example, in the knee, changes in the infrapatellar fat pad are most strongly related with changes in pain [25]. On the other hand, it has been reported that mononuclear cell infiltrates into the synovial tissue and the presence of lymphoid aggregates are not necessarily associated with clinical signs of inflammation like heat, pain, redness, and/or effusion [27,29].

These points should all be taken into account, as well as the variable character over the course of disease (early versus late, chronic versus acute, and flares), together with variable changes in synovial activity over time. As such, synovial inflammatory activity in osteoarthritis is not only variable between patients, but also between joints and within joints with different relations to tissue damage and clinical symptoms, all being variable over time. Therefore, it should be recognized that data from specific studies cannot simply be translated at all times to the role of synovitis in osteoarthritis in general.

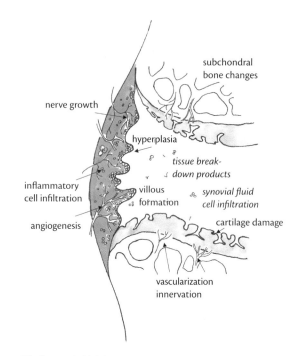

Figure 6.2 Osteoarthritic joint.

Synovial reaction

Chronic synovitis is associated with synovial changes like hyperplasia as a result of proliferation and recruitment of synovial and inflammatory cells, angiogenesis, and nerve growth [30–32] (Figure 6.2). Acute synovitis may be apparent in osteoarthritis, but increasingly subclinical and low-grade clinical, more chronic inflammation is being recognized to be a driving force in the osteoarthritic process as well [33]. Acute synovitis, or flares, not only occur in non-inflamed joints but can also be superimposed upon chronic inflammatory activity [34]. The most common finding in synovitis is hyperplasia of the synovial lining with slender villous formation and limited layers of synovial membrane cells, which is already found early in the disease [31]. Actual inflammation with clear villi and thickening of the synovial membrane, in addition to hyperplasia, characterized by infiltration of inflammatory cells and hypervascularization, is seen in more advanced disease [35].

Synovial cells

Synovitis consists of the activation and proliferation of the synovial lining cells and the infiltration of inflammatory cells into the sublining tissue, with both contributing to thickening (hyperplasia) of the synovial membrane. Synovitis is characterized by an infiltration of mononuclear cells, predominantly macrophages and T cells but also infiltration of neutrophils, dendritic cells, NK cells, and even B cells have been reported [32,36,37]. These inflammatory cells have been shown to add to angiogenesis by the production of angiogenic factors, and as such might be involved in the (early) induction of angiogenesis [29]. In combination with the production of chemokines by many of these cells [38], inflammation is enhanced in an autocrine manner (Figure 6.3).

Neutrophils have been found in acute synovitis in which removal of an irritant as a host response is suggested [5,29]. In case of acute inflammatory flares seen in osteoarthritis, these cells are suggested

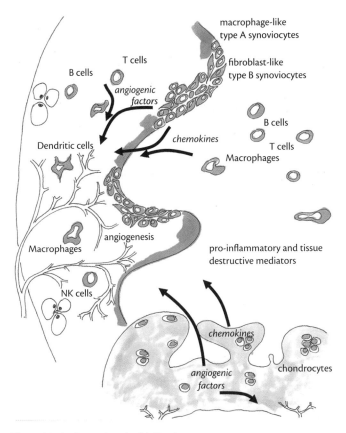

Figure 6.3 Angiogenesis and cell infiltration.

to be involved as well [39]. On the other hand, other researchers suggest that neutrophils are not found in the synovial joint [40].

Macrophages are abundantly present in (chronically) inflamed osteoarthritis synovium and exhibit an activated phenotype, substantiated by the production of inflammatory mediators (e.g. tumour necrosis factor alpha (TNFA) and interleukin 1 beta (IL1B)), angiogenic factors (e.g. vascular endothelial growth factor (VEGF) and macrophage inflammatory protein 1 alpha (MIP1A)), as well as proteases [30,41,42]. Moreover, macrophages can stimulate other cells like endothelial cells and fibroblasts to produce proinflammatory mediators, angiogenic factors, and proteases, resulting in increased synovitis and tissue destruction [43].

Dendritic cells have also been reported to be present in low numbers in osteoarthritic synovium of humans and rodents [44,45], probably playing a role in T-cell antigen presentation in addition to macrophages providing this function.

T cells are of CD4 as well as CD8 origin and express markers of immune activation such as major histocompatibility complex class II and have a Th1 polarized (proinflammatory) phenotype [46]. These T cells are also found in osteoarthritic synovial fluid, the majority of them being CD4+ T cells with a memory phenotype [32,47]. The T-cell response may potentially be directed against a common joint tissue-related antigen based on the T-cell receptor arrangement and oligoclonal expansion [23,48]. Also T cells add to neo-vascularization of the synovial tissue by producing pro-angiogenic factors [29].

NK cells in limited [27] as well as high [49] numbers with elevated receptor expression for chemokines [50] have been reported in the osteoarthritic joint, although not many research groups have

been studying these cells in this low-grade inflammatory disease. They have been reported to express a quiescent phenotype consistent with post-activation exhaustion [38], possibly related to a role in the early phase under certain conditions in the disease.

The knowledge of the role of *B cells* in osteoarthritis is still limited. In general, these cells are rarely described [23], although it has also been reported that they can be detected in half of the osteoarthritis patients tested [51]. Interestingly, if B cells are found in osteoarthritic joints, they are in an activated state [23]. Autoantibodies against breakdown products of collagen in osteoarthritis joints have been reported in the older literature, but such observations have not been reported recently [52,53].

It is important to notice that not only mononuclear cells from the synovial tissue and in the synovial fluid are involved in the inflammatory activity. The cartilage chondrocytes are also able to produce most of the factors produced by these inflammatory cells including the inflammatory cytokines, chemokines, and angiogenic factors [23] (Figure 6.3).

Angiogenesis

The synovium is highly vascularized under healthy conditions to supply the cartilage with nutrients [30]. In osteoarthritis, angiogenesis and inflammation of the synovium are closely integrated processes and affect synovitis and related clinical symptoms [30,39,54]. Angiogenesis, neo-vascularization, the formation of new blood vessels, may be most important in potentiating inflammation rather than initiating it [29].

Angiogenesis is a complex process, initiated via several pathways, in which in the end endothelial cells produce VEGF and angiopoietins, ensuring vessel stability [29,55–57]. Apart from being a potent stimulator of angiogenesis, VEGF also contributes to inflammation via plasma extravasation [58,59]. Also vascular regression is observed which does not lead to a decrease in vascular density, in fact, there is a redistribution of synovial vessel and a change towards a more immature phenotype [60]. A fully functional microvasculature is formed by the differentiation of the newly formed vessels into arterioles, capillaries, and venules. An inflammatory response is maintained by the supply of inflammatory cells through these new vessels. Angiogenesis can indirectly promote itself by increasing inflammatory cell infiltration, and increasing angiogenic factor release [29,61]. Also hypoxia, acting via hypoxia-inducible factor 1 alpha (HIF1A) can be involved in angiogenesis, HIF1A is to be co-localized with microvascularity in osteoarthritic synovium.

Synovial angiogenesis is found in all stages of osteoarthritis [30] but could contribute to the transition from acute to chronic synovitis by potentiating inflammatory pathways [29,61]. Synovial tissue from early osteoarthritis patients contains higher levels of angiogenic factors, suggesting a more active angiogenesis in early osteoarthritic synovium [34]. Importantly, angiogenic activity in osteoarthritis is also regulated through changes in the articular cartilage by promoting the expression and release of angiogenic factors from chondrocytes [62]. Release of these factors may also lead to ingrowth of blood vessels from the bone into cartilage at the bone–cartilage interface [63]. Angiogenesis in the synovium is associated with histological synovitis, but not clearly with cartilage changes, whereas vascular density at the osteochondral junction is more clearly associated with changes in the cartilage but not with histological synovitis [64]. In more severe osteoarthritis, vascular breaching of the tidemark to the cartilage is observed [61]. In this way, inflammation-related mediators from the bone (and vice versa) can also enter and influence cartilage damage (Figure 6.3).

Intracapsular fat pads

Fat pads are intracapsular, extrasynovial-located adipose tissues within joints, found most prominently in the knee but also in other joints. Adipose tissue in general secretes different adipokines, cytokines, and other inflammatory mediators contributing to inflammation [65]. In addition to adipocytes, the intra-articular fat pads in osteoarthritic joints contain a connective tissue matrix, nerve fibres, vascular cells, and immune cells [66] (Figure 6.4). The fat pads contain, in between the large adipocytes, macrophages, T cells, B cells, and mast cells. In the stromal vascular cell fraction of the osteoarthritic intra-articular adipose tissue, the T cells show a Th1 proinflammatory phenotype, whereas macrophages are of an M1 (proinflammatory) as well as M2 (anti-inflammatory) phenotype. Mast cells are more abundantly present in intra-articular adipose tissue than in subcutaneous fat, which might be related to angiogenesis, where vascularization of intra-articular adipose tissue is reported to be higher than that of subcutaneous tissue [67]. In addition to multiple adipokines produced by the adipocytes, the intra-articular adipocytes and the embedded inflammatory cells produce multiple proinflammatory cytokines including TNFA and IL6, the latter in higher levels than in subcutaneous fat [65]. As such, the intra-articular adipose tissue is considered to play an important role in joint inflammation as well.

The adipose tissue outside the joint is suggested to be systemically related to osteoarthritis. Specifically in cases of obesity, it produces and secretes large amounts of inflammatory mediators such as proinflammatory cytokines and adipokines, of which the

production is changed in the presence of osteoarthritis [20,68,69]. As such the relation between obesity and osteoarthritis clearly goes beyond the influence of enhanced joint loading and the excessive fat is suggested to add to low-grade systemic inflammation adding to the osteoarthritic process [70]. Also there is an interplay and autocrine stimulation between adipokines, proinflammatory mediators, and angiogenic factors, the different cell types influencing each other [20,71], contributing to low-grade inflammatory activity systemically [72].

Moreover, obesity is associated with a disturbed lipid metabolism, leading to changes in the levels of high-density lipoproteins and levels of free fatty acids, triglycerides, and oxidized low-density lipoproteins [73,74] suggested to play a role in osteoarthritis as well [75,76], although so far this has been less extensively studied.

Clinical impact

Symptoms

Osteoarthritis is characterized by structural changes in bone and cartilage, muscle, and tendon weakness and/or contracture, as well as (low-grade/intermittent) synovial tissue inflammation with possible joint effusion. All influence each other at a mechanical and biochemical level, and result in joint stiffness and most importantly pain. Pain is intermittent and typically intense during weight-bearing activities like walking and stair climbing [77]. The relationship between pain and the actual structural changes is not very clear yet. Subchondral bone changes seem to provide the best correlation, but also (changes in) synovitis and effusion as seen on magnetic resonance imaging (MRI) have been reported to correlate with knee pain [25,78,79] and functional outcomes [80].

Synovitis relates to progression of disease

It is inevitable that synovitis in whatever way, low-grade chronic or intermittent flares, adds to the severity and progression of disease. Synovial inflammation (synovitis and effusion) is related to more cartilage pathology years later [24,81] and effusion assessed by ultrasound (US) evaluation predicts joint replacement [82]. More synovitis (higher synovial volume) is related to a higher Kellgren–Lawrence grade, representing more joint damage and also the proportion of patients with synovitis increases with the progress of tissue damage [83]. However, molecular cross-talk between the synovium, cartilage, and the other adjacent tissues can influence the final impact of synovitis on joint changes [84,85].

Detecting synovitis

There are various ways to detect and characterize (score) synovitis: clinical evaluation, histochemistry of synovial tissue biopsies, arthroscopy, US, MRI, and even measurement of biochemical markers [23,86].

Clinical evaluation

The cardinal signs of inflammation are redness, pain, heat, swelling, and restriction of motion [87]. The restriction of passive motion can be the first and only physical sign of osteoarthritis [77]. Palpable joint swelling due to thickening of the synovium or synovial fluid effusion is considered to indicate synovial inflammation [88]. Joint enlargement, resulting from joint effusion, bony swelling, or both, is present during osteoarthritic flares, but can also be present during chronic osteoarthritis [77].

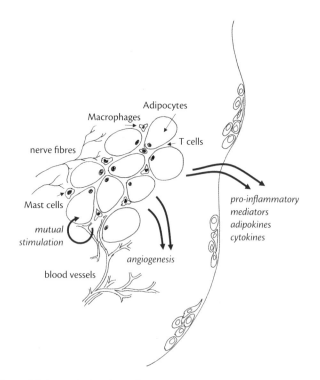

Figure 6.4 Intra-articular adipose tissue.

Histochemistry of biopsies

The synovial changes in osteoarthritis as described above, such as cell composition and vascularization, are predominantly based upon histological changes in synovial composition analysed from synovial tissue biopsies either taken by needle biopsies, during arthroscopic evaluation, at surgery (such as during meniscus treatment), or in the end at joint replacement surgery. Scoring histology in early osteoarthritis is difficult, since synovial tissue changes are often focal and can easily be missed by random biopsies [89].

Arthroscopy

For orthopaedics, arthroscopy is the gold standard for imaging of cartilage damage and synovial abnormalities. Arthroscopy has been used to show the association between knee effusion and synovitis [23,24]. Arthroscopic studies suggest synovial thickening to be associated with inflammatory changes in 50% of patients with osteoarthritis, and the presence of synovitis detected by arthroscopy is associated with more severe chondropathy [23]. Using a standardized macroscopic description of the synovial appearance, a distinction could be made between reactive and inflammatory synovium in which inflammatory synovium was suggested to have a direct effect on adjacent cartilage [24]. Arthroscopy is suggested to be used as a monitoring tool as well as a diagnostic or therapeutic procedure [90]. This is made possible by the development of arthroscopic scoring systems for determining the severity of synovial lesions (e.g. the Synovitis Score, a composite index incorporating intensity, extent, and location of synovial abnormalities) [90]. However, arthroscopy is not comprehensive for assessment of overall synovitis and severity depends on the underlying cause [90]. Not all compartments of a joint can be fully visualized and not all joints are easily accessible.

Imaging modalities

Magnetic resonance imaging

MRI has good potential to objectively quantify the morphology and integrity of the synovium, however it has been predominantly used for evaluation of other joint tissues [91] and clearly more for the knee than for the smaller hand joints [92]. A comprehensive review has recently been provided by Guermazi et al. describing advances and limitations, acquisition sequences, and relations with severity and symptoms of disease for knee, hip, and hand joints [92]. Limitations are the acquisition time, complexity of the more advanced techniques, as well as the costs [77] and often but not necessarily the use of contrast agent [93]. Synovial scoring by MRI is mainly based on synovial thickening and joint effusion graded collectively ('effusion synovitis'); distinguishing between synovial fluid and synovial tissue needs the use of contrast. Different scoring methods have been described for knee, hands, and hips [25,83,94–98].

Characteristics of the synovium on MRI correlate with histopathology of synovium biopsies, especially in early disease [28,47,99–101]. Severity of synovitis (enhanced synovial volume) correlates with increased severity of the disease on radiographs [88,92]. Synovitis can precede the development of radiographic knee osteoarthritis [102]. Longitudinally, synovial changes on MRI relate to cartilage loss over time [25,103]. Knee joint effusion synovitis and knee cartilage defects are correlated cross-sectionally and longitudinally [104]. However, others have found that synovitis does not relate to severity of cartilage damage [28]. It has been reported that 75% of patients with less than 4 years of osteoarthritis symptoms present with synovial thickening on MRI [47] and 37% in elderly persons without radiographic osteoarthritis [105].

Ultrasonography

US has the ability to image synovium in several planes using grey scale, representing effusion and synovial hypertrophy, and additionally power Doppler as a measure for vascularization of the tissue, representing more active inflammation [106–109]. It does not require a contrast agent and allows for real-time visualization. The penetration depth of the signal limits the tissue that can be assessed. As such, the technique is specifically suitable for the smaller joints affected by osteoarthritis, but is used for larger joints as well. A drawback is that US outcome is very dependent on the experience of the observer [110]. Several studies have been published over the years. Synovial involvement (synovitis and effusion) by US is found in 47% of patients with painful knee osteoarthritis [111]. The presence of knee effusion evaluated by US in addition to other parameters predicted the need for joint replacement surgery [82]. Inflammatory features evaluated by US, especially when persistently present, are associated with radiological progression of hand osteoarthritis [112]. Clearly synovial abnormalities on US are more common in osteoarthritic joints but the associations with severity and symptoms are not conclusive [81,113,114].

Biochemical markers

Synovial tissue metabolism and inflammation can be assessed with biochemical markers. The more and the larger the joints involved, the higher the chance of detecting such markers in the peripheral compartment. A cluster of biochemical markers has been related to low-grade synovitis in osteoarthritis [115]. Serum cartilage oligomeric matrix protein (sCOMP) is present in synovial tissue, is produced by synoviocytes, and is associated with synovitis and/or effusion. Serum hyaluronan and serum N-propeptides of collagen type III are two non-specific markers of synovial activity, segregated with sCOMP, all found to be associated with clinical synovitis [115,116]. General markers of inflammation are found to be raised in osteoarthritis including high-sensitivity C-reactive protein (related to IL6 and YKL40 levels) [117] and to be related to synovial cell infiltration [118] and to progression in early osteoarthritis [119]. However, correction of potential confounders such as body mass index decreases such relations. Recently it was suggested that evaluation of biochemical markers in the joint synovial fluid instead of the peripheral compartment is worthwhile to consider since better relationships with tissue changes are found [120]. Also systemic or local adipokines might be relevant markers of synovial (intra-articular adipose tissue) activity of knee and hand osteoarthritis [121,122]. Although promising, there are still some bridges to cross before such markers become of relevance to clinical practice.

Pathways that promote synovitis

There are numerous mediators involved in synovial activity, among them angiogenic factors, cytokines, chemokines, and proteases. Clearly, the number and diversity of these mediators in osteoarthritic joints, the complex roles and interactions of these molecules in inflammation, extracellular matrix (ECM) damage and repair, changes over time, and the physiological roles of most of these

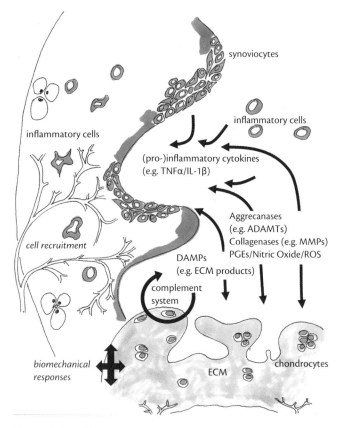

Figure 6.5 Synovitis perpetuation.

mediators in normal ECM turnover and 'healthy' immunological defence, makes it virtually impossible to provide a comprehensive and still convenient overview of these molecules and their pathways.

Even in the absence of classical (overt) inflammation, healthy cartilage chondrocytes and (within normal physiology) 'surveilling' synovial cells, express mediators (stimulators as well as inhibitors) of inflammation including classical cytokines (such as IL1B, TNFA, and IL6), proteases (such as collagenases (including metalloproteinases; MMPs) and aggrecanases (such as a disintegrin and metalloproteinase with thrombospondin motifs; ADAMTS)) as well as other mediators (such as cyclooxygenase (COX), and nitric oxide (NO) as a result of mechanical or oxidative stress) [123] all being part of normal ECM turnover (Figure 6.5).

During the process of osteoarthritis, many of these mediators are upregulated. This upregulation may be restricted to the cartilage tissue, driven by biomechanical processes, and for a long period of time remain clinically unnoticed. Alternatively (or coinciding), synovial tissue inflammation can develop after (sub)acute, or chronic joint injury including mechanical derangement by, for example, meniscal extrusion or tears, joint overuse, hypermobility, mal-alignment, or ligament rupture [124,125]. Although an acute trauma may result in an acute inflammatory response, this inflammatory response is most often transient, demonstrated by a transient increase in inflammatory mediators in the synovial fluid [126]. However, even such acute responses may be critical in a degenerative process later on [127]. This initial response can also lead to a vicious cycle by which acute local tissue damage leads to

acute synovial inflammation, which in turn leads to more chronic tissue damage and repair, resulting in a chronic inflammatory tissue destructive processes [128]. This may result in the intermittent or chronic low-grade inflammation in osteoarthritis.

Innate immune system

More recently, the networks of diverse innate inflammatory danger signals have gained attention in osteoarthritis research. Damage-associated molecular patterns (DAMPs), including alarmins (S100 proteins), high-mobility group box (HMGB) protein 1, ECM proteins (e.g. collagen, fibronectin, and proteoglycan), and free fatty acids and their receptors (pattern-recognition receptors; PRR), such as toll-like receptors (TLRs) and receptors of advanced glycation end-products (RAGEs), as well as elements of the complement system are elevated in the osteoarthritic joint and have become molecules of interest. Synoviocytes (specifically macrophages) as well as chondrocytes express a variety of TLRs and RAGEs, which are upregulated by tissue damage and inflammation in osteoarthritis [129,130]. Ligands for these receptors including over-expressed S100 proteins [131], HMGB proteins, elevated levels of cartilage ECM components [130] such as tenascin C [132], fibronectin isoforms [133], small-molecular-weight species of hyaluronic acid [134] and biglycan [135], but also certain plasma proteins [136] can activate the TLR cascade, stimulating the nuclear factor kappa B (NFKB) pathway and subsequent production of chemokines and cytokines. These in turn recruit and activate macrophages, and lymphocytes leading to downstream activation of inflammatory and catabolic processes in the synovium as well as the cartilage, processes which in their turn perpetuate the upregulation of DAMPs [137,138]. The consequent induction and amplification of synovitis and chondrocyte-related inflammatory processes (including PPR activation [139]) amplify the catabolic processes of joint damage and thus osteoarthritis progression [140]. But clearly, the book of DAMPs and their PPRs is not closed because protective roles of TLRs have also been described; knockout of TLR2 in a murine model results in more severe disease, suggesting a protective as well as destructive role of TLR [141] (Figure 6.5).

Complement activation is also considered a factor in disease progression in osteoarthritis [137]. The complement cascade is a major player in the activation of the immune system. In osteoarthritic joints, complement can be activated by DAMPs (including cartilage matrix constituents), but also by cell debris, by crystals (e.g. hydroxyapatite and calcium pyrophosphate dehydrate), and by cartilage ECM components such as aggrecan and fibromodulin [137,142]. Increased expression and activity of manifold effector molecules of the complement pathways including formation of membrane attack complex (MAC) occurs in early human osteoarthritis, and synovial expression of multiple complement inhibitors are decreased in human disease [136,137,143,144]. Activation of the cascade, resulting in MAC is essential for removal of many pathogens, however improper regulation can lead to tissue damage, as may be the case in osteoarthritis. Activated complement components accumulate in cartilage and change chondrocyte activity. MAC can directly lyse cells through formation of pores in the cellular membrane, and induce sub-lytic inflammatory signalling pathways that further promotes cartilage damage and results in an increase of ECM breakdown products, perpetuating the cycle of complement activation [42].

Cytokine-related processes

Proinflammatory cytokines like IL1B, TNFA, IL6, IL8, IL17, their natural regulators such as the IL1Ra (receptor antagonist) and anti-inflammatory cytokines such as IL4, IL10, IL13 as well as proteases (collagenases and aggrecanases) and many other soluble components (NO prostaglandins (PGEs), etc.) involved in inflammation are released during the inflammatory process by synovial (inflammatory) cells as well as chondrocytes and are found (in general elevated) in the osteoarthritic joint [145–147]. These mediators play a pivotal role in initiating, perpetuating, and progression of osteoarthritis [148,149] (Figure 6.5; Table 6.1). For a more comprehensive overview of the additional inflammatory mediators see Table 6.1. During cartilage degradation, in both early and advanced osteoarthritis, synovial cells phagocytize ECM waste products released in the synovial cavity, and the synovial membrane releases proinflammatory mediators [23]. These in turn lead to increased cartilage breakdown and synovial inflammation, and an excess in the production of proteolytic enzymes.

IL1B and TNFA

IL1B and TNFA are the two major cytokines (but clearly not the only ones) involved in the pathogenesis of osteoarthritis, mainly

Table 6.1 Important inflammatory mediators in osteoarthritis

Mediator	Description	References
IL1B	Proinflammatory cytokine elevated in synovial fluid/membrane, subchondral bone, and cartilage. Supresses type II collagen and aggrecan expression. Stimulates the release of MMP1, MMP3, MMP13, NO, PGE2. Induces the production of IL6, IL8, MCP1, and CCL5 (RANTES)	[136,151,152, 221–223]
IL1RA	Anti-inflammatory cytokine that inhibits IL1B and PGE2 release	[223,224]
IL4	Anti-inflammatory cytokine that is elevated in osteoarthritis (OA) tissue. Inhibits IL1B, TNFA, proteases, PGE2 release and apoptosis of synoviocytes. Upregulates IL1Ra and TIMP	[223,225,226]
IL6	Ambivalent cytokine, pro/anti-inflammatory effects, found elevated in synovial fluid and in supranatural amounts in the synovium. Upregulates MMP1 and MMP13 in combination with IL1B and oncostatin. Activates B cells and T cells, and mediates recruitment of inflammatory cells to site of infiltration. IL6 also induces synovial fibroblasts to produce angiogenic factors and stimulates chondrocytes and synovial fibroblasts to release chemokines like IL8 Reduces expression of type II collagen. Induces the production of TIMP, but not MMPs, involved in feedback mechanism that limits proteolytic damage. Reduces proteoglycan loss in acute phase OA, but enhances osteophyte formation in the chronic phase of OA. Stimulates proliferation of chondrocytes	[43,223,227]
IL8	Proinflammatory chemokine synthesized by monocytes, macrophages, chondrocytes, and fibroblasts, and is found to be elevated in OA tissue. Induces iNOS, MMP1, IL1B, TNFA and IL6, and stimulates proteoglycan depletion	[228]
IL10	Anti-inflammatory cytokine elevated in OA tissue. Inhibits IL1B, TNFA, MMPs, and PGE2 release, and upregulates IL1RA and TIMP. Modulates TNFA by increasing release of TNFsr, downregulating receptor surface expression	[223,229]
IL13	Anti-inflammatory cytokine elevated in OA tissue. Inhibits IL1B, TNFA, MMPs, and PGE2 release, and apoptosis of synoviocytes. Upregulates IL1RA and TIMP	[223,230]
IL15	Proinflammatory cytokine elevated in synovial fluid in early OA (more than advanced OA). Closely associated with MMP1 and MMP3. IL15 receptor is present on the synovial lining layer and the endothelium. Involved in recruitment and survival of CD8+ T cells	[128,223,231]
IL17	Proinflammatory cytokine that induces IL1B, TNF, and IL6 production. IL17 also upregulates NO and MMPs and downregulates proteoglycan levels	[223,232]
IL18	Proinflammatory cytokine elevated in human OA chondrocytes. Acts through IL1 dependent and IL1 independent pathways	[223,233]
IL21	Proinflammatory cytokine, elevated the synovium during early OA	[231]
TNFA	Proinflammatory cytokine elevated in synovial fluid/membrane, in subchondral bone and in cartilage. Supresses the synthesis of proteoglycan, link protein, and type II collagen in chondrocytes. Stimulates the release of MMP1, MMP3, MMP13, NO, and PGE2. Induces production of IL6, IL8, MCP1, and CCL5	[136,223,234,235]
RANTES	Proinflammatory cytokine, also known as CCL5, elevated in OA tissue. Induces iNOS, MMP1, and IL6, and stimulates proteoglycan depletion	[236]
TGFβ/VEGF	Vascular growth factors, inducing angiogenesis	[30,237]
Adiponectin	Protein hormone predominantly secreted by differentiated adipocytes, but also by synovial fibroblasts. Adiponectin receptors on synovial fibroblasts lead to an increased production of MMPs, cytokines, and PGE2	[238,239]
Leptin/visfatin	Proinflammatory adipokines	[240,241]

(continued)

Table 6.1   Continued

Mediator	Description	References
Resistin	Proinflammatory adipokine that induces cartilage destruction and synovial inflammation. Upregulates IL6 and TNFA in macrophages and synovial fluid cells	[242]
PGE2	Prostaglandin that causes hyperalgesia, upregulated by IL1B and TNFA	[243]
NO/NOS/iNOS	Mainly produced by IL1B and TNFA. NO activates NFKB in peripheral blood mononuclear cells, an important transcription factor in iNOS gene expression in response to inflammation, and contributes to cartilage degradation	[163]
MCP1	Elevated in OA tissue. Induces iNOS, MMP1, and IL6. Stimulates proteoglycan depletion	[244]
ICAM1	Intercellular cell adhesion protein 1 is an adhesion molecule that mediates monocyte adhesion and regulates movement of mononuclear cells into inflammatory sites	[245]
VCAM1	Vascular cell adhesion protein 1 is an adhesion molecule that mediates monocyte adhesion and regulates movement of mononuclear cells into inflammatory sites	[246,247]
MMP1/3/9/13	Chemokine enzymes capable of degrading ECM. Involved in catabolic process and remodelling of ECM. MMP1 is produced by fibroblasts, chondrocytes and synovial fibroblasts at sites of synovial attachment to articular cartilage. MMP1 is capable of degrading type I/II/III collagens	[248,249]
Substance-P	Neurotransmitter that mediates proinflammatory signals, vasodilatation and contributes to pain. Located in subintimal portion of synovial membrane and in areas with osteophytes and cartilage erosions. Induces PGE2 and collagenases by synoviocytes and induces proliferation of synoviocytes	[5,87]
LIF	Leukaemia inhibitory factor (LIF) is a cytokine elevated in OA synovial membrane/fluid. LIF is upregulated by IL1B and TNFA. LIF stimulates cartilage proteoglycan degradation/resorption, MMP synthesis and NO production.	[23,250]
	LIF induces acute-phase protein synthesis, lipoprotein lipase activity and the expression of collagenase and stromelysin, but not TIMP	
	Enhances IL1B and IL8 in chondrocytes and IL1B and TNFA in synovial fibroblasts. Regulates connective tissue such as cartilage and bone	
CXCL13	Attracts activated B cells in synovial membrane lymphoid aggregates	[251]
COX2	Upregulates PGE2, and is upregulated by TNFA, IL6, IL1B, and via TLR4 stimulation	[173]
Bradykinin	A neuropeptide generated in the synovium. Initiates and maintains inflammation and allows for excitation and sensitization of nerve fibres	[23,252]
TIMP	Tissue inhibitor of metalloproteinases	[234]

produced by activated synoviocytes, and mononuclear cells; but also chondrocytes themselves are capable of producing these cytokines that induce inflammation and cartilage degradation [150]. Patients with osteoarthritis have increased levels of IL1B and TNFA in the synovial membrane and synovial fluid, but also elevated levels in subchondral bone and cartilage. Both IL1B and TNFA have been found in higher concentrations in patients with early osteoarthritis than patients with advanced osteoarthritis [34]. These cytokines not only induce cartilage catabolism; osteoarthritic progression is also stimulated by suppression of anabolic processes by inhibition of cartilage ECM formation including production of aggrecan and collagen type II, the major ECM constituents of articular cartilage [151,152].

In healthy individuals, IL1B is not produced as much as its natural antagonist, IL1RA; in osteoarthritis a disturbed balance is an additional enhancer to the catabolic effects of IL1B [153]. Activation of cells by IL1B is mediated through the receptor IL1r, extensively expressed on synovial cells and chondrocytes. IL1B can also bind to a second specific (decoy) receptor that is unable to transduce a signal. IL1RA is produced by several cells including synovial fibroblasts and chondrocytes and is capable of binding to both receptors, as such providing anti-inflammatory properties [153]. TNFA has

two receptors, TNFR55 and TNFR75, the latter only responding to membrane-bound TNF. Their expression is modulated by, among others, both IL1B and TNFA. IL1B and TNFA can independently initiate and propagate inflammation in osteoarthritis joints, however, it has been shown that a simultaneous injection leads to more cartilage destruction than either cytokine alone in animal models [154,155]. Both IL1B and TNFA can upregulate their own production, via the activation of NFKB [156]. Additionally, synovial fibroblasts are capable of upregulating IL1B and TNFA upon stimulation of their IL1B and TNFA receptors [157], in turn activating synovial cell activation [158]. IL1B and TNFA can stimulate chondrocytes and synovial cells to produce many of the other inflammatory mediators [159].

Oxidative stress

IL1B and TNFA also induce the production of NO and reactive oxygen species (ROS) (mostly the superoxide anion), generating radicals capable of cartilage degradation [160]. Downregulation of antioxidant enzyme expression by IL1B and TNFA reduces the amount of ROS and NO that can be cleared, thus increasing the damaging potential of ROS and NO on cartilage [161]. NO has a major role in the modulation of chondrocyte function in osteoarthritis. NO is upregulated in the inflammatory osteoarthritic joint. In the affected joint, free radicals like NO and ROS are mediators of inflammation and tissue destruction contributing to disease progression [160,162].

ROS are chemically reactive molecules originating from conversion of oxygen [163]. They are formed as a by-product of normal metabolism, and are increased during osteoarthritic conditions. ROS are involved in the regulation of biochemical factors that are involved in cartilage degradation and joint inflammation and influence certain intracellular signalling pathways [162,163]. ROS can directly cause damage to all matrix components, either by a direct attack, or indirectly by reducing matrix components synthesis by apoptosis of the cells or by latent activation of MMPs. ROS can regulate the activity of transcription factors through oxidative modifications of, for example, cysteines. ROS involvement in inflammation, fibrosis control, and nociception has been reported as well [163]. However, whilst the effect of ROS on synovial inflammation is clearly proinflammatory, ROS have also been shown to downregulate the expression of proinflammatory genes in chondrocytes [164].

Epigenetic changes

At all different levels within the osteoarthritic joint and clearly also in the synovial membrane, epigenetic changes such as post-translational methylations, as well as the role of microRNAs are becoming a new area of research. Such changes, like in many diseases, are sure to be found to be of influence in the disease process, causative, and/or epiphenomenal [165,166].

Pain related to synovitis

Pain is the defining reason why most people seek care. Current pain management of osteoarthritis falls short of patients' needs in terms of providing adequate and sustained pain relief. Osteoarthritis-associated joint pain has a strong mechanical component, triggered by specific activities and relieved by rest [167]. The joint is a heavily innervated organ, and its sensory innervation is organized predominantly towards proprioception and nociception. Nociceptive fibres are located in the joint capsule, synovium, meniscus, bone marrow, periarticular ligaments, periosteum, subchondral bone, and the marrow cavity of osteophytes [68,168]. Consequently pain can originate from many articular tissues. Intra-articular local anaesthetics abolish knee osteoarthritis pain [169] suggesting that these structures are in contact with the intra-articular environment as well. As cartilage is an aneural and avascular tissue, it is often considered as non-participatory in joint pain. However, osteoarthritic cartilage is potentially a large source of mediators that can act as nociceptive mediators, including cytokines, other mediators, and possibly extracellular fragments. Moreover, it has been demonstrated that nociceptors express TLRs, which are PRRs that recognize a large array of DAMPs released during tissue injury and contribute to pain generation [170–172]. In osteoarthritis, no information on the role of TLRs on nociceptors and pain generation currently exists, but TLRs play a clear role in synovitis in osteoarthritis as described above [128,173]. This indicates that TLRs contribute to pain in osteoarthritis indirectly by activating synovial fibroblasts and macrophages [128], and potentially directly by sensitizing nociceptors.

Inflammation plays a critical role in the initial increase and processing of nociceptive input [174]. Many of the substances involved with inflammation are also neuroactive. These substances stimulate chemosensitive nociceptors and can be categorized into three groups [175] (Table 6.2). However, it is unclear to what extent the low and often varying level of inflammation in osteoarthritis can actually produce this enhanced nociceptive receptor sensitivity. Mediators related to tissue destruction might be involved, as well

Table 6.2 Stimulation of chemosensitive nociceptors, subdivided by the release origin

Origin	Mediators	Description	References
Damaged cells	Hydrogen ions (H$^+$)	These factors are released by damaged tissue and activate the nociceptors, previously excited directly by the causal stimulus itself	[253,254]
	Adenosine triphosphate (ATP)		
Inflammatory cells	Bradykinin	Bradykinin increases capillary permeability and is among the most potent pain-producing substances identified to date. The factors in this group exert specific effects and sensitize the receptors to other factors. They cause primary hyperalgesia, a nociceptive stimulus that produces pain that is disproportionately severe compared to the intensity of the stimulus	[215,253–256]
	Prostaglandins		
	Leukotrienes		
	Proinflammatory cytokines: ◆ TNFA ◆ IL1B ◆ IL6 ◆ IL17 ◆ High-mobility group protein B1 (HMGB1)		
	Anti-inflammatory cytokines: ◆ IL4 ◆ IL10	Anti-inflammatory cytokines suppress pro-inflammatory cytokine expression, and macrophage/microglial activation. These cytokines provide strong pain inhibition, but even more so with the combined IL4–10 synerkine	
	Nerve growth factor (NGF)		
Nociceptors	Substance-P	Released by the nociceptor itself and can activate these receptors either directly or indirectly. These mechanisms result in a vicious circle of pain stimulation	[182,183,253]

as sensitization by a vicious cycle of mediators. That explains why patients with osteoarthritis can react in a more exaggerated way to innocuous stimuli.

Synovitis induces the release of prostaglandins, neuropeptides, and cytokines. These mediators are capable of causing hyperalgesia by activating threshold receptors or by sensitizing fine unmyelinated sensory nerves in the osteoarthritic joint. For example, TNFA and IL6 can cause prolonged mechanical hypersensitivity, whereas IL17 sensitizes joint nociceptors to mechanical stimuli [176]. The proinflammatory cytokines TNFA and IL1B can affect sensory neurons directly, but also indirectly by the downstream activation of other cytokines, chemokines, prostanoids, neurotrophins, NO, lipids, and via the complement and NFKB pathways [176,177].

Persisting stimulation of nociceptors by these substances will lead to heightened neuronal activity; second-order neurons in the spinal cord increase their firing rate, enhancing the pain transmission and intensifying the pain sensation [87]. Joint damage can lead to joint inflammation and subsequent pain. However, reverse causality holds true as well, sensitization and heightened nociception can lead to an increase in inflammation, and thus an increase in joint damage. This happens at the same time as turnover within the synovial tissue and neurological restructuring of the joint. This means that cell activation, proliferation, and infiltration due to synovitis is accompanied by growth as well as retraction of nerve endings, associated with enhanced pain sensation [178–18]. Peripheral nerves do not proliferate, they grow by neurite extension or arborization, which is the terminal branching of nerve fibres in a treelike pattern [181,182]. This change in innervation pattern of the synovial layer is also demonstrated in osteoarthritis. Synovial material obtained at knee joint replacement with and without inflammation exhibited a similar vascular and neuronal network. However, the inflamed synovium had a decreased number of nerve fibres reaching the synovial lining layer depending on the degree of inflammation. The deeper areas (e.g. the capsule) were less affected [183].

Moreover, the joint is innervated by postganglionic sympathetic efferents, but also by sensory fibres, that are distinguished based on their anatomic features [184,185], and stimulation of these fibres is associated with a specific kind of pain. Different types of fibres can be identified in the joint:

◆ Aβ fibres (group II): thick myelinated nerves, innervating the capsule, fat pad, ligaments, menisci, and periosteum. These nerves may mediate sudden pain on movement or pressure.

◆ Aδ fibres (group III): thin nerves with myelin sheath that disappear in the terminal region, innervating capsule, ligaments, menisci, periosteum, and mineralized bone. These nerves may mediate sudden pain on movement or pressure.

◆ C fibres (group IV): thin unmyelinated nerves, innervating capsule, ligaments, menisci, periosteum and mineralized bone. These nerves may mediate slow, burning pain as described by many patients with osteoarthritis.

Inflammatory mediators can also stimulate nerves in the absence of mechanical stimulation. Over a period of hours or days, upregulation of genes within the synovium and recruitment of inflammatory cells enhance peripheral sensitization, that is, reduction of the pain threshold, whilst neuronal plasticity contributes to central sensitization, increasing the excitability of neurons within the central nervous system, resulting in multiple amplification of the pain sensation [29]. This is supported by the indications that hip osteoarthritis patients have a lower pain threshold compared to healthy controls [186]. In addition, there is also a tendency to note sensitivity to innocuous warmth and cold in patients with hip osteoarthritic pain [187]. The pain becomes more constant over time, from shorter periods of aching and throbbing to continuous periods of intense pain [176].

Angiogenesis has proven to be a major contributor to inflammation and in a wide variety of tissues unmyelinated (C fibres) nerve growth follows angiogenesis [181,182]. However, the exact role of angiogenesis in pain is less established. In addition to the growth of these fibres and presence of classic nociceptors, there are also fibres present that only become active after damage or inflammation, called silent nociceptors. They can have a substantial contribution to pain sensation in osteoarthritis.

Before joint pain is reported, radiographic evidence of joint damage can be observed. Moreover, the extent of joint damage has little relation to the amount of pain experienced, especially in knee osteoarthritis [188,189]. However, more recent studies indicate stronger associations between structural changes and pain severity. For instance, radiographic osteoarthritis and individual radiographic characteristics were demonstrated to be strongly associated with knee pain [190]. Remarkably, especially joint space narrowing was more strongly associated with pain than were osteophytes [191]. Using imaging modalities like MRI, it has been shown that bone marrow lesions [192], subarticular bone attribution [78], effusion [25], and synovitis are associated with knee pain [192]. In OA patients, more severe disease leads to worse structural outcome, which makes it difficult to determine the contribution of the individual tissue changes, but research has shown that changes in subchondral bone and synovial changes seem to predominate [193].

Therapeutic approach to treat synovitis

Treatment of synovial inflammation in osteoarthritis is hampered by the fact that inflammation is, in general, low grade and variable over time. Treatment needs to be provided over a very long time period because of the chronic character of the disease with often several comorbidities such as obesity and diabetes. Since multiple joints are involved, there is a need for systemic treatment. This all makes anti-inflammatory treatment for osteoarthritis a real challenge. Irrespectively, targeting synovitis may hold promise specifically for those patients in whom synovitis dominates the disease.

General anti-inflammatory treatment

General systemic and local anti-inflammatory treatment limiting synovial tissue activity in osteoarthritis such as non-steroidal anti-inflammatory drugs (NSAIDs) and selective COX2 inhibitors as well as effects of corticoid-steroid injections and other supposedly inflammation controlling intra-articular injections will be discussed elsewhere, as will be the potential disease-modifying OA drugs. More recently, approaches with the anti-rheumatic drug methotrexate (MTX) have been dared [194]. However, because MTX is cytotoxic and has potential serious life-threatening side effects its use cannot be justified simply for treatment of the, in general, low-grade synovial inflammation in osteoarthritis.

Anti-angiogenic treatment

Targeting angiogenesis, and with that synovitis, could prevent disease progression and alleviate symptoms. Anti-angiogenic strategies have been implemented especially in the oncological field. Although the mechanism/initiation of angiogenesis differs between osteoarthritis and oncology, this does not mean that therapies efficient in one cannot be efficient in another. Broad inhibition of angiogenesis and inflammation with the use of drugs may however not easily be applicable due to potential toxicity of these drugs modifying biologically important physiological processes [29].

Targeted anti-inflammatory (antibody) treatment

As has become clear from the above-discussed complexity of mediators involved, there are limitations in the ability to control inflammatory mediators in osteoarthritis collectively. This resulted in great interest in identifying and targeting the specific inflammatory mediators and pathways that contribute to the disease and through that developing an anti-cytokine therapy for osteoarthritis [147]. Strategies aimed at preventing excessive proinflammatory cytokine production, signalling, and downstream NFKB activation, by the use of highly specific drugs, small interfering RNAs (siRNAs), or other biological inhibitors [195], are the focus of current osteoarthritis research. Animal models show hopeful results, however, as all these mediators are mutually interacting in human disease, clinical treatment is a challenge. Clearly these biological therapies will not be suitable for all types of osteoarthritis [196], and biological therapies targeting single cytokines that are increased in osteoarthritis joint tissues (e.g. IL1B and TNFA) have not yet resulted in either effective or pragmatic treatment in human osteoarthritis [153].

Anti-TNF to control synovitis

Thus far, despite compelling evidence suggesting the role of TNFA in the degenerative nature of osteoarthritis, no agents targeting the TNF family have been approved for osteoarthritis treatment. Small studies, in the case of clear inflammatory hand osteoarthritis injections of anti-TNFs, did not appear to be exclusively successful. Treatment with adalimumab (subcutaneously applied) did not significantly improve the signs and symptoms of erosive hand osteoarthritis [197]. Adalimumab had no clear effect in erosive hand osteoarthritis but only appeared to slow down progression of joint damage in the most progressive subpopulation [198]. Adalimumab was not superior to placebo in patients with hand osteoarthritis not responding to analgesics and NSAIDs [199]. With infliximab, symptomatic effects were obtained in erosive hand osteoarthritis but disease-modifying action was not significant [200]. In a single case of knee osteoarthritis, in addition to treatment with a COX2 inhibitor, adalimumab seemed to alleviate symptoms of pain [201]. In an open uncontrolled study, patients with knee effusions treated with adalimumab showed promising short-term clinical benefit [202].

Preclinical studies also suggest that monoclonal antibodies and single-chain antibodies against TNFA can potently inhibit inflammation and prevent cartilage damage [203]. In contrast to full antibodies, these smaller antibodies also penetrate into cartilage and might reverse the TNFA-induced catabolic state of articular cartilage in addition to targeting synovial TNFA-driven inflammation.

Anti-IL1 to control synovitis

In mouse models, the effects of ILRA have demonstrated promising results [149,204,205]. Also with use of gene therapy, where the IL1RA gene has been successfully transferred into synovial cells, the consequent increase in IL1RA in the joint protects the joint from IL1B-induced joint damage. This was proven to be protective in rabbit, dog, and horse models of osteoarthritis [206]. Overexpression of the decoy IL1 receptor prevents production of multiple proinflammatory tissue destructive signals [207]. However, an important issue for human gene approaches is safety, especially when applied in a non-fatal disease like osteoarthritis.

Also for anti-IL treatment, clinical studies were not conclusively positive. Treatment of knee osteoarthritis with the IL1RA anakinra was not associated with improvements in osteoarthritic symptoms compared with placebo [208]. A case series of three patients with erosive hand osteoarthritis treated subcutaneously with anakinra showed relief of pain [209]. Systemic administration of AMG108, a monoclonal antibody against IL1R in patients with knee osteoarthritis, showed minimal, if any, clinical benefit [210]. Treatment very early in the disease, where temporary high levels of IL1 are found, may be slightly more promising, at least in the short term, as two small studies reported [211,212].

Pro-anabolic treatment

Instead of reduction of proinflammatory mediators, it is also an option to stimulate the production and activity of anti-inflammatory mediators. Along this line of thought, recombinant human IL4 (rhIL4) has been created and tested on osteoarthritic synovial tissue, showing evident IL1B or TNFA reduction [213]. IL13 has been shown experimentally to be useful by testing on human synovial membranes from osteoarthritis patients. A combination of IL4 and IL10 has been proven to be chondroprotective in mouse models [214]. A combined molecule (IL4–10 synerkine) has also proven to protect cartilage from blood-induced damage [215]. This synerkine has been developed to overcome the low bioavailability of the separate cytokines, and shows improved inhibitory activities (as compared to the combination of IL4 and IL10 monotherapy) [215]. However of all these anti-inflammatory cytokine approaches, IL10 is the only one currently in clinical trials for treatment of rheumatoid arthritis [153].

Summary

Synovium is an integrated tissue of the diarthrodial joints which interacts with all the other joint tissues and specifically is important in nourishment and lubrication of the articular cartilage, removal of waste products, and immunological surveillance. Much knowledge about the synovium and its numerous mediators in the healthy condition and during the degenerative process of osteoarthritis has been gained over the past decades. Chronic as well as recurrent low-grade synovial inflammation definitely contributes to progression and symptoms of certain patients with osteoarthritis. Low-grade inflammation may even be causative in the disease. The challenge is that osteoarthritis is a heterogeneous disorder with inflammation not only of the synovial tissue but with its mediators also present in cartilage and bone. Therefore, despite the presence of inflammatory mediators, in some cases synovitis may be seen as a bystander and not as a driving force in pathogenesis [216]. Further studies are needed to obtain a comprehensive understanding of its role in such a way that it is of use for routine diagnosis, prognosis, and specifically treatment of the disease [40,217].

Anti-inflammatory therapy may have benefits for some phenotypes of the disease. The presence of 'systemic inflammation' in osteoarthritis of some patients may even provide a rationale for more aggressive anti-inflammatory drugs including biological therapy. Future research must be directed towards defining the risk-to-benefit ratio for biological therapy, especially if the purpose of the therapy is to target mediators of low-grade inflammation. This will be extremely challenging, because mediators of low-grade inflammation are likely to have important physiological effects on other organ systems. The representation of several subtypes with potentially certain specific set of cytokines, could allow for personalized anti-inflammatory medicine, thus increasing therapeutic efficiency [218]. Better stratification might also become possible using imaging modalities like MRI and US [93,219,220]. To develop highly efficient therapies we will probably need innovations in delivery systems, locally or such as nanotechnology, to selectively and safely target joints in a durable manner.

The absence of a clear effect of most anti-inflammatory therapies may be caused by treatment of a general osteoarthritis population, not taking into account subtypes of the disease with, for example, specific TNFA or IL1B involvement or involvement of certain inflammatory cell subsets, if existing. It might, on the other hand, suggest that in addition to the inflammatory component perpetuating the disease, a degenerative biomechanically driven component is able to drive the disease independently of inflammation (at least in certain phenotypes).

References

1. Brandt KD, Smith GN, Simon LS. Intraarticular injection of hyaluronan as treatment for knee osteoarthritis: what is the evidence? *Arthritis Rheum* 2000; 43:1192–203.
2. Bao J-P, Chen W-P, Wu L-D. Lubricin: a novel potential biotherapeutic approaches for the treatment of osteoarthritis. *Mol Biol Rep* 2011; 38:2879–85.
3. Hui A, McCarty W. A systems biology approach to synovial joint lubrication in health, injury, and disease. Wiley Interdiscip Rev Syst Biol Med 2012; 4(1):15–37.
4. Rhee D, Marcelino J. The secreted glycoprotein lubricin protects cartilage surfaces and inhibits synovial cell overgrowth. *J Clin Invest* 2005; 115:622–31.
5. Sutton S, Clutterbuck A, Harris P, et al. The contribution of the synovium, synovial derived inflammatory cytokines and neuropeptides to the pathogenesis of osteoarthritis. *Vet J* 2009; 179:10–24.
6. Bannuru RR, Natov NS, Obadan IE, et al. Therapeutic trajectory of hyaluronic acid versus corticosteroids in the treatment of knee osteoarthritis: a systematic review and meta-analysis. *Arthritis Rheum* 2009; 61:1704–11.
7. Li J, Gorski DJ, Anemaet W, et al. Hyaluronan injection in murine osteoarthritis prevents TGFbeta 1-induced synovial neovascularization and fibrosis and maintains articular cartilage integrity by a CD44-dependent mechanism. *Arthritis Res Ther* 2012; 14:R151.
8. Dahl LB, Dahl IM, Engström-Laurent A, Granath K. Concentration and molecular weight of sodium hyaluronate in synovial fluid from patients with rheumatoid arthritis and other arthropathies. *Ann Rheum Dis* 1985; 44:817–822.
9. Mathieu P, Conrozier T, Vignon E, Rozand Y, Rinaudo M. Rheologic behavior of osteoarthritic synovial fluid after addition of hyaluronic acid: a pilot study. *Clin Orthop Relat Res* 2009; 467:3002–9.
10. Goldberg RL, Huff JP, Lenz ME, et al. Elevated plasma levels of hyaluronate in patients with osteoarthritis and rheumatoid arthritis. *Arthritis Rheum* 1991; 34:799–807.
11. Izumisawa Y, Yamaguchi M. Equine synovial villi: distinctive structural organization of vasculature and novel nerve endings. *J Vet Med Sci* 1996; 58(12):1193–204.
12. Bartok B, Firestein GS. Fibroblast-like synoviocytes: key effector cells in rheumatoid arthritis. *Immunol Rev* 2010; 233:233–55.
13. Edwards J, Willoughby D. Demonstration of bone marrow derived cells in synovial lining by means of giant intracellular granules as genetic markers. *Ann Rheum Dis* 1982; 41:177–82.
14. Matsubara T, Spycher M. The ultrastructural localization of fibronectin in the lining layer of rheumatoid arthritis synovium: the synthesis of fibronectin by type B lining cells. *Rheumatol Int* 1983; 3:75–79.
15. Jones EA, Crawford A, English A, et al. Synovial fluid mesenchymal stem cells in health and early osteoarthritis: detection and functional evaluation at the single-cell level. *Arthritis Rheum* 2008; 58:1731–40.
16. Mastbergen SC, Saris DB, Lafeber FP. Functional articular cartilage repair: here, near, or is the best approach not yet clear? *Nat Rev Rheumatol* 2013; 9:277–90.
17. Seok J, Warren HS, Cuenca AG, et al. Genomic responses in mouse models poorly mimic human inflammatory diseases. *Proc Natl Acad Sci U S A* 2013; 110:3507–12.
18. Kobezda T, Ghassemi-Nejad S, Mikecz K, Glant TT, Szekanecz Z. Of mice and men: how animal models advance our understanding of T-cell function in RA. *Nat Rev Rheumatol* 2014; 10:160–70.
19. Fang H, Beier F. Mouse models of osteoarthritis: modelling risk factors and assessing outcomes. *Nat Rev Rheumatol* 2014; 10:413–21.
20. Ushiyama T, Chano T, Inoue K, Matsusue Y. Cytokine production in the infrapatellar fat pad: another source of cytokines in knee synovial fluids. *Ann Rheum Dis* 2003; 62:108–12.
21. Bijlsma J, Lafeber F. Glucosamine sulfate in osteoarthritis: the jury is still out. *Ann Intern Med* 2008; 148(4):315–16.
22. Kortekaas MC, Kwok W-Y, Reijnierse M, Huizinga TWJ, Kloppenburg M. In erosive hand osteoarthritis more inflammatory signs on ultrasound are found than in the rest of hand osteoarthritis. *Ann Rheum Dis* 2013; 72:930–4.
23. Sellam J, Berenbaum F. The role of synovitis in pathophysiology and clinical symptoms of osteoarthritis. *Nat Rev Rheumatol* 2010; 6:625–35.
24. Ayral X, Pickering EH, Woodworth TG, Mackillop N, Dougados M. Synovitis: a potential predictive factor of structural progression of medial tibiofemoral knee osteoarthritis—results of a 1 year longitudinal arthroscopic study in 422 patients. *Osteoarthritis Cartilage* 2005; 13:361–7.
25. Hill CL, Hunter DJ, Niu J, et al. Synovitis detected on magnetic resonance imaging and its relation to pain and cartilage loss in knee osteoarthritis. *Ann Rheum Dis* 2007; 66:1599–603.
26. Lambert C, Dubuc JE, Montell E, et al. Gene expression pattern of cells from inflamed and normal areas of osteoarthritis synovial membrane. *Arthritis Rheumatol (Hoboken, NJ)* 2014; 66:960–8.
27. Moradi B, Rosshirt N, Tripel E, et al. Unicompartmental and bicompartmental knee osteoarthritis show different patterns of mononuclear cell infiltration and cytokine release in the affected joints. *Clin Exp Immunol* 2014; 180(1):143–54.
28. Loeuille D, Chary-Valckenaere I, Champigneulle J, et al. Macroscopic and microscopic features of synovial membrane inflammation in the osteoarthritic knee: correlating magnetic resonance imaging findings with disease severity. *Arthritis Rheum* 2005; 52:3492–501.
29. Bonnet CS, Walsh DA. Osteoarthritis, angiogenesis and inflammation. *Rheumatology* 2005; 44:7–16.
30. Haywood L, McWilliams DF, Pearson CI, et al. Inflammation and angiogenesis in osteoarthritis. *Arthritis Rheum* 2003; 48:2173–7.
31. Oehler S, Neureiter D, Meyer-Scholten C, Aigner T. Subtyping of osteoarthritic synoviopathy. *Clin Exp Rheumatol* 2002; 20:633–40.
32. Haynes MK, Hume EL, Smith JB. Phenotypic characterization of inflammatory cells from osteoarthritic synovium and synovial fluids. *Clin Immunol* 2002; 105:315–25.
33. Spector TD, Hart DJ, Nandra D, et al. Low-level increases in serum C-reactive protein are present in early osteoarthritis of the knee and predict progressive disease. *Arthritis Rheum* 1997; 40:723–7.
34. Benito MJ, Veale DJ, FitzGerald O, van den Berg WB, Bresnihan B. Synovial tissue inflammation in early and late osteoarthritis. *Ann Rheum Dis* 2005; 64:1263–7.
35. Ayral X, Dougados M. Viability of chondroscopy as a means of cartilage assessment. *Ann Rheum Dis* 1995; 54:613–14.

36. Roach HI, Aigner T, Soder S, Haag J, Welkerling H. Pathobiology of osteoarthritis: pathomechanisms and potential therapeutic targets. *Curr Drug Targets* 2007; 8:271–82.

37. De Clerck LS, De Gendt CM, Bridts CH, Van Osselaer N, Stevens WJ. Expression of neutrophil activation markers and neutrophil adhesion to chondrocytes in rheumatoid arthritis patients: relationship with disease activity. *Res Immunol* 1995; 146:81–7.

38. Haseeb A, Haqqi TM. Immunopathogenesis of osteoarthritis. *Clin Immunol* 2013; 146:185–96.

39. Lingen MWM. Role of leukocytes and endothelial cells in the development of angiogenesis in inflammation and wound healing. *Arch Pathol Lab Med* 2001; 125:67–71.

40. Goldring M, Otero M. Inflammation in osteoarthritis. *Curr Opin Rheumatol* 2011; 23:471–8.

41. Martel-Pelletier J, Pelletier JP. Is osteoarthritis a disease involving only cartilage or other articular tissues? *Eklem Hastalik Cerrahisi* 2010; 21:2–14.

42. Martel-Pelletier J, Alaaeddine N, Pelletier JP. Cytokines and their role in the pathophysiology of osteoarthritis. *Front Biosci* 1999; 4:D694–703.

43. Bondeson J, Wainwright SD, Lauder S, Amos N, Hughes CE. The role of synovial macrophages and macrophage-produced cytokines in driving aggrecanases, matrix metalloproteinases, and other destructive and inflammatory responses in osteoarthritis. *Arthritis Res Ther* 2006; 8:R187.

44. Pettit A, MacDonald K. Differentiated dendritic cells expressing nuclear RelB are predominantly located in rheumatoid synovial tissue perivascular mononuclear cell aggregates. *Arthritis Rheum* 2000; 43:791–800.

45. Cao Y, Cao Y, Meng H, et al. Dendritic cells of synovium in experimental model of osteoarthritis of rabbits. *Cell Physiol Biochem* 2012; 30(1):23–32.

46. Sakkas LI, Platsoucas CD. The role of T cells in the pathogenesis of osteoarthritis. *Arthritis Rheum* 2007; 56:409–24.

47. Fernandez-Madrid F, Karvonen RL, Teitge RA, et al. Synovial thickening detected by MR imaging in osteoarthritis of the knee confirmed by biopsy as synovitis. *Magn Reson Imaging* 1995; 13:177–83.

48. Nakamura H, Yoshino S, Kato T. T-cell mediated inflammatory pathway in osteoarthritis. *Osteoarthritis Cartilage* 1999; 7:401–2.

49. Huss RS, Huddleston JI, Goodman SB, Butcher EC, Zabel B. Synovial tissue-infiltrating natural killer cells in osteoarthritis and periprosthetic inflammation. *Arthritis Rheum* 2010; 62:3799–805.

50. Campbell JJ, Qin S, Unutmaz D, et al. Unique subpopulations of CD56+ NK and NK-T peripheral blood lymphocytes identified by chemokine receptor expression repertoire. *J Immunol* 2001; 166:6477–82.

51. Dar WA, Knechtle SJ. CXCR3-mediated T-cell chemotaxis involves ZAP-70 and is regulated by signalling through the T-cell receptor. *Immunology* 2007; 120:467–85.

52. Jasin H. Autoantibody specificities of immune complexes sequestered in articular cartilage of patients with rheumatoid arthritis and osteoarthritis. *Arthritis Rheum* 1985; 28(3):241–8.

53. Cooke TD, Bennett EL, Ohno O. The deposition of immunoglobulins and complement in osteoarthritic cartilage. *Int Orthop* 1980; 4:211–7.

54. Walsh DA, Haywood L. Angiogenesis: a therapeutic target in arthritis. *Curr Opin Investig Drugs* 2001; 2:1054–63.

55. Ashraf S, Walsh DA. Angiogenesis in osteoarthritis. *Curr Opin Rheumatol* 2008; 20:573–80.

56. Hasegawa M, Segawa T, Maeda M, Yoshida T, Sudo A. Thrombin-cleaved osteopontin levels in synovial fluid correlate with disease severity of knee osteoarthritis. *J Rheumatol* 2011; 38:129–34.

57. Liekens S, De Clercq E, Neyts J. Angiogenesis: regulators and clinical applications. *Biochem Pharmacol* 2001; 61:253–70.

58. Ferrara N. Role of vascular endothelial growth factor in regulation of physiological angiogenesis. *Am J Physiol Cell Physiol* 2001; 280:C1358–66.

59. Van Hinsbergh VW, Koolwijk P, Hanemaaijer R. Role of fibrin and plasminogen activators in repair-associated angiogenesis: in vitro studies with human endothelial cells. *EXS* 1997; 79:391–411.

60. Stevens CR, Blake DR, Merry P, Revell PA, Levick JR. A comparative study by morphometry of the microvasculature in normal and rheumatoid synovium. *Arthritis Rheum* 1991; 34:1508–13.

61. Walsh DA, Bonnet CS, Turner EL, et al. Angiogenesis in the synovium and at the osteochondral junction in osteoarthritis. *Osteoarthritis Cartilage* 2007; 15:743–51.

62. Smith JO, Oreffo ROC, Clarke NMP, Roach HI. Changes in the antiangiogenic properties of articular cartilage in osteoarthritis. *J Orthop Sci* 2003; 8:849–57.

63. Suri S, Walsh DA. Osteochondral alterations in osteoarthritis. *Bone* 2012; 51:204–11.

64. Mapp PI, Walsh DA. Mechanisms and targets of angiogenesis and nerve growth in osteoarthritis. *Nat Rev Rheumatol* 2012; 8:390–8.

65. Klein-Wieringa IR, Kloppenburg M, Bastiaansen-Jenniskens YM, et al. The infrapatellar fat pad of patients with osteoarthritis has an inflammatory phenotype. *Ann Rheum Dis* 2011; 70:851–7.

66. Frayn KN, Karpe, F, Fielding BA, Macdonald IA, Coppack SW. Integrative physiology of human adipose tissue. *Int J Obes Relat Metab Disord* 2003; 27:875–88.

67. Liu J, Divoux A, Sun J, et al. Genetic deficiency and pharmacological stabilization of mast cells reduce diet-induced obesity and diabetes in mice. *Nat Med* 2009; 15:940–5.

68. Suri S, Gill SE, Massena de Camin S, et al. Neurovascular invasion at the osteochondral junction and in osteophytes in osteoarthritis. *Ann Rheum Dis* 2007; 66:1423–8.

69. Pottie P, Presle N, Terlain B, et al. Obesity and osteoarthritis: more complex than predicted! *Ann Rheum Dis* 2006; 65:1403–5.

70. Clockaerts S, Bastiaansen-Jenniskens YM, et al. The infrapatellar fat pad should be considered as an active osteoarthritic joint tissue: a narrative review. *Osteoarthritis Cartilage* 2010; 18:876–82.

71. Fain JN. Release of interleukins and other inflammatory cytokines by human adipose tissue is enhanced in obesity and primarily due to the nonfat cells. *Vitam Horm* 2006; 74:443–77.

72. Iwata M, Ota KT, Duman RS. The inflammasome: pathways linking psychological stress, depression, and systemic illnesses. *Brain Behav Immun* 2013; 31:105–14.

73. Klop B, Elte JWF, Cabezas MC. Dyslipidemia in obesity: mechanisms and potential targets. *Nutrients* 2013; 5:1218–40.

74. Thijssen E, van Caam A, van der Kraan PM. Obesity and osteoarthritis, more than just wear and tear: pivotal roles for inflamed adipose tissue and dyslipidaemia in obesity-induced osteoarthritis. *Rheumatology (Oxford)* 20145; 54(4):588–600.

75. Sturmer T, Sun Y, Sauerland S, et al. Serum cholesterol and osteoarthritis. The baseline examination of the Ulm Osteoarthritis Study. *J Rheumatol* 1998; 25:1827–32.

76. Triantaphyllidou I-E, Kalyvioti E, Karavia E. Perturbations in the HDL metabolic pathway predispose to the development of osteoarthritis in mice following long-term exposure to western-type diet. *Osteoarthritis Cartilage* 2013; 21:322–30.

77. Bijlsma JWJ, Berenbaum F, Lafeber FPJG. Osteoarthritis: an update with relevance for clinical practice. *Lancet* 2011; 377:2115–26.

78. Torres L, Dunlop DD, Peterfy C, et al. The relationship between specific tissue lesions and pain severity in persons with knee osteoarthritis. *Osteoarthritis Cartilage* 2006; 14:1033–40.

79. Dougados M. Clinical assessment of osteoarthritis in clinical trials. *Curr Opin Rheumatol* 1995; 7:87–91.

80. Sowers M, Karvonen-Gutierrez CA, Jacobson JA, Jiang Y, Yosef M. Associations of anatomical measures from MRI with radiographically defined knee osteoarthritis score, pain, and physical functioning. *J Bone Joint Surg Am* 2011; 93:241–51.

81. Roemer FW, Kassim Javaid M, Guermazi A, et al. Anatomical distribution of synovitis in knee osteoarthritis and its association with joint effusion assessed on non-enhanced and contrast-enhanced MRI. *Osteoarthritis Cartilage* 2010; 18:1269–74.

82. Conaghan PG, D'Agostino MA, Le Bars M, et al. Clinical and ultrasonographic predictors of joint replacement for knee osteoarthritis: results from a large, 3-year, prospective EULAR study. *Ann Rheum Dis* 2010; 69:644–7.

83. Krasnokutsky S, Belitskaya-Lévy I, Bencardino J, et al. Quantitative magnetic resonance imaging evidence of synovial proliferation is associated with radiographic severity of knee osteoarthritis. *Arthritis Rheum* 2011; 63:2983–91.

84. Scanzello CR, Goldring SR. The role of synovitis in osteoarthritis pathogenesis. *Bone* 2012; 51:249–57.

85. Martelpelletier J. Pathophysiology of osteoarthritis. *Osteoarthritis Cartilage* 2004; 12:31–33.

86. Brandt KD, Dieppe P, Radin E. Etiopathogenesis of osteoarthritis. *Med Clin North Am* 2009; 93:1–24.

87. Hunter DJ, McDougall JJ, Keefe FJ. The symptoms of osteoarthritis and the genesis of pain. *Med Clin North Am* 2009; 93:83–100.

88. Krasnokutsky S, Attur M, Palmer G, Samuels J, Abramson SB. Current concepts in the pathogenesis of osteoarthritis. *Osteoarthritis Cartilage* 2008; 16(Suppl 3):S1–3.

89. Krenn V, Morawietz L, Burmester GR, et al. Synovitis score: discrimination between chronic low-grade and high-grade synovitis. *Histopathology* 2006; 49:358–64.

90. Ayral X, Ravaud P, Bonvarlet JP, et al. Arthroscopic evaluation of post-traumatic patellofemoral chondropathy. *J Rheumatol* 1999; 26:1140–7.

91. Hayashi D, Roemer FW, Katur A, et al. Imaging of synovitis in osteoarthritis: current status and outlook. *Semin Arthritis Rheum* 2011; 41:116–30.

92. Guermazi A, Hayashi D, Roemer FW, et al. Synovitis in knee osteoarthritis assessed by contrast-enhanced magnetic resonance imaging (MRI) is associated with radiographic tibiofemoral osteoarthritis and MRI-detected widespread cartilage damage: the MOST study. *J Rheumatol* 2014; 41:501–8.

93. Pelletier JP, Raynauld JP, Abram F, et al. A new non-invasive method to assess synovitis severity in relation to symptoms and cartilage volume loss in knee osteoarthritis patients using MRI. *Osteoarthritis Cartilage* 2008; 16(Suppl 3):S8–13.

94. Peterfy CG, Guermazi A, Zaim S, et al. Whole-Organ Magnetic Resonance Imaging Score (WORMS) of the knee in osteoarthritis. *Osteoarthritis Cartilage* 2004; 12:177–90.

95. Fotinos-Hoyer AK, Guermazi A, Jara H, et al. Assessment of synovitis in the osteoarthritic knee: Comparison between manual segmentation, semiautomated segmentation, and semiquantitative assessment using contrast-enhanced fat-suppressed T1-weighted MRI. *Magn Reson Med* 2010; 64:604–9.

96. Rhodes LA, Grainger AJ, Keenan AM, et al. The validation of simple scoring methods for evaluating compartment-specific synovitis detected by MRI in knee osteoarthritis. *Rheumatology* 2005; 44:1569–73.

97. Haugen IK, Østergaard M, Eshed I, et al. Iterative development and reliability of the OMERACT Hand Osteoarthritis MRI Scoring System. *J Rheumatol* 2014; 41:386–91.

98. Roemer FW, Crema MD, Trattnig S, Guermazi A. Advances in imaging of osteoarthritis and cartilage. *Radiology* 2011; 260:332–54.

99. Ostergaard, M. Different approaches to synovial membrane volume determination by magnetic resonance imaging: manual versus automated segmentation. *Br J Rheumatol* 1997; 36:1166–77.

100. De Lange-Brokaar BJE, Ioan-Facsinay A, Yusuf E, et al. Degree of synovitis on MRI by comprehensive whole knee semi-quantitative scoring method correlates with histologic and macroscopic features of synovial tissue inflammation in knee osteoarthritis. *Osteoarthritis Cartilage* 2014; 22:1606–13.

101. Loeuille D, Rat AC, Goebel JC, et al. Magnetic resonance imaging in osteoarthritis: which method best reflects synovial membrane inflammation?. Correlations with clinical, macroscopic and microscopic features. *Osteoarthritis Cartilage* 2009; 17:1186–92.

102. Atukorala I, Kwoh CK, Guermazi A, et al. Synovitis in knee osteoarthritis: a precursor of disease? *Ann Rheum Dis* 2016; 75(2):390–5.

103. Roemer FW, Zhang Y, Niu J, et al. Tibiofemoral joint osteoarthritis: risk factors for MR-depicted fast cartilage loss over a 30-month period in the multicenter osteoarthritis study. *Radiology* 2009; 252:772–80.

104. Wang X, Blizzard L, Halliday A, et al. Association between MRI-detected knee joint regional effusion-synovitis and structural changes in older adults: a cohort study. *Ann Rheum Dis* 2016; 75(3):519–25.

105. Guermazi A, Niu J, Hayashi D, et al. Prevalence of abnormalities in knees detected by MRI in adults without knee osteoarthritis: population based observational study (Framingham Osteoarthritis Study). *BMJ* 2012; 345:e5339–9.

106. Mancarella L, Magnani M, Addimanda O, et al. Ultrasound-detected synovitis with power Doppler signal is associated with severe radiographic damage and reduced cartilage thickness in hand osteoarthritis. *Osteoarthritis Cartilage* 2010; 18:1263–8.

107. Hall M, Doherty S, Courtney P, et al. Synovial pathology detected on ultrasound correlates with the severity of radiographic knee osteoarthritis more than with symptoms. *Osteoarthritis Cartilage* 2014; 22:1627–33.

108. Keen HI, Wakefield RJ, Grainger AJ, et al. Can ultrasonography improve on radiographic assessment in osteoarthritis of the hands? A comparison between radiographic and ultrasonographic detected pathology. *Ann Rheum Dis* 2008; 67:1116–20.

109. Guermazi A, Roemer FW, Crema MD, Englund M, Hayashi D. Imaging of non-osteochondral tissues in osteoarthritis. *Osteoarthritis Cartilage* 2014; 22:1590–605.

110. Wakefield RJ, D'Agostino MA, Iagnocco A, et al. The OMERACT Ultrasound Group: status of current activities and research directions. *J Rheumatol* 2007; 34:848–51.

111. D'Agostino MA, Conaghan P, Le Bars M, et al. EULAR report on the use of ultrasonography in painful knee osteoarthritis. Part 1: prevalence of inflammation in osteoarthritis. *Ann Rheum Dis* 2005; 64:1703–9.

112. Kortekaas MC, Kwok W-Y, Reijnierse M, Kloppenburg M. Inflammatory ultrasound features show independent associations with progression of structural damage after over 2 years of follow-up in patients with hand osteoarthritis. *Ann Rheum Dis* 2015; 74(9):1720–4.

113. Iagnocco A. Imaging the joint in osteoarthritis: a place for ultrasound? *Best Pract Res Clin Rheumatol* 2010; 24:27–38.

114. Hall M, Doherty S, Courtney P, et al. Synovial pathology detected on ultrasound correlates with the severity of radiographic knee osteoarthritis more than with symptoms. *Osteoarthritis Cartilage* 2014; 22:1627–33.

115. Van Spil WE, Jansen NW, Bijlsma JW, et al. Clusters within a wide spectrum of biochemical markers for osteoarthritis: data from CHECK, a large cohort of individuals with very early symptomatic osteoarthritis. *Osteoarthritis Cartilage* 2012; 20:745–54.

116. Garnero P, Aronstein WS, Cohen SB, et al. Relationships between biochemical markers of bone and cartilage degradation with radiological progression in patients with knee osteoarthritis receiving risedronate: the Knee Osteoarthritis Structural Arthritis randomized clinical trial. *Osteoarthritis Cartilage* 2008; 16:660–6.

117. Conrozier T, Carlier MC, Mathieu P, et al. Serum levels of YKL-40 and C reactive protein in patients with hip osteoarthritis and healthy subjects: a cross sectional study. *Ann Rheum Dis* 2000; 59:828–31.

118. Pearle AD, Scanzello CR, George S, et al. Elevated high-sensitivity C-reactive protein levels are associated with local inflammatory findings in patients with osteoarthritis. *Osteoarthritis Cartilage* 2007; 15:516–23.

119. Stürmer T, Brenner H, Koenig W, Günther K-P. Severity and extent of osteoarthritis and low grade systemic inflammation as assessed

by high sensitivity C reactive protein. *Ann Rheum Dis* 2004; 63:200–5.

120. Lafeber FPJG, van Spil WE. Osteoarthritis year 2013 in review: biomarkers; reflecting before moving forward, one step at a time. *Osteoarthritis Cartilage* 2013; 21:1452–64.

121. De Boer TN, van Spil WE, Huisman AM, et al. Serum adipokines in osteoarthritis; comparison with controls and relationship with local parameters of synovial inflammation and cartilage damage. *Osteoarthritis Cartilage* 2012; 20:846–53.

122. Yusuf E, Ioan-Facsinay A, Bijsterbosch J, et al. Association between leptin, adiponectin and resistin and long-term progression of hand osteoarthritis. *Ann Rheum Dis* 2011; 70:1282–4.

123. Heinegård D, Saxne T. The role of the cartilage matrix in osteoarthritis. *Nat Rev Rheumatol* 2011; 7:50–6.

124. Andriacchi TP, Mündermann A, Smith RL, et al. A framework for the in vivo pathomechanics of osteoarthritis at the knee. *Ann Biomed Eng* 2004; 32:447–57.

125. Englund M, Guermazi A, Gale D, et al. Incidental meniscal findings on knee MRI in middle-aged and elderly persons. *N Engl J Med* 2008; 359:1108–15.

126. Lohmander LS, Englund PM, Dahl LL, Roos EM. The long-term consequence of anterior cruciate ligament and meniscus injuries: osteoarthritis. *Am J Sports Med* 2007; 35:1756–69.

127. Lotz MK, Kraus VB. Correction: Posttraumatic osteoarthritis: pathogenesis and pharmacological treatment options. *Arthritis Res Ther* 2010; 12:408.

128. Scanzello CR, Plaas A, Crow MK. Innate immune system activation in osteoarthritis: is osteoarthritis a chronic wound? *Curr Opin Rheumatol* 2008; 20:565–72.

129. Ishijima M, Watari T, Naito K, et al. Relationships between biomarkers of cartilage, bone, synovial metabolism and knee pain provide insights into the origins of pain in early knee osteoarthritis. *Arthritis Res Ther* 2011; 13:R22.

130. Janeway CA, Medzhitov R. Innate immune recognition. *Annu Rev Immunol* 2002; 20:197–216.

131. Foell D, Wittkowski H, Vogl T, Roth J. S100 proteins expressed in phagocytes: a novel group of damage-associated molecular pattern molecules. *J Leukoc Biol* 2007; 81:28–37.

132. Midwood K, Sacre S, Piccinini AM, et al. Tenascin-C is an endogenous activator of Toll-like receptor 4 that is essential for maintaining inflammation in arthritic joint disease. *Nat Med* 2009; 15:774–80.

133. Lasarte JJ, Casares N, Gorraiz M, et al. The extra domain A from fibronectin targets antigens to TLR4-expressing cells and induces cytotoxic T cell responses in vivo. *J Immunol* 2007; 178:748–56.

134. Taylor KR, Trowbridge JM, Rudisill JA, et al. Hyaluronan fragments stimulate endothelial recognition of injury through TLR4. *J Biol Chem* 2004; 279:17079–84.

135. Schaefer L, Babelova A, Kiss E, et al. The matrix component biglycan is proinflammatory and signals through Toll-like receptors 4 and 2 in macrophages. *J Clin Invest* 2005; 115:2223–33.

136. Sohn D, Sokolove J, Sharpe O, et al. Plasma proteins present in osteoarthritic synovial fluid can stimulate cytokine production via Toll-like receptor 4. *Arthritis Res Ther* 2012; 14:R7.

137. Wang Q, Rozelle AL, Lepus CM, et al. Identification of a central role for complement in osteoarthritis. *Nat Med* 2011; 17:1674–9.

138. Liu-Bryan R, Terkeltaub R. The growing array of innate inflammatory ignition switches in osteoarthritis. *Arthritis Rheum* 2012; 64:2055–8.

139. Blom AB, van Lent PL, Libregts S, et al. Crucial role of macrophages in matrix metalloproteinase-mediated cartilage destruction during experimental osteoarthritis: Involvement of matrix metalloproteinase 3. *Arthritis Rheum* 2007; 56:147–57.

140. Loeser R, Goldring S. Osteoarthritis: a disease of the joint as an organ. *Arthritis Rheumatol* 2012; 64:1697–707.

141. Abdollahi-Roodsaz S, Joosten LA, Koenders MI, et al. Stimulation of TLR2 and TLR4 differentially skews the balance of T cells in a mouse model of arthritis. *J Clin Invest* 2008; 118:205–16.

142. Sjöberg AP, Manderson GA, Mörgelin M, et al. Short leucine-rich glycoproteins of the extracellular matrix display diverse patterns of complement interaction and activation. *Mol Immunol* 2009; 46:830–9.

143. Gobezie R, Kho A, Krastins B, et al. High abundance synovial fluid proteome: distinct profiles in health and osteoarthritis. *Arthritis Res Ther* 2007; 9:R36.

144. Lepus CM, Song JJ, Wang Q, et al. Brief report: carboxypeptidase B serves as a protective mediator in osteoarthritis. *Arthritis Rheumatol (Hoboken, NJ)* 2014; 66:101–6.

145. O'Dell JR. Rheumatoid arthritis: the clinical picture. In Koopman WJ (ed) *Arthritis and Allied Conditions: A Textbook of Rheumatology*. Philadelphia, PA: Lippincott Williams & Wilkins, 2001:1153–74.

146. Goldring MB. The role of cytokines as inflammatory mediators in osteoarthritis: lessons from animal models. *Connect Tissue Res* 1999; 40:1–11.

147. Goldring MB. Anticytokine therapy for osteoarthritis. *Expert Opin Biol Ther* 2001; 1:817–29.

148. Van de Loo FAJ, Joosten LAB, Van Lent PLEM, Arntz OJ, Van den Berg WB. Role of interleukin-1, tumor necrosis factor alpha, and interleukin-6 in cartilage proteoglycan metabolism and destruction: effect of in situ blocking in murine antigen- and zymosan-induced arthritis. *Arthritis Rheum* 1995; 38:164–72.

149. Caron JP, Fernandes JC, Martel-Pelletier J, et al. Chondroprotective effect of intraarticular injections of interleukin-1 receptor antagonist in experimental osteoarthritis. Suppression of collagenase-1 expression. *Arthritis Rheum* 1996; 39:1535–44.

150. Steenvoorden MMC, Bank RA, Ronday HK, et al. Fibroblast-like synoviocyte-chondrocyte interaction in cartilage degradation. *Clin Exp Rheumatol* 2007; 25:239–45.

151. Pfander D, Heinz N, Rothe P, Carl H-D, Swoboda B. Tenascin and aggrecan expression by articular chondrocytes is influenced by interleukin 1beta: a possible explanation for the changes in matrix synthesis during osteoarthritis. *Ann Rheum Dis* 2004; 63:240–4.

152. Goldring MB, Birkhead J, Sandell LJ, Kimura T, Krane SM. Interleukin 1 suppresses expression of cartilage-specific types II and IX collagens and increases types I and III collagens in human chondrocytes. *J Clin Invest* 1988; 82:2026–37.

153. Fernandes JC, Martel-Pelletier J, Pelletier J-P. The role of cytokines in osteoarthritis pathophysiology. *Biorheology* 2002; 39:237–46.

154. Page Thomas DP, King B, Stephens T, Dingle JT. In vivo studies of cartilage regeneration after damage induced by catabolin/interleukin-1. *Ann Rheum Dis* 1991; 50:75–80.

155. Henderson B, Pettipher ER. Arthritogenic actions of recombinant IL-1 and tumour necrosis factor alpha in the rabbit: evidence for synergistic interactions between cytokines in vivo. *Clin Exp Immunol* 1989; 75:306–10.

156. Attur MG, Pate I, Patel RN, Abramson SB, Amin AR. Autocrine production of IL-1 beta by human osteoarthritis-affected cartilage and differential regulation of endogenous nitric oxide, IL-6, prostaglandin E2, and IL-8. *Proc Assoc Am Physicians* 1998; 110:65–72

157. Westacott CI, Barakat AF, Wood L, et al. Tumor necrosis factor alpha can contribute to focal loss of cartilage in osteoarthritis. *Osteoarthritis Cartilage* 2000; 8:213–21.

158. Alaaeddine N, DiBattista JA, Pelletier JP, et al. Osteoarthritic synovial fibroblasts possess an increased level of tumor necrosis factor-receptor 55 (TNF-R55) that mediates biological activation by TNF-alpha. *J Rheumatol* 1997; 24:1985–94.

159. Kapoor M, Martel-Pelletier J, Lajeunesse D, Pelletier J-P, Fahmi H. Role of proinflammatory cytokines in the pathophysiology of osteoarthritis. *Nat Rev Rheumatol* 2011; 7:33–42.

160. Afonso V, Champy R, Mitrovic D, Collin P, Lomri A. Reactive oxygen species and superoxide dismutases: role in joint diseases. *Joint Bone Spine* 2007; 74:324–9.

161. Scott JL, Gabrielides C, Davidson RK, et al. Superoxide dismutase downregulation in osteoarthritis progression and end-stage disease. *Ann Rheum Dis* 2010; 69:1502–10.

162. Gibson JS, Milner PI, White R, Fairfax TPA, Wilkins RJ. Oxygen and reactive oxygen species in articular cartilage: modulators of ionic homeostasis. *Pflugers Arch Eur J Physiol* 2008; 455:563–73.

163. Henrotin YE, Bruckner P, Pujol JPL. The role of reactive oxygen species in homeostasis and degradation of cartilage. *Osteoarthritis Cartilage* 2003; 11:747–55.

164. Mathy-Hartert M, Martin G, Devel P, et al. Reactive oxygen species downregulate the expression of pro-inflammatory genes by human chondrocytes. *Inflamm Res* 2003; 52:111–18.

165. Vrtačnik P, Marc J, Ostanek B. Epigenetic mechanisms in bone. *Clin Chem Lab Med* 2014; 52:589–608.

166. Barter MJ, Bui C, Young DA. Epigenetic mechanisms in cartilage and osteoarthritis: DNA methylation, histone modifications and microRNAs. *Osteoarthritis Cartilage* 2012; 20:339–49.

167. Felson DT. Developments in the clinical understanding of osteoarthritis. *Arthritis Res Ther* 2009; 11:203.

168. Felson DT. The sources of pain in knee osteoarthritis. *Curr Opin Rheumatol* 2005; 17:624–8.

169. Creamer P, Hunt M, Dieppe P. Pain mechanisms in osteoarthritis of the knee: effect of intraarticular anesthetic. *J Rheumatol* 1996; 23:1031–6.

170. Acosta C, Davies A. Bacterial lipopolysaccharide regulates nociceptin expression in sensory neurons. *J Neurosci Res* 2008; 86:1077–86.

171. Kim D, You B, Lim H, Lee SJ. Toll-like receptor 2 contributes to chemokine gene expression and macrophage infiltration in the dorsal root ganglia after peripheral nerve injury. *Mol Pain* 2011; 7:74.

172. Liu T, Gao Y-J, Ji R-R. Emerging role of Toll-like receptors in the control of pain and itch. *Neurosci Bull* 2012; 28:131–44.

173. Sokolove J, Lepus CM. Role of inflammation in the pathogenesis of osteoarthritis: latest findings and interpretations. *Ther Adv Musculoskelet Dis* 2013; 5:77–94.

174. Schaible HG, Grubb BD. Afferent and spinal mechanisms of joint pain. *Pain* 1993; 55:5–54.

175. Coutaux A, Adam F, Willer JC, Le Bars D. Hyperalgesia and allodynia: peripheral mechanisms. *Jt Bone Spine* 2005; 72:359–71.

176. Malfait A-M, Schnitzer TJ. Towards a mechanism-based approach to pain management in osteoarthritis. *Nat Rev Rheumatol* 2013; 9:654–64.

177. Yu C-J, Ko CJ, Hsieh CH, et al. Proteomic analysis of osteoarthritic chondrocyte reveals the hyaluronic acid-regulated proteins involved in chondroprotective effect under oxidative stress. *J Proteomics* 2014; 99:40–53.

178. Mapp PI, Kidd BL, Gibson SJ, et al. Substance P-, calcitonin gene-related peptide- and C-flanking peptide of neuropeptide Y-immunoreactive fibres are present in normal synovium but depleted in patients with rheumatoid arthritis. *Neuroscience* 1990; 37:143–53.

179. Buma P, Verschuren C, Versleyen D, Van der Kraan P, Oestreicher AB. Calcitonin gene-related peptide, substance P and GAP-43/B-50 immunoreactivity in the normal and arthrotic knee joint of the mouse. *Histochemistry* 1992; 98:327–39.

180. Mayer DJ, Mao J, Holt J, Price DD. Cellular mechanisms of neuropathic pain, morphine tolerance, and their interactions. *Proc Natl Acad Sci U S A* 1999; 96:7731–6.

181. Walsh DA, Hu DE, Mapp PI, et al. Innervation and neurokinin receptors during angiogenesis in the rat sponge granuloma. *Histochem J* 1996; 28:759–69.

182. Fortier LA, Nixon AJ. Distributional changes in substance P nociceptive fiber patterns in naturally osteoarthritic articulations. *J Rheumatol* 1997; 24:524–30.

183. Eitner A, Pester J, Nietzsche S, Hofmann GO, Schaible H-G. The innervation of synovium of human osteoarthritic joints in comparison with normal rat and sheep synovium. *Osteoarthritis Cartilage* 2013; 21:1383–91.

184. Dray A, Read SJ. Arthritis and pain. Future targets to control osteoarthritis pain. *Arthritis Res Ther* 2007; 9:212.

185. McDougall JJ. Arthritis and pain. Neurogenic origin of joint pain. *Arthritis Res Ther* 2006; 8:220.

186. Ordeberg G. Characterization of joint pain in human OA. *Novartis Found Symp* 2004; 260:105–15.

187. Bradley LA, Kersh BC, DeBerry JJ, et al. Lessons from fibromyalgia: abnormal pain sensitivity in knee osteoarthritis. *Novartis Found Symp* 2004; 260:258–70.

188. Bedson J, Croft PR. The discordance between clinical and radiographic knee osteoarthritis: a systematic search and summary of the literature. *BMC Musculoskelet Disord* 2008; 9:116.

189. Hannan MT, Felson DT, Pincus T. Analysis of the discordance between radiographic changes and knee pain in osteoarthritis of the knee. *J Rheumatol* 2000; 27:1513–17.

190. Duncan R, Peat G, Thomas E, et al. Symptoms and radiographic osteoarthritis: not as discordant as they are made out to be? *Ann Rheum Dis* 2007; 66:86–91.

191. Neogi T, Felson D, Niu J, et al. Association between radiographic features of knee osteoarthritis and pain: results from two cohort studies. *BMJ* 2009; 339:b2844–b2844.

192. Felson DT, Chaisson CE, Hill CL, et al. The association of bone marrow lesions with pain in knee osteoarthritis. *Ann Intern Med* 2001; 134:541–9.

193. Lo GH, McAlindon TE, Niu J, et al. Bone marrow lesions and joint effusion are strongly and independently associated with weight-bearing pain in knee osteoarthritis: data from the osteoarthritis initiative. *Osteoarthritis Cartilage* 2009; 17:1562–9.

194. Wenham CYJ, Grainger AJ, Hensor EM, et al. Methotrexate for pain relief in knee osteoarthritis: An open-label study. *Rheumatol (United Kingdom)* 2013; 52:888–92.

195. Marcu KB, Otero M, Olivotto E, Borzi RM, Goldring MB. NF-kappa B signaling: multiple angles to target OA. *Curr Drug Targets* 2010; 11:599–613.

196. Mobasheri A. The future of osteoarthritis therapeutics: emerging biological therapy. *Curr Rheumatol Rep* 2013; 15:385.

197. Magnano MD, Chakravarty EF, Broudy C, et al. A pilot study of tumor necrosis factor inhibition in erosive/inflammatory osteoarthritis of the hands. *J Rheumatol* 2007; 34:1323–7.

198. Verbruggen G, Wittoek R, Vander Cruyssen B, Elewaut D. Tumour necrosis factor blockade for the treatment of erosive osteoarthritis of the interphalangeal finger joints: a double blind, randomised trial on structure modification. *Ann Rheum Dis* 2012; 71:891–8.

199. Chevalier X, Ravaud P, Maheu E, et al. Adalimumab in patients with hand osteoarthritis refractory to analgesics and NSAIDs: a randomised, multicentre, double-blind, placebo-controlled trial. *Ann Rheum Dis* 2015; 74(9):1697–705.

200. Fioravanti A, Fabbroni M, Cerase A, Galeazzi M. Treatment of erosive osteoarthritis of the hands by intra-articular infliximab injections: a pilot study. *Rheumatol Int* 2009; 29:961–5.

201. Grunke M, Schulze-Koops H. Successful treatment of inflammatory knee osteoarthritis with tumour necrosis factor blockade. *Ann Rheum Dis* 2006; 65:555–6.

202. Maksymowych WP, Russell AS, Chiu P, et al. Targeting tumour necrosis factor alleviates signs and symptoms of inflammatory osteoarthritis of the knee. *Arthritis Res Ther* 2012; 14:R206.

203. Urech DM, Feige U, Ewert S, et al. Anti-inflammatory and cartilage-protecting effects of an intra-articularly injected anti-TNF{alpha} single-chain Fv antibody (ESBA105) designed for local therapeutic use. *Ann Rheum Dis* 2010; 69:443–9.

204. Pelletier JP, Caron JP, Evans C, et al. In vivo suppression of early experimental osteoarthritis by interleukin-1 receptor antagonist using gene therapy. *Arthritis Rheum* 1997; 40:1012–9.

205. Chevalier X, Eymard F, Richette P. Biologic agents in osteoarthritis: hopes and disappointments. *Nat Rev Rheumatol* 2013; 9:400–10.

206. Baragi VM, Renkiewicz RR, Jordan H, et al. Transplantation of transduced chondrocytes protects articular cartilage from interleukin 1-induced extracellular matrix degradation. *J Clin Invest* 1995; 96:2454–60.

207. Attur MG, Dave MN, Leung MY, et al. Functional genomic analysis of type II IL-1beta decoy receptor: potential for gene therapy in human arthritis and inflammation. *J Immunol* 2002; 168:2001–10.

208. Chevalier X, Goupille P, Beaulieu AD, et al. Intraarticular injection of anakinra in osteoarthritis of the knee: a multicenter, randomized, double-blind, placebo-controlled study. *Arthritis Rheum* 2009; 61:344–52.

209. Bacconnier L, Jorgensen C, Fabre S. Erosive osteoarthritis of the hand: clinical experience with anakinra. *Ann Rheum Dis* 2009; 68:1078–9.

210. Chevalier X, Conrozier T, Richette P. Desperately looking for the right target in osteoarthritis: the anti-IL-1 strategy. *Arthritis Res Ther* 2011; 13:124.

211. Brown C, Toth A, Magnussen R. Clinical benefits of intra-articular anakinra for persistent knee effusion. *J Knee Surg* 2011; 24:61–5.

212. Kraus VB, Birmingham J, Stabler TV, et al. Effects of intraarticular IL1-Ra for acute anterior cruciate ligament knee injury: a randomized controlled pilot trial (NCT00332254). *Osteoarthritis Cartilage* 2012; 0:271–8.

213. Bendrups A, Hilton A, Meager A, Hamilton JA. Reduction of tumor necrosis factor a and interleukin-1b levels in human synovial tissue by interleukin-4 and glucocorticoid. *Rheumatol Int* 1993; 12:217–20.

214. Van Roon JA, Lafeber FP, Bijlsma JW. Synergistic activity of interleukin-4 and interleukin-10 in suppression of inflammation and joint destruction in rheumatoid arthritis. *Arthritis Rheum* 2001; 44:3–12.

215. Hartgring S, Steen-Louws C, Hack C, et al. IL4–10 Synerkine: a novel immunoregulatory drug to prevent immunopathology in rheumatic diseases. *Arthritis Rheum* 2013; 65(Suppl 1):1763.

216. Vlad SC, Neogi T, Aliabadi P, Fontes JDT, Felson DT. No association between markers of inflammation and osteoarthritis of the hands and knees. *J Rheumatol* 2011; 38:1665–70.

217. Van der Kraan PM, van den Berg WB. Chondrocyte hypertrophy and osteoarthritis: role in initiation and progression of cartilage degeneration? *Osteoarthritis Cartilage* 2012; 20:223–32.

218. Blagojevic M, Jinks C, Jeffery A, Jordan KP. Risk factors for onset of osteoarthritis of the knee in older adults: a systematic review and meta-analysis. *Osteoarthritis Cartilage* 2010; 18:24–33.

219. Li W, Abram F, Pelletier JP, et al. Fully automated system for the quantification of human osteoarthritic knee joint effusion volume using magnetic resonance imaging. *Arthritis Res Ther* 2010; 12:R173.

220. Raynauld JP, Kauffmann C, Beaudoin G, et al. Reliability of a quantification imaging system using magnetic resonance images to measure cartilage thickness and volume in human normal and osteoarthritic knees. *Osteoarthr Cartil* 2003; 11:351–60.

221. Meszaros E, Malemud CJ. Prospects for treating osteoarthritis: enzyme-protein interactions regulating matrix metalloproteinase activity. *Ther Adv Chronic Dis* 2012; 3:219–29.

222. Shakibaei M, Schulze-Tanzil G, John T, Mobasheri A. Curcumin protects human chondrocytes from IL-1β-induced inhibition of collagen type II and β1-integrin expression and activation of caspase-3: an immunomorphological study. *Ann Anat* 2005; 187:487–97.

223. Wojdasiewicz P, Poniatowski AA, Szukiewicz D. The role of inflammatory and anti-inflammatory cytokines in the pathogenesis of osteoarthritis. *Mediators Inflamm* 2014; 2014:561459.

224. Palmer G, Guerne P-A, Mezin F, et al. Production of interleukin-1 receptor antagonist by human articular chondrocytes. *Arthritis Res* 2002; 4:226–31.

225. Van Meegeren ME, Roosendaal G, Jansen NWD, et al. IL-4 alone and in combination with IL-10 protects against blood-induced cartilage damage. *Osteoarthritis Cartilage* 2012; 20(7):764–72.

226. Yorimitsu M, Nishida K, Shimizu A, et al. Intra-articular injection of interleukin-4 decreases nitric oxide production by chondrocytes and ameliorates subsequent destruction of cartilage in instability-induced osteoarthritis in rat knee joints. *Osteoarthr Cartil* 2008; 16:764–71.

227. Distel E, Cadoudal T, Durant S, Poignard A, Chevalier X, Benelli C. The infrapatellar fat pad in knee osteoarthritis: an important source of interleukin-6 and its soluble receptor. *Arthritis Rheum* 2009; 60(11):3374–7.

228. Chauffier K, Laiguillon MC, Bougault C, et al. Induction of the chemokine IL-8/Kc by the articular cartilage: possible influence on osteoarthritis. *Jt Bone Spine* 2012; 79:604–9.

229. Alaaeddine N, Di Battista JA, Pelletier J, et al. Inhibition of tumor necrosis factor alpha-induced prostaglandin E2 production by the antiinflammatory cytokines interleukin-4, interleukin-10, and interleukin-13 in osteoarthritic synovial fibroblasts. *Arthritis Rheum* 1999; 42(4):710–18.

230. Hart PH, Ahern MJ, Smith MD, Finlay-Jones JJ. Comparison of the suppressive effects of interleukin-10 and interleukin-4 on synovial fluid macrophages and blood monocytes from patients with inflammatory arthritis. *Immunology* 1995; 84:536–42.

231. Scanzello CR, Umoh E, Pessler F, et al. Local cytokine profiles in knee osteoarthritis: elevated synovial fluid interleukin-15 differentiates early from end-stage disease. *Osteoarthritis Cartilage* 2009; 17:1040–8.

232. Honorati MC, Bovara M, Cattini L, Piacentini A, Facchini A. Contribution of interleukin 17 to human cartilage degradation and synovial inflammation in osteoarthritis. *Osteoarthritis Cartilage* 2002; 10:799–807.

233. Dinarello CA. Overview of the interleukin-1 family of ligands and receptors. *Semin Immunol* 2013; 25:389–93.

234. Lefebvre V, Peeters-Joris C, Vaes G. Modulation by interleukin 1 and tumor necrosis factor alpha of production of collagenase, tissue inhibitor of metalloproteinases and collagen types in differentiated and dedifferentiated articular chondrocytes. *Biochim Biophys Acta* 1990; 1052:366–78.

235. El Mansouri FE, Chabane N, Zayed N, et al. Contribution of H3K4 methylation by SET-1A to interleukin-1-induced cyclooxygenase 2 and inducible nitric oxide synthase expression in human osteoarthritis chondrocytes. *Arthritis Rheum* 2011; 63(1):168–79.

236. Hsu YH, Hsieh MS, Liang YC, et al. Production of the chemokine eotaxin-1 in osteoarthritis and its role in cartilage degradation. *J Cell Biochem* 2004; 93:929–39.

237. Blaney Davidson EN, van der Kraan PM, van den Berg WB. TGF-beta and osteoarthritis. *Osteoarthritis Cartilage* 2007; 15:597–604.

238. Chen H-T, Tsou H-K, Chen J-C, Shih JM-K, Chen Y-J, Tang C-H. Adiponectin enhances intercellular adhesion molecule-1 expression and promotes monocyte adhesion in human synovial fibroblasts. *PLoS One* 2014; 9(3):e92741.

239. Qatanani M, Szwergold NR, Greaves DR, Ahima RS, Lazar MA. Macrophage-derived human resistin exacerbates adipose tissue inflammation and insulin resistance in mice. *J Clin Invest* 2009; 119:531–9.

240. Chen W-P, Bao J-P, Feng J, Hu P-F, Shi Z-L, Wu L-D. Increased serum concentrations of visfatin and its production by different joint tissues in patients with osteoarthritis. *Clin Chem Lab Med* 2010; 48:1141–5.

241. Dumond H, Presle N, Terlain B, et al. Evidence for a key role of leptin in osteoarthritis. *Arthritis Rheum* 2003; 48:3118–29.

242. Koskinen A, Vuolteenaho K, Moilanen T, Moilanen E. Resistin as a factor in osteoarthritis: synovial fluid resistin concentrations correlate positively with interleukin 6 and matrix metalloproteinases MMP-1 and MMP-3. *Scand J Rheumatol* 2014; 43(3):249–53.

243. Ricciotti E, FitzGerald G. Prostaglandins and inflammation. *Arterioscler Thromb* 2011; 31(5):986–1000.

244. Thomas Vangsness J, Burke WS, Narvy SJ, MacPhee RD, Fedenko AN. Human knee synovial fluid cytokines correlated with grade

of knee osteoarthritis: a pilot study. *Bull NYU Hosp Jt Dis* 2011; 69(2):122–7.

245. Lavigne P, Benderdour M, Lajeunesse D, Shi Q, Fernandes JC. Expression of ICAM-1 by osteoblasts in healthy individuals and in patients suffering from osteoarthritis and osteoporosis. *Bone* 2004; 35:463–70.

246. Smith MD, Triantafillou S, Parker A, Youssef PP, Coleman M. Synovial membrane inflammation and cytokine production in patients with early osteoarthritis. *J Rheumatol* 1997; 24:365–71.

247. Shibakawa A, Aoki H, Masuko-Hongo K, et al. Presence of pannus-like tissue on osteoarthritic cartilage and its histological character. *Osteoarthritis Cartilage* 2003; 11:133–40.

248. Rübenhagen R, Schüttrumpf JP, Stürmer KM, Frosch K-H. Interleukin-7 levels in synovial fluid increase with age and MMP-1 levels decrease with progression of osteoarthritis. *Acta Orthop* 2012; 83(1):59–64.

249. Ribbens C, Andre B, Kaye O, et al. Synovial fluid matrix metalloproteinase-3 levels are increased in inflammatory arthritides whether erosive or not. *Rheumatology (Oxford)* 2000; 39:1357–65.

250. Jiang Y, Xiao Q, Hu Z, et al. Tissue levels of leukemia inhibitory factor vary by osteoarthritis grade. *Orthopedics* 2014; 37(5):e460–e464.

251. Shi K, Hayashida K, Kaneko M, et al. Lymphoid chemokine B cell-attracting chemokine-1 (CXCL13) is expressed in germinal center of ectopic lymphoid follicles within the synovium of chronic arthritis patients. *J Immunol* 2001; 166:650–5.

252. Meini S, Maggi CA. Knee osteoarthritis: a role for bradykinin? *Inflamm Res* 2008; 57:351–61.

253. Austin PJ, Moalem-Taylor G. The neuro-immune balance in neuropathic pain: Involvement of inflammatory immune cells, immune-like glial cells and cytokines. *J Neuroimmunol* 2010; 229:26–50.

254. Gold MS, Gebhart GF. Nociceptor sensitization in pain pathogenesis. *Nat Med* 2010; 16:1248–57.

255. Barthel C, Yeremenko N, Jacobs R, et al. Nerve growth factor and receptor expression in rheumatoid arthritis and spondyloarthritis. *Arthritis Res Ther* 2009; 11:R82.

256. Qin Y, Chen Y, Wang W, et al. HMGB1-LPS complex promotes transformation of osteoarthritis synovial fibroblasts to a rheumatoid arthritis synovial fibroblast-like phenotype. *Cell Death Dis* 2014; 5:e1077.

CHAPTER 7

The innervation of the joint and its role in osteoarthritis pain

Jason J. McDougall and Joel A. Vilensky

Introduction

Joint sensory nerves were originally thought only to fire orthodromically transmitting nociceptive (pain) and proprioceptive (position sense) information from articular tissues towards the central nervous system (CNS). However, there is now established evidence to show that articular afferent nerves can fire antidromically contributing to joint inflammation in OA [1]. Sympathetic efferent nerves can also control joint vasomotor tone by reducing synovial blood flow although their effectiveness is reduced with arthritis [2]. Thus, both the sensory and sympathetic nervous systems are strongly involved in regulating joint perfusion.

In addition to controlling joint vasomotor control, the nervous system regulates muscle contraction to prevent abnormal movements which may lead to the development of OA. However, data from humans with neuropathies and from deafferentation studies in animals suggest that ipsilateral afferent nerves are probably not solely responsible for maintaining joint stability during normal activities. Rather, central neural networks appear capable of protecting normal joints by limiting their range of motion within 'safe' boundaries without concurrent peripheral sensory input.

Joint innervation

The nerves supplying diarthrodial joints are primarily nociceptive. The posterior articular nerve of the rat, for example, is composed of 400 axons of which 80% are unmyelinated [3]. Of these unmyelinated fibres, one-third are type IV afferents with the remaining two-thirds being sympathetic efferents. The remaining 20% of joint nerves are myelinated and the vast majority of those are type III afferents. The conduction velocity of the nociceptors is relatively slow (<20 m/s) which is in part due to their small diameter (<5 µm). The peripheral terminals of joint nociceptors are always unmyelinated and occur as 'free' nerve endings which are exquisitely sensitive to the joint microenvironment.

The larger-diameter myelinated nerves are involved in proprioception and possess specialized nerve endings including Pacinian corpuscles, spray-like Ruffini endings, or fusiform Golgi–Mazzoni apparatus [4]. The Ruffini receptors are thought to function as stretch receptors, whereas Pacini receptors appear to be stimulated by compression (Figures 7.1 and 7.2 and see [5], for more details about these receptors). Although the physiological properties of these receptors are well defined, their role in joint biomechanics is not. The difficulty in defining that role is due partly to the relative

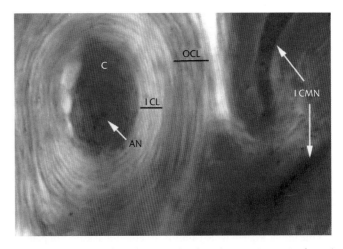

Figure 7.1 Large type II (Pacini) nerve ending from the posterior meniscofemoral ligament of the canine knee. This ending is folded on itself. AN, axis neurite (unmyelinated); C, central core; ICL, inner circumferential lamella; ICMN, intracapsular myelinated axon; OCL, outer circumferential lamella. Gold chloride stain. Original ×320.

scarcity of these receptors. For example, the entire anterior cruciate ligament (ACL) of a 3-year-old child was found to contain only 17 mechanoreceptors [6]. The majority of these proprioceptive nerves are found in the joint capsule and in the epiligament, particularly at the insertion sites of ligament into bone [4].

Nociceptive neurons may be broadly divided into two main categories: (1) nociceptors that stain positive for isolectin B4 (IB4) which are non-peptidergic neurons, and (2) neuropeptide-containing sensory nerves. In joints, very few of the nociceptors are IB4 positive [7,8] with the majority of afferents expressing neuropeptides such as substance P (SP), calcitonin gene-related peptide (CGRP), vasoactive intestinal peptide (VIP), and endomorphin-1 [9–12]. Levels of these neuropeptides are elevated in arthritic joints [13–16] suggesting that peptidergic neurons are involved in modulating joint inflammation.

Joint nociception and osteoarthritis

The 'free' nerve endings of joint nociceptors possess mechanogated ion channels that open during joint movement [17]. Opening of these ion channels leads to small generator potentials in the nerve ending which escalates until a threshold potential is reached at

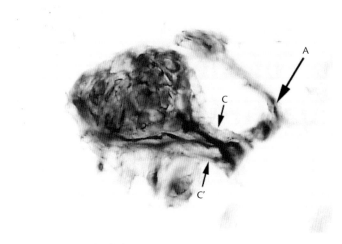

Figure 7.2 A type I (Ruffini) nerve ending from the medial collateral ligament of knee of a cat. A, node of Ranvier of parent axon; C, C', capsule surrounding three myelinated terminal intracapsular axons. Original ×320.

which point the nerve terminal depolarizes and an action potential is produced. This electrochemical signal is transmitted to the CNS where it activates specific regions of the somatosensory cortex and the sensation of movement is perceived. As the movement becomes increasingly noxious, more mechanogated ion channels are opened and a bombardment of action potentials is relayed to the CNS [17]. The thalamus distributes the encoded electrical activity to specific regions of the brain to produce the overall feeling of joint pain. These brain areas include the somatosensory cortex which gives the perception of pain, the prefrontal cortex which contextualizes the pain, and the limbic system which affords the emotional aspect of pain.

Theoretically, joint pain can arise from nociceptors residing in all joint tissues except articular cartilage, which is aneural. Dieppe proposed that the severe joint pain associated with OA may originate primarily from the nerves located within the subchondral bone, which are stimulated by increased intraosseous pressure [18]. Electrophysiological recording from knee joint afferents in preclinical models of OA indicate that fibres with receptive fields in the joint capsule and extra-articular ligaments are also likely sources of joint pain [19,20]. Although only a small quantity of synovial fluid can be aspirated from the normal human knee, large quantities can often be aspirated from diseased joints. This increase in volume is associated with an increase in intra-articular pressure (as much as 20 mmHg in arthritic joints, compared to −2 to −10 mmHg in normal joints [21–23]. This increase in intra-articular pressure increases the firing rate of joint afferents leading to the sensation of joint pain [24,25].

A perplexing aspect of OA is the tenuous relationship between joint pathology and the extent of pain being reported by the patient [26,27]. Some patients describe excruciating pain yet have normal looking joints, while other OA patients have highly degenerated joints but report little to no pain. Various psychosocial factors (e.g. coping versus catastrophizing) and limitations in pain-reporting questionnaires may account for some of this discrepancy (see Chapter 14); however, phenotypic changes in the peripheral nervous system also appear to be involved. Electrophysiological recordings from OA guinea pig knee joint afferents found no correlation between nociception and joint destruction [28] providing the first objective evidence that pain is a poor predictor of OA severity.

Peripheral sensitization

Inflammation greatly accentuates the transmission of pain sensation from a joint [29]. In the presence of inflammation, articular afferent fibres exhibit increased sensitivity. Under these conditions, normally innocuous movements generate increased neural activity, which is perceived as pain. The increase in neural impulses is due to the heightened activity of the mechanosensory nerves that normally respond to innocuous movements, and by the activation of nociceptors, which normally do not respond to these movements [29–31]. Additionally, joints appear to contain 'silent nociceptors' that become active in the presence of local inflammation. Pain is often induced or increased when the diseased joint is loaded (weight bearing), or with movement, although spontaneous nociceptor hyperactivity may occur in OA joints at rest [28]. Since inflammatory mediators are primarily responsible for peripheral sensitization [32], identification of the algogens involved in this process would greatly enhance the development of novel drug entities that aim to inhibit or silence sensitized nociceptors.

Inflammatory mediators

A variety of inflammatory mediators are known to accumulate in the synovial fluid of diseased joints which contribute to arthritis pain (see also Chapter 13) [33]. A major family of inflammatory chemicals are the eicosanoids (prostaglandins, thromboxanes, leukotrienes) which are produced by the oxidation of arachidonic acid by cyclooxygenase (COX) enzymes. Non-steroidal anti-inflammatory drugs (NSAIDs) inhibit COX activity thereby reducing the accumulation of eicosanoids, in particular prostaglandin E2. Within the joint, prostaglandins induce and perpetuate inflammation by causing vasodilation and permitting an influx of additional inflammatory mediators. In addition, they sensitize joint pain receptors [34]. NSAIDs have been shown to reduce the levels of prostaglandins and interleukin 6 (a pro-inflammatory cytokine) in the synovial fluid of OA knees [35]. This likely results in a decrease in joint pain by reducing the hypersensitivity of afferent fibres in the joint. Since COX inhibitors can also reduce neuronal activity in the spinal cord [36], systemic administration of NSAIDs can diminish the magnitude of joint pain by blocking central sensitization and possibly referred pain.

The COX enzyme exists in two distinct isoforms viz. COX1 and COX2. Although these two isoforms have 60% homology and have similar catabolic mechanisms, they differ in how they become activated. COX1 is a constitutive enzyme that is present throughout the body and maintains normal homeostasis (e.g. renal perfusion and gastrointestinal cytoprotection). In contrast, COX2 is an inducible enzyme that is only transiently 'switched on' following tissue injury or inflammation. This inherent disparity of the COX enzymes led to the development of selective COX2 inhibitors (COXIBs) the rationale being that these targeted blockers would inhibit pathological eicosanoid synthesis while leaving the production of physiological eicosanoids unhindered. There is still great debate surrounding the relative safety of COXIBs versus standard NSAIDs. The general consensus is that there are believed to be fewer gastrointestinal complications (bleeding, ulceration) with COXIBs; however, there is an increased risk of cardiovascular events with long-term usage. The American Heart Association, therefore, recommends that (1) the lowest dose of COXIBs required to control pain be used, (2) that only patients with a low risk of thromboembolisms be prescribed COXIBs, and (3) patients should also take low-dose aspirin (81 mg per day) and a proton pump inhibitor [37].

It is clear that NSAIDs are not effective in relieving joint pain in all patients with OA. Even with full therapeutic doses of NSAIDs, a substantial amount of residual pain often remains. The reasons for this are unknown. The addition of the analgesic, acetaminophen, in OA patients receiving an NSAID may further reduce the level of pain, consistent with the view that the mechanisms of action of NSAIDs and acetaminophen are different. Indeed, acetaminophen is deacetylated in the liver to *p*-aminophenol which upon entering the brain elevates the accumulation of endocannabinoids which ultimately reduce inflammatory pain [38].

Sympathetic nervous system

Joints are innervated with postganglionic sympathetic nerve fibres, which regulate blood flow in articular arterioles. Blood flow to the joint increases after sympathectomy [39] and decreases when sympathetic nerves are electrically stimulated [40]. Furthermore, recent evidence suggests that this neuronal regulation is perhaps more important in joints than in other body structures. In rabbit knees, McDougall et al. [41] demonstrated an absence of the expected reactive hyperaemia after release from 5 minutes of femoral artery occlusion. Additionally, changes in systemic blood pressure produced by intravenous infusions or by exsanguination caused a directly proportional change in blood flow to the knee joint, implying that articular arteries cannot autoregulate their tone and are therefore wholly dependent on endogenous vasoactive mediators.

The role of vasomotor control on joint blood flow has been investigated in relation to joint injury. McDougall et al. [1] found that after ACL transection, rabbit knees became hyperaemic, in association with the early development of OA. Because prior denervation of the articular nerve supply prevented this hyperaemia, the vascular changes that occur after ACL transection appeared to be neurogenically mediated. Similar events have been demonstrated in chronically inflamed knees where the loss of sympathetic vasoconstriction was due to a disruption in α-adrenoceptor function [2,42].

Inflammatory neuropeptides

Afferent fibres containing inflammatory neuropeptides are commonly found in articular tissues, particularly in association with vascular structures. Peripheral release of substance P, CGRP, and VIP into joints causes synovial vasodilatation [43–45], protein extravasation [46,47], and pain [48,49] in a process termed 'neurogenic inflammation' [50]. Lam and Ferrell [51] found that the severity of experimentally induced acute joint inflammation was reduced by 44% (as indicated by the quantity of plasma proteins in the joint capsule; an index of vascular permeability) in animals pretreated with capsaicin, which depletes substance P from nerve endings, and by 93% after pre-treatment with a substance P antagonist.

As described above, the presence of these neuropeptides sensitizes joint afferents, thereby increasing joint pain. It has been demonstrated that, in contrast to those neuropeptides that increase joint afferent sensitization, other neuropeptides decrease sensitization. In normal and acutely inflamed knee joints of rats, endomorphin 1 (an endogenous μ-opioid receptor peptide ligand) was shown to decrease the response of articular nerves to noxious movements [52]. The antinociceptive effect of this neuropeptide, however, was abrogated in chronically inflamed joints due to downregulation of

μ-opioid receptors. Thus, we may hypothesize that the mechanosensitivity of articular afferents in normal joints may be regulated by a balance between pro-inflammatory neuropeptides, such as substance P, and anti-inflammatory peptides, such as endomorphin 1. In the inflamed joint, the pro-inflammatory peptides predominate, suggesting that the application of endomorphin 1 or its synthetic analogues could be used clinically to reduce acute inflammation and the associated pain.

Proteases and protease-activated receptors

Proteolytic enzymes orchestrate numerous physiological processes such as blood clotting and tissue repair. In arthritis, various proteases accumulate in diseased joints where they cause the progressive breakdown of articular tissues by hydrolysing long chain proteins [53,54]. In addition to this enzymatic activity, proteases can also cleave a group of G protein-coupled receptors called the protease-activated receptors (PARs). There are currently four PARs each with their own distinct cleavage site in the N-terminal domain of the receptor. Specific proteases are able to slice off the extracellular N-terminus revealing a tethered ligand which can now bind to the second extracellular loop of the PAR leading to receptor activation and downstream signalling. All four PARs have been identified in synovial joints and their activation leads to tissue inflammation and pain modulation [55]. PAR2 and PAR4 have been localized on joint primary afferents and activation of these receptors leads to neuronal sensitization and pain [56–58]. The sensitizing effect of PAR2 is mediated through the opening of transient receptor potential vanilloid-1 ion channels with the subsequent release of pro-inflammatory neuropeptides [59,60]. Conversely, the pain producing effects following PAR4 activation involve the secondary release of bradykinin from synovial mast cells and the stimulation of neuronal bradykinin B2 receptors [58,61]. The role of PAR1 in controlling joint pain is unclear, but it is thought to be anti-nociceptive and involves an opioidergic mechanism [62].

Current research is aiming to identify the specific PAR-cleaving proteases that are released into inflamed joints. Thus far thrombin has been shown to cleave PAR1 on synovial fibroblasts [63], PAR2 is activated by neutrophil elastase [64], mast cell tryptase [65], and matriptase [66], while PAR4 is cleaved by cathepsin G [67]. Selective protease inhibitors or PAR antagonists offer exciting possibilities in treating arthritis not only by inhibiting tissue degradation, but also by silencing joint nociceptor activity.

Neuropathic osteoarthritis pain

A significant number of OA patients do not respond to classical NSAIDs or other treatments that are typically used to manage inflammatory pain. The pain these patients describe often has a 'pins and needles' quality to it, may be sharp and shooting, or feels like an electric shock. These pain descriptors are characteristic of sensory nerve damage indicating that some OA patients suffer from neuropathic pain. Clinical assessment studies using a modified pain questionnaires have identified a subpopulation of OA patients that present with neuropathic-like pain symptoms [68]. The proportion of OA patients reporting neuropathic pain ranges anywhere from 5% to 45% [69,70] highlighting the subjective limitation of the questionnaires used.

Emerging preclinical data also support the concept of a neuropathic component to OA pain [33,71]. Following joint injury, the peripheral nerves innervating rabbit knees undergo a dramatic shift in their phenotype. Around the time early-onset OA develops in this model, the joint nerves become truncated, tortuous, and filled with neuropeptides consistent with a peripheral neuropathy [4,72]. The sensory nerves innervating guinea pig OA joints fire spontaneously in the absence of any external stimulation suggesting damage to the peripheral nervous system and a source of neuropathic pain [28]. In other animal models of OA, there is increased expression of a pan-neuronal marker of nerve injury (activating transcription factor 3) [73], while drugs that are used to treat neuropathic pain have been found to be effective in alleviating nociception in arthritic rodents [74,75].

The molecular entities responsible for the generation of neuropathic OA pain are still under investigation although some promising candidates are coming to light. A subset of voltage-gated sodium channels (NaV) are exclusively expressed on nociceptors and are upregulated following nerve injury. NaV1.3, NaV1.7 and NaV1.8 have all been found to accumulate in the injured area of painful neuromas where they cause neuronal hyperexcitability [76,77]. More recently it has been found that pharmacological blockade of articular NaV1.8 ion channels in OA knees reduced nociceptor activity and pain [78]. Similarly, spinal inhibition of the voltage gated calcium channel CaV2.2 reduced pain transmission in OA animals while having no effect in sham controls [79]. These findings indicate that cation channels present on joint nociceptors may be an effective way of targeting neuropathic OA pain and avoid the unwanted side effects of local anaesthetics or complete nerve blocks.

Summary

Despite being highly prevalent in the general population, relatively little is known about the mechanisms and mediators involved in the generation of OA pain. The source of OA pain undoubtedly starts in the joint, although the specific joint tissues from which joint pain originates in OA patients are uncertain. The transmission of nociceptive impulses by articular nerves is accentuated in the presence of inflammatory mediators (e.g. substance P), so that normally innocuous movements of the OA joint may be painful. In addition, substance P and other inflammatory neuropeptides are released by the nerves themselves, contributing to 'neurogenic inflammation.' However, other neuropeptides (e.g. endomorphin 1) are anti-inflammatory, offering the possibility of novel approaches to treat joint pain and inflammation. The lack of a correlation between the severity of joint damage and the amount of pain reported by some OA patients certainly complicates clinical assessment studies. The use of objective measures (e.g. electrophysiology) in preclinical models of OA is helping us to sort out the neuronal pathways involved in joint pain perception. The realization that not all OA pain is created equal and that some patients may have a neuropathic or significant inflammatory component to their pain will improve our understanding of the disease and help us to develop more personalized treatments directed towards specific patient subgroups.

References

1. McDougall JJ, Ferrell WR, Bray RC. Neurogenic origin of articular hyperemia in early degenerative joint disease. *Am J Physiol* 1999; 276:R345–52.
2. McDougall JJ, Karimian SM, Ferrell WR. Prolonged alteration of sympathetic vasoconstrictor and peptidergic vasodilator responses in rat knee joints by adjuvant-induced arthritis. *Exp Physiol* 1995; 80:349–57.
3. Hildebrand C, Oqvist G, Brax L, Tuisku F. Anatomy of the rat knee joint and composition of a major articular nerve. *Anat Rec* 1991; 229:545–55.
4. McDougall JJ, Bray RC, Sharkey KA. A morphological and immunohistochemical examination of nerves in normal and injured collateral ligaments of rat, rabbit and human knee joints. *Anat Rec* 1997; 248:29–39.
5. Hogervorst T, Brand RA. Mechanoreceptors in joint function. *J Bone Joint Surg* 1998; 80-A:1365–78.
6. Krauspe R, Schmitz F, Zoller G, Drenckhahn D. Distribution of neurofilament-positive nerve fibres and sensory endings in the human anterior cruciate ligament. *Arch Orthop Trauma Surg* 1995; 114:194–8.
7. Ivanavicius SP, Blake DR, Chessell IP, Mapp PI. Isolectin B4 binding neurons are not present in the rat knee joint. *Neuroscience* 2004; 128:555–60.
8. Kuniyoshi K, Ohtori S, Ochiai N, et al. Characteristics of sensory DRG neurons innervating the wrist joint in rats. *Eur J Pain* 2007; 11:323–8.
9. Grönblad M, Konttinen YT, Korkala O, et al. Neuropeptides in the synovium of patients with rheumatoid arthritis and osteoarthritis. *J Rheumatol* 1988; 15:1807–10.
10. Hokfelt T, Kellerth JO, Nilsson G, Pernow B. Experimental immunohistochemical studies on the localisation and distribution of substance P in the cat primary sensory neurones. *Brain Res* 1975; 100:235–52.
11. Mapp PI, Kidd BL, Gibson SJ, et al. Neuropeptides are found in normal and inflamed synovium. *Br J Rheumatol* 1989; 28(Suppl 3):8.
12. McDougall JJ, Baker CL, Hermann PM. Attenuation of knee joint inflammation by peripherally administered endomorphin-1. *J Mol Neurosci* 2004; 22, 125–37.
13. Devillier P, Weill B, Renoux M, Menkes C, Pradelles, P. Elevated levels of tachykinin-like immunoreactivity in joint fluids from patients with inflammatory diseases. *N Engl J Med* 1981; 314:1323.
14. Lygren I, Østensen M, Burhol PG, Husby G. Gastrointestinal peptides in serum and synovial fluid from patients with inflammatory joint disease. *Ann Rheum Dis* 1986; 45:637–40.
15. Marshall KW, Chiu B, Inman RD. Substance P and arthritis: analysis of plasma and synovial fluid levels. *Arthritis Rheum* 1990; 33:87–90.
16. McDougall JJ, Barin AK, McDougall CM. Loss of vasomotor responsiveness to the m-opioid receptor ligand endomorphin-1 in adjuvant monoarthritic rat knee joints. *Am J Physiol Regul Integr Comp Physiol* 2004; 286:R634–41.
17. Heppelmann B, McDougall JJ. Inhibitory effect of amiloride and gadolinium on fine afferent nerves in the rat knee: evidence of mechano-gated ion channels in joints. *Exp Brain Res* 2005; 167:114–18.
18. Dieppe P. Subchondral bone should be the main target for the treatment of pain and disease progression in osteoarthritis. *Osteoarthritis Cartilage* 1999; 7:325–6.
19. Schuelert N, McDougall JJ. Electrophysiological evidence that the vasoactive intestinal peptide receptor antagonist VIP(6-28) reduces nociception in an animal model of osteoarthritis. *Osteoarthritis Cartilage* 2006; 14:1155–62.
20. Schuelert N, McDougall JJ. Grading of monosodium iodoacetate-induced osteoarthritis reveals a concentration-dependent sensitization of nociceptors in the knee joint of the rat. *Neurosci Lett* 2009; 465:184–8.
21. Jayson MI, St Dixon AJ. Intra-articular pressure in rheumatoid arthritis of the knee. I. Pressure changes during passive joint distension. *Ann Rheum Dis* 1970; 29:261–5.
22. Levick JR. An investigation into the validity of subatmospheric pressure recordings from synovial fluid and their dependence on joint angle. *J Physiol* 1979; 289:55–67.
23. Reeves B. Negative pressures in knee joints. *Nature* 1966; 212:1046.
24. Andrew BL, Dodt E. The deployment of sensory nerve endings at the knee joint of the cat. *Acta Physiol Scand* 1953; 28:8287–96.
25. Ferrell WR, Nade S, Newbold PJ. The interrelation of neural discharge, intra-articular pressure, and joint angle in the knee of the dog. *J Physiol* 1986; 373:353–65.

26. Hannan MT, Felson DT, Pincus T. Analysis of the discordance between radiographic changes and knee pain in osteoarthritis of the knee. *J Rheumatol* 2000; 27:1513–17.

27. Lethbridge-Cejku M, Scott WW Jr, Reichle R, et al. Association of radiographic features of osteoarthritis of the knee with knee pain: data from the Baltimore Longitudinal Study of Aging. *Arthritis Care Res* 1995; 8:182–8.

28. McDougall JJ, Andruski B, Schuelert N, Hallgrimsson B, Matyas JR. Unravelling the relationship between age, nociception and joint destruction in naturally occurring osteoarthritis of Dunkin Hartley guinea pigs. *Pain* 2009; 141:222–32.

29. Schaible HG, Schmidt RF. Time course of mechanosensitivity changes in articular afferents during a developing experimental arthritis. *J Neurophysiol* 1988; 60:2180–95.

30. Coggeshall RE, Hong KA, Langford LA, Schaible HG, Schmidt RF. Discharge characteristics of fine medial articular afferents at rest and during passive movements of inflamed knee joints. *Brain Res* 1983; 272:185–8.

31. Grigg P, Schaible HG, Schmidt RF. Mechanical sensitivity of group III and IV afferents from posterior articular nerve in normal and inflamed cat knee. *J Neurophysiol* 1986; 55:635–43.

32. McDougall JJ. Arthritis and pain. Neurogenic origin of joint pain. *Arthritis Res Ther* 2006; 8:220–9.

33. Krustev E, Rioux D, McDougall JJ. Mechanisms and mediators that drive arthritis pain. *Curr Osteoporos Rep* 2015; 13:216–24.

34. Schaible HG, Schmidt RF. Excitation and sensitization of fine articular afferents from cat's knee joint by prostaglandin E2. *J Physiol* 1988; 403:91–104.

35. Schumacher HR Jr, Meng Z, Sieck M, et al. Effect of a nonsteroidal antiinflammatory drug on synovial fluid in osteoarthritis. *J Rheumatol* 1996; 23:1774–7.

36. Malmberg AB, Yaksh TL. Antinociceptive actions of spinal nonsteroidal anti-inflammatory agents on the formalin test in the rat. *J Pharmacol Exp Ther* 1992; 263:136–46.

37. Antman EM, Bennett JS, Daugherty A, et al. Use of nonsteroidal antiinflammatory drugs: an update for clinicians: a scientific statement from the American Heart Association. *Circulation* 2007; 115:1634–42.

38. Mallet C, Daulhac L, Bonnefont J, et al. Endocannabinoid and serotonergic systems are needed for acetaminophen-induced analgesia. *Pain* 2008; 139:190–200.

39. Levine JD, Dardick SJ, Roizen MF, Helms C, Basbaum AI. Contribution of sensory afferents and sympathetic efferents to joint injury in experimental arthritis. *J Neurosci* 1986; 6:3423–9.

40. McDougall JJ, Karimian SM, Ferrell WR. Alteration of substance P-mediated vasodilatation and sympathetic vasoconstriction in the rat knee joint by adjuvant-induced inflammation. *Neurosci Lett* 1994; 174:127–9.

41. McDougall JJ, Ferrell WR, Bray RC. Spatial variation in sympathetic influences on the vasculature of the synovium and medial collateral ligament of the rabbit knee joint. *J Physiol* 1997; 503:435–43.

42. McDougall JJ. Abrogation of α-adrenergic vasoactivity in chronically inflamed rat knee joints. *Am J Physiol Regul Integr Comp Physiol* 2001; 281:R821–7.

43. Lam FY, Ferrell WR. Capsaicin suppresses substance P-induced joint inflammation in the rat. *Neurosci Lett* 1989; 105:155–88.

44. Lam FY, Ferrell WR. CGRP modulates nerve-mediated vasoconstriction of rat knee joint blood vessels. *Regul Peptides* 1991; 34:118.

45. McDougall JJ, Barin AK. The role of joint nerves and mast cells in the alteration of vasoactive intestinal peptide (VIP) sensitivity during inflammation progression in rats. *Br J Pharmacol* 2005; 145:104–13.

46. Karimian SM, Ferrell WR. Plasma protein extravasation into the rat knee joint induced by calcitonin gene-related peptide. *Neurosci Lett* 1994; 166:39–42.

47. Scott DT, Lam FY, Ferrell WR. Time course of substance P-induced protein extravasation in the rat knee joint measured by microturbidimetry. *Neurosci Lett* 1991; 129:74–6.

48. McDougall JJ, Schuelert N. Age alters the ability of substance P to sensitize joint nociceptors in guinea pigs. *J Mol Neurosci* 2007; 31:289–96.

49. McDougall JJ, Watkins L, Li Z. Vasoactive intestinal peptide (VIP) is a modulator of joint pain in a rat model of osteoarthritis. *Pain* 2006; 123:98–105.

50. Levine JD, Moskowitz MA, Basbaum AI. The contribution of neurogenic inflammation in experimental arthritis. *J Immunol* 1985; 135:843s–7s.

51. Lam FY, Ferrell WR. Inhibition of carrageenan-induced joint inflammation by substance P antagonist. *Ann Rheum Dis* 1989; 48:928–32.

52. Li Z, Proud D, Zhang C, Wiehler S, McDougall JJ. Chronic arthritis downregulates peripheral mu-opioid receptor expression with concomitant loss of endomorphin-1 anti-nociception. *Arthritis Rheum* 2005; 52:3210–19.

53. Lavery JP, Lisse JR. Preliminary study of the tryptase levels in the synovial fluid of patients with inflammatory arthritis. *Ann Allergy* 1994; 72:425–7.

54. Nakano S, Ikata T, Kinoshita I, Kanematsu J, Yasuoka S. Characteristics of the protease activity in synovial fluid from patients with rheumatoid arthritis and osteoarthritis. *Clin Exp Rheumatol* 1999; 17:161–70.

55. Russell FA, McDougall JJ. Proteinase activated receptor (PAR) involvement in mediating arthritis pain and inflammation. *Inflamm Res* 2009; 58:119–26.

56. McDougall JJ, Zhang C, Cellars L, et al. Triggering of proteinase-activated receptor 4 leads to joint pain and inflammation in mice. *Arthritis Rheum* 2009; 60:728–37.

57. Russell FA, Schuelert N, Veldhoen VE, Hollenberg MD, McDougall JJ. Proteinase-activated receptor-2 (PAR(2)) activation sensitises primary afferents and causes leukocyte rolling and adherence in the rat knee joint. *Br J Pharmacol* 2012; 167(8):1665–78.

58. Russell FA, Veldhoen VE, Tchitchkan D, McDougall JJ. Proteinase-activated receptor-4 (PAR4) activation leads to sensitization of rat joint primary afferents via a bradykinin B2 receptor-dependent mechanism. *J Neurophysiol* 2010; 103:155–63.

59. Amadesi S, Nie J, Vergnolle N, et al. Protease-activated receptor 2 sensitizes the capsaicin receptor transient receptor potential vanilloid receptor 1 to induce hyperalgesia. *J Neurosci* 2004; 24:4300–12.

60. Helyes Z, Sándor K, Borbély E, et al. Involvement of transient receptor potential vanilloid 1 receptors in protease-activated receptor-2-induced joint inflammation and nociception. *Eur J Pain* 2010; 14:351–8.

61. Russell FA, Zhan S, Dumas A, et al. The pronociceptive effect of proteinase-activated receptor-4 stimulation in rat knee joints is dependent on mast cell activation. *Pain* 2011; 152:354–60.

62. Martin L, Augé C, Boué J, et al. Thrombin receptor: an endogenous inhibitor of inflammatory pain, activating opioid pathways. *Pain* 2009; 146:121–9.

63. Hirano F, Kobayashi A, Hirano Y, et al. Thrombin-induced expression of RANTES mRNA through protease activated receptor-1 in human synovial fibroblasts. *Ann Rheum Dis* 2002; 61:834–7.

64. Muley MM, Reid AR, Botz B, et al. Neutrophil elastase induces inflammation and pain in mouse knee joints via activation of proteinase-activated receptor-2. *Br J Pharmacol* 2016; 173(4):766–77.

65. Palmer HS, Kelso EB, Lockhart JC, et al. Protease-activated receptor 2 mediates the proinflammatory effects of synovial mast cells. *Arthritis Rheum* 2007; 56:3532–40.

66. Milner JM, Patel A, Davidson RK, et al. Matriptase is a novel initiator of cartilage matrix degradation in osteoarthritis. *Arthritis Rheum* 2010; 62:1955–66.

67. Russell FA, Schuelert N, Veldhoen VE, McDougall JJ. Cathepsin G has an anti-nociceptive effect in normal rat knee joints. *Inflamm Res* 2011; 60(Suppl 1):S293–S295.

68. Hochman JR, Gagliese L, Davis AM, Hawker GA. Neuropathic pain symptoms in a community knee OA cohort. *Osteoarthritis Cartilage* 2011; 19:647–54.

69. Hochman JR, Davis AM, Elkayam J, Gagliese L, Hawker GA. Neuropathic pain symptoms on the modified painDETECT correlate

with signs of central sensitization in knee osteoarthritis. *Osteoarthritis Cartilage* 2013; 21:1236–42.

70. Ohtori S, Orita S, Yamashita M, et al. Existence of a neuropathic pain component in patients with osteoarthritis of the knee. *Yonsei Med J* 2012; 53:801–5.

71. McDougall JJ, Linton P. Neurophysiology of arthritis pain. *Curr Pain Headache Rep* 2012; 16:485–91.

72. McDougall JJ, Yeung G, Leonard CA, Bray RC. A role for calcitonin gene-related peptide in rabbit knee joint ligament healing. *Can J Physiol Pharmacol* 2000; 78:535–40.

73. Ivanavicius SP, Ball AD, Heapy CG, et al. Structural pathology in a rodent model of osteoarthritis is associated with neuropathic pain: increased expression of ATF-3 and pharmacological characterisation. *Pain* 2007; 128:272–82.

74. Fernihough J, Gentry C, Malcangio M, et al. Pain related behaviour in two models of osteoarthritis in the rat knee. *Pain* 2004; 112:83–93.

75. Hanesch U, McDougall JJ, Pawlak M. Inhibitory effects of gabapentin on rat articular afferent mechanosensitivity. *Regul Peptides* 2000; 89:63.

76. Black JA, Liu S, Tanaka M, Cummins TR, Waxman SG. Changes in the expression of tetrodotoxin-sensitive sodium channels within dorsal root ganglia neurons in inflammatory pain. *Pain* 2004; 108:237–47.

77. Black JA, Nikolajsen L, Kroner K, Jensen TS, Waxman SG. Multiple sodium channel isoforms and mitogen-activated protein kinases are present in painful human neuromas. *Ann Neurol* 2008; 64:644–53.

78. Schuelert N, McDougall JJ. Involvement of Nav 1.8 sodium ion channels in the transduction of mechanical pain in a rodent model of osteoarthritis. *Arthritis Res Ther* 2012; 14:R5.

79. Rahman W, Patel R, Dickenson AH. Electrophysiological evidence for voltage-gated calcium channel 2 (Cav2) modulation of mechano- and thermosensitive spinal neuronal responses in a rat model of osteoarthritis. *Neuroscience* 2015; 305:76–85.

SECTION 3

Epidemiology

CHAPTER 8

Epidemiology

Nigel Arden and Michael C. Nevitt

Introduction

Osteoarthritis (OA) is the most common joint disorder in the industrialized world. In industrialized populations, radiographic evidence of OA occurs in the majority of people by 65 years of age, and in about 80% of those aged over 75 years. In the United States, it is second only to ischaemic heart disease as a cause of work disability in men over 50 years of age, and accounts for more hospitalizations than rheumatoid arthritis (RA) each year. It is associated with considerable costs to individuals and to health service providers and accounts for over 90% of lower limb joint replacements performed in the western healthcare systems [1]. More recently, OA has been demonstrated to be associated with an increased mortality, especially from cardiovascular causes [2,3].

Despite the impact of OA on patients and the health service, OA remains an *elusive* condition to define and treat. Traditionally, OA has been diagnosed using radiographs and more recently magnetic resonance imaging (MRI); however, the last 20 years of research has changed our thinking about the disease and its treatment. We know today that OA takes up to 10–15 years to develop, has a range of risk factors, and that there is a considerable discordance between symptoms and structural signs, such that new classifications and definitions are moving away from structural criteria to combined structure and pain definitions. In this chapter we will review the definition and classification of OA and its prevalence, incidence, and natural history.

Definition and classification

Definition

OA is a heterogeneous disease, which involves all of the synovial joint tissues and is defined by a combination of joint symptoms and structural pathology (e.g. on X-ray). The primary symptoms include joint pain and stiffness. The joint pathology is diverse, involving all joint tissues, and includes focal damage and loss of articular cartilage, abnormal remodelling and attrition of subchondral bone, osteophytes (bone growth at the joint margins), ligamentous laxity, meniscal damage, muscle weakness, and synovial inflammation [4,5]. OA is now regarded as a failure of joint repair in an organ in response to trauma and mechanical stress and the pathological observations in the advance to disease are as much a product of attempted repair as of the primary insult or damage which contributed to initiation of the process (Figure 8.1). We should, however, not forget that pain as well as other symptoms are modulated by central and peripheral central nervous system processes and as such, painful OA should be regarded as a whole-person disease [6].

Radiographs have traditionally been utilized to diagnose and classify OA, most commonly graded using the criteria of Kellgren and Lawrence (KL) [7] (see Chapter 16). The main limitations of radiographs are their insensitivity to early pathological changes and relatively poor association with symptoms. A significant proportion of patients with classic radiographic features of OA will not experience clinically significant symptoms. Up to 50% of patients with radiographic knee OA, defined by KL grade 2 or above, do not experience regular pain. A similar proportion of patients with knee pain suggestive of OA do not have radiographic features of OA [8]. The use of MRI in OA research, which can detect cartilage degradation, bone marrow lesions, synovitis, and meniscal abnormalities, has identified abnormalities in a large proportion of radiographically normal joints [9]. Despite the greater sensitivity of MRI in detecting joint damage, its clinical relevance remains under investigation [10]. Indeed, in a large study of participants without radiographic signs of OA and without symptoms, MRI abnormalities thought to be associated with OA were detected in 89% of knees. OA should therefore be defined as structural OA, as defined earlier in this section, with the additional presence of symptoms that are relevant to the patient.

Diagnostic criteria

The most widely used diagnostic criteria were developed by the American College of Rheumatology (ACR) [11,12]. These criteria identify subjects with clinical OA using joint pain for most days of the prior month as the major inclusion criteria. This contrasts with the use of radiographic changes alone wherein many subjects do not report joint pain. The algorithms for classification were developed by comparing patients with clinically diagnosed OA and controls who had joint pain due to other arthritic or musculoskeletal diseases. Table 8.1 illustrates the criteria for hand, knee, and hip. They are useful for clinical studies and randomized controlled trials of new interventions to enhance comparison between studies. Despite the clinical relevance of these definitions, their use in population-based research is less clearly defined and prevalence estimates using the ACR case definitions are likely to be substantially lower than those based on traditional radiographic criteria.

International groups are currently producing criteria for the diagnosis of early OA, which will standardize research in this important area of disease for secondary prevention and early treatment trials. Hopefully these will be published in the near future.

Classification

Osteoarthritis can be classified in several ways: traditionally it has been classified into either primary or secondary OA. Several

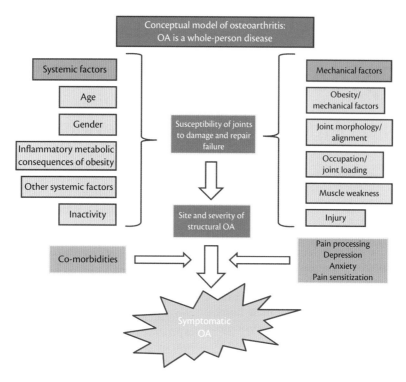

Figure 8.1 Conceptual model of osteoarthritis: OA is a whole-person disease.

disorders are well recognized as causes of secondary OA. They can be divided into four main categories [13] (Box 8.1). However, the distinction between primary and secondary OA is not always clear, as there is evidence that a significant proportion of subjects who develop secondary OA have some generalized predisposition to the disorder, on the one hand, and that mechanical factors, trauma, and other local factors determine which joints develop OA in people with a generalized disposition [14].

Several other features of OA have been used in attempts to subset the disorder. For example, the term *inflammatory OA* is sometimes used for patients with obvious inflammation and multiple joint involvement [15,16]. This should be differentiated from the high prevalence of inflammation in knee OA, which often results in secondary inflammation due to intra-articular cartilage debris [17]. Some patients develop erosions of their interphalangeal joints, leading to the classification of the subset of erosive OA [18,19]. This disorder tends to occur in middle-aged women, presents acutely with features of marked inflammation and pain, and subsides over a period of months to years, leaving joint erosions, deformity, and occasional ankylosis. Similarly, atrophic (without marginal osteophytes) and destructive forms of OA probably represent ends of the spectrum of disease rather than separate entities. Finally, insights into OA are provided by a variety of rare or geographically localized diseases, which are associated with the development of premature disease. Examples include dysplastic conditions such as Blount disease [20] or Mseleni disease [21], and unusual forms of arthritis like Kashin–Beck disease [21].

Prevalence and incidence

The joints most commonly affected by OA are the knee, hip, hand, foot, and spine, with the wrists, shoulders, and ankles less frequently

involved [22]. Hip and knee OA have the greatest impact, on both patients and healthcare providers, as they are commonly affected and are associated with substantial pain and stiffness, often leading to significant problems with mobility and to disability requiring expensive surgical treatments [23]. OA accounts for over 90% of hip and knee replacement performed in industrialized countries [1]. In the United Kingdom alone, the combined number of knee and hip joint replacements performed is in excess of 170 000 annually [24].

Prevalence

The prevalence of pathological features of OA has been assessed in systematic autopsy studies. In a series of 1000 cases in 1926, Heine documented almost universal evidence of cartilage damage in people aged over 65 years. More recent studies, report the presence of cartilage erosions, subchondral bone changes, and osteophyte in the knees of 60% of men and 70% of women who died in their 60s and 70s. Prevalence estimates from such studies tend to be higher than those from radiographic surveys, partly because relatively mild pathological change is not apparent on radiographs, and also because pathological studies examine the whole joint surface and tissues not visualized by radiograph. Furthermore, we do not know whether the cases identified in these studies were associated with the current or future important clinical symptoms of pain and disability. More recently, MRI has been used to study 701 individuals with neither radiographic signs of OA nor symptoms in the knee. MRI abnormalities thought to be associated with knee OA were detected in 89% of knees, again calling into question the clinical relevance of these findings [9].

The majority of currently available information on the prevalence of OA comes from population-based radiographic surveys, without reference to pain. More recently, good data is being published on the clinically relevant outcomes of joint pain, symptomatic

Table 8.1 ACR criteria for OA of the hand, hip, and knee

		OA is present if the items present are:
Hand	**Clinical**	
	1. Hand pain, aching or stiffness for most days or prior month	1, 2, 3, 4 or 1, 2, 3, 5
	2. Hard tissue enlargement of ≥2 of 10 selected hand joints[a]	
	3. MCP swelling in ≤2 joints	
	4. Hard tissue enlargement of ≥2 DIP joints	
	5. Deformity of ≥1 of 10 selected hand joints	
Hip	**Clinical and radiographic**	
	1. Hip pain for most days of the prior month	1, 2, 3 or 1, 2, 4 or 1, 3, 4
	2. ESR ≤20mm/h (laboratory)	
	3. Radiograph femoral and/or acetabular osteophytes	
	4. Radiograph hip joint-space narrowing.	
Knee	**Clinical**	
	1. Knee pain for most days of prior month	1, 2, 3, 4 or 1, 2, 5 or 1, 4, 5
	2. Crepitus on active joint motion	
	3. Morning stiffness ≤ 30 min in duration	
	4. Age ≥ 38 years	
	5. Bony enlargement of the knee on examination	
Knee	**Clinical and radiographic**	
	1. Knee pain for most days of prior month	1, 2 or 1, 3, 5, 6 or 1, 4, 5, 6
	2. Osteophytes at joint margins (radiograph)	
	3. Synovial fluid typical of OA (laboratory)	
	4. Age ≥ 40 years	
	5. Morning stiffness ≤ 30 min	
	6. Crepitus on active joint motion	

[a]Ten selected hand joints include bilateral second and third PIP joints, second and third PIP joints and first CMC joints.

radiographic OA, and joint arthroplasty. The prevalence of radiographic OA rises with age at all joint sites (see Chapter 10 and Figure 8.2).

Radiographic knee OA
The prevalence of radiographic OA in the tibiofemoral joint of the knee increases with age, especially in postmenopausal women. The prevalence rates are 4% in women aged 35–44 and 5.6% in men of the same age [25]. However, the rates in the over 65s shows a female excess: 49.1% versus 26.4% respectively. Other population-based studies have also reported consistent figures: the Chingford Study published prevalence rates of 13.7% in women aged 45–64 years [26]. The Framingham study reported rates of 30.8% in men and 34.8% in women aged 65 and over [27]. Rates in Asian populations have recently been studied: in the Beijing Study, rates in men and

Box 8.1 Classification of osteoarthritis

Primary
1. Idiopathic
   - Peripheral
   - Spinal apophyseal joints.

Secondary
1. Metabolic—examples include:
   - Ochronosis
   - Acromegaly
   - Haemochromatosis
   - Calcium crystal deposition.
2. Anatomical—examples include:
   - Slipped femoral epiphysis
   - Epiphyseal dysplasias
   - Blount's disease
   - Legg–Perthes disease
   - Congenital dislocation of the hip
   - Leg-length inequality
   - Hypermobility syndromes.
3. Traumatic—examples include:
   - Major joint trauma
   - Fracture through a joint or osteonecrosis
   - Joint surgery (e.g. meniscectomy)
   - Chronic injury (occupational arthropathies).
4. Inflammatory—examples include:
   - Any inflammatory arthropathy
   - Septic arthritis.
5. Neuropathic
   - Charcot joints.

Classification by the presence of specific features
- Inflammatory OA
- Erosive OA
- Atrophic or destructive OA
- OA with chondrocalcinosis
- Others.

women aged 65 and over were 27.6% and 47.6% respectively [27]. In the ROAD study from Japan, a remarkably high 47.0% of men and 70.2% of women aged 60 and over had radiographic knee OA [28]. At present, there is little population-based data on the prevalence of radiographic OA in the patellofemoral joint.

Radiographic hip OA
Fewer population-based data are available on radiographic hip OA prevalence among those aged 50 and over compared to the knee,

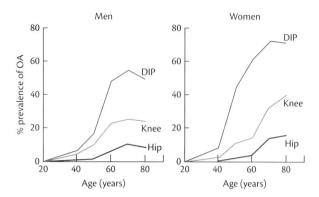

Figure 8.2 Estimates for the prevalence of radiographic OA affecting the DIP joint, knee, and hip in a large Dutch population sample.

van Saase JL, van Romunde LK, Cats A, Vandenbroucke JP, Valkenburg HA. Epidemiology of osteoarthritis: Zoetermeer survey. Comparison of radiological osteoarthritis in a Dutch population with that in 10 other populations. *Ann Rheum Dis* 1989; 48(4):271–80.

and the estimates vary widely, from less than 5% in the United States as a whole [29], to nearly 20% in a US urban population [30] and 28% in a southern US rural population [31]. Some, but not all, studies find a higher prevalence in men than in women. In contrast to knee OA, there are important, documented racial differences in the occurrence of hip OA. Although there have been few population-based studies of OA in Chinese or other Asian populations, the studies that do exist suggest that while knee OA is as prevalent or more prevalent as in elderly white people, the prevalence of hip OA appears to be much lower among Asians [32–35] The most rigorous comparative population study to date found that radiographic hip OA was 80–90% less frequent in urban Chinese than in white people in the United States, and symptomatic hip OA was practically non-existent in the Chinese.

Radiographic hand OA

Data from the United States using the NHES/NHANES survey demonstrated a prevalence of hand OA of 29.5% in subjects aged over 25 years [36]. A study from the Netherlands [37] included 6585 inhabitants randomly selected from the population of a Dutch village: 75% of women aged 60–70 years had OA of their distal interphalangeal (DIP) joints, and even by 40 years of age, 10–20% of subjects had evidence of severe radiographic disease of their hands or feet. The Beijing Study compared the age-standardized prevalence of radiographic hand OA between Chinese and US white people aged 60 and over. Among white people, 85.0% of women and 75.2 of men had OA; while in Chinese people the corresponding prevalences were 44.5% and 47.0% [38].

Prevalence of joint pain and symptomatic osteoarthritis

Although the majority of studies have focused on the prevalence of radiographic changes of OA, there is an increasing amount of research into the prevalence of joint pain and symptomatic OA in older adults in the community. This information is essential to allow accurate planning of the needs and options for healthcare of patients. In most studies, the prevalence of symptomatic OA (the combination of pain plus radiographic findings in the same joint) at the knee, hip, and hand in men is less than one-quarter, and in women less than one-third, of the prevalence of radiographic OA in the same population [27,28,30,38]. The prevalence of self-reported knee pain in the United Kingdom in adults at least 40 years of age is between 20% and 28% with approximately 50% reporting disability

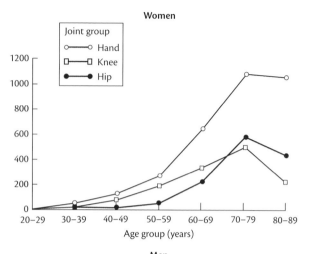

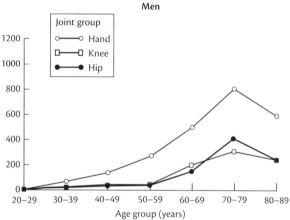

Figure 8.3 Incidence per 100,000 of symptomatic osteoarthritis of the hand, knee, and hip. Data from the Fallon Community Health Plan.

Kwoh CK. Epidemiology of osteoarthritis. In: Newman A, Cauley JA, editors. *The Epidemiology of Aging.* Springer Netherlands; 2012.

as a result of their knee pain (Figure 8.3) [39]. Of patients with knee pain, roughly 50% will have radiographic changes of OA and can therefore be classified as symptomatic OA. A primary care-based study of patients over 55 years from England found that 18.1% of patients registered with the practice had a clinical diagnosis of knee OA [40]. Symptomatic OA of the hip is less common than at the knee with prevalence estimates of between 0.7% and 4.4% [29,41,42] with estimates for the hand of roughly 2.5%.

Incidence

The epidemiological studies of the incidence of OA are summarized in Table 8.2. In a population-based incidence study of symptomatic hip and knee OA from Rochester, Minnesota, United States, age- and sex-adjusted rates for OA of the hip and knee were found to be 47.3 per 100 000 person-years and 163.8 per 100 000 person-years respectively [43]. The most recent data to characterize the incidence of symptomatic hand, hip, and knee OA were obtained from the Fallon Community Health Plan, a health maintenance organization located in the north-east United States [44] (Figure 8.3). In this study, the age- and sex-standardized incidence rate of hand OA was 100 per 100 000 person-years (95% confidence interval (CI) 86–115); for hip OA, 88 per 100 000 person-years; and for knee OA, 240 per 100 000 person-years. The incidence of

Table 8.2 Epidemiological studies of incidence of OA

Study	Site	Sex	Incidence rates (per 100 000)
Wilson et al. [43]	Hip OA	M + F	47.3
	Knee OA	M + F	163.8
Kallman et al. [71]	Hand OA	M	100
Oliveria et al. [108]	Hip OA	M + F	88
	Knee OA	M + F	240
	Hand OA	M + F	100
Cooper et al. [109]	Knee OA	M + F	250

F, female; M, male.

hand, hip, and knee disease increased with age and women had higher rates than men, especially after the age of 50 years. A levelling off occurred for both groups at all joint sites around the age of 80 years. By the age of 70–89 years, the incidence of symptomatic knee OA among women approached 1% per year. Comparison of these data with age- and sex-adjusted arthroplasty rates in the northern United States suggests that the rate of surgery is beginning to match the incidence rate of severe hip disease, but that a considerable shortfall exists between surgical treatment and disease incidence for knee OA.

Lifetime risk

Murphy et al. [45,46] used data from the Johnston County study to estimate that of people who lived to age 85, 25% would develop symptomatic hip OA and 45% would develop symptomatic knee OA. An even more useful metric for explaining risk of disease to patients, and also for healthcare planners and others interested in understanding the costs and benefits of treatments and interventions, is to estimate an individual's risk at a certain age, usually 50 years old, of developing OA or requiring a joint replacement during the remainder of their life. Lifetime risks have now been published for a number of important outcomes in OA. The lifetime risk for receiving a total hip replacement (THR) was estimated using the UK General Practice Research Database (GPRD) [47]. The estimated lifetime risk for a 50-year-old man was 7.1% and for women 11.6%. The corresponding figure for total knee replacement (TKR) was 8.1% and 10.8% respectively. It is estimated that over 90% of THRs and 95% of TKRs were performed with OA as the indication [1]. The lifetime risk of these operations increased significantly between 1991 and 2005.

Natural history

Knee osteoarthritis

Knee OA in mid to late life is typically a slowly developing process occurring over decades from first onset of joint tissue lesions and symptoms to advanced joint impairment (structural damage, persistent and severe pain), functional limitation, disablement, and joint death (knee replacement) [40,48–50]. However, evidence from both older [48,51–54] and more recent [26, 49,55–62] cohort studies shows that while all domains of knee OA outcome change slowly on average, there is substantial heterogeneity in trajectories, with the possible existence of a subset of more rapidly developing or steadily progressing disease at one end of the spectrum [63] in addition to large groups at all stages of disease characterized by a slowly progressive or a relatively stable course (Table 8.3).

Table 8.3 Studies of the natural history of knee OA

Study	No. of subjects	Measure	Follow-up (years)	Proportion (%) deteriorated
Hernborg (1977) [51]	84 knees	C	15	55
		R	15	56
Danielsson (1970) [112]	106 knees	R	15	33
Massardo (1989) [54]	31	R	8	62
Dougados (1991) [113]	353	C	1	28
		R	1	29
Schouten (1992) [110]	142	R	12	34
Spector (1992) [53]	63	R	11	33
Spector (1994) [111]	58	R	2	22
Ledingham (1995) [116]	350 knees	R	2	72
McAlindon (1999) [117]	470	R	4	11[a]
Cooper et al. (2000) [109]	354	R	5	22

C, clinical; R, radiographic.

[a]Incident OA.

Older studies of knee OA patients with 8–15 years of follow-up, although lacking the frequent standardized measurements of contemporary cohort studies [48], are informative in showing that one- to two-thirds of knees with symptomatic OA have cumulative structural worsening indicated by joint space narrowing (which reflects loss of articular cartilage and damage to the meniscus) [64] and KL grades (based on both joint space narrowing and osteophytes) [65], changes that are almost always irreversible. Similarly, these studies suggest an overall trend for pain worsening, with half or more of clinic patients with knee OA having worsening pain or undergoing major surgery [48,49,51–54,66]. But more recent cohort studies with repeated measurements using state of the art standardized instruments have found that pain and function change little, on average, during 3–5 years with conflicting evidence for an overall worsening in these outcomes [55–62,67,68]. One reason for an appearance of stability is that in contrast to the cumulative and largely irreversible nature of damage to cartilage and meniscus, variability over time in symptoms and functional limitation includes periods of improvement as well as deterioration and stability. Improvement in pain and function is about as common as worsening, with 15–25% changing in both directions over 3–5 years [57,58,60–62,67,69–71].

While many studies have documented the course of pain and physical function in knee OA, there is limited data on the risk of disability and variability over time in this domain [72–75]. Cohort studies of knee OA often focus on younger populations and responsive measures of pain and function, with the assumption that limitations in these domains eventually threaten independent living and full participation in life and eventually lead to disability. The lack of data may reflect a relatively low risk of disability in these cohorts, the long time frame over which disability develops, and the ability of joint replacement and behavioural adaptations to alter the disablement process [74–78]. In older populations with a variety of chronic conditions, recurring episodes of functional limitation and disability are common, with more frequent episodes potentially contributing to a greater risk of a chronic poor outcome [79,80], but whether this is the case for knee OA is uncertain [76].

Hip osteoarthritis

The natural history of hip OA is also very variable. Many cases that come to surgery have a relatively short history of severe symptoms, suggesting that a rapidly progressive phase lasting between 3 months and 3 years may often precede the advanced stages of OA. There are fewer prospective studies of hip OA than of knee OA (Table 8.3). In a Danish follow-up study of 121 hips over three decades ago, the majority (65%) showed radiographic deterioration over a 10-year follow-up period [81]. Symptomatic improvement in this series was surprisingly common, occurring in the majority of patients. This is at variance with the results of another longitudinal study, which documented frequent deterioration in the clinical course of hip OA patients [66]. In a Dutch study of patients identified from the general population who had established OA in one or both hips, 29% of the subjects showed a worsening of their radiographic scores over a 12-year follow-up period. Nonetheless, unlike knee OA, a few patients with hip OA can experience clear-cut radiological and symptomatic recovery [67]. This appears to occur most often among patients who have marked osteophytosis and in those with concentric disease. Osteonecrosis is the major complication of hip OA and tends to occur late in the natural history. Rapidly progressive hip OA can lead to an unusual appearance with extensive bone destruction and a wide interbone distance. This appearance was initially observed among patients who ingested anti-inflammatory drugs and was termed analgesic hip [69,70]. However, it is now recognized to occur in groups of subjects who ingest few or no such agents.

Hand osteoarthritis

OA principally affects the DIP joints, proximal interphalangeal (PIP) joints, and thumb base in the hand. The evolution of hand OA is usually complete after a period of a few years. It has been studied both clinically and radiographically. The condition usually starts with aching in the affected joints and tends to have a remitting and relapsing course over the initial years. There is often clear evidence of inflammatory phases in which individual joints become warm and tender. Bony swelling develops during this phase and cysts may form. After a variable time period, often lasting several years, these flares and the pain tend to subside. The swellings become firm and fixed and joint movement becomes progressively reduced. The condition then appears to enter a stable phase during the seventh and eighth decades of life. Imaging studies show this evolution of change to be accompanied by sequential changes in joint anatomy and physiology. Kallman and colleagues reported that among men with DIP joint OA, more than 50% experienced progression of radiographic disease over 10 years [71]. The progression was fastest in the DIP joints and was slower in PIP joints and the thumb

base. The presence of joint space narrowing at baseline increased the risk that subjects would develop subsequent osteophytes, and joints with severe radiographic changes at baseline had slower progression rates than joints with milder radiographic changes. The rates of OA progression in individual subjects paralleled the rate of progression hinted at by cross-sectional studies in which subjects are studied at different ages. A further 10-year follow-up study of 59 men and women with hand OA demonstrated that 48% developed new DIP osteophytes and at either DIP, PIP, or first carpometacarpal (CMC) joint roughly 50% deteriorated over the period; 97% of patients deteriorated when all joint scores were added together [72].

Predicting the incidence and progression of osteoarthritis

OA is a heterogeneous disease with multiple risk factors and variable rates of progression. As such, in the era of preventative medicine, it would be helpful to have a clinical tool to identify a subject's risk of developing OA in order to target prevention strategies. Furthermore a tool to predict progression in those with existing disease would be ideal and allow physicians to target treatments to the correct patients. An example of such a tool is the FRAX tool used to predict fracture, which has gained acceptance and is in regular use around the world [82].

When producing a predictive tool it is important to consider a number of points. Firstly, who is the target audience? A model to be useful in primary care must include clinical tests easily available in that setting, whereas a model for secondary care can include detailed imaging and biomarkers. Secondly, the outcome of interest must be specified, preferably onset or progression of clinical OA rather than simply radiographic OA. Thirdly, the period of interest must be specified and 5 years would seem to be a clinically useful term for OA. Fourthly, the model should not only predict the risk of OA or disease worsening, but also make clear the factors that are driving the risk so that clinicians can target appropriate interventions. Fifthly, the use of the model must be specified; it is highly likely that a model to predict incidence and progression of OA will be different from a model predicting response to treatment.

Studies of risk factors for worsening of knee OA have identified few robust predictors of progression [83], attributed, in part, to methodological challenges in the study of disease prognosis [84,85]. Studying the effects of risk factors on outcomes in individuals with disease must address the potential for collider stratification bias (a form of selection bias) when the risk factors of interest are also causes of factors that are important stratifying variables or covariates [86,87]. For example, determining the effect of obesity on clinical outcomes stratifying by stage of disease or controlling for knee pain is susceptible to this bias. Finally, to be useful for guiding interventions, prediction models must identify causal risk factors.

Although there is no currently validated OA risk prediction tool available, a number of groups have published predictive models that confirm the viability of this approach in OA [88,89]. Kerkhof produced a model to predict the risk of incident radiographic knee OA using data form the Rotterdam cohorts with external validation of the model in the Chingford Cohort [88]. The model had areas under the curve (AUCs) of 0.75–0.86, which are acceptable for a tool to be used in clinical practice. Zhang and colleagues produced a model using data form primary care with validation in GOAL and the OAI

[89]. They produced separate models for radiographic knee OA and symptomatic knee OA. The model was reasonably predictive in the original cohort with AUC values of 0.69 for radiographic knee OA and 0.70 for symptomatic knee OA. The validation in the GOAL cohort was promising with AUCs of 0.74 and 0.79 respectively; however, when the model was tested for transportability to the United States-based Osteoarthritis Initiative risk factor-enriched cohort, the tool did not perform well with AUCs of 0.60 for both models.

Thomas and colleagues assessed the ability to predict radiographic hip OA and the need for a THR in the Chingford cohort [90]. Using clinical variables alone was not particularly predictive with AUCs of 0.58 and 0.64 respectively; however, the additional measures of hip morphology using the Hip Morf tool increased the AUCs considerably to 0.67 and 0.83 respectively.

Burden of disease

Morbidity worldwide

OA is among the top ten non-communicable causes of years lived with disability [91]. Hip and knee OA specifically account for 10% of all years lived with disability due to musculoskeletal disorders [92]. Knee OA has been estimated to account for over 5 million quality-adjusted life years lost in Americans age 50 to 84, and the burden is especially great among the two-thirds of women with knee OA who are also obese [93].

Costs

The overall cost of OA in developed countries is estimated to be between 1% and 3% of gross domestic product [94]. Knee and hip OA have an especially large impact on the healthcare costs of musculoskeletal disease. Knee and hip pain, functional limitation, and disability are key factors in the need for joint replacement [95,96], whose dramatically increasing rates and contribution to costs [97–99] will continue to soar without effective interventions to prevent poor clinical outcomes in this disease.

Mortality

There is an increasing body of research supporting an increased risk of premature mortality in patients with OA, but there is a paucity of high-quality population-based longitudinal studies with adequate follow-up and adjustment for important confounders, such as comorbidity. A systematic review found that the evidence for an association between OA and increased mortality was moderate, with the strongest evidence for death from acute cardiovascular and gastrointestinal causes [100], but noted methodological shortcomings across these studies, including lack of accounting for potential confounders, samples that were not population based, short follow-up times, and insufficient statistical power. One of the first studies published in this area was by Cerhan et al. in 1995. They found that radiographic OA is associated with decreased survival of middle-aged women, assessed at 55 joints, who worked in the radium dial-painting industry [101]. An increasing number of joints affected by OA was associated with early mortality (hazard ratio (HR) 1.45; 95% CI 1.12–1.87) for each three additional joints groups affected. Further studies have examined joint specific mortality.

Hip and knee

Nüesch and colleagues utilized a large selected population-based sample of men and women with symptomatic radiographic knee and/or hip OA and compared mortality to general population statistics after a median of 14 years' follow-up [2,3,102–105]. They reported a significant excess in all-cause mortality (standardized mortality ratio 1.55; 95% CI 1.41–1.70). There was a high risk of cardiovascular disease (CVD)- and dementia-related mortality (standardized mortality ratio 1.71; 95% CI 1.49–1.98, and 1.99; 95% CI 1.22–3.25, respectively). Hawker and colleagues examined the contribution of baseline OA symptoms severity to all-cause mortality and CVD outcomes, within a cohort of patients with OA [3]. They showed that worse walking disability, use of a walking aid, and poor baseline function is independently associated with excess all-cause mortality.

Kluzek and colleagues have recently reported data from the Chingford study of women with a median of 21.7 years of follow up [106]. Women with symptomatic, radiographic knee OA had an increased risk of all-cause mortality (HR 1.97; 95% CI, 1.23–3.17) and CVD-specific mortality (HR 3.57; 95% CI, 1.53–8.34). Knee pain was associated with an increased CVD-specific mortality (HR 2.93; 95% CI 1.47–5.85), but not all cause mortality (HR 1.44; 95% CI 0.99–2.08).

Barbour and colleagues reported mortality data from the Study of Osteoporotic Fractures [107]. Over a median follow-up of 16.1 years, radiographic hip OA was associated with a small increased risk of all-cause mortality (HR 1.14; 95% CI 1.05–1.24), and a modest increased risk of CVD-specific mortality (HR 1.24; 95% CI 1.09–1.41). The excess mortality was at least partially explained by the effect of hip OA on physical function.

Hand

The association between any hand OA and mortality is unclear. Haara and colleagues demonstrated no overall association in Finnish adults, but did identify a small increased risk of CVD mortality in men with severe disease. Haara and colleagues also demonstrated that symmetrical DIP OA in women, but not men, predicted premature CVD mortality during a 15- to 17-year follow-up [102,103]. These results stand in contrast to more recent publication from the Framingham Study showing no association with an excess mortality in either radiographic or symptomatic hand OA [104]. This is also consistent with recent results from the Chingford cohort which demonstrated no association for either radiographic or symptomatic hand OA [106]. Overall, it would appear that any association of hand OA with mortality is, at most, modest.

Other or multiple joints

Patients with symptomatic primary OA of hand, spine, or lower limb OA were not found to have a higher risk of death than the general population [105]. Mortality in men and women from two different cohorts of patients consulting health professionals for OA at the hip, knee, or hand, were compared with general population mortality data. The lack of an increase in mortality could be explained by the heterogeneity of OA groups, including the fact that all subjects had self-referred to the physicians; and the use of national population data as controls, which by definition will include a large number of cases of OA.

In summary, OA is associated with an increased risk of mortality, the greatest risk being at the knee. The effect is strongest for symptomatic OA, with much smaller associations for radiographic OA.

References

1. Culliford DJ, Maskell J, Beard DJ, et al. Temporal trends in hip and knee replacement in the United Kingdom: 1991 to 2006. *J Bone Joint Surg Br* 2010; 92(1):130–5.

2. Nuesch E, Dieppe P, Reichenbach S, et al. All cause and disease specific mortality in patients with knee or hip osteoarthritis: population based cohort study. *BMJ* 2011; 342:d1165.

3. Hawker GA, Croxford R, Bierman AS, et al. All-cause mortality and serious cardiovascular events in people with hip and knee osteoarthritis: a population based cohort study. *PLoS One* 2014; 9(3):e91286.

4. Hutton CW. Osteoarthritis: the cause not result of joint failure? *Ann Rheum Dis* 1989; 48(11):958–61.

5. Roemer FW, Kassim Javaid M, Guermazi A, et al. Anatomical distribution of synovitis in knee osteoarthritis and its association with joint effusion assessed on non-enhanced and contrast-enhanced MRI. *Osteoarthritis Cartilage* 2010; 18(10):1269–74.

6. Neogi T. The epidemiology and impact of pain in osteoarthritis. *Osteoarthritis Cartilage* 2013; 21(9):1145–53.

7. Kellgren JH, Lawrence JS. Radiological assessment of osteo-arthrosis. *Ann Rheum Dis* 1957; 16(4):494–502.

8. Bedson J, Croft PR. The discordance between clinical and radiographic knee osteoarthritis: a systematic search and summary of the literature. *BMC Musculoskelet Disord* 2008; 9:116.

9. Guermazi A, Niu J, Hayashi D, et al. Prevalence of abnormalities in knees detected by MRI in adults without knee osteoarthritis: population based observational study (Framingham Osteoarthritis Study). *BMJ* 2012; 345:e5339.

10. Hunter DJ, Guermazi A, Roemer F, Zhang Y, Neogi T. Structural correlates of pain in joints with osteoarthritis. *Osteoarthritis Cartilage* 2013; 21(9):1170–8.

11. Altman R, Alarcon G, Appelrouth D, et al. The American College of Rheumatology criteria for the classification and reporting of osteoarthritis of the hand. *Arthritis Rheum* 1990; 33(11):1601–10.

12. Altman R, Alarcon G, Appelrouth D, et al. The American College of Rheumatology criteria for the classification and reporting of osteoarthritis of the hip. *Arthritis Rheum* 1991; 34(5):505–14.

13. Arden N, Nevitt M. Osteoarthritis—Epidemiology. *Best Pract Res Clin Rheumatol* 2006; 20(1):1–2.

14. Sharma L. Local factors in osteoarthritis. *Curr Opin Rheumatol* 2001; 13(5):441–6.

15. Berenbaum F. Osteoarthritis as an inflammatory disease (osteoarthritis is not osteoarthrosis!). *Osteoarthritis Cartilage* 2013; 21(1):16–21.

16. Ehrlich GE. Inflammatory osteoarthritis—I. The clinical syndrome. *J Chronic Dis* 1972; 25(6–7):317–28.

17. Evans CH, Mazzocchi RA, Nelson DD, Rubash HE. Experimental arthritis induced by intraarticular injection of allogenic cartilaginous particles into rabbit knees. *Arthritis Rheum* 1984; 27(2):200–7.

18. Utsinger PD, Resnick D, Shapiro RF, Wiesner KB. Roentgenologic, immunologic, and therapeutic study of erosive (inflammatory) osteoarthritis. *Arch Internal Med* 1978; 138(5):693–7.

19. Verbruggen G, Goemaere S, Veys EM. Systems to assess the progression of finger joint osteoarthritis and the effects of disease modifying osteoarthritis drugs. *Clin Rheumatol* 2002; 21(3):231–43.

20. Zayer M. Osteoarthritis following Blount's disease. *Int Orthop* 1980; 4(1):63–6.

21. Sokoloff L. Endemic forms of osteoarthritis. *Clinics Rheum Dis* 1985; 11(2):187–202.

22. Newman AB, Haggerty CL, Goodpaster B, et al. Strength and muscle quality in a well-functioning cohort of older adults: the Health, Aging and Body Composition Study. *J Am Geriatr Soc* 2003; 51(3):323–30.

23. Guccione AA, Felson DT, Anderson JJ, et al. The effects of specific medical conditions on the functional limitations of elders in the Framingham Study. *Am J Public Health* 1994; 84(3):351–8.

24. Culliford D, Maskell J, Judge A, et al. Future projections of total hip and knee arthroplasty in the UK: Results From The Uk Clinical Practice Research Datalink. *Osteoarthritis Cartilage* 2015; 23(4):594–600.

25. Lawrence JS, Bremner JM, Bier F. Osteo-arthrosis. Prevalence in the population and relationship between symptoms and x-ray changes. *Ann Rheum Dis* 1966; 25(1):1–24.

26. Leyland KM, Hart DJ, Javaid MK, et al. The natural history of radiographic knee osteoarthritis: a fourteen-year population-based cohort study. *Arthritis Rheum* 2012; 64(7):2243–51.

27. Zhang Y, Xu L, Nevitt MC, et al. Comparison of the prevalence of knee osteoarthritis between the elderly Chinese population in Beijing and whites in the United States: The Beijing Osteoarthritis Study. *Arthritis Rheum* 2001; 44(9):2065–71.

28. Muraki S, Oka H, Akune T, et al. Prevalence of radiographic knee osteoarthritis and its association with knee pain in the elderly of Japanese population-based cohorts: the ROAD study. *Osteoarthritis Cartilage* 2009; 17(9):1137–43.

29. Lawrence RC, Felson DT, Helmick CG, et al. Estimates of the prevalence of arthritis and other rheumatic conditions in the United States. Part II. *Arthritis Rheum* 2008; 58(1):26–35.

30. Kim C, Linsenmeyer KD, Vlad SC, et al. Prevalence of radiographic and symptomatic hip osteoarthritis in an urban United States community: the Framingham osteoarthritis study. *Arthritis Rheumatol* 2014; 66(11):3013–7.

31. Jordan JM, Linder GF, Renner JB, Fryer JG. The impact of arthritis in rural populations. *Arthritis Care Res* 1995; 8(4):242–50.

32. Shichikawa K, Mayeda A, Komatsubara Y, et al. Rheumatic complaints in urban and rural populations in Osaka. *Ann Rheum Dis* 1966; 25(1):25–31.

33. Hoaglund FT, Yau AC, Wong WL. Osteoarthritis of the hip and other joints in southern Chinese in Hong Kong. *J Bone Joint Surg Am.* 1973; 55(3):545–57.

34. Hoaglund FT, Oishi CS, Gialamas GG. Extreme variations in racial rates of total hip arthroplasty for primary coxarthrosis: a population-based study in San Francisco. *Ann Rheum Dis* 1995; 54(2):107–10.

35. Lau EM, Lin F, Lam D, Silman A, Croft P. Hip osteoarthritis and dysplasia in Chinese men. *Ann Rheum Dis* 1995; 54(12):965–9.

36. Lawrence RC, Helmick CG, Arnett FC, et al. Estimates of the prevalence of arthritis and selected musculoskeletal disorders in the United States. *Arthritis Rheum* 1998; 41(5):778–99.

37. van Saase JL, van Romunde LK, Cats A, Vandenbroucke JP, Valkenburg HA. Epidemiology of osteoarthritis: Zoetermeer survey. Comparison of radiological osteoarthritis in a Dutch population with that in 10 other populations. *Ann Rheum Dis* 1989; 48(4):271–80.

38. Zhang Y, Xu L, Nevitt MC, et al. Lower prevalence of hand osteoarthritis among Chinese subjects in Beijing compared with white subjects in the United States: the Beijing Osteoarthritis Study. *Arthritis Rheum* 2003; 48(4):1034–40.

39. Felson DT. The course of osteoarthritis and factors that affect it. *Rheum Dis Clin North Am* 1993; 19(3):607–15.

40. Ettinger B, Davis MA, Neuhaus JM, Mallon K. Long term functioning in knee osteoarthritis: effects of comorbid conditions. *J Clin Epidemiol* 1994; 47:809–15.

41. Tepper S, Hochberg MC. Factors associated with hip osteoarthritis: data from the First National Health and Nutrition Examination Survey (NHANES-I). *Am J Epidemiol* 1993; 137(10):1081–8.

42. Jordan JM, Helmick CG, Renner JB, et al. Prevalence of hip symptoms and radiographic and symptomatic hip osteoarthritis in African Americans and Caucasians: the Johnston County Osteoarthritis Project. *J Rheumatol* 2009; 36(4):809–15.

43. Wilson MG, Michet CJ, Jr, Ilstrup DM, Melton LJ, 3rd. Idiopathic symptomatic osteoarthritis of the hip and knee: a population-based incidence study. *Mayo Clinic Proc* 1990; 65(9):1214–21.

44. Kwoh CK. Epidemiology of osteoarthritis. In Newman AB, Cauley JA (eds) *The Epidemiology of Aging.* Dordrecht: Springer; 2012:523–36.

45. Murphy L, Schwartz TA, Helmick CG, et al. Lifetime risk of symptomatic knee osteoarthritis. *Arthritis Rheum* 2008; 59(9):1207–13.

46. Murphy LB, Helmick CG, Schwartz TA, et al. One in four people may develop symptomatic hip osteoarthritis in his or her lifetime. *Osteoarthritis Cartilage* 2010; 18(11):1372–9.

47. Culliford DJ, Maskell J, Kiran A, et al. The lifetime risk of total hip and knee arthroplasty: results from the UK general practice research database. *Osteoarthritis Cartilage* 2012; 20(6):519–24.

48. Felson DT. The course of osteoarthritis and factors that affect it. *Rheum Dis Clin North Am* 1993; 19:607.

49. Wolfe F, Lane NE. The longterm outcome of osteoarthritis: rates and predictors of joint space narrowing in symptomatic patients with knee osteoarthritis. *J Rheumatol* 2002; 29(1):139–46.

50. Kwoh CK. Epidemiology of osteoarthritis. In Newman AB, Cauley JA (eds) *The Epidemiology of Aging*. Dordrecht: Springer; 2012:523–36.

51. Hernborg JS, Nilsson BE. The natural course of untreated osteoarthritis of the knee. *Clin Orthop* 1977; 123:130–7.

52. Odenbring S, Lindstrand A, Egund N, Larsson J, Heddson B. Prognosis for patients with medial gonarthrosis. A 16-year follow-up study of 189 knees. *Clin Orthop Related Res* 1991(266):152–5.

53. Spector TD, Dacre JE, Harris PA, Huskisson EC. Radiological progression of osteoarthritis: an 11 year follow up study of the knee. *Ann Rheum Dis* 1992; 51:1107–10.

54. Massardo L, Watt I, Cushnaghan J, Dieppe P. Osteoarthritis of the knee joint: an eight year prospective study. *Ann Rheum Dis* 1989; 48(11):893–7.

55. van Dijk GM, Dekker J, Veenhof C, van den Ende CH. Course of functional status and pain in osteoarthritis of the hip or knee: a systematic review of the literature. *Arthritis Rheum* 2006; 55(5):779–85.

56. van Dijk GM, Veenhof C, Spreeuwenberg P, et al. Prognosis of limitations in activities in osteoarthritis of the hip or knee: a 3-year cohort study. *Arch Phys Med Rehabil* 2010; 91(1):58–66.

57. Wesseling J, Bierma-Zeinstra SM, Kloppenburg M, Meijer R, Bijlsma JW. Worsening of pain and function over 5 years in individuals with 'early' OA is related to structural damage: data from the Osteoarthritis Initiative and CHECK (Cohort Hip & Cohort Knee) study. *Ann Rheum Dis* 2015; 74(2):347–53.

58. Jinks C, Jordan K, Croft P. Osteoarthritis as a public health problem: the impact of developing knee pain on physical function in adults living in the community: (KNEST 3). *Rheumatology (Oxford)* 2007; 46(5):877–81.

59. Mallen CD, Peat G, Thomas E, Dunn KM, Croft PR. Prognostic factors for musculoskeletal pain in primary care: a systematic review. *Br J Gen Pract* 2007; 57(541):655–61.

60. Muller S, Thomas E, Peat G. The effect of changes in lower limb pain on the rate of progression of locomotor disability in middle and old age: evidence from the NorStOP cohort with 6-year follow-up. *Pain* 2012; 153(5):952–9.

61. Pisters MF, Veenhof C, van Dijk GM, et al. The course of limitations in activities over 5 years in patients with knee and hip osteoarthritis with moderate functional limitations: risk factors for future functional decline. *Osteoarthritis Cartilage* 2012; 20(6):503–10.

62. Ayis S, Dieppe P. The natural history of disability and its determinants in adults with lower limb musculoskeletal pain. *J Rheumatol* 2009; 36(3):583–91.

63. Holla JF, van der Leeden M, Heymans MW, et al. Three trajectories of activity limitations in early symptomatic knee osteoarthritis: a 5-year follow-up study. *Ann Rheum Dis* 2014; 73(7):1369–75.

64. Hunter DJ, Zhang YQ, Tu X, et al. Change in joint space width: hyaline articular cartilage loss or alteration in meniscus? *Arthritis Rheum* 2006; 54(8):2488–95.

65. Kellgren JH, Empire Rheumatism Council. *The Epidemiology of Chronic Rheumatism. The Atlas of Standard Radiographs*, Vol. 2. Oxford: Blackwell Scientific; 1963.

66. Dieppe P, Cushnaghan J, Tucker M, Browning S, Shepstone L. The Bristol 'OA500 study': progression and impact of the disease after 8 years. *Osteoarthritis Cartilage* 2000; 8(2):63–8.

67. Mallen CD, Peat G, Thomas E, Lacey R, Croft P. Predicting poor functional outcome in community-dwelling older adults with knee pain: prognostic value of generic indicators. *Ann Rheum Dis* 2007; 66(11):1456–61.

68. Soni A, Kiran A, Hart DJ, et al. Prevalence of reported knee pain over twelve years in a community-based cohort. *Arthritis Rheum* 2012; 64(4):1145–52.

69. Thomas E, Dunn KM, Mallen C, Peat G. A prognostic approach to defining chronic pain: application to knee pain in older adults. *Pain* 2008; 139(2):389–97.

70. Sharma L, Cahue S, Song J, et al. Physical functioning over three years in knee osteoarthritis: role of psychosocial, local mechanical, and neuromuscular factors. *Arthritis Rheum* 2003; 48(12):3359–70.

71. Kallman DA, Wigley FM, Scott WWJr, Hochberg MC, Tobin JD. The longitudinal course of hand osteoarthritis in a male population. *Arthritis Rheum* 1990; 33(9):1323–32.

72. Jordan KP, Wilkie R, Muller S, Myers H, Nicholls E. Measurement of change in function and disability in osteoarthritis: current approaches and future challenges. *Curr Opin Rheumatol* 2009; 21(5):525–30.

73. Keysor JJ, Jette AM, LaValley MP, et al. Community environmental factors are associated with disability in older adults with functional limitations: the MOST study. *J Gerontol A Biol Sci Med Sci* 2010; 65(4):393–9.

74. Wilkie R, Peat G, Thomas E, Croft P. Factors associated with restricted mobility outside the home in community-dwelling adults ages fifty years and older with knee pain: an example of use of the International Classification of Functioning to investigate participation restriction. *Arthritis Rheum* 2007; 57(8):1381–9.

75. Davis AM, Perruccio AV, Ibrahim S, et al. The trajectory of recovery and the inter-relationships of symptoms, activity and participation in the first year following total hip and knee replacement. *Osteoarthritis Cartilage* 2011; 19(12):1413–21.

76. Wilkie R, Thomas E, Mottram S, Peat G, Croft P. Onset and persistence of person-perceived participation restriction in older adults: a 3-year follow-up study in the general population. *Health Qual Life Outcomes* 2008; 6:92.

77. Maxwell JL, Keysor JJ, Niu J, et al. Participation following knee replacement: the MOST cohort study. *Phys Ther* 2013; 93(11):1467–74.

78. Jette AM, Keysor JJ. Disability models: implications for arthritis exercise and physical activity interventions. *Arthritis Rheum* 2003; 49(1):114–20.

79. Gill TM. Disentangling the disabling process: insights from the precipitating events project. *Gerontologist* 2014; 54(4):533–49.

80. Hardy SE, Allore HG, Guo Z, Dubin JA, Gill TM. The effect of prior disability history on subsequent functional transitions. *J Gerontol A Biol Sci Med Sci* 2006; 61(3):272–7.

81. Kellgren J, Jeffrey M, Ball J. *The Epidemiology of Chronic Rheumatism. Volume II: Atlas of Standard Radiographs of Arthritis.* Oxford: Blackwell Scientific Publications; 1963.

82. Kanis JA, Johnell O, Oden A, Johansson H, McCloskey E. FRAX and the assessment of fracture probability in men and women from the UK. *Osteoporos Int* 2008; 19(4):385–97.

83. Belo JN, Berger MY, Reijman M, Koes BW, Bierma-Zeinstra SM. Prognostic factors of progression of osteoarthritis of the knee: a systematic review of observational studies. *Arthritis Rheum* 2007; 57(1):13–26.

84. Zhang Y, Niu J, Felson DT, et al. Methodologic challenges in studying risk factors for progression of knee osteoarthritis. *Arthritis Care Res (Hoboken)* 2010; 62(11):1527–32.

85. Zhang Y, Neogi T, Hunter D, Roemer F, Niu J. What effect is really being measured? An alternative explanation of paradoxical phenomena in studies of osteoarthritis progression. *Arthritis Care Res (Hoboken)* 2014; 66(5):658–61.

86. Hernan MA, Hernandez-Diaz S, Robins JM. A structural approach to selection bias. *Epidemiology* 2004; 15(5):615–25.

87. Glymour MM. Invited commentary: when bad genes look good—APOE*E4, cognitive decline, and diagnostic thresholds. *Am J Epidemiol* 2007; 165(11):1239–46.

88. Kerkhof HJ, Bierma-Zeinstra SM, Arden NK, et al. Prediction model for knee osteoarthritis incidence, including clinical, genetic and biochemical risk factors. *Ann Rheum Dis* 2014; 73(12):2116–21.

89. Zhang W, McWilliams DF, Ingham SL, et al. Nottingham knee osteoarthritis risk prediction models. *Ann Rheum Dis* 2011; 70(9):1599–604.

90. Thomas GE, Palmer AJ, Batra RN, et al. Subclinical deformities of the hip are significant predictors of radiographic osteoarthritis and joint replacement in women. A 20 year longitudinal cohort study. *Osteoarthritis Cartilage* 2014; 22(10):1504–10.

91. Murray CJ, Vos T, Lozano R, et al. Disability-adjusted life years (DALYs) for 291 diseases and injuries in 21 regions, 1990-2010: a systematic analysis for the Global Burden of Disease Study 2010. *Lancet* 2012; 380(9859):2197–223.

92. March L, Smith EU, Hoy DG, et al. Burden of disability due to musculoskeletal (MSK) disorders. *Best Pract Res Clin Rheumatol* 2014; 28(3):353–66.

93. Losina E, Walensky RP, Reichmann WM, et al. Impact of obesity and knee osteoarthritis on morbidity and mortality in older Americans. *Ann Internal Med* 2011; 154(4):217–26.

94. Hiligsmann M, Bruyère O, Reginster JY, et al. Health economics in the field of osteoarthritis: an Expert's consensus paper from the European Society for Clinical and Economic Aspects of Osteoporosis and Osteoarthritis (ESCEO). *Semin Arthritis Rheum* 2013; 43(3):303–13.

95. Boutron I, Rannou F, Jardinaud-Lopez M, et al. Disability and quality of life of patients with knee or hip osteoarthritis in the primary care setting and factors associated with general practitioners' indication for prosthetic replacement within 1 year. *Osteoarthritis Cartilage* 2008; 16(9):1024–31.

96. Gossec L, Paternotte S, Maillefert JF, et al. The role of pain and functional impairment in the decision to recommend total joint replacement in hip and knee osteoarthritis: an international cross-sectional study of 1909 patients. Report of the OARSI-OMERACT Task Force on total joint replacement. *Osteoarthritis Cartilage* 2011; 19(2):147–54.

97. Kim S. Changes in surgical loads and economic burden of hip and knee replacements in the US: 1997-2004. *Arthritis Rheum* 2008; 59(4):481–8.

98. Weinstein AM, Rome BN, Reichmann WM, et al. Estimating the burden of total knee replacement in the United States. *J Bone Joint Surg Am.* 2013; 95(5):385–92.

99. Losina E, Paltiel AD, Weinstein AM, et al. Lifetime medical costs of knee osteoarthritis management in the United States: impact of extending indications for total knee arthroplasty. *Arthritis Care Res (Hoboken)* 2015; 67(2):203–15.

100. Hochberg MC. Mortality in osteoarthritis. *Clin Exp Rheumatol* 2008; 26(5 Suppl 51):S120–4.

101. Cerhan JR, Wallace RB, el-Khoury GY, Moore TE, Long CR. Decreased survival with increasing prevalence of full-body, radiographically defined osteoarthritis in women. *Am J Epidemiol* 1995; 141(3):225–34.

102. Haara MM, Heliovaara M, Kroger H, et al. Osteoarthritis in the carpometacarpal joint of the thumb. Prevalence and associations with disability and mortality. *J Bone Joint Surg Am* 2004; 86-A(7):1452–7.

103. Haara MM, Manninen P, Kroger H, et al. Osteoarthritis of finger joints in Finns aged 30 or over: prevalence,

determinants, and association with mortality. *Ann Rheum Dis* 2003; 62(2):151–8.

104. Haugen IK, Ramachandran VS, Misra D, et al. Hand osteoarthritis in relation to mortality and incidence of cardiovascular disease: data from the Framingham Heart Study. *Ann Rheum Dis* 2015; 74(1):74–81.

105. Liu R, Kwok W, Vliet Vlieland T, et al. Mortality in osteoarthritis patients. *Scand J Rheumatol* 2014:1–4.

106. Kluzek S, Sanchez-Santos MT, Leyland KM, et al. Painful knee but not hand osteoarthritis is an independent predictor of mortality over 23 years follow-up of a population-based cohort of middle-aged women. *Ann Rheum Dis* 2015 [Epub ahead of print] doi: 10.1136/annrheumdis-2015-208056.

107. Barbour KE, Lui LY, Nevitt MC, et al. Hip osteoarthritis and the risk of all-cause and disease-specific mortality in older women: a population-based cohort study. *Arthritis Rheumatol* 2015; 67(7):1798–805.

108. Oliveria SA, Felson DT, Reed JI, et al. Incidence of symptomatic hand, hip, and knee osteoarthritis among patients in a health maintenance organization. *Arthritis Rheum* 1995; 38(8):1134–41.

109. Cooper C, Snow S, McAlindon TE, et al. Risk factors for the incidence and progression of radiographic knee osteoarthritis. *Arthritis Rheum* 2000; 43(5):995–1000.

110. Schouten JSAG, van den Ouweland FA & Valkenburg HA. A 12 year follow up study in the general population on prognostic factors of cartilage loss in osteoarthritis of the knee. *Ann Rheum Dis* 1992; 51:932–7.

111. Spector TD, Hart DJ & Doyle DV. Incidence and progression of osteoarthritis in women with unilateral knee disease in the general population: the effect of obesity. *Ann Rheum Dis* 1994; 53(9):565–8.

112. Danielsson L, Hernborg J. Clinical and roentgenologic study of knee joints with osteophytes. *Clin Orthop Relat Res* 1970; 69:302–12.

113. Dougados M, Gueguen A, Nguyen M, Thiesce A, Listrat V, Jacob L, Nakache JP, Gabriel KR, Lequesne M, Amor B. Longitudinal radiologic evaluation of osteoarthritis of the knee. *J Rheumatol* 1992; 19(3):378–84.

114. Schouten JSAG, van den Ouweland FA & Valkenburg HA. A 12 year follow up study in the general population on prognostic factors of cartilage loss in osteoarthritis of the knee. *Ann Rheum Dis* 1992; 51:932–7.

115. Spector TD, Hart DJ & Doyle DV. Incidence and progression of osteoarthritis in women with unilateral knee disease in the general population: the effect of obesity. *Ann Rheum Dis* 1994; 53(9):565–8.

116. Ledingham J, Regan M, Jones A, Doherty M. Factors affecting radiographic progression of knee osteoarthritis. *Ann Rheum Dis* 1995; 54(1):53–8.

117. McAlindon TE, Wilson PW, Aliabadi P, Weissman B, Felson DT. Level of physical activity and the risk of radiographic and symptomatic knee osteoarthritis in the elderly: the Framingham study. *Am J Med* 1999; 106(2):151–7.

SECTION 4

Risk factors

CHAPTER 9

Genetics

Ana M. Valdes

Introduction

Osteoarthritis (OA) is the most common human arthritis and as such it has a considerable global impact. The total economic burden for arthritis is estimated to be 1–2.5% of the gross national product in Western countries [1]. This burden is predicted to rise substantially as the prevalence of OA increases with a greater proportion of the population living longer. Epidemiological studies have demonstrated that OA is a complex trait with numerous environmental and genetic risk factors. A great deal of effort has been spent elucidating these risk factors and progress has been made. It is clear, however, that the causes behind the development and progression of OA continue to remain largely elusive.

Identification of those genes that, in conjunction with environmental factors, predispose to OA severity will lead to a better understanding of the mechanisms underlying disease development and thus promote improved health strategies for prevention. An understanding of the molecular signalling pathways involved in the initiation and progression of the disease will improve clinical diagnosis and help identify improved, tailored treatment regimens.

Heritability of osteoarthritis

The extent to which OA runs in families can be measured by assessing how much higher the risk is of developing OA among relatives of an affected person compared to the risk seen in the population at large. This risk ratio for a relative, such as a sibling, of an affected individual to that of the general population prevalence is termed the recurrence-risk ratio [2] and for affected siblings the recurrence-risk ratio is called the lambda sib (λs). The occurrence of OA has been tested in siblings of subjects with OA severe enough to lead to a total joint replacement (TJR) and compared to the general population it has been found that siblings have a significantly higher prevalence of OA. The sibling recurrence-risk ratio for radiographic knee OA has been estimated to be 2.08–3.21 and for radiographic hip OA between 4.27 and 5.07. For total knee replacement, estimates ranging between 2.8 and 4.8 have been reported and for total hip replacement, between 1.78 and 8.5 [3]. However, these estimates do not take into account the fact that some of the similarities between siblings may be due to a shared environment and similar lifestyle choices of individuals within the same family. A more accurate way of assessing the actual genetic contribution to OA is through the use of classical twin studies, which enable investigators to quantify the environmental and genetic factors that contribute to a trait or disease. Comparing the similarity of genetically identical twins for a trait or disease with the resemblance of

Table 9.1 Heritability of large-joint osteoarthritis-related traits in twin and family studies

Trait	Heritability (h^2)	Data from reference
Radiographic knee osteoarthritis	39%	[56]
Radiographic hip osteoarthritis	60%	[57]
Generalized osteoarthritis	42%	[58]
Knee pain reporting	44–46%	[4,59]
Radiographic progression	69%	[17]
Cartilage volume	77–85%	[60]
Changes muscle strength in lower limb	64%	[4]

non-identical twins offers the best estimate of the extent to which genetic variation determines variation of that trait or 'heritability'. The heritability of OA has been calculated in twin sets after adjustment of the data for other known risk factors such as age, sex, and body mass index (BMI). Heritability has also been investigated using variance component methods in pedigrees (e.g. [4]). Such findings show that the influence of genetic factors in radiographic OA of the hand, hip, and knee in women is between 30% and 65%, independent of known environmental or demographic confounding factors. Classical twin studies and family studies have also investigated the genetic contribution to cartilage volume, progression of disease, change in lower limb muscle strength, and pain reporting as summarized in Table 9.1.

Known genetic risk factors for osteoarthritis

Over the last 10–15 years, efforts have focused on the search for loci that predispose to the disease. The approaches followed have reflected the concurrent status quo of complex disease genetics: candidate gene studies (testing variants in genes already hypothesized to be involved in OA), genome-wide linkage scans (testing ~400 genetic markers in the genome to assess differences in segregation in families with members affected by OA), small-scale (<100 000 genetic variants) genome-wide association studies (GWASs), and more recently large-scale GWASs (testing >100 000 genetic variants).

A candidate gene association study is limited in that it relies upon a priori understanding of the aetiology of OA and allows for only very small regions of the genome to be targeted for investigation.

Consequently, many important genes have probably been overlooked using this method. As described below, this approach has identified a number of important genes such *ASPN* (asporin, a cartilage protein involved in chondrogenesis), *FRZB* (frizzled secreted protein, important in WNT signalling, a crucial pathway for cartilage metabolism), and *PTGS2* (prostaglandin-endoperoxide synthase 2, an important mediator in inflammation) that continue to be compelling targets for functional studies and further genetic replication in independent populations.

The candidate gene association method identified the polymorphism rs143383 within the 5′ untranslated region (UTR) of the gene *GDF5*. This is still the most robustly replicated polymorphism to be associated with OA and the only locus to successfully replicate across diverse Asian and European populations. Whilst very few genes meet the strict criteria of replication, even fewer have also demonstrated functional significance. Among these, some of the most compelling are *ASPN* [5], the gene encoding growth differentiation factor 5, *GDF5* [6–8], and the *SMAD3* gene [9]. These three genes have in common being part of the bone morphogenetic protein (BMP) signalling pathway. Another interesting gene identified first by linkage analysis and later by association, is the deiodinase iodothyronine type II gene (*DIO2*) [10]. *DIO2* encodes an intracellular enzyme in the thyroid pathway, responsible for the local bioavailability of thyroid hormone in specific tissues, including the growth plate. The active thyroid hormone, triiodothyronine (T_3), plays an essential role in the control of chondrocyte proliferation and differentiation, inhibiting BMP2-induced growth of mouse rib.

Notwithstanding these findings, it is now widely recognized that candidate gene approaches may not be the optimal strategies for dissecting the genetic aetiology of common complex disorders. In fact, a recent study [11] explored the association between 199 candidate genes as defined by the Human Genome Epidemiology (HuGE) Navigator in a large dataset. The study was sufficiently powered having studied 5636 patients with knee OA and 16 972 control subjects, and 4349 patients with hip OA and 17 836 control subjects of European ancestry and further replication in 5921 people. Only variants of two of the candidate genes, *COL11A1* and *VEGF*, reached the significance level after adjustment for multiple tests ($p < 1.58 \times 10^{-5}$). The remaining 197 genes were not associated. These data confirm that at least for OA, variants located in candidate genes based on current knowledge of joint biology are unlikely to contribute substantially to the risk of OA [11].

Traits and outcomes studied in the genetics of osteoarthritis

For both epidemiological and genetic studies the definition of OA which is used most often is a radiographic one, usually based on the Kellgren/Lawrence (K/L) grade [12]. In addition, several studies have focused on 'clinical OA' defined as radiographic OA in the presence of pain or other American College of Rheumatology criteria and some studies use TJR with a primary indication of OA as a surrogate for severe clinical OA [13]. The merit of these definitions has been discussed elsewhere [13], but it is worth noting that OA represents a group of disorders and the inter- and intra-articular patterns of OA have distinct risk factor profiles and disease courses [14]. In fact, genetic variation may be contributing to

risk of OA through different mechanisms and molecular pathways (Figure 9.1).

In a genetic association study, the selection of a correct phenotype is critical for the interpretation of the study as well as for the power to find true significant and plausible results. Previous efforts using multiple dichotomous-composed definitions in GWASs of OA yielded few genomic loci. Reasons for this include low power in the discovery phase of the GWAS and phenotypic heterogeneity. Phenotypic heterogeneity can substantially reduce power in GWASs [15] and it is clear that OA suffers from this; for example, in the case of hip OA, some cases only exhibit joint space narrowing and not osteophyte formation. A way to decrease phenotypic heterogeneity is through the use of intermediate phenotypes and endophenotypes. Endophenotypes are stable phenotypes that can be more reliably phenotyped and quantified and additionally, they might be closer to what is encoded in the DNA sequence. To separate and define these subphenotypes it is therefore desirable to investigate the components that define different forms of OA, such as radiographic severity, extent of cartilage loss, presence/absence of synovitis, pain and functional severity of the disease, and generalized versus non-generalized disease. The genetic contribution to some of these factors is only beginning to be addressed.

Cartilage loss and disease progression

Cartilage loss is one of the main traits evidencing OA. Twin and sibling studies have indicated that the heritability of cartilage volume is very high [16]. Using longitudinal X-ray data, heritability estimates of 62% for progression of osteophytes and 72% for progression of JSN of the knee, independent of age and BMI, have been reported (63%) [17]. A genetic influence on radiographic disease progression over 2 years was also assessed in a sibling-pair design in a separate study on generalized symptomatic OA (the GARP study) [18]. These results highlight a strong genetic influence on progression of OA and provide a logical basis for the next step to identify specific genetic factors responsible for both incidence and progression of OA. To date, no genome-wide association scans on progression have been reported.

Radiographic severity

The most common definition of OA for genetic studies has been a radiographic one, usually based on the K/L system [19] which assigns a value from 0 to 4 with the aid of atlas reproductions; the cut-off of 2, corresponding to definite osteophytes and possible joint space narrowing, is the norm. However, the presence of osteophytes is extremely common in the general population [19] and a K/L grade of 2 is not necessarily of clinical concern. An important aspect is therefore to investigate the extent to which genetic variation influences radiographic severity. A study in the United States showed that haplotypes in the interleukin 1 receptor antagonist (*IL1RN*) gene were associated with greater radiographic knee OA severity [20] and this was later confirmed by a much larger European study [21]. These data suggest that one of the pathways contributing to radiographic severity may be related to inflammation.

Minimal joint space width (mJSW) is an endophenotype that represents cartilage thickness. The principal advantage of mJSW as an endophenotype is the focus on one structure of the joint (cartilage) and it is primarily 'state independent' (measurable in an individual

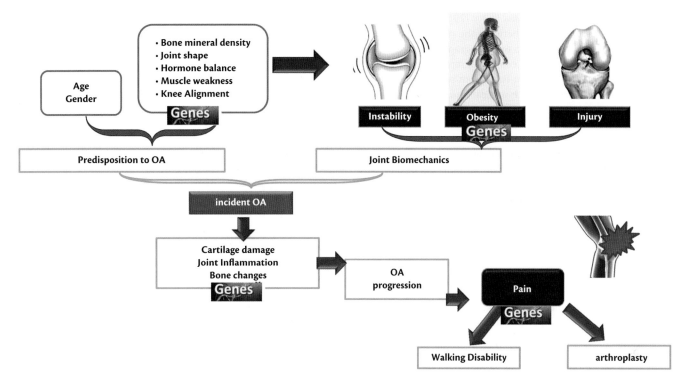

Figure 9.1 Schematic diagram of the various mechanisms whereby genetic variation may contribute to the risk of OA. External factors, such as age, gender, injury, and lifestyle, along with genetic variation affect an individual's risk of developing incident OA and of OA progressing to a severe stage. These risk factors can also influence molecular, physiological, and morphological features which in turn influence the risk of both incidence and progression of OA. The genes identified to date with genome-wide significance in either Asian or Caucasian populations to influence risk of OA are shown.

whether or not the illness is active). Additionally, gradual narrowing of the joint space width is part of the definition of OA and it is seen during the progression of hip OA on radiographs with a very good reliability [22]. The use of a definition based on the joint space width as an endophenotype was shown to be a successful approach to identify genes responsible for cartilage thickness (development and/or maintenance) and OA. In addition, the use of a quantitative trait such as mJSW to discover signals implicated in hip OA has some advantages. Quantitative traits are more powerful than dichotomous traits, especially when the accuracy of the measure is better for the quantitative trait [23]. Quantitative traits are traits with a continuous distribution in natural populations, with population variation often approximating a statistical normal distribution on an appropriate scale.

Joint morphology

Another trait related to OA that has been investigated genetically is joint shape. Developmental hip disorders (DHDs) such as developmental dysplasia of the hip, slipped capitis femoris epiphysis, and femoroacetabular impingement may cause symptoms and disability in adulthood or earlier as a result of altered joint morphology. DHDs share a common mechanism of local cumulative mechanical overload and damage of joint structures that may cause hip OA [24]. Some groups have assessed whether genetic factors affecting hip morphology can be identified and whether they relate to risk of hip OA. To date, two such reports have been published: Baker et al. [25] found that variants in the WNT antagonist *FRZB* gene were associated with hip shape and Waarsing et al. [26] reported that variants in the *DIO2* gene were significantly associated with hip shape. Both of these variants had previously been reported to

be associated with risk of hip OA. To date, no GWAS has been published on hip morphology traits, presumably because of the relatively small number of individuals available with both hip shape measures and genome-wide genotyping. However, as with mJSW, this type of analysis may uncover further genes implicated in both risk of OA and skeletal morphogenesis.

Synovitis

There is a growing body of evidence that synovial inflammation is implicated in many of the signs and symptoms of OA, including joint swelling and effusion. Histologically, the OA synovium shows hyperplasia with an increased number of lining cells and a mixed inflammatory infiltrate consisting mainly of macrophages [27]. Low-grade OA synovitis is cytokine driven; tumour necrosis factor alpha and interleukin 1 have been suggested as key players. While multiple factors are likely active in this process, recent evidence has implicated the innate immune system, the older or more primitive part of the body's immune defence mechanisms. The roles of some of the components of the innate immune system have been tested in OA models *in vivo* including the roles of synovial macrophages and the complement system [27]. To date, no studies on the genetic contribution to synovitis in OA have been published.

Pain

Pain, not tissue damage to the joint, is the main clinical outcome of OA. Relief from severe chronic OA pain remains an unmet medical need and a major reason for seeking surgical intervention, resulting in 100 000 TJRs every year in the United Kingdom [28] and over 500 000 TJRs in the United States [29]. There is extensive literature reporting discordance between the presence and severity of symptoms and the degree of radiographic structural OA (e.g. [30]). The relationship between radiographic changes of OA and pain experienced by a patient is far from perfect and remains weak once the influence of psychological and social factors and comorbidity have been taken into account [31]. The mechanisms involved in pain due to OA are only poorly understood and the molecular aetiology of pain in OA has yet to be fully understood. The current lack of understanding of the mechanisms underlying chronic pain in general, and chronic pain associated with OA in particular, accounts for the general ineffectiveness of currently available treatment options. Human genetics of OA pain can help understand the molecular pathogenesis of OA nociception as it represents a non-invasive way of testing relevant clinical populations. Genetic variants implicated in pain sensitivity have been shown to be significantly different between asymptomatic radiographic cases of OA and symptomatic cases. These included amino acid change variants in the catechol-O-methyltransferase protein (COMT), the voltage gated sodium channel Nav1.7 protein (SCN9A), and the transient receptor potential cation channel, subfamily V, member 1 protein (TRPV1). For the SCN9A variant, a replication study using three independent cohorts failed to find any association between this variant and symptomatic OA and between this variant and pain scores in OA cases [32]. On the other hand, an amino acid change in TRPV1 has been shown to influence both risk of symptomatic OA versus controls (odds ratio (OR) = 0.75, 95% confidence interval (CI) 0.64–0.88) and risk of symptomatic OA versus non-painful OA (OR = 0.73, 95% CI 0.57–0.94) after adjustment for age, sex, BMI, and radiographic severity in the study of seven independent cohorts [33]. These results indicate that the genetic contribution to pain sensitivity influences genetic risk of clinical OA.

Variation in other proteins has also been implicated in OA pain. The Val158Met variant of COMT is known to be responsible for differential pain sensitivity in humans [34]. Van Meurs et al. found that carriers of the variant Met allele had an almost threefold higher risk of hip pain compared to the wildtype genotype [34] although the results were not replicated in independent cohorts. Neogi and co-workers combined data from eight cohorts from the United Kingdom, the United States, and Australia (n = 10 715) but found only a very modest increase in the risk of painful knee OA (OR = 1.10, p < 0.2) which failed to reach statistical significance [35].

Another gene that has been implicated in pain in OA is the PCSK6 (also called PACE4) gene which encodes a pro-protein convertase that activates the main enzymes involved in degradation of human OA cartilage. A candidate gene study investigating variants in this gene failed to find any association with radiographic OA but found a strong association between the frequency of an intronic variant and the prevalence of symptomatic knee OA. Replication in three additional cohorts confirmed that the minor allele at rs900414 was consistently increased among asymptomatic compared to symptomatic radiographic knee OA cases in all four cohorts. A fixed-effects meta-analysis yielded an OR = 1.35 (95% CI 1.17–1.56, p = 4.3 × 10⁻⁵) and no significant between-study heterogeneity. Studies in mice revealed that Pcsk6 knockout mice were significantly protected against pain in a battery of algesiometric assays [36].

Genome-wide association studies

The completion of the Human Genome Project, coupled with a greater understanding of the correlation between single nucleotide polymorphisms (SNPs) (linkage disequilibrium, LD) brought about by the International HapMap Project (whose aim was to describe the common patterns of human DNA sequence variation), provided the opportunity to systematically search across the genome, testing large numbers of common genetic variants or markers for association with disease. GWASs have become accepted as the way forward in the search for susceptibility loci for common diseases.

Genome-wide association studies for osteoarthritis

Several GWASs for OA have been carried out (see Table 9.2). Initially, small-scale studies of approximately 100 000 SNPs were reported with small discovery populations and larger-scale replication populations. Such a study identified DVWA (double von Willebrand factor type A domain) to be associated with OA in Asian populations [37]. Later, a United Kingdom GWAS using pooled DNA from 357 cases and 285 controls reported the identification of a signal (rs4140564) between PTGS2 and PLA2G4A [38].

Since then, several large-scale GWASs for OA and OA-related traits have been published, including studies from the Netherlands, the United Kingdom, Japan, and the United States.

The Japanese study involved a standard approach employing 899 cases and 3396 controls. Replication increased the size to 1879 cases and 4814 controls. Two SNPs located within a small region of the human leucocyte antigen (HLA) locus on chromosome 6p were identified to be associated with knee OA, with p < 7 × 10⁻⁸ [39]. However, replication was not achieved in European cohorts and, surprisingly, a population of Han Chinese [40]. More recently, a large-scale replication study of 36 408 controls and 5749 knee OA cases from European descent showed that the SNPs identified by Nakajima and co-workers [39] are conclusively not associated in European populations [41]. The same study showed that in Japanese individuals these SNPs are in strong LD (r² = 0.86) with the HLA class II haplotype DRB1*1502 DQA1*0103 DQB1*0601 (frequency in Japanese 8%) which would be protective for knee OA. In Caucasian and Chinese samples, the SNPs identified by the Japanese GWAS are not in LD with that haplotype (r² < 0.07), and the HLA haplotype in question is also much rarer (0.8% and 2.3% respectively) than in Japanese samples. Thus, although the HLA class II region may be implicated in the risk of knee OA, the results to date do not allow a generalization to European populations.

In terms of the GWAS in European descent samples, the GWAS from Rotterdam also utilized a relatively small discovery cohort of 1341 cases and 3496 controls from the Netherlands. Replication involved additional European cohorts and North Americans of European descent. This produced a respectably powered study of 14 934 cases and 39 000 controls. A signal (p < 8 × 10⁻⁸, OR = 1.14) was identified in a region on chromosome 7q22 that included a large LD block extending over 500 kb associated with knee and hand OA. The addition of several more cohorts to the original study increased the evidence for the veracity of this signal. However, the LD block contains six genes, all of which are equally good candidates for association with OA. These include PRKAR2B (protein kinase, cAMP-dependent, regulatory, type II, beta), GPR22 (G protein-coupled receptor 22), and COG5 (component of oligomeric Golgi complex 5). Additional investigation intriguingly

Table 9.2 Genetic associations with large-joint osteoarthritis and related traits derived from genome-wide association studies with $p < 1 \times 10^{-7}$

SNP ID	Gene	Ethnic group	Trait	p-value	Putative or known function	Reference
rs11718863	DVWA	Asians	Knee OA	7×10^{-11}	Cartilage-specific tubulin binding	[37]
rs11177	GLN3/GLT8D1	Caucasians	Hip or knee OA	7×10^{-11}	Cell cycle control, tumorigenesis, and cellular senescence	[47]
rs4836732	ASTN2	Caucasians	THR	6.1×10^{-10}	Glial neuronal migration	[47]
rs9350591	FILIP1/SENP6	Caucasians	THR	2×10^{-9}	Various genes	[47]
rs10947262	BTNL2	Asians	Knee OA	5×10^{-9}	Immunomodulatory function, T-cell response	[39]
rs4730250	COG5/GPR22/DUS4L/HBP1	Caucasians	Knee OA	9×10^{-9}	Various genes	[43]
rs11842874	MCF2L	Caucasians	Knee or hip OA	9×10^{-9}	Cell motility	[44]
rs10492367	PTHLH	Caucasians	Hip OA	1.5×10^{-8}	Chondrogenic regulator	[47]
rs835487	CHST11	Caucasians	THR	2×10^{-8}	Chondroitin sulfotransferase involved in cartilage metabolism	[47]
rs7775228	HLA–DQB1	Asians	Knee OA	2×10^{-8}	Immune response (antigen presentation)	[39]
rs12107036	TP63	Caucasians	TKR in women	7×10^{-8}	Member of the p53 family of transcription factors	[47]
rs8044769	FTO	Caucasians	TKR in women	7×10^{-8}	Control of energy homeostasis	[47]
rs10948172	SUPT3H/RUNX2	Caucasians	OA (hip or knee) in men	8×10^{-8}	Probable transcriptional activator	[47]
rs6094710	NCOA3	Caucasians	Hip OA	7.9×10^{-9}	Nuclear receptor	[49]
rs788748	IGFBP3	Caucasians	Hip OA	2×10^{-8}	Cartilage catabolism and osteogenic differentiation	[50]
rs12982744	DOT1L	Caucasians	Hip OA	8.8×10^{-8}	WNT signalling	[52]

OA, osteoarthritis; THR, total hip replacement; TKR, total knee replacement.

revealed an expression quantitative trait locus within *GPR22* in high LD with the identified association signal [42]. A subsequent meta-analysis which included 6709 cases of knee OA cases and 44 439 controls showed conclusively that this signal is associated with genome-wide significance in European descent samples with OR = 1.17 (95% CI 1.11–1.24) and a p-value of 9.2×10^{-9}, but not in Asian populations, where the OR was 1.03 (95% CI 0.85–1.25; not significant) [43].

The arcOGEN (arc Osteoarthritis Genetics) study is a United Kingdom-based consortium based around seven collection centres. This group generated 1000 Genomes Project-based imputation [45] on 3177 knee and hip OA cases and 4894 population controls. This type of analysis involves using whole-genome sequence data from the 1000 Genomes Project and the genotype data generated to infer the likely genotype at millions of polymorphic DNA sites, vastly expanding the number of variants tested. These inferred or 'imputed' data were then used to detect previously unidentified risk

loci. Through large-scale replication, which included radiographic knee and hip OA in addition to TJR cases, it was possible to establish robust association with SNPs in the MCF.2 cell line-derived transforming sequence-like (*MCF2L*) gene [44]. The top signal rs11842874 reached a combined OR = 1.17 (95% CI 1.11–1.23, $p = 2.1 \times 10^{-8}$) across a total of 19 041 OA cases and 24 504 controls of European descent.

MCF2L is a rho-specific guanine nucleotide exchange factor. In humans, MCF2L regulates neurotrophin 3-induced cell migration in Schwann cells [45]. Neurotrophin 3 is a member of the nerve growth factor (NGF) family and binds to two specific NGF receptors, TRKB and TRKC. Recently, treatment of knee OA patients with a humanized monoclonal antibody that inhibits NGF has been found to be associated with joint pain reduction and an improvement in function [46]. This exciting result supports the relevance of nociceptive molecular pathways in genetic susceptibility to OA. It also clearly exemplifies the power of imputation techniques and highlights the need for more extensive coverage than that of the medium-size arrays (e.g. 600 000 SNPs) as this variant was only one identified when many more variants were tested, via imputation.

The most promising signals were replicated in an independent set of up to 7473 cases and 42 938 controls, from studies in Iceland, Estonia, the Netherlands, and the United Kingdom. This study has identified several new genetic loci associated with large-joint OA (Table 9.2) which we discuss in the following paragraphs.

The most significant association signal resided on chromosome 3 and was followed up by two SNPs in perfect LD with each other: rs11177 is a DNA change that results in an amino acid change within exon three of GNL3, coding for nucleostemin (OR = 1.12 [95% CI 1.08–1.16], p = 1.25×10^{-10}) and rs6976 situated in the 3′ UTR of the GLT8D1 gene. Interestingly, the authors also reported that whereas nucleostemin was barely detectable in cultured chondrocytes from control subjects, it was clearly detectable in cultured chondrocytes from osteoarthritic patients and was significantly upregulated in OA versus control chondrocytes, indicating a role for nucleostemin in OA cartilage degradation [47].

All of the remaining four genome-wide significant signals emanated from hip OA: rs4836732 located within intron 18 of the ASTN2 gene (OR = 1.18 [1.12–1.25], p = 2.42×10^{-9}); rs9350591 located 38 kb upstream of FILIP1 and 70 kb upstream of SENP6; rs10492367 (OR = 1.14 [1.09–1.20], p = 1.48×10^{-8}) 59 kb downstream of KLHDC5 and 96 kb downstream of PTHLH; and rs835487 (OR = 1.13 [1.09–1.18], p = 1.64×10^{-8}; total hip replacement) located within intron 2 of CHST11.

Three additional signals approached genome-wide significance: rs12107036 was associated with OA in females with total knee replacement (TKR) and resides within intron 12 of TP63 (tumour protein p63). Association with rs8044769 was strongest in the female OA stratum (allele C: OR = 1.11 [1.07–1.15], p = 6.85×10^{-8}), within intron 1 of the fat mass and obesity-associated (FTO) gene. The final signal was seen in the male OA stratum at rs10948172 (OR = 1.14 [1.09–1.20], p = 7.92×10^{-8}), situated in the vicinity of the SUPT3H gene [47]. For the most part, the role of these molecules on OA pathogenesis remains to be elucidated.

One noteworthy variant to arise from this GWAS of OA maps to the FTO gene. Subsequent to the GWAS, this variant was typed in seven independent cohorts from the United Kingdom and Australia and its association with OA was investigated in case–control analyses with and without BMI adjustment and in analyses matched for BMI category. A Mendelian randomization approach was employed using the FTO variant as the instrumental variable to evaluate the role of overweight on OA. In a meta-analysis of all overweight (BMI ≥ 25) samples versus normal-weight controls irrespective of OA status the association of rs8044769 with overweight was, as expected, highly significant (OR [CIs] for allele G = 1.14 [01.08–1.19], p = 7.5×10^{-7}). A significant association with knee OA is present in the analysis without BMI adjustment (OR [CIs] = 1.08 [1.02–1.14], p = 0.009) but the signal fully attenuated after BMI adjustment (OR [CIs] = 0.99[0.93–1.05], p = 0.666). This Mendelian randomization approach confirms the causal role of overweight on OA and that the association of the FTO gene with OA is mediated via obesity [48].

Two GWASs in the past 2 years have focused specifically on hip OA. The study by Evangelou and co-workers [49] performed a GWAS meta-analysis for hip OA on over 78 000 participants. One locus, at 20q13, represented by rs6094710 (minor allele frequency (MAF) 4%) near the nuclear receptor coactivator 3 (NCOA3) gene, reached genome-wide significance level with p = 7.9×10^{-9} and OR = 1.28 (95% CI 1.18–1.39) in the combined analysis of discovery (p = 5.6×10^{-8}) and follow-up studies (p = 7.3×10^{-4}). We showed that this gene is expressed in articular cartilage and its expression was significantly reduced in OA-affected cartilage. Moreover, two loci remained suggestive of association; rs5009270 at 7q31 (MAF 30%, p = 9.9×10^{-7}, OR = 1.10) and rs3757837 at 7p13 (MAF 6%, p = 2.2×10^{-6}, OR = 1.27 in male-specific analysis).

Another recent GWAS [50] selected hip OA cases from the Osteoporotic Fractures in Men (MrOS) Study and the Study of Osteoporotic Fractures (SOF) (654 cases and 4697 controls, combined) and was replicated in five independent studies (3243 cases and 6891 controls, combined). The A allele of rs788748, located 65 kb upstream of the IGFBP3 gene, was associated with lower risk of hip OA (OR = 0.71, p = 2×10^{-8}). The association replicated in five studies (OR = 0.92, p = 0.020), but the joint analysis of discovery and replication results was not of genome-wide significant (p = 1×10^{-6}). The rs788748 A allele was also associated with lower circulating IGFBP3 protein levels (p = 4×10^{-13}). Chondrocyte hypertrophy, a deleterious event in OA pathogenesis, was largely prevented upon IGFBP3 knockdown in chondrocytes. Furthermore, IGFBP3 overexpression induced cartilage catabolism and osteogenic differentiation.

Castaño-Betancourt and colleagues [51] carried out a GWAS on cartilage thickness in the hip in the Rotterdam study and identified a SNP in the DOT1L gene to be strongly associated with mJSW on a radiograph [51]. This result was replicated in independent cohorts from the United Kingdom and overall achieved a genetic effect size (expressed as the regression coefficient beta) of 0.09 mm/allele; p = 1.1×10^{-11}. Experimental work by the same authors showed that this gene plays a role in chondrogenic bone development via regulation of WNT signalling [51]. The association was replicated with an overall meta-analysis p-value of 1.1×10^{-11}. The SNP is located in the DOT1L gene, which is an evolutionarily conserved histone methyltransferase, recently identified as a potentially dedicated enzyme for WNT target gene activation in leukaemia. Immunohistochemical staining of DOT1L protein in mouse limbs supports a role for DOT1L in chondrogenic differentiation and adult articular cartilage. DOT1L is also expressed in osteoarthritic articular chondrocytes. Silencing of mouse Dot1l inhibited chondrogenesis in vitro.

The allele at this SNP associated with lower mJSW was later shown to be associated with a 10% increased risk for hip OA overall (p = 8.8×10^{-8}) which achieved genome-wide statistical significance and a larger effect size in males (OR 1.17, 95% CI 1.11–1.23, p = 7.8×10^{-9}) and was only nominally significant in women with an OR = 1.05, consistent with the sexual dimorphism seen for some forms of hip OA [52].

What genome-wide association studies have taught us about the pathogenesis of osteoarthritis

Combining a number of GWASs in a meta-analysis has proven to be very fruitful. However, there are many pitfalls that beset a badly thought out meta-analysis and can result in spurious results. The main problem is heterogeneity between the studies or populations. This can be as a result of population differences, such as groups of different ethnic backgrounds, that can make combining Asian and European populations problematic.

However, inconsistent criteria for inclusion into the study can also prove to be a problem.

Clinical relevance

One of the criticisms raised against genetic studies is that they are far removed from clinical practice. However, as genetic knowledge progresses, genetic studies are informing our understanding of the pathogenesis of the disease. For example, OA has traditionally been subdivided between idiopathic and post-traumatic OA [53]. A number of studies have shown substantial differences in the characteristics of post-traumatic knee OA patients and idiopathic ones in terms of age, gender, BMI, and radiographic characteristics. However, in spite of such striking differences, individuals with a history of trauma had nonetheless the same genetic contribution, or even slightly higher, than individuals with idiopathic knee OA. These results point to a clear susceptibility to OA which is merely exacerbated by the exposure to an injury and not to a different molecular pathogenesis [54]. Similarly, genetic studies have pointed to different molecular pathogenesis overall between generalized and non-generalized forms of large-joint OA [14].

The rise in the prevalence of OA and the associated increased health and economic burden have intensified the need for disease-modifying pharmacological treatments for OA, a task that has proven extremely challenging possibly due to the vast heterogeneity of OA. Established OA is a heterogeneous disease with multiple subsets of patients of which some are more amenable for treatment than others. In addition, only a subset of patients with a specified degree of radiographic OA progress to more severe OA within a time framework reasonable for a randomized clinical trial. Moreover, the effective application of any developed treatments depends on the ability to apply them in early stages of the disease before the joint is irremediably damaged. In order to do so, several things need to happen: (1) identify groups of patients likely to respond to a given pharmacotherapy (e.g. antiresorptants [55]), (2) identify groups of patients likely to progress within a reasonable time frame to reduce the costs of clinical development, and (3) identify and diagnose early stages of OA. Genetic markers, in combination with imaging and biochemical markers, have the potential to assist in all three of these tasks. In order for this to become a reality, however, a much larger number of genetic variants able to explain a larger proportion of the genetic contribution to OA is needed.

Conclusion

The identification of genes involved in the initiation and progression of OA is clearly of paramount importance. It would be of major benefit in the identification of the molecular mechanisms involved and may even lead to the development of novel therapeutics. So far, most attempts to identify predisposing genetic variants have been frustrating. It has been a long and at times exasperating journey, but as more cohorts with OA phenotyping are genotyped with GWAS arrays, it is becoming increasingly possible to identify consistent signals and it is likely that the next year or two will see a much larger number of genes implicated in OA being discovered, as is already being reported at various international conferences. Looking towards the future, with the advent of next-generation sequencing technologies it will become feasible to directly assess the role of all the genetic variation in the genome in disease risk.

Acknowledgements

This work was supported by a EULAR project grant (grant number 108239).

References

1. Bitton R. The economic burden of osteoarthritis. *Am J Manag Care* 2009; 15(8 Suppl):S230–5.
2. Risch N. Linkage strategies for genetically complex traits. II. The power of affected relative pairs. *Am J Hum Genet* 1990; 46(2):229–41.
3. Valdes AM, Spector TD. Genetic epidemiology of hip and knee osteoarthritis. *Nat Rev Rheumatol* 2011; 7(1):23–32.
4. Zhai G, Ding C, Stankovich J, et al. The genetic contribution to longitudinal changes in knee structure and muscle strength: a sibpair study. *Arthritis Rheum* 2005; 52:2830–4.
5. Kizawa H, Kou I, Iida A, et al. An aspartic acid repeat polymorphism in asporin inhibits chondrogenesis and increases susceptibility to osteoarthritis. *Nat Genet* 2005; 37(2):138–44.
6. Miyamoto Y, Mabuchi A, Shi D, et al. functional polymorphism in the 5' UTR of GDF5 is associated with susceptibility to osteoarthritis. *Nat Genet* 2007; 39(4):529–33.
7. Valdes AM, Evangelou E, Kerkhof HJ, et al. The GDF5 rs143383 polymorphism is associated with osteoarthritis of the knee with genome-wide statistical significance. *Ann Rheum Dis* 2011; 70:873–5.
8. Chapman K, Takahashi A, Meulenbelt I, et al. A meta-analysis of European and Asian cohorts reveals a global role of a functional SNP in the 5' UTR of GDF5 with osteoarthritis susceptibility. *Hum Mol Genet* 2008; 17(10):1497–504.
9. Valdes AM, Spector TD, Tamm A, et al. Genetic variation in the SMAD3 gene is associated with hip and knee osteoarthritis. *Arthritis Rheum* 2010; 62(8):2347–52.
10. Meulenbelt I, Min JL, Bos S, et al. Identification of DIO2 as a new susceptibility locus for symptomatic osteoarthritis. *Hum Mol Genet* 2008; 17(12):1867–75.
11. Rodriguez-Fontenla C, Calaza M, Evangelou E, et al. Assessment of osteoarthritis candidate genes in a meta-analysis of nine genome-wide association studies. *Arthritis Rheumatol* 2014; 66(4):940–9.
12. Sharma L, Kapoor D. Epidemiology of osteoarthritis. In Moskowitz RW, Altman RD, Hochberg MC, Buckwalter JA, Goldberg VM (eds) *Osteoarthritis: Diagnosis and Medical/Surgical Management*, 4th ed. Philadelphia: Lippincott Williams & Wilkins; 2007:3–26.
13. Kerkhof HJ, Meulenbelt I, Akune T, et al. Recommendations for standardization and phenotype definitions in genetic studies of osteoarthritis: the TREAT-OA consortium. *Osteoarthritis Cartilage* 2011; 19(3):254–64.
14. Valdes AM, McWilliams D, Arden NK, et al. Involvement of different risk factors in clinically severe large joint osteoarthritis according to the presence of hand interphalangeal nodes. *Arthritis Rheum* 2010; 62(9):2688–95.
15. Ioannidis JP. Calibration of credibility of agnostic genome-wide associations. *Am J Med Genet B Neuropsychiatr Genet* 2008; 147B:964–72.
16. Hunter DJ, Snieder H, March L, et al. Genetic contribution to cartilage volume in women: a classical twin study. *Rheumatology* 2003; 42:1495–500.
17. Zhai G, Hart DJ, Kato BS, MacGregor A, Spector TD. Genetic influence on the progression of radiographic knee osteoarthritis: a longitudinal twin study. *Osteoarthritis Cartilage* 2007; 15(2):222–5.
18. Botha-Scheepers SA, Watt I, Slagboom E, et al. Influence of familial factors on radiologic disease progression over two years in siblings with osteoarthritis at multiple sites: a prospective longitudinal cohort study. *Arthritis Rheum* 2007; 57(4):626–32.
19. Altman RD, Hochberg M, Murphy WAJr, Wolfe F, Lequesne M. Atlas of individual radiographic features in osteoarthritis. *Osteoarthritis Cartilage* 1995; 3(Suppl A):3–70.

20. Attur M, Wang HY, Kraus VB, et al. Radiographic severity of knee osteoarthritis is conditional on interleukin 1 receptor antagonist gene variations. *Ann Rheum Dis* 2010; 69(5):856–61.

21. Kerkhof HJ, Doherty M, Arden NK, et al. Large-scale meta-analysis of interleukin-1 beta and interleukin-1 receptor antagonist polymorphisms on risk of radiographic hip and knee osteoarthritis and severity of knee osteoarthritis. *Osteoarthritis Cartilage* 2011; 19(3):265–71.

22. Conaghan PG, Hunter DJ, Maillefert JF, Reichmann WM, Losina E. Summary and recommendations of the OARSI FDA osteoarthritis Assessment of Structural Change Working Group. *Osteoarthritis Cartilage* 2011; 19(5):606–10.

23. Mackay TF. Q&A: Genetic analysis of quantitative traits. *J Biol* 2009; 8(3):23.

24. Hogervorst T, Eilander W, Fikkers JT, Meulenbelt I. Hip ontogenesis: how evolution, genes, and load history shape hip morphotype and cartilotype. *Clin Orthop Relat Res* 2012; 470(12):3284–96.

25. Baker-Lepain JC, Lynch JA, Parimi N, et al. Variant alleles of the WNT antagonist FRZB are determinants of hip shape and modify the relationship between hip shape and osteoarthritis. *Arthritis Rheum* 2012; 64(5):1457–65.

26. Waarsing JH, Kloppenburg M, Slagboom PE, et al. Osteoarthritis susceptibility genes influence the association between hip morphology and osteoarthritis. *Arthritis Rheum* 2011; 63(5):1349–54.

27. Orlowsky EW, Kraus VB. The role of innate immunity in osteoarthritis: when our first line of defense goes on the offensive. *J Rheumatol* 2015; 42(3):363–71.

28. Culliford D, Maskell J, Judge A, et al. Future projections of total hip and knee arthroplasty in the UK: results from The UK Clinical Practice Research Datalink. *Osteoarthritis Cartilage* 2015 23(4):594–600.

29. Losina E, Walensky RP, Kessler CL, et al. Cost-effectiveness of total knee arthroplasty in the United States: patient risk and hospital volume. *Arch Intern Med* 2009; 169(12):1113–21.

30. Hannan MT, Felson DT, Pincus T. Analysis of discordance between radiographic change and knee pain in osteoarthritis of the knee. *J Rheumatol* 2000; 27:1513–17.

31. Ayis S, Dieppe P. The natural history of disability and its determinants in adults with lower limb musculoskeletal pain. *J Rheumatol* 2009; 36(3):583–91.

32. Valdes AM, Arden NK, Vaughn FL, et al. Role of the Na(V)1.7 R1150W amino acid change in susceptibility to symptomatic knee osteoarthritis and multiple regional pain. *Arthritis Care Res (Hoboken)* 2011; 63(3): 440–4.

33. Valdes AM, De Wilde G, Doherty SA, et al. The Ile585Val TRPV1 variant is involved in risk of painful knee osteoarthritis. *Ann Rheum Dis* 2011; 70(9):1556–61.

34. van Meurs JB, Uitterlinden AG, Stolk L, et al. A functional polymorphism in the catechol-O-methyltransferase gene is associated with osteoarthritis-related pain. *Arthritis Rheum* 2009; 60(2):628–9.

35. Neogi T, Soni A, Doherty SA, et al. Contribution of the COMT Val158Met variant to symptomatic knee osteoarthritis. *Ann Rheum Dis* 2014; 73(1):315–17.

36. Malfait AM, Seymour AB, Gao F, et al. A role for PACE4 in osteoarthritis pain: evidence from human genetic association and null mutant phenotype. *Ann Rheum Dis* 2012; 71(6):1042–8.

37. Miyamoto Y, Shi D, Nakajima M, et al. Common variants in DVWA on chromosome 3p24.3 are associated with susceptibility to knee osteoarthritis. *Nat Genet* 2008; 40(8):994–8.

38. Valdes AM, Loughlin J, Timms KM, et al. Genome-wide association scan identifies a prostaglandin-endoperoxide synthase 2 variant involved in risk of knee osteoarthritis. *Am J Hum Genet* 2008; 82(6):1231–40.

39. Nakajima M, Takahashi A, Kou I, et al. New sequence variants in HLA class II/III region associated with susceptibility to knee osteoarthritis identified by genome-wide association study. *PLoS One* 2010; 5(3):e9723.

40. Shi D, Zheng Q, Chen D, et al. Association of single-nucleotide polymorphisms in HLA class II/III region with knee osteoarthritis. *Osteoarthritis Cartilage* 2010; 18(11):1454–7.

41. Valdes AM, Styrkarsdottir U, Doherty M, et al. Large scale replication study of the association between HLA class II/BTNL2 variants and osteoarthritis of the knee in European-descent populations. *PLoS One* 2011; 6(8):e23371.

42. Kerkhof HJ, Lories RJ, Meulenbelt I, et al. A genome-wide association study identifies an osteoarthritis susceptibility locus on chromosome 7q22. *Arthritis Rheum* 2010; 62:499–510.

43. Evangelou E, Valdes AM, Kerkhof HJ, et al. Meta-analysis of genome-wide association studies confirms a susceptibility locus for knee osteoarthritis on chromosome 7q22. *Ann Rheum Dis* 2011; 70(2):349–55.

44. Day-Williams AG, Southam L, Panoutsopoulou K, et al. A variant in MCF2L is associated with osteoarthritis *Am J Hum Genet* 2011; 89(3):446–50.

45. Liu Z, Adams HC3rd, Whitehead IP. The rho-specific guanine nucleotide exchange factor Dbs regulates breast cancer cell migration. *J Biol Chem* 2009; 284:15771–80.

46. Lane NE, Schnitzer TJ, Birbara CA, et al. Tanezumab for the treatment of pain from osteoarthritis of the knee. *N Engl J Med* 2010; 363(16):1521–31.

47. Zeggini E, Panoutsopoulou K, Southam L, et al. Identification of new susceptibility loci for osteoarthritis (arcOGEN): a genome-wide association study. *Lancet* 2012; 380(9844):815–23.

48. Panoutsopoulou K, Metrustry S, Doherty SA, et al. The effect of FTO variation on increased osteoarthritis risk is mediated through body mass index: a Mendelian randomisation study. *Ann Rheum Dis* 2014; 73(12):2082–6.

49. Evangelou E, Kerkhof HJ, Styrkarsdottir U, et al. A meta-analysis of genome-wide association studies identifies novel variants associated with osteoarthritis of the hip. *Ann Rheum Dis* 2014; 73(12):2130–6.

50. Evans DS, Cailotto F, Parimi N, et al. Genome-wide association and functional studies identify a role for IGFBP3 in hip osteoarthritis. *Ann Rheum Dis* 2015; 74(10):1861–7.

51. Castaño Betancourt MC, Cailotto F, Kerkhof HJ, et al. Genome-wide association and functional studies identify the DOT1L gene to be involved in cartilage thickness and hip osteoarthritis. *Proc Natl Acad Sci U S A* 2012; 109(21):8218–23.

52. Evangelou E, Valdes AM, Castano-Betancourt MC, et al. The DOT1L rs12982744 polymorphism is associated with osteoarthritis of the hip with genome-wide statistical significance in males. *Ann Rheum Dis* 2013; 72(7):1264–5.

53. Swärd P, Kostogiannis I, Neuman P, et al. Differences in the radiological characteristics between post-traumatic and non-traumatic knee osteoarthritis. *Scand J Med Sci Sports* 2010; 20(5):731–9.

54. Valdes AM, Doherty SA, Muir KR, et al. The genetic contribution to severe post-traumatic osteoarthritis. *Ann Rheum Dis* 2013; 72(10):1687–90.

55. Karsdal MA, Bay-Jensen AC, Lories RJ, et al. The coupling of bone and cartilage turnover in osteoarthritis: opportunities for bone antiresorptives and anabolics as potential treatments? *Ann Rheum Dis* 2014; 73(2):336–48.

56. Spector TD, Cicuttini F, Baker J, et al. Genetic influences on osteoarthritis in women: a twin study. *BMJ* 1996; 312:940–3.

57. MacGregor AJ, Antoniades L, Matson M, et al. The genetic contribution to radiographic hip osteoarthritis in women: results of a classic twin study. *Arthritis Rheum* 2000; 43:2410–16.

58. Nelson AE, Smith MW, Golightly YM, Jordan JM. 'Generalized osteoarthritis': a systematic review. *Semin Arthritis Rheum* 2014; 43(6):713–20.

59. Williams FM, Spector TD, MacGregor AJ. Pain reporting at different body sites is explained by a single underlying genetic factor. *Rheumatology (Oxford)* 2010; 49(9):1753–5.

60. Zhai G, Stankovich J, Ding C, et al. The genetic contribution to muscle strength, knee pain, cartilage volume, bone size, and radiographic osteoarthritis: a sibpair study. *Arthritis Rheum* 2004; 50(3):805–10.

CHAPTER 10

Age, gender, race/ethnicity, and socioeconomic status in osteoarthritis and its outcomes

Joanne M. Jordan, Kelli D. Allen, and Leigh F. Callahan

Introduction

Osteoarthritis (OA) is the most common joint condition worldwide, affecting 27 million people in the United States in 2005 [1]. OA typically affects the knee, hip, hand, great toe, and spine and frequently occurs in multiple joints. As a result of this joint distribution, it can impair mobility and result in significant disability, need for total joint replacement (TJR), and healthcare utilization [2,3]. Given that it is more common in older individuals and in those with overweight or obesity, each increasing in our society, it is estimated that the demand for total knee replacement (TKR) will have risen approximately 600% between 2010 and 2030 to almost 3.5 million procedures annually in the United States [4] (Figure 10.1).

OA is unusual in those younger than age 40, then commonly the result of an underlying metabolic disorder or a prior joint injury [2]. Some geographic and racial/ethnic variation exists in the prevalence and incidence of OA for specific joints, likely due to variation in genetics, anatomy, and environmental exposures (Box 10.1). Many OA outcomes vary by socioeconomic status (SES) and other social factors [5–8] (Box 10.2). This chapter will describe demographic and social determinants of knee, hip, and hand OA, including how these factors impact radiographic (rOA) and symptomatic OA (sxOA), OA-related pain and function, and its treatment.

For the purposes of this narrative, rOA typically refers to OA defined by Kellgren and Lawrence (KL) grade of 2 or greater [9], and severe rOA to KL grades 3 and 4; sxOA refers to a joint with both rOA and symptoms, usually defined by pain, aching, or stiffness.

Osteoarthritis and ageing

OA of all joints is strongly related to increasing age [2]. Although rOA of the hand, for example, may be almost universal in older individuals, OA is not an inevitable consequence of ageing. Age tends to place joint tissues at higher risk of oxidative damage and renders them less responsive to anabolic factors; altered biomechanics with age-related sarcopenia and diminishing strength and function may further contribute to age-related joint risk [10,11].

Whether OA continues to increase in the oldest old has been open to question. Issues, such as depletion of susceptible individuals and death by competing causes present challenges to answering

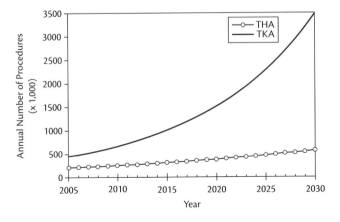

Figure 10.1 The projected number of primary total hip arthroplasty (THA) and total knee arthroplasty procedures in the United States from 2005 to 2030. Steven Kurtz et al. *J Bone Joint Surg Am* 2007; 89:780–785.

> **Box 10.1** Summary of key racial and gender differences in OA
>
> ◆ Greater prevalence, severity, and progression of knee OA in African Americans than Caucasians. Also racial differences in specific radiographic features of knee OA
>
> ◆ Lower prevalence of hip OA among Chinese than US Caucasians
>
> ◆ Greater prevalence of knee OA in Chinese women than US Caucasian women
>
> ◆ Possible lower risk of hip OA among African Americans compared with Caucasians
>
> ◆ Lower prevalence of self-reported arthritis among Hispanics than Caucasians in United States
>
> ◆ Worse pain and function among African Americans than Caucasians with knee OA
>
> ◆ Lower rates of total joint replacement among African Americans than Caucasians with OA; also higher rates among women than men with OA, though women may receive procedure at more advanced age.

> **Box 10.2** Summary of key SES differences in OA
>
> ♦ Greater prevalence of radiographic and self-reported knee and hip OA in individuals with lower levels of educational attainment and household income in US and European studies
>
> ♦ Greater prevalence of radiographic knee and hip OA in individuals living in a community of high household poverty rate in US studies
>
> ♦ Greater prevalence of self-reported hand OA in individuals with lower household educational attainment and income in Danish study
>
> ♦ Greater prevalence of self-reported OA associated with poorer individual and community SES measures in European, US, and Australian studies
>
> ♦ Increased pain and poorer function associated with poorer individual and community SES measures in US and European studies.

this question [2]. Data from the Johnston County Osteoarthritis Project (JoCo OA), a population-based cohort of OA in African Americans and Caucasians aged 45 and older in North Carolina, United States, have recently shown that incidence rates of knee symptoms, radiographic knee OA (rKOA) and severe rKOA, symptomatic knee OA (sxKOA) and severe sxKOA, were highest among those aged 75 years or older compared to those who were aged 45–54 years at baseline approximately 5–7 years earlier [12]. Incidence of hip symptoms and symptomatic hip OA (sxHOA) increased with increasing age and were highest in those aged 75 and over, although the largest increase in incidence of radiographic hip OA (rHOA) was seen in those 55–64 years and levelled out for the older age groups [13].

Gender and racial differences in osteoarthritis prevalence, incidence, and radiographic features

Knee osteoarthritis

Several US-based studies have found racial/ethnic differences in the prevalence of KOA between African Americans and Caucasians [14–16]. In the Third National Health and Nutrition Examination Survey (NHANES-III), African Americans were 50–65% more likely to have rKOA and sxKOA than Caucasians, with no significant differences between Mexican Americans and Caucasians [14]. In JoCo OA, African Americans had greater prevalence of severe rKOA (13.9% vs 6.6%) than Caucasians [16] and greater risk of rKOA progression [17].

Differences in OA prevalence between African Americans and Caucasians may vary by gender, but results have been conflicting. In NHANES-I, African American women were twice as likely to have rKOA than Caucasian women, with no gender differences among men [18]. In JoCo OA, however, although both African American men and women were about 35% more likely than Caucasians to have rKOA, after adjustment for demographic and clinical factors, this racial difference persisted only for men [19]. Further, incidence of knee symptoms, sxKOA, and severe sxKOA, but not rKOA or

severe rKOA, were slightly higher in women than men, but these differences were not statistically significant for either African Americans or Caucasians [12].

Studies have also compared the prevalence of rKOA in the Beijing Osteoarthritis Study and Caucasians in the US-based Framingham Osteoarthritis Study [20, 21]. While the prevalence of rKOA was similar between Chinese and Caucasian men, Chinese women had about 45% higher prevalence of rKOA and sxKOA, and twice the prevalence of bilateral rKOA, compared with Caucasian women [21]. Medial rKOA was less prevalent among Chinese men than Caucasian men, while lateral rKOA was more common among both Chinese men and women [20].

With regard to specific radiographic features of KOA, data from JoCo OA identified several racial differences [19]: compared with Caucasians, African Americans had more severe tibiofemoral rKOA, higher prevalence of tricompartmental rKOA, greater prevalence and severity of osteophytes and joint space narrowing (JSN), and higher likelihood of sclerosis. Racial differences in some features tended to be more pronounced in the lateral tibiofemoral compartment. Analyses from the Osteoarthritis Initiative (OAI) showed that African Americans were more likely than Caucasians to have valgus thrust during walking, and this could contribute to the greater risk of lateral knee OA in African Americans [22].

Hip osteoarthritis

Although some indirect comparisons have indicated that black people in Africa and the Caribbean have lower rates of rHOA than Caucasians [23–25], comparisons of rHOA prevalence in African Americans and Caucasians in cross-sectional US cohorts have not identified substantial differences [26–29]. However, African Americans did have lower risk of incident rHOA and sxHOA [13,17], but were as likely as Caucasians to have it progress [17], potentially explaining differences between cross-sectional and longitudinal results.

Data from the JoCo OA cohort also identified some racial differences in specific radiographic features of hip OA, which varied by gender. Among women, African Americans were more likely than Caucasians to have superior and medial JSN, moderate or severe axial JSN, medial or lateral osteophytes, and subchondral cysts. Among men, African Americans were more likely than Caucasians to have superior or medial JSN and lateral osteophytes, but less likely to have axial JSN [28].

One study showed that Chinese women in the Beijing Osteoarthritis Study had a significantly lower age-standardized prevalence of rHOA compared with Caucasian women in the US-based Study of Osteoporotic Fractures and NHANES-I [30]. The same result obtained for Chinese men compared with Caucasian men in NHANES-I.

Hand osteoarthritis

In the NHANES-III cohort, the prevalence of symptomatic hand OA (sxHaOA) was similar among Caucasians, African Americans, and Mexican Americans (7–10%) [31]. However, there were larger differences in the prevalence of asymptomatic hand OA (based on physical examination): Caucasians = 40%, African Americans = 22.9%, Mexican Americans = 30.8%. In a cohort of pre- and perimenopausal women, there were no significant differences in the prevalence of rHaOA in at least one joint between African Americans and Caucasians, but after adjustment for demographic and clinical factors, African American women had a higher prevalence of metacarpophalangeal OA (11.7% vs 2.6%, respectively, p = 0.001) [15]. In contrast, African American men and women in JoCo OA were much less likely to have rHaOA and multijoint combinations that included hand OA (hand + knee, hand + hip, hand + knee + hip) than Caucasians [32]. Both rHaOA and sxHaOA were more prevalent among participants in the Beijing Osteoarthritis Study than in the Framingham Osteoarthritis Study [33].

Self-reported osteoarthritis and arthritis

Some studies have also examined racial differences in self-reported OA or arthritis. In the US National Health Interview Survey, the age-adjusted prevalence of self-reported doctor-diagnosed arthritis was lower for Hispanics (14.4%) than for Caucasians (21.9%) or African Americans (22.3%) [34]. Data from a large sample of older Mexican Americans also showed a substantially lower prevalence of self-reported arthritis compared with the general population [35,36]. However, among a cohort of older adults (age ≥70), the age and sex-adjusted prevalence of self-reported arthritis was higher among both Hispanics (52.3%) and African Americans (47.0%) compared with Caucasians (31.9%) [37]. In the Women's Health Initiative, the adjusted odds of self-reported OA was significantly lower among Asians than Caucasians [38].

Gender and racial differences in pain and function in osteoarthritis

Many studies have identified racial and gender differences in OA-related outcomes, particularly pain and function [34,39–48]. Among JoCo OA participants with rKOA (but without rHOA), African American men and women reported significantly worse pain, stiffness, and function [40]. Among OAI participants with sxKOA, non-white race was associated with a trajectory of increased pain severity over a 6-year period [49]. In another sample of individuals with KOA, 6-minute walk distances were lower among African Americans than Caucasians [44]. Importantly, following weight loss and physical activity programmes, 6-minute walk distances improved for both African Americans and Caucasians, and there was no longer a significant racial difference.

Studies have also reported differences in pain sensitivity among individuals with OA [50,51], consistent with prior findings observed in the context of other pain-related conditions. For example, in a sample of patients with sxKOA, African Americans exhibited greater sensitivity to both mechanical and heat-induced pain [51]. Interestingly, study results also suggested these racial differences may have been mediated by lower vitamin D levels among African Americans.

Gender and racial differences in osteoarthritis treatment

There are well established racial/ethnic differences in the use of TJR surgery among individuals with OA, with African Americans and those with lower SES receiving this procedure less often than Caucasians and those with higher SES, respectively [52–57]. Racial differences in use of TJR have not been attributed to clinical appropriateness [58,59], nor provider referrals or communication about TJR [60,61]. However, in several studies, African Americans expected poorer outcomes from TJR and were less willing to consider TJR if recommended [45,62–70]. White and African American women with KOA were less willing to have TKR than men in a study from Pittsburgh, Pennsylvania, United States [57], but no gender difference was seen in willingness in the JoCo OA [70]. Recent data suggest that women in general may receive joint replacements more commonly than men [56,71], although they may be older than men are when they undergo the procedure [71].

There is some evidence that African Americans with OA receive opioid medications less frequently than Caucasians, consistent with patterns in other pain-related conditions [72]. Another study found that both Hispanics and African Americans with OA were prescribed fewer days' supply of non-steroidal anti-inflammatory drugs compared with Caucasians [73]. Studies also highlight the need to disseminate behavioural interventions among minorities with OA. Specifically, when compared to Caucasians with OA, African Americans are more commonly overweight or obese, less physically active, and more likely to utilize pain coping skills that are associated with worse outcomes [40,41,74,75].

Socioeconomic status differences in osteoarthritis prevalence and radiographic features

A number of SES measures, including educational attainment (most commonly), occupation, income, and proxy measures for community SES or deprivation (social context) have been examined in relation to OA [5–8].

Knee osteoarthritis

In the early 1990s, significant associations were reported between rKOA (odds ratio (OR) 1.53, 95% confidence interval (CI) 1.05–2.23) and knee pain (OR 1.34, 95% CI 1.09–01.65) with educational attainment of 8 or fewer years compared to 13 or more years in the NHANES-I [76]. The associations between knee pain with low educational attainment remained significant after adjustment for age, race, sex, smoking, body mass index (BMI), and knee injury (OR 1.52, 95% CI 1.2–1.93), while the rKOA and education associations did not remain in women, but did in men (OR 2.08, 95% CI 1.05–4.11).

In 2004, a population survey in Norway showed that individuals with 9 or fewer years or 9–12 years of education were 25–30% more likely to have age- and sex-adjusted self-reported, doctor- or X-ray-diagnosed KOA, compared to those with 12 or more years of education [77].

Associations between low educational attainment and rKOA have also been observed in JoCo OA [78, 79]. The first study examined associations of low educational attainment (<12 years vs ≥12 years) with four rKOA outcomes (rKOA, bilateral rKOA, sxKOA, and bilateral sxKOA) in men, women, and a subset of postmenopausal women [78]. After adjusting for age, race, occupation, lifestyle and clinical variables, in the total group of women, those with lower educational attainment were 50–85% more likely to have each of the four rKOA outcomes [78]. In the subset of postmenopausal women, these observations were partly explained by hormone replacement therapy. In the men, unadjusted analyses revealed significant associations between low educational attainment and rKOA, bilateral rKOA, and sxKOA, but after adjustment, only the association with sxKOA remained significant (OR 1.86, 95% CI 1.20–2.87) [78].

Further analyses in JoCo OA examined independent associations of educational attainment (<12 years vs ≥12 years), occupation (non-managerial or not) and Census block group household community poverty rate with the four knee OA outcomes examined above [79]. When all three SES variables were analysed simultaneously in adjusted models, low educational attainment was significantly associated with rKOA (OR 1.44, 95% CI 1.20–1.73), bilateral rKOA (OR 1.43, 95% CI 1.13–1.81), and sxKOA (OR 1.66, 95% CI 1.34–2.06). Independently, living in a community of high household poverty rate was associated with rKOA (OR 1.83, 95% CI 1.43–2.36), bilateral rKOA (OR 1.56, 95% CI 1.12–2.16), and sxKOA (OR 1.36, 95% CI 1.00–1.83). There was no significant independent association between occupation and the outcomes when analysed with education and community poverty [79]. Low educational attainment was also associated with incident rKOA and severe rKOA, statistically significantly so after adjustment, only for severe rKOA. Similar associations were seen between annual household income and incident knee symptoms [12].

In a Danish study, national register data were linked to OA hospital contacts in a cohort of 4.6 million Danes [80]. The influence of the highest educational attainment and income of the household on OA risk overall as well as anatomical sites was examined. Educational attainment of the household was significantly associated with the risk of KOA in women, with those living in a household whose highest level of education was basic attainment compared to vocational having a relative risk of 1.13 (95% CI 1.11–1.16) [80]. As the household educational attainment level increased, the risk was reduced. For men, highest household educational attainment of vocational was the highest risk for KOA. The risk of KOA was also related to income per adult in a household in both men and women, with higher risk associated with less income [80].And, in a retrospective ecological study using an area-based SES deprivation measure in analyses of medical database records for more than 5 million individuals in Catalonia (Spain), higher rates of KOA were found in the most deprived areas [81].

Hip osteoarthritis

Associations between educational attainment (≤12 years vs >12 years) and rHOA prevalence were examined in NHANES-I [26]. Although bivariable logistic regression analyses suggested that higher educational level was significantly associated with rHOA (OR 1.69, 95% CI 1.01–2.81), a multivariable model determined that this relationship was of borderline statistical significance (OR 1.64, 95% CI 0.95–2.85); NHANES-I data are characterized by very low prevalence of rHOA, which may have limited the ability to examine these issues [26]. Family income was not significantly associated with rHOA in unadjusted or adjusted models.

In addition to associations between low educational attainment and KOA, both the 2004 population survey from Norway and the Danish national register study (discussed earlier, see 'Knee osteoarthritis') revealed significantly increased prevalence of HOA among individuals with lower levels of educational attainment [77,80], the Danish study also showing associations with income. Additionally, the study from Catalonia showed increased HOA in deprived areas [81], and an Australian study reported a non-significant U-shaped association of total hip replacement (THR) surgery with SES defined as the Index of Relative Socioeconomic Disadvantage of the census district where one lived [82].

Independent associations of educational attainment (<12 years vs ≥12 years), occupation (non-managerial or not), and Census block group household community poverty rate with rHOA and sxHOA were examined in the JoCo OA Project in a manner similar to the analyses with KOA discussed earlier [83]. Those with lower educational attainment were 45% more likely to have sxHOA and 90% more likely to have bilateral sxHOA than those with higher education, after adjustment for all SES measures and other covariates simultaneously [83]. Living in a community with a high household poverty rate also showed independent associations with rHOA (OR 1.50, 95% CI 1.18–1.92) and bilateral rHOA (OR 1.87. 95% CI 1.32–2.66). No significant associations were noted between occupation and rHOA outcomes [83].

Hand osteoarthritis

Both the Norway and Danish studies described earlier also examined associations between educational attainment and HaOA [77,80]. Significant associations were not noted between lower levels of educational attainment and HaOA in this Norwegian study [77], but were seen in both men and women in the Danish national registry data [80]. And, generally findings held for income per adult in the Danish households, with economic affluence associated with reduced likelihood of HaOA [80]. The Catalonia study described previously also noted increased rates of HaOA in areas of deprivation [81].

Self-reported osteoarthritis and arthritis

SES differences in the prevalence of common diseases were examined in pooled microlevel data from non-standardized surveys conducted in eight European countries in the 1990s [84]. OA was one of the 17 conditions examined. Those with low levels of education, defined as no education and primary versus secondary and above, were approximately 35% more likely to report OA [84] in the pooled data, and this association remained statistically significant when stratified by age and sex. In an Australian study examining SES associations with self-reported arthritis in indigenous and non-indigenous individuals aged 18–64, more disadvantaged positions of education, employment status, housing, income, and area-level SES were significantly associated with reporting OA in non-indigenous respondents [85]. Among indigenous respondents, only area-level SES disadvantage was associated. Similar to findings noted for self-reported KOA and HOA in the Danish national registry study, lower household educational attainment and income were associated with higher likelihood of reporting OA overall [85].

In the United States, cohort studies of self-report of any type of arthritis (where OA is likely the majority of the arthritis) have noted associations between lower levels of a person's current individual and community SES and arthritis [86], as well as their childhood SES [87].

Socioeconomic status and pain and function in osteoarthritis

In addition to differences reported in the prevalence or incidence of OA according to individual and community-level SES, a number of studies have identified differences in health-related outcomes, particularly pain and disability, among people with OA [5,88]. In a study of participants with rKOA in NHANES-III, lower income level was associated with fair or poor self-reported health status in multivariable models adjusted for age, race, comorbidities, sex, and BMI [88]. In those with KOA and in those with HOA in JoCo OA, low educational attainment and living in a community with a higher poverty rate were both significantly associated with worse pain and function [83,89].

Socioeconomic status and outcomes following total hip replacement

Several studies have examined associations between SES with outcomes in THR [90,91]. In analyses of the Dresden Hip Registry and the Swedish Hip Arthroplasty Register, poorer SES parameters were independent predictors of poorer pain, function, and quality of life outcomes after THR [90,91]. In analyses examining the effect of social deprivation, measured by the Carstairs index, on the Oxford hip score 1 year after THR, the patients who were most deprived underwent surgery at an earlier age, were less satisfied with their outcome, and had an increased risk of dislocation and mortality [92].

Conclusions

Age, gender, race/ethnicity, and SES variations in OA and its outcomes are well established around the globe, but reasons for these differences vary. It can be particularly difficult to separate some factors from each other, particularly gender, race/ethnicity, and SES, especially when comparing different healthcare systems. While genetic and anatomical explanations may explain some variations in OA outcomes, lifestyle factors and occupational and environmental differences associated with SES and demographics may explain OA variations in others. Future research needs to move past mere description of disparities to explanations and informed interventions to address them.

Acknowledgement

The authors would like to acknowledge Antoine Baldassari for his help with the production of the manuscript.

References

1. Lawrence RC, Felson DT, Helmick CG, et al. Estimates of the prevalence of arthritis and other rheumatic conditions in the United States: Part II. *Arthritis Rheum* 2008; 58(1):26–35.
2. Neogi T, Zhang Y. Epidemiology of osteoarthritis. *Rheum Dis Clin N Am* 2013; 39(1):1–19.
3. United States Bone and Joint Initiative. *The Burden of Musculoskeletal Diseases in the United States*, 3rd ed. 2014. Available at: http://www.boneandjointburden.org.
4. Kurtz S, Ong K, Lau E, Mowat F, Halpern M. Projections of primary and revision hip and knee arthroplasty in the United States from 2005 to 2030. *J Bone Joint Surg Am* 2007; 89(4):780–5.
5. Luong MLN, Cleveland RJ, Nyrop KA, Callahan LF. Social determinants and osteoarthritis outcomes. *Aging Health* 2012; 8(4):413–37.
6. Guillemin F, Carruthers E, Li LC. Determinants of MSK health and disability – social determinants of inequities in MSK health. *Best Pract Res Clin Rheumatol* 2014; 28(3):411–33.
7. Burke NJ, Joseph G, Pasick RJ, Barker JC. Theorizing social context: rethinking behavioral theory. *Health Educ Behav* 2009; 36(5 Suppl):55S–70S.
8. Oakes JM, Kaufman JS. *Methods in Social Epidemiology*, Vol. 1. New York: John Wiley & Sons; 2006.
9. Kellgren J, Lawrence J. *Atlas of Standard Radiographs (Department of Rheumatology and Medical Illustrations, University of Manchester)*. Oxford: Blackwell Press; 1963.
10. Lotz M, Loeser RF. Effects of aging on articular cartilage homeostasis. *Bone* 2012; 51(2):241–8.
11. Vo N, Niedernhofer LJ, Nasto LA, et al. An overview of underlying causes and animal models for the study of age-related degenerative disorders of the spine and synovial joints. *J Orthop Res* 2013; 31(6):831–7.
12. Murphy LB, Moss S, Do BT, et al. Annual incidence of knee symptoms and four knee osteoarthritis outcomes in the Johnston County Osteoarthritis Project. *Arthritis Care Res* 2016; 68(1):55–65.
13. Moss AS, Murphy LB, Helmick CG, et al. Annual incidence rates of hip symptoms and three hip oa outcomes from a U.S. population-based cohort study: The Johnston County Osteoarthritis Project. *Osteoarthritis Cartilage* 2016 Apr pii: S1063-4584(16)30031-0. doi: 10.1016/j.joca.2016.04.012. [Epub ahead of print].
14. Dillon CF, Rasch EK, Gu Q, Hirsch R. Prevalence of knee osteoarthritis in the United States: arthritis data from the Third National Health and Nutrition Examination Survey 1991–1994. *J Rheumatol* 2006; 33:2271–9.
15. Sowers M, Lachance L, Hochberg M, Jamadar D. Radiographically defined osteoarthritis of the hand and knee in young and middle-aged African American and Caucasian women. *Osteoarthritis Cartilage* 2000; 8:69–77.
16. Jordan JM, Helmick CG, Renner JB, et al. Prevalence of knee symptoms and radiographic and symptomatic knee osteoarthritis in African Americans and Caucasians: the Johnston County Osteoarthritis Project. *J Rheumatol* 2007; 31(4):172–80.
17. Kopec JA, Sayre EC, Schwartz TA, et al. Occurrence of radiographic osteoarthritis of the knee and hip among African Americans and whites: a population-based prospective cohort study. *Arthritis Care Res (Hoboken)* 2013; 65(6):928–35.
18. Anderson JJ, Felson DT. Factors associated with osteoarthritis of the knee in the first National Health and Nutrition Examination Survey (HANES I). *Am J Epidemiol* 1988; 128(1):179–89.
19. Braga L, Renner JB, Schwartz TA, et al. Differences in radiographic features of knee osteoarthritis in African Americans and Caucasians: the Johnston County Osteoarthritis Project. *Osteoarthritis Cartilage* 2009; 17:1554–61.
20. Felson DT, Nevitt MC, Zhang Y, et al. High prevalence of lateral knee osteoarthritis in Beijing Chinese compared with Framingham Caucasian subjects. *Arthritis Rheum* 2002; 46(5):1217–22.
21. Zhang Y, Xu L, Nevitt MC, et al. Comparison of the prevalence of knee osteoarthritis between the elderly Chinese population in Beijing and whites in the United States: the Beijing Osteoarthritis Study. *Arthritis Rheum* 2001; 44:2065–71.
22. Chang A, Hochberg M, Song J, et al. Frequency of varus and valgus thrust and factors associated with thrust presence in persons with or at higher risk for knee osteoarthritis. *Arthritis Rheum* 2010; 62(5):1403–11.
23. Ali-Gombe A, Croft PR, Silman AJ. Osteoarthritis of the hip and acetabular dysplasia in Nigerian men. *J Rheumatol* 1996; 23(3):512–15.
24. Solomon L, Beighton P, Lawrence JS. Rheumatic disorders in the South African Negro. Part II. Osteo-arthritis. *S Afr Med J* 1975; 49:1737–40.
25. Lawrence JS, Sebo M. The geography of osteoarthritis. In Nuki GK (ed) *The Aetiopathogeneis of Osteoarthritis*. London: Pitman; 1980:155–83.
26. Tepper S, Hochberg MC. Factors associated with hip osteoarthritis: data from the first national health and nutrition examination survey (NHANES-1). *Am J Epidemiol* 1993; 137(10):1081–8.
27. Jordan JM, Helmick CG, Renner JB, et al. Prevalence of hip symptoms and radiographic and symptomatic hip osteoarthritis in African Americans and Whites: the Johnston County Osteoarthritis Project. *J Rheumatol* 2009; 36(4):809–15.
28. Nelson AE, Braga L, Renner JB, et al. Characterization of individual radiographic features of hip osteoarthritis in African American and

White women and men: the Johnston County Osteoarthritis Project. *Arthritis Care Res* 2010; 62(2):190–7.

29. Murphy LB, Helmick CG, Schwartz TA, et al. One in four people may develop symptomatic hip osteoarthritis in his or her lifetime *Osteoarthritis Cartilage* 2010; 18(11):1372–9.

30. Nevitt MC, Xu L, Zhang Y, et al. Very low prevalence of hip osteoarthritis among Chinese elderly in Beijing, China, compared with whites in the United States: the Beijing osteoarthritis study. *Arthritis Rheum* 2002; 46(7):1773–9.

31. Dillon CF, Hirsch R, Rasch EK, Gu Q. Symptomatic hand osteoarthritis in the United States: prevalence and functional impairment estimates from the third U.S. National Health and Nutrition Examination Survey, 1991–1994. *Am J Phys Med Rehabil* 2007; 86(1):12–21.

32. Nelson AE, Renner JB, Schwartz TA, et al. Differences in multi-joint radiographic osteoarthritis phenotypes among African Americans and Caucasians: the Johnston County Osteoarthritis Project. *Arthritis Rheum* 2011; 63(12):3843–52.

33. Zhang Y, Xu L, Nevitt MC, et al. Lower prevalence of hand osteoarthritis among Chinese subjects in Beijing compared with white subjects in the United States: the Beijing Osteoarthritis Study. *Arthritis Rheum* 2003; 48(4):1034–40.

34. Centers for Disease Control and Prevention, Racial/ethnic differences in the prevalence and impact of doctor-diagnosed arthritis—United States, 2002. *MMWR Morb Mortal Wkly Rep* 2005; 54:119–23.

35. al Snih S, Markides KS, Ray L, Freeman JL, Goodwin JS. Prevalence of arthritis in older Mexican Americans. *Arthritis Care Res* 2000; 13(6):409–16.

36. al Snih S, Ray L, Markides KS. Prevalence of self-reported arthritis among elders from Latin American and the Caribbean and among Mexican Americans from the southwest United States. *J Aging Health* 2006; 18:207–23.

37. Dunlop DD, Manheim LM, Song J, Chang RW. Arthritis prevalence and activity limitations in older adults. *Arthritis Rheum* 2001; 44:212–21.

38. Wright NC, Riggs GK, Lisse JR, et al. Self-reported osteoarthritis, ethnicity, body mass index, and other associated risk factors in postmenopausal women—results from the Women's Health Initiative. *J Am Geriatr Soc* 2008; 56:1736–43.

39. Sims EL, Keefe FJ, Kraus VB, et al. Racial differences in gait mechanics associated with knee osteoarthritis. *Aging Clin Exp Res* 2009; 21(6):463–9.

40. Allen KD, Helmick CG, Schwartz TA, et al. Racial differences in self-reported pain and function among individuals with radiographic hip and knee osteoarthritis: the Johnston County Osteoarthritis Project. *Osteoarthritis Cartilage* 2009; 17(9):1132–6.

41. Allen KD, Oddone EZ, Coffman CJ, et al. Racial differences in osteoarthritis pain and function: potential explanatory factors. *Osteoarthritis Cartilage* 2010; 18:160–7.

42. Golightly YM, Dominick KL. Racial variations in self-reported osteoarthritis symptom severity among veterans. *Aging Clin Exp Res* 2005; 17:264–9.

43. Burns R, Graney MJ, Lummus AC, et al. Differences in self-reported osteoarthritis disability and race. *J Natl Med Assoc* 2007; 99(9):1046–51.

44. Foy CG, Penninx BW, Shumaker SA, et al. Long-term exercise therapy resolves ethnic differences in baseline health status in older adults with knee osteoarthritis. *J Am Geriatr Soc* 2005; 53(9):1469–57.

45. Groeneveld PW, Kwoh CK, Mor MK, et al. Racial differences in expectations of joint replacement surgery outcomes. *Arthritis Rheum* 2008; 59(5):730–7.

46. Song J, Chang HJ, Tirodkar M, et al. Racial/ethnic differences in activities of daily living disability in older adults with arthritis: a longitudinal study. *Arthritis Care Res* 2007; 57(6):1058–66.

47. Shih VC, Song J, Chang RW, Dunlop DD. Racial differences in activities of daily living limitation onset in older adults with arthritis: a national cohort study. *Arch Phys Med Rehabil* 2005; 86:1521–6.

48. Theis KA, Murphy L, Hootman JM, Helmick CG, Yelin E. Prevalence and correlates of arthritis-attributable work limitation in the US

population among persons ages 18-64: 2002 National Health Interview Survey data. *Arthritis Care Res* 2007; 57(3):355–63.

49. Collins JE, Katz JN, Dervan EE, Losina E. Trajectories and risk profiles of pain in persons with radiographic, symptomatic knee osteoarthritis: data from the osteoarthritis initiative. *Osteoarthritis Cartilage* 2014; 22(5):622–30.

50. Cruz-Almeida Y, Sibille KT, Goodin BR, et al. Racial and ethnic differences in older adults with knee osteoarthritis. *Arthritis Rheumatol* 2014; 66(7):1800–10.

51. Glover TL, Goodin BR, Horgas AL, et al. Vitamin D, race, and experimental pain sensitivity in older adults with knee osteoarthritis. *Arthritis Rheum* 2012; 64(12):3926–35.

52. Skinner J, Weinstein JN, Sporer SM, Wennberg JE. Racial, ethnic, and geographic disparities in rates of knee arthroplasty among Medicare patients. *N Engl J Med* 2003; 349(14):1350–9.

53. Dunlop DD, Manheim LM, Song J, et al. Age and racial/ethnic disparities in arthritis-related hip and knee surgeries. *Med Care* 2008; 46(2):200–8.

54. Hoaglund FT, Oishi CS, Gialamas GG. Extreme variations in racial rates of total hip arthroplasty for primary coxarthrosis: a population-based study in San Francisco. *Ann Rheum Dis* 1995; 54:107–10.

55. Centers for Disease Control and Prevention. Racial disparities in total knee replacement among Medicare enrollees—United States, 2000–2006. *MMWR Morb Mortal Wkly Rep* 2009; 58:133–8.

56. Mahomed NN, Barrett J, Katz JN, et al. Epidemiology of total knee replacement in the United States Medicare population. *J Bone Joint Surg Am* 2005; 87(6):1222–8.

57. Vina ER, Cloonan YK, Ibrahim SA, et al. Race, sex, and total knee replacement consideration: role of social support. *Arthritis Care Res (Hoboken)* 2013; 65(7):1103–11.

58. Ang DC, Tahir N, Hanif H, et al. African Americans and whites are equally appropriate to be considered for total joint arthroplasty. *J Rheumatol* 2009; 36:1971–6.

59. Ang DC, James G, Stump TE. Clinical appropriateness and not race predicted referral for joint arthroplasty. *Arthritis Care Res* 2009; 61(12):1677–85.

60. Hausmann LR, Hanusa BH, Kresevic DM, et al. Orthopedic communication about osteoarthritis treatment: does patient race matter? *Arthritis Care Res* 2011; 63(5):635–42.

61. Hausmann LRM, Mor M, Hanusa BH, et al. The effect of patient race on total joint replacement recommendations and utilization in the orthopedic setting. *J Gen Intern Med* 2010; 25(9):982–8.

62. Ang DC, Ibrahim SA, Burant CJ, et al. Ethnic differences in the perception of prayer and consideration of joint arthroplasty. *Med Care* 2002; 40(6):471–6.

63. Ibrahim SA, Siminoff LA, Burant CJ, Kwoh CK. Differences in expectations of outcome mediate African American/white patient differences in 'willingness' to consider joint replacement. *Arthritis Rheum* 2002; 46(9):2429–35.

64. Kroll TL, Richardson M, Sharf BF, Suarez-Almazor ME. 'Keep on truckin' or 'It's got you in this little vacuum': race-based perceptions in decision-making for total knee arthroplasty. *J Rheumatol* 2007; 34:1069–75.

65. Suarez-Almazor ME, Souchek J, Kelly PA, et al. Ethnic variation in knee replacement: Patient preferences or uninformed disparity? *Arch Intern Med* 2005; 165:1117–24.

66. Byrne MM, Souchek J, Richardson M, Suarez-Almazor M. Racial/ethnic differences in preference for total knee replacement surgery. *J Clin Epidemiol* 2006; 59:1078–86.

67. Gandhi R, Razak F, Davey JR, Mahomed NN. Ethnicity and patient's perception of risk in joint replacement surgery. *J Rheumatol* 2008; 35:1664–7.

68. Ang DC, Monahan PO, Cronan TA. Understanding ethnic disparities in the use of total joint arthroplasty: application of the Health Belief Model. *Arthritis Care Res* 2008; 59(1):102–8.

69. Blum MA, Ibrahim SA. Race/ethnicity and use of elective joint replacement in the management of end-stage knee/hip osteoarthritis: a review of the literature. *Clin Geriatr Med* 2012; 28(3):521–32.

70. Allen KD, Golightly YM, Callahan LF, et al. Race and sex differences in willingness to undergo total joint replacement: the Johnston County Osteoarthritis Project. *Arthritis Care Res (Hoboken)* 2014; 66(8):1193–202.

71. Culliford DJ, Maskell J, Beard DJ, et al. Temporal trends in hip and knee replacement in the United Kingdom: 1991 to 2006. *Bone Joint Surg Br* 2010; 92: 130–5.

72. Dominick KL, Bosworth HB, Dudley TK, et al. Patterns of opioid analgesic prescription among patients with osteoarthritis. *J Pain Palliat Care Pharmacother* 2004; 18(1):31–46.

73. Dominick KL, Bosworth HB, Jeffreys AS, et al. Racial/ethnic variations in nonsteroidal anti-inflammatory drug (NSAID) use among patients with osteoarthritis. *Pharmacoepidemiol Drug Saf* 2004; 13:683–94.

74. Song J, Hochberg MC, Chang RW, et al. Racial and ethnic differences in physical activity guidelines attainment among people at high risk of or having knee osteoarthritis. *Arthritis Care Res (Hoboken)* 2013; 65(2):195–202.

75. Jones AC, Kwoh CK, Groeneveld PW, et al. Investigating racial differences in coping with chronic osteoarthritis pain. *J Cross Cultural Gerontol* 2008; 23:339–47.

76. Hannan MT, Anderson JJ, Pincus T, Felson DT. Educational attainment and osteoarthritis: differential associations with radiographic changes and symptom reporting. *J Clin Epidemiol* 1992; 45(2):139–47.

77. Grotle M, Hagen KB, Natvig B, et al. Prevalence and burden of osteoarthritis: results from a population survey in Norway. *J Rheumatol* 2008; 35(4):677–84.

78. Callahan LF, Shreffler J, Siaton BC, et al. Limited educational attainment and radiographic and symptomatic knee osteoarthritis: a cross-sectional analysis using data from the Johnston County (North Carolina) Osteoarthritis Project. *Arthritis Res Ther* 2010; 12(2):R46.

79. Callahan LF, Cleveland RJ, Shreffler J, et al. Associations of educational attainment, occupation and community poverty with knee osteoarthritis in the Johnston County (North Carolina) osteoarthritis project. *Arthritis Res Ther* 2011; 13(5):R169.

80. Jørgensen K, Pedersen BV, Nielsen NM, et al. Socio-demographic factors, reproductive history and risk of osteoarthritis in a cohort of 4.6 million Danish women and men. *Osteoarthritis Cartilage* 2011; 19(10):1176–82.

81. Reyes C, Garcia-Gil M, Elorza JM, et al. Socioeconomic status and the risk of developing hand, hip or knee osteoarthritis: a region-wide ecological study. *Osteoarthritis Cartilage* 2015; 23(8):1323–9.

82. Brennan SL, Stanford T, Wluka AE, et al. Cross-sectional analysis of association between socioeconomic status and utilization of primary total hip joint replacements 2006–7: Australian Orthopaedic Association National Joint Replacement Registry. *BMC Musculoskelet Disord* 2012; 13(1):63.

83. Cleveland RJ, Luong ML, Knight JB, et al. Independent associations of socioeconomic factors with disability and pain in adults with knee osteoarthritis. *BMC Musculoskelet Disord* 2013; 14:297.

84. Dalstra JA, Kunst AE, Borrell C, et al. Socioeconomic differences in the prevalence of common chronic diseases: an overview of eight European countries. *Int J Epidemiol* 2005; 34(2):316–26.

85. Cunningham J. Socioeconomic disparities in self-reported arthritis for Indigenous and non-Indigenous Australians aged 18–64. *Int J Public Health*, 2011; 56(3):295–304.

86. Callahan LF, Shreffler J, Mielenz T, et al. Arthritis in the family practice setting: associations with education and community poverty. *Arthritis Care Res* 2008; 59(7):1002–8.

87. Baldassari AR, Cleveland RJ, Callahan LF. Independent associations of childhood and current socioeconomic status with risk of self-reported doctor-diagnosed arthritis in a family-medicine cohort of North-Carolinians. *BMC Musculoskelet Disord* 2013; 14(1):327.

88. Reichmann WM, Katz JN, Kessler CL, Jordan JM, Losina E. Determinants of self-reported health status in a population-based sample of persons with radiographic knee osteoarthritis. *Arthritis Care Res* 2009; 61(8):1046–53.

89. Knight JB, Callahan LF, Luong ML, et al. The association of disability and pain with individual and community socioeconomic status in people with hip osteoarthritis. *Open Rheumatol J* 2011; 5:51.

90. Greene ME, Rolfson O, Nemes S, et al. Education attainment is associated with patient-reported outcomes: findings from the Swedish Hip Arthroplasty Register. *Clin Orthop Relat Res* 2014; 472(6):1868–76.

91. Schäfer T, Krummenauer F, Mettelsiefen J, Kirschner S, Günther KP. Social, educational, and occupational predictors of total hip replacement outcome. *Osteoarthritis Cartilage* 2010; 18(8):1036–42.

92. Clement, N, Muzammil A, Macdonald D, Howie CR, Biant LC. Socioeconomic status affects the early outcome of total hip replacement. *J Bone Joint Surge Br* 2011; 93(4):464–9.

CHAPTER 11

Morphology

Richard Aspden and Jenny Gregory

Introduction

Every archaeologist knows that bone morphology tells the story of how someone lived. Whether it is the oversized radii of the archers on the Mary Rose or the twisted spine of Richard III found under a car park in Leicester, the shapes of our bones reflect not only our genes but what we ate, our activity, and the injuries and diseases we suffered during our lifetime. The current shape of our bones reflects this and gives clues to our risk of musculoskeletal diseases, making them useful biomarkers. Over the last few years this has become an active area of research in osteoarthritis (OA), particularly with the increased use of statistical shape modelling (SSM).

Joint shape and osteoarthritis

OA alters the shape and structure of joints, with both deformation of existing structures and extra tissue in the form of osteophytes. These and other features are recognized within grading schemes such as Kellgren–Lawrence Grading (KLG) [1]. Quantitative joint morphometry has the potential to develop sensitive measures of progression and risk that could one day be used in clinical trials alongside, or instead of, established measures such as joint space width.

Geometry

Many geometrical measures have been used to describe joint morphology (Figure 11.1a). Some are well established, such as the alpha and CE angles which are indicators of impingement and an increased risk of hip OA [2–4]. More recently, software tools such as Hip Morf or knee images digital analysis (KIDA) collect multiple anatomical measurements [3,5]. Geometrical measures are also used in the calculation of engineering-based calculations, such as hip structural analysis, which was developed to predict fracture risk in osteoporosis but has been applied to OA [6].

Statistical shape modelling

SSM, which includes active shape modelling (ASM) [7], is a powerful tool for measuring joint morphology. First used for radiographic hip OA by Gregory et al. in 2007 [8], it has been widely adopted for investigating joint shape in OA, primarily from radiographs, but also magnetic resonance imaging (MRI) or dual energy X-ray absorptiometry (DXA) scans. Shape modelling can be used either as a segmentation tool, to aid calculation of geometrical measures and cartilage thickness, for planning or evaluating surgery, or as an outcome measure [9,10].

In SSM, sets of points are placed on each image in a dataset to identify features of interest (Figure 11.1b). From these points, new variables (modes of variation) are created that quantify the variation within the dataset. The steps are summarized in Figure 11.2. Firstly, the outlines are matched as closely as possible without distorting the proportions using a technique called Procrustes analysis. Next, principal components analysis (PCA) is applied to the aligned points to identify the correlations in the dataset and extract

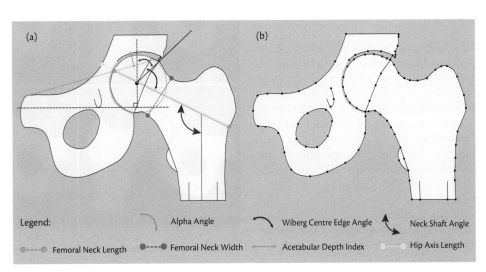

Figure 11.1 A comparison of (a) common geometric measures used for investigation of hip osteoarthritis and (b) the design of a statistical shape model (SSM) for the hip joint.

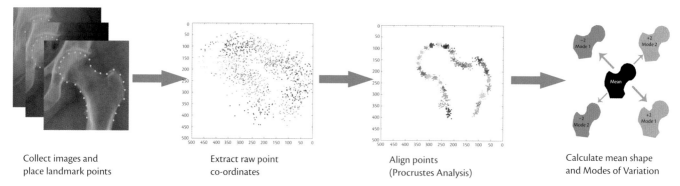

Collect images and
place landmark points

Extract raw point
co-ordinates

Align points
(Procrustes Analysis)

Calculate mean shape
and Modes of Variation

Figure 11.2 Flow chart showing the steps involved in generating a SSM.

orthogonal modes which quantify and describe the shape of each bone relative to the sample population. ASM developer Tim Cootes and colleagues in Manchester, United Kingdom, used these statistical models to guide an automated search enabling fast segmentation of images [7] and in recent years, the accuracy of these search algorithms has been further improved with the use of random forest algorithms [11,12]. The mode scores can be used as output scores for clinical assessment and have been applied to many joint structures.

Morphometry by joint

Spine

Spine OA is common but links between joint morphometry using SSM and OA have not been directly addressed. SSM has been used, however, in MRI studies, which discovered that the cervical spine straightens remarkably when singing high notes. Professional singers commonly experience neck problems and links between this and OA have yet to be explored [13]. SSM of the thoracic and lumbar spine can automatically identify vertebral fractures (many of which are missed in standard assessment) [14]. Studies of the lumbar spine have found that each person has an intrinsic shape, identifiable in all postures, which affects how we adapt to loadbearing [15,16]. This may have implications for OA and low back pain research.

Hip

The hip is the joint most extensively studied for links between morphology and OA and geometrical measures, especially angles, have been used for many years. Hip dysplasia, an under-coverage of the femoral head, is quantified using measures such as acetabular depth index, or the CE angle, which can also be used to identify pincer impingement; an over-coverage of the femoral head [17]. One of the strongest geometrical risk factors is the alpha angle which measures femoral head asphericity (cam impingement) and is markedly more prevalent in men than women and those participating in high-impact sport [18,19]. Both Chingford and CHECK cohorts found the alpha angle the strongest predictor of end-stage OA [20,21] and combined analysis gave recommended thresholds of 60° for normal and 78° for pathological angles, based on the receiver operating characteristic curve (0.69) [22].

SSM has recently become popular and a range of templates have been proposed (Figure 11.3). The smallest used a limited section of the proximal femur [8], the most common extends this to the

lesser trochanter with varying numbers of points [23–27]. Barr et al. included osteophytes and part of the acetabulum to try to capture OA severity and impingement/dysplasia [28], whilst others have included more of the pelvis [29,30]. Model design is driven by both practical considerations, for example, the visibility of features, and more philosophical ones, such as hypothesis and study design.

Hip SSM studies have primarily been performed in two dimensions, using radiographs or DXA. DXA, usually used for diagnosing osteoporosis, opens the possibility of combining studies of OA in studies of osteoporosis, allowing investigation of the interaction of these disorders [30], even including bone density distribution in the SSM [31].

Hip shape can predict total hip replacement (THR) independently of KLG [29,32] and the incidence of radiographic [8,24,26], though perhaps not clinical, OA [29]. It is not yet clear whether the shapes identified are a consequence of early (pre-radiographic) OA or are pre-existing, placing those individuals at greater risk of developing OA. Longitudinal studies of joint shape and its associations

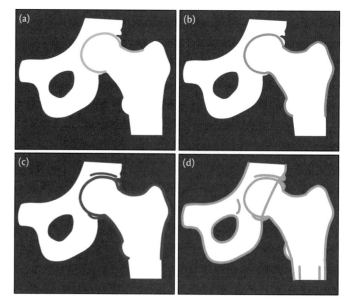

Figure 11.3 Schematic illustrating the coverage of the hip joint used by different SSM designs. From (a) a small section of the proximal femur [1], to (b) including the lesser trochanter [2–6], (c) including osteophytes and the acetabulum [7], and finally (d) incorporating much of the pelvis [8,9].

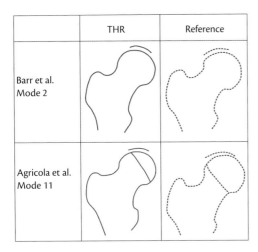

	THR	Reference
Barr et al. Mode 2		
Agricola et al. Mode 11		

Figure 11.4 Sketch showing the proximal femur and acetabular shapes based on models from two studies predicting THR [8,10]. Although models from different studies cannot easily be quantitatively compared, similarities in modes are visually apparent.

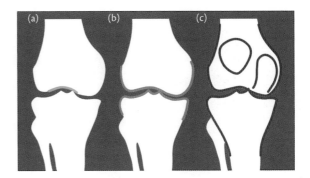

Figure 11.5 Schematic illustrating the coverage of the knee joint used by different SSM designs, from the intercondylar notch (a), through to the whole knee joint (c).

with genetic factors may help to clarify this. Two studies have identified interactions between genetics, hip SSM and radiographic OA with single nucleotide polymorphisms (SNPs) in *FRZB* and *DIO2* genes [33,34]. A third, studying unaffected hips from a population with unilateral hip OA identified three other SNPs associated with femur shape previously linked to hip OA [35]. Three-dimensional models have also been used to model impingement in Legg–Calvé–Perthes disease [36].

Comparison of study results is not trivial. Modes represent only the shape variation within the population studied and consequently differ between studies. Visual comparisons of modes, however, can show strong similarities in the shapes associated with OA or THR (Figure 11.4). Geometrical measures, capturing single- rather than whole-bone changes, make comparisons between studies or between an individual and a typical population more straightforward. Although specialized software such as Hip Morf or KIDA makes measurements easier and more reliable, with care they can be measured on any suitable image. Since they only capture one aspect of morphometry, geometrical measures can be easier to understand and interpret than the SSM modes. However, shape models may pick up more information by including features missed by direct measures but, ideally, will need a reference population in order to report repeatable outcome measures. In research, the combination of both approaches can provide a 'best of both worlds' scenario, sometimes done using SSM points to calculate geometry though this is not always practical [22,23].

Knee

Knees are the most commonly studied joints in OA clinical studies, although SSM has rarely been used apart from aiding cartilage segmentation [10].

Like the hip, many different model designs have been applied (Figure 11.5). Two-dimensional SSMs using photographs from archaeological studies found changes in knee shape, particularly the intercondylar notch, associated with OA [37]. Intercondylar notch shape was also highlighted by a radiographic study which found that knee shape predicted clinical outcome following ACL rupture [38]. Haverkamp et al. found three SSM modes associated with

radiographic OA (KLG ≥ 2), but whilst all were significantly associated with osteophytes, they had differing associations with joint deformity, joint space narrowing, cartilage lesions, and pain [39].

In three dimensions, data from the Osteoarthritis Initiative have provided a valuable source for knee SSM. Using it, Neogi et al. showed differences in bone shape, with development of osteophytic ridges, between OA and control knees (Figure 11.6) and found knee shape predicted incident radiographic OA 12 months later, with the strongest prediction coming from the whole joint (femur, tibia, and patella) rather than individual bones [40]. Bredbenner et al. found differences in the shape of the femur and tibia, though not their alignment, between people in the control and incidence groups [41]. Finally Zhang et al. showed not only how the size and shape of the lateral meniscus varies between individuals but how this affects the contact area, possibly leading to greater cartilage stresses in people with higher body mass index (BMI) [42].

Geometrically, the femorotibial angle has been used to investigate incident radiographic OA and identify clusters according to disease progression using KIDA [43,44]. Whilst the link between femorotibial angle and OA progression seems strong, findings linking angle and incidence of OA have been mixed; some reporting a relationship between malalignment and development of knee OA, particularly in the obese [45], others finding no association with incidence and consider malalignment is most likely a marker of disease severity [46,47]. Interestingly, tibial bone area has been shown to predict total knee replacement and cartilage volume loss after adjustment for age, sex, BMI and other factors [48,49].

Ankle and foot

Models of ankle and foot structure have been developed, but so far only published in abstract format. Milliken et al. found clear differences in foot shape between osteoarthritic, hallux valgus and control subjects [50], whilst Schaefer et al., using geometrical measures, found osteoarthritic ankles had flatter, less stable ankle joints with reduced support compared to controls [51].

Upper limbs

Three-dimensional SSMs of the shoulder have been used both for measuring glenoid version and bone loss in OA [52,53]. In the hands, modelling of the carpometacarpal and trapeziometacarpal joints using computed tomography have shown clear patterns related to OA of the thumb [54,55]; however, whole-hand skeletal

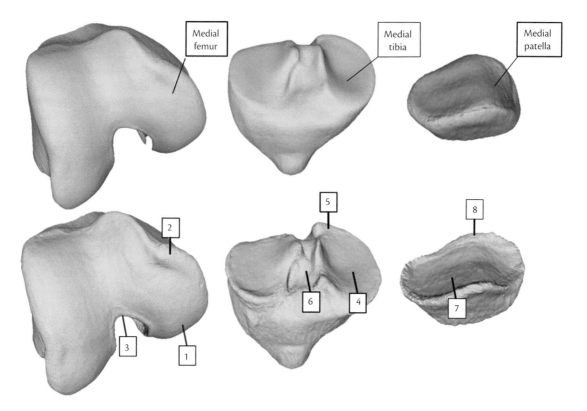

Figure 11.6 Knee SSM model from Neogi et al. [11] showing three-dimensional shape differences between control (top) and OA knees (bottom). OA bones showed wider, flatter condyles in the femur (1) and tibia (4) and increased cartilage plate size in the patella (7) and ridges of osteophytic growth in each bone (2, 5, and 8) with a narrowing of both the notch (3) and tibial spines (6).

Neogi T, Bowes MA, Niu J, De Souza KM, Vincent GR, Goggins J, et al. Magnetic resonance imaging-based three-dimensional bone shape of the knee predicts onset of knee osteoarthritis: data from the osteoarthritis initiative. *Arthritis & Rheumatism* 2013; 65(8):2048–58.

structure has generally been used as a segmentation tool to guide other assessments, such as RapidScore software to guide Sharp-van der Heijde scoring (56).

Discussion

SSM has clearly shown that hip morphology plays an important role in OA. At their most basic, measures of shape or morphology can differentiate between healthy bones and those with differing severities of disease, equivalent to a quantitative KLG. Further, they can identify those at greatest risk of incident or fast-progressing OA which may benefit clinical trials in the future by allowing stratification of patient groups.

Joint shape will affect the local biomechanical environment but may reflect wider musculoskeletal factors. Cluster analysis explored multiple joint OA [57] and found metabolic factors related to obesity may also direct multiple joint morphology [58]. Using SSM and geometry, two studies have found that shape of the hip was associated with ipsilateral lateral and medial compartment knee OA [59,60].

Conclusion

SSM is a quantitative and versatile tool for structural analysis of musculoskeletal disorders, particularly OA. With increasing speed and accuracy of automated point placement it has potential to

provide real clinical benefit for assessment of OA in all the joints of the body.

References

1. Kellgren JH, Lawrence JS. Radiological assessment of osteoarthritis. *Ann Rheum Dis* 1957; 16:494–502.
2. Agricola R, Heijboer MP, Ginai AZ, et al. A cam deformity is gradually acquired during skeletal maturation in adolescent and young male soccer players: a prospective study with minimum 2-year follow-up. *Am J Sports Med* 2014; 42(4):798–806.
3. Thomas GE, Palmer AJ, Batra RN, et al. Subclinical deformities of the hip are significant predictors of radiographic osteoarthritis and joint replacement in women. A 20 year longitudinal cohort study. *Osteoarthritis Cartilage* 2014; 22(10):1504–10.
4. Doherty M, Courtney P, Doherty S, et al. Nonspherical femoral head shape (pistol grip deformity), neck shaft angle, and risk of hip osteoarthritis: a case-control study. *Arthritis Rheum* 2008; 58(10):3172–82.
5. Marijnissen AC, Vincken KL, Vos PA, et al. Knee Images Digital Analysis (KIDA): a novel method to quantify individual radiographic features of knee osteoarthritis in detail. *Osteoarthritis Cartilage* 2008; 16(2):234–43.
6. Javaid MK, Lane NE, Mackey DC, et al. Changes in proximal femoral mineral geometry precede the onset of radiographic hip osteoarthritis: the study of osteoporotic fractures. *Arthritis Rheum* 2009; 60(7):2028–36.
7. Cootes TF, Taylor CJ, Cooper DH, Graham J. Active shape models – their training and application. *Comp Vis Image Understand* 1995; 61(1):38–59.

8. Gregory JS, Waarsing JH, Day J, et al. Early identification of radiographic osteoarthritis of the hip using an active shape model to quantify changes in bone morphometric features: can hip shape tell us anything about the progression of osteoarthritis? *Arthritis Rheum* 2007; 56(11):3634–43.

9. Fripp J, Crozier S, Warfield SK, Ourselin S. Automatic segmentation of the bone and extraction of the bone-cartilage interface from magnetic resonance images of the knee. *Phys Med Biol* 2007; 52(6):1617–31.

10. Williams TG, Holmes AP, Waterton JC, et al. Anatomically corresponded regional analysis of cartilage in asymptomatic and osteoarthritic knees by statistical shape modelling of the bone. *IEEE Trans Med Imaging* 2010; 29(8):1541–59.

11. Lindner C, Thiagarajah S, Wilkinson JM, Wallis GA, Cootes TF. Development of a fully automatic shape model matching (FASMM) system to derive statistical shape models from radiographs: application to the accurate capture and global representation of proximal femur shape. *Osteoarthritis Cartilage* 2013; 21(10):1537–44.

12. Lindner C, Wallis GA, Cootes TF. Increasing shape modelling accuracy by adjusting for subject positioning: an application to the analysis of radiographic proximal femur symmetry using data from the Osteoarthritis Initiative. *Bone* 2014; 61:64–70.

13. Miller NA, Gregory JS, Aspden RM, Stollery PJ, Gilbert FJ. Using active shape modeling based on MRI to study morphologic and pitch-related functional changes affecting vocal structures and the airway. *J Voice* 2014; 28(5):554–64.

14. Roberts M, Cootes T, Pacheco E, Adams J. Quantitative vertebral fracture detection on DXA images using shape and appearance models. *Acad Radiol* 2007; 14(10):1166–78.

15. Meakin JR, Gregory JS, Aspden RM, Smith FW, Gilbert FJ. The intrinsic shape of the human lumbar spine in the supine, standing and sitting postures: characterisation using an active shape model. *J Anat* 2009; 215(2):206–11.

16. Pavlova AV, Meakin JR, Cooper K, Barr RJ, Aspden RM. The lumbar spine has an intrinsic shape specific to each individual that remains a characteristic throughout flexion and extension. *Eur Spine J* 2014; 23 Suppl 1:S26–32.

17. Harris-Hayes M, Royer NK. Relationship of acetabular dysplasia and femoroacetabular impingement to hip osteoarthritis: a focused review. *PM R* 2011; 3(11):1055–67.e1.

18. Hack K, Di Primio G, Rakhra K, Beaule PE. Prevalence of cam-type femoroacetabular impingement morphology in asymptomatic volunteers. *J Bone Joint Surg Am* 2010; 92(14):2436–44.

19. Siebenrock KA, Behning A, Mamisch TC, Schwab JM. Growth plate alteration precedes cam-type deformity in elite basketball players. *Clin Orthop Relat Res* 2013; 471(4):1084–91.

20. Agricola R, Heijboer MP, Bierma-Zeinstra SMA, et al. Cam impingement causes osteoarthritis of the hip: a nationwide prospective cohort study (CHECK). *Ann Rheum Dis* 2013; 72(6):918–23.

21. Nicholls AS, Kiran A, Pollard TC, et al. The association between hip morphology parameters and nineteen-year risk of end-stage osteoarthritis of the hip: a nested case-control study. *Arthritis Rheum* 2011; 63(11):3392–400.

22. Agricola R, Waarsing JH, Thomas GE, et al. Cam impingement: defining the presence of a cam deformity by the alpha angle: data from the CHECK cohort and Chingford cohort. *Osteoarthritis Cartilage* 2014; 22(2):218–25.

23. Gregory JS, Testi D, Stewart A, et al. A method for assessment of the shape of the proximal femur and its relationship to osteoporotic hip fracture. *Osteoporos Int* 2004; 15 (1):5–11.

24. Lynch JA, Parimi N, Chaganti RK, Nevitt MC, Lane NE. The association of proximal femoral shape and incident radiographic hip OA in elderly women. *Osteoarthritis Cartilage* 2009; 17(10):1313–18.

25. Lindner C, Thiagarajah S, Wilkinson JM, Wallis GA, Cootes TF. Fully automatic segmentation of the proximal femur using random forest regression voting. *IEEE Trans Med Imaging* 2013; 32(8):1462–72.

26. Nelson AE, Liu F, Lynch JA, et al. Association of incident symptomatic hip osteoarthritis with differences in hip shape by active shape modeling: the Johnston County osteoarthritis project. *Arthritis Care Res* 2014; 66(1):74–81.

27. Lindner C, Thiagarajah S, Wilkinson JM, et al. Accurate bone segmentation in 2D radiographs using fully automatic shape model matching based on regression-voting. *Med Image Comput Comput Assist Interv* 2013; 16(Pt 2):181–9.

28. Barr RJ, Gregory JS, Reid DM, et al. Predicting OA progression to total hip replacement: can we do better than risk factors alone using active shape modelling as an imaging biomarker? *Rheumatology* 2012; 51(3):562–70.

29. Agricola R, Reijman M, Bierma-Zeinstra SMA, et al. Total hip replacement but not clinical osteoarthritis can be predicted by the shape of the hip: a prospective cohort study (CHECK). *Osteoarthritis Cartilage* 2013; 21(4):559–64.

30. Goodyear SR, Barr RJ, McCloskey E, et al. Can we improve the prediction of hip fracture by assessing bone structure using shape and appearance modelling? *Bone* 2013; 53(1):188–93.

31. Waarsing JH, Rozendaal RM, Verhaar JA, Bierma-Zeinstra SM, Weinans H. A statistical model of shape and density of the proximal femur in relation to radiological and clinical OA of the hip. *Osteoarthritis Cartilage* 2010; 18(6):787–94.

32. Barr RJ, Gregory JS, Reid DM, et al. Predicting OA progression to total hip replacement: can we do better than risk factors alone using active shape modelling as an imaging biomarker? *Rheumatology (Oxford)* 2012; 51(3):562–70.

33. Waarsing JH, Kloppenburg M, Slagboom PE, et al. Osteoarthritis susceptibility genes influence the association between hip morphology and osteoarthritis. *Arthritis Rheum* 2011; 63(5):1349–54.

34. Baker-LePain JC, Lynch JA, Parimi N, et al. Variant alleles of the Wnt antagonist FRZB are determinants of hip shape and modify the relationship between hip shape and osteoarthritis. *Arthritis Rheum* 2012; 64(5):1457–65.

35. Lindner C, Thiagarajah S, Wilkinson JM, et al. Investigation of association between hip osteoarthritis susceptibility loci and radiographic proximal femur shape. *Arthritis Rheumatol* 2015; 67(8):2076–84.

36. Chan EF, Farnsworth CL, Koziol JA, Hosalkar HS, Sah RL. Statistical shape modeling of proximal femoral shape deformities in Legg-Calvé-Perthes disease and slipped capital femoral epiphysis. *Osteoarthritis Cartilage* 2013; 21(3):443–9.

37. Shepstone L, Rogers J, Kirwan JR, Silverman BW. Shape of the intercondylar notch of the human femur: a comparison of osteoarthritic and non-osteoarthritic bones from a skeletal sample. *Ann Rheum Dis* 2001; 60(10):968–73.

38. Eggerding V, Van Kuijk KSR, Van Meer BL, et al. Knee shape might predict clinical outcome after an anterior cruciate ligament rupture. *Bone Joint J* 2014; 96 B(6):737–42.

39. Haverkamp DJ, Schiphof D, Bierma-Zeinstra SM, Weinans H, Waarsing JH. Variation in joint shape of osteoarthritic knees. *Arthritis Rheum* 2011; 63(11):3401–7.

40. Neogi T, Bowes MA, Niu J, et al. Magnetic resonance imaging-based three-dimensional bone shape of the knee predicts onset of knee osteoarthritis: data from the osteoarthritis initiative. *Arthritis Rheum* 2013; 65(8):2048–58.

41. Bredbenner TL, Eliason TD, Potter RS, et al. Statistical shape modeling describes variation in tibia and femur surface geometry between Control and Incidence groups from the Osteoarthritis Initiative database. *J Biomech* 2010; 43(9):1780–6.

42. Zhang KY, Kedgley AE, Donoghue CR, Rueckert D, Bull AMJ. The relationship between lateral meniscus shape and joint contact parameters in the knee: a study using data from the Osteoarthritis Initiative. *Arthritis Res Ther* 2014; 16(1).

43. Kinds MB, Marijnissen AC, Vincken KL, et al. Evaluation of separate quantitative radiographic features adds to the prediction of incident radiographic osteoarthritis in individuals with recent onset of knee pain: 5-year follow-up in the CHECK cohort. *Osteoarthritis Cartilage* 2012; 20(6):548–56.

44. Kinds MB, Marijnissen AC, Viergever MA, et al. Identifying phenotypes of knee osteoarthritis by separate quantitative radiographic features may improve patient selection for more targeted treatment. *J Rheumatol* 2013; 40(6):891–902.

45. Brouwer GM, van Tol AW, Bergink AP, et al. Association between valgus and varus alignment and the development and progression of radiographic osteoarthritis of the knee. *Arthritis Rheum* 2007; 56(4):1204–11.

46. Hunter DJ, Niu J, Felson DT, et al. Knee alignment does not predict incident osteoarthritis: the Framingham osteoarthritis study. *Arthritis Rheum* 2007; 56(4):1212–18.

47. Zhai G, Ding C, Cicuttini F, Jones G. A longitudinal study of the association between knee alignment and change in cartilage volume and chondral defects in a largely non-osteoarthritic population. *J Rheumatol* 2007; 34(1):181–6.

48. Ding C, Martel-Pelletier J, Pelletier JP, et al. Two-year prospective longitudinal study exploring the factors associated with change in femoral cartilage volume in a cohort largely without knee radiographic osteoarthritis. *Osteoarthritis Cartilage* 2008; 16(4):443–9.

49. Cicuttini FM, Jones G, Forbes A, Wluka AE. Rate of cartilage loss at two years predicts subsequent total knee arthroplasty: a prospective study. *Ann Rheum Dis* 2004; 63(9):1124–7.

50. Milliken N, Menz HB, Roddy E, et al. Foot morphology in osteoarthritis and hallux valgus. *Osteoarthritis Cartilage* 2014; 22:S302.

51. Schaefer KL, Sangeorzan BJ, Fassbind MJ, Ledoux WR. The comparative morphology of idiopathic ankle osteoarthritis. *J Bone Joint Surg Am* 2012; 94(24):e181.

52. Scalise JJ, Bryan J, Polster J, Brems JJ, Iannotti JP. Quantitative analysis of glenoid bone loss in osteoarthritis using three-dimensional computed tomography scans. *J Shoulder Elbow Surg* 2008; 17(2):328–35.

53. Scalise JJ, Codsi MJ, Bryan J, Iannotti JP. The three-dimensional glenoid vault model can estimate normal glenoid version in osteoarthritis. *J Shoulder Elbow Surg* 2008; 17(3):487–91.

54. Halilaj E, Moore DC, Laidlaw DH, et al. The morphology of the thumb carpometacarpal joint does not differ between men and women, but changes with aging and early osteoarthritis. *J Biomech* 2014; 47(11):2709–14.

55. van de Giessen M, de Raedt S, Stilling M, et al. Localized component analysis for arthritis detection in the trapeziometacarpal joint. *Med Image Comput Comput Assist Interv* 2011; 14(Pt 2):360–7.

56. Thodberg HH, Kreiborg S, Juul A, Pedersen KD. The BoneXpert method for automated determination of skeletal maturity. *IEEE Trans Med Imaging* 2009; 28(1):52–66.

57. Nelson AE, Elstad E, DeVellis RF, et al. Composite measures of multi-joint symptoms, but not of radiographic osteoarthritis, are associated with functional outcomes: the Johnston County Osteoarthritis Project. *Disabil Rehabil* 2014; 36(4):300–6.

58. Aspden RM. Obesity punches above its weight in osteoarthritis. *Nat Rev Rheumatol* 2011; 7(1):65–8.

59. Wise BL, Kritikos L, Lynch JA, et al. Proximal femur shape differs between subjects with lateral and medial knee osteoarthritis and controls: the Osteoarthritis Initiative. *Osteoarthritis Cartilage* 2014; 22(12):2067–73.

60. Boissonneault A, Lynch JA, Wise BL, et al. Association of hip and pelvic geometry with tibiofemoral osteoarthritis: Multicenter Osteoarthritis Study (MOST). *Osteoarthritis Cartilage* 2014; 22(8):1129–35.

CHAPTER 12

Lifestyle

Jos Runhaar and Sita M. A. Bierma-Zeinstra

Introduction

Modern lifestyles put a great burden on the human musculoskeletal system. Since 1980, the worldwide prevalence of obesity has tripled in many European countries [1]. Obesity is known to affect both weight-bearing and non-weight-bearing joints due to a combination of mechanical overload and systemic inflammation. Mechanical load on weight-bearing and non-weight-bearing joints is also influenced by occupational use of the musculoskeletal system. With an ageing population and hence longer occupational careers, the exposure to occupational joint loading rises, although mechanization offers some relief in certain occupational fields. On the other hand, both to combat the obesity pandemic and to increase or maintain the quality of life, physical activity and sports are encouraged next to a healthy diet. Although both have a positive influence on cardiovascular risk factors, physical activity and especially sporting activities do lead to increased loading of the active joints and increased risk for joint injuries, which might lead to osteoarthritis (OA) development.

This chapter will provide an overview of the current knowledge on lifestyle risk factors for the development and progression of OA as published in recent systematic reviews, complemented with several narrative reviews.

Risk factors for osteoarthritis development

Sports and physical activity

Being physically active and participating regularly in sporting activities is highly recommended by the authorities. Thirty minutes of moderate physical activity for 5 days each week (or equivalent) is globally set as a norm, since it is known to reduce the incidence of diseases such as ischaemic heart disease, diabetes, and breast and colon cancer. It also positively affects the risk of stroke, hypertension, and depression [1]. Despite these recommendations and health benefits, physical activity and certainly sporting activities put major loads on the active joints and hence stress the joint cartilage and other passive structures, such as the joint capsule. Given the known involvement of these structures in the osteoarthritic disease, it is not surprising that physical activity and sports have been discussed as potential risk factors for OA development.

Based on a series of available systematic reviews [2–7], it is obvious that there is very little uniformity between the studies evaluating the association between physical activity or sports and the development of OA. This is mainly caused by the large variation in definitions used for sports and physical activity and the exposure to these factors, but also study design of the included studies troubled

uniform conclusions. Systematic reviews including retrospective, cross-sectional, and prospective studies [5,6] find conflicting evidence for an association between physical and sports activities and the subsequent development of both radiographic and clinical knee and hip OA. Systematic reviews limiting inclusion of studies to longitudinal studies still call for more uniformity in definitions used for quantifying and qualifying sports and physical activities and in definitions of OA development, but generally are able to combine study results. These studies conclude there is moderate evidence for a positive relationship between general physical sporting activities and development of hip OA, with an odds ratio (OR) of approximately 2 [4,7] (Table 12.1). Although Vignon et al. [7] report that the association does not differ for clinical and radiographic measures of hip OA, data presented by Lievense and co-workers suggest this association is only present for clinical measures of hip OA, not radiographic hip OA [4]. Breaking the sports and physical activities down into specific activities only resulted in moderate evidence for increased hip OA development for running, again when OA was clinically assessed [4]. Two systematic reviews studying the development of radiographic and clinical knee OA conclude there is an increased risk of knee OA development among those who exercise more regularly or intensely [2,7]. On the other hand, Hart and co-workers [3] found the diversity between the studies included in their systematic review too large to make an overall judgement in favour or against physical activity as a risk factor for OA development. Overall, the current literature is insufficient to discriminate between specific sporting activities [7]. This limits the possibilities to evaluate whether certain sports are more harmful than others or whether low-impact activities such as golf, swimming, and cycling even have protective effects on future OA development and to distinguish between the development of clinical signs or radiographic features of OA.

A strong factor troubling the interpretation of studies on the relationship between physical activity and OA development is joint trauma, such as meniscal tears and anterior cruciate ligament (ACL) rupture [4,6]. Sports and physical activity, especially those with longer duration and at higher intensity, are major risk factors for joint trauma. Subsequently, joint trauma is one of the strongest risk factors for OA development [8,9]. For several of the studies included in the previously mentioned systematic reviews, it is unclear whether adjustment for joint trauma has taken place. Among studies with explicit adjustment for joint trauma, a positive relationship between sports and physical activity and OA development seems to be only present in highly active and elite athletes [4,6]. When comparing the risk for joint trauma among different sporting activities, it is obvious that non-contact and

Table 12.1 The relation between physical activity/sports and the development of knee, hip, and hand OA based on systematic reviews including only longitudinal studies

	Risk factor	Outcome	Conclusion
Blagojevic et al. [2]	'Physical activity, running and exercise'	Onset of knee OA, knee pain, knee disability or physical limitations related to knee or radiographic knee OA	'Higher quality studies generally suggested an increased risk of knee OA in those who exercise more regularly or intensely'
Vignon et al. [7]	'Sport and recreational activity'	All clinical and radiographic manifestations of OA of the knee and hip	'A high degree of scientific evidence that sport is a risk factor for knee and hip OA and that the risk correlates with intensity and duration of the level of exposure'
Hart et al. [3]	'Physical activity/exercise'	Incidence and progression of hip, knee, and hand OA	'The case for or against physical activity as a risk factor for OA remains complex and controversial'
Lievense et al. [4]	'Physical sporting activities'	Development of clinical or radiological hip OA	'There is moderate evidence for a positive relationship between physical sporting activities in general and hip OA', but 'a stronger association in the clinically as compared with radiographically assessed hip OA' was found

non-elite sporting activities do not raise the risk for joint trauma [10,11], while contact sports such as soccer and rugby strongly increase the risk for acute meniscal tears [10] and ACL rupture [11] at any level.

On the other end of the spectrum, physical inactivity might also be regarded as a possible risk factor for OA development. A large part of this association will be explained by overweight/obesity (see later in this chapter), caused by an imbalance between energy intake and expenditure. Nevertheless, at least for knee and hand OA, there seems a relation between reduced muscle strength of the muscles affecting these joints and the incidence of OA symptoms [7,12]. Together with the fact that there is strong evidence that the risk for knee and hip OA is lower for physical activity than it is for overweight and joint trauma [7], mild to moderate levels of sports and physical activity in order to prevent overweight/obesity and muscle weakness, when minimizing the risk of joint trauma, seems recommendable for joint and overall health.

Occupational activities

Like physical activity, the term occupational activities covers a wide range of occupations, physical tasks, and possible harmful exposures. Nevertheless, the current literature on the risk of occupational activities on subsequent OA development is far less scattered than it is for sports and physical activities.

The majority of studies on the association between occupational activities and OA development focuses on the hip and knee joints [2,6,7,13–19], but also studies on the development of hand OA in relation to occupational activities are available [20,21]. There is strong and convincing evidence that physically demanding occupations and occupational activities are an independent risk factor for the development of hip and knee OA. Heavy lifting, squatting, kneeling, and climbing stairs are identified as specific task increasing the risk for future radiographic and clinical knee OA development [2,6,7,13,16,17,19]. From all occupations wherein employees are exposed to high loads, farmers, construction workers, loggers, miners, floor-layers, and physical educational teachers are identified as having an increased risk for knee OA development [2,7,13,16,19]. For both clinical and radiographic hip OA, only lifting heavy loads [7,14,15,18] is consistently identified as a risk behaviour, while only farming is identified as occupation at risk [7,14,15].

Although it is generally not defined as occupational load, Vignon and colleagues [7] also evaluated the risk of activities of daily living such as housekeeping, gardening, shopping, and do-it-yourself projects. They found that there is moderate evidence that activities of daily living are a risk factor for future knee OA, with ORs adjusted for age, sex, and obesity ranging from 1.7 to 3.3, and that the risk increases with intensity and duration of these activities. Data on the association between activities of daily living and hip OA development or to discriminating between clinical and radiographic OA were too limited to draw conclusions from [7].

According to estimations, that do not seem to have been updated since the mid 1990s, approximately 5–30% of all knee and hip OA might result from occupational loading [22–24]. Thereby, it is approximately as strong a risk factor of future OA development as obesity [7].

Based on 19 observational studies, Hammer and co-workers found an association between pinch grip work and radiographic OA in the first proximal interphalangeal and metacarpophalangeal joints, but not with the other thumb joints or the wrist joint [20]. Hand grip work and exposure to hand–arm vibrations were not associated with radiographic finger or wrist OA. Unfortunately, most included studies were cross-sectional, so the meta-analysis only provided limited evidence for the relation between occupational hand loading and finger and wrist OA. A systematic review on factors associated with hand pain and function, not specified as being OA related, was also limited due to the lack of prospective observational studies [21].

Overweight/obesity

According to the World Health Organization, the prevalence of obesity has tripled in many European countries since the 1980s and the numbers of those affected continue to rise [1]. Besides being linked to cardiovascular diseases, cancer, and diabetes, overweight/obesity is also strongly linked to the development of OA throughout the literature. Although the absolute risk for subsequent OA is higher for joint injuries, the combination with the very high prevalence makes overweight/obesity the greatest risk factor for OA nowadays. In general, the link between overweight/obesity and OA development is attributed to higher/altered loading of the weight-bearing joints [25,26] and to systemic low-grade inflammation [27].

Overweight and obesity are generally defined based on cut-off values of the body mass index (BMI). Despite the fact that different cut-off scores are used in the literature, while others use BMI as a continuous measure, the general picture is very clear: the higher the BMI, the higher the risk for OA development. For the knee OA development, multiple systematic reviews showed increased ORs for individuals with higher BMI or in the higher BMI categories [2,6,28–31] (Table 12.2). Depending on the comparison tested and the duration of follow-up, the risk for knee OA development for overweight individuals is in the range of 1.6–2.2 times higher [2,31], while obesity increases the risk by a factor of 2.6–8.1 ([2,30,31]. These reviews did not differentiate between forms of knee OA diagnoses and selected either clinical or radiographic outcomes or combined both outcomes. Whether there is a linear association between BMI and knee OA development is uncertain. In a meta-analysis using data from 18 studies including nearly 900 000 subjects, Jiang and co-workers [29] showed that a 5-unit increase in BMI was associated with an increased risk for knee OA development of 35%. On the other hand, Zhou and colleagues [31] showed a significant non-linear dose–response

association for BMI and knee OA development. The point estimate for a BMI of 25 kg/m^2 showed a modest risk with an OR of 1.6 (95% confidence interval (CI) 1.3–1.8), compared to reference (BMI 22.5 kg/m^2). A BMI of 30 kg/m^2 and of 35 kg/m^2 showed higher risks with ORs of 3.6 (95% CI 2.5–5.1) and 7.5 (95% CI 4.2–13.1), respectively [31].

Multiple systematic reviews are available on the association between overweight/obesity and the development of hip OA [6,28,32,33]. Despite the fact that the hip joint is generally less studied than the knee joint in OA research, Jiang and colleagues were able to combine data from 11 studies, including over 2 000 000 subjects in their meta-analysis [32]. They found that a 5-unit increase in BMI was associated with an increased risk for hip OA development of 11% when combining radiographic and clinical outcomes. Earlier, Lievense and co-workers found an increased OR of approximately 2 for obesity on clinical hip OA development in six high-quality studies, while the one high-quality study using a radiological outcome showed no significant association with obesity [33]. Although the risk for future hip OA development due to overweight/obesity seems a bit lower than it is for knee OA and

Table 12.2 The relation between overweight/obesity and OA development

	Risk factor	Outcome	Conclusion
Zhou et al. [31]	BMI 25.0 kg/m^2 vs 22.5 kg/m^2	Incidence of radiographic knee OA	Pooled OR (95% CI): 1.59 (1.34–1.81)
	BMI 30.0 kg/m^2 vs 22.5 kg/m^2		Pooled OR (95% CI): 3.55 (2.51–5.11)
	BMI 35.0 kg/m^2 vs 22.5 kg/m^2		Pooled OR (95% CI): 7.45 (4.19–13.13)
Jiang et al. 2012 [29]	5-unit increase in BMI	Incidence of radiographic and/or clinical knee OA	Pooled OR (95% CI): 1.25 (1.17–1.35)
Lee and Kean 2012 [30]	BMI ≥ 30 kg/m^2	Incidence of radiographic and/or clinical and/or joint surgery for knee OA	ORs ranged from 2.81 to 8.1
Blagojevic et al. [2]	Overweight vs normal weight	Onset of knee OA, knee pain, knee disability, or physical limitations related to knee or radiographic knee OA	Pooled OR (95% CI): 2.18 (1.86–2.55)
	Obesity vs normal weight		Pooled OR (95% CI): 2.63 (2.28–3.05)
	Overweight or obesity vs normal weight		Pooled OR (95% CI): 2.96 (2.56–3.43)
Richmond et al. [6]	Overweight or obesity vs normal weight	Presence or development of knee and/or hip OA	ORs ranged from 1.6 to 15.4
	5-unit increase in BMI	Surgery for knee and/or hip OA	Pooled OR (95% CI): 1.54 (1.29–1.83)
Guh et al. 2009 [28]	Overweight vs normal weight	Knee and/or hip joint replacement due to OA	Pooled risk estimates (95% CI) for men: 2.76 (2.05–3.70) Pooled risk estimates (95% CI) for women: 1.75 (1.35–2.26)
	Obesity vs normal weight		Pooled risk estimates (95% CI) for men: 4.20 (2.76–6.41) Pooled risk estimates (95% CI) for women: 2.19 (1.77–2.71)

evidence for radiographic hip OA development is scarce, still the risk is significantly increased compared to normal weight [6,34].

In the only available systematic review on the effect of overweight/obesity on hand OA development, moderate evidence for a positive association was found for radiographic with or without clinical hand OA, with a pooled risk ratio of 1.9. Separating radiographic from clinical hand OA resulted in limited and conflicting evidence, respectively [35]. The significant association between overweight/obesity and hand OA development highlights the fact that apart from mechanical factors, systemic factors also play a role in the development of OA in overweight/obese individuals, since mechanical load on the hand joints is generally regarded as limited. Adipose tissue is known to secrete adipokines, which are thought to be partly responsible for the association between overweight/obesity and OA development, but the evidence is scarce [34,36]. On the other hand, studies have also suggested a role of cardiovascular risk factors, such as hypertension, high cholesterol, and high blood glucose levels, in the development of OA [2,36]. Since overweight/obesity is one of the strongest risk factors for these factors [28], a causal path from overweight/obesity through these factors on OA development is suggested, but strong evidence for causality is lacking [36].

Nutrition

There is a lot of theoretical knowledge on the possible link between nutrition and OA development. For instance, observational studies show that OA patients have a low intake of vitamin D and vitamin E [37]. Since it is known that these vitamins are essential for cartilage metabolism, a causal link between these nutritional factors and OA development was suggested [37]. Even polymorphisms of the vitamin D receptor have been found to be associated with risk for OA [38,39]. Nevertheless, the current evidence for a true causal relationship between nutrition and OA development is scarce [34]. Only a few longitudinal studies on different nutritional factors and their relation to OA development in different joints are available [9,34,40]. Based on these studies, the evidence for the relationship between vitamins D, C, E, and K, and selenium and incidence of OA is limited and often conflicting [9,34,40,41]. Based on the evidence available in basic science for a role of nutritional factors in the pathway of OA development, more clinical research into this field seems warranted [9,40].

Smoking

Although smoking is seen as a major risk factor for conditions as cancer, diabetes, and cardiovascular diseases, it has been reported to be protective for Alzheimer and Parkinson diseases and OA [42]. A large systematic review of 48 observational studies indeed showed a protective effect of smoking on OA development among the included case–control studies which were mainly hospital based. In these studies, controls were selected from populations where smoking-related conditions are more present, so the control groups had a higher exposure to smoking, which led to a negative association with OA development [42,43]. Because the preventive effect was nullified among cohort studies, especially in community-based settings, the authors conclude that the association is false negative [42]. This result is supported by another systematic review that also found no association in the cohort studies [2], which are scientifically higher ranked than case–control studies. When

---

Box 12.1 Lifestyle risk factors for knee and hip OA development

Strong evidence for an association:

◆ Overweight/obesity

◆ High occupational loads.

Inconclusive evidence for an association:

◆ Sports and physical activity

◆ Nutritional factors.

Strong evidence for no association:

◆ Smoking.

---

stratifying these analysis to OA site, a preventive effect was found only for knee OA, not hip, hand, or spine OA, but again only in the case–control studies [42].

A second possible form of bias of the protective effect of smoking on OA development is the association with BMI. Smokers tend to have a lower BMI and might therefore be at lower risk for future OA development. This form of bias was confirmed in the subgroup meta-analysis of the large systematic review; among studies not controlling for BMI a protective effect was found for smoking on OA development (OR 0.87, 95% CI 0.76–0.99), while this effect was neutral among studies adjusting for BMI (OR 0.93, 95% CI 0.82–1.06) [42].

Conclusions

Clearly, lifestyle is a factor to account for when assessing the risk for OA development in different joints (Box 12.1). There is strong and convincing evidence that both a high BMI and high occupational loads are related to the development of knee, hip, and hand OA, although limited efforts have been put into discriminating the risks for radiographic and clinical OA development. Both a high BMI and high occupational loads seem possible targets for preventive interventions. Given the lack of effective treatment options for OA, the international acknowledgement of the importance of preventive measures rises [44].

When limited to mild to moderate levels of sports and physical activity, the positive effects on health measures exceed the increased risk for OA development due to increased joint loads. Especially when the risk for joint trauma is minimized, practising sports and physical activities of mild to moderate intensity in order to prevent or treat overweight/obesity and muscle weakness seems recommendable for joint and overall health.

Despite indications of an association between nutritional factors and OA development, mainly in basic science, there is only limited evidence for a causal relation in observational studies. Contrary to this, recent evaluation of the association between smoking and OA development does provide uniform results and no further studies seem required; high-quality observational studies, with proper confounder adjustments, show smoking not to be related to OA development.

Prognostic lifestyle factors for osteoarthritis progression

Longitudinal observational studies evaluating risk factors for OA development include subjects with no OA at baseline and test the association between baseline risk factors and subsequent OA development. In contrast, longitudinal observational studies evaluating risk factors for OA progression are limited to subjects with OA at baseline. Although this might only look like a difference in the selection of subjects, the latter form of study design has some methodological concerns [45]. Given the fact that several risk factors studied for their effects on the progression of OA were probably already present before OA even developed (e.g. high BMI, malalignment, or genetic factors), limiting the analysis to subjects already having the disease might lead to biased estimations [45]. Ideally, the change in the risk factor after the baseline measurement, and hence after OA has developed, is tested for its effects on OA progression. Unfortunately, these insights were only introduced into OA literature recently, so most longitudinal observational studies on risk factors for OA progression have not taken these concerns into account [45].

Sports and physical activity

Based on the high-quality studies included in two available systematic reviews, there is strong evidence that there is no association between physical activity or moderate participation in sports and the progression of radiographic [46,47] and clinical [47] knee OA. It seems that knee OA patients can continue to engage in regular sporting activities as long as these activities do not cause pain, but avoiding sports with high risk for joint trauma, such as soccer/football, rugby, and volleyball [48] seems recommendable [7]. These results are supported by the substantial evidence for positive effects of exercise therapy on knee OA complaints from a large number of randomized controlled trials [49]. Two recent systematic reviews from the Cochrane library showed pooled effect sizes of −0.38 (95% CI −0.55 to −0.20) and 0.38 (95% CI −0.54 to −0.05) for exercise therapy on hip pain and hip function [50] and −0.49 (95% CI −0.59 to −0.39) and −0.52 (95% CI −0.64 to −0.39) for exercise therapy on knee pain and function [49], respectively. Nevertheless, follow-up duration of these trials is generally short and no effects of exercise therapy on structural changes are found. Therefore, the effect of physical activity and sports on the progression of structural abnormalities in already affected knees is less well known. Moreover, the strong evidence for no association between strength of the upper leg and radiographic [46,47] and clinical [47] knee OA progression, shows that the mechanisms behind the effect of exercise therapy and therewith the aetiology of knee OA progression in combination with physical exercise is largely unknown.

There is very little evidence available on the effects of physical activity and sports on the progression of hip OA. Despite the fact that exercise therapy for hip OA patients is proven to be effective on a symptom level [50], this might be only a placebo effect [51] and again no long-term effects on structural changes have been evaluated.

Occupational activities

Occupational load as a risk factor for OA progression has been studied far less than for the incidence of OA. Only one systematic review, reporting on three observational studies (two cross-sectional, one longitudinal study) on the progression of structural features of knee OA, is available [17]. Pooled risk estimates presented for the progression of knee OA among these studies ranged from 1.16 to 1.52, but only one estimate, of a cross-sectional study, was actually statistically significant [17]. The one longitudinal study showed no effect of squatting, kneeling, or crawling, or of lifting heavy loads on joint space narrowing over 12 years among individuals with radiologic knee OA (Kellgren and Lawrence grade ≥ 2) at baseline [52]. Hence, there is limited evidence for the association between occupational activities and the progression of structural features of knee OA and none regarding the progression of clinical signs. More longitudinal observational data, not only focusing on the knee joint or structural progression, is necessary in order to provide evidence for clinicians who treat and inform patients with physically high demanding jobs suffering from OA.

Overweight/obesity

Contrary to the strong evidence for an association between overweight and obesity and knee and hip OA development, the evidence for an association with OA progression is less convincing. Systematic reviews on progression of radiographic knee OA report conflicting evidence for an association between BMI [46,47,53]. While systematic reviews on progression of clinical knee OA report either conflicting evidence [47] or evidence for a positive association with BMI [54]. However, when limited to studies with a follow-up duration of 3 years or more, Chapple and co-workers also found strong evidence for a positive association between BMI and radiographic or clinical knee OA progression [47]. A best evidence synthesis of six observational studies on the relationship between body weight or BMI and progression of radiographic hip OA showed strong evidence for no association [55].

Given the counterintuitive character of these results, together with the earlier described methodological issues for observational studies including only subjects with OA, the discussion on whether the absence of an association between overweight/obesity and OA progression is a true finding is still ongoing [34,45]. In order to elucidate the true relationship between high body weight and OA progression, the association between weight gain during the follow-up period and the concurrent OA progression should be studied over a substantial follow-up period in subjects with definite OA at baseline. Only then can the true association between overweight or obesity and OA progression be established [45].

Nutrition

Several nutritional factors are linked to the progression of OA, in several joints. For instance, the Framingham study showed a threefold reduction in the risk for knee OA progression for subjects in the middle and highest tertile of vitamin C intake [56]. On the other hand, high levels of vitamin D intake also showed a protective effect for hip OA progression [57]. In contrast, two recent randomized controlled trials showed opposite effects of vitamin D intake on pain and function among subject with knee OA [58,59]. For more details on this, see Chapter 31 which discusses nutraceuticals.

Despite the high number of nutritional factors that are suggested to play a role in the progression of OA in several joints, there are only few factors tested in high-quality longitudinal observational studies. Therefore, at best, there is only limited evidence for their involvement in knee OA progression [46,47]. In summary, there is limited evidence that there is an association between the progression of knee OA and low serum levels and low dietary intake of vitamin D, and low intake of vitamin C, limited evidence for no association between progression of knee OA and low intake of beta carotene, and vitamin B1 and B6, and conflicting evidence regarding vitamin E intake [46,47].

Smoking

The role of smoking on OA progression has always been controversial. Several studies showed that smoking had a protective effect on OA progression [60,61], but this was not supported by other studies [62]. Contrary to other systematic reviews that searched the literature for all available risk factors for OA progression and where only one study was identified [46,47], a recent systematic review focused solely on smoking as a risk factor and the authors were able to include 16 observational studies with a total of 12 883 OA patients [43]. The meta-analysis showed a non-significant association between smoking and radiographic or clinical (by means of joint replacement) OA progression, with an OR of 0.92 (95% CI 0.83–1.02). Although several subgroup analyses showed significant effects (e.g. community-based studies and radiographic OA studies), these effects were only marginal and were no longer statistically significant in the meta-regression analysis when multiple covariates were adjusted [43]. Hence, it should be concluded that there is no effect of smoking on OA progression.

Conclusions

For knee OA, there is strong evidence that there is no association between physical activity or moderate participation in sports and the progression of radiographic and clinical knee OA (Box 12.2). However, as for OA development, avoiding joint trauma seems important. The association between physical activity and sports and progression of hip OA is less well studied. Here, too little data is available to make proper recommendations.

The same is true for occupational activities and nutritional factors as risk factors for OA progression. For both factors, theoretical and basic science evidence is available, but high-quality observational studies distinguishing between radiographic and clinical OA progression are lacking.

Contrary to the strong evidence for an increased risk for OA development among overweight and obese subjects, the evidence for an increased risk for OA progression is far weaker. Given the recent proposed concerns regarding the methodology of observational studies for OA progression [45], the discussion on the true effect of overweight and obesity on OA progression will probably continue. Updated analyses should be performed in observational studies, accounting for the potential epidemiologic limitations.

Despite early claims of a preventive effect of smoking on OA progression, a recent extensive meta-analysis shows there is no significant association between smoking and OA progression.

Box 12.2 Prognostic lifestyle factors for knee and hip OA progression

Inconclusive evidence for an association:

+ High occupational loads
+ Nutritional factors
+ Overweight/obesity.

Strong evidence for no association:

+ Sports and physical activity
+ Smoking.

References

1. World Health Organization. *Global Status Report on Noncommunicable Diseases 2010*. Geneva: World Health Organization; 2010.
2. Blagojevic M, Jinks C, Jeffery A, Jordan KP. Risk factors for onset of osteoarthritis of the knee in older adults: a systematic review and meta-analysis. *Osteoarthritis Cartilage* 2010; 18(1):24–33.
3. Hart LE, Haaland DA, Baribeau DA, Mukovozov IM, Sabljic TF. The relationship between exercise and osteoarthritis in the elderly. *Clin J Sport Med* 2008; 18(6):508–21.
4. Lievense AM, Bierma-Zeinstra SM, Verhagen AP, et al. Influence of sporting activities on the development of osteoarthritis of the hip: a systematic review. *Arthritis Rheum* 2003; 49(2):228–36.
5. Papavasiliou KA, Kenanidis EI, Potoupnis ME, Kapetanou A, Sayegh FE. Participation in athletic activities may be associated with later development of hip and knee osteoarthritis. *Phys Sportsmed* 2011; 39(4):51–9.
6. Richmond SA, Fukuchi RK, Ezzat A, et al. Are joint injury, sport activity, physical activity, obesity, or occupational activities predictors for osteoarthritis? A systematic review. *J Orthop Sports Phys Ther* 2013; 43(8):515–B19.
7. Vignon E, Valat JP, Rossignol M, et al. Osteoarthritis of the knee and hip and activity: a systematic international review and synthesis (OASIS). *Joint Bone Spine* 2006; 73(4):442–55.
8. Muthuri SG, McWilliams DF, Doherty M, Zhang W. History of knee injuries and knee osteoarthritis: a meta-analysis of observational studies. *Osteoarthritis Cartilage* 2011; 19(11):1286–93.
9. Hunter DJ, March L, Sambrook PN. Knee osteoarthritis: the influence of environmental factors. *Clin Exp Rheumatol* 2002; 20(1):93–100.
10. Snoeker BA, Bakker EW, Kegel CA, Lucas C. Risk factors for meniscal tears: a systematic review including meta-analysis. *J Orthop Sports Phys Ther* 2013; 43(6):352–67.
11. Moses B, Orchard J, Orchard J. Systematic review: annual incidence of ACL injury and surgery in various populations. *Res Sports Med* 2012; 20(3–4):157–79.
12. Segal NA, Glass NA. Is quadriceps muscle weakness a risk factor for incident or progressive knee osteoarthritis? *Phys Sportsmed* 2011; 39(4):44–50.
13. Jensen LK. Knee osteoarthritis: influence of work involving heavy lifting, kneeling, climbing stairs or ladders, or kneeling/squatting combined with heavy lifting. *Occup Environ Med* 2008; 65(2):72–89.
14. Jensen LK. Hip osteoarthritis: influence of work with heavy lifting, climbing stairs or ladders, or combining kneeling/squatting with heavy lifting. *Occup Environ Med* 2008; 65(1):6–19.
15. Lievense A, Bierma-Zeinstra S, Verhagen A, Verhaar J, Koes B. Influence of work on the development of osteoarthritis of the hip: a systematic review. *J Rheumatol* 2001; 28(11):2520–8.
16. McMillan G, Nichols L. Osteoarthritis and meniscus disorders of the knee as occupational diseases of miners. *Occup Environ Med* 2005; 62(8):567–75.
17. McWilliams DF, Leeb BF, Muthuri SG, Doherty M, Zhang W. Occupational risk factors for osteoarthritis of the knee: a meta-analysis. *Osteoarthritis Cartilage* 2011; 19(7):829–39.
18. Sulsky SI, Carlton L, Bochmann F, et al. Epidemiological evidence for work load as a risk factor for osteoarthritis of the hip: a systematic review. *PLoS One* 2012; 7(2):e31521.
19. Ezzat AM, Li LC. Occupational physical loading tasks and knee osteoarthritis: a review of the evidence. *Physiother Can* 2014; 66(1):91–107.
20. Hammer PE, Shiri R, Kryger AI, Kirkeskov L, Bonde JP. Associations of work activities requiring pinch or hand grip or exposure to hand-arm vibration with finger and wrist osteoarthritis: a meta-analysis. *Scand J Work Environ Health* 2014; 40(2):133–45.
21. Nicholls EE, van der Windt DA, Jordan JL, Dziedzic KS, Thomas E. Factors associated with the severity and progression of self-reported hand pain and functional difficulty in community-dwelling older adults: a systematic review. *Musculoskeletal Care* 2012; 10(1):51–62.

22. Heliovaara M, Makela M, Impivaara O, et al. Association of overweight, trauma and workload with coxarthrosis. A health survey of 7,217 persons. *Acta Orthop Scand* 1993; 64(5):513–8.

23. Olsen O, Vingard E, Koster M, Alfredsson L. Etiologic fractions for physical work load, sports and overweight in the occurrence of coxarthrosis. *Scand J Work Environ Health* 1994; 20(3):184–8.

24. Cooper C, McAlindon T, Coggon D, Egger P, Dieppe P. Occupational activity and osteoarthritis of the knee. *Ann Rheum Dis* 1994; 53(2):90–3.

25. Andriacchi TP, Mundermann A, Smith RL, Alexander EJ, Dyrby CO, Koo S. A framework for the in vivo pathomechanics of osteoarthritis at the knee. *Ann Biomed Eng* 2004; 32(3):447–57.

26. Runhaar J, Koes BW, Clockaerts S, Bierma-Zeinstra SM. A systematic review on changed biomechanics of lower extremities in obese individuals: a possible role in development of osteoarthritis. *Obes Rev* 2011; 12(12):1071–82.

27. Bijlsma JW, Berenbaum F, Lafeber FP. Osteoarthritis: an update with relevance for clinical practice. *Lancet* 2011; 377(9783):2115–26.

28. Guh DP, Zhang W, Bansback N, Amarsi Z, Birmingham CL, Anis AH. The incidence of co-morbidities related to obesity and overweight: a systematic review and meta-analysis. *BMC Public Health* 2009; 9:88.

29. Jiang L, Tian W, Wang Y, et al. Body mass index and susceptibility to knee osteoarthritis: a systematic review and meta-analysis. *Joint Bone Spine* 2012; 79(3):291–7.

30. Lee R, Kean WF. Obesity and knee osteoarthritis. *Inflammopharmacology* 2012; 20(2):53–8.

31. Zhou ZY, Liu YK, Chen HL, Liu F. Body mass index and knee osteoarthritis risk: a dose-response meta-analysis. *Obesity (Silver Spring)* 2014; 22(10):2180–5.

32. Jiang L, Rong J, Wang Y, et al. The relationship between body mass index and hip osteoarthritis: a systematic review and meta-analysis. *Joint Bone Spine* 2011; 78(2):150–5.

33. Lievense AM, Bierma-Zeinstra SM, Verhagen AP, et al. Influence of obesity on the development of osteoarthritis of the hip: a systematic review. *Rheumatology (Oxford)* 2002; 41(10):1155–62.

34. Neogi T, Zhang Y. Epidemiology of osteoarthritis. *Rheum Dis Clin North Am* 2013; 39(1):1–19.

35. Yusuf E, Nelissen RG, Ioan-Facsinay A, et al. Association between weight or body mass index and hand osteoarthritis: a systematic review. *Ann Rheum Dis* 2010; 69(4):761–5.

36. Litwic A, Edwards MH, Dennison EM, Cooper C. Epidemiology and burden of osteoarthritis. *Br Med Bull* 2013; 105:185–99.

37. Clark KL. Nutritional considerations in joint health. *Clin Sports Med* 2007; 26(1):101–18.

38. Uitterlinden AG, Burger H, van Duijn CM, et al. Adjacent genes, for COL2A1 and the vitamin D receptor, are associated with separate features of radiographic osteoarthritis of the knee. *Arthritis Rheum* 2000; 43(7):1456–64.

39. Uitterlinden AG, Fang Y, Bergink AP, et al. The role of vitamin D receptor gene polymorphisms in bone biology. *Mol Cell Endocrinol* 2002; 197(1–2):15–21.

40. McAlindon TE, Biggee BA. Nutritional factors and osteoarthritis: recent developments. *Curr Opin Rheumatol* 2005; 17(5):647–52.

41. Garstang SV, Stitik TP. Osteoarthritis: epidemiology, risk factors, and pathophysiology. *Am J Phys Med Rehabil* 2006; 85(11 Suppl):S2–11.

42. Hui M, Doherty M, Zhang W. Does smoking protect against osteoarthritis? Meta-analysis of observational studies. *Ann Rheum Dis* 2011; 70(7):1231–7.

43. Pearce F, Hui M, Ding C, Doherty M, Zhang W. Does smoking reduce the progression of osteoarthritis? Meta-analysis of observational studies. *Arthritis Care Res (Hoboken)* 2013; 65(7):1026–33.

44. Neogi T, Zhang Y. Osteoarthritis prevention. *Curr Opin Rheumatol* 2011; 23(2):185–91.

45. Zhang Y, Niu J, Felson DT, et al. Methodologic challenges in studying risk factors for progression of knee osteoarthritis. *Arthritis Care Res (Hoboken)* 2010; 62(11):1527–32.

46. Belo JN, Berger MY, Reijman M, Koes BW, Bierma-Zeinstra SM. Prognostic factors of progression of osteoarthritis of the knee: a systematic review of observational studies. *Arthritis Rheum* 2007; 57(1):13–26.

47. Chapple CM, Nicholson H, Baxter GD, Abbott JH. Patient characteristics that predict progression of knee osteoarthritis: a systematic review of prognostic studies. *Arthritis Care Res (Hoboken)* 2011; 63(8):1115–25.

48. Hootman JM, Dick R, Agel J. Epidemiology of collegiate injuries for 15 sports: summary and recommendations for injury prevention initiatives. *J Athl Train* 2007; 42(2):311–9.

49. Fransen M, McConnell S, Harmer AR, et al. Exercise for osteoarthritis of the knee. *Cochrane Database Syst Rev* 2015; 1:CD004376.

50. Fransen M, McConnell S, Hernandez-Molina G, Reichenbach S. Exercise for osteoarthritis of the hip. *Cochrane Database Syst Rev* 2014; 4:CD007912.

51. Bennell KL, Egerton T, Martin J, et al. Effect of physical therapy on pain and function in patients with hip osteoarthritis: a randomized clinical trial. *JAMA* 2014; 311(19):1987–97.

52. Schouten JS, van den Ouweland FA, Valkenburg HA. A 12 year follow up study in the general population on prognostic factors of cartilage loss in osteoarthritis of the knee. *Ann Rheum Dis* 1992; 51(8):932–7.

53. Bastick AN, Belo JN, Runhaar J, Bierma-Zeinstra SM. What are the prognostic factors for radiographic progression of knee osteoarthritis? A meta-analysis. *Clin Orthop Relat Res* 2015; 473(9):2969–89.

54. Bastick AN, Runhaar J, Belo JN, Bierma-Zeinstra SM. Prognostic factors for progression of clinical osteoarthritis of the knee: a systematic review of observational studies. *Arthritis Res Ther* 2015; 17:152.

55. Lievense AM, Bierma-Zeinstra SM, Verhagen AP, Verhaar JA, Koes BW. Prognostic factors of progress of hip osteoarthritis: a systematic review. *Arthritis Rheum* 2002; 47(5):556–62.

56. McAlindon TE, Jacques P, Zhang Y, et al. Do antioxidant micronutrients protect against the development and progression of knee osteoarthritis? *Arthritis Rheum* 1996; 39(4):648–56.

57. Lane NE, Gore LR, Cummings SR, et al. Serum vitamin D levels and incident changes of radiographic hip osteoarthritis: a longitudinal study. Study of Osteoporotic Fractures Research Group. *Arthritis Rheum* 1999; 42(5):854–60.

58. McAlindon T, LaValley M, Schneider E, et al. Effect of vitamin D supplementation on progression of knee pain and cartilage volume loss in patients with symptomatic osteoarthritis: a randomized controlled trial. *JAMA* 2013; 309(2):155–62.

59. Sanghi D, Mishra A, Sharma AC, et al. Does vitamin D improve osteoarthritis of the knee: a randomized controlled pilot trial. *Clin Orthop Relat Res* 2013; 471(11):3556–62.

60. Sandmark H, Hogstedt C, Lewold S, Vingard E. Osteoarthrosis of the knee in men and women in association with overweight, smoking, and hormone therapy. *Ann Rheum Dis* 1999; 58(3):151–5.

61. Liu B, Balkwill A, Banks E, et al. Relationship of height, weight and body mass index to the risk of hip and knee replacements in middle-aged women. *Rheumatology (Oxford)* 2007; 46(5):861–7.

62. Wilder FV, Hall BJ, Barrett JP. Smoking and osteoarthritis: is there an association? The Clearwater Osteoarthritis Study. *Osteoarthritis Cartilage* 2003; 11(1):29–35.

SECTION 5

Pain

CHAPTER 13

Neurobiology of pain in osteoarthritis

Philip Mease

Introduction

Pain is the principal clinical dimension of osteoarthritis (OA) and is the primary focus of OA non-surgical treatment. Our understanding of the neurobiology of the pain experience in OA has deepened, revealing a complex interplay of peripheral and central nervous system (CNS) mechanisms, influenced by genetic, emotional, and sociocultural elements. Through elucidation of these mechanisms, and developing methods to determine their activity in a given patient, we have the potential to more effectively target currently available therapies, often in combination fashion, as well as develop new targeted therapies.

Peripheral mechanisms of pain in osteoarthritis

OA is a disorder of cartilage and adjacent bone degeneration and remodelling, with some degree of inflammatory response. As cartilage degenerates and thins, there are also changes occurring in the joint synovium, fibrocartilage, and periarticular ligaments, tendon, and bones [1,2]. Cartilage itself is an aneural structure, but the adjacent tissues are innervated.

A principal function of sensory input from the normal joint is to advise the body of position in space and movement. This type of sensory input is not typically consciously perceived; pain is the primary sensation that is consciously perceived [2]. Joints are innervated directly from nerve cell bodies or branches of nerves supplying periosteum, skin, or muscle. Three types of nerves include thick myelinated Aβ, thin myelinated Aδ, and unmyelinated C fibres that are sensory afferents or sympathetic efferents [2–4]. Aβ fibres terminate in the joint menisci, capsule, ligaments, and periosteum. These fibres have a low threshold of response and primarily conduct innocuous mechanical and thermal tactile stimuli and are involved in reflex responses [4]. Aδ and C fibres terminate in the same tissues as well as fatty tissue and synovium. These fibres are primarily nociceptive and have a higher threshold of activation, thus serving their role to alert regarding more noxious mechanical, thermal, or chemical stimuli that may lead to tissue injury [4].

Stimulus information transfer to the CNS is coded based on the firing frequency and duration of the action potential in these fibres, which in turn is controlled by activation of ion channels in the afferent nerve [2,4]. Ion channels involved in noxious mechanoreceptor function include the degenerin epithelial sodium channel group and the acid-sensing channel. Noxious thermal stimuli, including capsaicin and mustard oil, involve members of the transient receptor potential (TRP) family, members of which have different thermal thresholds and chemical activators [4]. There are a number of voltage-gated sodium channels (VGSCs), proteins composed of an α and two smaller β subunits, that are important for action potential generation in peripheral nociceptive neurons, with significant specificity of roles. Abnormal activity, oedema, or presence of inflammatory mediators in synovial fluid, affecting VGSC behaviour may result in hyperalgesia. VGSCs open with depolarizing stimuli and may remain open depending on conformational changes, rendering them inactive (i.e. not transmitting sodium ions). The effect of potential therapeutic agents designed to block these channels depend upon whether the channel is inactive (preferred) or closed. Mutations of genes which encode VGSCs result in both increased and decreased pain sensitivity. Non-selective sodium channel blockade (e.g. with topical lidocaine) can reduce pain but also reduce ability to discern tactile sensory stimuli important to detect noxious injurious movements. Thus, developing effective yet safe sodium channel-blocking therapeutics will likely involve more selective blockade [4].

Peripheral sensitization

Key neuropeptides involved in nociceptive signalling in joint afferents include substance P, calcitonin gene-related peptide (CGRP), somatostatin, neurokinin A, galanin, neuropeptide Y, and encephalin, many of which are generated in inflammatory states [2]. Some sensory neurons, particularly of the Aδ and C types, may be mechanoinsensitive during normal states but when inflammation is present, become mechanosensitive and have a lowered threshold for transmitting noxious signal. Also, fibres may fire more strongly as they transition along the spectrum of innocuous to noxious stimulation. Whereas it is recognized that inflammation increases mechanosensitization, leading not only to pain experience with lighter pressure and in the normal range of motion, but also in the resting state. This has been most clearly demonstrated in models of inflammatory arthritis. With the more recent recognition of inflammatory changes in the osteoarthritic joint, this can be present in OA as well. In the mono-iodoacetate (MIA) rodent model of chemically induced OA, an increased dose of MIA was correlated with increased mechanosensitivity of joint afferents, suggesting that such an increase could occur related to a worsening course of OA.

However, this correlation was not observed in an old guinea pig model of more slowly occurring spontaneous OA [2,3].

An example of the role of peripheral mediation of central sensitization can be seen with activation of the neurotrophin, nerve growth factor (NGF). NGF is produced in the setting of tissue injury. Among several cellular targets, it acts directly on C-fibre high-affinity NGF receptor tyrosine kinase (TRKA) and low-affinity neurotrophin receptor, p75 [5]. TRKA activation induces downstream signalling pathways such as phospholipase C (PLC), mitogen-activated protein kinase (MAPK), and phosphoinositide 3 kinase (PI3K). This leads to potentiation of proteins at the peripheral nociceptor terminal, particularly TRPV1, which in turn leads to changes in cellular heat sensitivity [5]. Additionally, NGF is retrogradely transported to the nociceptor cell nucleus, where it induces increased expression of substance P, TRPV1, and Nav1.8 sodium channel subunit [5]. Additively, these events enhance nociceptor excitability in a rapid and variably sustained manner. Inhibition of NGF has been shown to reduce pain in OA [6].

Cytokines

Tissue injury also leads to increased expression of a variety of pro-inflammatory cytokines such as interleukin (IL)-1B, IL6, and tumour necrosis factor alpha (TNFA). These can have a direct effect on nociceptor stimulation but also activate immune cells to produce prostaglandins, NGF, bradykinin, and other pro-nociceptive mediators. Inhibition of these cytokines can decrease pain either directly via decrease of nociceptor activation or indirectly by decreasing inflammation in joints [5,7,8]. Schaible et al. describe animal data for TNFA and IL6 effect on nociceptors and diminution of nociceptor activation/sensitization with inhibition of these cytokines, marshalling evidence for direct effect on these cells independent of the immunomodulatory/anti-inflammatory effect of such inhibition [7]. Examples include the co-localization of TRPV1 and TNFR1 receptors on dorsal root ganglia neurons and increase of TRV1 receptor expression with incubation with TNFA, as well as decreased mechanosensitivity of C fibres post exposure to a TNF inhibitor.

Synovitis

The role of synovitis in osteoarthritis has been reviewed by Goldring and Otero [8]. Previously considered a prototype non-inflammatory arthritis, there is evidence that a low-grade synovitis can be present, replete with cellular proliferation of immune cells and the production of pro-inflammatory cytokines, documented histologically and supported by synovial fluid and magnetic resonance imaging (MRI) evidence [8–10]. Chondrocytes are capable of responding to mechanical injury by increasing the production of pro-inflammatory cytokines and collagen-degrading proteinases such as metalloproteinases (MMPs). Aggrecanases of the ADAMTS (a disintegrin and metalloproteinase with thrombospondin 1 motifs) family of proteinases which have a specific role in cartilage degradation in OA are upregulated by inflammatory stimuli. IL1 and TNFA induce synthesis of prostaglandin E2, by stimulating the gene expression of cyclooxygenase (COX)-2, upregulate the production of nitric oxide, and other prostanoids and phospholipases which contribute to nociceptor sensitization and activation. Mechanical stress and inflammatory mediators induce signalling pathways in chondrocytes, including the nuclear factor kappa B and MAPK pathways, which in turn activate chondrocytes to produce inflammatory cytokines, chemokines, and transcription factors which regulate genes responsible for catabolic and inflammatory activity [8].

Spinal cord pathways of osteoarthritis pain

An afferent nerve from a joint projects to several spinal cord segments via multilevel dorsal horns (Figure 13.1). In the dorsal horn, peripherally generated action potentials cause neurotransmitter release from central axon terminals. Some neurons, particularly Aβ fibres, are activated by innocuous pressure for the purpose of transmission of positional sense whereas others, particularly Aδ and C fibres, are high threshold and require noxious pressure (e.g. higher frequency stimulus intensity) to transmit pain [2,4]. These neurons use glutamate as a fast neurotransmitter. Glutamate binds to α-amino-3-hydroxy-5-methyl-4-isoxazolaepropionic acid (AMPA), N-methyl-D-aspartic acid (NMDA), and glutamate receptors in postsynaptic terminals in the dorsal horn [4,11]. The AMPA receptor is involved in the baseline response to a noxious stimulus whereas the NMDA receptor increases and extends the pain response [11]. These receptors produce postsynaptic potentials which signal the intensity, duration, and location of peripheral noxious stimuli. More intense C-fibre stimulation leads to expression of neuropeptides such as substance P and CGRP [2]. The afferent neurons project to either intraspinal interneurons and motoneurons or to extraspinal sites such as the cerebellum, hypothalamus, thalamus, and ventral forebrain. Functional imaging studies in humans suggest that principal pain processing areas include the primary and secondary somatosensory cortex, the insula, the anterior cingulate gyri, and the prefrontal cortices. Location and intensity are discerned in the primary somatosensory cortex, whereas type of noxious stimulus is determined in the secondary somatosensory cortex. The affective-motivational component of pain is processed in the limbic system, displeasurable, suffering aspects in the anterior cingulate cortex, and emotional eversion and autonomic reaction are centred in the insula [2].

Central sensitization

It is now recognized that OA, as well as other forms of chronic joint pain and inflammation, can generate central sensitization. Central sensitization is defined as a state in which neurons activated by nociceptive stimuli are sensitized by such stimuli and become hyperresponsive to subsequent stimuli to the neuron's receptor fields [12]. Intense, repeated, or prolonged signalling from peripheral nociceptors (e.g. from OA joints) modulates spinal cord nociceptive neurons, leading to decreased activation thresholds, increased synaptic excitability, and increased firing thresholds. Peripheral inflammatory mediators include inflammatory cytokines such as TNF, chemokines such as CCL3, proteases such as tryptase and trypsin, kinins, prostaglandins, and NGF [2,4]. These mediators peripherally sensitize the nerve terminal in such a way that innocuous stimuli are now perceived as painful.

That there are multiple mediators makes it more difficult to achieve therapeutic benefit from a blocker of a single mediator. A variety of kinases, including calcium-dependent protein kinase C (PKC), cyclic-AMP-dependent protein kinase A (PKA), PI3K, MAPK, extracellular signal-regulated kinase (ERK) and June kinase are intracellular signalling kinases involved in activating sodium channels, TRP family channels, and receptors in neurons resulting in excitation that outlasts the stimulus, part of central sensitization [4]. Further, NMDA receptor phosphorylation results in increased

The synovial membrane

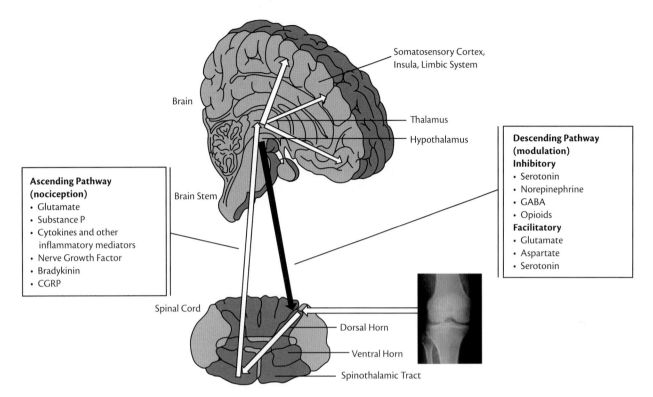

Brain

Ascending Pathway
(nociception)
• Glutamate
• Substance P
• Cytokines and other
  inflammatory mediators
• Nerve Growth Factor
• Bradykinin
• CGRP

Brain Stem

Spinal Cord

Somatosensory Cortex,
Insula, Limbic System

Thalamus

Hypothalamus

Descending Pathway
(modulation)
Inhibitory
• Serotonin
• Norepinephrine
• GABA
• Opioids
Facilitatory
• Glutamate
• Aspartate
• Serotonin

Dorsal Horn

Ventral Horn

Spinothalamic Tract

Figure 13.1 Neurological pain pathways and associated neurotransmitters thought to be active in pain perception associated with osteoarthritis. Ascending pathways are nociceptive. Descending pathways modulate the response to painful stimuli at the dorsal horn. Modulating fibres can either facilitate or inhibit pain signalling through the ascending pathway.

Illustration is modified from original, provided courtesy of Patrick J. Lynch, medical illustrator; C. Carl Jaffe, MD, cardiologist. http://commons.wikimedia.org/wiki/File:Skull_and_sagittal_brain.svg?uselang=fr.html#globalusage

receptor distribution in the cell membrane and increased responsiveness to glutamate [4]. Central sensitization of neurons in the dorsal horn can occur rapidly and be sustained for hours; transcription-dependent changes may last for days. Upregulation of gene expression with resultant increases of COX, substance P and its receptor, neurokin 1, and dynorphin may yield greater chronicity as well as hyperalgesia and allodynia [4]. Central sensitization is characterized by reduced thermal and mechanical thresholds in a diffuse distribution, reflecting enlarged spinal cord receptive fields [11]. The phenomenon of temporal summation occurs, in which pain increases with repeated stimulation even as the stimulus remains the same, a phenomenon that can be inhibited by NMDA antagonists [11].

Microglia

Glial cells (e.g. microglia) which serve as resident macrophages in the CNS, may contribute to central sensitization. Post-nerve injury, microglia cluster in the dorsal horn and release proinflammatory cytokines which enhance central sensitization and pain [5]. P2-type purinergic receptors on microglia are activated by ATP. Animal studies suggest that microglial activation can serve a disinhibition role, leading to gamma aminobutyric acid (GABA)-induced depolarization rather than hyperpolarization, that is, increased neuronal sensitization [5]. Toll-like receptors, part of the innate immune system response to injury or pathogens, appear to be implicated in microglial activation [5].

Descending inhibitory pathways

Afferent spinal cord neurons that have joint input can be inhibited by descending modulatory systems. Neurons from brain centres such as the insula, frontal cortex, amygdala, and the hypothalamus project through the periaqueductal grey and indirectly project to the dorsal horn via the rostral ventromedial medulla and pontomesencephalic region [4]. Descending inhibitory neurotransmitters include GABA, cannabinoid receptor 1 and 2, three opioid receptors, μ, δ, and κ, norepinephrine, and serotonin, which may also have some facilitatory function [2,4] (Figure 13.1). GABAergic or glycinergic inhibitory neurons are present in the superficial dorsal horn and are fundamentally important for the 'gate control' theory of pain, that is, that decrease or loss of function of these interneurons results in increased pain [13]. Disinhibition contributes to NMDA-influenced central sensitization, resulting in mechanical allodynia [5]. Therapies which boost the quantity and function of these inhibitory neurotransmitters demonstrate analgesic benefit in various pain conditions, including OA [14], and this is an avenue for future therapy development. Experimental evidence in animal models demonstrates that interference with descending inhibition will decrease neuronal threshold for mechanostimulation and increase response and receptor field size [2]. Also, external noxious stimuli from a different part of the body may inhibit nociceptive neuronal activity in the cord, a process known as diffuse noxious inhibitory control [2].

At a population level, OA pain intensity correlates poorly with degree of joint damage assessed by radiographic changes [15], although within individuals, pain severity is associated with radiographic damage and the presence of bone marrow lesions on MRI [1,16,17]. The variability of these findings suggest that central sensitization may have a significant role in the pain experience of OA, particularly when considering those with significant pain despite little evidence of radiographic damage. Quantitative sensory testing studies demonstrate that OA patients are more sensitive to experimental pain stimuli than healthy controls, both at sites close to affected OA joints but also distant from these sites (e.g. the contralateral joint or even the forehead) [11,18,19]. In knee OA patients compared to controls, Imamura et al. demonstrated increased subcutaneous, myotomal, and sclerotomal hyperalgesia at multiple dermatomal levels in OA, hypothesizing the importance of peripheral mechanisms in earlier stages of OA and central mechanisms in later stages [20]. In a classic study by Kosek and Ordeberg, abnormal diffuse pain responses in subjects with hip OA were noted to be reversible after hip replacement surgery, achieving thresholds similar to healthy controls 6–14 months post surgery [21]. A controlled study of 48 knee OA patients compared to 24 age- and sex-matched controls demonstrated greater loss of descending analgesic activity and greater temporal summation in the OA patients [19].

Neuroimaging

Neuroimaging studies corroborate the above-noted findings. Gwilym et al. performed functional MRI of the brain of OA patients compared to controls undergoing quantitative sensory testing [18]. Enhanced activity in the periaqueductal grey matter was interpreted as an increase in descending facilitatory pathways. More recently, this same group compared patients with painful hip OA to age- and sex-matched controls by brain MRI with voxel-based morphometry. They found a significant decrease in grey matter volume of the contralateral thalamus, and to a lesser extent, the ipsilateral thalamus, in OA patients compared to controls prior to hip arthroplasty. Nine months post hip surgery and decreased pain, the thalamic volume changes had reversed and were similar to healthy controls [22]. This type of grey matter volume change has been noted in other chronic pain conditions [23,24]. This apparent anatomical change has been theorized to represent blood flow changes or cellular changes and change after improvement of pain is considered to be consistent with CNS neuroplasticity.

Kulkarni et al. assessed knee OA patients with positron emission tomography of the brain using ^{18}F-fluorodeoxyglucose. Scanning was performed during three different states: arthritic knee pain, experimental knee pain (heat pain stimuli to the skin overlying the knee), and pain-free [25]. The two pain states were associated with increased activity in the pain 'matrix', including the somatosensory cortex, perigenual cingulate cortex, insula, primary motor cortex, orbitofrontal cortex, inferior parietal cortex, putamen, left thalamus, and right prefrontal cortex. However, the arthritis pain state additionally showed increased activity in the cingulate cortex, left thalamus, and amygdala, areas considered to be involved in the processing of fear, emotion, and aversive conditioning.

Genetics

Genetic influences in the experience of OA pain have also been explored, in parallel with a growing awareness of genetic influences on other chronic pain conditions. Van Meurs et al. [26] studied a large OA database, and noted the usual lack of correlation between radiographic changes and symptomatology, but a strong association between female carriers of the 158Met variant of catechol-O-methyltransferase (COMT) as compared to carriers of the Val/Val COMT genotype. This joined observations by a variety of researchers, including Zubieta et al. [27] and Diatchenko et al. [28], as reviewed by Clauw and Witter [29], on the important role played by gene variants that encode neurotransmitter function and differentially affect pain sensitivity.

Concomitant fibromyalgia

Noting the prominent role of central sensitization and the activation of pro-nociceptive neurons and mediators in the spinal cord and brain, in addition to the periphery in the OA pain experience, it is pertinent to query the prevalence of fibromyalgia (FM) in OA patients given the overlapping pathogenic neurobiology of these conditions, if such a demarcation is possible to discern [11,14,30,31]. FM is a term which describes patients with a chronic pain syndrome characterized by central sensitization [31], possibly some element of peripheral sensitization [32], as well as chronic fatigue, sleep disturbance and variably other somatic symptoms. The neurobiology of the condition shares many of the same central mechanisms as discussed above [32–34]. Up to 10% of OA patients may have concomitant FM [35,36] in observed cohorts of OA patients. Phillips and Clauw have noted that a significant proportion of OA patients express fatigue and sleep disturbance as prominent symptoms [31]. Determining whether to attribute a broader symptom complex of more widespread pain, fatigue, and sleep problems, which occurs in some OA patients, to the pathogenic neurobiology of OA, concomitant FM, or other aetiologies, including psychosocial factors, is not a trivial challenge. Centrally acting drugs such as the serotonin-norepinephrine reuptake inhibitor duloxetine have been demonstrated to improve knee OA pain [37], presumably acting by improving descending inhibitory signalling in OA. It may well be that such approaches can also impact the broader neurobiological pathology of concomitant OA and FM.

Conclusion

The neurobiological pathogenesis of pain in OA represents a continuum from the peripheral joint to the spinal cord and brain and back. Peripheral nociceptors become activated by mechanical, neurotransmitter, and inflammatory signals which generate both acute pain experienced in the CNS as well as the phenomenon of central sensitization, especially with prolonged duration and greater severity of disease. Intermittent pain experience becomes continuous and more impactful. Greater understanding of the neurobiology of pain, its complex signalling pathways, receptor mechanisms, and array of neurotransmitters, cytokines, and other mediators continues to provide avenues for development of targeted pain modulatory therapies.

References

1. Felson DT. Developments in the clinical understanding of osteoarthritis. *Arthritis Res Ther* 2009; 11(1):203.
2. Schaible HG. Joint pain: basic mechanisms. In McMahon SB, Kolzenburg M, Tracey I, Turk DC (eds) *Wall and Melzack's Textbook of Pain*, 6th ed. Philadelphia, PA: Elsevier/Saunders; 2013:609–19.
3. Schaible HG. Mechanisms of chronic pain in osteoarthritis. *Curr Rheumatol Rep* 2012; 14(6):549–56.

4. Bingham B, Ajit SK, Blake DR, et al. The molecular basis of pain and its clinical implications in rheumatology. *Nat Clin Pract Rheumatol* 2009; 5(1):28–37.

5. Basbaum AI, Bautista DM, Scherrer G, et al. Cellular and molecular mechanisms of pain. *Cell* 2009; 139(2):267–84.

6. Lane NE, Schnitzer TJ, Birbara CA, et al. Tanezumab for the treatment of pain from osteoarthritis of the knee. *N Engl J Med* 2010; 363(16):1521–31.

7. Schaible HG, von Banchet GS, Boettger MK, et al. The role of proinflammatory cytokines in the generation and maintenance of joint pain. *Ann N Y Acad Sci* 2010; 1193:60–9.

8. Goldring MB, Otero M. Inflammation in osteoarthritis. *Curr Opin Rheumatol* 2011; 23(5):471–8.

9. Sellam J, Berenbaum F. The role of synovitis in pathophysiology and clinical symptoms of osteoarthritis. *Nat Rev Rheumatol* 2010; 6(11):625–35.

10. Hayashi D, Roemer FW, Katur A, et al. Imaging of synovitis in osteoarthritis: current status and outlook. *Semin Arthritis Rheum* 2011; 41(2):116–30.

11. Lee YC, Nassikas NJ, Clauw DJ. The role of the central nervous system in the generation and maintenance of chronic pain in rheumatoid arthritis, osteoarthritis and fibromyalgia. *Arthritis Res Ther* 2011; 13(2):211.

12. Latremoliere A, Woolf CJ. Central sensitization: a generator of pain hypersensitivity by central neural plasticity. *J Pain* 2009; 10(9):895–926.

13. Melzack R, Wall PD. Pain mechanisms: a new theory. *Science* 1965; 150(3699):971–9.

14. Mease PJ, Hanna S, Frakes EP, et al. Pain mechanisms in osteoarthritis: understanding the role of central pain and current approaches to its treatment. *J Rheumatol* 2011; 38(8):1546–51.

15. Bedson J, Croft PR. The discordance between clinical and radiographic knee osteoarthritis: a systematic search and summary of the literature. *BMC Musculoskelet Disord* 2008; 9:116.

16. Neogi T, Felson D, Niu J, et al. Association between radiographic features of knee osteoarthritis and pain: results from two cohort studies. *BMJ* 2009; 339:b2844.

17. Zhang Y, Nevitt M, Niu J, et al. Fluctuation of knee pain and changes in bone marrow lesions, effusions, and synovitis on magnetic resonance imaging. *Arthritis Rheum* 2011; 63(3):691–9.

18. Gwilym SE, Keltner JR, Warnaby CE, et al. Psychophysical and functional imaging evidence supporting the presence of central sensitization in a cohort of osteoarthritis patients. *Arthritis Rheum* 2009; 61(9):1226–34.

19. Arendt-Nielsen L, Nie H, Laursen MB, et al. Sensitization in patients with painful knee osteoarthritis. *Pain* 2010; 149(3):573–81.

20. Imamura M, Imamura ST, Kaziyama HH, et al. Impact of nervous system hyperalgesia on pain, disability, and quality of life in patients with knee osteoarthritis: a controlled analysis. *Arthritis Rheum* 2008; 59(10):1424–31.

21. Kosek E, Ordeberg G. Abnormalities of somatosensory perception in patients with painful osteoarthritis normalize following successful treatment. *Eur J Pain* 2000; 4(3):229–38.

22. Gwilym SE, Filippini N, Douaud G, et al. Thalamic atrophy associated with painful osteoarthritis of the hip is reversible after arthroplasty: a longitudinal voxel-based morphometric study. *Arthritis Rheum* 2010; 62(10):2930–40.

23. Apkarian AV, Sosa Y, Sonty S, et al. Chronic back pain is associated with decreased prefrontal and thalamic gray matter density. *J Neurosci* 2004; 24(46):10410–5.

24. May A. Chronic pain may change the structure of the brain. *Pain* 2008; 137(1):7–15.

25. Kulkarni B, Bentley DE, Elliott R, et al. Arthritic pain is processed in brain areas concerned with emotions and fear. *Arthritis Rheum* 2007; 56(4):1345–54.

26. van Meurs JB, Uitterlinden AG, Stolk L, et al. A functional polymorphism in the catechol-O-methyltransferase gene is associated with osteoarthritis-related pain. *Arthritis Rheum* 2009; 60(2):628–9.

27. Zubieta JK, Heitzeg MM, Smith YR, et al. COMT val158met genotype affects mu-opioid neurotransmitter responses to a pain stressor. *Science* 2003; 299(5610):1240–3.

28. Diatchenko L, Nackley AG, Slade GD, et al. Catechol-O-methyltransferase gene polymorphisms are associated with multiple pain-evoking stimuli. *Pain* 2006; 125(3):216–24.

29. Clauw DJ, Witter J. Pain and rheumatology: thinking outside the joint. *Arthritis Rheum* 2009; 60(2):321–4.

30. Staud R. Evidence for shared pain mechanisms in osteoarthritis, low back pain, and fibromyalgia. *Curr Rheumatol Rep* 2011; 13(6):513–20.

31. Phillips K, Clauw DJ. Central pain mechanisms in chronic pain states—maybe it is all in their head. *Best Pract Res Clin Rheumatol* 2011; 25(2):141–54.

32. Staud R. Peripheral pain mechanisms in chronic widespread pain. *Best Pract Res Clin Rheumatol* 2011; 25(2):155–64.

33. Ablin K, Clauw DJ. From fibrositis to functional somatic syndromes to a bell-shaped curve of pain and sensory sensitivity: evolution of a clinical construct. *Rheum Dis Clin North Am* 2009; 35(2):233–51.

34. Russell IJ, Larson AA. Neurophysiopathogenesis of fibromyalgia syndrome: a unified hypothesis. *Rheum Dis Clin North Am* 2009; 35(2):421–35.

35. Haliloglu S, Carlioglu A, Akdeniz D, et al. Fibromyalgia in patients with other rheumatic diseases: prevalence and relationship with disease activity. *Rheumatol Int* 2014; 34(9):1275–80.

36. Wolfe F, Cathey MA. Prevalence of primary and secondary fibrositis. *J Rheumatol* 1983; 10(6):965–8.

37. Chappell AS, Ossanna MJ, Liu-Seifert H, et al. Duloxetine, a centrally acting analgesic, in the treatment of patients with osteoarthritis knee pain: a 13-week, randomized, placebo-controlled trial. *Pain* 2009; 146(3):253–60.

CHAPTER 14

Contextual aspects of pain: why does the patient hurt?

David A. Walsh

Introduction

Osteoarthritis (OA) pain is both a sensory and emotional experience, determined not only by pathology within the joint, but also moderated by the central nervous system, and interpreted within a psychosocial context. To hurt is to 'suffer pain' [1], emphasizing pain's emotional context. Pain-related suffering combines depression, anxiety, frustration, fear, and anger [2], and is affected both by personality traits and demographic factors, as well as by pain's sensory and emotional dimensions. Context (Table 14.1) has both internal and external dimensions. Genetic variation, gender, age, comorbidities, psychological factors, and neuronal sensitization each contributes to the individual's internal context. Ethnicity, social and work interactions, and healthcare provision contribute to external context. Context not only influences pain interpretation, but also modulates central processing and thereby modifies pain's sensory and emotional components. Understanding contextual aspects of pain helps us to appreciate why not all patients with apparently the same severity of disease report the same pain. Context modulates treatment responses, and importantly determines the actions that people take in response to suffering OA pain. Context can pose threats to successful treatment outcomes, but also provides opportunities to improve arthritis pain.

Internal and external context

Contextual factors that have been prospectively associated with worse OA pain include more severe structural change and pain severity at baseline, medical comorbidities, anxiety and depression, inactivity, non-white race, lower educational achievement or social class, and the presence of OA at additional sites [3–6]. Being overweight or obese is associated with increased risk of future OA pain severity and disability [6–8], and, reciprocally, OA pain can interfere with successful weight loss behaviours such as increasing physical activity and reducing caloric consumption [9,10]. Fatigue and disability also predicted worsening OA [11]. Similar factors contribute to increased functional limitation, both mediated by and in parallel to increased pain [12].

Internal context

Genetic context

Genetic risk factors point to constitutional influences on chronic OA pain (Figure 14.1). Biomechanical factors resulting from variations

Table 14.1 Contextual factors contributing to OA pain. Contextual factors that might modulate pain experience attributed to concurrent OA, or predict worse pain outcomes in prospective studies. Most published research has not tested for inter-dependence or mediation between factors, and primary associations between context and OA pain remain uncertain. Genetic polymorphisms might interact with social factors to explain some of the variation in pain reporting between sexes or ethnic populations. Classification of fibromyalgia as a comorbidity remains controversial, and an alternative model proposes that fibromyalgianess might represent a continuum of symptoms that might either precede or result from OA pain. People with OA pain typically display low or moderate levels of psychological distress (low mood or anxiety), and associations with pain severity or poor outcome might often reflect variation within the normal range rather than clinically comorbid depression or anxiety

Demographic factors	Genetic variation
	Gender
	Age
	Lower educational achievement
Comorbidities	OA at additional sites
	Overweight or obese
	Medical comorbidities
	Fibromyalgia
	Clinical anxiety/depression
	Fatigue
Psychological factors	Personality traits
	Low mood
	Anxiety/fear
	Expectations
	Acceptance
Neuronal sensitization	Peripheral
	Central
Physical activity	Inactivity
	Disability
Social factors	Ethnicity
	Social class
	Social and work interactions
	Dependence on physical ability
	Healthcare provision and access

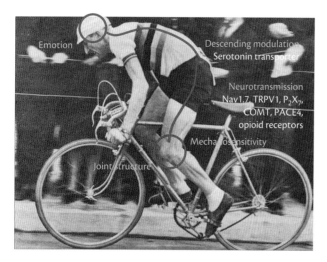

Figure 14.1 Genetic influences on OA pain. Genetic polymorphisms might affect pain transduction, transmission, and experience at multiple levels in pain pathways, as well as by modulating other contextual factors such as comorbidities. Photograph: Marcel Kint, 1938 world road racing champion wearing his rainbow jersey to a stage win in the 1939 Tour de France. His brother, Léon Kint, won the Gent-Leper road race in 1939.
Photograph from *Le Miroir des Sports*, 1939; 1081:9.

in joint shape might mediate some genetic effects on OA pain [13]. Other genetic effects might differ from those predicting structural OA, involving pain neurotransmission through variations in ion channels Nav1.7 and TRPV1, P_2X_7 purinergic receptors, catecholamine O-methyl transferase (COMT), and paired amino acid converting enzyme 4 (PACE4) [14,15]. COMT [16] and opioid receptor [17–19] polymorphisms might contribute to variability in sensitivities to mechanical stimuli. Genetic variation might underpin differences in emotional modulation of pain [20], and serotonin transporter polymorphisms might influence descending pain modulation [21].

Gender

Genetic factors might interact with hormonal and social factors to mediate observed associations between female gender and worse OA pain [3,4]. Emotional responses might, in part, mediate higher reported pain and lower pain tolerance during quantitative sensory testing in women [22], although more successful use by women of strategies that counteract adverse emotional responses to pain might have a greater impact on OA pain than does gender itself [23].

Age

Both radiographic OA and painful OA increase in prevalence with increasing age [3–5]. Older people often see OA as a part of normal ageing, requiring acceptance rather than treatment [24], and consider themselves healthy despite painful joints, particularly if they remain able to continue with everyday activities and social roles [25]. Indeed, acceptance is key in adapting to life with chronic OA pain [26]. By contrast, younger people might experience more distress and frustration in managing OA, seeing it as a condition that is associated with advancing age [24].

Comorbidities and fibromyalgia

The prevalence of comorbidities is higher in people with OA than would be expected of age- and sex-matched non-arthritic controls [27], and comorbidities augment the impact of OA pain on participation in social and domestic life, mainly through further increasing

locomotor disability and depression [28,29]. Fibromyalgia might exacerbate the OA pain experience when it precedes OA onset [3,30], and pain sensitivity can increase as arthritis persists and progresses. Arthritis leads both to peripheral and central sensitization of nociceptive inputs, both those arising from the affected joint and more widespread affecting distant articular and non-articular structures [31,32]. Reversal of changes to pain processing by the central nervous system following successful pain relief from arthroplasty further supports a causal contribution from arthritis to central sensitization [33].

Psychological factors

Chronic pain predisposes to depressed mood [11], and people with OA report worse pain if they display higher levels of depressive symptoms [34]. Worse OA pain has also been associated with lower acceptance [35], lower self-efficacy [36], and higher external locus of control [37]. These cognitive factors might moderate the effects of pain severity on mood. For example, higher levels of pain acceptance can buffer the expected increase in negative affect during pain exacerbations [35]. Chronic OA pain might be more distressing than is acute experimental pain, in part due to expectations that pain will be permanent or deteriorate, lower acceptance, and higher functional impact.

Catastrophizing

Catastrophizing describes an excessive worry about pain, linked to beliefs that pain will be permanent or deteriorating, is beyond personal control and necessarily indicates physical harm, and will prevent valued activities [38]. The tendency to catastrophize might be a personal trait, pre-existing before the onset of OA [39], or might develop as a part of the OA condition, particularly after deterioration in pain [40]. Higher catastrophizing might partially explain differences in pain reporting between men and women [39].

Catastrophizing is associated with more severe OA pain [22,41,42], and is associated with worse physical function [41–44], anxiety and mood disturbance [42,44], and poorer sleep quality [44]. Pain catastrophizing not only varies between individuals, but also from day to day within an individual, and both stable and varying levels of catastrophizing mediate relationships between pain and negative affect [45].

As well as being associated with current pain severity, high pain catastrophizing is associated with worse outcomes for pain and function, both following usual care [5,36], and after psychological or surgical interventions [42]. Catastrophizing is associated with pain that might persist after arthroplasty [46], interacting with other contextual factors, including age, comorbid low back pain and anxiety, and acute postoperative pain severity, to influence post-arthroplasty outcome [42,47]. Relationships between pain sensation, unpleasantness, and suffering are in part mediated by catastrophizing, and unpleasantness and catastrophizing each contribute independently to the hurt of OA pain [2]. Interventions that reduce catastrophizing might therefore directly reduce suffering.

Catastrophizing is not only a psychological response to OA pain, but also might augment central OA pain processing. Catastrophizing is associated with pain qualities often associated with neuropathic pain [48], and with lower pressure pain thresholds in people with OA [22]. Greater pain anticipation might mediate some of the undesirable effects of catastrophizing, and common brain mechanisms might underlie both suffering and catastrophizing [49,50]. Depression and anxiety also modulate pain signalling through alterations in descending inhibitory and excitatory pathway activities [51], and catastrophizing might share underlying mechanisms with the hopelessness and fear that contribute to psychological distress.

External context

Social and work interactions and healthcare provision contribute to external context. These external influences add to information from media and campaign groups and personal experiences to form an individual's beliefs about pain and its treatment. External context influences expectations about OA and its treatment. The prevalence of musculoskeletal pain might vary little between different parts of the world, although healthcare utilization and sickness absence for musculoskeletal pain varies widely [2]. Increased burden of OA pain in areas of socioeconomic deprivation might not be explained by differences in the prevalence of radiographic OA [52], but might be mediated by a greater dependence on physical ability for financial independence, variations in access to healthcare, or by other risk factors for chronic pain.

Effects of context on pain assessment

Context not only affects the individual's experience of pain, but also how they communicate it. In assessing pain in others, we instinctively integrate verbal and non-verbal cues with our beliefs about other possible explanations for these behaviours, including cultural norms and the purpose of the encounter. A clinical consultation can have various objectives. Patients might seek advice, treatment, or endorsement of their illness. Attendance at a consultation might aim to satisfy the expectations of family, employers, or a referring healthcare professional. Pain reporting should be viewed within its context, whether to a healthcare professional, to an employer or benefits agency, or to a researcher.

Contextual effects on question responses

Effects of context on pain reporting are apparent both in face-to-face consultations and using questionnaires. Responses to questions administered together might be inter-correlated, independent of the questions asked, suggesting influences from person-level characteristics and from contextual information, including content of other questions. Questions used to determine eligibility for specific treatment or for financial benefit, might elicit responses emphasizing the severity and impact of pain, whereas one used to determine eligibility to continue treatment, or to evaluate a valued service might emphasize pain improvements.

Questionnaires used with people suffering arthritis pain were developed in other pain groups, and might be interpreted differently by people with OA [53]. The painDETECT questionnaire performs well to classify people with back pain with or without sciatica (neuropathic pain) [54]. PainDETECT generally displays internal consistency in OA populations [53], except that the item about pain that comes and goes during the day might be interpreted as referring to pain on activities such as walking or standing, which is characteristic of mechanical or nociceptive rather than neuropathic pain. Questionnaires might be adapted to focus on OA knee pain by modifying item or introductory wording, incorporating within questionnaire booklets alongside other knee-specific items, or use in studies or clinics that overtly address knee OA. Such contextual modifications might be expected to alter responses. Patients presenting with knee pain might hesitate to mention pains at other locations, and might understate psychological symptoms which they believe are irrelevant to the presenting problem. Such concealment might aim to avoid invalidating the specific and organic nature of their problem. However, widespread pain and psychosocial factors influence treatment responses, and it is important to recognize reporting biases during assessment.

Quantitative sensory testing

Quantitative sensory testing has also pointed to contextual effects on pain assessment. These psychophysical techniques depend on patient-reported sensory experiences in response to standardized stimuli. Variation in pain-related measurements might be due either or both to alterations in reporting and in pain experience [55].

Pressure pain detection thresholds (PPTs) are elicited by a standardized ramped blunt pressure stimulus which is halted at the point at which the participant experiences pain rather than pressure. Interobserver variability in PPT measurements might partly be attributable to social interactions between participant and assessor, and to cognitive distractions [56,57]. A concurrent painful stimulation at a site distant from the test stimulus can increase PPTs (reduce sensitivity), a phenomenon now referred to as conditioned pain modulation [58,59]. Pain intensity reported in response to a standard stimulus might increase following repeated stimulation with a periodicity of seconds, the phenomenon of temporal summation. Temporal summation is associated with sensitivity to physical activity, as indicated by increasing pain during a walk test of constant intensity [44]. Psychological factors such as expectations, anxiety, fear, and low mood [44] are associated with lower PPTs (more sensitive).

Treatment context

Treatment context is a key influence on responses to specific interventions (Figure 14.2). Treatment context is a key mediator of placebo effects in randomized controlled trials, and meta-analyses indicate that approximately half of the reduction in reported OA pain in trials of medical analgesics might be attributable to contextual, rather than pharmacological effects [60]. Optimizing treatment context therefore has great potential to improve quality of life. Key aspects of treatment context are patient expectations and qualities of the therapeutic environment. Patients' beliefs might or might not reflect the treatment contexts provided by different healthcare systems and professional groups, which are based on a range of disease models, research evidence, or professional experience. Clinicians should acknowledge the validity of the patient's perspective whilst raising additional treatment possibilities.

Treatment expectations

Treatment expectations, based on underlying beliefs, are informed by prior experience and information obtained both within and outside of the clinic [61,62]. Treatment beliefs might be either treatment-specific or general. For example, invasive and expensive interventions by expert specialists might be expected to have greater benefit than self-administered treatments. Expectations might be subconsciously modulated, for example according to the colour or size of a tablet. Treatments that previously have been found effective by the patient or an acquaintance might seem more likely to be successful. Flare designs have been used in clinical trials of non-steroidal anti-inflammatory drugs (NSAIDs), selectively recruiting participants whose arthritis pain flares following NSAID withdrawal

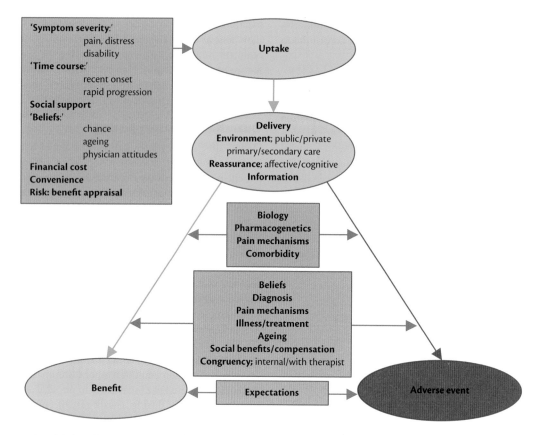

Figure 14.2 Contextual modulation of treatment outcome. The presumed ideal that people with OA pain will access, receive, and benefit from treatment is modulated by a range of factors. Not all people will choose to seek or accept treatment, and the balance between treatment benefit and harm is influenced by biological factors, patient beliefs, and expectancy. A range of diverse factors influence treatment uptake. The context in which treatment is delivered has potential to influence both treatment adherence and effects. Beliefs and expectancy influence not only placebo responses that might enhance treatment effects, but simultaneously determine nocebo responses that might be barriers to patient benefit. Experience of benefit or adverse events will further challenge or reinforce beliefs that can modulate future treatment context.

in order to increase likelihood of response to a subsequent NSAID [63]. Correspondingly, previous treatment failure might predict failure of a subsequent intervention, due to overlapping modes of action between successive treatments or to reduced patient expectations. Treatment expectations affect pain at least in part by effects on central pain processing [64,65], dependent both on the nature of the intervention and individual characteristics of the OA sufferer [66].

Congruency between treatment and pain mechanism

Greater benefit might be expected when a treatment's mode of action is congruent with the cause of pain. OA pain viewed as a biomechanical problem might be expected to respond to biomechanical interventions. Centrally augmented pain might be expected to respond to centrally acting drugs, whereas peripherally driven pain might respond better to local treatments. However, even though older people might view their OA as being normal 'wear and tear', this need not necessarily lead them to restrict their physical activity, considering instead that it is important to keep joints moving in order to maintain independence [25].

Adverse events

Treatments can bring adverse events as well as benefits. Adverse events can counteract analgesic benefit, due both to compounding of pain bothersomeness by comorbid symptoms and to associated alterations in pain processing [67]. Adverse events in people

receiving 'inactive' interventions in clinical trials (nocebo response) reflect those experienced by people receiving active treatment, highlighting the role of expectation [68]. Expectations might be simultaneously both positive and negative; treatments with a greater risk of adverse events might be seen as stronger, and therefore more likely to be effective. Belief that the patient is being offered a suboptimal treatment, for example, due to cost, or being allocated to a waiting list or usual care control treatment in a randomized trial might be associated with worse outcomes. Withdrawal of treatments previously found helpful by the patient can cause particular distress. Differences in beliefs between patients and healthcare professionals create a non-empathic environment that can be a barrier to effective treatment [69].

Treatment uptake

Ultimately a treatment can only have biological effects if it is taken up by the patient, and treatment uptake is also influenced by beliefs about the likely benefits and risks of treatment.

Uptake of primary care treatments

Primary care access for OA treatment is determined only partially by pain severity and recent onset [25], psychological distress, and disability [56,70–72]. Many people do not consult despite severely disabling OA pain [71]. Social factors such as not being in a partnership and prior receipt of medical prescriptions [70], and beliefs that chance determines health [37] each can influence primary healthcare utilization for OA. Believing that OA is an inevitable part of older age about which nothing can be done, negative attitudes from the general practitioner [55], and costs of interventions [73] each have been associated with lower primary care consultation.

Uptake of arthroplasty

People seek arthroplasty often after years of OA pain and previous primary care utilization [70]. Decisions about surgery are influenced by pain severity, rate of deterioration, activity limitations, psychological distress, perceptions about joint replacement surgery, and convenience [62,72,74–76]. A decision to proceed with surgery might be influenced more by beliefs about likely benefits and risks than by pain severity [76,77]. Different treatment expectations might contribute to widely varying arthroplasty rates across geographic regions, and between ethnic groups [61,78,79].

Treatment risk evaluation

Different people evaluate specific benefits and risks differently. Some patients wait until their symptoms are no longer bearable, whereas others seek surgery pre-emptively, before symptoms get worse [62]. People appraise risk differently in response to verbal, statistical, or pictorial information [80]. The risk of an adverse event might be weighted more strongly, irrespective of its statistical probability, if it has been experienced previously either by the patient or through an acquaintance. In one study, nearly one-quarter of people with OA were unwilling to accept any additional risks of heart attack or stroke for only a 2-point reduction in pain on a 10-point scale, whereas risk of stomach bleed appeared more acceptable [81].

Adjusting context to improve arthritis pain

Aspects of context that seem most amenable to healthcare interventions include the clinician–patient interaction, treatment of risk factors or comorbidities, and provision of synergistic treatments. Adjusting aspects of physical environment and interactions with family, colleagues, and employers often requires multidisciplinary interventions delivered by several agencies.

Methodological considerations in studies of contextual interventions

Methodologies for optimizing treatment context or determining the effects of specific contextual interventions suffer limitations. Study designs developed for complex interventions are appropriate in the investigation of the multiple interactions that characterize contextual interventions [82]. The double-blind, randomized controlled clinical trial creates its own specific context. Inviting informed consent modifies participants' understanding of their condition and its possible treatment, by using written information sheets that describe both the rationale and content of interventions. Assessment tools such as questionnaires might also raise expectations or alter understanding. Control groups are not context-free, so might be considered to be exposed to a form of active treatment, and nocebo effects in control groups might be inadvertently augmented. Trial participants allocated to 'usual care' might perceive that they are receiving less than in the active comparator treatment,

in contrast to optimal clinical practice where the patient might expect to receive the best available treatment. Some of these contextual effects might be avoided by concealing the design of clinical trials, but this raises ethical concerns of deception and lack of informed consent. Cohort studies might better reflect 'real-world' clinical practice, but tend to overestimate effect sizes compared to randomized controlled trials.

Cognitive and affective reassurance

Key aspects of clinician–patient interactions centre on reassurance. A systematic review has emphasized the importance of cognitive reassurance, providing constructive information that meets the needs of the individual [69]. Affective reassurance requires empathy with the patient, listening and responding positively to their problems and concerns. Affective reassurance in the absence of cognitive reassurance might not be valued, and indeed might be unhelpful to patients. However, affective reassurance might be a prerequisite for successful cognitive reassurance, encouraging the patient to engage in appropriate reflection on new information. Providing information alone might have little effect on beliefs, even when offered by someone who holds respect as an expert in the field. Instead, structured approaches might be more successful through which the clinician explores patients' beliefs and previous experience and presents alternative models that fit both with the patient's previous experience and are congruent with the proposed treatment.

Investigation

Clinical examination and investigations contribute to the treatment context. Radiographic findings have some predictive value for treatment responses. Lower degrees of tibiofemoral joint space narrowing predicts less analgesic benefit from total knee arthroplasty, although its predictive value is too low to alone determine clinical decisions [83]. Imaging can perhaps best be seen as a part of the treatment context, endorsing the importance of the patient's problem, and supporting an explanation of that problem that is consistent with the treatment that is to be offered. Conversely, not undertaking investigations might conflict with the patient's expectations, undermine confidence, and reduce treatment benefits.

Targeting risk factors for poor outcomes

Although joint replacement surgery is effective for most, up to 20% of people continue to suffer pain and disability after surgery [84]. Worse pain outcomes following joint arthroplasty have been associated with worse preoperative mental health and pain, preoperative catastrophizing [85], and higher numbers of comorbid conditions [86] including obesity [87], and with early postoperative complications [87]. However, even combinations of risk factors explain only a small proportion of treatment outcome [83], and baseline risk factors should not alone be used to determine treatment allocation. Any effect of obesity is small compared to the likely benefit from surgery, even in obese patients [88]. Risk factors, however, might offer therapeutic opportunities through which primary treatment outcomes might be improved.

Combination therapies

Concurrent treatments contribute to treatment context and combinations of specific treatments acting through discrete mechanisms might be expected to be more effective than any single agent in treating the diverse aspects of OA pain. However, evidence of effectiveness of combination strategies is often lacking in randomized controlled trials due to the complexity, logistic difficulties, and expense of such studies. In practice, medical and physical interventions are often provided by different professionals at different times and changes to the organization of healthcare delivery might be necessary both to investigate and to optimize potential synergy between treatments.

Weight reduction strategies, and psychological and physiotherapeutic interventions

Weight reduction strategies have been associated with significant improvements in OA knee pain in people with obesity, although their effect sizes for knee pain are small [89,90]. Benefit might be limited by low effectiveness of weight reduction strategies in treating obesity, although weight reduction is only one possible analgesic mechanism of these interventions. Combining weight reduction strategies with psychological or physiotherapeutic interventions in overweight and obese people with OA might further improve pain outcomes [89,90].

People receiving both pain coping skills training and lifestyle behavioural weight management demonstrated better pain and weight reduction, and improved functional and psychological outcomes than did those receiving either treatment alone or usual care [90]. The combination of weight reduction strategies plus exercise reduced pain more effectively than either intervention alone [89]. However, in trials of complex combined interventions, augmented analgesic benefit might be influenced by other contextual factors such as perceived intervention intensity and patient contact time.

Conclusion

The context in which OA pain is experienced moderates and, to an extent, mediates its severity and impact. Treatment contexts moderate and mediate therapeutic effectiveness. Understanding the nature and consequences of context helps explain heterogeneity between different people with OA pain, and opens avenues for potentially powerful interventions that could improve their quality of life.

References

1. Hurt. In *Oxford Dictionaries*. Oxford University Press; n.d. http://www.oxforddictionaries.com/definition/english/hurt.
2. Wade JB, Riddle DL, Price DD, Dumenci L. Role of pain catastrophizing during pain processing in a cohort of patients with chronic and severe arthritic knee pain. *Pain* 2011; 152:314–9.
3. Juhakoski R, Malmivaara A, Lakka TA, et al. Determinants of pain and functioning in hip osteoarthritis—a two-year prospective study. *Clin Rehabil* 2013; 27:281–7.
4. Collins JE, Katz JN, Dervan EE, Losina E. Trajectories and risk profiles of pain in persons with radiographic, symptomatic knee osteoarthritis: data from the osteoarthritis initiative. *Osteoarthritis Cartilage* 2014; 22:622–30.
5. Alschuler KN, Molton IR, Jensen MP, Riddle DL. Prognostic value of coping strategies in a community-based sample of persons with chronic symptomatic knee osteoarthritis. *Pain* 2013; 154:2775–81.
6. Zeni JA, Jr, Higginson JS. Differences in gait parameters between healthy subjects and persons with moderate and severe knee

7. osteoarthritis: a result of altered walking speed? [Erratum appears in *Clin Biomech* 2009; 24(6):532]. *Clin Biomech* 2009; 24:372–8.
7. Spector TD, Hart DJ, Doyle DV. Incidence and progression of osteoarthritis in women with unilateral knee disease in the general population: the effect of obesity. *Ann Rheum Dis* 1994; 53:565–8.
8. Jordan JM, Luta G, Renner JB, et al. Self-reported functional status in osteoarthritis of the knee in a rural southern community: the role of sociodemographic factors, obesity, and knee pain. *Arthritis Care Res* 1996; 9:273–8.
9. Der Ananian C, Wilcox S, Watkins K, Saunders R, Evans AE. Factors associated with exercise participation in adults with arthritis. *J Aging Phys Activity* 2008; 16:125–43.
10. Rosemann T, Kuehlein T, Laux G, Szecsenyi J. Factors associated with physical activity of patients with osteoarthritis of the lower limb. *J Eval Clin Pract* 2008; 14:288–93.
11. Hawker GA, Gignac MA, Badley E, et al. A longitudinal study to explain the pain-depression link in older adults with osteoarthritis. *Arthritis Care Res* 2011; 63:1382–90.
12. Pisters MF, Veenhof C, van Dijk GM, et al. The course of limitations in activities over 5 years in patients with knee and hip osteoarthritis with moderate functional limitations: risk factors for future functional decline. *Osteoarthritis Cartilage* 2012; 20:503–10.
13. Kalichman L, Zhu Y, Zhang Y, et al. The association between patella alignment and knee pain and function: an MRI study in persons with symptomatic knee osteoarthritis. *Osteoarthritis Cartilage* 2007; 15:1235–40.
14. Thakur M, Dawes JM, McMahon SB. Genomics of pain in osteoarthritis. *Osteoarthritis Cartilage* 2013; 21:1374–82.
15. Bratus A, Aeschlimann A, Russo G, Sprott H. Candidate gene approach in genetic epidemiological studies of osteoarthritis-related pain. *Pain* 2014; 155:217–21.
16. Martinez-Jauand M, Sitges C, Rodriguez V, et al. Pain sensitivity in fibromyalgia is associated with catechol-O-methyltransferase (COMT) gene. *Eur J Pain* 2013; 17:16–27.
17. Fillingim RB, Kaplan L, Staud R, et al. The A118G single nucleotide polymorphism of the mu-opioid receptor gene (OPRM1) is associated with pressure pain sensitivity in humans. *J Pain* 2005; 6:159–67.
18. Huang CJ, Liu HF, Su NY, et al. Association between human opioid receptor genes polymorphisms and pressure pain sensitivity in females. *Anaesthesia* 2008; 63:1288–95.
19. Sato H, Droney J, Ross J, et al. Gender, variation in opioid receptor genes and sensitivity to experimental pain. *Mol Pain* 2013; 9:20.
20. Palit S, Sheaff RJ, France CR, et al. Serotonin transporter gene (5-HTTLPR) polymorphisms are associated with emotional modulation of pain but not emotional modulation of spinal nociception. *Biol Psychol* 2011; 86:360–9.
21. Lindstedt F, Berrebi J, Greayer E, et al. Conditioned pain modulation is associated with common polymorphisms in the serotonin transporter gene. *PLoS ONE* 2011; 6:e18252.
22. France CR, Keefe FJ, Emery CF, et al. Laboratory pain perception and clinical pain in post-menopausal women and age-matched men with osteoarthritis: relationship to pain coping and hormonal status. *Pain* 2004; 112:274–81.
23. Affleck G, Tennen H, Keefe FJ, et al. Everyday life with osteoarthritis or rheumatoid arthritis: independent effects of disease and gender on daily pain, mood, and coping. *Pain* 1999; 83:601–9.
24. Gignac MA, Davis AM, Hawker G, et al. 'What do you expect? You're just getting older': a comparison of perceived osteoarthritis-related and aging-related health experiences in middle- and older-age adults. *Arthritis Rheum* 2006; 55:905–12.
25. Grime J, Richardson JC, Ong BN. Perceptions of joint pain and feeling well in older people who reported being healthy: a qualitative study. *Br J Gen Pract* 2010; 60:597–603.
26. Koyama Y, Miyashita M, Kazuma K, et al. Preparing a version of the Nottingham Adjustment Scale (for psychological adjustment) tailored to osteoarthritis of the hip. *J Orthop Sci* 2006; 11:359–64.

27. Schram MT, Frijters D, van de Lisdonk EH, et al. Setting and registry characteristics affect the prevalence and nature of multimorbidity in the elderly. *J Clin Epidemiol* 2008; 61:1104–12.

28. Wilkie R, Blagojevic-Bucknall M, Jordan KP, Lacey R, McBeth J. Reasons why multimorbidity increases the risk of participation restriction in older adults with lower extremity osteoarthritis: a prospective cohort study in primary care. *Arthritis Care Res* 2013; 65:910–9.

29. Xie H, Xu F, Chen R, et al. Image formation of brain function in patients suffering from knee osteoarthritis treated with moxibustion. *J Tradit Chin Med* 2013; 33:181–6.

30. Juhakoski R, Tenhonen S, Anttonen T, Kauppinen T, Arokoski JP. Factors affecting self-reported pain and physical function in patients with hip osteoarthritis. *Arch Phys Med Rehabil* 2008; 89:1066–73.

31. Malfait AM, Schnitzer TJ. Towards a mechanism-based approach to pain management in osteoarthritis. *Nat Rev Rheumatol* 2013; 9:654–64.

32. Suokas AK, Walsh DA, McWilliams DF, et al. Quantitative sensory testing in painful osteoarthritis: a systematic review and meta-analysis. *Osteoarthritis Cartilage* 2012; 20:1075–85.

33. Gwilym SE, Filippini N, Douaud G, Carr AJ, Tracey I. Thalamic atrophy associated with painful osteoarthritis of the hip is reversible after arthroplasty: a longitudinal voxel-based morphometric study. *Arthritis Rheum* 2010; 62:2930–40.

34. Rosemann T, Gensichen J, Sauer N, Laux G, Szecsenyi J. The impact of concomitant depression on quality of life and health service utilisation in patients with osteoarthritis. *Rheumatol Int* 2007; 27:859–63.

35. Kratz AL, Davis MC, Zautra AJ. Pain acceptance moderates the relation between pain and negative affect in female osteoarthritis and fibromyalgia patients. *Ann Behav Med* 2007; 33:291–301.

36. Rayahin JE, Chmiel JS, Hayes KW, et al. Factors associated with pain experience outcome in knee osteoarthritis. *Arthritis Care Res* 2014; 66:1828–35.

37. Cross MJ, March LM, Lapsley HM, Byrne E, Brooks PM. Patient self-efficacy and health locus of control: relationships with health status and arthritis-related expenditure. *Rheumatology (Oxford)* 2006; 45:92–6.

38. Rosenstiel AK, Keefe FJ. The use of coping strategies in chronic low back pain patients: relationship to patient characteristics and current adjustment. *Pain* 1983; 17:33–44.

39. Keefe FJ, Lefebvre JC, Egert JR, et al. The relationship of gender to pain, pain behavior, and disability in osteoarthritis patients: the role of catastrophizing. *Pain* 2000; 87:325–34.

40. Peat G, Thomas E. When knee pain becomes severe: a nested case-control analysis in community-dwelling older adults. *J Pain* 2009; 10:798–808.

41. Sinikallio SH, Helminen EE, Valjakka AL, Vaisanen-Rouvali RH, Arokoski JP. Multiple psychological factors are associated with poorer functioning in a sample of community-dwelling knee osteoarthritis patients. *J Clin Rheumatol* 2014; 20:261–7.

42. Sullivan M, Tanzer M, Stanish W, et al. Psychological determinants of problematic outcomes following total knee arthroplasty. *Pain* 2009; 143:123–9.

43. Riddle DL, Jensen MP. Construct and criterion-based validity of brief pain coping scales in persons with chronic knee osteoarthritis pain. *Pain Med* 2013; 14:265–75.

44. Wideman TH, Finan PH, Edwards RR, et al. Increased sensitivity to physical activity among individuals with knee osteoarthritis: relation to pain outcomes, psychological factors, and responses to quantitative sensory testing. *Pain* 2014; 155:703–11.

45. Sturgeon JA, Zautra AJ, Arewasikporn A. A multilevel structural equation modeling analysis of vulnerabilities and resilience resources influencing affective adaptation to chronic pain. *Pain* 2014; 155:292–8.

46. Hirakawa Y, Hara M, Fujiwara A, Hanada H, Morioka S. The relationship among psychological factors, neglect-like symptoms and postoperative pain after total knee arthroplasty. *Pain Res Manag* 2014; 19:251–6.

47. Masselin-Dubois A, Attal N, Fletcher D, et al. Are psychological predictors of chronic postsurgical pain dependent on the surgical model?

48. A comparison of total knee arthroplasty and breast surgery for cancer. *J Pain* 2013; 14:854–64.

48. Hochman JR, Davis AM, Elkayam J, Gagliese L, Hawker GA. Neuropathic pain symptoms on the modified painDETECT correlate with signs of central sensitization in knee osteoarthritis. *Osteoarthritis Cartilage* 2013; 21:1236–42.

49. Gracely RH, Geisser ME, Giesecke T, et al. Pain catastrophizing and neural responses to pain among persons with fibromyalgia. *Brain* 2004; 127:835–43.

50. Seminowicz DA, Davis KD. Cortical responses to pain in healthy individuals depends on pain catastrophizing. *Pain* 2006; 120:297–306.

51. de Souza JB, Potvin S, Goffaux P, Charest J, Marchand S. The deficit of pain inhibition in fibromyalgia is more pronounced in patients with comorbid depressive symptoms. *Clin J Pain* 2009; 25:123–7.

52. Cleveland RJ, Luong ML, Knight JB, et al. Independent associations of socioeconomic factors with disability and pain in adults with knee osteoarthritis. *BMC Musculoskelet Disord* 2013; 14:297.

53. Moreton BJ, Tew V, das Nair R, et al. Pain phenotype in patients with knee osteoarthritis: classification and measurement properties of pain-DETECT and self-report Leeds assessment of neuropathic symptoms and signs scale in a cross-sectional study. *Arthritis Care Res* 2015; 67:519–28.

54. Freynhagen R, Baron R, Gockel U, Tolle TR. painDETECT: a new screening questionnaire to identify neuropathic components in patients with back pain. *Curr Med Res Opin* 2006; 22:1911–20.

55. Paskins Z, Sanders T, Hassell AB. What influences patients with osteoarthritis to consult their GP about their symptoms? A narrative review. *BMC Fam Pract* 2013; 14:195.

56. Schreiber KL, Campbell C, Martel MO, et al. Distraction analgesia in chronic pain patients: the impact of catastrophizing. *Anesthesiology* 2014; 121:1292–301.

57. Martinsen S, Flodin P, Berrebi J, et al. Fibromyalgia patients had normal distraction related pain inhibition but cognitive impairment reflected in caudate nucleus and hippocampus during the Stroop Color Word Test. *PLoS ONE* 2014; 9:e108637.

58. Graven-Nielsen T, Wodehouse T, Langford RM, Arendt-Nielsen L, Kidd BL. Normalization of widespread hyperesthesia and facilitated spatial summation of deep-tissue pain in knee osteoarthritis patients after knee replacement. *Arthritis Rheum* 2012; 64:2907–16.

59. Kosek E, Ordeberg G. Lack of pressure pain modulation by heterotopic noxious conditioning stimulation in patients with painful osteoarthritis before, but not following, surgical pain relief. *Pain* 2000; 88:69–78.

60. Zhang W, Robertson J, Jones AC, Dieppe PA, Doherty M. The placebo effect and its determinants in osteoarthritis: meta-analysis of randomised controlled trials. *Ann Rheum Dis* 2008; 67:1716–23.

61. Ibrahim SA, Siminoff LA, Burant CJ, Kwoh CK. Understanding ethnic differences in the utilization of joint replacement for osteoarthritis: the role of patient-level factors. *Med Care* 2002; 40:I44–51.

62. Sansom A, Donovan J, Sanders C, et al. Routes to total joint replacement surgery: patients' and clinicians' perceptions of need. *Arthritis Care Res* 2010; 62:1252–7.

63. Trijau S, Avouac J, Escalas C, Gossec L, Dougados M. Influence of flare design on symptomatic efficacy of non-steroidal anti-inflammatory drugs in osteoarthritis: a meta-analysis of randomized placebo-controlled trials. *Osteoarthritis Cartilage* 2010; 18:1012–8.

64. Carlino E, Frisaldi E, Benedetti F. Pain and the context. *Nat Rev Rheumatol* 2014; 10:348–55.

65. Kong J, Gollub RL, Polich G, et al. A functional magnetic resonance imaging study on the neural mechanisms of hyperalgesic nocebo effect. *J Neurosci* 2008; 28:13354–62.

66. Kong J, Spaeth R, Cook A, et al. Are all placebo effects equal? Placebo pills, sham acupuncture, cue conditioning and their association. *PLoS ONE* 2013; 8:e67485.

67. Geuter S, Buchel C. Facilitation of pain in the human spinal cord by nocebo treatment. *J Neurosci* 2013; 33:13784–90.

68. Faasse K, Petrie KJ. The nocebo effect: patient expectations and medication side effects. *Postgrad Med J* 2013; 89:540–6.

69. Pincus T, Holt N, Vogel S, et al. Cognitive and affective reassurance and patient outcomes in primary care: a systematic review. *Pain* 2013; 154:2407–16.

70. Rosemann T, Joos S, Szecsenyi J, Laux G, Wensing M. Health service utilization patterns of primary care patients with osteoarthritis. *BMC Health Serv Res* 2007; 7:169.

71. Bedson J, Mottram S, Thomas E, Peat G. Knee pain and osteoarthritis in the general population: what influences patients to consult? *Fam Pract* 2007; 24:443–53.

72. Mitchell HL, Carr AJ, Scott DL. The management of knee pain in primary care: factors associated with consulting the GP and referrals to secondary care. *Rheumatology (Oxford)* 2006; 45:771–6.

73. Jinks C, Ong BN, O'Neill T. 'Well, it's nobody's responsibility but my own.' A qualitative study to explore views about the determinants of health and prevention of knee pain in older adults. *BMC Public Health* 2010; 10:148.

74. Dosanjh S, Matta JM, Bhandari M, Anterior THARC. The final straw: a qualitative study to explore patient decisions to undergo total hip arthroplasty. *Arch Orthop Trauma Surg* 2009; 129:719–27.

75. Hall M, Migay AM, Persad T, et al. Individuals' experience of living with osteoarthritis of the knee and perceptions of total knee arthroplasty. *Physiother Theory Pract* 2008; 24:167–81.

76. Hawker GA, Guan J, Croxford R, et al. A prospective population-based study of the predictors of undergoing total joint arthroplasty. *Arthritis Rheum* 2006; 54:3212–20.

77. Rudan JF, Harrison MM, Grant HJ. Determining patient concerns before joint arthroplasty. *J Arthroplasty* 2009; 24:1115–9.

78. Suarez-Almazor ME, Souchek J, Kelly PA, et al. Ethnic variation in knee replacement: patient preferences or uninformed disparity? *Arch Intern Med* 2005; 165:1117–24.

79. Groeneveld PW, Kwoh CK, Mor MK, et al. Racial differences in expectations of joint replacement surgery outcomes. *Arthritis Rheum* 2008; 59:730–7.

80. Flynn D, Ford GA, Stobbart L, et al. A review of decision support, risk communication and patient information tools for thrombolytic treatment in acute stroke: lessons for tool developers. *BMC Health Serv Res* 2013; 13:225.

81. Richardson CG, Chalmers A, Llewellyn-Thomas HA, et al. Pain relief in osteoarthritis: patients' willingness to risk medication-induced gastrointestinal, cardiovascular, and cerebrovascular complications. *J Rheumatol* 2007; 34:1569–75.

82. Medical Research Council. *Developing and Evaluating Complex Interventions: New Guidance.* Medical Research Council; 2007. http://www.mrc.ac.uk/documents/pdf/developing-and-evaluating-complex-interventions/.

83. Valdes AM, Doherty SA, Zhang W, et al. Inverse relationship between preoperative radiographic severity and postoperative pain in patients with osteoarthritis who have undergone total joint arthroplasty. *Semin Arthritis Rheum* 2012; 41:568–75.

84. Beswick AD, Wylde V, Gooberman-Hill R, Blom A, Dieppe P. What proportion of patients report long-term pain after total hip or knee replacement for osteoarthritis? A systematic review of prospective studies in unselected patients. *BMJ Open* 2012; 2:e000435.

85. Riddle DL, Wade JB, Jiranek WA, Kong X. Preoperative pain catastrophizing predicts pain outcome after knee arthroplasty. *Clin Orthop* 2010; 468:798–806.

86. Lingard EA, Katz JN, Wright EA, Sledge CB, Kinemax Outcomes Group. Predicting the outcome of total knee arthroplasty. *J Bone Joint Surg Am* 2004; 86-A:2179–86.

87. Nunez M, Lozano L, Nunez E, et al. Total knee replacement and health-related quality of life: factors influencing long-term outcomes. *Arthritis Rheum* 2009; 61:1062–9.

88. Judge A, Batra RN, Thomas GE, et al. Body mass index is not a clinically meaningful predictor of patient reported outcomes of primary hip replacement surgery: prospective cohort study. *Osteoarthritis Cartilage* 2014; 22:431–9.

89. Messier SP, Loeser RF, Miller GD, et al. Exercise and dietary weight loss in overweight and obese older adults with knee osteoarthritis: the Arthritis, Diet, and Activity Promotion Trial. *Arthritis Rheum* 2004; 50:1501–10.

90. Somers TJ, Blumenthal JA, Guilak F, et al. Pain coping skills training and lifestyle behavioral weight management in patients with knee osteoarthritis: a randomized controlled study. *Pain* 2012; 153:1199–209.

SECTION 6

Clinical assessment

CHAPTER 15

Clinical assessment: signs, symptoms, and patient perceptions in osteoarthritis

Margreet Kloppenburg

Introduction

Osteoarthritis (OA) is a highly prevalent disorder that can cause significant suffering and disability for patients, at great individual and societal costs. To facilitate correct diagnosing, differentiating OA from other musculoskeletal disorders and optimizing treatment, recognition of symptoms and signs due to OA, insight in their prevalence, and underlying pathophysiological mechanisms are crucial.

Patient perspective

Patients with OA are most important in understanding which symptoms play a role in OA, and what their impact and consequences are. Examples of patient-reported symptoms are depicted in Box 15.1. Qualitative research, using patient interviews with open-ended questions and focus groups, has been performed for this purpose. Pain, physical disability, and fatigue are regarded as highly important [1–6].

Box 15.1 Osteoarthritic symptoms reported by patients with osteoarthritis as examples of the patient perspective

- Pain
- Physical disability
- Fatigue
- Stiffness
- Joint cracking or clicking
- Limping
- Joint swelling
- Reduced strength
- Aesthetic changes
- Effect on social, leisure, and household activities, work
- Difficulty getting dressed
- Psychosocial consequences.

Pain is a multidimensional symptom with respect to quality ('sharp', 'throbbing', 'aching', 'tenderness', 'itching', 'like fever', 'tearing'), intensity ('like knife cutting', 'as electric shock'), frequency, duration, time of day or season, regular (starting pains) versus unpredictable, at rest versus related to activity, location, relation to triggering factors (weather), and its psychological impact [1,3,7–9]. A group of 143 patients with hip and knee OA from four English-speaking countries reported two distinct types of pain: 'a dull, aching pain, which become more constant over time, punctuated increasingly with short episodes of a more intense, often unpredictable, emotionally draining pain' [10]. The intermittent, variable pain was also identified by a group in 28 patients with hip and knee OA [11]; the latter group of patients also reported that pain is inextricable from function and that their experience of joint pain is influenced by pain elsewhere in the body [11]. The majority of a group of 123 patients with symptomatic knee or hip OA from the community reported night pain [12]. Remarkably, night pain was experienced regardless of stage of OA, although its severity increased as the disease progressed. Night pain was felt to be predicted by daytime activity or the weather and to be related to sleep disturbances.

The majority of a group of 46 patients with knee and hip OA from a population-based cohort indicated that they had experienced fatigue. Mental health was identified as both affecting and being affected by fatigue. Fatigue had a substantial impact on their lives by influencing physical function, ability to participate in in social activities, and to do household chores [2].

Other important domains identified by patients with OA are stiffness, joint cracking or clicking, limping, and swelling [1–6]. Hand OA patients from five European countries reported as additional domains reduced strength and aesthetic changes [9]. Embarrassment due to the appearance of their hands was also recognized in another study in patients with hand OA [13]. Patients with foot OA reported as specific issues the importance of footwear and foot appearance, especially in women, and difficulty for patients to recognize and prioritize foot symptoms [14].

Patients with OA experience great impact and consequences from their condition; they report an effect on social and leisure activities, such as recreational and sportive activities, work, and household activities [1,4–6,9]. Hand OA patients report difficulty getting dressed [9]. Loss of these activities was experienced as very upsetting and having important psychological consequences [3,5,9].

Although most studies have been performed in a Western socio-cultural context, a focus group study in 41 Asian patients with knee OA from different ethnic backgrounds showed that similar domains are involved among Asian and Western OA patients [5]. However, the latter study showed also that between ethnic groups differences can be observed with respect to impact of OA on social activities and psychological consequences.

General osteoarthritis symptoms and signs, and their underlying pathogenesis

Pain, stiffness, disability, and fatigue are indicative for all subtypes of OA (Table 15.1). However, their prevalence and severity vary widely between patients. Patients in different setting, such as from primary, secondary, or tertiary care, report different levels of symptoms and signs and therefore the setting has to be taken in account when studying symptoms and signs. For example, in a Spanish population-based study, individuals with symptomatic hand OA did not report a reduced health-related quality of life when compared to healthy controls [15], whereas patients with hand OA collected from a hospital-based rheumatology outpatient clinic did; the health-related quality of life of the latter was even similar to patients with rheumatoid arthritis [16]. Furthermore, symptoms reported by patients with elbow OA, a rare OA subtype, are severe; however, these patients represent end-stage disease from secondary or tertiary care [17–19].

Pain

Pain is multidimensional and varies throughout the day [20,21]. Usually, pain aggravates during the day with use and activities of the OA joint and declines at the end of the day [22,23]. Pain can be located in the OA joint or beyond, and has many origins.

An important type of OA pain is locally felt by patients in the OA joint. Local pain can be ascribed to structural changes and local processes in the OA joint, so-called nociceptive pain. Hyaline articular cartilage is not innervated and cartilage deterioration in itself cannot generate pain, but the other joint tissues synovium, subchondral bone, joint capsule, and periosteum, can. Mild synovial inflammation is prevalent in OA and could lead to pain via inflammatory mediators such as cytokines and prostaglandins, as

is also supported by magnetic resonance imaging (MRI) and ultrasonography studies [24,25]. Another local source of pain is the subchondral bone, where processes of fibrosis and trabecular bone turnover visualized as 'bone marrow lesions' on MRI are associated with pain [25]; also bony enlargements at the joint margins are suggested to be associated with pain [26,27]. Local nociceptive pain can also be generated or aggravated by extra-articular structures that are secondary to OA, such as bursitis, tendinitis, or tension on ligaments.

Another type of pain, originating from changes in the central nervous system—so-called central pain—is recognized to be frequent in OA. In the process of central sensitization, nociceptive stimuli are amplified by the spinal cord or other central mechanisms that result in enhancement or modulation of perception of pain. Central pain is characterized by its multifocal or widespread character, diffuse hyperalgesia, allodynia, lower thresholds for pain, and the association with other centrally mediated factors, such as fatigue, sleep disturbance, and depression [28]. Central pain is familial and genetic factors seems to be involved [29,30].

Stiffness

The majority of patients with OA experiences stiffness [7,31]. Stiffness occurs after awakening in the morning (morning stiffness) and in general its duration is relatively short. In studies in 100 and 50 patients with knee or hip OA and hand OA, respectively, that investigated the multidimensionality of discomfort in OA patients the mean duration of morning stiffness was 14.5 minutes (range 1–120) and 38 minutes respectively [7,31]. Furthermore, stiffness occurs frequently after prolonged inactivity, such as sitting or lying [7,31]. Stiffness in OA often follows a circadian rhythm, with highest levels in the morning [32], suggesting an inflammatory influence [33]. Stiffness after inactivity is considered to be mechanically driven, although association between self-reported stiffness and radiographic OA severity is relatively poor, as is also the case for the association with other self-reported symptoms.

Disability

Pain and deformities in the joint and surrounding tissues through the OA process result in loss of functioning. A wide spectrum of problems can be observed in patients with OA, depending on the joints affected and on stage of the condition. The International Classification of Function, Disability and Health (ICF) approved by the World Health Organization offers a multidimensional framework to define this spectrum of typical problems in functioning of patients with OA [34]. For OA, preliminary ICF core sets (comprehensive and brief sets) have been defined that have been validated [35,36]. Impairments due to OA are decreased joint mobility, malalignment, dislocation, decreased strength, abnormal muscle function, and abnormal gait pattern (limping). As a consequence, execution of tasks and actions (activities) can be limited and have a negative impact on participation and involvement in life situations. Domains (categories) that can be limited in patients with OA are mobility (lifting and carrying objects, changing and maintaining body position, fine hand use, walking, moving around, using transportation, and driving), self-care (washing, toileting, dressing), domestic life (doing household, assisting others), intimate relationships, remunerative employment, community life, and recreation and leisure (http://www.who.int/classification/icf). The ICF framework reflects that the impact OA has on a patient's life depends not

Table 15.1 General and joint-specific osteoarthritic symptoms and signs

General symptoms and signs	Joint-specific symptoms and signs
Pain	Bony enlargement
Morning and inactivity stiffness	Malalignment and/or deformity
Disability	Decreased range of motion
Joint tenderness	Soft tissue swelling with(out) effusion and/or warmth
Fatigue and sleep disturbances	Crepitus
	Clicking
	Instability
	Muscle weakness
	Decreased performance
	Alterations in gait

only on the condition itself but also of the interaction with environmental and personal factors, so-called contextual factors.

The societal impact of OA disability is illustrated by the Global Burden of Disease 2010 Study showing that musculoskeletal conditions are the second cause of the total years lived with disability worldwide [37]; within this group of musculoskeletal conditions OA has a significant contribution [38].

Joint tenderness

Joint tenderness is the result of pressure or joint movement during physical examination. Pressure on the knee—also called bony tenderness—is part of the classification criteria set for knee OA [39]. An index for joint tenderness has been developed by Doyle and colleagues [40], which was a modification of the widely used Ritchie index for rheumatoid arthritis [41]. The Doyle index assesses 48 joints or joint groups, based on the pattern of joint involvement in OA. Tenderness is graded by pressure on the lateral joint margin or by passive joint movement on a four-point scale; the total score ranges from 0 to 144 (Table 15.2). Joints with prosthesis are not graded and not included in the score. Reliability of the score is good and it is easy to perform; performance takes an average of

Table 15.2 The Doyle Index pain is graded 0–3 (0 = no pain, 1 = patient complaints of pain, 2 = patient complaints of pain and winces, and 3 = patient complaints of pain, winces, and withdraws joint) in 48 joints or joint groups by palpation or passive movement

Joint	Method of testing	Number of units
DIP II–V (individually)	Pressure	8
PIP II–V, IP I (individually)	Pressure	10
MCP II–V	Pressure	2
MCP I	Pressure	2
CMC I	Pressure	2
Wrist	Pressure	2
Elbow	Pressure	2
Shoulder	Pressure	2
Acromioclavicular	Pressure	1
Sternoclavicular	Pressure	1
Cervical spine	Movement	1
Lumbar spine	Movement	1
Hip	Movement	2
Knee	Pressure	2
Ankle	Movement	2
Talocalcaneal	Movement	2
Midtarsal	Movement	2
MTP I	Pressure	2
MTP II–V	Pressure	2
Total		48

CMC-1, first carpometacarpal joints; DIP, distal interphalangeal joints; IP-1, first interphalangeal joint; MCP, metacarpal joints; MTP, metatarsal joints; PIP, proximal interphalangeal joints.

5 minutes [40,42]. Modifications of the Doyle index, only incorporating the hands or knees and hips, have been investigated [42]. The correlations of the Doyle index score with self-reported pain levels are only moderate [42], suggesting that other aspects of the disease than self-reported pain are captured [42–44]. Doyle et al. suggested that joint tenderness reflects inflammatory pain since the Doyle index decreased statistically significant after receiving an anti-inflammatory treatment, but not after a simple analgesic [40].

Fatigue and sleep disturbances

Patients experience considerable amounts of fatigue with an important impact on their lives [2,9]. Clinical relevant levels of fatigue are reported by 40–66% of patients with knee or hip OA consulting outpatient clinics [45,46]. OA-related fatigue have been linked with older age [47], greater pain [45,46,48], worse health status [46], psychological factors, such as depression [46,47,49] and physical function [45,47]. In two studies women with knee or hip OA were assessed for fatigue, pain and physical activity several times/day over 5 days; objective physical activity was assessed by an accelerometer. In the first study it was shown that fatigue, more than pain, was negatively associated with physical activity, and that fatigue escalated throughout each day. This escalation was steeper and of higher severity than in matched controls [50]. The negative association between clinically relevant fatigue and physical activity was confirmed in the second study in OA patients [51]. Additional analyses suggested that functional mobility (Timed Up and Go) moderated the relationship between fatigue and activity, especially in patients with high functional mobility.

Individuals with OA often suffer from poor sleep. In a community-based cohort of knee and hip OA patients, 70% reported poor sleep [52,53]. Sleep disturbances included both difficulty in falling asleep, interruption of sleep, and early morning awakening [54]. Poor sleep was associated with (nocturnal) pain, greater OA severity [53,55], and psychosocial factors [52,53], and is an important contributor to fatigue [46,53].

Measurement of patient-reported pain and disability

Multiple measures are available to assess patient-reported pain and function [56–59]. Some are specific for OA, whereas others are generic or developed for other rheumatic diseases than OA. The supporting evidence for their metric properties, including reliability, validity, and feasibility, varies. There is also large variability in their content, time and way of acquisition (patient self-administered or doctor administered), and availability in the public domain. At the moment it is impossible to recommend the use of one measure over another, since all have their own strengths and weaknesses. Which is the most suitable depends on the purpose of measurement, for instance, a clinical trial or patient care.

For pain at different joint sites the generic one-dimensional measures visual analogue scale (VAS) and numerical rating scale (NRS) are widely used. This single-item scale is self-administered by the patient and relatively easy to perform; the actual question and timeframe can differ [57]. The Intermittent and Constant Osteoarthritis Pain (ICOAP) questionnaire can be used to capture the multiple dimensions of pain in knee or hip OA; an 11-item OA-specific measure evaluating intensity and frequency of constant pain and pain that 'comes and goes', and their impact on mood, sleep, and quality of life [10]. The ICOAP is freely available in many languages [60]. Other widely used OA-specific pain measures are the subscales of Knee Injury and Osteoarthritis Outcome Score (KOOS) [61] or Western Ontario and McMaster University OA Index (WOMAC) [43], and Australian/Canadian OA Hand Index (AUSCAN) [44].

Patient Acceptable Symptom State

From the patient perspective, symptoms can be defined following the concept of whether the patient 'feels well' given the current level of symptoms, the Patient Acceptable Symptom State (PASS). This concept is especially developed in the context of clinical trials to assess patient-reported outcomes [62], but is also used in evaluating management in daily practice [63]. In a study in five chronic rheumatic diseases, including 602 patients with OA of the knees, hips, and hands participating in a clinical trial studying non-steroidal anti-inflammatory drugs, a PASS of 40 or 4 was defined as outcome measures on 0–100 VAS or on 0–10 NRS, respectively [64]. In a study in 2414 patients with painful knee or/and hip OA, the PASS after 7 days of usual treatment was 4 (on a NRS 0–10) for pain at rest and 5 for pain at movement [63]. Which factors affect the PASS differs between studies and need further study.

Psychosocial factors and their role in symptoms and signs

Numerous studies have shown that the relationship between objective measures of OA damage, such as radiographic signs of structural damage, and subjective measures of OA, such as pain and disability that are reported by the patients, is poor [65,66]. These observations are in line with the recognition that health outcomes of OA, as also for other chronic illnesses, are determined not only by medical, but also by non-medical factors, such as personal and environmental factors, supporting a biopsychosocial model to understand pain and disability in OA [67–69].

Patients' perceptions about osteoarthritis

The perceptions people have about their illness are of importance, since they influence health outcomes as disability and healthcare use, and affect the strategies people use to cope with their disease [68–70]. Several models have been proposed to understand this link concerning self-regulation processes that mediate between the disease, pain, disability, and psychological adjustment. According to Leventhal's Common Sense Model of self-regulation (CSM), people's cognitive representations of the illness determine emotional responses and guide coping efforts. Patients create mental representations of their disease, based on illness-related beliefs, knowledge, experience, and information from other people, in order to make sense of and manage the health problem [68,70]. Illness representations address different aspects of patients' beliefs and ideas about their condition: such as about its nature and associated symptoms, about its likely cause(s), its duration, about its consequences (severity and impact on functioning), and whether patients can make sense of their illness experience, patients' belief their condition can be treated or controlled, and whether patients generate negative emotions due to their condition [70–72]. Another patient belief described by Bandura is 'their capabilities to manage environmental demands'—self-efficacy—'which affect the courses of

action they choose to pursue, how much effort they put forth in a given endeavour, how long they persevere in the face of obstacles an failure experiences, how much anxiety and depression they experience in coping with stressors' [73].

In a study of 61 patients over 60 years of age with OA from a rheumatology practice, the majority viewed their OA as 'a fairly serious condition that is painful, chronic, and incurable but susceptible to control though one or more of the aspects of treatment recommended by their health-care practitioner' [74]. Negative emotional responses are mentioned [13]. Elderly people above 70 years of age with knee or hip OA regarded their OA more often as a natural part of growing old, than patients aged between 50 to 59 years [75]. However, illness perceptions vary considerably between individuals with OA. Especially the beliefs about the nature of OA and its symptoms (report of experience of number of common symptoms and belief these symptoms associate to their OA), and about the consequences of their OA, were associated with health outcome, such as poorer disability [76,77], worse pain [78], poorer quality of life [74], utilization of medical services [74,78], and negative mood [74,79]; these illness perceptions were also associated with more passive coping and negative mood in a longitudinal study in 82 elderly from the community [80]. Furthermore, the perceived duration of OA by patients as chronic was associated with pain [78] and disability [77], and negative emotional representations were associated with disability [77] and healthcare use [78] in cross-sectional studies. In a longitudinal study in 241 OA patients, illness perceptions about OA changed. They perceived their OA as more chronic and less controllable, believed to have better understanding of their disease and experienced less negative emotions due to OA after 6 years [81]. Patients identified as sharing a similar profile of negative changes in illness perceptions had significantly worse functioning, independent of measures of OA severity [82].

In a systematic review of longitudinal studies there was strong evidence that higher levels of self-efficacy predict reduced levels of disability at follow-up [76]. In 480 community-dwelling elderly with knee pain, the level of certainty that a patient could complete and repeat a stair climb task (self-efficacy) was associated with the stair climb task and with self-reported disability after 30 months, after adjustment for demographics and disease variables [83]. Self-efficacy as protective factor for disability after 3 years was confirmed in 257 community-acquired knee OA patients [84]. Several cross-sectional studies support these findings [85–87]. Self-efficacy is also associated with pain [85,88].

Coping strategies

In a model by Lazarus and Folkman, the role of cognitive and behavioural coping strategies in the psychological adjustment to disease is described from the perspective of emotional stressors, such as pain. Coping strategies that focus on problems or on emotions are discriminated [80,89].

A wide variety of coping strategies are used by patients with OA [13]. In 4719 patients with knee or hip OA with a mean age of 67 years consulting primary care, both active pain coping strategies, being pain transformation, distraction, and reducing demands, and passive coping strategies, retreating, worrying, and resting, were used [90]. Coping strategy scores were higher in patients with both knee and hip involvement than for patients with OA at one site, and in women compared with men.

Several studies have investigated the association between coping strategies and mood or depression, showing different results [76,80,91–93]. The use of the passive coping strategies, worrying and resting, was correlated with more severe impairment; lower correlations were observed with pain intensity [90]. The number of longitudinal studies in patients with OA investigating coping strategies and pain and function outcomes is scarce. In a longitudinal study in 926 patients with knee and hip complaints, the passive coping strategy of worrying was associated with less disability in patients with knee pain after 2 years, while no associations of coping strategies with disability in patients with hip pain was seen [94]. In general it is assumed that passive coping strategies, such as catastrophizing and worrying, and resting and guarding, are maladaptive and associated with more pain or worse function [80,87,90,95–97]. In a longitudinal sub-study in 797 patients from the Osteoarthritis Initiative with knee OA, 22.5% and 7.3% of variance in change in pain and function after 1-year of follow-up could be explained by coping strategies. The coping strategies praying/hoping, pain catastrophizing, and increased behavioural activities were prognostic for pain outcome and praying/hoping and ignoring pain were prognostic for function outcome [98].

Depression and anxiety

The prevalence of depression among elderly people with OA is high. Nineteen per cent of 1021 patients diagnosed in general practice with knee and hip had at least a moderately severe depression [99]. In another large cohort of patients with symptomatic knee or hip OA, over 21% had a depressed mood [49]. Many studies in patients with OA have been performed to understand which factors contribute to depression, and these have shown that a variety of factors, including age, female sex, pain, physical disability, fatigue, co-morbidities, stressful life events, and lack of social support and contacts, are associated with depression [46,99–103]. Longitudinal studies have been performed to understand how pain, physical disability, and depression are linked in symptomatic knee and hip OA [100,101]. In 184 community-dwelling adults 55 years of age and older, physical symptoms were associated with participation after 18 months, which was partially mediated by activity limitations and depressive symptoms. In another study in 529 patients with painful knee and hip OA, pain had its effect on depressed mood after 2 years through its effect on disability and fatigue, which in turn led to worsening of pain and disability.

Since depression, chronic pain, and disability in OA are so linked to each other, meaning that patients with depression experience more chronic pain and disability, whereas patients with chronic pain and disability often experience a depression, these relationships could easily result in a vicious circle. As a result, concomitant depression in OA aggravates the burden of OA and has been shown to increase health service utilization [104].

The effect of multi-morbidities on symptoms

Many patients in the elderly population, especially women with lower social economic status, seem to suffer from multi-morbidity [105]. The most common multi-morbidity pattern consists of OA with cardiometabolic disorders [105]. Co-morbidities, including also obesity and low back pain, have unfavourable effects on symptoms, such as pain or disability, in patients with OA [106–109]. However, rheumatic and cardiovascular co-morbidities do not seem to have a more than additive effect on outcomes as sick leave or work disability in workers [110]. OA as a co-morbid condition in patients with cardiovascular disease seems to be associated with poor outcome, such as chest pain or shortness of breath; although the size of its effect is not clear, but seems to be less than additive [111–113].

Joint-specific symptoms and clinical signs

OA can affect any joint in the body, and is especially prevalent in the hands, knees, hips, facet joints, and big toes. Many symptoms or signs are joint specific (see Table 15.1), such as bony enlargements, malalignment and deformity, decreased range of motion, and decreased performance, the presence of soft tissue swelling with or without effusion or warmth.

Knee osteoarthritis

Within the knee, the patellofemoral, medial, and lateral tibiofemoral compartments can be distinguished. Most studies address the tibiofemoral joint or knee joint as a whole. However, OA in the patellofemoral compartment can occur in isolation [114,115]. Knee OA often co-occur with OA in the contralateral joint or with hand OA.

Knee pain and disability

Knee pain in early OA is experienced during activities, as walking, stair climbing, and bending. In more advanced stages, knee OA is also experienced at rest. Patients with knee OA experience limitations in function, such as in getting out of a chair, ascending and descending stairs, walking, kneeling, or squatting [7]. These symptoms and signs can be the result of OA in the different compartments of the knee; both isolated tibiofemoral and patellofemoral OA are associated with pain and decreased function. However, symptoms and signs do not seem to be specific for patellofemoral or tibiofemoral OA. In a population-based study in 745 adults 50 years of age or older with knee pain, it was not possible to make a diagnosis of isolated patellofemoral OA, isolated tibiofemoral, or combined patellofemoral/tibiofemoral OA, despite the assessment of a large number of symptoms and signs [114]. Also in a recent study in patients with knee pain, commonly used questions, such as anterior knee pain, pain with stairs, or walking on level ground could not distinguish patients with isolated patellofemoral or tibiofemoral OA [116].

Patterns and localization of knee pain in OA are rather unclear. A knee pain map was developed to assess knee pain in more detail [117]. A study using the interviewer-administered knee pain map showed that in most painful knees with OA or at risk for OA, the pain is localized (pointed out by one or two fingers), especially at the medial joint line, patella, or lateral joint line; regional or diffuse knee pain is less frequent [117]. Especially regional knee pain is reported by women, diffuse knee pain by people with a higher body mass index (BMI), and localized knee pain by younger individuals [118].

Crepitus

Crepitus in the knee is an audible grinding noise or palpable vibration in the knee that is detected by the hand of the examiner on the knee of the patient. Crepitus can be assessed during active motion of the knee (i.e. with weight bearing, such as squatting) or during passive flexion/extension of the knee. Crepitus on active motion of the knee is one of the clinical signs required to classify knee OA [39]. Crepitus can be assessed specifically for different compartments of the knee, being the patella, medial and lateral tibiofemoral joints, or as general crepitus [119]. The reliability to assess crepitus differs considerably between studies [119–122]. In a study by Cibere and colleagues investigating the reliability of different forms of crepitus, general passive crepitus was most reliable [119].

Crepitus on active motion assessed with the hand of the examiner on the patella was present in 44.2% of 891 participants aged 45 years or older from the community [123]. Crepitus seems especially associated with patellofemoral OA, although its value to diagnose patellofemoral OA is unclear [114,123].

Bony enlargement, decreased range of motion, and fixed flexion deformity

Bony enlargement and decreased range of motion (restricted movement), together with crepitus, are among the most useful signs to diagnose knee OA [39,124]. Bony enlargement can be palpated at the joint line during physical examination. It can be assessed fairly reliable [119]. The underlying origin for bony enlargement is not so clear, since it has been scarcely investigated. In a recent study comparing physical examination with structural abnormalities on radiographs or MRI, no associations with bony enlargements were found [125].

Knee flexion in knee OA is decreased. In a community-dwelling elderly population, restricted knee flexion was associated with knee pain, female sex, and BMI [126]. In a cohort of patients with early symptomatic knee OA impaired knee flexion was associated with severe pain on knee flexion, bony enlargement, medial tibiofemoral osteophytes, crepitus, and BMI [127]. Range of motion can be assessed by a goniometer. In more advanced stages of knee OA, a flexion contracture or fixed knee flexion deformity can be found; the knee cannot fully extent to 0° which results in a leg length difference. Fixed flexion deformity will affect muscle function and gait. A flexion contracture can be reliably assessed [119].

Malalignment

Alignment of the knee is defined by the line from hip (mid femoral head) to (mid) ankle. Varus alignment is represented by a line that passes medial to the knee, whereas valgus alignment is represented by a line lateral of the knee. Both varus and valgus malalignment are prevalent signs. In a population-based study in elderly patients, radiographic varus and valgus alignment was observed in 26% and 36% of knees, respectively [128]. Alignment is an important biomechanical factor of loading; a shift from a neutral alignment disturbs the load distribution of the knee.

Static alignment is seldom measured clinically, although it has been shown that alignment can be measured by a goniometer, at inspection or by condylar distance in a reliable way [119]. Usually, it is assessed on radiographs, preferably on full-limb radiographs, but alternatively on AP radiographs.

Longitudinal studies have shown that radiographically defined malalignment is associated with development and progression of knee OA [128,129]. Varus malalignment in particular plays an unfavourable role in overweight and obese people.

Instability

Instability of the knee is the sudden loss of postural support across the knee at the time of weight bearing and this experience by patients is assessed by their self-report of 'giving way, buckling or shifting of their knee' [130]. In the community it is reported by 10% of the adults, especially in those with radiographic signs of knee OA, knee pain, or decreased quadriceps strength [130]. In patients with knee OA, the prevalence is higher and reported by the majority [131,132]. Knee instability contributes to decreased physical function [130–132].

Effusion and warmth

Effusion and warmth can be found during physical examination, and are thought to reflect inflammation or a 'flare' in the OA knee joint [133]. During a 'flare' these signs are often accompanied by increases in pain and morning stiffness. In a European study of 600 patients with painful knee OA, 34% had joint effusion during physical examination [134]. Studies investigating the reliability to assess effusion and soft tissue swelling during physical exam are variable: some report moderate reliability between observers [122,135], whereas others show good reliability [119]. Effusion assessed during physical exam is associated with effusion assessed with ultrasonography [134]. Warmth is less well studied and appears less reliable [119,122].

Gait, varus thrust, and muscle function

OA in the knee results in alterations in gait. Walking speed is decreased and limping occurs. For detailed gait analysis, a three-dimensional quantitative kinematic or kinetic analysis can be done, although currently their value is not clear [136]. In some patients, during gait or stance phase a worsening (or onset) of varus malalignment occurs, with an increase of load across the medial tibiofemoral joint. During lift off and swing phase the varus malalignment improves (back to neutral). This phenomenon is called varus thrust. Varus thrust can be observed visually during walking and is associated with knee progression [137].

Knee joint mobility also depends on muscle function, especially of the quadriceps muscle [138].

Quadriceps muscle weakness is frequently observed in knee OA and associated with pain and disability. However, quadriceps strength assessment cannot be done during physical examination but requires special equipment, such as a dynamometer. Muscle atrophy is less well studied, but can be present and is suggested to be assessed in a reliable manner [119].

Questionnaires and performance tests

To measure knee pain or physical function in knee OA many questionnaires are available, some more used than others (for review see [56,58]). The most widely used are the KOOS (freely available at http://www.koos.nu [61,139]) and the subscales of the WOMAC [43].

Multiple single- and multi-activity measures exist to assess actual physical function in patients with knee OA. However, not all these tests have been evaluated sufficiently for their metric properties. In a systematic review summarizing performance-based tests for evaluation of patients with either knee or hip OA, best evidence was found for the 40-metre self-paced walk test, the 30-second chair–stand test, and the Timed Up and Go test [140]. The best-rated multi-activity measures were the Stratford Battery, Physical

Activity Restrictions, and the Functional Assessment System [140]. The recommended minimal set by OARSI includes the 30-second chair–stand test, 40-metre fast-paced walk test, and a stair-climb test [141].

Hip osteoarthritis

Hip OA is a relatively frequent subtype of OA that is often bilateral; it can co-occur with OA in the knee, but its co-occurrence with hand OA is more prevalent.

Hip pain and disability

Hip OA can result in pain at rest and on movement in the hip region and can have an intermittent or constant character, as described above. However, due to its deep location and the presence of many extra-articular structures in the pelvic and inguinal region as potential causes of pain, it can be difficult to distinguish intra-articular pain that results from OA in the hip joint. Pain in the groin and thigh region is generally considered as associated with hip OA [142–145]. Pain in the knee or lower leg, and in the buttock [144,146], can also be the result of hip OA—referred pain— although alternative explanations, such as lumbosacral spondylosis [147] or knee OA, have to be considered.

Specific symptoms and signs of functional disability due to hip OA are limitations, such as with joint mobility (limping), walking, stair climbing, bending to floor, and putting on socks [7].

Decreased range of motion, muscle weakness, and deformity

Hip OA results in imitations in all movements of the hip joint [142,148]; limitations in internal rotation and flexion are used to classify OA [149]. Active or passive movement of the hip joint may be painful [40]. Hip movement in healthy elderly patients depends on sex, BMI, and ethnicity [126], and also varies between individuals. Therefore comparison of left to right in a patient is helpful to assess decreased range of motion. Range of motion can be assessed with a two-arm goniometer. Reliability of the measurement of range of motion differs between studies [119,150–152]; internal rotation and flexion are considered as the most reliable measures. Deformities in end-stage hip OA result in fixed flexion with exorotation, accompanied by a shortening of the affected extremity.

Decreased muscle strength, as assessed by a dynamometer, of the affected extremity is seen in hip OA, also with muscle atrophy. Knee and hip extensors and flexors especially are involved and to a lesser extent hip adductors and abductors [153]. In severe hip OA a positive Trendelenburg sign can be seen.

Both decreased range of motion and muscle weakness add to disability in hip OA.

Questionnaires and performance tests

To measure hip pain and physical function in OA many questionnaires are available, some more used than others (for review see [59]). The most widely used for hip OA are the Hip Injury Osteoarthritis Outcome Score-short form (HOOS-PS) (freely available at http://www.koos.nu [61,139]) and the subscales of the WOMAC [43].

The recommended performance-based tests to evaluate actual physical function in patients with hip OA are similar to those recommended to evaluate knee OA [140,141].

Hand osteoarthritis

In general, hand OA is a polyarticular disease, which affects distal interphalangeal joints (DIPJs) most frequently, less frequently first carpometacarpal joints (CMCJs) and proximal interphalangeal joints (PIPJs), and the least frequently metacarpophalangeal (MCPJs) [154,155,156,157]. OA in the wrist is rarely seen. The involvement follows a specific pattern: clustering is seen primarily symmetrically and by row (DIPJ, PIPJs, MCPJs), and to a lesser extent by ray [155] OA in the thumb base, the first CMCJ with or without scaphotrapezoid joint OA, can co-occur with other joints in the first ray: the first interphalangeal joint (IPJ), first MCPJ, first CMCJ and scaphotrapezoid joint [158], or with OA at other sites in the hand [159,160].

Hand pain and disability

Important symptoms in hand OA are hand pain and decrease in physical function, affecting daily activities such as writing, carrying, household activities, and handling small objects. The severity of these symptoms differs between subsets of hand OA. In community-based studies, people with erosive OA had more pain [161,162] and more hand disability [162] than people with non-erosive radiographic hand OA. Patients with erosive OA also experience worse hand mobility and less satisfaction with hand function and aesthetics than those with non-erosive hand OA. Both erosions and nodes seem to contribute to this high clinical burden [163].

The contribution of thumb base OA to hand pain and disability is controversial. Patients, from both primary and secondary care, with combined finger and thumb base OA report most pain and disability [158,164]. Moreover, hand pain and reduced grip strength were especially associated with radiographic thumb base OA, when compared with OA in other hand joint groups [154,165]. However, in a study comparing functional disability and grip strength in patients with clinical hand OA who had more symptomatic thumb base OA (67 patients) or more symptomatic IPJ OA (49 patients), no differences were shown between the two patient groups [166]. In contrast, in a study of 308 patients with symptomatic hand OA, which took into account the co-occurrence of IPJ and first CMC OA and the number of joints involved, presence of first CMCJ OA contributes more to pain and disability than IPJ OA [164].

Nodes and deformities

Bony enlargements and/or nodes and deformities (e.g. see Figure 15.1), being lateral deviation of IPJs or subluxation and adduction of the first CMCJs, are typical clinical hallmarks of hand OA [167,168]. These signs occur with or without symptoms. Nodes have been associated with underlying structural abnormalities, such as osteophytes on radiographs [169,170,171]. Several hypotheses about their formation in hand OA are available [169], such as the notion that these nodes are traction spurs, which can fuse with osteophytes. Bony enlargements in DIPJs and PIPJs—Heberden's and Bouchard's nodes, respectively—can be reliably assessed during physical examination [172].

Hand strength, mobility, and joint swelling

In hand OA, hand strength, as assessed by grip strength or pinch grip strength, and hand mobility are decreased [31,44,173–175]. Also clinical signs of synovitis can be found in hand OA, especially in erosive or inflammatory hand OA, with soft tissue swelling and overlying redness accompanied by pain [176,177].

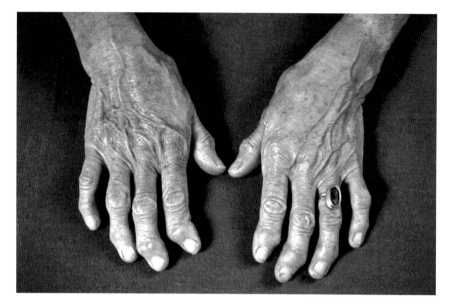

Figure 15.1 Nodes or bony enlargements with deformities in hand osteoarthritis.

Diagnostic and performance tests

To diagnose thumb base OA, the grind test (compressing the joint axially whilst rotating the thumb) was suggested; the reliability for confirming or excluding the diagnosis was moderate (specificity 80%, sensitivity 53%) [178].

To assess hand pain or physical function in hand OA several questionnaires are available (for review see [56,58]). The most widely used for hand pain is the AUSCAN pain subscale [44] and for function the Functional Index for Hand OA (FIHOA) [179] and the AUSCAN function subscale [44].

Multiple tests exist to assess the performance of the hands in patients with OA, such as the Grip Ability Test, Moberg Pickup Test, Arthritis Hand Function Test, and the Jebsen–Taylor Hand Function Test. The metric properties of these tests are not extensively tested in patients with hand OA [58].

Facet joint osteoarthritis

OA in the synovial facet joints is associated with other degenerative processes in the spine, being degeneration of the disc and formation of vertebral osteophytes (for review see [180,181]). Degenerative abnormalities in the spine are highly prevalent and especially seen in the cervical and lumbar region.

Low back pain and neck pain

Low back pain and neck pain are highly prevalent with high impact, as evidenced by their position in the top ten of causes of living with disability in the Global Burden of Disease Study 2010 [37]. Low back pain and neck pain are complex disorders, and can be the result of many causes, such as muscular and ligamental disorders, malignancies, vertebral fractures, inflammatory disorders as spondyloarthropathies, spinal infections, and degenerative disorders. In a recent systematic review with meta-analysis, radiographic disc degeneration and to a lesser extent radiographic vertebral osteophytes were shown to be associated with low back pain [182]. However, in the same review no association with radiographic

facet joint OA was seen. Epidemiological studies using computed tomography scanning, which is better suited to visualize facet joint OA, in the community, had equivocal results [183,184]. However, facet joints are well innervated and studies using irritating injections in the facet joints of normal volunteers and injections with anaesthetics to block pain in patients with painful facet joint OA, suggest that facet joint OA is associated with pain in the neck or lower back with some degree of radiation into the upper or lower limbs [180].

Osteophytes and deformities at the facet joint can cause impingement of spinal nerve roots, which can result in radicular pain or neurogenic claudication. Pain resulting from neurogenic claudication is especially seen with walking or extending of the back and relieved by bending of the waist, such as during bicycling.

Diagnostic tests

No examinations or tests are available that are specific predictors for pain due to facet joint OA [185], although experts have proposed several indicators of low back pain due to facet joint OA [186]. However, several of the suggested indicators require injections and can therefore not be easily performed; moreover these indicators have to be validated.

Shoulder and elbow osteoarthritis

OA in the shoulder can affect the acromioclavicular and glenohumeral joints especially in the elderly and lead to self-reported shoulder pain (in acromioclavicular OA superiorly) and joint tenderness on palpation. Glenohumeral OA is associated with crepitus, decreased range of motion (flexion and external rotation) [187], and altered scapulohumeral rhythm [188]. Shoulder pain is associated with decreased range of motion [187,189]. In acromioclavicular OA, pain can be elicited by the cross-body adduction test.

OA in the elbow joint—humeroulnar, humeroradial, or radioulnar—is rare, and especially seen in middle-aged men. In the literature, case series of patients with elbow OA are presented, mostly to evaluate surgical procedures [17–19]. Patients report pain on use, during motion or in full extension or flexion [17–19], and morning and inactivity stiffness [18]. In an early stage, loss of terminal extension develops, and later on, flexion and extension are further restricted; supination and pronation can be restricted as well [17–19]. Locking during movement [17] and crepitus can be experienced [18]. Clinical signs of synovitis can be seen [18]. In end stages, patients report paraesthesia in the small and ring fingers, indicative of irritation of the ulnar nerve or decreased sensibility and weakness due to ulnar neuropathy [17,19].

Ankle and foot osteoarthritis

OA in the foot is highly frequent and results in foot pain, aggravated by walking, and disability [14,190]. It preferentially affects the first metatarsophalangeal joints (MTPJ), often bilateral, and less frequently the other MTPJs, PIPJs, and midfoot; the latter often in conjunction with pes planes. Bony enlargements at the first MTPJ can be palpated accompanied by decreased range of motion (hallux rigidus). Hallux valgus (e.g. see Figure 15.2), an angulation of the big toe, is highly frequent and suggested to be a component of generalized OA [191,192]. Bony enlargements and malalignment can lead to a bunion or bursitis overlying the first MTPJ at the medial site due to pressure from shoes.

Ankle OA is rare and mostly secondary to trauma. Symptoms include pain, stiffness, and disability. Signs are gait abnormalities, limping, hindfoot malalignment (varus or valgus) [193,194], and decreased dorsal and plantar flexion and decreased inversion

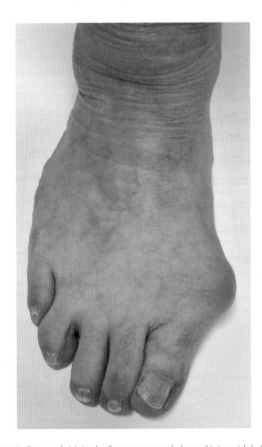

Figure 15.2 Osteoarthritis in the first metatarsophalangeal joint with hallux valgus.

Table 15.3 American College of Rheumatology classification criteria sets for knee osteoarthritis

Clinical and laboratory	Clinical and radiographic	Clinical
Knee pain +	Knee pain +	Knee pain +
At least 5 of 9:	At least 1 of 3:	At least 3 of 6:
◆ Age > 50 years	◆ Age > 50 years	◆ Age > 50 years
◆ Stiffness < 30 min	◆ Stiffness < 30 min	◆ Stiffness < 30 min
◆ Crepitus	◆ Crepitus	◆ Crepitus
◆ Bony tenderness	+ Osteophytes	◆ Bony tenderness
◆ Bony enlargement		◆ Bony enlargement
◆ No palpable warmth		◆ No palpable warmth
◆ ESR < 40 mm/hour		
◆ RF < 1:40		
◆ SF OA		

ESR, erythrocyte sedimentation rate; RF, rheumatoid factor; SF OA, synovial fluid signs of osteoarthritis (clear, viscous or white blood cell count < 2000/mm^3).

and eversion [194]. In addition, decreased standing balance [195] and lower muscle atrophy [196] are suggested. Finally, deviations in ankle joint alignment due to knee OA resulting in changed ankle mechanics can be seen [197].

Temporomandibular osteoarthritis

OA in the temporomandibular joint is part of the temporomandibular disorders. Reported symptoms are jaw pain during chewing or jaw opening and painful clicking. Furthermore coarse crepitus on opening or closing is observed with restricted jaw motion [198].

Value of symptoms and signs to diagnose or to classify osteoarthritis

OA is a clinical diagnosis. The European League Against Rheumatism (EULAR) evidence-based recommendations show that for diagnosing knee OA the symptoms of persistent knee pain, limited morning stiffness, reduced function, and the signs of crepitus, restricted movement, and bony enlargements are the most useful. Assuming a background prevalence of 12.5% of knee OA in adults aged 45 years or older, the estimated probability of having

Table 15.4 American College of Rheumatology classification criteria for hand osteoarthritis

Clinical
Pain, aching or stiffness +
3 of 4 of the following features:
◆ Hard tissue enlargements of 2 or more of 10 selected joints
◆ Hard tissue enlargements of 2 or more DIP joints
◆ Fewer than 3 swollen MCP joints
◆ Deformity of at least 1 of 10 selected joints

DIP, distal interphalangeal; MCP, metacarpal phalangeal.

Ten selected joints are bilateral second and third distal interphalangeal, second and third proximal interphalangeal and first carpometacarpal joints.

Table 15.5 American College of Rheumatology classification criteria sets for hip osteoarthritis

Clinical and laboratory	Clinical, laboratory and radiogaphic
Hip pain +	Hip pain +
◆ Hip internal rotation < 15°	at least 2 of the following 3 features:
◆ ESR ≤ 45 mm/hour (if not available, substitute hip flexion ≤ 115°)	◆ ESR < 20 mm
	◆ Radiographic femoral or acetabular osteophytes
OR	◆ Radiographic joint space narrowing (superior, axial and/or medial)
◆ Hip internal rotation ≥ 15°	
◆ Pain on hip internal rotation	
◆ Morning stiffness of the hip ≤ 60 min	
◆ Age > 50 years	

ESR, erythrocyte sedimentation rate.

radiographic knee OA increased with increasing number of positive features, to 99% when all six symptoms and signs were present [124]. Also for hand OA a composite of several symptoms and signs have to be available to make the diagnosis, as illustrated by the EULAR evidence-based recommendations [168]. Pain on usage, mild morning or inactivity stiffness, and bony nodes of DIPJs or PIPJs, have limited value as a single diagnostic marker. However, a composite of multiple symptoms and signs greatly increased the chance of the diagnosis [168]. The value of signs and symptoms is also reflected by their role in classifying OA. The presence of the symptoms 'pain', and to a lesser extent, 'stiffness' is crucial in the widely used classification criteria developed by the American College of Rheumatology (see Table 15.3). For classifying knee or hand OA the presence of specific symptoms or signs is even sufficient (see Tables 15.3 and 15.4) [39,199]. For classifying hip OA, additional laboratory or radiographic signs are required (see Table 15.5) [149].

Summary and conclusion

Patients with OA show a variety of general and joint-specific symptoms and signs enabling a correct diagnosis, often without the necessity for supporting radiographic or laboratory test results. However, signs and symptoms are not pathognomonic so differentiating OA from other musculoskeletal disorders can be a challenge. The reliability of the assessment of some signs is unclear or limited, requiring more research. Moreover, psychosocial factors, patients' perceptions about their illness, and their coping strategies are of importance for the symptoms and signs patients experience. They should be taken in account when making a diagnosis and optimizing treatment.

References

1. Gignac MA, Davis AM, Hawker G, et al. 'What do you expect? You're just getting older': A comparison of perceived osteoarthritis-related and aging-related health experiences in middle- and older-age adults. *Arthritis Rheum* 2006; 55(6):905–12.
2. Power JD, Badley EM, French MR, Wall AJ, Hawker GA. Fatigue in osteoarthritis: a qualitative study. *BMC Musculoskelet Disord* 2008; 9:63.
3. Tallon D, Chard J, Dieppe P. Exploring the priorities of patients with osteoarthritis of the knee. *Arthritis Care Res* 2000; 13(5):312–9.
4. Witteveen AG, Hofstad CJ, Breslau MJ, Blankevoort L, Kerkhoffs GM. The impact of ankle osteoarthritis. The difference of opinion between patient and orthopedic surgeon. *Foot Ankle Surg* 2014; 20(4):241–7.
5. Xie F, Li SC, Fong KY, et al. What health domains and items are important to patients with knee osteoarthritis? A focus group study in a multiethnic urban Asian population. *Osteoarthritis Cartilage* 2006; 14(3):224–30.
6. Xie F, Li SC, Thumboo J. Do health-related quality-of-life domains and items in knee and hip osteoarthritis vary in importance across social-cultural contexts? A qualitative systematic literature review. *Semin Arthritis Rheum* 2005; 34(6):793–804.
7. Bellamy N, Buchanan WW. A preliminary evaluation of the dimensionality and clinical importance of pain and disability in osteoarthritis of the hip and knee. *Clin Rheumatol* 1986; 5(2):231–41.
8. Cedraschi C, Delezay S, Marty M, et al. 'Let's talk about OA pain': a qualitative analysis of the perceptions of people suffering from OA. Towards the development of a specific pain OA-Related questionnaire, the Osteoarthritis Symptom Inventory Scale (OASIS). *PLoS One* 2013; 8(11): e79988.
9. Stamm T, van der Giesen F, Thorstensson C, et al. Patient perspective of hand osteoarthritis in relation to concepts covered by instruments measuring functioning: a qualitative European multicentre study. *Ann Rheum Dis* 2009; 68(9):1453–60.
10. Hawker GA, Stewart L, French MR, et al. Understanding the pain experience in hip and knee osteoarthritis—an OARSI/OMERACT initiative. *Osteoarthritis Cartilage* 2008; 16(4):415–22.
11. Gooberman-Hill R, Woolhead G, Mackichan F, et al. Assessing chronic joint pain: lessons from a focus group study. *Arthritis Rheum* 2007; 57(4):666–71.
12. Woolhead G, Gooberman-Hill R, Dieppe P, Hawker G. Night pain in hip and knee osteoarthritis: a focus group study. *Arthritis Care Res (Hoboken)* 2010; 62(7):944–9.
13. Hill S, Dziedzic KS, Ong BN. The functional and psychological impact of hand osteoarthritis. *Chronic Illn* 2010; 6(2):101–10.
14. Thomas MJ, Moore A, Roddy E, Peat G. 'Somebody to say "come on we can sort this"': a qualitative study of primary care consultation among older adults with symptomatic foot osteoarthritis. *Arthritis Care Res (Hoboken)* 2013; 65(12):2051–5.
15. Carmona L, Ballina J, Gabriel R, Laffon A. The burden of musculoskeletal diseases in the general population of Spain: results from a national survey. *Ann Rheum Dis* 2001; 60(11):1040–5.
16. Slatkowsky-Christensen B, Mowinckel P, Loge JH, Kvien TK. Health-related quality of life in women with symptomatic hand osteoarthritis: a comparison with rheumatoid arthritis patients, healthy controls, and normative data. *Arthritis Rheum* 2007; 57(8):1404–9.
17. Antuna SA, Morrey BF, Adams RA, O'Driscoll SW. Ulnohumeral arthroplasty for primary degenerative arthritis of the elbow: long-term outcome and complications. *J Bone Joint Surg Am* 2002; 84-A(12):2168–73.
18. Doherty M, Preston B. Primary osteoarthritis of the elbow. *Ann Rheum Dis* 1989; 48(9):743–7.
19. Wada T, Isogai S, Ishii S, Yamashita T. Debridement arthroplasty for primary osteoarthritis of the elbow. *J Bone Joint Surg Am* 2004; 86-A(2):233–41.
20. Bellamy N, Sothern RB, Campbell J. Rhythmic variations in pain perception in osteoarthritis of the knee. *J Rheumatol* 1990; 17(3):364–72.
21. Bellamy N, Sothern RB, Campbell J, Buchanan WW. Rhythmic variations in pain, stiffness, and manual dexterity in hand osteoarthritis. *Ann Rheum Dis* 2002; 61(12):1075–80.
22. Allen KD, Coffman CJ, Golightly YM, Stechuchak KM, Keefe FJ. Daily pain variations among patients with hand, hip, and knee osteoarthritis. *Osteoarthritis Cartilage* 2009; 17(10):1275–82.
23. Focht BC, Ewing V, Gauvin L, Rejeski WJ. The unique and transient impact of acute exercise on pain perception in older, overweight,

or obese adults with knee osteoarthritis. *Ann Behav Med* 2002; 24(3):201–10.

24. Kortekaas MC, Kwok WY, Reijnierse M, et al. Pain in hand osteoarthritis is associated with inflammation: the value of ultrasound. *Ann Rheum Dis* 2010; 69(7):1367–9.

25. Yusuf E, Kortekaas MC, Watt I, Huizinga TW, Kloppenburg M. Do knee abnormalities visualised on MRI explain knee pain in knee osteoarthritis? A systematic review. *Ann Rheum Dis* 2011; 70(1):60–7.

26. Kortekaas MC, Kwok WY, Reijnierse M, Huizinga TW, Kloppenburg M. Osteophytes and joint space narrowing are independently associated with pain in finger joints in hand osteoarthritis. *Ann Rheum Dis* 2011; 70(10):1835–7.

27. Neogi T, Felson D, Niu J, et al. Association between radiographic features of knee osteoarthritis and pain: results from two cohort studies. *BMJ* 2009; 339): b2844.

28. Phillips K, Clauw DJ. Central pain mechanisms in the rheumatic diseases: future directions. *Arthritis Rheum* 2013; 65(2):291–302.

29. Thakur M, Dawes JM, McMahon SB. Genomics of pain in osteoarthritis. *Osteoarthritis Cartilage* 2013; 21(9):1374–82.

30. Zhai G, Stankovich J, Ding C, et al. The genetic contribution to muscle strength, knee pain, cartilage volume, bone size, and radiographic osteoarthritis: a sibpair study. *Arthritis Rheum* 2004; 50(3):805–10.

31. Bellamy N, Campbell J, Haraoui B, et al. Dimensionality and clinical importance of pain and disability in hand osteoarthritis: Development of the Australian/Canadian (AUSCAN) Osteoarthritis Hand Index. *Osteoarthritis Cartilage* 2002; 10(11):855–62.

32. Bellamy N, Sothern RB, Campbell J, Buchanan WW. Rhythmic variations in pain, stiffness, and manual dexterity in hand osteoarthritis. *Ann Rheum Dis* 2002; 61(12):1075–80.

33. Berenbaum F. Osteoarthritis: when chondrocytes don't wake up on time. *Arthritis Rheum* 2013; 65(9):2233–5.

34. Dreinhofer K, Stucki G, Ewert T, et al. ICF Core Sets for osteoarthritis. *J Rehabil Med* 2004; (44 Suppl):75–80.

35. Oberhauser C, Escorpizo R, Boonen A, Stucki G, Cieza A. Statistical validation of the brief International Classification of Functioning, Disability and Health Core Set for osteoarthritis based on a large international sample of patients with osteoarthritis. *Arthritis Care Res (Hoboken)* 2013; 65(2):177–86.

36. Xie F, Thumboo J, Fong KY, et al. Are they relevant? A critical evaluation of the international classification of functioning, disability, and health core sets for osteoarthritis from the perspective of patients with knee osteoarthritis in Singapore. *Ann Rheum Dis* 2006; 65(8):1067–73.

37. Vos T, Flaxman AD, Naghavi M, et al. Years lived with disability (YLDs) for 1160 sequelae of 289 diseases and injuries 1990-2010: a systematic analysis for the Global Burden of Disease Study 2010. *Lancet* 2012; 380(9859):2163–96.

38. Hoy DG, Smith E, Cross M, et al. Reflecting on the global burden of musculoskeletal conditions: lessons learnt from the global burden of disease 2010 study and the next steps forward. *Ann Rheum Dis* 2015; 74(1):4–7.

39. Altman R, Asch E, Bloch D, et al. Development of criteria for the classification and reporting of osteoarthritis. Classification of osteoarthritis of the knee. Diagnostic and Therapeutic Criteria Committee of the American Rheumatism Association. *Arthritis Rheum* 1986; 29(8):1039–49.

40. Doyle DV, Dieppe PA, Scott J, Huskisson EC. An articular index for the assessment of osteoarthritis. *Ann Rheum Dis* 1981; 40(1):75–8.

41. Ritchie DM, Boyle JA, McInnes JM, et al. Clinical studies with an articular index for the assessment of joint tenderness in patients with rheumatoid arthritis. *Q J Med* 1968; 37(147):393–406.

42. Bijsterbosch J, Wassenaar MJ, le Cessie S, et al. Doyle Index is a valuable additional pain measure in osteoarthritis. *Osteoarthritis Cartilage* 2010; 18(8):1046–50.

43. Bellamy N, Buchanan WW, Goldsmith CH, Campbell J, Stitt LW. Validation study of WOMAC: a health status instrument for measuring clinically important patient relevant outcomes to antirheumatic drug therapy in patients with osteoarthritis of the hip or knee. *J Rheumatol* 1988; 15(12):1833–40.

44. Bellamy N, Campbell J, Haraoui B, et al. Clinimetric properties of the AUSCAN Osteoarthritis Hand Index: an evaluation of reliability, validity and responsiveness. *Osteoarthritis Cartilage* 2002; 10(11):863–9.

45. Snijders GF, van den Ende CH, Fransen J, et al. Fatigue in knee and hip osteoarthritis: the role of pain and physical function. *Rheumatology (Oxford)* 2011; 50(10):1894–900.

46. Wolfe F, Hawley DJ, Wilson K. The prevalence and meaning of fatigue in rheumatic disease. *J Rheumatol* 1996; 23(8):1407–17.

47. Stebbings S, Herbison P, Doyle TC, Treharne GJ, Highton J. A comparison of fatigue correlates in rheumatoid arthritis and osteoarthritis: disparity in associations with disability, anxiety and sleep disturbance. *Rheumatology (Oxford)* 2010; 49(2):361–7.

48. Wolfe F. Determinants of WOMAC function, pain and stiffness scores: evidence for the role of low back pain, symptom counts, fatigue and depression in osteoarthritis, rheumatoid arthritis and fibromyalgia. *Rheumatology (Oxford)* 1999; 38(4):355–61.

49. Sale JE, Gignac M, Hawker G. The relationship between disease symptoms, life events, coping and treatment, and depression among older adults with osteoarthritis. *J Rheumatol* 2008; 35(2):335–42.

50. Murphy SL, Smith DM, Clauw DJ, Alexander NB. The impact of momentary pain and fatigue on physical activity in women with osteoarthritis. *Arthritis Rheum* 2008; 59(6):849–56.

51. Murphy SL, Alexander NB, Levoska M, Smith DM. Relationship between fatigue and subsequent physical activity among older adults with symptomatic osteoarthritis. *Arthritis Care Res (Hoboken)* 2013; 65(10):1617–24.

52. Chen CJ, McHugh G, Campbell M, Luker K. Subjective and objective sleep quality in individuals with osteoarthritis in Taiwan. *Musculoskeletal Care* 2015; 13(3):148–59.

53. Hawker GA, French MR, Waugh EJ, et al. The multidimensionality of sleep quality and its relationship to fatigue in older adults with painful osteoarthritis. *Osteoarthritis Cartilage* 2010; 18(11):1365–71.

54. Wilcox S, Brenes GA, Levine D, Sevick MA, Shumaker SA, Craven T. Factors related to sleep disturbance in older adults experiencing knee pain or knee pain with radiographic evidence of knee osteoarthritis. *J Am Geriatr Soc* 2000; 48(10):1241–51.

55. Sasaki E, Tsuda E, Yamamoto Y, et al. Nocturnal knee pain increases with the severity of knee osteoarthritis, disturbing patient sleep quality. *Arthritis Care Res (Hoboken)* 2014; 66(7):1027–32.

56. Collins NJ, Misra D, Felson DT, Crossley KM, Roos EM. Measures of knee function: International Knee Documentation Committee (IKDC) Subjective Knee Evaluation Form, Knee Injury and Osteoarthritis Outcome Score (KOOS), Knee Injury and Osteoarthritis Outcome Score Physical Function Short Form (KOOS-PS), Knee Outcome Survey Activities of Daily Living Scale (KOS-ADL), Lysholm Knee Scoring Scale, Oxford Knee Score (OKS), Western Ontario and McMaster Universities Osteoarthritis Index (WOMAC), Activity Rating Scale (ARS), and Tegner Activity Score (TAS). *Arthritis Care Res (Hoboken)* 2011; 63 Suppl 11: S208–28.

57. Hawker GA, Mian S, Kendzerska T, French M. Measures of adult pain: Visual Analog Scale for Pain (VAS Pain), Numeric Rating Scale for Pain (NRS Pain), McGill Pain Questionnaire (MPQ), Short-Form McGill Pain Questionnaire (SF-MPQ), Chronic Pain Grade Scale (CPGS), Short Form-36 Bodily Pain Scale (SF-36 BPS), and Measure of Intermittent and Constant Osteoarthritis Pain (ICOAP). *Arthritis Care Res (Hoboken)* 2011; 63 Suppl 11: S240–52.

58. Poole JL. Measures of hand function: Arthritis Hand Function Test (AHFT), Australian Canadian Osteoarthritis Hand Index (AUSCAN), Cochin Hand Function Scale, Functional Index for Hand Osteoarthritis (FIHOA), Grip Ability Test (GAT), Jebsen Hand Function Test (JHFT), and Michigan Hand Outcomes Questionnaire (MHQ). *Arthritis Care Res (Hoboken)* 2011; 63(Suppl 11): S189–99.

59. Nilsdotter A, Bremander A. Measures of hip function and symptoms: Harris Hip Score (HHS), Hip Disability and Osteoarthritis Outcome Score (HOOS), Oxford Hip Score (OHS), Lequesne

Index of Severity for Osteoarthritis of the Hip (LISOH), and American Academy of Orthopedic Surgeons (AAOS) Hip and Knee Questionnaire. *Arthritis Care Res (Hoboken)* 2011; 63 Suppl 11): S200-S207.

60. Maillefert JF, Kloppenburg M, Fernandes L, et al. Multi-language translation and cross-cultural adaptation of the OARSI/OMERACT measure of intermittent and constant osteoarthritis pain (ICOAP). *Osteoarthritis Cartilage* 2009; 17(10):1293–6.

61. Roos EM, Roos HP, Lohmander LS, Ekdahl C, Beynnon BD. Knee Injury and Osteoarthritis Outcome Score (KOOS)—development of a self-administered outcome measure. *J Orthop Sports Phys Ther* 1998; 28(2):88–96.

62. Tubach F, Ravaud P, Baron G, et al. Evaluation of clinically relevant states in patient reported outcomes in knee and hip osteoarthritis: the patient acceptable symptom state. *Ann Rheum Dis* 2005; 64(1):34–7.

63. Perrot S, Bertin P. 'Feeling better' or 'feeling well' in usual care of hip and knee osteoarthritis pain: determination of cutoff points for patient acceptable symptom state (PASS) and minimal clinically important improvement (MCII) at rest and on movement in a national multi-center cohort study of 2414 patients with painful osteoarthritis. *Pain* 2013; 154(2):248–56.

64. Tubach F, Ravaud P, Martin-Mola E, et al. Minimum clinically important improvement and patient acceptable symptom state in pain and function in rheumatoid arthritis, ankylosing spondylitis, chronic back pain, hand osteoarthritis, and hip and knee osteoarthritis: results from a prospective multinational study. *Arthritis Care Res (Hoboken)* 2012; 64(11):1699–707.

65. Claessens AA, Schouten JS, van den Ouweland FA, Valkenburg HA. Do clinical findings associate with radiographic osteoarthritis of the knee? *Ann Rheum Dis* 1990; 49(10):771–4.

66. Dahaghin S, Bierma-Zeinstra SM, Hazes JM, Koes BW. Clinical burden of radiographic hand osteoarthritis: a systematic appraisal. *Arthritis Rheum* 2006; 55(4):636–47.

67. Creamer P, Lethbridge-Cejku M, Costa P, et al. The relationship of anxiety and depression with self-reported knee pain in the community: data from the Baltimore Longitudinal Study of Aging. *Arthritis Care Res* 1999; 12(1):3–7.

68. Pimm TJ, Weinman J. Applying Leventhal's self regulation model to adaptation and intervention in rheumatic diseases. *Clin Psychol Psychother* 1998; 5:62–75.

69. Keefe FJ, Smith SJ, Buffington AL, et al. Recent advances and future directions in the biopsychosocial assessment and treatment of arthritis. *J Consult Clin Psychol* 2002; 70(3):640–55.

70. Leventhal H, Weinman J, Leventhal EA, Phillips LA. Health Psychology: the Search for Pathways between Behavior and Health. *Annu Rev Psychol* 2008; 59):477–505.

71. Hampson SE. Personal models and management of chronic illness: a comparison of diabetes and osteoarthritis. *Eur J Pers* 1997; 11:401–14.

72. Moss-Morris R, Weinman J, Petrie KJ, et al. The revised illness perception questionnaire (IPQ-R). *Psychol Health* 2002; 17(1):1–16.

73. Bandura A. Comments on the crusade against the causal efficacy of human thought. *J Behav Ther Exp Psychiatry* 1995; 26(3):179–90.

74. Hampson SE, Glasgow RE, Zeiss AM. Personal models of osteoarthritis and their relation to self-management activities and quality of life. *J Behav Med* 1994; 17(2):143–58.

75. Appelt CJ, Burant CJ, Siminoff LA, Kwoh CK, Ibrahim SA. Arthritis-specific health beliefs related to aging among older male patients with knee and/or hip osteoarthritis. *J Gerontol A Biol Sci Med Sci* 2007; 62(2):184–90.

76. Benyon K, Hill S, Zadurian N, Mallen C. Coping strategies and self-efficacy as predictors of outcome in osteoarthritis: a systematic review. *Musculoskeletal Care* 2010; 8(4):224–36.

77. Botha-Scheepers S, Riyazi N, Kroon HM, et al. Activity limitations in the lower extremities in patients with osteoarthritis: the modifying effects of illness perceptions and mental health. *Osteoarthritis Cartilage* 2006; 14(11):1104–10.

78. Hill S, Dziedzic K, Thomas E, Baker SR, Croft P. The illness perceptions associated with health and behavioural outcomes in people with musculoskeletal hand problems: findings from the North Staffordshire Osteoarthritis Project (NorStOP). *Rheumatology (Oxford)* 2007; 46(6):944–51.

79. Orbell S, Johnston M, Rowley D, Espley A, Davey P. Cognitive representations of illness and functional and affective adjustment following surgery for osteoarthritis. *Soc Sci Med* 1998; 47(1):93–102.

80. Hampson SE, Glasgow RE, Zeiss AM. Coping with osteoarthritis by older adults. *Arthritis Care Res* 1996; 9(2):133–41.

81. Bijsterbosch J, Scharloo M, Visser AW, et al. Illness perceptions in patients with osteoarthritis: change over time and association with disability. *Arthritis Rheum* 2009; 61(8):1054–61.

82. Kaptein AA, Bijsterbosch J, Scharloo M, et al. Using the common sense model of illness perceptions to examine osteoarthritis change: a 6-year longitudinal study. *Health Psychol* 2010; 29(1):56–64.

83. Rejeski WJ, Miller ME, Foy C, Messier S, Rapp S. Self-efficacy and the progression of functional limitations and self-reported disability in older adults with knee pain. *J Gerontol B Psychol Sci Soc Sci* 2001; 56(5): S261–5.

84. Sharma L, Cahue S, Song J, et al. Physical functioning over three years in knee osteoarthritis: role of psychosocial, local mechanical, and neuromuscular factors. *Arthritis Rheum* 2003; 48(12):3359–70.

85. Lorig K, Chastain RL, Ung E, Shoor S, Holman HR. Development and evaluation of a scale to measure perceived self-efficacy in people with arthritis. *Arthritis Rheum* 1989; 32(1):37–44.

86. Maly MR, Costigan PA, Olney SJ. Self-efficacy mediates walking performance in older adults with knee osteoarthritis. *J Gerontol A Biol Sci Med Sci* 2007; 62(10):1142–6.

87. McKnight PE, Afram A, Kashdan TB, Kasle S, Zautra A. Coping self-efficacy as a mediator between catastrophizing and physical functioning: treatment target selection in an osteoarthritis sample. *J Behav Med* 2010; 33(3):239–49.

88. Wright LJ, Zautra AJ, Going S. Adaptation to early knee osteoarthritis: the role of risk, resilience, and disease severity on pain and physical functioning. *Ann Behav Med* 2008; 36(1):70–80.

89. Folkman S, Lazarus RS. The relationship between coping and emotion: implications for theory and research. *Soc Sci Med* 1988; 26(3):309–17.

90. Perrot S, Poiraudeau S, Kabir M, et al. Active or passive pain coping strategies in hip and knee osteoarthritis? Results of a national survey of 4,719 patients in a primary care setting. *Arthritis Rheum* 2008; 59(11):1555–62.

91. Keefe FJ, Affleck G, France CR, et al. Gender differences in pain, coping, and mood in individuals having osteoarthritic knee pain: a within-day analysis. *Pain* 2004; 110(3):571–7.

92. Affleck G, Tennen H, Keefe FJ, et al. Everyday life with osteoarthritis or rheumatoid arthritis: independent effects of disease and gender on daily pain, mood, and coping. Pain 1999; 83(3):601–9.

93. Blalock SJ, Devellis BM, Giorgino KB. The relationship between coping and psychological well-being among people with osteoarthritis: a problem-specific approach. *Ann Behav Med* 1995; 17(2):107–15.

94. Holla JF, Steultjens MP, Roorda LD, et al. Prognostic factors for the two-year course of activity limitations in early osteoarthritis of the hip and/or knee. *Arthritis Care Res (Hoboken)* 2010; 62(10):1415–25.

95. Steultjens MP, Dekker J, Bijlsma JW. Coping, pain, and disability in osteoarthritis: a longitudinal study. *J Rheumatol* 2001; 28(5):1068–72.

96. Murphy SL, Kratz AL, Williams DA, Geisser ME. The association between symptoms, pain coping strategies, and physical activity among people with symptomatic knee and hip osteoarthritis. *Front Psychol* 2012; 3:326.

97. Somers TJ, Keefe FJ, Pells JJ, et al. Pain catastrophizing and pain-related fear in osteoarthritis patients: relationships to pain and disability. *J Pain Symptom Manage* 2009; 37(5):863–72.

98. Alschuler KN, Molton IR, Jensen MP, Riddle DL. Prognostic value of coping strategies in a community-based sample of persons with chronic symptomatic knee osteoarthritis. *Pain* 2013; 154(12):2775–81.

99. Rosemann T, Backenstrass M, Joest K, et al. Predictors of depression in a sample of 1,021 primary care patients with osteoarthritis. *Arthritis Rheum* 2007; 57(3):415–22.

100. Hawker GA, Gignac MA, Badley E, et al. A longitudinal study to explain the pain-depression link in older adults with osteoarthritis. *Arthritis Care Res (Hoboken)* 2011; 63(10):1382–90.

101. Machado GP, Gignac MA, Badley EM. Participation restrictions among older adults with osteoarthritis: a mediated model of physical symptoms, activity limitations, and depression. *Arthritis Rheum* 2008; 59(1):129–35.

102. McIlvane JM, Schiaffino KM, Paget SA. Age differences in the pain-depression link for women with osteoarthritis. Functional impairment and personal control as mediators. *Womens Health Issues* 2007; 17(1):44–51.

103. Skoldenberg OG, Salemyr MO, Boden HS, Ahl TE, Adolphson PY. The effect of weekly risedronate on periprosthetic bone resorption following total hip arthroplasty: a randomized, double-blind, placebo-controlled trial. *J Bone Joint Surg Am* 2011; 93(20):1857–64.

104. Rosemann T, Gensichen J, Sauer N, Laux G, Szecsenyi J. The impact of concomitant depression on quality of life and health service utilisation in patients with osteoarthritis. *Rheumatol Int* 2007; 27(9):859–63.

105. Violan C, Foguet-Boreu Q, Flores-Mateo G, et al. Prevalence, determinants and patterns of multimorbidity in primary care: a systematic review of observational studies. *PLoS One* 2014; 9(7):e102149.

106. Collins JE, Katz JN, Dervan EE, Losina E. Trajectories and risk profiles of pain in persons with radiographic, symptomatic knee osteoarthritis: data from the osteoarthritis initiative. *Osteoarthritis Cartilage* 2014; 22(5):622–30.

107. Geryk LL, Carpenter DM, Blalock SJ, DeVellis RF, Jordan JM. The impact of co-morbidity on health-related quality of life in rheumatoid arthritis and osteoarthritis patients. *Clin Exp Rheumatol* 2015; 33:366–74.

108. Weiss E. Knee osteoarthritis, body mass index and pain: data from the Osteoarthritis Initiative. *Rheumatology (Oxford)* 2014; 53(11):2095–9.

109. Wesseling J, Welsing PM, Bierma-Zeinstra SM, et al. Impact of self-reported comorbidity on physical and mental health status in early symptomatic osteoarthritis: the CHECK (Cohort Hip and Cohort Knee) study. *Rheumatology (Oxford)* 2013; 52(1):180–8.

110. van der Burg LR, Boonen A, van Amelsvoort LG, et al. Effects of cardiovascular comorbidities on work participation in rheumatic diseases: a prospective cohort study among working individuals. *Arthritis Care Res (Hoboken)* 2014; 66(1):157–63.

111. Hosseini K, Gaujoux-Viala C, Coste J, et al. Impact of co-morbidities on measuring indirect utility by the Medical Outcomes Study Short Form 6D in lower-limb osteoarthritis. Best Pract Res *Clin Rheumatol* 2012; 26(5):627–35.

112. Prior JA, Jordan KP, Kadam UT. Associations between cardiovascular disease severity, osteoarthritis co-morbidity and physical health: a population-based study. *Rheumatology (Oxford)* 2014; 53(10):1794–802.

113. Rushton CA, Kadam UT. Impact of non-cardiovascular disease comorbidity on cardiovascular disease symptom severity: a population-based study. *Int J Cardiol* 2014; 175(1):154–61.

114. Peat G, Duncan RC, Wood LR, Thomas E, Muller S. Clinical features of symptomatic patellofemoral joint osteoarthritis. *Arthritis Res Ther* 2012; 14(2): R63.

115. Stefanik JJ, Niu J, Gross KD, et al. Using magnetic resonance imaging to determine the compartmental prevalence of knee joint structural damage. *Osteoarthritis Cartilage* 2013; 21(5):695–9.

116. Stefanik JJ, Neogi T, Niu J, et al. The diagnostic performance of anterior knee pain and activity-related pain in identifying knees with structural damage in the patellofemoral joint: the Multicenter Osteoarthritis Study. *J Rheumatol* 2014; 41(8):1695–702.

117. Thompson LR, Boudreau R, Hannon MJ, et al. The knee pain map: reliability of a method to identify knee pain location and pattern. *Arthritis Rheum* 2009; 61(6):725–31.

118. Thompson LR, Boudreau R, Newman AB, et al. The association of osteoarthritis risk factors with localized, regional and diffuse knee pain. *Osteoarthritis Cartilage* 2010; 18(10):1244–9.

119. Cibere J, Bellamy N, Thorne A, et al. Reliability of the knee examination in osteoarthritis: effect of standardization. *Arthritis Rheum* 2004; 50(2):458–68.

120. Cushnaghan J, Cooper C, Dieppe P, et al. Clinical assessment of osteoarthritis of the knee. *Ann Rheum Dis* 1990; 49(10):768–70.

121. Hart DJ, Spector TD, Brown P, et al. Clinical signs of early osteoarthritis: reproducibility and relation to x ray changes in 541 women in the general population. *Ann Rheum Dis* 1991; 50(7):467–70.

122. Jones A, Hopkinson N, Pattrick M, Berman P, Doherty M. Evaluation of a method for clinically assessing osteoarthritis of the knee. *Ann Rheum Dis* 1992; 51(2):243–5.

123. Schiphof D, van MM, de Klerk BM, et al. Crepitus is a first indication of patellofemoral osteoarthritis (and not of tibiofemoral osteoarthritis). *Osteoarthritis Cartilage* 2014; 22(5):631–8.

124. Zhang W, Doherty M, Peat G, Bierma-Zeinstra MA, Arden NK, Bresnihan B, et al. EULAR evidence-based recommendations for the diagnosis of knee osteoarthritis. *Ann Rheum Dis* 2010; 69(3):483–9.

125. Knoop J, Dekker J, Klein JP, et al. Biomechanical factors and physical examination findings in osteoarthritis of the knee: associations with tissue abnormalities assessed by conventional radiography and high-resolution 3.0 Tesla magnetic resonance imaging. *Arthritis Res Ther* 2012; 14(5): R212.

126. Escalante A, Lichtenstein MJ, Dhanda R, Cornell JE, Hazuda HP. Determinants of hip and knee flexion range: results from the San Antonio Longitudinal Study of Aging. *Arthritis Care Res* 1999; 12(1):8–18.

127. Holla JF, Steultjens MP, van der Leeden M, et al. Determinants of range of joint motion in patients with early symptomatic osteoarthritis of the hip and/or knee: an exploratory study in the CHECK cohort. *Osteoarthritis Cartilage* 2011; 19(4):411–9.

128. Brouwer GM, van Tol AW, Bergink AP, et al. Association between valgus and varus alignment and the development and progression of radiographic osteoarthritis of the knee. *Arthritis Rheum* 2007; 56(4):1204–11.

129. Sharma L, Song J, Felson DT, et al. The role of knee alignment in disease progression and functional decline in knee osteoarthritis. *JAMA* 2001; 286(2):188–95.

130. Felson DT, Niu J, McClennan C, et al. Knee buckling: prevalence, risk factors, and associated limitations in function. *Ann Intern Med* 2007; 147(8):534–40.

131. Fitzgerald GK, Piva SR, Irrgang JJ. Reports of joint instability in knee osteoarthritis: its prevalence and relationship to physical function. *Arthritis Rheum* 2004; 51(6):941–6.

132. Knoop J, van der Leeden M, van der Esch M, Thorstensson CA, Gerritsen M, Voorneman RE, et al. Association of lower muscle strength with self-reported knee instability in osteoarthritis of the knee: results from the Amsterdam Osteoarthritis cohort. *Arthritis Care Res (Hoboken)* 2012; 64(1):38–45.

133. Baddour VT, Bradley JD. Clinical assessment and significance of inflammation in knee osteoarthritis. *Curr Rheumatol Rep* 1999; 1(1):59–63.

134. D'Agostino MA, Conaghan P, Le Bars M, et al. EULAR report on the use of ultrasonography in painful knee osteoarthritis. Part 1: prevalence of inflammation in osteoarthritis. *Ann Rheum Dis* 2005; 64(12):1703–9.

135. Hauzeur JP, Mathy L, De M, V. Comparison between clinical evaluation and ultrasonography in detecting hydrarthrosis of the knee. *J Rheumatol* 1999; 26(12):2681–3.

136. Ornetti P, Maillefert JF, Laroche D, et al. Gait analysis as a quantifiable outcome measure in hip or knee osteoarthritis: a systematic review. *Joint Bone Spine* 2010; 77(5):421–5.

137. Chang A, Hayes K, Dunlop D, et al. Thrust during ambulation and the progression of knee osteoarthritis. *Arthritis Rheum* 2004; 50(12):3897–903.

138. Bennell KL, Wrigley TV, Hunt MA, Lim BW, Hinman RS. Update on the role of muscle in the genesis and management of knee osteoarthritis. *Rheum Dis Clin North Am* 2013; 39(1):145–76.

139. Davis AM, Perruccio AV, Canizares M, et al. The development of a short measure of physical function for hip OA HOOS-Physical Function Shortform (HOOS-PS): an OARSI/OMERACT initiative. *Osteoarthritis Cartilage* 2008; 16(5):551–9.

140. Dobson F, Hinman RS, Hall M, et al. Measurement properties of performance-based measures to assess physical function in hip and knee osteoarthritis: a systematic review. *Osteoarthritis Cartilage* 2012; 20(12):1548–62.

141. Dobson F, Hinman RS, Roos EM, et al. OARSI recommended performance-based tests to assess physical function in people diagnosed with hip or knee osteoarthritis. *Osteoarthritis Cartilage* 2013; 21(8):1042–52.

142. Bierma-Zeinstra SM, Oster JD, Bernsen RM, et al. Joint space narrowing and relationship with symptoms and signs in adults consulting for hip pain in primary care. *J Rheumatol* 2002; 29(8):1713–8.

143. Birrell F, Croft P, Cooper C, et al. Radiographic change is common in new presenters in primary care with hip pain. PCR Hip Study Group. *Rheumatology (Oxford)* 2000; 39(7):772–5.

144. Khan AM, McLoughlin E, Giannakas K, Hutchinson C, Andrew JG. Hip osteoarthritis: where is the pain? *Ann R Coll Surg Engl* 2004; 86(2):119–21.

145. Sakamoto J, Morimoto Y, Ishii S, et al. Investigation and macroscopic anatomical study of referred pain in patients with hip disease. *J Phys Ther Sci* 2014; 26(2):203–8.

146. Hattori Y, Doi K, Sakamoto S, Hoshino S, Dodakundi C. Capsulectomy and debridement for primary osteoarthritis of the elbow through a medial trans-flexor approach. *J Hand Surg Am* 2011; 36(10):1652–8.

147. de Schepper EI, Damen J, Bos PK, et al. Disk degeneration of the upper lumbar disks is associated with hip pain. *Eur Spine J* 2013; 22(4):721–6.

148. Birrell F, Croft P, Cooper C, et al. Predicting radiographic hip osteoarthritis from range of movement. *Rheumatology (Oxford)* 2001; 40(5):506–12.

149. Altman R, Alarcon G, Appelrouth D, et al. The American College of Rheumatology criteria for the classification and reporting of osteoarthritis of the hip. *Arthritis Rheum* 1991; 34(5):505–14.

150. Croft PR, Nahit ES, Macfarlane GJ, Silman AJ. Interobserver reliability in measuring flexion, internal rotation, and external rotation of the hip using a plurimeter. *Ann Rheum Dis* 1996; 55(5):320–3.

151. Poulsen E, Christensen HW, Penny JO, et al. Reproducibility of range of motion and muscle strength measurements in patients with hip osteoarthritis—an inter-rater study. *BMC Musculoskelet Disord* 2012; 13):242.

152. Pua YH, Wrigley TV, Cowan SM, Bennell KL. Intrarater test-retest reliability of hip range of motion and hip muscle strength measurements in persons with hip osteoarthritis. *Arch Phys Med Rehabil* 2008; 89(6):1146–54.

153. Loureiro A, Mills PM, Barrett RS. Muscle weakness in hip osteoarthritis: a systematic review. *Arthritis Care Res (Hoboken)* 2013; 65(3):340–52.

154. Dahaghin S, Bierma-Zeinstra SM, Ginai AZ, et al. Prevalence and pattern of radiographic hand osteoarthritis and association with pain and disability (the Rotterdam study). *Ann Rheum Dis* 2005; 64(5):682–7.

155. Egger P, Cooper C, Hart DJ, et al. Patterns of joint involvement in osteoarthritis of the hand: the Chingford Study. *J Rheumatol* 1995; 22(8):1509–13.

156. Kalichman L, Li L, Batsevich V, Malkin I, Kobyliansky E. Prevalence, pattern and determinants of radiographic hand osteoarthritis in five Russian community-based samples. *Osteoarthritis Cartilage* 2010; 18(6):803–9.

157. Toba N, Sakai A, Aoyagi K, et al. Prevalence and involvement patterns of radiographic hand osteoarthritis in Japanese women: the Hizen-Oshima Study. *J Bone Miner Metab* 2006; 24(4):344–8.

158. Marshall M, van der Windt D, Nicholls E, et al. Radiographic hand osteoarthritis: patterns and associations with hand pain and function in a community-dwelling sample. *Osteoarthritis Cartilage* 2009; 17(11):1440–7.

159. Cooper C, Egger P, Coggon D, et al. Generalized osteoarthritis in women: pattern of joint involvement and approaches to definition for epidemiological studies. *J Rheumatol* 1996; 23(11):1938–42.

160. Marshall M, van der Windt D, Nicholls E, Myers H, Dziedzic K. Radiographic thumb osteoarthritis: frequency, patterns and associations with pain and clinical assessment findings in a community-dwelling population. *Rheumatology (Oxford)* 2011; 50(4):735–9.

161. Haugen IK, Englund M, Aliabadi P, et al. Prevalence, incidence and progression of hand osteoarthritis in the general population: the Framingham Osteoarthritis Study. *Ann Rheum Dis* 2011; 70(9):1581–6.

162. Kwok WY, Kloppenburg M, Rosendaal FR, et al. Erosive hand osteoarthritis: its prevalence and clinical impact in the general population and symptomatic hand osteoarthritis. *Ann Rheum Dis* 2011; 70(7):1238–42.

163. Bijsterbosch J, van Bemmel JM, Watt I, et al. Systemic and local factors are involved in the evolution of erosions in hand osteoarthritis. *Ann Rheum Dis* 2011; 70(2):326–30.

164. Bijsterbosch J, Visser W, Kroon HM, et al. Thumb base involvement in symptomatic hand osteoarthritis is associated with more pain and functional disability. *Ann Rheum Dis* 2010; 69(3):585–7.

165. Dominick KL, Jordan JM, Renner JB, Kraus VB. Relationship of radiographic and clinical variables to pinch and grip strength among individuals with osteoarthritis. *Arthritis Rheum* 2005; 52(5):1424–30.

166. Spacek E, Poiraudeau S, Fayad F, et al. Disability induced by hand osteoarthritis: are patients with more symptoms at digits 2-5 interphalangeal joints different from those with more symptoms at the base of the thumb? *Osteoarthritis Cartilage* 2004; 12(5):366–73.

167. Kloppenburg M, Kwok WY. Hand osteoarthritis—a heterogeneous disorder. *Nat Rev Rheumatol* 2012; 8(1):22–31.

168. Zhang W, Doherty M, Leeb BF, et al. EULAR evidence-based recommendations for the diagnosis of hand osteoarthritis: report of a task force of ESCISIT. *Ann Rheum Dis* 2009; 68(1):8–17.

169. Alexander CJ. Heberden's and Bouchard's nodes. *Ann Rheum Dis* 1999; 58(11):675–8.

170. Cicuttini FM, Baker J, Hart DJ, Spector TD. Relation between Heberden's nodes and distal interphalangeal joint osteophytes and their role as markers of generalised disease. *Ann Rheum Dis* 1998; 57(4):246–8.

171. Thaper A, Zhang W, Wright G, Doherty M. Relationship between Heberden's nodes and underlying radiographic changes of osteoarthritis. *Ann Rheum Dis* 2005; 64(8):1214–6.

172. Myers HL, Thomas E, Hay EM, Dziedzic KS. Hand assessment in older adults with musculoskeletal hand problems: a reliability study. *BMC Musculoskelet Disord* 2011; 12):3.

173. Allen KD, Jordan JM, Renner JB, Kraus VB. Relationship of global assessment of change to AUSCAN and pinch and grip strength among individuals with hand osteoarthritis. *Osteoarthritis Cartilage* 2006; 14(12):1281–7.

174. Jones G, Cooley HM, Bellamy N. A cross-sectional study of the association between Heberden's nodes, radiographic osteoarthritis of the hands, grip strength, disability and pain. *Osteoarthritis Cartilage* 2001; 9(7):606–11.

175. Kjeken I, Dagfinrud H, Slatkowsky-Christensen B, et al. Activity limitations and participation restrictions in women with hand osteoarthritis: patients' descriptions and associations between dimensions of functioning. *Ann Rheum Dis* 2005; 64(11):1633–8.

176. Ehrlich GE. Inflammatory osteoarthritis. I. The clinical syndrome. *J Chronic Dis* 1972; 25(6):317–28.

177. Peter JB, Pearson CM, Marmor L. Erosive osteoarthritis of the hands. *Arthritis Rheum* 1966; 9(3):365–88.

178. Merritt MM, Roddey TS, Costello C, Olson S. Diagnostic value of clinical grind test for carpometacarpal osteoarthritis of the thumb. *J Hand Ther* 2010; 23(3):261–7.

179. Dreiser RL, Maheu E, Guillou GB, Caspard H, Grouin JM. Validation of an algofunctional index for osteoarthritis of the hand. *Rev Rhum Engl Ed* 1995; 62(6 Suppl 1):43S–53S.

180. Gellhorn AC, Katz JN, Suri P. Osteoarthritis of the spine: the facet joints. *Nat Rev Rheumatol* 2013; 9(4):216–24.

181. Kalichman L, Hunter DJ. Lumbar facet joint osteoarthritis: a review. *Semin Arthritis Rheum* 2007; 37(2):69–80.

182. Raastad J, Reiman M, Coeytaux R, Ledbetter L, Goode AP. The association between lumbar spine radiographic features and low back pain: a systematic review and meta-analysis. *Semin Arthritis Rheum* 2015; 44(5):571–85.

183. Kalichman L, Li L, Kim DH, et al. Facet joint osteoarthritis and low back pain in the community-based population. *Spine (Phila Pa 1976)* 2008; 33(23):2560–5.

184. Suri P, Hunter DJ, Rainville J, Guermazi A, Katz JN. Presence and extent of severe facet joint osteoarthritis are associated with back pain in older adults. *Osteoarthritis Cartilage* 2013; 21(9):1199–206.

185. Schwarzer AC, Wang SC, Bogduk N, McNaught PJ, Laurent R. Prevalence and clinical features of lumbar zygapophysial joint pain: a study in an Australian population with chronic low back pain. *Ann Rheum Dis* 1995; 54(2):100–6.

186. Wilde VE, Ford JJ, McMeeken JM. Indicators of lumbar zygapophyseal joint pain: survey of an expert panel with the Delphi technique. *Phys Ther* 2007; 87(10):1348–61.

187. Kobayashi T, Takagishi K, Shitara H, et al. Prevalence of and risk factors for shoulder osteoarthritis in Japanese middle-aged and elderly populations. *J Shoulder Elbow Surg* 2014; 23(5):613–9.

188. Fayad F, Roby-Brami A, Yazbeck C, et al. Three-dimensional scapular kinematics and scapulohumeral rhythm in patients with glenohumeral osteoarthritis or frozen shoulder. J Biomech 2008; 41(2):326–32.

189. Kircher J, Morhard M, Magosch P, et al. How much are radiological parameters related to clinical symptoms and function in osteoarthritis of the shoulder? *Int Orthop* 2010; 34(5):677–81.

190. Rao S, Baumhauer JF, Nawoczenski DA. Is barefoot regional plantar loading related to self-reported foot pain in patients with midfoot osteoarthritis. *Osteoarthritis Cartilage* 2011; 19(8):1019–25.

191. Dufour AB, Casey VA, Golightly YM, Hannan MT. Characteristics associated with hallux valgus in a population-based foot study of older adults. *Arthritis Care Res (Hoboken)* 2014; 66(12):1880–6.

192. Roddy E, Zhang W, Doherty M. Prevalence and associations of hallux valgus in a primary care population. *Arthritis Rheum* 2008; 59(6):857–62.

193. Queen RM, Carter JE, Adams SB, et al. Coronal plane ankle alignment, gait, and end-stage ankle osteoarthritis. *Osteoarthritis Cartilage* 2011; 19(11):1338–42.

194. Valderrabano V, Horisberger M, Russell I, Dougall H, Hintermann B. Etiology of ankle osteoarthritis. *Clin Orthop Relat Res* 2009; 467(7):1800–6.

195. McDaniel G, Renner JB, Sloane R, Kraus VB. Association of knee and ankle osteoarthritis with physical performance. *Osteoarthritis Cartilage* 2011; 19(6):634–8.

196. Valderrabano V, von Tscharner V, Nigg BM, et al. Lower leg muscle atrophy in ankle osteoarthritis. *J Orthop Res* 2006; 24(12):2159–69.

197. Hubbard TJ, Hicks-Little C, Cordova M. Changes in ankle mechanical stability in those with knee osteoarthritis. *Arch Phys Med Rehabil* 2010; 91(1):73–7.

198. Wiese M, Svensson P, Bakke M, et al. Association between temporomandibular joint symptoms, signs, and clinical diagnosis using the RDC/TMD and radiographic findings in temporomandibular joint tomograms. *J Orofac Pain* 2008; 22(3):239–51.

199. Altman R, Alarcon G, Appelrouth D, et al. The American College of Rheumatology criteria for the classification and reporting of osteoarthritis of the hand. *Arthritis Rheum* 1990; 33(11):1601–10.

CHAPTER 16

Radiography and computed tomography imaging of osteoarthritis

Daichi Hayashi, Ali Guermazi, and Frank W. Roemer

Introduction

Imaging is essential for assessing structural joint damage and disease progression of osteoarthritis (OA). Articular structures that are evaluated by imaging include hyaline cartilage, bone and bone marrow, menisci in the knee, labrum in the shoulder and hip, synovium, and various ligaments. Conventional radiography is still the basis for diagnosis and the most commonly used imaging modality. Magnetic resonance imaging (MRI) is widely applied in epidemiological studies and clinical trials, which is discussed in detail in Chapter 18. Computed tomography (CT) is an important additional tool that offers insight into high-resolution anatomical details and allows three-dimensional (3D) post-processing of imaging data, which is of particular importance for orthopaedic surgery planning. This chapter describes the roles and limitations of both conventional radiography and CT, including CT arthrography, in clinical practice and OA research. The emphasis will be on OA of the knee, but other joints will also be mentioned where appropriate.

Conventional radiography

Role of radiography in imaging of osteoarthritis

Radiography is the simplest, least expensive, and most widely available imaging technique. It enables detection of bony features associated with OA including marginal osteophytes, subchondral sclerosis, attrition, and subchondral cysts [1]. The presence of these features can be observed in any joint that is affected by OA. Unlike rheumatoid arthritis, bony erosion is not a common feature of OA, although it can be seen in erosive OA, typically in the interphalangeal joints of the hands. In addition to subjective assessment of joint space narrowing (JSN), radiography allows quantitative measurement of joint space width (JSW), an indirect surrogate of cartilage thickness and meniscal integrity in the knee, although precise and direct assessment of each of these articular structures is not possible with radiography [2]. Nevertheless, progression of JSN is the most commonly used end point for the assessment of OA progression and complete loss of JSW characterized by bone-on-bone contact indicates so-called end-stage OA, which is considered one of the indications for joint replacement.

Semi-quantitative assessment of knee OA features

The severity of OA can be estimated using semi-quantitative scoring systems. Published atlases provide image examples that represent specific grades [1]. The Kellgren and Lawrence (KL) classification [3] is a widely accepted scheme used for defining the presence or absence of radiographic OA using grade 2 disease as the threshold for a diagnosis of radiographic OA. The KL scheme is a composite measure comprising the presence or absence of marginal osteophytes and JSN. Figure 16.1 shows examples of the different grades of the KL scheme. Patients with clinical signs and symptoms of OA with a KL grade of 0 or 1 may fulfil the clinical criteria of OA but will be considered as having 'pre-radiographic' OA from a structural viewpoint. A modified, simplified version of the KL grading scheme is summarized in Table 16.1. However, KL grading has its limitations; in particular KL grade 3 includes all degrees of JSN, regardless of the actual extent. Figures 16.2 and 16.3 show typical examples of definite radiographic progression that cannot be coded by the KL scoring system. Recently, a modification of KL grading was suggested to improve the sensitivity to change in longitudinal knee OA studies including the addition of JSN to the radiographic diagnosis of knee OA [4]. For OA progression, the authors recommend focusing on JSN alone using either a semi-quantitative [5] or quantitative approaches.

The Osteoarthritis Research Society International (OARSI) atlas [1] takes a different approach and grades tibiofemoral JSN and osteophytes separately for each compartment of the knee (Box 16.1). In contrast to the KL scheme, the OARSI atlas does not provide specific definitions but displays specific image examples to illustrate the different grades for each compartment. This compartmental scoring appears to be more sensitive to longitudinal radiographic changes than KL grading. In addition, the importance of centralized radiographic assessment in regard to observer reliability needs to be emphasized, as even expert readers apply different thresholds when scoring JSN [6]. Figure 16.4 shows typical examples of semi-quantitative assessment according to the KL and OARSI grading schemes. Note that semi-quantitative scoring is applied not only to the knee joint but also to other joints, particularly the hip and the interphalangeal joints of the hands as is shown in Figure 16.5.

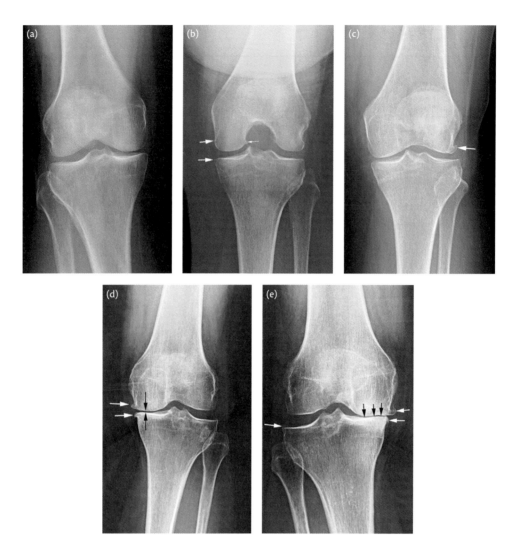

Figure 16.1 The Kellgren–Lawrence (KL) classification is a composite scale of OA severity taking into account primarily the radiographic OA features of marginal osteophytes and joint space narrowing in the anteroposterior radiograph. (a) KL grade 0. No signs of joint space narrowing and no marginal osteophytes are observed. (b) KL grade 1. Minimal, equivocal osteophytes are observed at the medial joint margins (large arrows). Note that so-called notch osteophytes at the centre of the joint (small arrow) are not considered in the KL scale. (c) KL grade 2 is characterized by presence of at least one definite marginal osteophyte (arrow) without evidence of joint space narrowing. (d) KL grade 3 knees exhibit signs of definite joint space narrowing (black arrows) and marginal osteophytes (white arrows). KL grade 3 knees with joint space narrowing but only minimal osteophytes are considered to represent the so-called atrophic phenotype of knee OA. (e) KL grade 4 is defined by bone-to-bone contact and complete obliteration of the joint space (black arrows). Note definite marginal osteophytes in addition (white arrows).

Table 16.1 Description of Kellgren and Lawrence and modified Kellgren and Lawrence grading systems for knee OA

	Original Kellgren and Lawrence classification	Modified Kellgren and Lawrence classification[a]	Radiographic osteoarthritis
Grade 0	No feature of osteoarthritis	No feature of osteoarthritis	No
Grade 1	Doubtful joint space narrowing and possible osteophytic lipping	Equivocal osteophyte	No
Grade 2	Definite osteophytes and possible joint-space narrowing	Unequivocal osteophyte	Yes
Grade 3	Moderate multiple osteophytes, definite joint space narrowing, and some sclerosis and possible deformity of bone ends	Joint-space narrowing	Yes
Grade 4	Large osteophytes, marked joint space narrowing, severe sclerosis, and definite deformity of bone ends	Bone-to-bone appearance	Yes

[a]Adapted from: Guermazi A, et al. *J Bone Joint Surg Am* 2009 Feb; 91 Suppl 1:54–62.

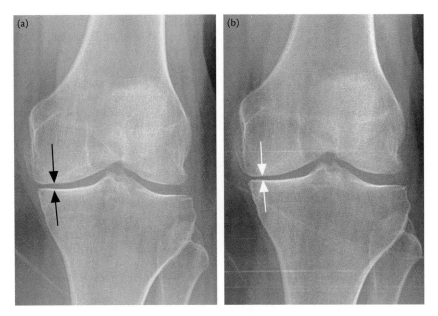

Figure 16.2 Example of progressive joint space narrowing and the insensitivity of radiographic scoring systems to change. (a) Baseline anteroposterior radiograph of the right knee, showing normal joint-space width in the lateral tibiofemoral compartment and OARSI grade 2 joint space narrowing in the medial tibiofemoral compartment at baseline (black arrows). The Kellgren–Lawrence (KL) grade is 3. (b) Follow-up radiograph of the same knee after 6 months, showing normal joint space width in the lateral compartment and unequivocally progressive medial tibiofemoral joint space narrowing at the time of follow-up (white arrows). However, according to the OARSI and KL scoring systems, there is no change in grade.

Quantitative assessments of joint space width and other articular features

Quantitative measures of JSW use a 'ruler', either a physical device or a software application, to measure the JSW as the distance between the projected femoral and tibial margins on the image. The femoral margin is defined as the projected edge of the bone, while the software usually determines the tibial margin as a bright band corresponding to the projection of the X-ray beam

through the radio-dense cortical shell at the base of the tibial plateau. Quantification of JSW using image processing software does require a digital version of the image which can be provided for plain films by a radiographic film digitizer, or files can be analysed directly if images were acquired in digital fashion primarily.

Measurement of JSW is the prerequisite for assessment of JSN in clinical trials. Prior to the development of automated and semi-automated methods, JSW was measured by using purely manual

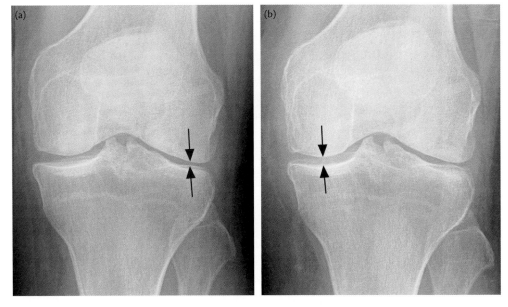

Figure 16.3 Example of the limitations of the Kellgren–Lawrence (KL) scoring system. (a) Baseline anteroposterior radiograph of the right knee. KL grade 3 was determined by the presence of definite lateral joint space narrowing (arrows). (b) Follow-up radiograph of the same knee after 6 months. Obvious narrowing of the medial tibiofemoral joint-space width from baseline to follow-up is observed (arrows—OARSI grade 1), but there is no change in the KL grade (grade 3) because no progressive narrowing of the lateral tibiofemoral joint-space width is observed.

Box 16.1 Osteoarthritis Research Society International (OARSI) grading system for knee OA features

Features and grading

◆ Medial femoral osteophyte: grade 0–3

◆ Medial tibial osteophyte: grade 0–3

◆ Lateral femoral osteophyte: grade 0–3

◆ Lateral tibial osteophyte: grade 0–3

◆ Medial tibiofemoral joint space narrowing: grade 0–3

◆ Lateral tibiofemoral joint space narrowing: grade 0–3.

methods [7,8]. Although manual methods offer simplicity of equipment and application and can be used to measure any linear distance, they are time-consuming, subjective, and labour intensive.

Automated and semi-automated techniques for use in clinical trials have been developed to provide rapid, objective, and precise measurements of JSW. Most of the work has been aimed at using automation to improve reproducibility of semi-quantitative scoring or manual measurements. Studies using these software methods have demonstrated improved precision over the manual methods and semi-quantitative scoring [9,10]. More recently, these methods have been evaluated using longitudinal studies to quantify the responsiveness to change [11]. Various degrees of responsiveness have been observed depending on the degree of OA severity, length of the follow-up, and the knee-positioning protocol [11–16].

Different measures of JSW have been introduced, including minimum JSW, mean JSW, joint space area, and location-specific JSW. Minimum JSW is defined as the shortest distance between the tibial and femoral margins of the joint space within the weight-bearing areas of the medial and lateral tibiofemoral compartments. In addition, newer methods, known as statistical shape models, have been introduced to segment the anatomy of the knee joint on radiographs [17,18]. This approach uses multivariate statistics to derive the allowable shape of an object from a set of examples.

Determination of mean JSW or joint space area has been studied in either a constant area or a region of interest, and its utility has been compared with that of minimum JSW. Minimum JSW was found to be more reproducible and more sensitive to change than is mean JSW or joint space area [19,20]. While the most commonly deployed and accepted outcome measurement to determine OA progression is minimum JSW, location-specific JSW measurement might offer advantages concerning reproducibility and responsiveness [8,11,21–23].

Measurements of JSW obtained from radiographs of knee OA have been found to be reliable especially when the study lasted longer than 2 years and when the radiographs were obtained with the knee in a standardized flexed position [24]. Studies of hip OA have shown conflicting results when correlating JSW and symptoms. However, studies have demonstrated that JSW can predict hip joint replacement [25].

A recently developed computer software called Knee Images Digital Analysis (KIDA) enables evaluation of JSW, osteophyte area, subchondral bone density, joint angle, and tibial eminence height as continuous variables [26]. Statistically significant correlations were found between KIDA parameters and OA severity as measured by the KL system. Moreover, significant differences were found between healthy and OA knees [26]. In the Cohort Hip & Cohort Knee (CHECK) cohort, these features progressed in severity at different times during follow-up: early (medial JSW, osteophyte area), late (minimum and lateral JSW, eminence height), and both early

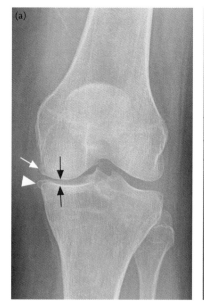 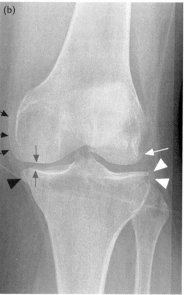

Figure 16.4 Examples of semi-quantitative radiographic assessment with use of the Kellgren–Lawrence (KL) and Osteoarthritis Research Society International (OARSI) grading schemes. (a) KL grade 3. No lateral femoral and tibial osteophytes are seen (OARSI grade 0). A medial femoral osteophyte OARSI grade 1 (white arrow), a medial tibial osteophyte OARSI grade 2 (white arrowhead), lateral tibiofemoral joint space width OARSI grade 0, and medial tibiofemoral joint space narrowing OARSI grade 2 (black arrows) are depicted. (b) KL grade 2. A lateral femoral osteophyte OARSI grade 2 (white arrow), a lateral tibial osteophyte OARSI grade 2 (white arrowheads), a medial femoral osteophyte OARSI grade 3 (black arrows), a medial tibial osteophyte OARSI grade 2 (black arrowhead), a normal lateral tibiofemoral joint space width (OARSI grade 0), and medial tibiofemoral joint space width (OARSI grade 1) (grey arrows) are shown.

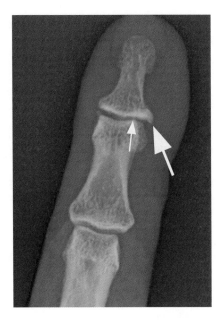

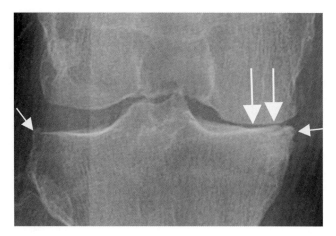

Figure 16.6 Atrophic OA. There is advanced medial joint space narrowing with almost bone-on-bone appearance (large arrows). However, despite advanced disease as reflected by the severity of joint space narrowing, there are only tiny tibial osteophytes present. Atrophic OA may be a reflection of more rapid progression, or decreased osteophyte formation due to systemic or local biomechanical factors.

Figure 16.5 Osteoarthritis of the distal interphalangeal joint. Anteroposterior radiograph shows definite ulnar joint space narrowing (OARSI grade 1—small arrow). In addition there is an OARSI grade 1 osteophyte at the ulnar joint margin at the base of the end phalanx (large arrow).

and late (varus angle, bone density), and correlations between different radiographic features varied between time points [27].

Limitations of radiography in imaging of OA

Because of inherent limitations of radiography for visualization of OA-related pathological changes, there is an ongoing debate regarding the potential inadequacy of radiographic measures to be applied as eligibility criteria or as outcome measures in OA clinical trials [28].

Recruitment of subjects to participate in knee OA trials is dependent on the radiographic definition of OA as defined by the KL grade [3]. However, despite having been stratified according to their KL grades, knees may have heterogeneous structural joint damage that cannot be visualized by radiography. As an example, a recent population-based observational study (Framingham OA study) [29], showed that osteophytes were detected by MRI in 524 (74%) of 710 knees with normal radiographs (KL grade 0), suggesting that radiography lacks sensitivity for the detection of early OA structural changes. Pathological features of OA that have been reported to be associated with pain include bone marrow lesions, synovitis, effusion, periarticular cystic lesions, and meniscal tears [30]. However, none of these joint pathologies can be visualized by radiography. In the above-mentioned study [29], the prevalence of bone marrow lesions, meniscal tears, and synovitis/effusion, respectively, was 52%, 24%, and 36% in radiographically normal knees. Another study also using the data from the Framingham OA study showed that pre-radiographic osteoarthritic changes were highly prevalent in the medial patella and medial posterior femur, that is, in locations that cannot be adequately assessed using the standard posterior–anterior radiograph of the knee joint [31]. These numbers imply that knees with a KL grade of 0 should not be automatically considered structurally normal and not necessarily be excluded from OA clinical trials.

It should also be noted that OA has multiple 'phenotypes' that are not apparent on radiography [32–34]. OA should be considered a complex and heterogeneous disease with multiple disease-triggering factors at the joint level and the systemic level, as well as a varied clinical course. Including patients with different phenotypes in the same clinical trial may increase the ambiguity of the results and hinder interpretation of results. Figure 16.6 represents an example of such a structural phenotype (i.e. atrophic OA) which is characterized by the presence of JSN with no or only tiny osteophytes.

Slowing of joint space loss is a widely used radiographic outcome measure [35]. Indeed, reduced loss of joint space as seen on radiography is the only imaging biomarker that has been included by the United States Food and Drug Administration in its draft recommendation, and also by the European Medicines Agency. JSW measurement by radiography is still recommended by the OARSI for clinical trials of structural modification [35]. However, radiography has several limitations to be used as a structural end point in OA disease-modifying OA drug (DMOAD) trials, as described below.

Firstly, focal cartilage loss or diffuse partial thickness loss in the tibiofemoral joint often does not produce a change in JSW. A study based on data from the Multicenter Osteoarthritis Study (MOST study) showed that 69 (42%) of 164 knees without JSN or definite osteophytes had focal or diffuse partial-thickness cartilage loss in the medial tibiofemoral joint as detected on MRI [36]. Secondly, radiography lacks sensitivity for detecting structural change over time [37]. OA is a very slow process. A recent study based on Osteoarthritis Initiative (OAI) data showed that only few knees in the large OAI cohort exhibited ongoing change while most were stable in regard to longitudinal structural progression. In stable knees, JSW remained the same for as long as 4 years [38]. In such knees, it would seem very difficult to test the efficacy of a drug, using radiographic outcome measures within the usual 1- or 2-year time frame that is the common time period for a clinical DMOAD trial.

Thirdly, joint space loss over time as seen on radiography lacks specificity, as such change may be due to any combination of cartilage loss, meniscal damage, or meniscal extrusion [39,40]. Adams and colleagues demonstrated in a small cohort that more than 50% of patients with radiographic JSN and meniscal extrusion (17 of 32) had no loss of cartilage as seen on MRI [41].

Lastly, due to its two-dimensional (2D) nature, the radiographic appearance of tibiofemoral joint space is heavily dependent on knee positioning and the angle of joint flexion. Unless exactly the same positioning and angulation are used at baseline and follow-up, measurement error may occur. A recent study showed that shifting the foot forward by 6 cm on a foot plate to simulate the varying extent of lower leg extension in a semi-flexed knee led to a statistically significant increase in the minimum JSW (+0.07 mm/cm of shift). This was clinically relevant when compared with a mean loss of JSW of 0.11 mm in knees with radiographic progression over 2 years [42].

Image acquisition techniques

It is paramount to guarantee standardization in radiographic acquisition especially in longitudinal studies. For decades, the extended-knee radiograph (i.e. bilateral weight-bearing anteroposterior view of both knees in full extension) has been the standard technique used for visualization of the tibiofemoral joint [43]. While the diagnostic utility of the extended-knee radiograph is established, this technique is limited in regard to reproducibility in longitudinal evaluation of JSW [44]. For this reason, several alternative protocols have been developed for standardized positioning of the knee. Common to all of these techniques is slight knee flexion, rather than extension, that provides contact between the tibia and the posterior aspect of the femoral condyle [45]. The protocols differ, however, with respect to the degree of flexion required, the angulation of the X-ray beam, and the parameter that is adjusted to meet the positioning standards of the examination. Fluoroscopy is used in some protocols to confirm satisfactory anatomic positioning of the medial tibial plateau prior to acquisition of the radiograph, while for others a non-fluoroscopic positioning standard is used (i.e. semi-flexed metatarsophalangeal and fixed flexion views) [46–49].

The advances in standardized knee radiography that have made clinical trials of DMOADs feasible can also benefit clinical practice. As mentioned above, the conventional extended-knee radiograph is still used in clinical practice to document evidence of marginal tibiofemoral osteophytes on which the diagnosis of knee OA is based. However, the radiographic severity of knee OA (i.e. the extent of JSN in the presence of marginal osteophytes) may not be apparent on the extended-knee view [44,50]. Most clinical radiology departments are capable of producing a posteroanterior radiograph of the knee in the Lyon–Schuss position with 10° caudad angulation of the X-ray beam (i.e. a fixed-flexion radiograph, with or without use of a positioning frame). A radiograph satisfying these standards would offer two distinct advantages over the conventional extended-knee view. Firstly, knee flexion is more likely to reveal cartilage loss that is common to the posterior aspect of the femur [45]. Secondly, the fixed-flexion view is more likely than the extended-knee view to represent the joint space in parallel or near-parallel alignment with the X-ray beam. These strengths promise greater accuracy in evaluation of the severity of structural changes of tibiofemoral OA and may result in an image of the knee that likely will be more reliably reproduced during repeated assessments of disease progression at a later time.

Recent applications of radiographic assessment in clinical studies

Despite the above-mentioned shortcomings, radiographic measurements are still commonly used in observational studies of knee OA. A prospective observational cohort study by Harvey and colleagues associated leg-length inequality of 1 cm or more with prevalent radiographic and symptomatic OA in the shorter leg, and described increased odds of progressive OA in the shorter leg over 30 months [51]. This study showed that leg-length inequality should be regarded as a modifiable risk factor for knee OA. Duryea and colleagues compared the responsiveness of radiographic JSW using automated software with MRI-derived measures of cartilage morphometry for OA progression [16]. Results demonstrated that measures of location-specific JSW using a software analysis of digital knee radiographic images were comparable to MRI in detecting OA progression. Although the limitations of radiography are known, the study showed that when the lower costs and greater accessibility of radiography are considered and compared to MRI, radiography still has a role to play in OA observational studies. A clinical trial by Mazzuca and colleagues showed varus malalignment of the lower limb negated the slowing of structural progression of medial JSN by doxycycline [52]. It remains to be seen if the same effect can be obtained on MRI-based evaluation of OA progression.

Using data from the CHECK study, Kinds and colleagues showed that measuring osteophyte area and minimum JSW in addition to demographic and clinical characteristics, improved the prediction of radiographic OA occurring 5 years later (area under curve receiver operating characteristic (ROC) = 0.74 vs 0.64 without radiographic features) in patients with knee pain but no OA at baseline [53]. A cross-sectional study based on the same cohort of patients showed that in patients with early symptomatic knee OA osteophytosis, bony enlargement, crepitus, pain, and higher body mass index (BMI) were associated with lower knee flexion [54]. JSN was associated with a lower range of motion in all planes. In addition, osteophytosis, flattening of the femoral head, femoral buttressing, pain, morning stiffness, male gender, and higher BMI were found to be associated with poorer range of motion in the hip, in two planes. Cam impingement is characterized by abnormal contact between the proximal femur and acetabulum caused by a non-spherical femoral head, known as a cam deformity. A cam deformity is usually quantified by the alpha angle with a larger alpha angle substantially increasing the risk for OA. Using the data from the aforementioned CHECK cohort as well as the Chingford cohort, a definite bimodal distribution of the alpha angle was found in both cohorts with a normal distribution up to 60°, indicating a clear distinction between normal and abnormal alpha angles [55]. A pathological threshold of 78° resulted in the maximum area under the ROC curve. Authors thus proposed alpha angle thresholds of 60° to define the presence of a cam deformity and 78° for a pathological cam deformity.

Two publications from a large-scale, Japanese population-based study demonstrated that occupational activities involving kneeling and squatting [56], as well as obesity, hypertension, and dyslipidaemia [57] were associated with lower medial minimum JSW when compared to controls. Another cross-sectional study found that a low level of vitamin D was associated with knee pain but not radiographic OA [58]. A longitudinal study by the same group showed accumulation of metabolic syndrome components (obesity, hypertension, dyslipidaemia, and impaired glucose tolerance) is significantly related to occurrence and progression of radiographic knee OA [59].

It is interesting to note that two older methods based on radiographic acquisition—that is, bone texture analysis and tomosynthesis—have experienced a revival lately. Bone texture analysis extracts 2D information from conventional radiography, that directly relates to 3D bone structure [60,61]. The authors of one study showed that bone texture may be a predictor of progression of tibiofemoral OA [62]. Whether bone texture correlates with other changes of subchondral bone such as MRI-detected bone marrow lesions or sclerosis remains to be seen. Tomosynthesis generates an arbitrary number of section images from a single pass of the X-ray tube. It has been shown that digital tomosynthesis improves sensitivity for depicting lesions in the chest, the breast, and in rheumatoid arthritis [63–66]. Hayashi et al. demonstrated that tomosynthesis is more sensitive to osteophytes and subchondral cysts than radiography, using 3T MRI as the reference [67]. Moreover, tomosynthesis seems to offer excellent intra-reader reliability regardless of reader experience [68]. A method for quantification of JSW using tomosynthesis has also been described [69]. The clinical availability of these systems is currently limited, but the potential of this technique for OA research might be worth exploring further.

Computed tomography and computed tomography arthrography

CT enables evaluation of osseous structures and soft tissue calcifications with much better anatomical details compared to radiography. A typical example of knee with OA as delineated by CT is shown in Figure 16.7. Relative strengths and limitations of radiography compared to CT and CT arthrography are summarized in Table 16.2. In clinical practice, CT is commonly used for preoperative planning of total joint arthroplasty thanks to its 3D capability. CT is rarely indicated in the routine evaluation of OA in clinical practice due to higher radiation dose and its relative lack of ability to delineate soft tissue changes compared to MRI. However, micro-CT has a long established role in animal-based studies of OA to assess trabecular and cortical microstructure [70,71].

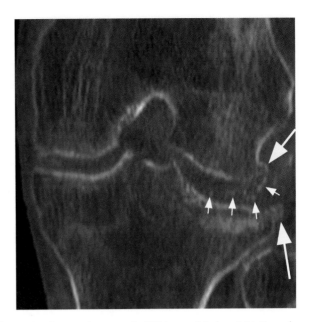

Figure 16.7 Computed tomography (CT) image of the knee joint. Coronal reformation. Image shows definite osteophytes at the lateral joint margin (large arrows) but no joint space narrowing. Note small intra-articular calcifications representing chondrocalcinosis of the lateral meniscus (small arrows). CT is highly sensitive for the depiction of calcifications. Overall, CT has lower contrast to visualize soft tissues, which is also seen in this example. The cruciate ligaments and the menisci are not seen.

CT also has an established role in assessing facet joint OA of the spine in both clinical and research settings [72]. An example of facet joint OA is presented in Figure 16.8. Using a CT-based semi-quantitative grading system of facet joint OA, a population-based study by Kalichman and colleagues showed a high prevalence of facet joint OA and that the prevalence of facet joint OA increases with age, with the highest prevalence at the L4–L5 spinal level [73]. In the same cohort of subjects, associations were observed for self-reported back pain with spinal stenosis [74], abdominal aortic calcification with facet joint OA [75], obesity with higher prevalence of facet joint OA [76], and increasing age with higher prevalence of disc narrowing, facet joint OA, and degenerative spondylolisthesis [76]. A recent animal study used micro-CT to

Table 16.2 Relative advantages and disadvantages of radiography, CT, and CT arthrography

	Radiography	CT	CT arthrography
Advantages	Low cost Wide availability Low radiation exposure Availability of established semi-quantitative grading schemes for osteoarthritis	High anatomical resolution and excellent depiction of bony structures 3D imaging with volumetric reconstruction	(In addition to advantages of CT) Accurate evaluation of focal cartilage defects Evaluation of meniscal tears and other intrinsic joint structures such as ligaments Potential to assess cartilage biochemical composition (to date only *ex vivo*)
Disadvantages	Projectional technique 2D imaging only Inability to visualize important OA-related pathologies including cartilage, bone marrow lesions, and synovitis Technical limitations including positioning of the joint and its reproducibility in longitudinal studies	Relative to X-ray higher costs Radiation exposure Inability to delineate soft tissue structures in detail	(In addition to disadvantages of CT) Highest cost due to the use of contrast Invasive—risk of pain, infection and haemorrhage post procedure

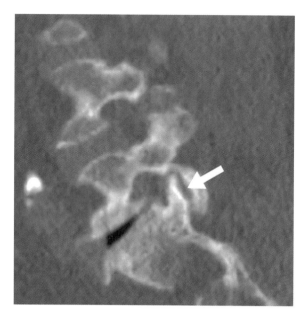

Figure 16.8 Sagittal computed tomography reformation of the lumbar spine. Image depicts osteoarthritic changes in the left facet joint of the L5/S1 level with joint space narrowing (arrow) and periarticular sclerosis. In addition, there is vacuum phenomenon in the intervertebral space (small arrow) and osteophytes at the neural foramen (arrowhead). Large foraminal osteophytes may cause nerve root irritation and typical associated clinical findings of ischialgia.

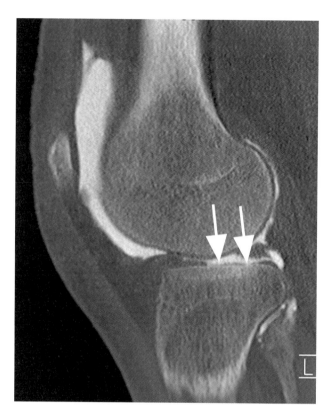

Figure 16.9 CT arthrography is considered the imaging gold standard for assessment of cartilage surface damage/integrity. Sagittal CT arthrogram of the knee joint shows hyperdense intra-articular contrast (asterisk) while cancellous bone is depicted with intermediate density. There is extensive full-thickness articular surface damage in the central weight-bearing parts of the lateral tibia reaching the subchondral plate (arrows).

assess cartilage alterations in the facet joint of rats, and showed that monosodium iodoacetate injection into facet joints provided a useful model for the study of OA changes in the facet [77].

CT arthrography enables evaluation of damage to articular cartilage with a high anatomical resolution in multiple planes, which is not possible by conventional arthrography since cartilage is radiolucent on fluoroscopy. CT arthrography can be performed using a single-contrast (iodine alone) or double-contrast (iodine and air) technique [78]. In general, the single-contrast technique is considered easier to perform with fewer side effects [79]. To avoid beam-hardening artefacts, the contrast material can be diluted with saline or local anaesthetics [78]. It has to be kept in mind that any arthrographic examination has a low risk of infection from the intra-articular injection [80]. Other risks include pain, vasovagal reactions, and systemic allergic reactions. A major disadvantage of CT arthrography is exposure of patients to higher radiation compared to radiography.

At present, CT arthrography is considered the most accurate method for assessing cartilage surface changes, which is shown in an exemplary fashion in Figure 16.9. It offers high spatial resolution and high contrast between the low attenuating cartilage and high attenuating superficial (contrast material filling the joint space) and deep (subchondral bone) boundaries [78]. Cadaveric studies have shown that CT arthrography is more accurate than MRI [81] or MR arthrography [82] for the assessment of cartilage thickness. For the hip joint, recent data indicates that MR arthrography seems similarly accurate compared to CT arthrography for the assessment of cartilage thickness [83].

Superficial focal cartilage lesions are well delineated by CT arthrography and appear as areas within the cartilage filled with the intra-articular contrast agent. CT arthrography offers high spatial resolution and high contrast between the cartilage and the intra-articular contrast agent leading to a high degree of confidence in depicting these lesions with a superior inter-reader reproducibility compared to MR arthrography [84]. In addition to delineating surface changes of cartilage, CT arthrography is able to delineate subchondral bone sclerosis, marginal osteophytes, and enables visualization of central osteophytes, which are associated with more severe changes of OA compared to marginal osteophytes [85].

Due to the high costs, invasive nature, and potential risks associated with intra-articular injection, arthrographic examinations are rarely used in large-scale clinical or epidemiological OA studies. However, arthrography has been used in small-scale clinical studies of post-traumatic OA [86]. Further high-resolution CT arthrography has been applied to examine the 3D progression pattern of acetabular cartilage damage in patients with hip dysplasia [87]. This study suggested that the cartilage thickness in the lateral zone divided by that in the medial zone may be a sensitive index for quantifying early cartilage damage associated with extent of labral disorders. Recently, Omoumi and colleagues evaluated a cohort of pre-total knee replacement OA knees using CT arthrography and demonstrated cartilage at the posterior aspect of the medial femoral condyle and at the anterior aspect of the lateral femorotibial compartment might be frequently preserved in advanced grades of knee OA [88]. Interestingly and not reported previously, another recent cross-sectional study utilizing CT arthrography of the knee showed that cartilage thickness at the most posterior aspect of the medial femoral condyle is increased in OA knees compared to non-OA knees, and this thickening was further associated with increasing KL grade [89]. More work is needed to confirm and understand the mechanism of these findings which are not well established in the literature.

Conclusion

Radiography is the most widely used first-line imaging modality for structural OA evaluation. Its inherent limitations should be noted, including lack of ability to directly visualize most OA-related pathological features in and around the joint, lack of sensitivity to longitudinal change and missing specificity of JSN, and technical difficulties regarding reproducibility of positioning of the joints in longitudinal studies. Modern CT allows detailed evaluation of anatomy with limitations in the assessment of soft tissue structures compared to MRI, which remains its major disadvantage. CT arthrography can be useful in evaluation of focal cartilage defects or meniscal tears; however, its applicability may be limited due to its invasive nature. Several detailed overviews of the most recent research endeavours dealing with topics discussed have been published that may add insight beyond what could be covered in this chapter [90–95].

References

1. Altman RD, Gold GE. Atlas of individual radiographic features in osteoarthritis, revised. *Osteoarthritis Cartilage* 2007; 15(Suppl A):A1–56.
2. Hunter DJ, Zhang YQ, Tu X, et al. Change in joint space width: hyaline articular cartilage loss or alteration in meniscus? *Arthritis Rheum* 2006; 54:2488–95.
3. Kellgren JH, Lawrence JS. Radiological assessment of osteo-arthrosis. *Ann Rheum Dis* 1957; 16:494–502.
4. Felson DT, Niu J, Guermazi A, Sack B, Aliabadi P. Defining radiographic incidence and progression of knee osteoarthritis: suggested modifications of the Kellgren and Lawrence scale. *Ann Rheum Dis* 2011; 70:1884–6.
5. Felson DT, Nevitt MC, Yang M, et al. A new approach yields high rates of radiographic progression in knee osteoarthritis. *J Rheumatol* 2008; 35:2047–54.
6. Guermazi A, Hunter DJ, Li L, et al. Different thresholds for detecting osteophytes and joint space narrowing exist between the site investigators and the centralized reader in a multicenter knee osteoarthritis study—data from the Osteoarthritis Initiative. *Skeletal Radiol* 2012; 41:179–86.
7. Lequesne M. Chondrometry. Quantitative evaluation of joint space width and rate of joint space loss in osteoarthritis of the hip. *Rev Rhum Engl Ed* 1995; 62:155–8.
8. Ravaud P, Chastang C, Auleley GR, et al. Assessment of joint space width in patients with osteoarthritis of the knee: a comparison of 4 measuring instruments. *J Rheumatol* 1996; 23:1749–55.
9. Duryea J, Li J, Peterfy CG, Gordon C, Genant HK. Trainable rule-based algorithm for the measurement of joint space width in digital radiographic images of the knee. *Med Phys* 2000; 27:580–91.
10. Marijnissen AC, Vincken KL, Vos PA, et al. Knee Images Digital Analysis (KIDA): a novel method to quantify individual radiographic features of knee osteoarthritis in detail. *Osteoarthritis Cartilage* 2008; 16:234–43.
11. Neumann G, Hunter D, Nevitt M, et al. Location specific radiographic joint space width for osteoarthritis progression. *Osteoarthritis Cartilage* 2009; 17:761–5.
12. Chu E, DiCarlo JC, Peterfy C, et al. Fixed-location joint space width measurement increases sensitivity to change in osteoarthritis. *Osteoarthritis Cartilage* 2007; 15:S192.
13. Duryea J, Hunter DJ, Nevitt MC, et al. Study of location specific lateral compartment radiographic joint space width for knee osteoarthritis progression: analysis of longitudinal data from the Osteoarthritis Initiative (OAI). *Osteoarthritis Cartilage* 2008; 16:S168.
14. Nevitt MC, Peterfy C, Guermazi A, et al. Longitudinal performance evaluation and validation of fixed-flexion radiography of the knee for detection of joint space loss. *Arthritis Rheum* 2007; 56:1512–20.
15. Benichou OD, Hunter DJ, Nelson DR, et al. One-year change in radiographic joint space width in patients with unilateral joint space narrowing: data from the Osteoarthritis Initiative. *Arthritis Care Res (Hoboken)* 2010; 62:924–31.
16. Duryea J, Neumann G, Niu J, et al. Comparison of radiographic joint space width with magnetic resonance imaging cartilage morphometry: analysis of longitudinal data from the Osteoarthritis Initiative. *Arthritis Care Res (Hoboken)* 2010; 62:932–7.
17. Cootes TF, Taylor CJ. Anatomical statistical models and their role in feature extraction. *Br J Radiol* 2004; 77(Spec No 2):S133–9.
18. Seise M, McKenna SJ, Ricketts IW, Wigderowitz CA. Learning active shape models for bifurcating contours. *IEEE Trans Med Imaging* 2007; 26(5):666–77.
19. Conrozier T, Lequesne M, Favret H, et al. Measurement of the radiological hip joint space width. An evaluation of various methods of measurement. *Osteoarthritis Cartilage* 2001; 9:281–6.
20. Vignon E. Radiographic issues in imaging the progression of hip and knee osteoarthritis. *J Rheumatol Suppl* 2004; 70:36–44.
21. Duryea J, Zaim S, Genant HK. New radiographic-based surrogate outcome measures for osteoarthritis of the knee. *Osteoarthritis Cartilage* 2003; 11(2):102–10.
22. Bruyère O, Henrotin YE, Honoré A, et al. Impact of the joint space width measurement method on the design of knee osteoarthritis studies. *Aging Clin Exp Res* 2003; 15:136–41.
23. Ratzlaff C, Van Wyngaarden C, Duryea J. Location-specific hip joint space width for progression of hip osteoarthritis—data from the Osteoarthritis Initiative. *Osteoarthritis Cartilage* 2014; 22:1481–7.
24. Reichmann WM, Maillefert JF, Hunter DJ, et al. Responsiveness to change and reliability of measurement of radiographic joint space width in osteoarthritis of the knee: a systematic review. *Osteoarthritis Cartilage* 2011; 19:550–6.
25. Chu Miow Lin D, Reichmann WM, Gossec L, et al. Validity and responsiveness of radiographic joint space width metric measurement in hip osteoarthritis: a systematic review. *Osteoarthritis Cartilage* 2011; 19:543–9.
26. Marijnissen AC, Vincken KL, Vos PA, et al. Knee Images Digital Analysis (KIDA): a novel method to quantify individual radiographic features of knee osteoarthritis in detail. *Osteoarthritis Cartilage* 2008; 16:234–43.
27. Kinds MB, Marijnissen AC, Bijlsma JW, et al. Quantitative radiographic features of early knee osteoarthritis: development over 5 years and relationship with symptoms in the CHECK cohort. *J Rheumatol* 2013; 40:58–65.
28. Guermazi A, Roemer FW, Felson DT, Brandt KD. Motion for debate: osteoarthritis clinical trials have not identified efficacious therapies because traditional imaging outcome measures are inadequate. *Arthritis Rheum* 2013; 65:2748–58.
29. Guermazi A, Niu J, Hayashi D, et al. Prevalence of abnormalities in knees detected by MRI in adults without knee osteoarthritis: population based observational study (Framingham Osteoarthritis Study). *BMJ* 2012; 345:e5339.
30. Yusuf E, Kortekaas MC, Watt I, Huizinga TW, Kloppenburg M. Do knee abnormalities visualised on MRI explain knee pain in knee osteoarthritis? A systematic review. *Ann Rheum Dis* 2011; 70:60–7.
31. Hayashi D, Felson DT, Niu J, Hunter DJ, Roemer FW, Aliabadi P, et al. Pre-radiographic osteoarthritic changes are highly prevalent in the medial patella and medial posterior femur in older persons: Framingham OA study. *Osteoarthritis Cartilage* 2014; 22:76–83.
32. Bijlsma JW, Berenbaum F, Lafeber FP. Osteoarthritis: an update with relevance for clinical practice. *Lancet* 2011; 377:2115–26.

33. Roemer FW, Guermazi A, Niu J, Zhang Y, Mohr A, Felson DT. Prevalence of magnetic resonance imaging–defined atrophic and hypertrophic phenotypes of knee osteoarthritis in a populationbased cohort. *Arthritis Rheum* 2012; 64:429–37.

34. Nelson AE, Renner JB, Schwartz TA, et al. Differences in multijoint radiographic osteoarthritis phenotypes among African Americans and Caucasians: the Johnston County Osteoarthritis Project. *Arthritis Rheum* 2011; 63:3843–52.

35. Conaghan PG, Hunter DJ, Maillefert JF, Reichmann WM, Losina E. Summary and recommendations of the OARSI FDA osteoarthritis Assessment of Structural Change Working Group. *Osteoarthritis Cartilage* 2011; 19:606–10.

36. Javaid MK, Lynch JA, Tolstykh I, et al. Pre-radiographic MRI findings are associated with onset of knee symptoms: the MOST study. *Osteoarthritis Cartilage* 2010; 18:323–8.

37. Amin S, LaValley MP, Guermazi A, et al. The relationship between cartilage loss on magnetic resonance imaging and radiographic progression in men and women with knee osteoarthritis. *Arthritis Rheum* 2005; 52:3152–9.

38. Felson D, Niu J, Sack B, et al. Progression of osteoarthritis as a state of inertia. *Ann Rheum Dis* 2013; 72:924–9.

39. Hunter DJ, Zhang YQ, Tu X, et al. Change in joint space width: hyaline articular cartilage loss or alteration in meniscus? *Arthritis Rheum* 2006; 54:2488–95.

40. Crema MD, Nevitt MC, Guermazi A, et al. Progression of cartilage damage and meniscal pathology over 30 months is associated with an increase in radiographic tibiofemoral joint space narrowing in persons with knee OA—the MOST study. *Osteoarthritis Cartilage* 2014; 22:1743–7.

41. Adams JG, McAlindon T, Dimasi M, Carey J, Eustace S. Contribution of meniscal extrusion and cartilage loss to joint space narrowing in osteoarthritis. *Clin Radiol* 1999; 54:502–6.

42. Kinds MB, Vincken KL, Hoppinga TN, et al. Influence of variation in semiflexed knee positioning during image acquisition on separate quantitative radiographic parameters of osteoarthritis, measured by Knee Images Digital Analysis. *Osteoarthritis Cartilage* 2012; 20:997–1003.

43. Leach RE, Gregg T, Siber FJ. Weight-bearing radiography in osteoarthritis of the knee. *Radiology* 1970; 97:265–8.

44. Mazzuca SA, Brandt KD, Katz BP. Is conventional radiography suitable for evaluation of a disease-modifying drug in patients with knee osteoarthritis? *Osteoarthritis Cartilage* 1997; 5:217–26.

45. Messieh SS, Fowler PJ, Munro T. Anteroposterior radiographs of the osteoarthritic knee. *J Bone Joint Surg Br* 1990; 72:639–40.

46. Buckland-Wright JC, Wolfe F, Ward RJ, Flowers N, Hayne C. Substantial superiority of semiflexed (MTP) views in knee osteoarthritis: a comparative radiographic study, without fluoroscopy, of standing extended, semiflexed (MTP), and schuss views. *J Rheumatol* 1999; 26:2664–74.

47. Peterfy C, Li J, Zaim S, et al. Comparison of fixed-flexion positioning with fluoroscopic semi-flexed positioning for quantifying radiographic joint-space width in the knee: test-retest reproducibility. *Skeletal Radiol* 2003; 32:128–32.

48. Buckland-Wright JC, Macfarlane DG, Williams SA, Ward RJ. Accuracy and precision of joint space width measurements in standard and macroradiographs of osteoarthritic knees. *Ann Rheum Dis* 1995; 54:872–80.

49. Mazzuca SA, Brandt KD, Buckland-Wright JC, et al. Field test of the reproducibility of automated measurements of medial tibiofemoral joint space width derived from standardized knee radiographs. *J Rheumatol* 1999; 26:1359–65.

50. Mazzuca SA, Brandt KD, Lane KA, Katz BP. Knee pain reduces joint space width in conventional standing anteroposterior radiographs of osteoarthritic knees. *Arthritis Rheum* 2002; 46:1223–7.

51. Harvey WF, Yang M, Cooke TD, et al. Association of leg-length inequality with knee osteoarthritis: a cohort study. *Ann Intern Med* 2010; 152:287–95.

52. Mazzuca SA, Brandt KD, Chakr R, Lane KA. Varus malalignment negates the structure-modifying benefits of doxycycline in obese women with knee osteoarthritis. *Osteoarthritis Cartilage* 2010; 18:1008–11.

53. Kinds MB, Marijnissen AC, Vincken KL, et al. Evaluation of separate quantitative radiographic features adds to the prediction of incident radiographic osteoarthritis in individuals with recent onset of knee pain: 5-year follow-up in the CHECK cohort. *Osteoarthritis Cartilage* 2012; 20:548–56.

54. Holla JF, Steultjens MP, van der Leeden M, et al. Determinants of range of joint motion in patients with early symptomatic osteoarthritis of the hip and/or knee: an exploratory study in the CHECK cohort. *Osteoarthritis Cartilage* 2011; 19:411–9.

55. Agricola R, Waarsing JH, Thomas GE, et al. Cam impingement: defining the presence of a cam deformity by the alpha angle: data from the CHECK cohort and Chingford cohort. *Osteoarthritis Cartilage* 2014; 22:218–25.

56. Muraki S, Oka H, Akune T, et al. Association of occupational activity with joint space narrowing and osteophytosis in the medial compartment of the knee: the ROAD study. *Osteoarthritis Cartilage* 2011; 19:840–6.

57. Yoshimura N, Muraki S, Oka H, Kawaguchi H, Nakamura K, Akune T. Association of knee osteoarthritis with the accumulation of metabolic risk factors such as overweight, hypertension, dyslipidemia, and impaired glucose tolerance in Japanese men and women: the ROAD study. *J Rheumatol* 2011; 38:921–30.

58. Muraki S, Dennison E, Jameson K, et al. Association of vitamin D status with knee pain and radiographic knee osteoarthritis. *Osteoarthritis Cartilage* 2011; 19:1301–6.

59. Yoshimura N, Muraki S, Oka H, et al. Accumulation of metabolic risk factors such as overweight, hypertension, dyslipidaemia, and impaired glucose tolerance raises the risk of occurrence and progression of knee osteoarthritis: a 3-year follow-up of the ROAD study. *Osteoarthritis Cartilage* 2012; 20:1217–26.

60. Pothuaud L, Benhamou CL, Porion P, et al. Fractal dimension of trabecular bone projection texture is related to three-dimensional microarchitecture. *J Bone Miner Res* 2000; 15:691–9.

61. Apostol L, Boudousq V, Basset O, et al. Relevance of 2D radiographic texture analysis for the assessment of 3D bone micro-architecture. *Med Phys* 2006; 33:3546–56.

62. Kraus VB, Feng S, Wang S, et al. Trabecular morphometry by fractal signature analysis is a novel marker of osteoarthritis progression. *Arthritis Rheum* 2009; 60:3711–22.

63. Dobbins JT, 3rd, McAdams HP. Chest tomosynthesis: technical principles and clinical update. *Eur J Radiol* 2009; 72:244–51.

64. Stevens GM, Birdwell RL, Beaulieu CF, Ikeda DM, Pelc NJ. Circular tomosynthesis: potential in imaging of breast and upper cervical spine—preliminary phantom and in vitro study. *Radiology* 2003; 228:569–75.

65. Canella C, Philippe P, Pansini V, et al. Use of tomosynthesis for erosion evaluation in rheumatoid arthritic hands and wrists. *Radiology* 2011; 258:199–205.

66. Duryea J, Dobbins JT, Lynch JA. Digital tomosynthesis of hand joints for arthritis assessment. *Med Phys* 2003; 30:325–33.

67. Hayashi D, Xu L, Roemer FW, et al. Detection of osteophytes and subchondral cysts in the knee with use of tomosynthesis. *Radiology* 2012; 263:206–15.

68. Hayashi D, Xu L, Gusenburg J, et al. Reliability of semiquantitative assessment of osteophytes and subchondral cysts on tomosynthesis images by radiologists with different levels of expertise. *Diagn Interv Radiol* 2014; 20:353–9.

69. Kalinosky B, Sabol JM, Piacsek K, et al. Quantifying the tibiofemoral joint space using x-ray tomosynthesis. *Med Phys* 2011; 38:6672–82.

70. Florea C, Malo MK, Rautiainen J, et al. Alterations in subchondral bone plate, trabecular bone and articular cartilage properties of rabbit femoral condyles at 4 weeks after anterior cruciate ligament transaction. *Osteoarthritis Cartilage* 2015; 23(3):414–22.

71. Intema F, Hazewinkel HA, Gouwens D, et al. In early OA, thinning of the subchondral plate is directly related to cartilage damage: results from a canine ACLT-meniscectomy model. *Osteoarthritis Cartilage* 2010; 18:691–8.

72. Hechelhammer L, Pfirmann CW, Zanetti M, et al. Imaging findings predicting the outcome of cervical facet joint blocks. *Eur Radiol* 2007; 17:959–64.

73. Kalichman L, Li L, Kim DH, et al. Facet joint osteoarthritis and low back pain in the community-based population. *Spine* 2008; 33:2560–5.

74. Kalichman L, Kim DH, Li L, et al. Computed tomography evaluated features of spinal degeneration: prevalence, intercorrelation, and association with self-reported low back pain. *Spine* 2010; 10:200–8.

75. Suri P, Katz JN, Rainville J, et al. Vascular disease is associated with facet joint osteoarthritis. *Osteoarthritis Cartilage* 2010; 18:1127–32.

76. Kalichman L, Guermazi A, Li L, et al. Association between age, sex, BMI and CT-evaluated spinal degeneration features. *J Back Musculoskelet Rehabil* 2009; 22:189–95.

77. Kim JS, Kroin JS, Buvanendran A, et al. Characterization of a new animal model for evaluation and treatment of back pain due to lumbar facet joint osteoarthritis. *Arthritis Rheum* 2011; 63:2966–73.

78. Omoumi P, Mercier GA, Lecouvet F, et al. CT arthrography, MR arthrography, PET and scintigraphy in osteoarthritis. *Radiol Clin North Am* 2009; 47:595–615.

79. Hall FM, Goldberg RP, Wyshak G, et al. Shoulder arthrography: comparison of morbidity after use of various contrast media. *Radiology* 1985; 154:339–41.

80. Berquist TH. Imaging of articular pathology: MRI, CT, arthrography. *Clin Anat* 1997; 10:1–13.

81. El-Khoury GY, Alliman KJ, Lundberg HJ, et al. Cartilage thickness in cadaveric ankles: measurement with double-contrast multi-detector row CT arthrography versus MR imaging. *Radiology* 2004; 233:768–73.

82. Wyler A, Bousson V, Bergot C, et al. Hyaline cartilage thickness in radiographically normal cadaveric hips: comparison of spiral CT arthrographic and macroscopic measurements. *Radiology* 2007; 242:441–9.

83. Wyler A, Bousson V, Bergot C, et al. Comparison of MR-arthrography and CT arthrography in hyaline cartilage-thickness measurement in radiographically normal cadaver hips with anatomy as gold standard. *Osteoarthritis Cartilage* 2009; 17:19–25.

84. Schmid MR, Pfirrmann CW, Hodler J, et al. Cartilage lesions in the ankle joint: comparison of MR arthrography and CT arthrography. *Skeletal Radiol* 2003; 32:259–65.

85. McCauley TR, Kornaat PR, Jee WH. Central osteophytes in the knee: prevalence and association with cartilage defects on MR imaging. *AJR Am J Roentgenol* 2001; 176:359–64.

86. Kraniotis P, Maragkos S, Tyllianakis M, et al. Ankle posttraumatic osteoarthritis: a CT arthrography study in patients with bi- and tri-malleolar fractures. *Skeletal Radiol* 2012; 41:803–9.

87. Tamura S, Nishii T, Shiomi T, et al. Three-dimensional patterns of early acetabular cartilage damage in hip dysplasia; a high-resolutional CT arthrography study. *Osteoarthritis Cartilage* 2012; 20:646–52.

88. Omoumi P, Michoux N, Thienpont E, Roemer FW, Vande Berg BC. Anatomical distribution of areas of preserved cartilage in advanced femorotibial osteoarthritis using CT arthrography (Part 1). *Osteoarthritis Cartilage* 2015; 23:83–7.

89. Omoumi P, Michoux N, Roemer FW, Thienpont E, Vande Berg BC. Cartilage thickness at the posterior medial femoral condyle is increased in femorotibial knee osteoarthritis: a cross-sectional CT arthrography study (Part 2). *Osteoarthritis Cartilage* 2015; 23:224–31.

90. Eckstein F, Wirth W, Nevitt MC. Recent advances in osteoarthritis imaging-the Osteoarthritis Initiative. *Nat Rev Rheumatol* 2012; 8:622–30.

91. Hayashi D, Guermazi A, Hunter DJ. Osteoarthritis year 2010 in review: imaging. *Osteoarthritis Cartilage* 2011; 19:354–60.

92. Hayashi D, Roemer FW, Guermazi A. Osteoarthritis year 2011 in review: imaging in OA—a radiologists' perspective. *Osteoarthritis Cartilage* 2012; 20:207–14.

93. Roemer FW, Guermazi A. Osteoarthritis year 2012 in review: imaging. *Osteoarthritis Cartilage* 2012; 20:1440–6.

94. Mosher TJ, Walker EA, Petscavage-Thomas J, Guermazi A. Osteoarthritis year 2013 in review: imaging. *Osteoarthritis Cartilage* 2013; 21:1425–35.

95. Roemer FW, Guermazi A. Osteoarthritis year in review 2014: imaging. *Osteoarthritis Cartilage* 2014; 22:2003–12.

CHAPTER 17

Ultrasound in osteoarthritis and crystal-related arthropathies

Walter Grassi, Tadashi Okano, and Emilio Filippucci

Introduction

Ultrasonography (US) is a safe and cheap imaging technique which in experienced hands allows for a multiplanar and multisite high-resolution assessment of both morphological and structural features of bone, cartilage, and intra- or periarticular soft tissues [1].

In daily clinical practice, conventional radiography is the standard imaging modality for assessing osteoarthritis (OA). However, it has low sensitivity for detecting early cartilage changes because it cannot provide a direct visualization of the joint cartilage [2]. US offers new insights to help in a better understanding of the cartilage status [3]. Moreover, US allows sensitive detection of several pathological changes in patients with OA including joint effusion, synovial hypertrophy, osteophyte formation, and meniscal protrusion.

Crystal identification using polarized light microscopy is the gold standard for the diagnosis of crystal-related arthropathies. Nevertheless, in the latest recommendations for the diagnosis and management of gout and calcium pyrophosphate dihydrate crystal deposition (CPPD) disease, the diagnostic potential of advanced imaging techniques, including US, has been recognized [4,5]. The potential applications of US in the management of patients with OA and crystal-related arthropathies are not only limited to diagnosis and monitoring.

A number of pilot studies have shown that the use of US as a guide for correct needle placement may increase the rate of successful aspiration of synovial fluid and visualize the spreading of the glucocorticoid or hyaluronic acid at the target area.

Osteoarthritis

Imaging plays a key role for diagnosis, prognosis, and follow-up in patients with OA. Although conventional X-ray is still the gold standard imaging technique in daily clinical practice, US has been revealed to be capable of detecting a wide spectrum of otherwise undetectable details. These include the following:

- Visualization of the chondrosynovial interface
- Analysis of cartilage echo-texture
- Quantitative assessment of cartilage thickness
- Visualization of bone–cartilage interface
- Detection of early/small osteophytes not visible on X-ray
- Detection of meniscal protrusion
- Visualization of fluid collection

- Highly sensitive depiction of inflammatory flares
- Guidance for aspiration and/or injection
- Short-term safe and cheap monitoring of tissue damage.

Joint damage in osteoarthritis

Joint space narrowing, subchondral osteosclerosis, osteophytes, and geodes are the most characteristic radiographic features of OA. However, conventional radiography is limited by its inability to directly visualize hyaline cartilage and menisci. Moreover, osteophytes that are placed perpendicularly to the X-ray beam are poorly detectable on plain radiography. Conversely, multiplanar US imaging acquisition allows for direct visualization of hyaline cartilage and 'hidden' osteophytes.

Hyaline cartilage involvement

Normal articular hyaline cartilage has characteristic US features (Figure 17.1a–c). It is bounded by an outer, well-defined chondrosynovial margin which is thinner than its equally sharp, deeper osteochondral counterpart. The echotexture is homogeneously anechoic or hypoechoic depending on the level of gain. The thickness of articular cartilage varies according to the size of the joint (0.1 mm at the head

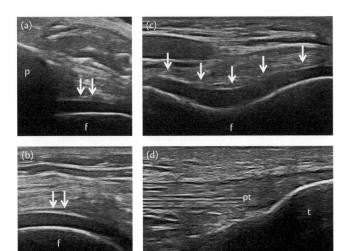

Figure 17.1 Healthy cartilage and tendon. (a–c) Normal femoral cartilage. White arrows show hyperechoic chondrosynovial margin in medial parapatellar transverse (a), longitudinal (b) and suprapatellar transverse (c) scans. Normal patellar tendon on longitudinal scan (d). f, femur; p, patella; pt, patella tendon; t, tibia.

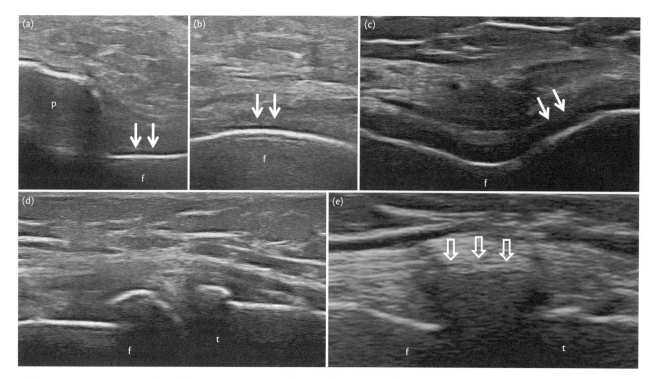

Figure 17.2 Joint damage in osteoarthritis. (a, b) Cartilage is almost lost (white arrows) in patient with severe OA in medial para-patellar transverse (a) and longitudinal (b) views. (c) Supra-patellar transverse scan shows cartilage damage of anteromedial femoral cartilage. (d) Medial longitudinal view shows osteophytes at both femur and tibia level. (e) A representative example of medial meniscal protrusion (open arrows) depicted using the medial longitudinal view. f, femur; p, patella; t, tibia.

of the middle phalanx to 2.6 mm at the medial femoral condyle) [6,7]. A wide spectrum of US changes can be detected in OA. The earliest structural changes seen with US include loss of the sharp definition of the chondrosynovial margin and microcleft formation. In more advanced stages of OA, US can detect the loss of the transparency together with thinning of cartilaginous layer (Figure 17.2a–c) [8]. The agreement between US and histological measurements of femoral cartilage thickness was found to be high, with the intraclass correlation coefficient ranging from 0.73 to 0.88 [9].

Osteophytes

Osteophytes can be considered one of the characteristic features of OA, detectable on conventional radiography at the joint margins. US can explore the bone surface and osteophytes appear as irregularities of the bony contour at the edge of the articular surface. There is evidence to support that US is more sensitive than conventional radiography in the detection of osteophytes [10]. The multiplanar capability and the high resolution can explain the higher sensitivity of US in the detection of osteophytes (Figure 17.2d).

Meniscal involvement

Meniscal subluxation is a prominent feature of knee OA and the presence of meniscal subluxation may affect proper meniscal function [11] (Figure 17.2e). US is able to assess the superficial portion of the meniscus in the supine non-weight-bearing position and also in the standing weight-bearing knees. A study using US to assess the subluxation of meniscus in the supine and weight-bearing positions showed that the medial meniscus was significantly displaced radially by weight bearing in control knees and in knees with Kellgren–Lawrence grades 1–3 [12]. Moreover, Malas et al. compared US meniscal bulging measurements and Kellgren–Lawrence radiographic grade and they found a positive correlation [13]. These results demonstrate that joint space

narrowing is often found to be secondary to meniscal bulging rather than loss of hyaline cartilage (Figure 17.3a–c). In order to correctly assess the damage of hyaline cartilage in knee OA, the assessment of menisci is important and US is able to visualize separately both hyaline cartilage and meniscal involvement.

Joint inflammation in osteoarthritis

The traditional X ray-based morphological assessment of OA is focused on bony changes that are characteristic of the established

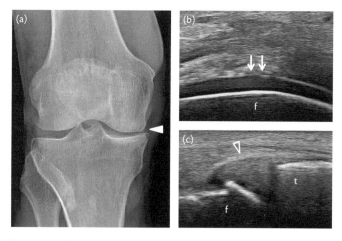

Figure 17.3 Discrepancy between radiographic and ultrasonographic findings. (a) Radiographic image shows definite joint space narrowing (white arrow head). (b) US image obtained in medial para-patellar view shows more than 2mm thick cartilage (white arrows) (c) The reason of joint space narrowing in radiograph is considered due to meniscal protrusion (open arrow head) as detected in medial longitudinal view by US. f, femur; t, tibia.

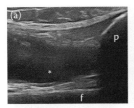 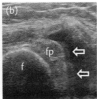 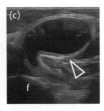

Figure 17.4 Joint inflammation in osteoarthritis. (a, b) Joint effusion (*) and proliferative synovitis (open arrows) of the knee in supra-patellar longitudinal (a) and transverse (b) scans. Proliferative synovial tissue is hypo-echoic with respect to fat pad. (c) Transverse posterior scan of the knee shows Baker's cyst (open arrow head). f, femur; fp, fat pad; p, patella.

disease. However, the spectrum of pathological changes in OA joints is consistently wider, also including fluid collection and synovial hypertrophy with or without increased blood perfusion. The detection of an even mild synovitis may be clinically relevant because it can affect the rate of both cartilage and bone damage. Thus, especially for a better understanding of the early disease, a careful evaluation of the joint cavity is required. US allows the detection of fluid collection and synovial hypertrophy that are related to the inflammatory flares in OA patients. This kind of information may affect the clinical decision-making process regarding the best tailored strategy of treatment.

Joint effusion

US is able to depict even minimal joint effusion, most commonly in the knee joint [14] (Figure 17.4a, b). US detected joint effusion in 55% of the symptomatic knees and 22% of the asymptomatic knees [15]. Typically the fluid is anechoic in OA, but it may appear inhomogeneous with particulate matter which may be due to proteinaceous material, debris, or calcified fragments [8].

Synovial hypertrophy

Synovial hypertrophy can be assessed as hypoechoic synovial hypertrophy in grey-scale mode (Figure 17.4b) and synovial hyperaemia can be detected and scored using power Doppler scanning methods. Both grey-scale and power Doppler mode were used for semi-quantitative scoring of hand OA features, but less commonly for knee OA. A good reliability for semi-quantitative US assessment of hand and knee OA was reported [16,17]. Klauser and colleagues used semi-quantitative assessment of synovial hyperemia (0–3 scale) by power-Doppler US to assess the efficacy of intra-articular hyaluronic acid injection in patients with hand OA [18]. This study demonstrated a correlation between a decrease in power Doppler score for hyperaemia and reduction in pain during the 4-week follow-up period.

Wu and colleagues investigated the association of US features with pain and the functional scores in patients with equal radiographic grades of OA in both knees [19]. US inflammatory features, including suprapatellar effusion and medial compartment synovitis, were positively and linearly associated with knee pain in motion. The severity of medial compartment synovitis was also associated with the degree of pain at rest and with the presence of medial knee pain. Moreover, Kortekaas and colleagues showed that signs of inflammation appear more frequently on US in patients with erosive hand OA than in those without erosive OA, not only in joints with erosive disease but also in those without bone erosions [20]. US-detected synovitis in patients with hand OA was associated with more severe radiological damage and reduced cartilage thickness [21].

Baker's cyst

Baker's cyst is a common finding in patients with knee OA (Figure 17.4c). It can induce some complications such as calf swelling, pseudo-thrombophlebitis, compartment syndrome, or pain. A Baker's cyst has been detected in 25% of the symptomatic knees and in 5% of the asymptomatic knees of patients with OA [15]. Clinical examination of the popliteal fossa doesn't allow a careful detection of Baker's cysts compared to US examination in subjects without knee pain [22].

Crystal-related arthropathies

Several recent investigations have shown that US can be considered a sensitive imaging technique to detect both monosodium urate (MSU) and pyrophosphate crystal aggregates. A wide spectrum of US findings may be detectable in patients with crystal-proven arthropathies including double-contour sign (Figure 17.5a), intra-articular sand-like crystals of uric acid (Figure 17.5c), intracartilaginous deposits (Figure 17.6b,c), intratendinous crystal clouds (Figures 17.5d and 17.6e), intra-articular, and/or intratendinous multiple hyperechoic dots (Figures 17.5c and 17.7a,b) [23–26]. In experienced hands, such US findings may change the standard diagnostic approach in patients with suspicion of crystal-related arthropathies.

The relevant diagnostic potential of US in detecting microcrystal arthropathies depends on the following characteristics:

- High-resolution power (<0.1 mm) at superficial tissues (targets not deeper than 1 cm)
- Multisite and multitissue assessment which allows for a quick panoramic view of the crystal deposits distribution
- Real-time imaging providing a safe guidance for the aspiration of even minimal synovial fluid collections
- Careful short-term monitoring of the tophi size in patients undertaking urate-lowering therapy.

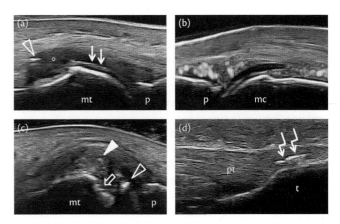

Figure 17.5 Gout. (a) Metatarsophalangeal joint on dorsal longitudinal scan shows double contour sign at the metatarsal head (white arrows) and hyperechoic bands generating acoustic shadows (open arrow head) in the dense fluid, urate sand (circle). (b) Acute gout attack in metacarpophalangeal joint on dorsal longitudinal scan. Note the intense intra-articular power Doppler signal. (c) Tophaceous deposits without (white arrow head) and with (open arrow head) posterior acoustic shadowing. Open white arrow indicates erosive changes of the metatarsal bone. (d) Patellar tendon on longitudinal scan showing MSU deposits appearing as subtle hyper-echoic lines (broken arrows). mc, metacarpal bone; mt, metatarsal bone; p, proximal phalanx; pt, patellar tendon; t, tibia.

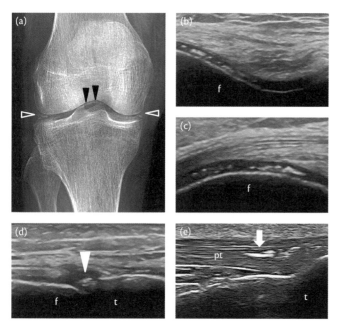

Figure 17.6 CPPD crystal deposition disease in the knee. (a) Conventional radiography showing meniscal calcifications (open arrowheads) and calcification of femoral hyaline cartilage (black arrowheads). Supra-patellar transverse (b) and longitudinal (c) scans showing hyper-echoic linear spots not generating acoustic shadowing, located within the hyaline cartilage of the lateral femoral condyle. (d) Calcified medial meniscus appears as homogeneously hyperechoic without acoustic shadowing (white arrowhead) on medial longitudinal scan. (e) Patellar tendon on longitudinal scan showing CPPD crystal deposition appearing as subtle hyper-echoic lines and spots (white arrow). f, femur: pt, patellar tendon; t, tibia.

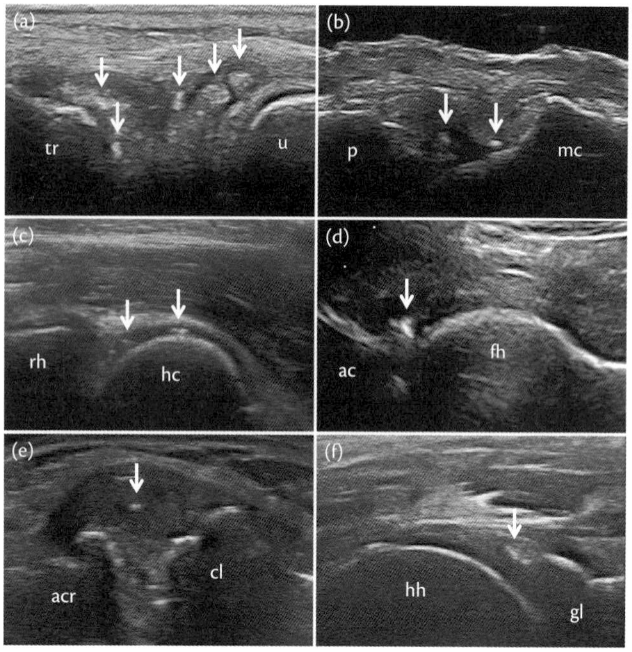

Figure 17.7 CPPD disease. (a–f) CPPD crystals can be detected in anatomic sites (white arrows). (a) Triangular fibrocartilage complex of the wrist. (b) Medial aspect of metacarpophalangeal joint. (c) Hyaline cartilage of elbow humeral capitellum. (d) Anterior acetabular labrum of hip joint. (e) Acromioclavicular joint. (f) Posterior glenoid labrum of glenohumeral joint. ac, acetabulum; acr, acromion; cl, clavicle; fh, femoral head; gl, glenoid; hc, humeral capitellum; hh, humeral head; mc, metacarpal bone; p, proximal phalanx; rh, radial head; tr, triquetrum; u, ulna.

Gout

Gout is a common disease caused by MSU crystal deposition, which is a consequence of the degree and duration of chronic hyperuricaemia [27]. Suspicion of gout is based on its typical clinical symptom (recurrent podagra) and laboratory findings (hyperuricaemia), while definitive diagnosis requires identification of MSU crystals in aspirated synovial fluid or tophi [28]. This procedure is easy to carry out in joints with inflammation during acute gout attacks or chronic gouty arthritis, but may not be feasible in joints without inflammation during intercritical periods.

US can show a wide spectrum of findings in patients with gout including fluid collection, joint cavity widening, peri- and intra-articular Doppler signal, and soft tissue oedema [29–33] (see also Chapter 43). Moreover, even in patients at their first attack, the sonographic features of the synovial fluid may be strongly evocative of gout, because of the high reflectivity of the MSU crystal aggregates that can be easily identified (Figure 17.5c). In patients with acute gouty arthritis, the Doppler signal may be highly intense both inside and around joints. Nevertheless, the Doppler signal is not directly related to symptoms being detectable also in asymptomatic joints with MSU crystal deposition.

Joint involvement

The double-contour sign is one of the most specific US findings in patients with gout (Figure 17.5a). It is generated by a homogenous linear deposition of crystal aggregates on the chondrosynovial interface of the hyaline cartilage. Naredo et al. reported a typical double-contour sign in 74.7% patients with gout [32]. A meta-analysis has

revealed that the pooled (95% confidence interval) sensitivity and specificity of the double-contour sign on US were 0.83 (0.72–0.91) and 0.76 (0.68–0.83), respectively [34]. Intra- and periarticular Doppler signal is always well evident during the acute attack (Figure 17.5b). It is not directly related to symptoms being detectable also in asymptomatic joints.

Figure 17.5c shows some representative examples of intra-articular MSU crystal aggregates that appear as hyperechoic dots. The broad spectrum of synovial fluid features in patients with acute gout may range from homogenous anechogenicity to a fully foggy echogenic material including multiple hyperechoic spots of various shape and size with or without posterior acoustic shadow.

Bone erosions are common, especially in patients with long-standing disease [35–37] (Figure 17.5c). In patients with gout, bone erosions may show some features that make them characteristic, such as microtophaceous aggregates inside the erosions (shining dots) and their shape and distribution.

Tophaceous gout is conventionally defined by the presence of tophi that are large enough to be visible on clinical examination. Tophi are traditionally regarded as a late clinical manifestation indicating a transition from acute intermittent gout to the chronic phase of the disease. US reveals the presence of tophi in unaffected first metatarsophalangeal (MTP) joints of patients with gout with a prevalence ranging from 27% to 42% [29,33]. Pineda et al. found intra-articular tophi in 16% of subjects with asymptomatic hyperuricaemia [38]. These preliminary data strongly suggest scanning the first MTP joints in all patients with suspected gout. US examination of the first MTP joint is feasible and fast, requiring no more than a few minutes.

Tendon involvement

Tendon involvement is frequent in gout (Figures 17.1d and 17.5d). Peri- and/or intratendinous MSU crystal aggregates of different size, shape, and echogenicity are frequently detectable in different anatomical regions. Patellar, triceps, and Achilles tendons are the most characteristic targets [32,39]. Intratendinous crystal aggregates may appear as isolated shining spots, clusters of punctate echoes (urate clouds), or large and compact depositions generating a posterior acoustic shadow. Their identification is easy because their presence deranges the typical fibrillary echotexture of the tendon. Most of them are asymptomatic at the moment of US examination. The main findings indicating acute gouty tendinopathy include focal hypoechoic thickening and intratendinous Doppler signal. Doppler signal has a variable distribution inside and outside the MSU aggregates. Intratendinous tophaceous deposition can be distinguished as 'cold' or 'hot' according to the absence or presence of surrounding Doppler signal. Tendinous tophi can be fully asymptomatic or may show spontaneous pain or pain on pressure.

Calcium pyrophosphate crystal deposition disease

Diagnosis of CPPD disease is generally based on the typical X-ray findings showing cartilage calcification (Figure 17.6a) or on the microscopic detection of CPPD crystals in the synovial fluid. A systematic study of the anatomical regions that could show CPPD crystal aggregates wouldn't be ethically acceptable using conventional radiography, while it is fast and easy to carry out by US. Moreover, there is a broad consensus among experts on considering US as a more sensitive diagnostic tool for CPPD disease than conventional radiography [40–42] (see also Chapter 51). Calcium pyrophosphate crystal deposits can be typically detected in the hyaline and meniscal fibrocartilage of the knee (Figure 17.6b–d), triangular fibrocartilage complex of the wrist (Figure 17.7a), and also in many other asymptomatic joints, including metacarpophalangeal joint (Figure 17.7b), elbow (Figure 17.7c), and hip (Figure 17.7d) [43–45]. The shoulder should also be regarded as another target area to scan in patients with CPPD disease (Figure 17.7e,f) [46].

Cartilage involvement

Hyaline cartilage is best assessed by US at the knee level where a wide portion of the femoral condyles can be easily scanned. Crystal deposits appear as hyperechoic spots or dots which may be isolated or aggregated in clusters, typically without acoustic shadowing and usually located in the middle third of the cartilage layer (Figure 17.6b,c). Such a distribution of the crystal aggregates differs from that of the MSU deposits which are on the cartilage surface [47]. Other anatomical sites where the hyaline cartilage can be explored by US include the humeral head, the humeral trochlea and capitellum, and the radial head at the elbow level, the metacarpal head, the femoral head, and the talus at the ankle joint.

Meniscal fibrocartilage is the most frequent anatomical target of CPPD disease. Crystal deposits appear as isolate or multiple hyperechoic spots usually not generating acoustic shadowing (Figure 17.6d). Meniscal calcification was found highly prevalent in patients with CPPD disease, being detected by US in at least one knee in 41 out of 42 patients [48]. Calcium pyrophosphate crystal aggregates can also be easily detected in the triangular fibrocartilage complex of the wrist and in the fibrocartilage of the acromion-clavicular joint [44].

Calcium pyrophosphate crystal aggregates are usually easy to detect. However, they must be distinguished from the MSU aggregates, osteochondral debris, and intra-articular air. While the detection of hyperechoic spots within the synovial fluid does not allow for a definite diagnosis, the typical calcified clouds at either the carpal triangular fibrocartilage complex or the knee menisci and intracartilaginous hyperechoic spots should be regarded as highly specific evidence of CPPD disease [40,47,48].

Tendon involvement

Calcifications in tendons are also characteristic imaging features of CPPD disease (Figure 17.6e) [49–54]. US is able to easily access and accurately evaluate both the tendon and the enthesis. Calcium pyrophosphate crystals aggregates appear as hyperechoic bands and spots, generally without posterior acoustic shadow [23,25]. Tendon calcifications appear as typical linear deposits, often distributed along the major axis of the tendon [48]. Excellent agreement between US and radiography in detecting calcifications and enthesophyte was found in a study of Achilles tendon and plantar fascia in patients with CPPD disease [55]. Achilles tendon and plantar fascia calcifications are frequent US findings in patients with CPPD. The sensitivity of US for detection of calcifications in Achilles tendon and plantar fascia was 57.9% and 15.8%, respectively, and the specificity was 100% for both [56]. Thus, US shows a wider distribution of the crystal deposits than traditionally thought in CPPD disease as in gout. Non-invasive, quick examination of multiple anatomical areas by US allows a detailed mapping of topography of crystal deposition in patients with CPPD disease.

Sonographic-guided procedures

US-guided procedures such as aspiration of synovial fluid, biopsy, and intra-articular injection of various drugs may play a key role in the management of patients with OA and crystal-related arthropathies. These procedures are traditionally performed using external anatomical landmarks without imaging guidance in daily practice. However, this kind of approach is often unsuccessful, especially for some targets such as small joints or synovial sheaths. US guidance allows the real-time visualization of the needle moving through different tissues and reaching the target to aspirate and/or inject (Figure 17.8a–c).

The correct placement of the tip of the needle plays a key role in improving efficacy and reducing side effects of the injection [57–60]. Several studies have demonstrated that US-guided injection provides a greater accuracy of glucocorticoid placement (Figure 17.8d) with improvement of clinical outcome [61,62]. Moreover, US-guided procedures reduce the pain of the patients. Sibbit et al. have reported that US-guided injection resulted in a 43% reduction in procedural pain and 58.5% reduction in absolute pain scores at the 2-week outcome compared with conventional anatomical-guided injection [61].

The accuracy of US-guided injection and correspondingly better clinical outcomes may also provide cost-effectiveness. Sibbit et al. found that US-guided injections modestly reduced the cost per patient per year by 8% relative to anatomical guidance [63]. More importantly, US guidance significantly reduced the cost per responder per year by 33% (p < 0.001). In their follow-up study, US-guided procedures reduced the costs of treating outpatients by 13%, particularly in responders by 58% [64].

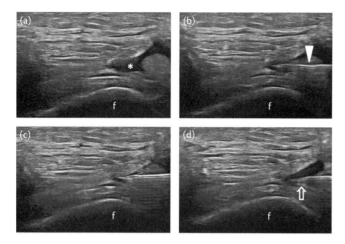

Figure 17.8 Sonographic guided procedures. (a) Joint effusion (*) of the knee in supra-patellar transverse scan. (b) The needle (arrowhead) is correctly placed at the target. (c) Joint effusion is completely aspirated. (d) Injection of the glucocorticoid appearing as echogenic material (empty white arrow). f, femur.

Conclusion

The principal indications for using US in OA include the detection of articular hyaline cartilage damage and the demonstration of synovial and adjacent soft tissue pathology. The great advantage of US is the direct visualization of the joint cartilage rather than a crude estimation of the possible cartilage thickness by radiographic measurements of joint space width. Moreover, multiplanar exploration allows a careful detection of even small and otherwise invisible osteophytes. US is also helpful for a better assessment of the joint because of its ability to show meniscal involvement and inflammatory changes including joint effusion, synovial hypertrophy, power Doppler technique, and Baker's cysts. US has also been proposed as a possible tool for monitoring the progression of OA.

US has demonstrated a relevant diagnostic potential in crystal-related arthropathies. The detection of highly evocative signs of gout and CPPD disease in asymptomatic subjects or in patients with equivocal clinical findings may have a deep impact on clinical decision-making processes, narrowing the differential diagnostic spectrum and avoiding other time-consuming and expensive diagnostic procedures. US differential diagnosis between gout and CPPD disease is based on the characteristics of crystal aggregates and their preferential localization in different anatomical areas. The double-contour sign is a highly specific finding for gout as well as the hyperechoic spots within the hyaline cartilage for CPPD disease.

Finally, US-guided procedures notably improve injection accuracy in the target intra- and periarticular joint space, even in small joints.

References

1. Grassi W, Cervini C. Ultrasonography in rheumatology: an evolving technique. *Ann Rheum Dis* 1998; 57(5):268–71.
2. Wang Y, Wluka AE, Jones G, Ding C, Cicuttini FM. Use magnetic resonance imaging to assess articular cartilage. *Ther Adv Musculoskelet Dis* 2012; 4(2):77–97.
3. Wick MC, Kastlunger M, Weiss RJ. Clinical imaging assessments of knee osteoarthritis in the elderly: a mini-review. *Gerontology* 2014; 60(5):386–94.
4. Sivera F, Andrés M, Carmona L, et al. Multinational evidence-based recommendations for the diagnosis and management of gout: integrating systematic literature review and expert opinion of a broad panel of rheumatologists in the 3e initiative. *Ann Rheum Dis* 2014; 73(2):328–35.
5. Zhang W, Doherty M, Bardin T, et al. European League Against Rheumatism recommendations for calcium pyrophosphate deposition. Part I: terminology and diagnosis. *Ann Rheum Dis* 2011; 70(4):563–70.
6. Grassi W, Lamanna G, Farina A, Cervini C. Sonographic imaging of normal and osteoarthritic cartilage. *Semin Arthritis Rheum* 1999; 28(6):398–403.
7. Grassi W, Filippucci E, Farina A. Ultrasonography in osteoarthritis. *Semin Arthritis Rheum* 2005; 34(6 Suppl 2):19–23.
8. Meenagh G, Filippucci E, Iagnocco A, et al. Ultrasound imaging for the rheumatologist VIII. Ultrasound imaging in osteoarthritis. *Clin Exp Rheumatol* 2007; 25(2):172–5.
9. Naredo E, Acebes C, Möller I, et al. Ultrasound validity in the measurement of knee cartilage thickness. *Ann Rheum Dis* 2009; 68(8):1322–7.
10. Haugen IK, Bøyesen P. Imaging modalities in hand osteoarthritis—and perspectives of conventional radiography, magnetic resonance imaging, and ultrasonography. *Arthritis Res Ther* 2011; 13(6):248.
11. Ko CH, Chan KK, Peng HL. Sonographic imaging of meniscal subluxation in patients with radiographic knee osteoarthritis. *J Formos Med Assoc* 2007; 106(9):700–7.
12. Kawaguchi K, Enokida M, Otsuki R, Teshima R. Ultrasonographic evaluation of medial radial displacement of the medial meniscus in knee osteoarthritis. *Arthritis Rheum* 2012; 64(1):173–80.
13. Malas F, Kara M, Kaymak B, Akıncı A, Özçakar L. Ultrasonographic evaluation in symptomatic knee osteoarthritis: clinical and radiological correlation. *Int J Rheum Dis.* 2014; 17(5):536–40.
14. D'Agostino MA, Conaghan P, Le Bars M, et al. EULAR report on the use of ultrasonography in painful knee osteoarthritis. Part 1: prevalence of inflammation in osteoarthritis. *Ann Rheum Dis* 2005; 64(12):1703–9.
15. Eşen S, Akarırmak U, Aydın FY, Unalan H. Clinical evaluation during the acute exacerbation of knee osteoarthritis: the impact of diagnostic ultrasonography. *Rheumatol Int* 2013; 33(3):711–7.
16. Iagnocco A, Conaghan PG, Aegerter P, et al. The reliability of musculoskeletal ultrasound in the detection of cartilage abnormalities at the metacarpo-phalangeal joints. *Osteoarthritis Cartilage* 2012; 20(10):1142–6.
17. Iagnocco A, Perricone C, Scirocco C, et al. The interobserver reliability of ultrasound in knee osteoarthritis. *Rheumatology (Oxford)* 2012; 51(11):2013–9.
18. Klauser AS, Faschingbauer R, Kupferthaler K, et al. Sonographic criteria for therapy follow-up in the course of ultrasound-guided intra-articular injections of hyaluronic acid in hand osteoarthritis. *Eur J Radiol* 2012; 81(7):1607–11.
19. Wu PT, Shao CJ, Wu KC, et al. Pain in patients with equal radiographic grades of osteoarthritis in both knees: the value of gray scale ultrasound. *Osteoarthritis Cartilage* 2012; 20(12):1507–13.
20. Kortekaas MC, Kwok WY, Reijnierse M, Huizinga TW, Kloppenburg M. In erosive hand osteoarthritis more inflammatory signs on ultrasound are found than in the rest of hand osteoarthritis. *Ann Rheum Dis* 2013; 72(6):930–4.
21. Mancarella L, Magnani M, Addimanda O, et al. Ultrasound-detected synovitis with power Doppler signal is associated with severe radiographic damage and reduced cartilage thickness in hand osteoarthritis. *Osteoarthritis Cartilage* 2010; 18(10):1263–8.
22. Akgul O, Guldeste Z, Ozgocmen S. The reliability of the clinical examination for detecting Baker's cyst in asymptomatic fossa. *Int J Rheum Dis.* 2014; 17(2):204–9.
23. Grassi W, Meenagh G, Pascual E, Filippucci E. 'Crystal clear'-sonographic assessment of gout and calcium pyrophosphate deposition disease. *Semin Arthritis Rheum* 2006; 36(3):197–202.
24. Thiele RG, Schlesinger N. Diagnosis of gout by ultrasound. *Rheumatology (Oxford)* 2007; 46(7):1116–21.
25. Frediani B, Filippou G, Falsetti P, et al. Diagnosis of calcium pyrophosphate dihydrate crystal deposition disease: ultrasonographic criteria proposed. *Ann Rheum Dis* 2005; 64(4):638–40.

26. Filippucci E, Di Geso L, Girolimetti R, Grassi W. Ultrasound in crystal-related arthritis. *Clin Exp Rheumatol* 2014; 32(1 Suppl 80):S42–7.

27. Richette P, Bardin T. Gout. *Lancet* 2010; 375(9711):318–28.

28. Zhang W, Doherty M, Pascual E, et al. EULAR evidence based recommendations for gout. Part I: Diagnosis. Report of a task force of the Standing Committee for International Clinical Studies Including Therapeutics (ESCISIT). *Ann Rheum Dis* 2006; 65(10):1301–11.

29. Howard RG, Pillinger MH, Gyftopoulos S, et al. Reproducibility of musculoskeletal ultrasound for determining monosodium urate deposition: concordance between readers. *Arthritis Care Res (Hoboken)* 2011; 63(10):1456–62.

30. Schueller-Weidekamm C, Schueller G, et al. Impact of sonography in gouty arthritis: comparison with conventional radiography, clinical examination, and laboratory findings. *Eur J Radiol* 2007; 62(3):437–43.

31. Filippucci E, Meenagh G, Delle Sedie A, et al. Ultrasound imaging for the rheumatologist XXXVI. Sonographic assessment of the foot in gout patients. *Clin Exp Rheumatol* 2011; 29(6):901–5.

32. Naredo E, Uson J, Jiménez-Palop M, et al. Ultrasound-detected musculoskeletal urate crystal deposition: which joints and what findings should be assessed for diagnosing gout? *Ann Rheum Dis* 2014; 73(8):1522–8.

33. Lamers-Karnebeek FB, Van Riel PL, Jansen TL. Additive value for ultrasonographic signal in a screening algorithm for patients presenting with acute mono-/oligoarthritis in whom gout is suspected. *Clin Rheumatol* 2014; 33(4):555–9.

34. Ogdie A, Taylor WJ, Weatherall M, et al. Imaging modalities for the classification of gout: systematic literature review and meta-analysis. *Ann Rheum Dis* 2015; 74(10):1868–74.

35. Carter JD, Kedar RP, Anderson SR, et al. An analysis of MRI and ultrasound imaging in patients with gout who have normal plain radiographs. *Rheumatology (Oxford)* 2009; 48(11):1442–6.

36. Rettenbacher T, Ennemoser S, Weirich H, et al. Diagnostic imaging of gout: comparison of high-resolution US versus conventional X-ray. *Eur Radiol* 2008; 18(3):621–30.

37. Wright SA, Filippucci E, McVeigh C, et al. High-resolution ultrasonography of the first metatarsal phalangeal joint in gout: a controlled study. *Ann Rheum Dis* 2007; 66(7):859–64.

38. Pineda C, Amezcua-Guerra LM, Solano C, et al. Joint and tendon subclinical involvement suggestive of gouty arthritis in asymptomatic hyperuricemia: an ultrasound controlled study. *Arthritis Res Ther* 2011; 13(1):R4.

39. de Ávila Fernandes E, Kubota ES, Sandim GB, et al. Ultrasound features of tophi in chronic tophaceous gout. *Skeletal Radiol* 2011; 40(3):309–15.

40. Filippucci E, Scirè CA, Delle Sedie A, et al. Ultrasound imaging for the rheumatologist. XXV. Sonographic assessment of the knee in patients with gout and calcium pyrophosphate deposition disease. *Clin Exp Rheumatol* 2010; 28(1):2–5.

41. Ellabban AS, Kamel SR, Omar HA, El-Sherif AM, Abdel-Magied RA. Ultrasonographic diagnosis of articular chondrocalcinosis. *Rheumatol Int* 2012; 32(12):3863–8.

42. Gutierrez M, Di Geso L, Filippucci E, Grassi W. Calcium pyrophosphate crystals detected by ultrasound in patients without radiographic evidence of cartilage calcifications. *J Rheumatol* 2010; 37(12):2602–3.

43. Barskova VG, Kudaeva FM, Bozhieva LA, et al. Comparison of three imaging techniques in diagnosis of chondrocalcinosis of the knees in calcium pyrophosphate deposition disease. *Rheumatology (Oxford)* 2013; 52(6):1090–4.

44. Kellner H, Zoller W, Herzer P. [Ultrasound findings in chondrocalcinosis]. *Z Rheumatol* 1990; 49(3):147–50.

45. Di Geso L, Tardella M, Gutierrez M, Filippucci E, Grassi W. Crystal deposition at elbow hyaline cartilage: the sonographic perspective. *J Clin Rheumatol* 2011; 17(6):344–5.

46. Filippucci E, Delle Sedie A, Riente L, et al. Ultrasound imaging for the rheumatologist. XLVII. Ultrasound of the shoulder in patients with gout and calcium pyrophosphate deposition disease. *Clin Exp Rheumatol* 2013; 31(5):659–64.

47. Filippucci E, Riveros MG, Georgescu D, Salaffi F, Grassi W. Hyaline cartilage involvement in patients with gout and calcium pyrophosphate deposition disease. An ultrasound study. *Osteoarthritis Cartilage* 2009; 17(2):178–81.

48. Filippou G, Filippucci E, Tardella M, et al. Extent and distribution of CPP deposits in patients affected by calcium pyrophosphate dihydrate deposition disease: an ultrasonographic study. *Ann Rheum Dis* 2013; 72(11):1836–9.

49. Gerster JC, Baud CA, Lagier R, Boussina I, Fallet GH. Tendon calcifications in chondrocalcinosis. A clinical, radiologic, histologic, and crystallographic study. *Arthritis Rheum* 1977; 20(2):717–22.

50. Gerster JC, Lagier R, Boivin G. Achilles tendinitis associated with chondrocalcinosis. *J Rheumatol* 1980; 7(1):82–8.

51. Kanterewicz E, Sanmartí R, Pañella D, Brugués J. Tendon calcifications of the hip adductors in chondrocalcinosis: a radiological study of 75 patients. *Br J Rheumatol* 1993; 32(9):790–3.

52. Yang BY, Sartoris DJ, Resnick D, Clopton P. Calcium pyrophosphate dihydrate crystal deposition disease: frequency of tendon calcification about the knee. *J Rheumatol* 1996; 23(5):883–8.

53. Foldes K, Lenchik L, Jaovisidha S, et al. Association of gastrocnemius tendon calcification with chondrocalcinosis of the knee. *Skeletal Radiol* 1996; 25(7):621–4.

54. Pereira ER, Brown RR, Resnick D. Prevalence and patterns of tendon calcification in patients with chondrocalcinosis of the knee: radiologic study of 156 patients. *Clin Imaging* 1998; 22(5):371–5.

55. Falsetti P, Frediani B, Acciai C, et al. Ultrasonographic study of Achilles tendon and plantar fascia in chondrocalcinosis. *J Rheumatol* 2004; 31(11):2242–50.

56. Ellabban AS, Kamel SR, Abo Omar HA, El-Sherif AM, Abdel-Magied RA. Ultrasonographic findings of Achilles tendon and plantar fascia in patients with calcium pyrophosphate deposition disease. *Clin Rheumatol* 2012; 31(4):697–704.

57. Balint PV, Kane D, Hunter J, et al. Ultrasound guided versus conventional joint and soft tissue fluid aspiration in rheumatology practice: a pilot study. *J Rheumatol* 2002; 29(10):2209–13.

58. Raza K, Lee CY, Pilling D, et al. Ultrasound guidance allows accurate needle placement and aspiration from small joints in patients with early inflammatory arthritis. *Rheumatology (Oxford)* 2003; 42(8):976–9.

59. Cunnington J, Marshall N, Hide G, et al. A randomized, double-blind, controlled study of ultrasound-guided corticosteroid injection into the joint of patients with inflammatory arthritis. *Arthritis Rheum* 2010; 62(7):1862–9.

60. Di Geso L, Filippucci E, Meenagh G, et al. CS injection of tenosynovitis in patients with chronic inflammatory arthritis: the role of US. *Rheumatology (Oxford)* 2012; 51(7):1299–303.

61. Sibbitt WL, Peisajovich A, Michael AA, et al. Does sonographic needle guidance affect the clinical outcome of intraarticular injections? *J Rheumatol* 2009; 36(9):1892–902.

62. Iagnocco A, Naredo E. Ultrasound-guided corticosteroid injection in rheumatology: accuracy or efficacy? *Rheumatology (Oxford)* 2010; 49(8):1427–8.

63. Sibbitt WL, Band PA, Chavez-Chiang NR, et al. A randomized controlled trial of the cost-effectiveness of ultrasound-guided intraarticular injection of inflammatory arthritis. *J Rheumatol* 2011; 38(2):252–63.

64. Sibbitt WL, Band PA, Kettwich LG, et al. A randomized controlled trial evaluating the cost-effectiveness of sonographic guidance for intra-articular injection of the osteoarthritic knee. *J Clin Rheumatol* 2011; 17(8):409–15.

CHAPTER 18

Imaging: magnetic resonance imaging

David J. Hunter and Frank W. Roemer

Introduction

The attractiveness of magnetic resonance imaging (MRI) as an imaging modality lies in part in its capacity to overcome many of the limitations associated with conventional radiography—the technique historically regarded as the gold standard in imaging of osteoarthritis (OA). MRI allows visualization of changes and pathologies in all joint tissues including cartilage and the menisci, the two tissue components responsible for the indirect radiographic marker of joint space narrowing; decreasing the length of time that must elapse before disease progression can be detected on less sensitive imaging modalities. Other elements of the joint—such as synovium, ligaments, and subchondral bone—can also be analysed simultaneously: a key development in the understanding of OA as a whole-joint disease.

The multitude of different pulse sequences available today allow optimized visualization of the different tissue types involved in the disease process [1]. Two-dimensional (2D) or multisection T1-weighted, T2-weighted, proton density-weighted, fast or turbo spin-echo (FSE), and several gradient-recalled echo (GRE) imaging techniques are now in routine use, and have proven efficacy in the quantitative assessment of articular cartilage morphology [1,2]. Newer techniques—most notably three-dimensional (3D) spin-echo (SE) and GRE sequences including dual-echo steady-state (DESS)-type methods—are likely to increase the accuracy of cartilage morphology assessments. Potentially significant from the standpoint of investigating OA pathogenesis has been the development of techniques that are able to identify and monitor cartilage composition including T2 relaxometry (also termed T2 mapping), delayed gadolinium-enhanced MRI of cartilage (dGEMRIC), diffusion-weighted and T1rho imaging techniques, and others [3]. Similarly, the use of contrast-enhanced MRI has led to an increased ability to detect alterations in subchondral bone and synovium respectively, that may be involved in osteoarthritic changes [4].

MRI therefore provides an ideal non-invasive means to investigate OA pathogenesis and pathophysiology: baseline and longitudinal differences in morphology and composition in various joint tissues can be used to both measure and predict disease progression, as well as clinical outcomes such as pain and function, potentially providing the identification of early indicators or biomarkers of disease. Indeed, a number of quantitative and qualitative MRI features—such as bone marrow lesions (BMLs), synovitis, and subchondral bone attrition—have already been identified that may be associated with OA disease progression, and more biomarkers will undoubtedly be identified as more long-term data become available [5–7].

In addition to providing insight into disease pathophysiology, biomarkers would also be particularly useful as a means of assessing the efficacy of potential disease- and structure-modifying interventions in clinical trials. Future disease-modifying or disease-preventing interventions would ideally take place quite some time before the onset of symptoms when structural joint damage might potentially still be reversible, given the long time-course of OA progression. This preventative trial strategy would make the use of clinical outcomes such as pain practically difficult, as the required follow-up for these studies would be somewhere in the vicinity of 10–20 years. The capacity to assess the disease-modifying impact of an intervention using MRI biomarkers would drastically reduce the time frame required for clinical trials, decreasing the costs involved and likely increasing the attractiveness to the industry of investing in the development of disease-modifying interventions and running clinical trials.

Despite its evident utility as a research tool, the relevance of MRI in clinical practice in the context of OA assessment is somewhat less clear. A diagnosis of OA is established based on clinical manifestations of the disease and can be confirmed by radiography, but does not rely on MRI. During the disease course, MRI might be helpful to characterize joint structural changes further, particularly in order to rule out other differential diagnoses of potential therapeutic relevance (such as avascular necrosis, pigmented villonodular synovitis, and osteochondritis dissecans) in cases when clinical symptoms show worsening. Before there is more widespread adoption, a number of issues must still be addressed: MRI remains expensive relative to radiography, there is a lack of standardization with regards to MRI systems (with significant differences reported between phased array coils and quadrature, for example), no well-established criteria exist for the diagnosis of OA using MRI, acquisition time can be unacceptably long for clinical use in some cases (up to 2 hours for dGEMRIC images), and in the absence of approved disease-modifying therapy its clinical utility in changing management is limited [3,8–10]. It is for these reasons that MRI remains—for the time being—almost exclusively the domain of clinical research.

This review therefore focuses on the utility of MRI in observational studies and clinical trials, detailing the available MRI techniques and quantitative/qualitative measurements, and their correlation with tissue damage. The possible future directions of

MRI in OA will also be discussed, with a view to its potential utility in identifying disease-modifying interventions.

MRI acquisition techniques

Although used to visualize a range of tissues from subchondral bone to synovium, the MRI techniques currently used to investigate cartilage in OA are broadly separated into two categories: those that assess cartilage morphology (encompassing parameters such as volume and thickness, as well as characterization of different types of cartilage lesions), and those that evaluate components of its biochemical composition (usually by using a surrogate to identify collagen content, glycosaminoglycan content, isotropy, and/or hydration) [3].

Morphology

The imaging techniques most commonly used in the context of OA assessment are 2D FSE sequences: either T1 weighted, T2 weighted, or proton density weighted with the water-sensitive sequences usually being fat suppressed to allow differentiation of bone marrow changes and increase the contrast between articular cartilage and subchondral bone [3]. Two-dimensional FSE sequences are generally regarded as providing good signal-to-noise ratio (SNR) and tissue delineation, with significantly shorter acquisition times (and therefore fewer motion artefacts than conventional SE sequences) due to the additional 180° refocusing radiofrequency pulses applied per 90° radiofrequency excitation [11]. T1-weighted images have been shown to provide good visualization of hyaline cartilage, but poor contrast between synovium and the cartilage surface, as well as other joint structures such as ligaments and menisci [11,12]. T2-weighted images, however, give excellent synovium–cartilage contrast, but poor visualization of internal cartilage pathology [3,13]. It is for these reasons that many institutions utilize intermediate-weighted FSE sequences with a mixed proton density and T2 weighting—with an echo time (TE) of 33–60 ms—to combine the synovial fluid–cartilage contrast associated with T2 weighting with improved internal cartilage signal, whilst avoiding the 'magic angle' effects that are problematic in proton density-weighted images [1,2]. Fat-suppression techniques are also often used in order to improve the subchondral bone-cartilage contrast. Fat saturation, the most commonly used technique, has been shown to increase the cartilage–bone contrast, but lengthens acquisition time and is susceptible to interference from objects such as metallic screws—clearly a common issue in imaging of the knee [14]. The recently developed IDEAL (iterative decomposition of water and fat with echo asymmetry and least squares estimation) and long-established STIR (short inversion time inversion recovery) techniques represent considerable improvements on standard fat saturation methods, with both techniques capable of obtaining good fat–water differentiation in the presence of magnetic field inhomogeneities [15,16].

Although FSE techniques show excellent sensitivity in the identification of cartilage lesions, the fact that they involve relatively thick slices and gaps between slices makes quantification of cartilage volume, a commonly applied strategy in OA research, particularly difficult [1,17,18]. Three-dimensional techniques are therefore quite attractive for segmentation and quantitative analysis, and 3D intermediate-weighted FSE sequences have recently gained increased usage in clinical assessment or scoring approaches [3].

Preliminary evidence suggests that 3D and multiplanar 2D intermediate-weighted FSE sequences provide similar accuracy for the evaluation of lesions of the articular cartilage and other knee tissues, though 3D methods may provide better quantification of cartilage volume and thickness [19,20].

Three-dimensional GRE sequences have the disadvantage of providing poor visualization of subchondral bone, making it difficult to determine the full extent of cartilage lesions, but are generally viewed as providing superior images of the cartilage surface [21,22]. Three-dimensional spoiled gradient-echo (SPGR) sequences make use of semi-random radiofrequency phase alterations to obtain high spatial resolution images that are ideal for the quantitative assessment of cartilage morphology using segmentation [18]. This ability to reliably quantify segmental cartilage changes makes SPGR a good candidate for use in longitudinal studies, as the effect of risk factors or biomarkers on cartilage morphology can be tracked for each joint region, and a number of large knee OA trials have included SPGR sequences in their protocols, making it the current 'standard' for quantitative morphological cartilage imaging [3,23]. Fast low-angle shot (FLASH) sequences employ a similar technique to SPGR, using random gradient pulses to spoil the steady state, and are also capable of obtaining good assessments of cartilage morphology, particularly with the addition of fat suppression [24]. SPGR and FLASH sequences both have a number of issues that limit their use in wider clinical scenarios: internal cartilage pathology is poorly visualized, they are vulnerable to susceptibility effects, the long acquisition time greatly increases the likelihood of motion artefacts, and there is relatively poor contrast between synovial fluid and cartilage [2].

DEFT (driven equilibrium Fourier transformation) imaging overcomes one of these difficulties by using direct return of magnetization to the z-axis with each excitation to greatly improve fluid–cartilage contrast [25]. Three-dimensional DESS imaging provides similarly good cartilage–fluid contrast, with the additional advantages of a shorter acquisition time and thinner sections with an improved resolution [26,27]. These benefits have contributed towards the high uptake of DESS sequences in several recent studies—most notably the Osteoarthritis Initiative (OAI)—utilizing 3D DESS imaging for the quantitative assessment of cartilage morphology [8]. Three-dimensional DESS imaging, in which data from multiple gradient echoes separated by a refocusing pulse are combined to form a reconstructed image, is therefore likely to be the imaging technique that is most clinically applicable for tracking cartilage morphology in the immediate future, especially using quantitative approaches [1,3]. Drawbacks, as is the case for all gradient echo sequences, are the decreased sensitivity for the detection of focal cartilage defects, likely to be one of the first manifestations of disease [28].

Three-dimensional bSSFP (balanced steady-state free precession)—also known as true FISP (fast imaging with steady-state progression), FIESTA (fast imaging employing steady state-acquisition), or balanced FFE (fast field echo), depending on the manufacturer of the machine—uses a similar principle to DESS sequences, with slightly different parameters [2,29]. bSSFP is particularly vulnerable, however, to off-resonance artefacts, and it provides comparatively poor resolution [3,18]. The combination of bSSFP with 3D radial k-space acquisition known as VIPR (vastly interpolated projection reconstruction imaging) produces particularly high signal–noise ratio in cartilage, as well as good contrast between multiple joint tissues, but without compromising the short acquisition time associated with DESS imaging [30]. This makes VIPR a potentially attractive option for clinical practice, but its utility in evaluating cartilage morphology has yet to be validated in large-scale clinical trials.

Composition

Hyaline articular cartilage is composed of approximately 70% water, with the remaining portion consisting largely of type II collagen fibres and glycosaminoglycans that together form the macromolecular framework [31]. Current MRI techniques measure a variety of mobile ions (such as gadolinium-based contrasts or sodium) that change distribution in response to the presence of proteoglycans, operating on the principle that the concentrations of these ions provide an indirect assessment of cartilage composition [3].

T2 mapping is the most widely available of the compositional imaging techniques in current usage. The method makes use of the fact that the T2 relaxation time of cartilage is largely determined by its water content, which is a close surrogate for the type II collagen concentration [32]. T2 mapping may therefore be ideal for usage in both cross-sectional studies and longitudinal studies aimed at tracking changes in collagen concentrations over time. Dunn et al. published the most significant study validating this idea, with areas of increased T2 associated with focal cartilage damage, and individuals with clinically diagnosed OA exhibiting generally higher T2 values, particularly within the medial compartment of the knee [33]. Reproducible differences in T2 values have also been observed in asymptomatic young adults, and it would certainly be interesting to see whether increased T2 values were associated with the long-term development of OA, as alterations in T2 would likely be evident before morphological cartilage changes, making it an ideal early biomarker of future disease [34]. No long-term studies have yet been conducted, however, and a correlation has not been shown between raised T2 values and clinical disease severity, so the utility of T2 mapping in monitoring disease progression is still unclear [35].

dGEMRIC imaging provides a measure of the proteoglycan content, rather than the collagen content, by assessing the varying concentration of the gadolinium (Gd)-based ions that distribute in accordance with proteoglycan concentration, with the negatively-charged Gd-DTPA^{2-} ions accumulating in regions proteoglycan depletion [18]. In the presence of Gd-DTPA^{2-} there is an approximately linear relationship between T1 and glycosaminoglycan content, so low dGEMRIC indices on T1 mapping are theoretically indicative of cartilage matrix depletion [36]. This has borne out well in several studies, with lower dGEMRIC indices associated with lower glycosaminoglycan content in histological and biochemical tests [37]. Importantly, dGEMRIC indices have also correlated well with Kellgren–Lawrence radiographic grading of OA severity making it a potentially attractive option for long-term monitoring of disease progression [38,39]. No trials have yet been conducted to assess whether a relationship exists between early dGEMRIC changes and later OA, however, so its usefulness as a biomarker for incident disease is unknown. The biggest drawbacks with the dGEMRIC technique limiting its usefulness in clinical settings are the need to administer contrast and the time required for the assessment; the 'delay' for the contrast to penetrate the cartilage (including movement of the joint post-contrast administration), and the lengthy T1 imaging means that the total time approaches 2 hours [3].

T1rho relaxation mapping has also been shown to effectively identify damaged hyaline cartilage, but is beset by similar time-related issues [40]. The technique involves applying an additional radiofrequency pulse after the magnetization is tipped into the transverse field, and provides information on motion-restricted water molecules and their surrounding macromolecular environment [41]. This is necessarily a time-consuming process, involving multiple datasets, and the pulse sequences required to perform it are generally only available at research institutions [3]. Unlike T2 mapping and dGEMRIC imaging, T1rho imaging also provides relatively non-specific information on macromolecular parameters, with factors such as collagen fibre orientation affecting values. These issues limit the clinical utility of T1rho mapping, and to date, no large clinical trials have made use of the technique.

Sodium imaging is based on the same principles of electrical charge as dGEMRIC, utilizing the idea that positively charged sodium ions will distribute in accordance with the abundance of the negatively charged proteoglycans [18,42]. Sodium imaging has shown promise in identifying proteoglycan depletion, and so may be useful in identifying early osteoarthritic changes, but is technically quite challenging [43,44]. The low concentration of sodium relative to hydrogen—as well as the lower gyromagnetic ratio and shorter T2 relaxation time—increase the SNR [18]. This decreases the resolution and necessitates the use of specialized hardware and high field strengths that are currently only available at a limited number of sites [3,18].

The development of chemical exchange saturation transfer (CEST) techniques may help solve this issue with resolution. CEST imaging is based on the principle that endogenous metabolites may be visualized through the detection of their exchangeable protons, with glycosaminoglycans (Gag) detectable by virtue of their high numbers of hydroxyl (-OH) groups [45]. A recent study reported a high correlation between GagCEST and sodium imaging in patellar cartilage, and the spatial resolution of GagCEST is inherently higher, making it a potentially ideal means of assessing glycosaminoglycan depletion in thin articular cartilage [46].

Diffusion-weighted imaging is a recently developed technique that involves applying multiple diffusion sensitive gradients, providing information on 3D diffusion of water molecules [18,47]. This could potentially give an insight into the cartilage composition and the actual cartilage architecture. Evidence suggests that the apparent diffusion coefficient (ADC)—a measurement that reflects that degree to which water molecules are restricted by cartilage matrix—correlates relatively well with proteoglycan content, and ADC mapping has shown promise in identifying regions of cartilage disruption [48–51]. Changes to the fractional anisotropy (FA)—an additional index describing the degree of directionality—theoretically reflect alterations to the structure of the collagen network itself, and FA values were recently shown to differ significantly in healthy and osteoarthritic knees [52,53]. Importantly, diffusion-weighted sequences are also very quick; no contrast is required and the acquisition time is usually less than 10 minutes. Diffusion-weighted imaging therefore provides the potential to rapidly and quantitatively assess both the proteoglycan and collagen components of the cartilage structure. This would obviously be ideal for clinical trials, but as yet, no large-scale longitudinal studies using diffusion-weighted imaging to track early cartilage changes have been conducted so its potential is largely unknown.

Grading of osteoarthritis using MRI

The parameters used in the quantitative measurements of cartilage changes are surprisingly varied, but most commonly include cartilage volume, cartilage thickness, cartilage surface area, total subchondral bone area, denuded bone area, cartilaginous subchondral bone area, and cartilage and bone surface curvature [54,55]. Quantitative grading has the advantage of being less reader-dependent than semi-quantitative systems, as well as being significantly easier to analyse statistically [54]. Despite this, the majority of clinical studies and trials use different methods of grading joint pathology that are semi-quantitative and multifactorial, employing measurements of cartilage morphology in addition to assessments of other joint structures (such as ligaments, menisci and subchondral bone).

The Whole-Organ Magnetic Resonance Imaging Score (WORMS) was the first widely utilized MRI-based knee OA grading system, and involves grading of eight articular features (cartilage, marrow abnormalities, bone cysts, bone attrition, osteophytes, menisci, ligaments, and synovitis) that may be compiled to give a total joint score. This is, however, rather difficult to interpret when making comparisons between knees, as the weighting and relevance of the different features with regard to disease progression are still unknown. The five features related to the articular surface (cartilage, marrow, cysts, attrition, and osteophytes) are further subdivided into 15 different regions on the basis of anatomical landmarks [56]. The WORMS scale has proven to be a reliable method of joint assessment, including high rates of inter-observer reproducibility [56,57], but has a number of issues related to cartilage scoring, namely the validity of compiling multiple factors like width, signal intensity, and depth into a single score.

The Boston–Leeds Osteoarthritis Knee Score (BLOKS) attempted to overcome this problem by using separate scores for the size and extent of cartilage loss, and also introduces a more extensive scoring system for BMLs that has a better association with pain severity. The BLOKS system also analyses eight articular features overall that are broadly similar to those assessed in WORMS, but regional segmentation involves only nine areas rather than the 15 used in WORMS (Table 18.1) [58].

Two extensive comparisons of the two methods performed in 2010 suggested the overall differences between the systems were modest; BML scoring in the WORMS system was superior to that used in the BLOKS system, though the reverse was true for meniscal scoring and neither system was clearly superior for assessing cartilage loss [57,59]. The BLOKS scale provided better detection of the effects of malalignment and a more intuitive linear scale, but the WORMS system showed better correlation with joint space narrowing [59]. Lynch et al. therefore recommended an amalgamation of the two methods be used for OA assessment.

To this end, the MRI OA knee score (MOAKS) system was developed in 2011 [60]. The MOAKS system includes seven articular features (BMLs and subchondral cysts, articular cartilage, osteophytes, synovitis/effusion, meniscus, ligaments/tendons and periarticular features) and 15 regions within the knee. Most notably, compared with BLOKS, the MOAKS method simplified BML and cartilage scoring (using regional delineation for both but removing measures of the adjacency of BMLs to the subchondral plate), added measures of meniscal morphology (hypertrophy and partial maceration) and added subluxation scoring [60] (Figures 18.1–5). Initial results suggesting that the method showed good reliability and inter-user agreement lead to its use in the OAI, and it is

Table 18.1 Comparison of the imaging features of the WORMS and MOAKS semi-quantitative scoring systems

MRI feature	WORMS system	MOAKS system
Cartilage	15 subregions, scored 0–6 based on depth and area of cartilage loss	12 subregions used, scores 0–3 for size and percentage of loss. No score for extent of cartilage loss
Bone marrow lesions	Scored 0–3 on the percentage of subregional bone volume occupied by the BML	Each subregion receives one size score based on thresholds. No score for BML percentage area
Osteophytes	Scored 0–7	Scored 0–3
Subchondral cysts	Scored 0–3 based on percentage of subregional bone volume	Scored with BMLs
Bone attrition	Scored 0–3	Not scored
Synovitis	Scored 0–3 (in combination with effusion)	Scored 0–3 for signal changes in Hoffa's fat pad as 'Hoffa synovitis'
Effusion	Score 0–3 (with synovitis)	Scored 0–3 as 'effusion synovitis'
Menisci	Scored 0–4 in six regions (anterior horn, body, posterior horn in medial/lateral menisci)	0–1 scoring for intrameniscal signal, vertical/complex/root tear, maceration, meniscal cyst, meniscal hypertrophy, partial maceration and progressive partial maceration in six regions
Meniscal extrusion	Not scored	Scored 0–3 as medial/lateral extrusion on coronal image, and anterior extrusion for medial/lateral meniscus on sagittal image
Ligaments	Cruciate and collateral ligaments scored as intact/torn	Cruciate ligaments scored as normal or complete tear, with insertional BMLs scored. Collateral ligaments not scored
Periarticular features	Scored 0–3; popliteal cysts, anserine bursitis, semimembranosus bursa, meniscal cyst, infrapatellar/prepatellar bursitis, tibiofibular cyst	Scored 0–1; patellar tendon signal, pes anserine bursitis, iliotibial band signal, popliteal cyst, infrapatellar bursa, ganglion cysts of tibiofibular joint, meniscus, semimembranosus, semitendinosus
Loose bodies	Scored 0–3	Scored as absent/present

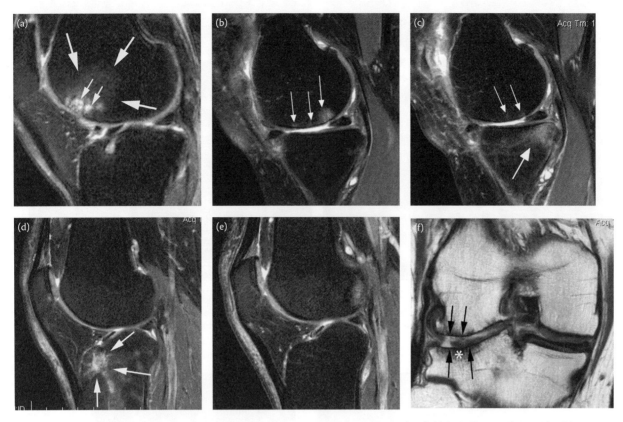

Figure 18.1 Examples of bone alterations in osteoarthritis (OA) as shown on magnetic resonance imaging (MRI). (a) Sagittal intermediate-weighted fat-suppressed image shows typical OA-related bone marrow lesion (BML). There is a subchondral cystic portion (small arrows) and a large surrounding ill-defined component of BML (large arrows). As cystic and non-cystic portions may have different clinical or structural relevance, measurement approaches should distinguish these from each other. Cystic lesions commonly develop in areas of pre-existing ill-defined BMLs. (b) A traumatic bone contusion (BML) due to direct anterior impact is seen in the anterior tibia in this sagittal fat-suppressed image. Traumatic BMLs commonly resolve completely without further sequelae as shown in image (c), a follow-up examination 5 months after trauma. (d) OA-related BMLs commonly fluctuate. Baseline image shows three distinct lesions in the central weight-bearing part of the medial femur (arrows). While the MOAKS and BLOKS scoring system differentiate individual lesions, both MOAKS and WORMS use a subregional approach of summing lesion volume in relation to total subregional volume. Note that no tibial BML is seen. (e) Follow-up image 12 months later shows regression of femoral BMLs with only two BMLs discernible (small arrows). Note that at the same time there is a large incident BML depicted in the posterior tibia (large arrow). Progression, regression, incidence and resolution of BMLs may all be observed in the same knee over time. (f) Advanced lateral tibiofemoral OA is shown in this coronal intermediate-weighted image. Note complete loss of lateral tibiofemoral articular cartilage. In addition there is flattening of the femoral surface and convexity of the tibial joint surface known as bone attrition, a feature of joint remodelling commonly observed in advanced stages of OA.

currently the most commonly used grading scheme for semi-quantitative assessment of OA.

Perhaps the biggest issue for semi-quantitative scoring systems lies in their lack of sensitivity relative to quantitative measurements [61]. This is particularly important for clinical trials with short follow-up times, leading to the introduction of 'within-grade' assessment for the coding of definite changes that do not fulfil the criteria for a full grade change. This may provide improved longitudinal sensitivity, and although within-grade changes are not currently part of the standard scoring systems, the fact that they have been shown to correlate well with OA risk factors and outcomes may mean that the technique will gain increased usage in future trials [61,62].

Linking MRI-identifiable tissue damage with osteoarthritis progression

Cartilage

The techniques available for the assessment of cartilage morphology and composition have already been discussed, but it is also necessary to include a brief outline of the relationship between the cartilage measurements and actual clinical outcomes. In accordance with the oft-cited disconnect between radiographic OA and clinical symptoms, the majority of morphological cartilage measures do not appear to be predictive of increased pain prevalence or severity [63,64]. Inconsistencies in the reporting of the exact metrics used, however, previously made it difficult to compare publications and results [54,65]. A study by Buck et al. reported that cartilage thickness, total subchondral bone area, and the denuded area of subchondral bone (but not cartilage volume) explained over 90% of the cross-sectional and longitudinal variation in the more comprehensive list of common morphological measures, and so may be regarded as the 'core' indicators of cartilage status [54,66]. Of these, the percentage denuded area of subchondral bone has shown the best correlation with clinical outcomes, with denuded areas associated with higher levels of both current and incident knee pain, particularly when the denuded areas lie within the medial or central weight-bearing areas [67,68]. Interestingly, despite the apparently weak association between cartilage changes and pain severity, the rate of cartilage loss does appear to correlate with the rate of total

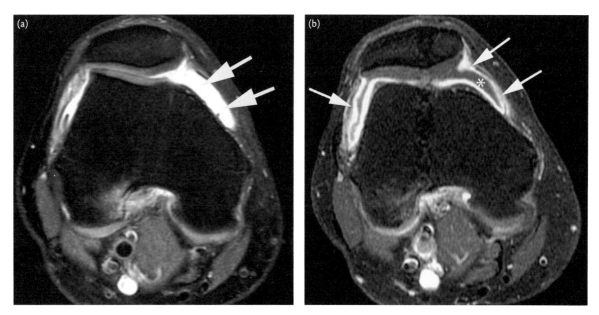

Figure 18.2 Synovitis and joint effusion. (a) Axial proton density-weighted fat-suppressed image show intra-articular hyperintensity consistent with joint effusion and synovitis. Note that joint fluid and synovial thickening cannot be distinguished using non-enhanced MRI. (b) Axial T1-weighted fat-suppressed image after intravenous contrast administration clearly delineates the enhancing synovium at the joint capsule (arrows) and visualizes intra-articular fluid as non-enhancing hypointensity (asterisk).

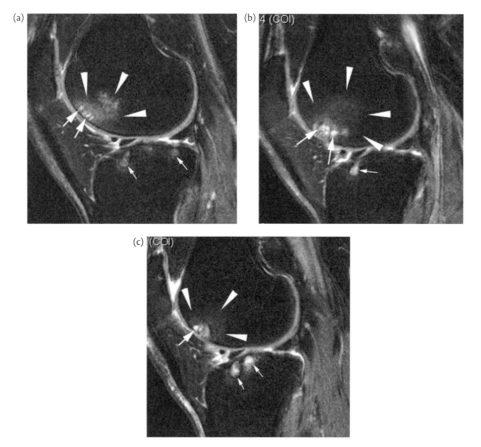

Figure 18.3 Bone marrow lesion (BML) assessment using semi-quantitative scoring. (a) Baseline sagittal intermediate-weighted fat-suppressed MRI shows a grade 2 MOAKS/grade 3 WORMS BML in the anterior lateral femur comprised of an ill-defined portion (arrowheads) and a cystic component (very small arrows). In addition, there are small cystic BMLs in the subchondral lateral tibia (small arrows). (b) Follow-up MRI 1 year later shows increase of overall lesion size (change from grade 2 to 3 for MOAKS, and within-grade change for WORMS) in the femur (arrowheads) plus an increase of size of femoral cystic component. While WORMS differentiates diffuse or ill-defined part of lesion from cystic portion as two distinct lesions, MOAKS takes both into account as one lesion. Note regression of posterior cystic lesion in the tibia and no change in size for cystic lesion in the anterior lateral tibia (arrow). (c) 2 years after baseline, decrease in overall femoral lesion size (arrowheads) is observed (now grade 2 by MOAKS and WORMS) while size of cystic portions of femoral BML remains stable (small arrow). There is an increase in tibial cystic lesion size with progression of anterior lesion and incident lesion in the central lateral tibia (very small arrows).

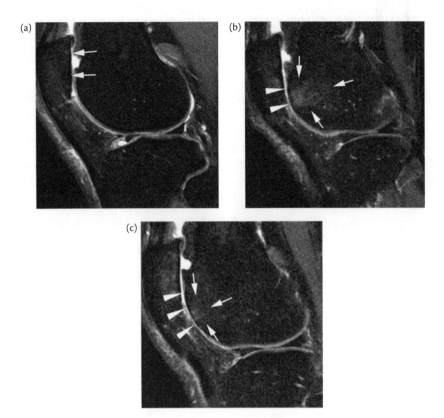

Figure 18.4 Evolution of cartilage damage over time. (a) Baseline fat-suppressed intermediate-weighted MRI shows an intact articular cartilage surface in the anterior lateral femur. There is diffuse full-thickness cartilage damage at the patella (arrows—WORMS 6, MOAKS 3.3). (b) 12 months later extensive full-thickness cartilage damage in the anterior lateral femur is observed that will be graded as a MOAKS 2.2 lesion (10–75% of subregion with any cartilage loss, 10–75% of subregion with full-thickness cartilage loss) and a grade 5 lesion using WORMS (arrowheads). Note adjacent subchondral ill-defined BML (grade 3 in WORMS and grade 2 in MOAKS). (c) Another 12 months later there is definite increase in area extent of lesion (arrowheads). Using MOAKS this lesion would now represent a grade 3.2 lesion (>75% of subregion with any cartilage loss, 10–75% of subregions showing full-thickness loss), in WORMS it would qualify as a grade 6 lesion (more than 75% of subregion affected by full-thickness cartilage loss), although there is still some cartilage preserved especially towards the more central part of the subregion. There is decease in size of the anterior lateral femoral BML (now WORMS grade 2, MOAKS grade 1).

knee arthroplasty (TKA). Cicuttini et al. reported that an increase in the rate of cartilage loss by 1% conveyed a 20% increased risk of TKA at 4 years, with an odds ratio of TKA for the highest–lowest tertiles of 7.1 [69]. Similarly, Eckstein et al. recently published data from the OAI indicating that cartilage loss accelerates in the 2 years prior to TKA [70]. The relative infancy of compositional measurements means that no large studies have yet been conducted assessing the longitudinal relationship between cartilage composition and pain/function, so the utility of composition in predicting clinical outcomes is as yet unknown.

Subchondral bone

BMLs, subchondral bone attrition, and subchondral bone marrow cysts are the features most commonly reported as being linked to disease progression, and examples of the subchondral bone marrow and articular surface changes are provided in Figures 18.1 and 18.3. BMLs are regions of diffuse signal abnormality within the trabecular bone that are best visualized on MRI as hyper-intense areas using fat-suppressed T2-weighted, proton density-weighted, short tau inversion recovery, or as hypointense areas on T1 imaging [4,71,72]. Traumatic BMLs must be distinguished from OA-related BMLs. These traumatic BMLs, also termed bone contusions or bone bruises, generally resolve within 6–12 months without long-term sequelae [73–75]. Traumatic BMLs with disruption of the articular

surface (or 'osteochondral injuries'), however, have previously been shown to be of relevance for the joint structure prognosis [76,77]. Importantly, they are also thought to be predictive of increased pain, lower IKDC (international knee documentation committee) clinical outcomes scores, and increased rates of arthroplasty [5,78,79].

Subchondral cyst-like lesions are regions of fluid-equivalent signal adjacent to the subchondral plate [72]. The cysts often occur concomitantly with ill-defined BMLs, and commonly develop in areas of diffuse, ill-delineated BMLs [80]. Although little is known about their impact on pain or functional outcomes, the presence of subchondral cysts does appear to convey an increased risk for TKA relative to BMLs alone [78,80].

Subchondral bone attrition is visualized on MRI as a flattening of the subchondral surface, and is thought to represent remodelling of the bone surface, potentially in response to altered loading patterns [4,6,81]. Attrition is commonly preceded by ill-defined BMLs, which supports the theory of subchondral structural bone changes, leading to altered biomechanics and consequent articular surface contour changes [82]. As well as being evident in advanced OA, bone attrition has been demonstrated in patients with mild symptomatic OA, before joint space narrowing was identified on radiography [6]. This is particularly interesting when viewed in the context of OA pathogenesis, as recently published results suggest that changes in bone curvature occur earlier than first thought

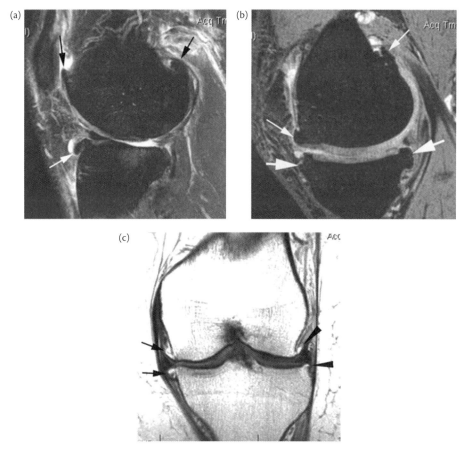

Figure 18.5 Osteophytes are one of the hallmark features of OA on imaging and part of the disease definition on X-rays. While WORMS uses a complex approach of osteophytes scoring on a 0–7 scale at 16 articular anatomical locations, MOAKS applies a somewhat simplified scheme on a 0–3 scale at only 12 different locations omitting the scores of the anterior and posterior medial and lateral tibia. (a) Sagittal fat-suppressed intermediate-weighted image of the lateral tibiofemoral compartment shows a moderate sized MOAKS grade 2/WORMS grade 4 osteophyte at the anterior femur, a MOAKS grade 3/WORMS grade 5 osteophyte at the posterior femur (black arrows) and a WORMS grade 5 osteophyte (white arrow) at the anterior lateral tibia (location not considered in MOAKS). Note diffuse cartilage loss at the central and posterior lateral tibia and femur and subchondral BML of the lateral tibial plateau, which shows moderate bone remodelling (attrition). (b) Sagittal dual-echo at steady-state (DESS) MRI of the medial tibiofemoral compartment shows moderate-sized (MOAKS grade 2/WORMS grade 3) osteophytes at the anterior and posterior medial femur (small arrows). At the tibia there is a tiny anterior osteophyte (WORMS grade 1—large arrow) and a moderate-to-large sized posterior osteophyte (WORMS grade 5—large arrow). Tibial locations are not scored in the sagittal plane using MOAKS. (c) Marginal osteophytes in the coronal plane are similarly considered in MOAKS and WORMS. Example shows medial femoral and tibial osteophytes (arrows—MOAKS grade 2/WORMS grade 4 femur and tibia) and small-to-moderate lateral osteophytes (arrowheads—MOAKS grade 2/WORMS grade 3 lateral femur and MOAKS grade 1/WORMS grade 1 lateral tibia).

following knee injury [83]. Bone curvature may therefore represent a useful biomarker for disease progression, especially considering its independent association with pain outcomes [84].

Synovium

Synovitis—defined as inflammation of the synovial membrane—has gained increasing attention recently as a potential driver of both disease progression and symptoms. Gadolinium-based contrast-enhanced imaging protocols are necessary to optimally visualize synovitis, with improved correlation between MRI-detected synovitis and histology, and better differentiation between synovitis and joint effusion than non-contrast enhanced imaging [7,18]. An example image illustrating the usefulness of contrast administration is presented in Figure 18.2. The differentiation of true synovitis and joint effusion appears to be important. Roemer et al. reported that in a cohort of patients with OA, synovitis was present in 96% of knees with effusion and 70% of those without effusion, suggesting that synovial inflammation is independent of joint effusion, and

may provide a better indication of pathology [85]. Atukorala et al. recently reported that the presence of effusion synovitis or Hoffa synovitis on MRI was strongly predictive of the development of radiographic OA over 4 years [86].

MRI-visualized synovitis also correlates particularly well with clinical outcomes, with a number of studies reporting that synovitis is predictive of pain in OA, and that higher grades of synovitis are associated with increased knee pain on the visual analogue scale [65,87]. Hill et al. actually managed to demonstrate that longitudinal fluctuations in synovitis were associated with matching changes in levels of knee pain, increasing the likelihood of a causal relationship [88]. Similarly, recently published results from the OAI highlighted a markedly increased risk for TKA the following year if either Hoffa synovitis or effusion synovitis was detectable on MRI, with odds ratios of 2.17 and 4.75, respectively [89]. It is therefore likely that the development of therapies targeting the pathways that promote synovitis in OA will be a major goal in OA research in the future [90]. The fact that magnetic resonance-based imaging has the ability to simultaneously assess synovitis as well as disease-defining cartilage changes makes it the ideal means of assessing the efficacy of novel interventions.

Menisci

The link between partial or complete meniscectomy and the long-term development of OA has been well documented, with numerous studies identifying partial and complete meniscectomy as a significant risk factor for OA and joint arthroplasty [91]. Similarly, meniscal lesions seem to be damaging to hyaline articular cartilage over the short term, with meniscal injury associated with a threefold increase in cartilage loss 2 years after the initial injury, and higher rates of total joint arthroplasty [92,93]. Despite this, the exact nature of the relationship between meniscal injury and articular cartilage damage has been rather harder to pin down, and it has been somewhat unclear whether the loss of meniscal function is the cause of articular cartilage damage, or merely a concurrent process [92].

Recent evidence suggests, however, that meniscal damage is likely involved in the pathogenesis of OA. Meniscal cells have been shown to increase their expression of inflammatory regulators interleukin 1 and inducible nitric oxide synthase in response to excessive compressive loading, and to express elevated levels of catabolic factors tumour necrosis factor alpha and matrix metalloproteinase 13 following anterior cruciate ligament (ACL) injury [94,95]. Similarly, meniscal injuries alter knee kinematics post injury, altering loading patterns across the joint and potentially contributing towards alterations in articular cartilage [96].

This increased understanding of the role of the menisci in OA pathogenesis heightens the need to adequately visualize and diagnose meniscal pathology. Proton density- or T1-weighted SE sequences in the sagittal and coronal planes are most commonly used, although axial planes may improve diagnostic sensitivity, particularly of radial or bucket-handle tears [97,98]. FSE sequences have not yet been shown to be superior to conventional SE sequences, with both systems returning similar sensitivity and specificity, but imaging at higher field strengths (3T) appears to greatly improve the SNR whilst maintaining the sensitivity and specificity [99].

T1rho and T2 mapping both demonstrate promise in identifying disease progression, with significant differences found between healthy subjects and patients with OA and measurements correlating well with increasing OA severity as determined using the Western Ontario and McMaster Arthritis Index (WOMAC) clinical pain and function scores [100]. Similarly, dGEMRIC mapping of the meniscus showed good correlation with dGEMRIC mapping of the articular cartilage, suggesting that destruction of the menisci and cartilage may be parallel processes [101]. Tracking meniscal composition using T1rho, T2 or dGEMRIC mapping may therefore represent a novel means of assessing OA progression, as the segmentation procedures required for menisci are much less cumbersome than those used for hyaline cartilage (which may take hours per knee) [100].

Ligaments

Rupture of the ACL is undoubtedly the best-studied ligamentous pathology in the context of OA. Osteoarthritic changes and related functional deficits have been reported as being present in approximately 50–70% of ACL-injured knees 10–15 years post injury; a figure that is particularly concerning given the majority of ACL

tears occur in active individuals within the 18–35-year age bracket, and the likelihood of the need for knee arthroplasty before the age of 50 [102–104]. The exact mechanism for this is yet to be elucidated, though recent evidence indicates that joint damage sustained at the time of ACL rupture—namely to articular cartilage, menisci, and subchondral bone—induces a series of inflammatory and biomechanical changes that ultimately result in OA.

This form of OA, aptly termed post-traumatic osteoarthritis (PTOA), represents an ideal model for the study of OA pathogenesis, as there is theoretically a definite 'start-point' from which changes to the joint may be tracked. Identifying ligament tears is therefore of great importance, and will likely become more so in the future as early interventions for PTOA are trialled. MRI is clearly the modality of choice for assessing ligament injuries, demonstrating excellent visualization of ligament structures and good accuracy in the identification of ligament tears [18]. A large meta-analysis by Smith et al. reported that the identification of complete ACL rupture on MRI in 53 studies was carried out with a sensitivity of 94.5% and a specificity of 95.3% [105]. The identification of partial tears, however, is significantly more difficult due to the non-specific diagnostic signs, and the values reported for sensitive and specificity are much lower [106,107]. The addition of oblique coronal or axial imaging and the use of 3T MRI machines improves diagnostic accuracy somewhat, though given that partial tears are still associated with significant morbidity—often progressing to complete tears or clinically-apparent knee laxity within a year—further improvement of assessment techniques will be necessary [108,109].

Utility of MRI in research

Observational studies

The broad aims of MRI-based studies investigating disease progression are to assess structural changes in joint tissues that are consistent with osteoarthritic damage, and correlate these changes with traditionally accepted markers of disease worsening, namely joint space narrowing and/or clinical signs and symptoms. The OAI, undoubtedly the largest trial assessing OA progression using MRI, makes use of both quantitative and semi-quantitative measurements, along with the MOAKS system for semi-quantitative scoring [8,110]. Pilot studies and preliminary published data from OAI subgroups suggest that the measurement techniques possess the required level of longitudinal sensitivity, and appear to correlate well with radiographic disease severity. Roemer et al., using data from the large MOST (Multicentre Osteoarthritis) trial, also found that scoring of within-grade changes provides a valid means of improving the longitudinal sensitive of semi-quantitative scoring systems [62].

Clinical trials

Despite the fact that MRI in OA is still in a relatively early developmental phase, it has been used quite successfully in a number of large-scale clinical trials. MRI utility in trials may be roughly classified into two types: the assessment of disease-modifying therapy (efficacy of intervention) and stratification of individuals into risk categories for future disease (prognostic biomarker). Each of these types requires a particular methodology, and the correct selection of MRI sequences and OA grading systems is vital to ensuring the findings are valid.

Quantitative cartilage measurements—most commonly thickness, volume, and denuded area—and semi-quantitative methods are the current methods of choice, and although any correlation with clinical outcomes has been rather difficult to identify, both methods have shown good cross-over with radiographic disease markers. Sequences focused on assessing cartilage morphology are therefore required, with 3D DESS and 3D FLASH sequences demonstrating the ideal properties [111].

The technical requirements of studies assessing potential disease-modifying agents are fairly similar to observational studies, though with one important distinction: the time period over which changes must be identified is significantly shorter. Joint space narrowing—the structural endpoint currently recommended by the European Medicines Agency and the US Food and Drug Administration guidelines for use in assessing the action of disease-modifying agents—has a lead time of at least 2 years, making the development and testing of possible agents both technically and financially unattractive. The fact that MRI has the capacity to detect structural changes significantly earlier than radiography makes it an attractive alternative. A reduced time-frame requires the measurements of joint damage to have improved longitudinal sensitivity, making quantitative and 'within-grade' analysis methods more suitable for use than broader semi-quantitative scoring systems [61]. Recent studies have supported this idea, with Wildi et al. and Stahl et al. reporting that quantitative measurements provide greater short-term sensitivity than semi-quantitative measurements [112,113].

The desire to develop and assess the efficacy of targeted interventions has also increased interest in the identification of imaging biomarkers: joint features visible on MRI that need not necessarily be involved in OA pathogenesis, but which are indicative of structural damage or increased future risk of disease. BMLs provide an ideal example of a possible biomarker as they increase risk of structural progression independently and in conjunction with concomitant localized tissue damage [79,114–116]. BMLs are easily visualized on MRI, and may represent a surrogate marker of osteoarthritic damage that is more rapidly identified and tracked than cartilage morphology. A particular difficulty for studies lies in the fact that sequences that are ideal for the visualization of a potential biomarker often differ from those necessary for assessing cartilage morphology and disease progress, meaning multiple sequences are required—a technical and financial hurdle. Another issue is a purely epidemiological one; some prognostic markers such as ligament tears may be relatively uncommon, so large subject numbers are required to properly evaluate their effect. The scale of the OAI (approximately 4800 subjects), and the fact that an unusually large number of sequences have been used, overcomes a number of these difficulties, and makes it ideal for assessing possible biomarkers. The FNIH (Foundation for the National Institutes of Health) OA Biomarkers Consortium project was recently started to leverage data from the OAI in order to investigate the ability of changes in several imaging and biochemical measures to predict clinical outcomes [117]. Importantly, the project has also developed a standard system for biomarker validation and qualification, facilitating a more coordinated approach to biomarker investigation for future studies.

Future possibilities for MRI in osteoarthritis

The development of novel acquisition techniques will undoubtedly continue to occur at a rapid rate, and a number of newly developed methods are worthy of mention.

Three-dimensional FSE imaging is an acquisition technique based on 3D fast SE sequencing that provides high T2-weighted contrast, with significantly improved SNR and SNR efficiency compared to other currently used 3D cartilage assessment techniques [118]. It may therefore provide an alternative to 2D FSE imaging, providing similar sensitivity and specificity for semi-quantitative scoring [119]. The drawbacks associated with the technique are mainly related to blurring, though the greatly reduced imaging time may justify its use in OA research [3].

Although 1.5T MRI systems are still the standard for clinical practice, the availability of 3T and even 7T machines is increasing. The SNR for a 3T magnet is approximately double that of a 1.5T machine, and the diagnostic performance in evaluating articular cartilage is slightly higher [3,120]. In addition, 3T machines provide practical advantages; the time required to obtain images of comparable quality and resolution shorter, meaning motion artefacts are reduced and patient turnover can be increased. The fact that 7T machines are currently only available in a few research centres has limited its use in large-scale trials, but several small studies have demonstrated its feasibility for cartilage assessment, and it is likely that 7T systems will provide significant benefits in the future [121,122].

Conclusion

The usefulness of MRI as an imaging modality in OA lies in its ability to accurately visualize multiple joint tissues, using a range of sequences and contrasts. This has led to an increased understanding of OA as a whole-joint disease, as specific changes in cartilage, subchondral bone, synovium, menisci, and ligaments can now be readily monitored. Improvements in techniques to measure short-term morphological and compositional alterations in cartilage will likely lead to the identification of biomarkers for osteoarthritic damage, as well as the capacity to rapidly assess the efficacy of disease-modifying interventions. It is hoped that this facilitate the development of potential disease-modifying agents, as the technical and financial hurdles that currently exist are reduced.

References

1. Gold GE, Chen CA, Koo S, Hargreaves BA, Bangerter NK. Recent advances in MRI of articular cartilage. *AJR Am J Roentgenol* 2009; 193(3):628.
2. Link TM, Stahl R, Woertler K. Cartilage imaging: motivation, techniques, current and future significance. *Eur Radiol* 2007; 17(5):1135–46.
3. Crema MD, Roemer FW, Marra MD, et al. Articular cartilage in the knee: current MR imaging techniques and applications in clinical practice and research 1. *Radiographics* 2011; 31(1):37–61.
4. Braun HJ, Gold GE. Diagnosis of osteoarthritis: imaging. *Bone*, 2012; 51(2):278–88.
5. Frobell R, Roos HP, Roos EM, et al. The acutely ACL injured knee assessed by MRI: are large volume traumatic bone marrow lesions a sign of severe compression injury? *Osteoarthritis Cartilage* 2008; 16(7):829–36.
6. Reichenbach S, Guermazi A, Niu J, et al. Prevalence of bone attrition on knee radiographs and MRI in a community-based cohort. *Osteoarthritis Cartilage* 2008; 16(9):1005–10.
7. Hayashi D, Roemer FW, Katur A, et al. Imaging of synovitis in osteoarthritis: current status and outlook. *Semin Arthritis Rheum* 2011; 41(2):116–30.
8. Eckstein F, Wirth W, Nevitt MC. Recent advances in osteoarthritis imaging—the Osteoarthritis Initiative. *Nat Rev Rheumatol* 2012; 8(10):622–30.

9. Menashe L, Hirko K, Losina E, et al. The diagnostic performance of MRI in osteoarthritis: a systematic review and meta-analysis. *Osteoarthritis Cartilage* 2012; 20(1):13–21.

10. Schneider E, Nevitt M, McCulloch C, et al. Equivalence and precision of knee cartilage morphometry between different segmentation teams, cartilage regions, and MR acquisitions. *Osteoarthritis Cartilage* 2012; 20(8):869–79.

11. Blackmon GB, Major NM, Helms CA. Comparison of fast spin-echo versus conventional spin-echo MRI for evaluating meniscal tears. *AJR Am J Roentgenol* 2005; 184(6):1740–43.

12. Vallotton J, Meuli RA, Leyvraz PF, Landry M. Comparison between magnetic resonance imaging and arthroscopy in the diagnosis of patellar cartilage lesions. *Knee Surg Sports Traumatol Arthrosc* 1995; 3(3):157–62.

13. Freeman DM, Bergman G, Glover G. Short TE MR microscopy: accurate measurement and zonal differentiation of normal hyaline cartilage. *Magn Reson Med* 1997; 38(1):72–81.

14. Disler D, McCauley TR, Kelman CG, et al. Fat-suppressed three-dimensional spoiled gradient-echo MR imaging of hyaline cartilage defects in the knee: comparison with standard MR imaging and arthroscopy. *AJR Am J Roentgenol* 1996; 167(1):127–32.

15. Jungius KP, Schmid MR, Zanetti M, et al. Cartilaginous defects of the femorotibial joint: accuracy of coronal Short inversion time inversion-recovery MR sequence 1. *Radiology* 2006; 240(2):482–8.

16. Gerdes CM, Kijowski R, Reeder SB. IDEAL imaging of the musculoskeletal system: robust water–fat separation for uniform fat suppression, marrow evaluation, and cartilage imaging. *AJR Am J Roentgenol* 2007; 189(5):W284–91.

17. Bredella M, Tirman PF, Peterfy CG, et al. Accuracy of T2-weighted fast spin-echo MR imaging with fat saturation in detecting cartilage defects in the knee: comparison with arthroscopy in 130 patients. *AJR Am J Roentgenol* 1999; 172(4):1073–80.

18. Shapiro LM, McWalter EJ, Son MS, et al. Mechanisms of osteoarthritis in the knee: MR imaging appearance. *J Magn Reson Imaging* 2014; 39(6):1346–56.

19. Kijowski R, Davis KW, Woods MA, et al. Knee joint: comprehensive assessment with 3D isotropic resolution fast spin-echo MR imaging—diagnostic performance compared with that of conventional MR imaging at 3.0 T 1. *Radiology* 2009; 252(2):486–95.

20. Ristow O, Steinbach L, Sabo G, et al. Isotropic 3D fast spin-echo imaging versus standard 2D imaging at 3.0 T of the knee—image quality and diagnostic performance. *Eur Radiol* 2009; 19(5):1263–72.

21. McGibbon CA, Trahan CA. Measurement accuracy of focal cartilage defects from MRI and correlation of MRI graded lesions with histology: a preliminary study. *Osteoarthritis Cartilage* 2003; 11(7):483–93.

22. Roemer FW, Guermazi A. MR imaging-based semiquantitative assessment in osteoarthritis. *Radiol Clin North Am* 2009; 47(4):633–54.

23. Disler DG, McCauley TR, Wirth CR, Fuchs MD. Detection of knee hyaline cartilage defects using fat-suppressed three-dimensional spoiled gradient-echo MR imaging: comparison with standard MR imaging and correlation with arthroscopy. *AJR Am J Roentgenol* 1995; 165(2):377–82.

24. Recht MP, Piraino DW, Paletta GA, Schils JP, Belhobek GH. Accuracy of fat-suppressed three-dimensional spoiled gradient-echo FLASH MR imaging in the detection of patellofemoral articular cartilage abnormalities. *Radiology* 1996; 198(1):209–12.

25. Gold GE, Fuller SE, Hargreaves BA, Stevens KJ, Beaulieu CF. Driven equilibrium magnetic resonance imaging of articular cartilage: initial clinical experience. *J Magn Reson Imaging* 2005; 21(4):476–81.

26. Moriya S, Miki Y, Yokobayashi T, Ishikawa M. Three-dimensional double-echo steady-state (3D-DESS) magnetic resonance imaging of the knee: contrast optimization by adjusting flip angle. *Acta Radiol* 2009; 50(5):507–11.

27. Staroswiecki E, Granlund KL, Alley MT, et al. Simultaneous estimation of T2 and apparent diffusion coefficient in human articular cartilage in vivo with a modified three-dimensional double echo steady state (DESS) sequence at 3 T. *Magn Reson Med* 2012; 67(4):1086–96.

28. Schaefer FK, Kurz B, Schaefer PJ, et al. Accuracy and precision in the detection of articular cartilage lesions using magnetic resonance imaging at 1.5 Tesla in an in vitro study with orthopedic and histopathologic correlation. *Acta Radiol* 2007; 48(10):1131–7.

29. Duerk JL, Lewin JS, Wendt M, Petersilge C. Invited. Remember true FISP? A high SNR, near 1-second imaging method for T2-like contrast in interventional MRI at 2 T. *J Magn Reson Imaging* 1998; 8(1):203–8.

30. Kijowski R, Blankenbaker DG, Klaers JL, et al. Vastly undersampled isotropic projection steady-state free precession imaging of the knee: diagnostic performance compared with conventional MR 1. *Radiology* 2009; 251(1):185–94.

31. Poole AR, Kojima T, Yasuda T, et al. Composition and structure of articular cartilage: a template for tissue repair. *Clinical Orthop Relat Res* 2001; 391:S26–33.

32. Liess C, Lüsse S, Karger N, Heller M, Glüer CC. Detection of changes in cartilage water content using MRI T 2-mapping in vivo. *Osteoarthritis Cartilage* 2002; 10(12):907–13.

33. Dunn TC, Lu Y, Jin H, Ries MD, Majumdar S. T2 relaxation time of cartilage at MR imaging: comparison with severity of knee osteoarthritis 1. *Radiology* 2004; 232(2):592–8.

34. Dardzinski BJ, Mosher TJ, Li S, Van Slyke MA, Smith MB. Spatial variation of T2 in human articular cartilage. *Radiology* 1997; 205(2):546–50.

35. Koff M, Amrami K, Kaufman K. Clinical evaluation of T2 values of patellar cartilage in patients with osteoarthritis. *Osteoarthritis Cartilage* 2007; 15(2):198–204.

36. Williams A, Gillis A, McKenzie C, et al. Glycosaminoglycan distribution in cartilage as determined by delayed gadolinium-enhanced MRI of cartilage (dGEMRIC): potential clinical applications. *AJR Am J Roentgenol* 2004; 182(1):167–72.

37. Bashir A, Gray ML, Hartke J, Burstein D. Nondestructive imaging of human cartilage glycosaminoglycan concentration by MRI. *Magn Reson Med* 1999; 41(5):857–65.

38. Williams A, Sharma L, McKenzie CA, Prasad PV, Burstein D. Delayed gadolinium-enhanced magnetic resonance imaging of cartilage in knee osteoarthritis: findings at different radiographic stages of disease and relationship to malalignment. *Arthritis Rheum* 2005; 52(11):3528–35.

39. Watanabe A, Wada Y, Obata T, et al. Delayed gadolinium-enhanced MR to determine glycosaminoglycan concentration in reparative cartilage after autologous chondrocyte implantation: preliminary results 1. *Radiology* 2006; 239(1):201–8.

40. Stahl R, Luke A, Li X, et al. T1rho, T2 and focal knee cartilage abnormalities in physically active and sedentary healthy subjects versus early OA patients—a 3.0-Tesla MRI study. *Eur Radiol* 2009; 19(1):132–43.

41. Wheaton AJ, Casey FL, Gougoutas AJ, et al. Correlation of T1rho with fixed charge density in cartilage. *J Magn Reson Imaging* 2004; 20(3):519–25.

42. Borthakur A, Shapiro EM, Beers J, et al. Sensitivity of MRI to proteoglycan depletion in cartilage: comparison of sodium and proton MRI. *Osteoarthritis Cartilage* 2000; 8(4):288–93.

43. Reddy R, Insko EK, Noyszewski EA, et al. Sodium MRI of human articular cartilage in vivo. *Magn Reson Med* 1998; 39(5):697–701.

44. Wheaton AJ, Borthakur A, Shapiro EM, et al. Proteoglycan loss in human knee cartilage: quantitation with sodium MR imaging—feasibility study 1. *Radiology* 2004; 231(3):900–5.

45. Kogan F, Hariharan H, Reddy R. Chemical exchange saturation transfer (CEST) imaging: description of technique and potential clinical applications. *Curr Radiol Rep* 2013; 1(2):102–14.

46. Schmitt B, Zbýn S, Stelzeneder D, et al. Cartilage quality assessment by using glycosaminoglycan chemical exchange saturation transfer and 23Na MR imaging at 7 T. *Radiology* 2011; 260(1):257–64.

47. Alexander AL, Lee JE, Lazar M, Field AS. Diffusion tensor imaging of the brain. *Neurotherapeutics* 2007; 4(3):316–29.

48. Burstein D, Gray ML, Hartman AL, Gipe R, Foy BD. Diffusion of small solutes in cartilage as measured by nuclear magnetic resonance (NMR) spectroscopy and imaging. *J Orthop Res* 1993; 11(4):465–78.

49. Mamisch TC, Menzel MI, Welsch GH, et al. Steady-state diffusion imaging for MR in-vivo evaluation of reparative cartilage after

matrix-associated autologous chondrocyte transplantation at 3 Tesla—preliminary results. *Eur J Radiol* 2008; 65(1):72–9.

50. Raya JG, Arnoldi AP, Weber DL, et al. Ultra-high field diffusion tensor imaging of articular cartilage correlated with histology and scanning electron microscopy. *MAGMA* 2011; 24(4):247–58.

51. Raya JG, et al. Change of diffusion tensor imaging parameters in articular cartilage with progressive proteoglycan extraction. *Invest Radiol* 2011; 46(6):401–9.

52. Dong Q, Welsh RC, Chenevert TL, et al. Clinical applications of diffusion tensor imaging. *J Magn Reson Imaging* 2004; 19(1):6–18.

53. Raya JG, Dettmann E, Notohamiprodjo M, et al. Feasibility of in vivo diffusion tensor imaging of articular cartilage with coverage of all cartilage regions. *Eur Radiol* 2014; 24(7):1700–6.

54. Eckstein F, Ateshian G, Burgkart R, et al. Proposal for a nomenclature for magnetic resonance imaging based measures of articular cartilage in osteoarthritis. *Osteoarthritis Cartilage* 2006; 14(10):974–83.

55. Eckstein F, Burstein D, Link TM. Quantitative MRI of cartilage and bone: degenerative changes in osteoarthritis. *NMR Biomed* 2006; 19(7):822–54.

56. Peterfy C, Guermazi A, Zaim S, et al. Whole-organ magnetic resonance imaging score (WORMS) of the knee in osteoarthritis. *Osteoarthritis Cartilage* 2004; 12(3):177–90.

57. Lynch JA, Roemer FW, Nevitt MC, et al. Comparison of BLOKS and WORMS scoring systems part I. Cross sectional comparison of methods to assess cartilage morphology, meniscal damage and bone marrow lesions on knee MRI: data from the osteoarthritis initiative. *Osteoarthritis Cartilage* 2010; 18(11):1393–401.

58. Hunter DJ, Lo GH, Gale D, et al. The development and reliability of a new scoring system for knee osteoarthritis MRI: BLOKS (Boston Leeds Osteoarthritis Knee Score). *Ann Rheum Dis* 2007; 67(2):206–11.

59. Felson DT, Lynch J, Guermazi A, et al. Comparison of BLOKS and WORMS scoring systems part II. Longitudinal assessment of knee MRIs for osteoarthritis and suggested approach based on their performance: data from the Osteoarthritis Initiative. *Osteoarthritis Cartilage* 2010; 18(11):1402–7.

60. Hunter D, Guermazi A, Lo GH, et al. Evolution of semi-quantitative whole joint assessment of knee OA: MOAKS (MRI Osteoarthritis Knee Score). *Osteoarthritis Cartilage* 2011; 19(8):990–1002.

61. Eckstein F, Guermazi A, Gold G, et al. Imaging of cartilage and bone: promises and pitfalls in clinical trials of osteoarthritis. *Osteoarthritis Cartilage* 2014; 22(10):1516–32.

62. Roemer FW, Nevitt MC, Felson DT, et al. Predictive validity of within-grade scoring of longitudinal changes of MRI-based cartilage morphology and bone marrow lesion assessment in the tibio-femoral joint–the MOST study. *Osteoarthritis Cartilage* 2012; 20(11):1391–8.

63. Raynauld P, Martel-Pelletier J, Berthiaume MJ, et al. Quantitative magnetic resonance imaging evaluation of knee osteoarthritis progression over two years and correlation with clinical symptoms and radiologic changes. *Arthritis Rheum* 2004; 50(2):476–87.

64. Phan CM, Link TM, Blumenkrantz G, et al. MR imaging findings in the follow-up of patients with different stages of knee osteoarthritis and the correlation with clinical symptoms. *Eur Radiol* 2006; 16(3):608–18.

65. Torres L, Dunlop DD, Peterfy C, et al. The relationship between specific tissue lesions and pain severity in persons with knee osteoarthritis. *Osteoarthritis Cartilage* 2006; 14(10):1033–40.

66. Buck RJ, Wyman BT, Le Graverand MP, et al. An efficient subset of morphological measures for articular cartilage in the healthy and diseased human knee. *Magn Reson Med* 2010; 63(3):680–90.

67. Moisio K, Eckstein F, Chmiel JS, et al. Denuded subchondral bone and knee pain in persons with knee osteoarthritis. *Arthritis Rheum* 2009; 60(12):3703–10.

68. Cotofana S, Wyman BT, Benichou O, et al. Relationship between knee pain and the presence, location, size and phenotype of femorotibial denuded areas of subchondral bone as visualized by MRI. *Osteoarthritis Cartilage* 2013; 21(9):1214–22.

69. Cicuttini FM, Jones G, Forbes A, Wluka AE. Rate of cartilage loss at two years predicts subsequent total knee arthroplasty: a prospective study. *Ann Rheum Dis* 2004; 63(9):1124–7.

70. Eckstein F, Boudreau RM, Wang Z, et al. Trajectory of cartilage loss within 4 years of knee replacement–a nested case–control study from the Osteoarthritis Initiative. *Osteoarthritis Cartilage* 2014; 22(10):1542–9.

71. Boks SS, Vroegindeweij D, Koes BW, et al. Follow-up of occult bone lesions detected at MR imaging: systematic review 1. *Radiology* 2006; 238(3):853–62.

72. Hunter D, Zhang W, Conaghan PG, et al. Systematic review of the concurrent and predictive validity of MRI biomarkers in OA. *Osteoarthritis Cartilage* 2011; 19(5):557–88.

73. Miller MD, Osborne JR, Gordon WT, Hinkin DT, Brinker MR. The natural history of bone bruises a prospective study of magnetic resonance imaging-detected trabecular microfractures in patients with isolated medial collateral ligament injuries. *Am J Sports Med* 1998; 26(1):15–19.

74. Bretlau T, Tuxøe J, Larsen L, et al. Bone bruise in the acutely injured knee. Knee Surgery, Sports Traumatology, *Arthroscopy* 2002; 10(2):96–101.

75. Boks SS, Vroegindeweij D, Koes BW, et al. Clinical consequences of posttraumatic bone bruise in the knee. *Am J Sports Med* 2007; 35(6):990–5.

76. Johnson DL, Urban WPJr, Caborn DN, Vanarthos WJ, Carlson CS. Articular cartilage changes seen with magnetic resonance imaging-detected bone bruises associated with acute anterior cruciate ligament rupture. *Am J Sports Med* 1998; 26(3):409–14.

77. Costa-Paz M, Muscolo DL, Ayerza M, et al. Magnetic resonance imaging follow-up study of bone bruises associated with anterior cruciate ligament ruptures. *Arthroscopy* 2001; 17(5):445–9.

78. Tanamas SK, Wluka AE, Pelletier JP, et al. Bone marrow lesions in people with knee osteoarthritis predict progression of disease and joint replacement: a longitudinal study. *Rheumatology* 2010; 49(12):2413–9.

79. Kijowski R, Sanogo ML, Lee KS, et al. Short-term clinical importance of osseous injuries diagnosed at MR imaging in patients with anterior cruciate ligament tear. *Radiology* 2012; 264(2):531–41.

80. Crema MD, Roemer FW, Zhu Y, et al. Subchondral cystlike lesions develop longitudinally in areas of bone marrow edema-like lesions in patients with or at risk for knee osteoarthritis: detection with MR imaging – The MOST Study 1. *Radiology* 2010; 256(3):855–62.

81. Coumas JM, Palmer WE. Knee arthrography: evolution and current status. *Radiol Clin North Am* 1998; 36(4):703–28.

82. Roemer FW, Neogi T, Nevitt MC, et al. Subchondral bone marrow lesions are highly associated with, and predict subchondral bone attrition longitudinally: the MOST study. *Osteoarthritis Cartilage* 2010; 18(1):47–53.

83. Hunter DJ, Lohmander LS, Makovey J, et al. The effect of anterior cruciate ligament injury on bone curvature: exploratory analysis in the KANON Trial. *Osteoarthritis Cartilage* 2014; 22(7):959–68.

84. Hernández-Molina G, Neogi T, Hunter DJ, et al. The association of bone attrition with knee pain and other MRI features of osteoarthritis. *Ann Rheum Dis* 2008; 67(1):43–7.

85. Roemer F, Kassim Javaid M, Guermazi A, et al. Anatomical distribution of synovitis in knee osteoarthritis and its association with joint effusion assessed on non-enhanced and contrast-enhanced MRI. *Osteoarthritis Cartilage* 2010; 18(10):1269–74.

86. Atukorala I, Kwoh CK, Guermazi A, et al. Synovitis in knee osteoarthritis: a precursor of disease? *Ann Rheum Dis* 2014; 75(2):390–5.

87. Baker K, Grainger A, Niu J, et al. Relation of synovitis to knee pain using contrast-enhanced MRIs. *Ann Rheum Dis* 2010; 69(10):1779–83.

88. Hill CL, Hunter DJ, Niu J, et al. Synovitis detected on magnetic resonance imaging and its relation to pain and cartilage loss in knee osteoarthritis. *Ann Rheum Dis* 2007; 66(12):1599–603.

89. Roemer FW, Kwoh CK, Hannon MJ, et al. Can structural joint damage measured with MR imaging be used to predict knee replacement in the following year? *Radiology* 2015; 274(3):810–20.

90. Scanzello CR, Goldring SR. The role of synovitis in osteoarthritis pathogenesis. *Bone* 2012; 51(2):249–57.

91. Roos, H, Laurén M, Adalberth T, et al. Knee osteoarthritis after meniscectomy: prevalence of radiographic changes after twenty-one years, compared with matched controls. *Arthritis Rheum* 1998; 41(4):687–93.

92. Murrell GA, Maddali S, Horovitz L, Oakley SP, Warren RF. The effects of time course after anterior cruciate ligament injury in correlation with meniscal and cartilage loss. *Am J Sports Med* 2001; 29(1):9–14.

93. Raynauld JP, Martel-Pelletier J, Haraoui B, et al. Risk factors predictive of joint replacement in a 2-year multicentre clinical trial in knee osteoarthritis using MRI: results from over 6 years of observation. *Ann Rheum Dis* 2011; 70(8):1382–8.

94. Gupta T, Zielinska B, McHenry J, Kadmiel M, Haut Donahue TL. IL-1 and iNOS gene expression and NO synthesis in the superior region of meniscal explants is dependent on magnitude of compressive strains. *Osteoarthritis Cartilage* 2008; 16(10):1213–9.

95. Brophy R, Rai MF, Zhang Z, Torgomyan A, Sandell LJ. Molecular analysis of age and sex-related gene expression in meniscal tears with and without a concomitant anterior cruciate ligament tear. *J Bone Joint Surg Am* 2012; 7(94):385–93.

96. Hosseini A, Li JS, Gill TJ4th, Li G. Meniscus injuries alter the kinematics of knees with anterior cruciate ligament deficiency. *Orthop J Sports Med* 2014; 2(8):2325967114547346.

97. Magee T, Williams D. Detection of meniscal tears and marrow lesions using coronal MRI. *AJR Am J Roentgenol* 2004; 183(5):1469–73.

98. Tarhan NC, Chung CB, Mohana-Borges AV, Hughes T, Resnick D. Meniscal tears: role of axial MRI alone and in combination with other imaging planes. *AJR Am J Roentgenol* 2004; 183(1):9–15.

99. Hopper M, Robinson P, Grainger A. Meniscal tear evaluation. Comparison of a conventional spin-echo proton density sequence with a fast spin-echo sequence utilizing a 512× 358 matrix size. *Clin Radiol* 2011; 66(4):329–33.

100. Rauscher I, Stahl R, Cheng J, et al. Meniscal measurements of T1ρ and T2 at MR imaging in healthy subjects and patients with osteoarthritis 1. *Radiology* 2008; 249(2):591–600.

101. Krishnan, N, Shetty SK, Williams A, et al. Delayed gadolinium-enhanced magnetic resonance imaging of the meniscus: an index of meniscal tissue degeneration? *Arthritis Rheum* 2007; 56(5):1507–11.

102. Lohmander L, Ostenberg A, Englund M, Roos H. High prevalence of knee osteoarthritis, pain and functional limitations in female soccer players twelve years after anterior cruciate ligament injury. *Arthritis Rheum* 2004; 50(10):3145–52.

103. Von Porat A, Roos EM, Roos H. High prevalence of osteoarthritis 14 years after an anterior cruciate ligament tear in male soccer players: a study of radiographic and patient relevant outcomes. *Ann Rheum Dis* 2004; 63(3):269–73.

104. Lohmander L, Englund PM, Dahl LL, Roos EM. The long-term consequence of anterior cruciate ligament and meniscus injuries: osteoarthritis. *Am J Sports Med* 2007; 35:1756–69.

105. Smith T, Lewis M, Song F, et al. The diagnostic accuracy of anterior cruciate ligament rupture using magnetic resonance imaging: a meta-analysis. *Eur J Orthop Surg Traumatol* 2012; 22(4):315–26.

106. Van Dyck, P, Vanhoenacker FM, Gielen JL, et al. Three tesla magnetic resonance imaging of the anterior cruciate ligament of the knee: can we differentiate complete from partial tears? *Skeletal Radiol* 2011; 40(6):701–7.

107. Van Dyck P, De Smet E, Veryser J, et al. Partial tear of the anterior cruciate ligament of the knee: injury patterns on MR imaging. *Knee Surg Sports Traumatol Arthrosc* 2012; 20(2):256–61.

108. Hong SH, Choi JY, Lee GK, et al. Grading of anterior cruciate ligament injury: diagnostic efficacy of oblique coronal magnetic resonance imaging of the knee. *J Comput Assist Tomogr* 2003; 27(5):814–9.

109. Ng AW, Griffith JF, Hung EH, Law KY, Yung PS. MRI diagnosis of ACL bundle tears: value of oblique axial imaging. *Skeletal Radiol* 2013; 42(2):209–17.

110. Eckstein F, Kwoh CK, Link TM. Imaging research results from the Osteoarthritis Initiative (OAI): a review and lessons learned 10 years after start of enrolment. *Ann Rheum Dis* 2014; 73(7):1289–300.

111. Wirth W, Nevitt M, Hellio Le Graverand MP, et al. Sensitivity to change of cartilage morphometry using coronal FLASH, sagittal DESS, and coronal MPR DESS protocols–comparative data from the Osteoarthritis Initiative (OAI). *Osteoarthritis Cartilage* 2010; 18(4):547–54.

112. Stahl R, Jain SK, Lutz J, et al. Osteoarthritis of the knee at 3.0 T: comparison of a quantitative and a semi-quantitative score for the assessment of the extent of cartilage lesion and bone marrow edema pattern in a 24-month longitudinal study. *Skeletal Radiol* 2011; 40(10):1315–27.

113. Wildi LM, Martel-Pelletier J, Abram F, et al. Assessment of cartilage changes over time in knee osteoarthritis disease-modifying osteoarthritis drug trials using semiquantitative and quantitative methods: pros and cons. *Arthritis Care Res* 2013; 65(5):686–94.

114. Frobell R, Le Graverand MP, Buck R, et al. The acutely ACL injured knee assessed by MRI: changes in joint fluid, bone marrow lesions, and cartilage during the first year. *Osteoarthritis Cartilage* 2009; 17(2):161–7.

115. Roemer FW, Felson DT, Wang K, et al. Co-localisation of non-cartilaginous articular pathology increases risk of cartilage loss in the tibiofemoral joint—the MOST study. *Ann Rheum Dis* 2013; 72(6):942–8.

116. Roemer FW, Guermazi A, Javaid MK, et al. Change in MRI-detected subchondral bone marrow lesions is associated with cartilage loss: the MOST Study. A longitudinal multicentre study of knee osteoarthritis. *Ann Rheum Dis* 2009; 68(9): 1461–5

117. Hunter DJ, Nevitt M, Losina E, Kraus V. Biomarkers for osteoarthritis: current position and steps towards further validation. *Best Pract Res Clin Rheumatol* 2014; 28(1):61–71.

118. Friedrich KM, Reiter G, Kaiser B, et al. High-resolution cartilage imaging of the knee at 3T: basic evaluation of modern isotropic 3D MR-sequences. *Eur J Radiol* 2011; 78(3):398–405.

119. Crema M, Nogueira-Barbosa MH, Roemer FW, et al. Three-dimensional (3D) intermediate weighted fast spin-echo magnetic resonance imaging (MRI) for semiquantitative whole organ assessment of knee osteoarthritis. *Osteoarthritis Cartilage* 2011; 19:S172.

120. Kijowski R, Blankenbaker DG, Davis KW, et al. Comparison of 1.5- and 3.0-T MR imaging for evaluating the articular cartilage of the knee joint 1. *Radiology* 2009; 250(3):839–48.

121. Wang L, Wu Y, Chang G, et al. Rapid isotropic 3D-sodium MRI of the knee joint in vivo at 7T. *J Magn Reson Imaging* 2009; 30(3):606–14.

122. Welsch GH, Apprich S, Zbyn S, et al. Biochemical (T2, T2* and magnetisation transfer ratio) MRI of knee cartilage: feasibility at ultra-high field (7T) compared with high field (3T) strength. *Eur Radiol* 2011; 21(6):1136–43.

CHAPTER 19

Laboratory tests

Leticia A. Deveza, Changhai Ding, Xingzhong Jin,
Xia Wang, Zhaohua Zhu, and David J. Hunter

Introduction

At this time, there are no laboratory tests that are diagnostic for osteoarthritis (OA) or considered reliable tools for its management. Several markers measured in serum, synovial fluid (SF), and urine are under investigation but no individual marker has accomplished these goals so far. In fact, extensive effort has been spent in ascertaining the utility of these biochemical markers to enable progress in the development of new disease-modifying drugs.

The role of laboratory tests in OA research has expanded significantly as the knowledge about the pathophysiology of the disease has increased. In this regard, progress has occurred in multiple areas such as the discovery of cytokines and adipocytokines involved in the OA process, the relationship between OA and dietary substances such as vitamin D, and the identification of novel genetic polymorphisms. Moreover, laboratory tests remain a useful part of the clinical armamentarium to investigate underlying diseases that may predispose to OA when suspected, and to aid in the distinction from other types of joint diseases, especially crystal-related and autoimmune causes. In this chapter, the most recent advances and implications related to laboratory tests in OA will be covered, as well as their utility in differential diagnosis and investigation of causative diseases.

Utility of laboratory tests

OA is a chronic joint disorder associated with ageing and with insidious onset. In this context, several conditions may present with similar clinical findings such as pseudogout, rheumatoid arthritis (RA), neuropathic arthropathy, and mycobacteria or fungal arthritis. Moreover, other diseases may have specific pathogenic mechanisms that, ultimately, also result in joint damage as observed in OA. Examples are metabolic diseases (haemochromatosis, haemoglobinopathy), endocrine diseases (acromegaly, diabetes mellitus), other types of bone diseases (Paget, osteopetrosis), and previous inflammatory arthritis. To date, no laboratory test is diagnostic of OA or useful for its management but they may be important tools for the differential diagnosis or when a specific underlying mechanism is suspected. Furthermore, laboratory tests may be helpful to detect genetic polymorphisms as a cause of hereditary OA (e.g. familial calcium pyrophosphate crystal deposition (CPPD) disease, chondrodysplasias, epiphyseal dysplasias, and osteochondrodysplasia) and to act as biochemical markers of the disease, helping to reveal underlying biological mechanisms that may lead to development of new therapeutic targets or contributing to early detection and risk stratification.

Exclusion of autoimmune and crystal-associated arthropathies

Although OA and autoimmune diseases have distinct features such as the presence of systemic involvement in the latter, laboratory tests are useful when the precise diagnosis cannot be established based only on history and physical examination, with or without radiographic evaluation. While inflammatory tests such as erythrocyte sedimentation rate (ESR) and C-reactive protein (CRP) are usually abnormal in autoimmune disorders and occasionally elevated in chronic crystal arthritis and superimposed flares, normal levels are observed in OA, except for mild elevations in high-sensitivity (hs)-CRP [1]. SF analysis also shows distinct patterns, with higher white blood cell (WBC) count and lower viscosity in autoimmune and crystal arthritis (see 'Synovial fluid analysis').

Serological testing for autoantibodies should be reserved for the cases in which an autoimmune disease is suspected. The specificity, sensitivity, and likelihood ratios of the tests should be considered when interpreting their results. For example, although 70–80% of patients with RA have increased levels of rheumatoid factor (RF), this test is not specific for this disease and may be positive in several other conditions (endocarditis, hepatitis C, systemic lupus erythematosus (SLE)) as well as in 5–6% of the normal elderly population. Anti-cyclic citrullinated peptide antibodies are more specific for the diagnosis of RA and are particularly useful when RF is negative in the appropriate clinical context [2].

Several autoimmune diseases test positive for antinuclear antibodies (ANAs) but the test alone should not be used to infer the presence of an autoimmune disorder as it can also be positive in 10–15% of the healthy population. However, the likelihood of an autoimmune disease is increased with high titres (≥1:320) and specific staining patterns (e.g. centromeric in systemic sclerosis and homogeneous in SLE). According to ANA patterns and clinical suspicion, further serological tests may be necessary. Similarly, the human leucocyte antigen B27 is a genetic predisposing factor for spondyloarthritis included in the Assessment of SpondyloArthritis international Society (ASAS) classification criteria and may be useful when the distinction of both axial and peripheral presentations and OA is not clear.

Synovial fluid analysis

The hallmark of SF in OA is its lower inflammatory characteristics compared to other joint pathologies. The fluid is usually clear, colourless, or slight yellow and the viscosity is normal or slightly reduced. Cellular content in OA is usually less than 2000 WBC/

mL. While cell count may reach higher than 10 000 WBC/mL in autoimmune diseases and higher than 50 000 WBC/mL in joint infection, normal SF usually contains fewer than 200 WBC/mL, showing that a low-grade inflammation is also present in OA. In the presence of crystals, however, an inflammatory effusion may occur and SF analysis will reveal a higher WBC count, predominance of polymorphonuclear leucocytes, and crystals under polarized light microscopy when calcium pyrophosphate or uric acid is present. Basic calcium phosphate crystals may also be present in SF and are better identified with alizarin red S stain. Calcium-containing crystals are commonly found in association of OA and may have a role in disease flares, precipitation of inflammation, and further joint damage [3].

Tests for metabolic diseases that predispose to osteoarthritis

Laboratory tests are useful to rule out or confirm the presence of underlying disorders or genetic predispositions leading to OA, within the proper clinical context. OA is a heterogeneous disorder with distinct risk factor profiles and disease courses. Some phenotypes are known to be associated with specific pathogenic mechanisms or clinical conditions (e.g. ochronosis and CPPD) while others are still under investigation (e.g. erosive hand OA and rapidly progressive forms of hip and knee OA).

Arthropathy due to haemochromatosis typically involves the second and third metacarpophalangeal joints with hook osteophytes, although any joint can be affected. It is most commonly manifest later in the disease course but it can be the first clinical presentation of iron overload [4]. Diagnosis is based on elevated serum transferrin saturation and ferritin concentration, followed by a genotype test to detect the *HFE* gene mutation on chromosome 6.

Joint complaints in acromegaly are frequent and may affect knees, hips, hands, spine, and jaws. The characteristics are bone enlargement, soft tissue prominence, widened joint spaces, and large marginal osteophyte formation [5]. Levels of insulin growth factor 1 (IGF-1) and growth hormone (GH) are required for diagnosis.

Ochronosis is a rare autosomal recessive hereditary metabolic disorder due to deficiency in the enzyme homogentisate 1,2-dioxygenase resulting in the accumulation of homogentisic acid. Deposition of homogentisic acid in cartilage and connective tissues leads to a black-grey pigmentation of nose, ears and sclerae and an arthropathy that affects the thoracolumbar spine and large joints, characteristically causing narrowing and calcification of the intervertebral discs with no or small osteophytes [6]. Diagnosis is confirmed by 24-hour urinary excretion of homogentisic acid.

A dietary disturbance caused by deficiency in selenium intake is also known to cause a rare form of joint degeneration known as Kashin–Beck disease. This disorder is endemic in China and usually causes joint symptoms early in life (5–15 years of age) and progressive joint dysfunction, enlargement, and deformity, affecting most commonly distal joints of upper and lower limbs.

Another condition closely associated to OA is the disease caused by deposition of basic calcium phosphate and pyrophosphate crystals in which crystals were shown to cause an inflammatory process that could contribute to joint damage [3]. These calcium-containing crystals are present in half of OA knees with effusion and are more prevalent in advanced radiographic stages of OA [7]. However, the question whether they act as factors in the pathogenesis of OA or

Table 19.1 Diseases or metabolic abnormalities that may predispose to OA and respective laboratory tests or gene associations

Condition	Laboratory test/associated gene
Ochronosis	24-hour urinary excretion of homogentisic acid
Acromegaly	*IGF-1*, growth hormone
Hypothyroidism	Thyroid stimulating hormone, free T3 and T4
Diabetes mellitus	Fast plasma glucose, A1C
Calcium-containing crystal disease	Polarized light microscopy for calcium pyrophosphate and alizarin red S stain for basic calcium phosphate (SF)
Haemochromatosis	Serum transferrin saturation and ferritin concentration, *HFE* mutation
Wilson disease	Serum ceruloplasmin, 24-hour urinary excretion of cooper
Hyperparathyroidism	Parathyroid hormone
Hypophosphatasia	Serum phosphorus
Hypomagnesaemia	Serum magnesium
Haemoglobinopathy	Haemoglobin electrophoresis
Gaucher disease	Acid beta-glucosidase activity in peripheral blood leucocytes
Familial CPPD	*ANKH*
Spondyloepiphyseal dysplasia; Stickler syndrome type I	*COL2A1*
Multiple epiphyseal dysplasia	*COMP, MATN3*
Metaphyseal chondrodysplasia	*COL10A1*
Spondyloepimetaphyseal dysplasia	*PAPSS2*
Otospondylomegaepiphyseal dysplasia; Stickler syndrome type III	*COL11A2*
Stickler syndrome type II; Marshall syndrome	*COL11A1*

are merely a consequence of more severe joint damage remains controversial [8]. Nevertheless, CPPD may occur in association with arthritis (pseudogout) and lead to joint degeneration. Numerous metabolic diseases are associated with CPPD such as hyperparathyroidism, haemochromatosis, hypomagnesaemia, hypophosphatasia, and Wilson disease [9]. Other laboratory tests that may be useful to investigate disorders associated with OA are shown in Table 19.1.

Hereditary osteoarthritis and genetic polymorphisms

The notable advances in molecular biology have allowed better understanding about genetic factors in the development of OA, even though the first description of a genetic component dates from more than 60 years ago [10]. Genetic factors are now estimated to be responsible for up to half of the risk for developing the disease. Monogenic disorders associated with OA have been described and an increasing number of other genetic polymorphisms are currently being determined [11] and are more comprehensively addressed in Chapter 9 of this book. An outline of the most common hereditary disorders along with the appropriate genetic test is included in Table 19.1. Early recognition of a hereditary cause is important as appropriate therapy may influence joint function and quality of life and prevent further joint damage. Unusual disease manifestations, presence of comorbidities, and early onset may be signs of this subset of disorders.

Vitamin D

Vitamin D comprises a group of fat-soluble secosteroids responsible for enhancing intestinal absorption of calcium, iron, phosphate, zinc, and magnesium. It has a significant role in calcium homeostasis and metabolism [12]. Vitamin D_2 (ergocalciferol) and vitamin D_3 (cholecalciferol) are the two major molecules in humans while $25(OH)_2D_3$ (calcitriol) is the biologically active form [13].

The inactive form 25-(OH)D is used to determine the vitamin D status in practice. Despite the lack of an absolute consensus, previous studies [14,15] have defined vitamin D deficiency as 25-(OH)D lower than 20 ng/mL (50 nmol/L), insufficiency as 25-(OH)D between 20 and 30 ng/ml (50–75 nmol/L) and higher than 30 ng/mL as recommended levels (Table 19.2). 25-(OH)D is considered toxic if greater than 200 ng/mL (500 nmol/L) [12,16,17].

Vitamin D deficiency, with a rate ranging from 50% to 80% [18,19], is very prevalent in the community and coexists frequently with OA in older people. The relationship between vitamin D and OA is still vague with some conflicting research findings. Insufficient serum vitamin D levels may be related to subchondral bone changes, since low serum vitamin D has been found to increase osteoblastic activity and bone turnover [20]. Improving the vitamin D status in the

Table 19.2 Summary table of laboratory markers in osteoarthritis and crystal arthropathies

Lab tests	Method	Description	Reference range
ESR, erythrocyte sedimentation rate	Westergren	Increased serum fibrinogen level causes red blood cells to clump	Male [71]: age 20, < 12 mm/h; age 55, < 14 mm/h; age 90, < 19 mm/h Female [71]: age 20, < 18 mm/h; age 55, < 21 mm/h; age 90, < 23 mm/h Newborn: 0~2 mm/h Neonatal to puberty: 3~13 mm/h
CRP, C-reactive protein, hs-CRP	Nephelometric assays, ELISA, rapid immunodiffusion, visual agglutination, immunoturbidimetry, laser nephelometry	Dead and dying cells phagocytized by macrophage cause increase in IL6, which promotes hepatic synthesis of CRP	Normal: 0~10 mg/L hs-CRP: <3 mg/L
Vitamin D	Competitive protein binding assays (CPBA) Immunoassay (IA, including radioimmunoassay & enzyme immunoassay) Liquid chromatography–mass spectrometry (LC-MS/MS)	First assay to measure vitamin D. Recognize 25-(OH)D$_2$ equally as well as 25(OH)D$_3$ Remains the predominant mode of measurement for 25-(OH)D. The method was used by many reference laboratories to establish reference ranges Overestimate 25(OH)D levels by approximately 10–20% Currently considered to be the gold standard but was not routinely used. Labour intensive and technically difficult but distinguish the various forms of vitamin D (vitamin D$_2$, vitamin D$_3$)	Preferred healthful level: 25-(OH)D >75 nmol/L Insufficient: 50–75 nmol/L Mild deficiency: 25–50 nmol/L Moderate deficiency: 12.5–25 nmol/L Severe deficiency: <12.5 nmol/L
IL1	Bioassays; ELISA; ELISPOT; flow cytometric-based immunofluorescence assays; immunohistochemistry; flow cytometry; antibody array assays; bead-based assays; *in situ* hybridization; limiting dilution analysis; RT-PCR	Produce fever; stimulate acute-phase protein; promote proliferation of Th2 cells	Blood or serum [72]: 0–5 pg/mL
IL6		Induce acute-phase protein synthesis, T-cell activation, IL2 production; stimulate B-cell IG production and haematopoietic progenitor cell growth	Blood or serum [72]: 5–15 pg/mL
TNFA		Involved in inflammatory response; activates endothelial cells and other cells of immune and non-immune systems; induces fever and septic shock; induces diapedesis	Blood or serum [72]: 0–16 pg/mL
Leptin		Regulates energy intake and expenditure at the hypothalamic level; pro-inflammatory and pro-catabolic factors	Blood or serum: It is recommended that each laboratory include its own panel of control sample in the assay
Adiponectin		Up-regulates IL10 in human macrophages; induced nitric oxide synthase type II and pro-inflammatory cytokines	Blood or serum [72]: 5–10 mcg/mL

elderly could protect against the development and worsening of knee OA [21]. In contrast to these positive findings, some studies reported that vitamin D status was unrelated to the risk of knee OA [22]. A recent systematic review, which included two randomized controlled trials (RCTs) and 13 observational studies, suggested that 25-(OH)D appeared to be implicated in structural changes rather than symptoms of knee OA [23]. Therefore, given the prevalence of deficiency in the community and its potential role in OA pathogenesis, our suggestion is that serum 25-(OH)D should be measured in knee OA patients as a regular test, particularly at the initial stage of disease.

According to a recent RCT study, 2-year vitamin D supplementation to bring serum 25-(OH)D levels into the normal range does not reduce knee pain, prevent cartilage loss, maintain physical function, or preserve radiographic joint space width compared with placebo. However, in those with low baseline 25-(OH)D (<15 ng/mL), vitamin D supplementation had larger effects on knee pain and change in cartilage volume than in those who received placebo, although these were not significant due to the small sample size [24]. In another RCT, knee OA patients with vitamin D deficiency were included and it was found that vitamin D supplementation significantly improved knee pain and function compared to placebo, but had no effect on progression of radiographic OA, possibly due to a short follow-up period [25]. A recent RCT in symptomatic knee OA patients with low 25-(OH)D, which addressed the limitations of the previous two RCTs, showed that vitamin D supplementation did not result in significant differences in change in MRI-measured tibial cartilage volume or knee pain over 2 years [26]. Given conflicting data it remains to be seen if vitamin D supplementation has a beneficial effect on knee OA.

Biochemical markers

The role of biochemical markers in osteoarthritis

Biomarkers are defined as characteristics that are objectively measured and evaluated as an indicator of normal biological processes, pathogenic processes, or pharmacology responses [27,28]. For OA, biomarkers are important tools to understand the pathophysiology of the disease as well as its distinct stages and phenotypes, develop drugs and other therapeutics, predict progression, and develop personalized evidence-based action plans. They encompass not only biochemical substances measured in blood, urine, and SF, but also gene-based and image markers especially from magnetic resonance such as cartilage thickness, synovitis, bone shape, and bone marrow lesions, which are beyond the scope of this chapter.

The use of biomarkers is well established in the field of osteoporosis in large part due to the therapeutic advances in the disease in the past years. Consequently, biomarkers have revealed the pathological events that lead to osteoporosis and assisted the development of the wide range of drugs that are currently available for its treatment [29]. In the field of OA, biochemical markers are undergoing significant progress and novel candidates are appearing as we gain a greater understanding of the pathophysiology of the disease [29]. At this point the specific interpretation and application of various biochemical markers in individuals requires further investigation before advocating their use in clinical practice.

The present section will cover the processes involved in biochemical biomarkers research from the discovery of a novel marker to its validation and qualification, the current classification and

nomenclature used to facilitate the study of biomarkers, potential applications in OA, and, finally, an outline about the most promising biochemical markers and their correlation to OA.

Steps for biomarkers validation and qualification

The ideal biochemical marker is one that represents a specific pathogenic process or treatment goal, is readily accessible in terms of sampling (e.g. blood, urine), has prompt available testing, and is stable in storage [30]. The advances in 'omics' research (proteomics, lipidomics, metabolomics, and genomics) revealed a wide range of new potential biomarkers, including not only proteins and fragments of proteins but also metabolites, carbohydrates, and genetic polymorphisms.

After the discovery of a potential biomarker, the validation process establishes its analytical performance, assessing parameters such as accuracy, stability, and precision. This process basically analyses whether the candidate is accurate and reliably measurable, as it is detailed in Table 19.3 [31,32]. The next step is the verification phase, in which the association of the biomarker with a given end point is investigated. One example of this process is the studies that determined the positive association of inflammatory markers with knee pain in OA [33]. Finally, the qualification phase analyses the test in a specific context (e.g. specific population, stage of disease or therapeutic intervention) and determines its clinical value and potential use as a surrogate end point in that context (clinical validation) [31]. To date, no biomarker has been qualified and recognized for systematic use.

Table 19.3 Biochemical biomarkers' characteristics assessed during the analytical performance verification

Performance	Description
Selectivity/ specificity	Ability to assess unequivocally the analyte in the presence of components that may be expected to be present [31]
Accuracy	Closeness of agreement between the value that is accepted either as the conventional true value or an accepted reference value and the value found [31]
Precision	Closeness of agreement between a series of measurements obtained from multiple sampling of the same homogeneous sample under the prescribed conditions [31]
Recovery	Extraction efficiency of an analytical process, reported as a percentage of the known amount of an analyte carried through the sample extraction and processing steps of the method [32]
Sensitivity	Lowest analyte concentration that can be measured specifically by an analytical procedure
Robustness	Capacity of a bioanalytical method to remain unaffected by small, but deliberate variations in method parameters and provides an indication of its reliability during normal usage [31]
Stability	The chemical stability of an analyte in a given matrix under specific conditions for given time intervals [32]
Linearity	Ability of an analytical procedure (within a given range) to obtain test results which are directly proportional to the concentration (amount) of analyte in the sample [31]

Classification and application of biochemical markers in osteoarthritis

According to the BIPED classification proposed by Bauer et al. in 2006 and later expanded to BIPEDS in 2011 [31,34], a biomarker can be classified into one or more categories according to its relevance (Table 19.4). This classification improves communication and application of biomarkers in the study of OA and is divided in to Burden of disease, Investigative, Prognostic, Efficacy of intervention, Diagnostic and Safety.

A 'burden of disease' biomarker assesses the severity of the disease in individuals with OA and is able to quantify the extent of involvement in all joints of the body. Investigative biomarkers are the ones not yet classified in any other category but which showed sufficient value for further research. In the field of diagnosis, one

Table 19.4 Summary of existing biochemical markers and their 'BIPEDS' classification for knee and hip

Biochemical marker	BIPEDS classification		ELISA assay type
	Knee	Hip	
Cartilage degradation:			
uCTX-II	BPED	BPD	Competitive-inhibition
s/uC1,2C	D(u)	None	Competitive-inhibition
s/uC2C	E (s); D (u)	B(s)	Competitive-inhibition
uColl2-1NO2	D (s); B,P (u)	D(s)	Competitive-inhibition
sCPII	D	B	Competitive-inhibition
sCOMP	BPD	BPD	Competitive-inhibition & sandwich
uHELIX-II	D	BPD	Competitive-inhibition
s/uColl 2-1	BP (u); D (s)	D(s)	Competitive-inhibition
uTIINE	BPE	None	Not commercially available
s/uPentosidine	BP (s)	None	HPLC
sKS	BPED	None	Competitive-inhibition
sYKL-40	BE	D	Not commercially available
sMMP3	E	None	Sandwich for total MMP3 assay
Cartilage synthesis:			
sPIIANP	BPD	None	Competitive-inhibition
sPIICP	None	B	Competitive-inhibition
sCS846	P	None	Competitive-inhibition
Bone degradation:			
s/uCTX-1	BP(u); D(s/u)	None	Competitive-inhibition
s/uNTX-1	PE(u)	P(s)	Competitive-inhibition
uPYD	BED	None	HPLC
uD-PYD	BED	None	HPLC
sICTP	None	BP	Sandwich
Bone synthesis:			
sBSP	D	B	Sandwich
sOC	BPED	None	ELISA
sPINP	DP	B	Sandwich
Synovial degradation:			
uGlc-Gal-PYD	BD	None	HPLC

(continued)

Table 19.4 Continued

Biochemical marker	BIPEDS classification		ELISA assay type
	Knee	Hip	
sHA	BPED	P	Sandwich protein binding assay
Synovial synthesis:			
sPIIINP	BD	None	Sandwich

B, burden of disease; P, prognostic; E, efficacy of intervention; D, diagnostic.

BSP, bone sialoprotein; C1,2C, collagenase-generated neoepitope of types I and II collagen collagenase; C2C, collagenase-generated neoepitope of type II collagen; CTX-I, carboxytelopeptide of type I collagen; CTX-II, carboxytelopeptide of type II collagen; COMP, cartilage oligomeric matrix protein; CS-846, aggrecan chondroitin sulphate 846 epitope; DPD, deoxy-pyridinoline; Glc-Gal-PYD, glucosyl-galactosyl-pyridinoline; HA, hyaluronan; HPLC, high-performance liquid chromatography; ICTP, carboxyterminal telopeptide of type I collagen; KS, keratan sulphate; NTX-I, MMP3, matrix metalloproteinases 3; N-telopeptide of type I collagen; OC, osteocalcin; PINP, procollagen I intact N-terminal; PYD, pyridinoline; PIIANP, type IIA procollagen amino propeptide; PIICP, type II procollagen carboxy-propeptide; PIIINP: procollagen III amino terminal propeptide; uTIINE, urinary type II collagen collagenase-generated neoepitope; YKL-40, human cartilage glycoprotein 39.

expected application of biomarkers is in detecting early stages of OA. The American College of Rheumatology (ACR) criteria for the diagnosis of OA are composed of clinical features with or without the addition of radiographic criteria [35]. They are highly sensitive but not useful to discern the early stages of OA from healthy subjects, a period of utmost importance for the prevention of further deterioration of the joint.

For the development of new drugs, biomarkers can be used to assess drug mechanism of action and efficacy, monitor safety, select drug candidates, predict clinical outcome, and assist with dose finding [29]. At present, the minority of participants included in clinical trials show progress of disease over time, which ultimately results in the need for a high number of participants and long duration of studies to evaluate clinical and/or radiological response [36]. By predicting those who are more likely to progress, biomarkers may allow the identification of more suitable participants for clinical trials, both increasing trial efficiency and also targeting participants who will benefit most from a potential structure modifying agent [37]. In this same scenario, they may play a key role in the development of a personalized plan of action for the management of OA, in which decision-making is based on an individual's specific tests rather than general recommendations [38]. This personalized approach is highlighted as a potential way to achieve better treatment results by recognizing the heterogeneity of OA, especially its different stages and phenotypes. To help illustrate this, it was recently shown that markers of bone turnover are different between early stages of knee and hip OA [39] and that markers of inflammation, cartilage degradation, and bone turnover are higher in erosive than non-erosive hand OA, possibly reflecting distinct pathogenic processes between these phenotypes [40].

Biochemical markers can also be categorized according to which process in OA pathogenesis they are related, such as bone remodelling, cartilage synthesis/degradation, and synovial activity [29, 41] (Figure 19.1).

Markers of cartilage degradation and synthesis

In general, the majority of studies have investigated the performance of biochemical markers in the OA knee followed by hip. Among all tests available, markers of cartilage degradation were the most extensively studied [42]. Markers of collagen turnover in cartilage may reflect collagen type II degradation (CTX-II, HELIX-II, C2C,

Coll 2-1, Coll 2-1NO2, and TIINE), synthesis (PIIANP and PIICP), or collagen type 1 and 2 degradation (C1,2C). There are a number of other biomarkers involved in cartilage metabolism such as non-collagenous proteins of cartilage (cartilage oligomeric matrix protein (COMP)), glycosaminoglycans (keratan sulphate (KS) and chondroitin sulphate 846 (CS846)), and metalloproteinases.

Among the most commonly investigated biomarkers, CTX-II, C2C, COMP, and PIIANP were associated with the presence of OA in knee and hip while CTX-II also showed a positive correlation to the total body burden of OA [43]. CTX-II was associated with low PIIANP levels in early stages of knee OA, highlighting the dissociation between collagen type II synthesis and degradation in this stage [44]. An increase in Coll 2-1 and Coll 2-1NO2 levels over 1 year was also able to predict progression in knee OA [45]. A few studies have shown a decrease in CTX-II levels after different interventions but its role as an indicator of treatment efficacy in the practice is yet to be defined [42,46–48].

Markers of synovial activity

This category includes PIIINP (synovium synthesis), hyaluronic acid and glycosil-galactosil pyridinolin (synovium degradation (Glc-Gal-Pyd)). Serum hyaluronic acid (sHA), serum PIIINP, and urinary Glc-Gal-Pyd were increased in OA patients compared to controls and urinary Glc-Gal-Pyd was associated with pain in knee OA, indicating the relationship between pain and synovitis [49]. Moreover, sHA was shown to be an indicator of the total body burden of the disease [43] and is associated with knee OA progression [50,51].

Markers of bone remodelling

Bone turnover has been characterized by three types of biomarkers: indicators of bone reabsorption (C- and N-terminal type I collagen telopeptides (CTX-1 and NTX-1, respectively)), bone formation (procollagen type I N-propeptide (P1NP)), and mineralization (osteocalcin). Serum P1NP has demonstrated diagnostic value and predicted OA progression in the early stages of knee OA, particularly progressive osteophytosis [52]. Furthermore, the combination of high levels of P1NP to increased markers of bone reabsorption enhanced the ability of P1NP to predict cartilage loss assessed by MRI [53], reflecting the role of high bone remodelling in OA progression. This same association was found for higher levels of osteocalcin and increased bone reabsorption markers.

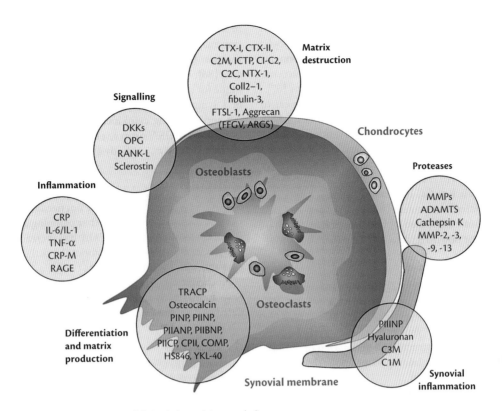

Figure 19.1 Potential biochemical markers in OA and their relation to joint metabolism.
Reproduced from *Annals of the Rheumatic Diseases*, Value of biomarkers in osteoarthritis: current status and perspectives, M Lotz et al., 72, copyright 2013 with permission from BMJ Publishing Group Ltd.

Another study has shown that CTX-1 and NTX-1 were elevated in progressive knee OA and not in non-progressors, suggesting that altered bone turnover may be a diagnostic and therapeutic target in patients with progressive OA [54]. Recently, the CHECK (Cohort Hip and Cohort Knee) study of early OA noted similarities between CTX-II and bone markers suggesting that CTX-II may reflect the metabolism of bone rather than cartilage [55].

Inflammatory mediators

Acute-phase reactants

ESR and CRP are the two most commonly used inflammatory markers in clinical practice. These two laboratory tests are usually used to detect inflammation when clinical symptoms are not obvious and they are commonly used to monitor disease activity over time and help evaluate the clinical response to therapeutic agents. Both ESR and CRP are non-specific inflammatory markers, in other words, they are not diagnostic of a particular disease.

ESR is the oldest inflammatory maker and was first described by the Polish pathologist Edmund Biernacki in 1897 [56]. The Westergren method is used most commonly. Of note, ESR is an indirect measure of acute-phase protein concentrations, with physiologically higher levels in females and increasing levels with age and in several other conditions such as anaemia and chronic kidney disease.

CRP is another longstanding laboratory test for inflammation and was discovered in 1930 [57]. It is an acute-phase protein that is produced by hepatocytes and regulated by the pro-inflammatory cytokine interleukin (IL)-6 in response to both acute and chronic inflammatory reactions. The name is derived from the fact that it reacts with the C-polysaccharide of *Pneumococcus* [58]. CRP rises

above 5 mg/L within 6 hours from the onset of inflammation and peaks at 48 hours. It has a constant half-life of 19 hours so the sole determinant for circulating CRP concentration is the synthesis rate [58]. The reference range of CRP in the healthy population is 3~10 mg/L. Many clinical laboratories use relatively insensitive nephelometric assays to measure CRP, yielding the actual value only when it is above 10 mg/L. As clinical research increased, semi- or fully automatic ELISA methods were introduced and CRP is predominately assayed under the term hs-CRP. A laser nephelometry method can detect hs-CRP levels as low as 0.2 mg/L [59], which allows hs-CRP to detect chronic low-grade inflammation.

OA has generally been perceived as a 'non-inflammatory' arthropathy. Inflammatory markers are usually normal in OA, including ESR (<20 mm/hour) and CRP levels (<3 mg/L). However, recent research suggests that inflammation may be both a primary event in OA and secondary to other aspects of the disease, such as biochemical changes within the cartilage [60]. In patients with OA, ESR is usually normal but CRP may be slightly elevated [1]. A recent systematic review of 32 studies concluded that serum hs-CRP levels were modestly higher in OA patient than healthy controls (mean difference 1.19 mg/L) and suggested that low-grade systemic inflammation was more associated with symptoms than progressive changes of the disease [61]. Testing for hs-CRP levels may be helpful in distinguishing certain OA phenotypes, such as erosive OA (EOA) of the hand [62].

Pro-inflammatory cytokines in osteoarthritis

OA is associated with cartilage destruction, subchondral bone remodelling, and soft tissue inflammation [63]. Pro-inflammatory cytokines secreted by inflammatory cells including infiltrating macrophages and adipocytes are now implicated in OA pathophysiology [64,65]. These cytokines induce the release of matrix anabolic enzymes and inhibit the synthesis of extracellular matrix components such as proteoglycan and type II collagen [66], subsequently accelerating cartilage degradation or inducing bone resorption in OA [67].

IL1B, tumour necrosis factor alpha (TNFA), and IL6 appear to be the major cytokines involved in the pathogenesis of OA, which makes them prime targets for therapeutic interventions. In OA patients, levels of both IL1B and TNF are increased in the SF, serum, subchondral bone, and cartilage [68]. Other pro-inflammatory cytokines including IL15, IL17, IL18, leukaemia inhibitory factor (LIF), and chemokines such as CC-chemokine ligand (CCL5), IL8, and monocyte chemoattractant protein (MCP)-1 are also elevated in OA and are significantly associated with increased matrix metalloproteinases (MMPs) or down-regulated proteoglycan levels [69].

Adipokines in osteoarthritis

White adipose tissue has emerged as a dynamic organ that releases inflammatory adipokines such as leptin, adiponectin, resistin, and visfatin that are involved in rheumatic diseases. Adipokines exert modulatory actions on cartilage, synovium, bone, and various cells, through directly inducing joint structural deterioration or regulating local inflammatory processes, leading to metabolic dysfunction in OA patients [70,71].

Leptin is produced predominantly in adipose tissue and has been reported to be positively correlated with body mass index, fat mass, and body weight among people with OA [72]. The strong synergistic relationship between leptin and pro-inflammatory cytokines has been discovered in OA, as leptin enhanced the expression of inducible nitric oxide synthase (iNOS), cyclooxygenase 2 (COX2), prostaglandin E2 (PGE2), IL6, and IL8 in cartilage [73]. The elevated expressions of leptin and its receptor isoform (Ob-Rb) have detrimental effects on chondrocyte proliferation by inducing MMPs and IL1B production [74], and are correlated with the degree of cartilage degradation [75]. The significant associations between obesity measures and osteoarthritic structural outcomes are largely mediated by leptin [76–78], suggesting it has a catabolic effect. It also exerts anabolic activity in chondrocytes by inducing the production of growth factors including insulin-like growth factor 1 (IGF1) and transforming growth factor beta (TGFβ) [79]. Furthermore, leptin is associated with increased biomarkers of bone formation, such as osteocalcin and N-terminal type I procollagen propeptide (PINP) in patients with knee OA [80].

Adiponectin is involved in cartilage homeostasis by increasing tissue inhibitor of metalloprotease (TIMP)-2 and decreasing IL1B-induced MMP3 [81]. Additionally, adiponectin up-regulates IL10 in human macrophages to increase TIMP1 levels and to prevent the extracellular matrix degradation [82]. On the other hand, adiponectin could induce nitric oxide synthase type II and pro-inflammatory cytokines in chondrocytes [83], and its plasma level was associated with increased OA radiographic severity [84]. These discrepancies may be due to the existence of different isoforms of adiponectin, which may have different effects on OA [85].

Laboratory tests for cytokines and adipokines

The utilization of accurate and sensitive methods for the measurement of cytokines and adipokines in body fluids is prerequisite for the proper use of these mediators in clinical practice. Various techniques such as enzyme-linked immunosorbent assay (ELISA),

in situ hybridization (ISH), immunohistochemistry, limiting dilution analysis, and single-cell reverse transcriptase polymerase chain reaction (RT-PCR) allow the enumeration of cytokine-producing cells [86]. In addition, flow cytometry is a powerful analytical technique for characterization of cytokine signatures of various subsets of T lymphocytes. The most commonly used methods of detecting and analysing cytokines or adipokines in a sample including traditional ELISA assays, enzyme-linked immunosorbent spot (ELISPOT) assays, antibody array assays, and bead-based assays.

Conclusion

In summary, laboratory tests are not needed for diagnosis of typical OA and are used to exclude other pathologies when indicated. The importance of these tests in OA has increased steeply in the last years, revealing new insights about the pathophysiology of the disease and with potential use in its early diagnosis and management.

Biochemical markers have a prominent role in research and will have an increased role in clinical practice once appropriately validated and qualified.

References

1. Wolfe F. The C-reactive protein but not erythrocyte sedimentation rate is associated with clinical severity in patients with osteoarthritis of the knee or hip. *J Rheumatol* 1997; 24(8):1486–8.
2. Whiting PF, Smidt N, Sterne JA, et al. Systematic review: accuracy of anti-citrullinated peptide antibodies for diagnosing rheumatoid arthritis. *Ann Intern Med* 2010; 152(7):456–W166.
3. Liu YZ, Jackson AP, Cosgrove SD. Contribution of calcium-containing crystals to cartilage degradation and synovial inflammation in osteoarthritis. *Osteoarthritis Cartilage* 2009; 17(10):1333–40.
4. Carroll GJ, Breidahl WH, Olynyk JK. Characteristics of the arthropathy described in hereditary hemochromatosis. *Arthritis Care Res (Hoboken)* 2012; 64(1):9–14.
5. Dons RF, Rosselet P, Pastakia B, Doppman J, Gorden P. Arthropathy in acromegalic patients before and after treatment: a long-term follow-up study. *Clin Endocrinol (Oxf)* 1988; 28(5):515–24.
6. Ventura-Rios L, Hernández-Díaz C, Gutiérrez-Pérez L, et al. Ochronotic arthropathy as a paradigm of metabolically induced degenerative joint disease. A case-based review. *Clin Rheumatol* 2016; 35(5):1389–95.
7. Nalbant S, Martinez JA, Kitumnuaypong T, et al. Synovial fluid features and their relations to osteoarthritis severity: new findings from sequential studies. *Osteoarthritis Cartilage* 2003; 11(1):50–4.
8. Olmez N, Schumacher Jr, HR. Crystal deposition and osteoarthritis. *Curr Rheumatol Rep* 1999; 1(2):107–11.
9. Jones AC, Chuck AJ, Arie EA, et al. Diseases associated with calcium pyrophosphate deposition disease. *Semin Arthritis Rheum* 1992; 22(3):188–202.
10. Stecher RM. Heberden's nodes: heredity in hypertrophic arthritis of the finger joints. *Am J Med Sci* 1941; 210:801–9.
11. Hochberg MC, Yerges-Armstrong L, Yau M, Mitchell BD. Genetic epidemiology of osteoarthritis: recent developments and future directions. *Curr Opin Rheumatol* 2013; 25(2):192–7.
12. Holick MF. High prevalence of vitamin D inadequacy and implications for health. *Mayo Clin Proc* 2006; 81(3):353–73.
13. Holick MF, Schnoes HK, DeLuca HF, Suda T, Cousins RJ. Isolation and identification of 1,25-dihydroxycholecalciferol. A metabolite of vitamin D active in intestine. *Biochemistry* 1971; 10(14):2799–804.
14. Malabanan AO, Turner AK, Holick MF. Severe generalized bone pain and osteoporosis in a premenopausal black female: effect of vitamin D replacement. *J Clin Densitom* 1998; 1(2):201–4.
15. Heaney RP. Vitamin D depletion and effective calcium absorption. *J Bone Miner Res* 2003; 18(7):1342.

16. von Domarus C, Brown J, Barvencik F, Amling M, Pogoda P. How much vitamin D do we need for skeletal health? *Clin Orthop Relat Res* 2011; 469(11):3127–33.

17. Bischoff-Ferrari HA, Giovannucci E, Willett WC, Dietrich T, Dawson-Hughes B. Estimation of optimal serum concentrations of 25-hydroxyvitamin D for multiple health outcomes. *Am J Clin Nutr* 2006; 84(1):18–28.

18. Cherniack EP, Florez H, Roos BA, Troen BR, Levis S. Hypovitaminosis D in the elderly: from bone to brain. *J Nutr Health Aging* 2008; 12(6):366–73.

19. Greene-Finestone LS, Berger C, de Groh M, et al. 25-Hydroxyvitamin D in Canadian adults: biological, environmental, and behavioral correlates. *Osteoporos Int* 2011; 22(5):1389–99.

20. Adams JS, Hewison M. Update in vitamin D. *J Clin Endocrinol Metab* 2010; 95(2):471–8.

21. Bergink AP, Uitterlinden AG, Van Leeuwen JP, et al. Vitamin D status, bone mineral density, and the development of radiographic osteoarthritis of the knee: The Rotterdam Study. *J Clin Rheumatol* 2009; 15(5):230–7.

22. Pettifor JM. Vitamin D and/or calcium deficiency rickets in infants and children: a concern for developing countries? *Indian Pediatr* 2007; 44(12):893–5.

23. Cao Y, Winzenberg T, Nguo K, et al. Association between serum levels of 25-hydroxyvitamin D and osteoarthritis: a systematic review. *Rheumatology (Oxford)* 2013; 52(7):1323–34.

24. McAlindon T, LaValley M, Schneider E, et al. Effect of vitamin D supplementation on progression of knee pain and cartilage volume loss in patients with symptomatic osteoarthritis: a randomized controlled trial. *JAMA* 2013; 309(2):155–62.

25. Sanghi D, Mishra A, Sharma AC, et al. Does vitamin D improve osteoarthritis of the knee: a randomized controlled pilot trial. *Clin Orthop Relat Res* 2013; 471(11):3556–62.

26. Jin X, Jones G, Cicuttini F, et al. Effect of vitamin d supplementation on tibial cartilage volume and knee pain among patients with symptomatic knee osteoarthritis: a randomized clinical trial. *JAMA* 2016; 315:1005–13.

27. Biomarkers Definitions Working Group. Biomarkers and surrogate endpoints: preferred definitions and conceptual framework. *Clin Pharmacol Ther* 2001; 69(3):89–95.

28. Wagner JA, Williams SA, Webster CJ. Biomarkers and surrogate end points for fit-for-purpose development and regulatory evaluation of new drugs. *Clin Pharmacol Ther* 2007; 81(1):104–7.

29. Lotz M, Martel-Pelletier J, Christiansen C, et al. Value of biomarkers in osteoarthritis: current status and perspectives. *Ann Rheum Dis* 2013; 72(11):1756–63.

30. Kraus VB. Do biochemical markers have a role in osteoarthritis diagnosis and treatment? *Best Pract Res Clin Rheumatol* 2006; 20(1):69–80.

31. Kraus VB, Burnett B, Coindreau J, et al. Application of biomarkers in the development of drugs intended for the treatment of osteoarthritis. *Osteoarthritis Cartilage* 2011; 19(5):515–42.

32. Food and Drug Administration. *Guidance for Industry: Bioanalytical Method Validation*, revised 1st ed. Silver Spring, MD: Food and Drug Administration; 2013.

33. Stannus OP, Jones G, Blizzard L, Cicuttini FM, Ding C. Associations between serum levels of inflammatory markers and change in knee pain over 5 years in older adults: a prospective cohort study. *Ann Rheum Dis* 2013; 72(4):535–40.

34. Bauer DC, Hunter DJ, Abramson SB, et al. Classification of osteoarthritis biomarkers: a proposed approach. *Osteoarthritis Cartilage* 2006; 14(8):723–7.

35. Altman R, Asch E, Bloch D, et al. Development of criteria for the classification and reporting of osteoarthritis. Classification of osteoarthritis of the knee. Diagnostic and Therapeutic Criteria Committee of the American Rheumatism Association. *Arthritis Rheum* 1986; 29(8):1039–49.

36. Kraus VB, Feng S, Wang S, et al. Subchondral bone trabecular integrity predicts and changes concurrently with radiographic and magnetic resonance imaging-determined knee osteoarthritis progression. *Arthritis Rheum* 2013; 65(7):1812–21.

37. Kraus VB, Blanco FJ, Englund M, et al. OARSI Clinical Trials Recommendations: soluble biomarker assessments in clinical trials in osteoarthritis. *Osteoarthritis Cartilage* 2015; 23(5):686–97.

38. Sawitzke AD. Personalized medicine for osteoarthritis: where are we now? *Ther Adv Musculoskelet Dis* 2013; 5(2):67–75.

39. Van Spil WE, Welsing PM, Bierma-Zeinstra SM, et al. The ability of systemic biochemical markers to reflect presence, incidence, and progression of early-stage radiographic knee and hip osteoarthritis: data from CHECK. *Osteoarthritis Cartilage* 2015; 23(8):1388–97.

40. Ramonda R, Lorenzin M, Modesti V, et al. Serological markers of erosive hand osteoarthritis. *Eur J Intern Med* 2013; 24(1):11–5.

41. Garnero P, Rousseau JC, Delmas PD. Molecular basis and clinical use of biochemical markers of bone, cartilage, and synovium in joint diseases. *Arthritis Rheum* 2000; 43(5):953–68.

42. van Spil WE, DeGroot J, Lems WF, Oostveen JC, Lafeber FP. Serum and urinary biochemical markers for knee and hip-osteoarthritis: a systematic review applying the consensus BIPED criteria. *Osteoarthritis Cartilage* 2010; 18(5):605–12.

43. Kraus VB, Kepler TB, Stabler T, Renner J, Jordan J. First qualification study of serum biomarkers as indicators of total body burden of osteoarthritis. *PLoS One* 2010; 5(3):e9739.

44. Garnero P, Ayral X, Rousseau JC, et al. Uncoupling of type II collagen synthesis and degradation predicts progression of joint damage in patients with knee osteoarthritis. *Arthritis Rheum* 2002; 46(10):2613–24.

45. Deberg MA, Labasse AH, Collette J, et al. One-year increase of Coll 2-1, a new marker of type II collagen degradation, in urine is highly predictive of radiological OA progression. *Osteoarthritis Cartilage* 2005; 13(12):1059–65.

46. Garnero P, Aronstein WS, Cohen SB, et al. Relationships between biochemical markers of bone and cartilage degradation with radiological progression in patients with knee osteoarthritis receiving risedronate: the Knee Osteoarthritis Structural Arthritis randomized clinical trial. *Osteoarthritis Cartilage* 2008; 16(6):660–6.

47. Christgau S, Henrotin Y, Tankó LB, et al. Osteoarthritic patients with high cartilage turnover show increased responsiveness to the cartilage protecting effects of glucosamine sulphate. *Clin Exp Rheumatol* 2004; 22(1):36–42.

48. Manicourt DH, Azria M, Mindeholm L, Thonar EJ, Devogelaer JP. Oral salmon calcitonin reduces Lequesne's algofunctional index scores and decreases urinary and serum levels of biomarkers of joint metabolism in knee osteoarthritis. *Arthritis Rheum* 2006; 54(10):3205–11.

49. Garnero P, Piperno M, Gineyts E, et al. Cross sectional evaluation of biochemical markers of bone, cartilage, and synovial tissue metabolism in patients with knee osteoarthritis: relations with disease activity and joint damage. *Ann Rheum Dis* 2001; 60(6):619–26.

50. Sharif M, George E, Shepstone L, et al. Serum hyaluronic acid level as a predictor of disease progression in osteoarthritis of the knee. *Arthritis Rheum* 1995; 38(6):760–7.

51. Georges C, Vigneron H, Ayral X, et al. Serum biologic markers as predictors of disease progression in osteoarthritis of the knee. *Arthritis Rheum* 1997; 40(3):590–1.

52. Kumm J, Tamm A, Lintrop M, Tamm A. Diagnostic and prognostic value of bone biomarkers in progressive knee osteoarthritis: a 6-year follow-up study in middle-aged subjects. *Osteoarthritis Cartilage* 2013; 21(6):815–22.

53. Berry PA, Maciewicz RA, Cicuttini FM, et al. Markers of bone formation and resorption identify subgroups of patients with clinical knee osteoarthritis who have reduced rates of cartilage loss. *J Rheumatol* 2010; 37(6):1252–9.

54. Bettica P, Cline G, Hart DJ, Meyer J, Spector TD. Evidence for increased bone resorption in patients with progressive knee osteoarthritis: longitudinal results from the Chingford study. *Arthritis Rheum* 2002; 46(12):3178–84.

55. van Spil WE, Drossaers-Bakker KW, Lafeber FP. Associations of CTX-II with biochemical markers of bone turnover raise questions on its tissue origin: data from CHECK, a cohort study of early osteoarthritis. *Ann Rheum Dis* 2013; 72(1):29–36.

56. Biernacki E. Samoistna sedymentacja krwi jako naukowa, praktyczno-kliniczna metoda badania. *Gaz Lek* 1987; 17(962):996.

57. Tillett WS, Francis T. Serological reactions in pneumonia with a non-protein somatic fraction of Pneumococcus. *J Exp Med* 1930; 52(4):561–71.

58. Pepys MB, Hirschfield GM. C-reactive protein: a critical update. *J Clin Invest* 2003; 111(12):1805–12.

59. Ledue TB, Rifai N. Preanalytic and analytic sources of variations in C-reactive protein measurement: implications for cardiovascular disease risk assessment. *Clin Chem* 2003; 49(8):1258–71.

60. Bonnet CS, Walsh DA Osteoarthritis, angiogenesis and inflammation. *Rheumatology (Oxford)* 2005; 44(1):7–16.

61. Jin X, Beguerie JR, Zhang W, et al. Circulating C reactive protein in osteoarthritis: a systematic review and meta-analysis. *Ann Rheum Dis* 2015; 74(4):703–10.

62. Punzi L, Ramonda R, Oliviero F, et al. Value of C reactive protein in the assessment of erosive osteoarthritis of the hand. *Ann Rheum Dis* 2005; 64(6):955–7.

63. Martel-Pelletier J, Lajeunesse D, Pelletier J-P, Etiopathogenesis of osteoarthritis. *Arthritis Allied Cond Textb Rheumatol* 2005; 15:2199–226.

64. Distel E, Cadoudal T, Durant S, et al. The infrapatellar fat pad in knee osteoarthritis: an important source of interleukin-6 and its soluble receptor. *Arthritis Rheum* 2009; 60(11):3374–7.

65. Iannone F, Lapadula G. Obesity and inflammation—targets for OA therapy. *Curr Drug Targets* 2010; 11(5):586–98.

66. Hashimoto M, Nakasa T, Hikata T, Asahara H. Molecular network of cartilage homeostasis and osteoarthritis. *Med Res Rev* 2008; 28(3):464–81.

67. Hoff P, Buttgereit F, Burmester GR, et al. Osteoarthritis synovial fluid activates pro-inflammatory cytokines in primary human chondrocytes. *Int Orthop* 2013; 37(1):145–51.

68. Koopman WJ, Mooreland LW (eds). *Arthritis and Allied Conditions: A Textbook of Rheumatology*. Philadelphia, PA: Lippincott Williams & Wilkins; 2005.

69. Kapoor M, Martel-Pelletier J, Lajeunesse D, Pelletier JP, Fahmi H. Role of proinflammatory cytokines in the pathophysiology of osteoarthritis. *Nat Rev Rheumatol* 2011; 7(1):33–42.

70. de Boer TN, van Spil WE, Huisman AM, et al. Serum adipokines in osteoarthritis; comparison with controls and relationship with local parameters of synovial inflammation and cartilage damage. *Osteoarthritis Cartilage* 2012; 20(8):846–53.

71. Gomez R, Conde J, Scotece M, et al. What's new in our understanding of the role of adipokines in rheumatic diseases? *Nat Rev Rheumatol* 2011; 7(9):528–36.

72. Koskinen A, Vuolteenaho K, Nieminen R, Moilanen T, Moilanen E. Leptin enhances MMP-1, MMP-3 and MMP-13 production in human osteoarthritic cartilage and correlates with MMP-1 and MMP-3 in synovial fluid from OA patients. *Clin Exp Rheumatol* 2011; 29(1):57–64.

73. Vuolteenaho K, Koskinen A, Kukkonen M, et al. Leptin enhances synthesis of proinflammatory mediators in human osteoarthritic cartilage—mediator role of NO in leptin-induced PGE2, IL-6, and IL-8 production. *Mediators Inflamm* 2009; 2009:345838.

74. Bao JP, Chen WP, Feng J, et al. Leptin plays a catabolic role on articular cartilage. *Mol Biol Rep* 2010; 37(7):3265–72.

75. Simopoulou T, Malizos KN, Iliopoulos D, et al. Differential expression of leptin and leptin's receptor isoform (Ob-Rb) mRNA between advanced and minimally affected osteoarthritic cartilage; effect on cartilage metabolism. *Osteoarthritis Cartilage* 2007; 15(8):872–83.

76. Ding C, Parameswaran V, Cicuttini F, et al. Association between leptin, body composition, sex and knee cartilage morphology in older adults: the Tasmanian older adult cohort (TASOAC) study. *Ann Rheum Dis* 2008; 67(9):1256–61.

77. Stannus OP, Cao Y, Antony B, et al. Cross-sectional and longitudinal associations between circulating leptin and knee cartilage thickness in older adults. *Ann Rheum Dis* 2015; 74(1):82–8.

78. Stannus OP, Jones G, Quinn SJ, et al. The association between leptin, interleukin-6, and hip radiographic osteoarthritis in older people: a cross-sectional study. *Arthritis Res Ther* 2010; 12(3):R95.

79. Dumond H, Presle N, Terlain B, et al. Evidence for a key role of leptin in osteoarthritis. *Arthritis Rheum* 2003; 48(11):3118–29.

80. Berry PA, Jones SW, Cicuttini FM, Wluka AE, Maciewicz RA. Temporal relationship between serum adipokines, biomarkers of bone and cartilage turnover, and cartilage volume loss in a population with clinical knee osteoarthritis. *Arthritis Rheum* 2011; 63(3):700–7.

81. Chen TH, Chen L, Hsieh MS, et al. Evidence for a protective role for adiponectin in osteoarthritis. *Biochim Biophys Acta* 2006; 1762(8):711–8.

82. Emanuela F, Grazia M, Marco de R, et al. Inflammation as a link between obesity and metabolic syndrome. *J Nutr Metab* 2012; 2012:476380.

83. Lago R, Gomez R, Otero M, et al. A new player in cartilage homeostasis: adiponectin induces nitric oxide synthase type II and pro-inflammatory cytokines in chondrocytes. *Osteoarthritis Cartilage* 2008; 16(9):1101–9.

84. Koskinen A, Juslin S, Nieminen R, et al. Adiponectin associates with markers of cartilage degradation in osteoarthritis and induces production of proinflammatory and catabolic factors through mitogen-activated protein kinase pathways. *Arthritis Res Ther* 2011; 13(6):R184.

85. Francin PJ, Abot A, Guillaume C, et al. Association between adiponectin and cartilage degradation in human osteoarthritis. *Osteoarthritis Cartilage* 2014; 22(3):519–26.

86. Bienvenu J, Monneret G, Fabien N, Revillard JP. The clinical usefulness of the measurement of cytokines. *Clin Chem Lab Med* 2000; 38(4):267–85.

SECTION 7

Management

CHAPTER 20

Introduction: the comprehensive approach

Michael Doherty, Johannes Bijlsma,
Nigel Arden, David J. Hunter, and Nicola Dalbeth

The importance of holistic assessment of the patient

The assessment and management of a person with osteoarthritis (OA) is a challenge to the clinical skills and judgement of any health professional. The main reasons why the person with OA seeks advice are pain and functional impairment. However, the correlation between pain severity, disability, and the extent of structural OA changes is not always strong, and the consequences of pain and impairment vary greatly from person to person, depending on factors such as personality, affect, occupational and recreational aspirations, other coexistent disease and disability, and the expectations of available healthcare delivery [1–3]. Therefore, assessing a person with symptomatic OA is potentially complex and must occur on at least two levels (Figure 20.1):

1. Assessment of *the joint*—for example, which joint or joints are involved, articular versus periarticular pain, degree of structural damage, presence of instability, degree of inflammation, restriction, and functional impairment

2. Assessment of *the person*—for example, impact and severity of pain and functional impairment, participation restriction, affect and level of distress, other medical problems, social support, quality of life, and illness perceptions and knowledge of arthritis and its treatment.

This requires a global, holistic approach if a successful individualized management plan with realistic goals is to be developed and agreed with the patient. Full account must be taken of the individual seeking advice, as well as of the severity of the OA afflicting their joints.

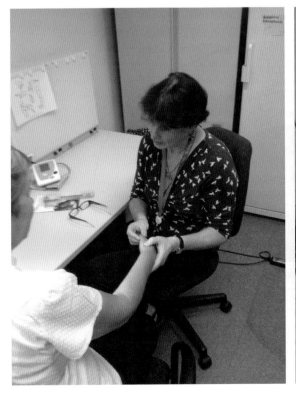 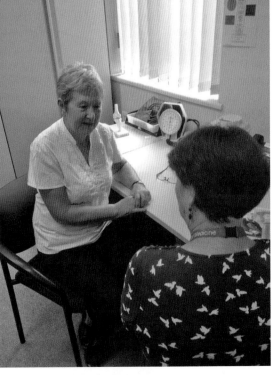

Figure 20.1 Holistic assessment of a patient with symptomatic OA is not just at the level of the joint but involves assessment of the person.

Management objectives

There is general agreement [4–11] that the central objectives of management are to:

- educate the person with OA about the condition and its treatment options and fully involve the informed patient in all decision-making relating to treatment
- control pain
- optimize function, reduce participation restriction, and improve quality of life
- beneficially modify the OA process.

These clearly interrelate and overlap. To achieve these aims, there are a wide variety of interventions from which to choose [4–11].

Principles of treatment selection

When considering the appropriate management strategy for an individual patient, the following general principles are pertinent:

1. Any management plan must be *individualized and patient-centred* with the *patient fully involved in decision-making*. The selection of treatments and the order in which they are tried is determined by the individual requirements and characteristics of the patient (the person and the joint, as above). The patient's perceptions and knowledge of OA and their preferences for certain forms of therapy require consideration and discussion. If the plan does not accord with the patient's beliefs, modified or not by the information they have received, adherence and a beneficial outcome are likely to be jeopardized [8,12,13].

2. The majority of treatments for OA have only small or modest effect sizes and although research evidence for combined interventions is very limited, in clinical practice a multifaceted *package of care*, rather than sequential monotherapy, is required [8,9].

Although management is highly individualized to each patient, certain evidence-based interventions which are safe, widely available, and often effective should be considered for every person with OA [8,9]. These core interventions (education, exercise, addressing adverse mechanical factors, weight loss if overweight or obese) are non-pharmacological and largely involve lifestyle changes. In addition, there are a wide range of additional treatment options that can be considered and discussed depending on individual patient requirements and the success of previous treatments. This '*core and options*' approach has particularly been emphasized by the National Institute for Health and Care Excellence (NICE) (Figure 20.2) [9].

3. In general, *simple and safe interventions are tried first*, before more complex, potentially injurious, treatments. In addition to the balance of safety and efficacy, the costs, local availability, logistics of delivery, and patient acceptability of individual treatments will also influence decision-making.

4. The *site of OA involvement* determines in part the selection of interventions. For example, some treatments such as topical creams and joint replacement surgery are limited in suitability or efficacy to one, or only a few, sites. However, most randomized controlled trials (RCTs) focus on knee OA and to a lesser extent hip and hand OA, and there is a paucity of research evidence for specific treatment approaches for OA at other sites such as the foot. Therefore many aspects of management need to involve a common-sense approach, with full involvement of the informed patient in decision-making.

5. Currently there are no approved disease-modifying OA drugs (DMOADs) and pharmacological treatments are primarily adjuncts to core treatments and prescribed for pain relief alone. For pain control, an *additive rather than substitutive* approach is recommended. That is, if the first option analgesic is insufficient, a second analgesic with a different mode of action is

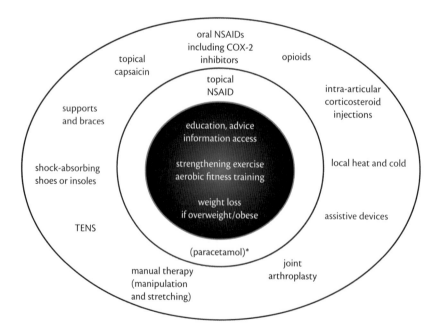

Figure 20.2 The core and options approach emphasized by NICE for recommended treatments available within the UK National Health Service [9]. Treatments to be considered for every patient are in the centre, 'first-line' analgesics to try are in the inner ring, and other options are in the outer ring. (*Note that the recommendation for paracetamol as the first-line oral analgesic is under review at present.)

added rather than given instead of the first (potentially a third or fourth may subsequently be added). This approach recognizes the complexity of pain processing and often the relatively modest effect of a single pharmacological agent used as monotherapy for chronic pain.

6. *Comorbidity* and concurrent medications are important and almost inevitable in the older population affected by OA. Such comorbidity may influence treatment selection for OA. For example, cardiovascular or renal disease might prevent the use of a particular treatment such as a non-steroidal anti-inflammatory drug (NSAID, including cyclooxygenase (COX)-2 selective inhibitors). Importantly, however, recognition and treatment of comorbidity such as non-restorative sleep or depression can alleviate the symptoms of OA and reduce the need for analgesia [8].

7. The wide variety of treatment approaches for this chronic condition may require the expertise of a number of different health professionals. A *coordinated multidisciplinary team approach* with *clear communication* is often required to deliver healthcare efficiently and to present coherent, rather than contradictory, management advice.

8. The status and requirements of the patient will change with time, usually slowly but sometimes more rapidly. This necessitates *regular review* and *readjustment of treatment options*, rather than the rigid continuation of a single plan.

Core treatments to consider in every person with osteoarthritis

Education and information access

This is the essential starting point (Figure 20.3). It is a primary responsibility of the doctor/health professional to inform patients (and/or their care givers) about:

♦ the nature of their condition

♦ its causes—especially those pertaining to the individual

♦ its prognosis

♦ any required investigations

♦ the available treatment options and their advantages and disadvantages.

Knowing about OA helps patients manage and cope with their condition and make informed choices between treatment options (see Chapter 21). However, in addition to being a professional responsibility, education itself improves the outcome. Being fully informed shifts the locus of control from the health professional to the patient, allows them to be fully involved in shared decision-making, and empowers them to subsequently 'self-manage' many of the agreed management components such as lifestyle modification. Although the exact mechanisms are unclear, provision of access to information and contact with a therapist may reduce pain and disability in patients with OA, improve self-efficacy, and reduce the frequency of primary care consultation and (in the United States) healthcare costs [8,14–16]. Such benefits are modest but long-lasting and safe [8].

The content and format of education requires discussion and tailoring to the individual, but can take many forms, including one-to-one discussion, group classes, regular telephone calls, educational literature, and interactive computer programmes [8]. Importantly, education should not be viewed as a one-off discrete element at the time the patient first seeks advice, but should be included in every aspect of management and be reinforced and developed at subsequent clinical encounters [8,9].

OA is often considered a uniformly progressive 'wear and tear' disease, the inevitable consequence of ageing, for which little can be done other than eventual surgical replacement of the worn-out joint. This negative and inaccurate perception is widespread not only in the community but also among doctors and other health professionals. In reality, however, OA is not inevitably progressive and many intervention strategies can reduce symptoms and improve function. An optimistic approach is therefore justified, and full information on OA personalized to the individual

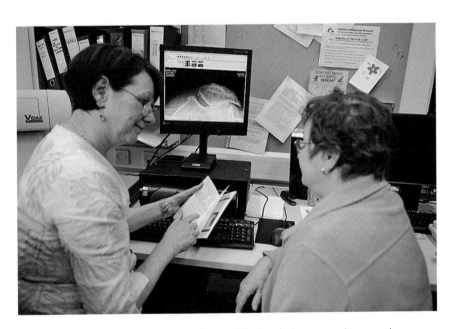

Figure 20.3 Providing education and information about OA is a professional responsibility but also improves patient-centred outcomes.

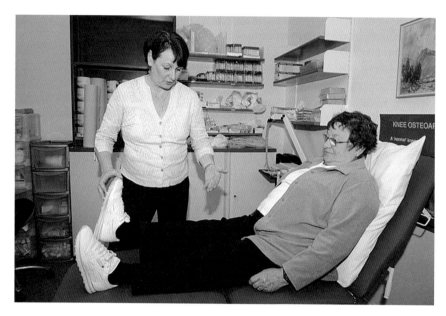

Figure 20.4 Simple initial quadriceps strengthening exercise (straight leg raise) being taught by a nurse to a patient with knee OA. Note the patient's footwear which she selected herself after being recommended to wear shoes with thick soft soles, no raised heel, sufficiently broad forefoot, and soft deep uppers.

(e.g. risk factors specific to them and the joint site involved) can counter negative misconceptions and enhance the benefits obtained through the patient's contextual response to receiving care [17].

Exercise

Many people with OA are concerned that continued physical activity may further damage their joints. The musculoskeletal system, however, is designed to move, and reduced activity is detrimental to the health of all its component tissues. OA can result in weakness and eventual wasting (type II atrophy) of all the muscles that act over the affected joint. Furthermore, poor aerobic fitness, a consequence of reduced activity, is associated with a low sense of 'well-being' and more reporting of pain and handicap from OA. Therefore, people with OA, irrespective of their age, should be encouraged to maintain activity and to undertake local neuromuscular training, strengthening and aerobic exercise using 'small amounts often' to increase general fitness, improve muscle strength, and maintain or increase the range of joint movement (see Chapter 22). There is good evidence that both strengthening and aerobic fitness exercise can reduce pain and disability from knee and hip OA [4–10,18,19]. Even simple, nurse-instructed exercise for knee OA undertaken at home can prove effective and safe in the long term (Figure 20.4) [20]. Such exercise not only reduces pain and disability but also improves the reduced muscle strength, proprioception, standing balance, and abnormal gait patterns associated with knee and hip OA, thus fundamentally influencing the physiological parameters of joint function [21–25].

In addition to its effects on pain and disability from OA, increased aerobic fitness encourages restorative (delta) sleep, improves psychological health, promotes functional independence, and benefits common co-morbidities such as obesity, diabetes, depression, chronic heart failure, and hypertension [22]. There are very few contraindications, even in elderly subjects, to a 'prescription of exercise' that combines stretching ('warm-up'), strengthening, and aerobic routines [22]. Tai chi, balneotherapy, and other forms of water-based exercise may additionally be considered as adjuncts to core exercise according to patient preference and availability [7,8,10].

Reduction of adverse mechanical factors, including weight loss if overweight

Since both high-impact acute injury and lower-impact repetitive micro-trauma are risk factors for OA [26,27], eliminating or reducing adverse mechanical factors is an accepted policy for primary prevention of OA in sports and occupational health. Similarly, avoiding or reducing adverse mechanical forces across a joint with OA may not only improve symptoms and function, but has obvious face validity in terms of secondary prevention, especially if these factors played a part in development of OA at that site.

Obesity is a common comorbidity and an important modifiable risk factor for knee OA (Figure 20.5), and to a lesser extent hip and hand OA. In randomized controlled trials (RCTs), obese or overweight patients with knee or hip OA who successfully lose weight show clear improvement in function and modest reduction in pain [8,9,28,29]. Reducing obesity is advised for many other health reasons and has obvious face validity with respect to both primary and secondary prevention of knee and hip OA (see Chapter 23). Assisting the patient to achieve and subsequently maintain weight reduction can be challenging, but in addition to full information and motivational discussion, successful weight loss programmes recommend an individualized programme that contains frequent self-monitoring, both diet and regular exercise, regular eating (three times daily), a good variety of food but reduced portion size, low (saturated) fat and sugar and high fruit and vegetable content, improved nutritional awareness through education, and modification of any individual eating triggers (e.g. stress) [8].

Another simple mechanical principle for OA at any joint site is to encourage patients to 'pace' their activities through the day rather than attempting too much at one go. Although it takes longer, this may allow them to achieve an activity without over-stressing their

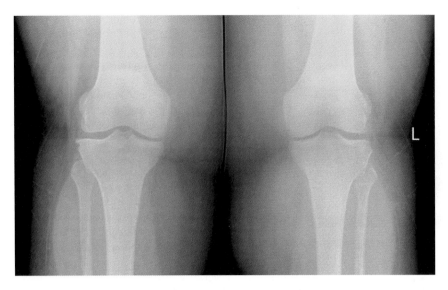

Figure 20.5 Standing radiograph of obese person with predominantly medial tibiofemoral OA. Weight loss in overweight and obese people is advised for many health reasons including primary and secondary prevention of OA and improved function, and to a lesser extent pain, in those with symptomatic knee OA.

OA joints. Patients with knee and hip OA also should be advised about appropriate footwear [8]. Shoes with thick but soft (e.g. air-filled) soles and no raised heels minimize rebound upward force transmission when walking, and it is also beneficial to have appropriate support for the arches and a broad enough forefoot size to allow comfortable spacing of the toes (Figure 20.4). Other simple devices can be considered for people with varus malalignment or patellofemoral OA, for example, wedged insoles or a selection of commercially available knee braces. The use of a walking stick or other walking aid (Figure 20.6) is a simple way of mechanically reducing symptoms from hip or knee OA [8,30]. Modification of the patient's home or work environment can further minimize external adverse mechanical factors and facilitate activities of daily living, for example, using a walk-in shower rather than a bath, raising the height of chairs, beds and toilet seats, or providing hand rails for stairs [8]. The patient may already be utilizing appropriate ways to cope with the consequences of their OA, but such strategies may be improved or new ones adopted with the assistance of a therapist.

Recommended first-line analgesics

Despite a very low effect size for pain relief in OA, paracetamol (acetaminophen) is traditionally the recommended oral analgesic of first choice and, if effective, is the preferred long-term analgesic for OA [4–11]. This is largely due to its perceived safety compared to other oral analgesics, as well as wide availability and low cost. However, the safety of paracetamol has recently come into question (Figure 20.7) because of growing evidence that it shares the same spectrum of side effects as oral NSAIDs, including gastrointestinal (GI) bleeding [31], hypertension, and renal impairment [32,33] (see Chapter 29). For example, in one community-based RCT [31], one in five participants with knee OA taking either paracetamol 1 g or ibuprofen 400 mg three times daily (i.e. usual over-the-counter doses) sustained a drop in haemoglobin of at least 1 g/dL at 3 months with reduced red cell indices and increased platelet count, presumably due to GI blood loss. Furthermore, the combination of the two caused this drop in 40% of participants, with 7%

showing drops of 2 g/dL or higher, which is a surrogate for a major GI bleed in many RCTs. The latter is particularly worrying given the recommended additive approach to analgesic prescribing and the large number of people who take both drugs on the mistaken premise [32] that paracetamol has no peripheral COX inhibition. Because of safety concerns such as this, as well as the growing realization that paracetamol hardly separates from placebo in OA

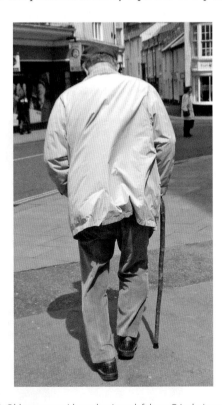

Figure 20.6 Older person with predominant left knee OA placing weight down his walking stick, held on the right side, while his left leg is in weight-bearing (stance) phase and his right leg is in swing-through phase. The appropriate height for the handle of a walking aid is determined by measuring the distance from the ulnar styloid to the ground, while standing.

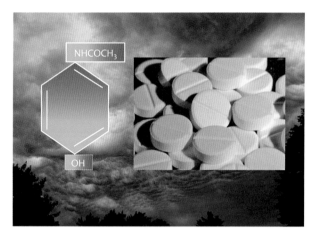

Figure 20.7 Paracetamol is a relatively insoluble metabolite of its more toxic precursor phenacetin (an antipyretic). Although perceived as a very safe, though weak analgesic for chronic pain, a storm is now brewing over paracetamol as there is increasing evidence to show that it shares the same potential side effects as oral NSAIDs but has a very small effect size that is below any minimum clinically important difference.

RCTs [10,34], it is possible that advice concerning paracetamol may change in forthcoming guideline updates. Indeed, paracetamol was not the first-line oral analgesic in the updated 2014 Osteoarthritis Research Society International guidelines [10], and in the recent NICE update (2014) [9] the recommendation to *not* prescribe paracetamol for OA created such controversy during stakeholder review that this advice was postponed pending a safety review by the Medicines and Healthcare products Regulatory Agency in the United Kingdom.

While a growing cloud hangs over paracetamol, in many guidelines the alternative first-line analgesic drug to try for painful peripheral joints with OA is a topical NSAID [4,6,9], especially

for those with comorbidity [10]. This can be as effective as an oral NSAID [9,35] but has little if any systemic toxicity, the only side-effect in practice being occasional local skin reactions (see Chapter 28). Topical treatments are very popular with patients and associate with good adherence, partly because it makes obvious sense to apply a pain relieving treatment directly to the site of symptoms (Figure 20.8). Indeed, in RCTs the mean effect size for pain relief is significantly higher for placebo topical NSAIDs (0.63, 95% confidence interval (CI) 0.47–0.80) than it is for placebo oral NSAIDs (0.49, 95% CI 0.34–0.63) supporting heightened expectancy from local treatment [36].

In most countries, paracetamol (up to 3 g daily), oral NSAIDs (e.g. lower doses of ibuprofen such as 600–1200 mg daily), and topical NSAIDs are available over the counter. One or all of these are likely to have been tried on an 'as-required' basis as part of self-management or following advice from a pharmacist, usually before seeking help from a medical practitioner. Other commonly tried self-medications are nutraceuticals (see Chapter 31) and a range of other natural health products, and the response and tolerability of the patient to any such self-medications need specific enquiry and discussion.

Other treatment options

A wide variety of other non-pharmacological, drug, and surgical interventions that may be considered as *additional options* are selected and added, as required, to the above core interventions (see Chapters 24–26 and 28–34). It is very difficult to rank treatments in order of OA 'severity' because of the numerous ways in which severity can be defined (e.g. X-ray change, pain, and disability) and the fact that different assessment measures do not necessarily progress in parallel. For example, relatively minor structural OA and modest pain in a single joint may be 'the final straw' and result in major participation restriction in an older person with

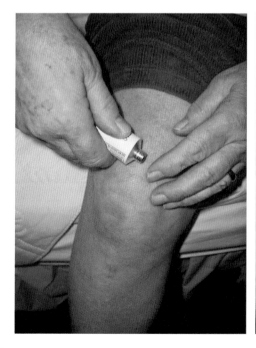
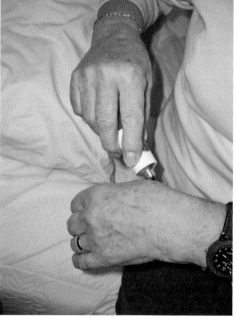

Figure 20.8 Topical NSAID being used by a patient for knee OA (left) and thumb-base OA (right).

other significant comorbidities. Pragmatically, therefore, the recommended core effective and safe treatments are given initial, equal priority for all patients irrespective of OA 'severity' and other treatments, especially more invasive ones, are considered second in order. Nevertheless, all decisions are made according to patient requirements. For example, at first consultation it may be appropriate to consider an intra-articular injection of the knee in an older patient with marked pain that has been unresponsive to self-medication and who wishes to attend her grand-daughter's wedding the following weekend. The expected improvement that she will experience may not only allow her to participate in a major family event, but is likely to increase her confidence in the rest of the agreed management plan. Thus there are no rigid algorithms to follow. Following a full patient assessment, practitioners need to apply common sense when selecting from their 'tool box' the most appropriate option for the job in hand.

Surgery, of course, is the 'final option' that is reserved for patients with persistent pain and disability that impacts significantly on their quality of life and which is refractory to conservative management [4–6,9] (see Chapter 33). Importantly, referral should be made before there is prolonged and established functional limitation and severe pain since this may compromise a good outcome following surgery.

The lives of patients who are severely incapacitated by hip or knee OA can be transformed by successful joint replacement (Figure 20.9). However, such major surgery is not without its risks, and it is not the 'ultimate answer' for everyone. For example, when assessed 3–4 years after surgery, up to 44% of people undergoing knee replacement and 27% undergoing hip replacement may be dissatisfied with their operation and continue to experience chronic, sometimes neuropathic-like, pain [37,38]. Furthermore, there are no rigid guidelines for deciding the timing of surgery or selecting those who might benefit most. As always, a global assessment is paramount, with patients actively involved in determining their own outcome.

The evidence for efficacy and the advantages and drawbacks of all currently available interventions for OA are fully discussed in Chapters 21–26 and 28–34. The exciting possibility of pharmacological modification of the OA process is considered in Chapter 35.

Stratified medicine and predictors of response to treatment

As explained in Chapter 1, attempts have been made to subdivide people within the spectrum of OA into certain subgroups according to their presumed main aetiological risk factor or sharing of certain phenotypic characteristics (clinical features, imaging, or other investigational biomarkers). This approach aligns with the aims of *stratified medicine* (also called *personalized* or *precision* medicine) which also seeks to subgroup according to a shared response to particular therapies. Indeed, the ultimate aim of stratified medicine is to help health professionals select the most appropriate treatment for a patient and to give 'the right treatment, for the right person, at the right time'. Although this may be advantageous in some conditions, it remains to be seen if a stratification approach will improve the care of people with a common complex disorder such as OA. This is because the suggested subgroups show considerable overlap, sometimes progress from one subset to another, and often coexist with other subsets at different sites within the same individual. Even if broad subgrouping were possible, the multifaceted and complex way in which OA can affect an individual makes it unlikely that discrete characteristics will accurately predict treatment response. The response of an individual to any treatment depends on many person-specific and context-specific factors, and

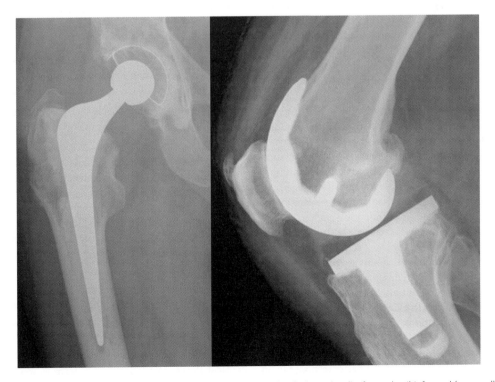

Figure 20.9 Examples of total joint replacements for the hip (left) and knee (right). Note that for knees 'total' refers to the tibiofemoral (not patellofemoral) articulations.

(a)   (b)

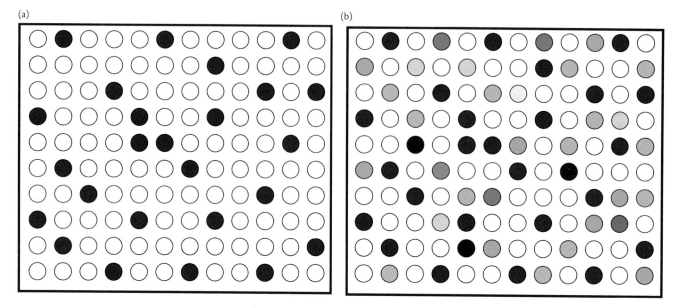

Figure 20.10 Most OA RCTs have multiple exclusion criteria which result in a relatively homogeneous sample from the whole population of people with OA (left). RCTs with fewer exclusions result in a more heterogeneous sample (right) which makes the results more generalizable to the whole population of people with OA and may also permit examination of predictors of treatment response. The second strategy requires more participants for randomization to distribute variation equally so is more expensive and less commonly undertaken.

it seems unlikely that one or a few factors shared in common by different people with OA will determine the degree of treatment response for patient-centred outcomes such as pain. Nevertheless, a full assessment of a person with OA will permit individualized characterization of that person with specific features (relating both to the joint(s) and the person) that are relevant to constructing an agreed management plan. With regular follow-up it is then possible to determine treatments that are working and those which may need adjustment or replacing with an alternative—the equivalent of an ongoing within person 'n-of-1' trial. This pragmatic 'individualized' medicine approach, based on individual rather than group characteristics, reflects many aspects of best practice and aligns well with current guidelines such as NICE [9].

This issue of stratified medicine is discussed in depth in Chapter 37.

Evidence regarding predictors of response in OA is sparse. A large number of exclusions usually apply in RCTs (e.g. degree of radiographic change, comorbidity, and concurrent medications) which conveniently produces a relatively homogeneous study population for factors that may influence outcome, thus restricting the number of patients required (Figure 20.10). However, this homogeneity of study populations means that possible predictors of response cannot be readily examined. Re-analysis of individual patient data in published RCTs, where this is feasible, is one way of trying to establish predictors of response, but ideally less exclusion criteria and a larger sample of heterogeneous participants is required in trials designed to allow this question to be addressed. Interestingly, when formally studied the evidence is not always what we might have predicted. For example, contrary to many people's expectation, the presence of clinical inflammation at the knee may not predict a better response to an oral NSAID [39,40], and presence of inflammation at the knee assessed clinically or by ultrasound (effusion and synovial hypertrophy) does not predict a better response to an intra-articular injection of corticosteroid [41,42]. This may reflect the complexity of the treatment response which is determined not just by joint-specific factors but also person-specific characteristics and contextual factors (see Chapter 27).

Translation of research evidence into practice

Although RCTs are the gold standard way of demonstrating efficacy and estimating the specific effect size of a treatment, there are several reasons why it is often difficult to extrapolate RCT or other research data on OA to routine clinical practice. For example:

♦ OA has different risk factors and outcomes at different joint sites. Though rarely studied, it is possible that treatment response also varies between sites. Extrapolation of RCT data from one site to another is often made, but may not be justified.

♦ A common selection bias is that participants are recruited from secondary care whereas the majority of OA patients are managed solely in primary care.

♦ As already mentioned, multiple exclusions in RCTs (e.g. having comorbidities or severe structural damage) often result in a relatively homogeneous sample of people with OA. Apart from reducing the ability to study predictors of response, this also means that trial participants may be unrepresentative of many people with OA in clinical practice and whether the study treatment will be as effective in more typical but complex patients is unanswered.

♦ An inclusion criterion for many analgesic drugs is for the patient to show significant worsening of symptoms following withdrawal of their current oral drugs. Such 'flare' designs have a selection bias towards drug-responsive participants and tend to inflate the treatment response and limit generalizability of the findings.

♦ Most RCTs are relatively short term (6 weeks to 6 months) and only a very few extend to 18–24 months. Many people with OA, however, have chronic symptoms and disability and more long-term efficacy and side effect data are needed. When available, long-term studies (e.g. for oral NSAID) are often far less positive than data from short-term studies [43,44].

♦ Most RCTs investigate monotherapy and very few examine the possible additive or interactive effects of combined treatments. In practice, however, several treatments are given concurrently as a package of care.

♦ The majority of trials in OA are of drug treatments, giving undue emphasis on pharmacological agents in the research base.

There are, of course, different forms of evidence. Short-term RCTs are not a good way to determine safety—large observational studies are required for this, although these are automatically assigned a lower grade of evidence in guideline development groups [45]. The incidence of side effects, costs, logistics of delivery, and personal experience of health professionals and patients all influence opinion concerning the overall clinical usefulness and effectiveness of specific treatments. In guidelines there is often discordance between the level of evidence and the strength of recommendation and level of agreement of expert clinicians [4–6]. It appears that our clinical practice is governed as much by our own experience, local situation, and personal bias as by the balance of published evidence.

There are a number of ways in which both the design and reporting of RCTs could improve the quality and clinical relevance of data obtained. One important example relates to the 'efficacy paradox' [46], when the reported effect of a treatment in an RCT differs markedly from the effect observed in clinical practice. The main reason for this is that the reporting of RCTs focuses on the difference between the outcome in the treatment group compared to that in the placebo group (i.e. the *specific effect* of the treatment) and it is this that is used to estimate the effect size ('strength') and the minimum clinically important difference of a treatment. However, in clinical practice it is the *overall treatment effect* that is observed, which includes both specific and non-specific contextual effects. Therefore, if a treatment has a large effect size but most of this is due to placebo/contextual effect (e.g. acupuncture), it may be not recommended in guidelines [9] but be seen to work well in clinical practice. Conversely, a treatment with a smaller overall treatment effect but which separates better from placebo may be supported in guidelines but be disappointing when used in practice. One way forward is for RCT results to emphasize not just the specific treatment effect, but also the overall treatment effect and the proportion attributable to contextual effects—the *proportional contextual effect* [47] (see Chapter 38). Such reporting more completely summarizes the trial evidence and should prove more helpful in guiding health

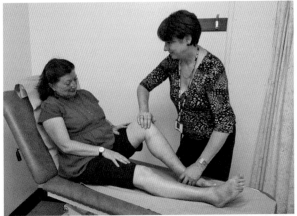
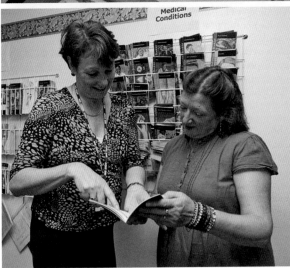
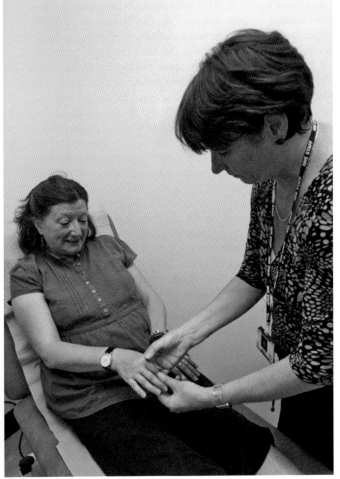

Figure 20.11 Thorough holistic assessment and good patient–practitioner interaction are central to the development of an appropriate individualized management plan.

professionals and guideline development groups than summaries based on specific treatment effect alone.

The importance of placebo (contextual) response in clinical care

The non-specific beneficial effects of treatment should not be underrated. It is noteworthy that the mean effect size of placebo analgesia in OA RCTs is in the moderate range (0.51, 95% CI 0.46–0.55) and is often greater than the specific effect size of the treatments used for OA [36]. Importantly, however, the positive effect that occurs when a participant believes they are receiving a treatment is not restricted to the context of an RCT—a non-specific 'contextual' or 'meaning' [48] response is an integral part of any clinical encounter and occurs when a patient receives active treatment. Expectancy is a key determinant of placebo and contextual response, and this is influenced by the illness perceptions and past experience of the patient as well as by a variety of contextual factors including the patient–practitioner interaction, the environment in which the treatment is received, the branding and colour of medications, the route of delivery of the treatment, and whether a treatment is new and expensive or old and cheap [17,49]. The benefits obtained through placebo and contextual responses are not simply 'a trick of the mind' but result from measurable biological changes within the patient [17,49] (see Chapter 27).

Unfortunately, whenever it has been audited, the management of OA often appears far from optimal [50]. Firstly, the core elements (education, exercise prescription, reduction of adverse mechanical factors) are often omitted and the most common treatment approach hinges upon drug treatments, predominantly NSAIDs. This discordance with current recommendations clearly needs to be addressed, and aspects relating to the organization and outcome of care are presented in Chapter 36 and the development and dissemination of guidelines are discussed in Chapter 37. Secondly, however, common patient complaints are that the doctor was 'too busy' to listen, they undertook only a superficial examination or no examination at all, they did not address key concerns, and they did not give a follow-up appointment (i.e. 'they did not want to see me again'). This also needs to be addressed. As health practitioners it is important that we appreciate the importance of this component of treatment and that we optimize the contextual aspects of care through a full, holistic patient assessment and good practitioner–patient interaction (Figure 20.11) [17] (see Chapter 27 for full discussion). These are components of recommended best practice but they also improve patient-centred outcomes [51]—the ultimate purpose of evidence-based care.

Conclusion

Management of the person with OA requires full assessment not just of the affected joints but also holistic assessment of the person. In line with current evidence-based guidelines, a package of care comprising core non-pharmacological treatments as well as other selected optional treatments should be agreed with full involvement of the informed patient and individualized to their specific needs. Drugs are adjuncts to assist pain control; currently topical NSAIDs are the safest effective analgesics to consider first for peripheral joint OA. It is essential to undertake regular follow-up to reassess the patient, reinforce and expand educational aspects, and to adjust the

management plan if required. A positive patient–practitioner interaction and optimization of contextual factors of care are also essential to management and can significantly improve patient-centred outcomes. There are caveats to interpreting research evidence and translating findings to clinical care, but in RCTs, the reporting of the overall treatment effect size and the proportion attributable to placebo could reduce the efficacy paradox.

References

1. Davis MA, Ettinger WH, Neuhas JM, Barclay JD, Segal MR. Correlates of knee pain among US adults with and without radiographic knee osteoarthritis. *J Rheumatol* 1992; 19:1943–9.
2. Hadler NM. Knee pain is the malady—not osteoarthritis. *Ann Intern Med* 1992; 116:598–9.
3. Creamer P, Lethbridge-Cejku M, and Hochberg MC. Factors associated with functional impairment in symptomatic knee osteoarthritis. *Rheumatology* 2000; 39:490–6.
4. Jordan KM, Arden NK, Doherty M, et al. EULAR Recommendations 2003: an evidence based approach to the management of knee osteoarthritis: Report of a Task Force of the Standing Committee for International Clinical Studies Including Therapeutic Trials (ESCISIT). *Ann Rheum Dis* 2003; 62(12):1145–55.
5. Zhang W, Doherty M, Arden N, et al. EULAR evidence based recommendations for the management of hip osteoarthritis: report of a task force of the EULAR Standing Committee for International Clinical Studies Including Therapeutics (ESCISIT). *Ann Rheum Dis* 2005; 64(5):669–81.
6. Zhang W, Doherty M, Leeb BF, et al. EULAR evidence based recommendations for the management of hand osteoarthritis: Report of a Task Force of the EULAR Standing Committee for International Clinical Studies Including Therapeutics (ESCISIT). *Ann Rheum Dis* 2007; 66(3):377–88.
7. Hochberg MC, Altman RD, April KT, et al. American College of Rheumatology 2012 recommendations for the use of nonpharmacologic and pharmacologic therapies in osteoarthritis of the hand, hip, and knee. *Arthritis Care Res* 2012; 64(4):465–74.
8. Fernandes L, Hagen KB, Bijlsma JW, et al. EULAR recommendations for the non-pharmacological core management of hip and knee osteoarthritis. *Ann Rheum Dis* 2013; 72(7):1125–35.
9. National Clinical Guideline Centre. *Osteoarthritis: Care and Management in Adults*. Clinical Guideline CG177. National Institute for Health and Care Excellence; 2014. https://www.nice.org.uk/guidance/cg177
10. McAlindon TE, Bannuru RR, Sullivan MC, et al. OARSI guidelines for the non-surgical management of knee osteoarthritis. *Osteoarthritis Cartilage* 2014; 22(3):363–88.
11. Nelson AE, Allen KD, Golightly YM, Goode AP, Jordan JM. A systematic review of recommendations and guidelines for the management of osteoarthritis: The Chronic Osteoarthritis Management Initiative of the U.S. Bone and Joint Initiative. *Sem Arthritis Rheum* 2014; 43(6):701–12.
12. Horne R. Patients' beliefs about treatment: the hidden determinant of treatment outcome? *J Psychosom Res* 1999; 47:491–5.
13. National Clinical Guideline Centre. *Medicines Adherence: Involving Patients in Decisions about Prescribed Medicines and Supporting Adherence*. Clinical Guideline CG76. National Institute for Health and Care Excellence; 2009. https://www.nice.org.uk/guidance/cg76
14. Weinberger M, Tierny WM, Booher P, Katz BP. Can the provision of information to patients with osteoarthritis improve functional status? *Arthritis Rheum* 1989; 32:1577–83.
15. Rene J, Weinberger M, Mazzuca SA, Brandt KD, Katz BP. Reduction of joint pain in patients with knee osteoarthritis who have received monthly telephone calls from lay personnel and whose medical regimens have remained stable. *Arthritis Rheum* 1992; 35:511–5.
16. Lorig KR, Mazonson PD, Holman HR. Evidence suggesting that health education for self-management in patients with chronic arthritis has

sustained health benefits while reducing health care costs. *Arthritis Rheum* 1993; 36:439–46.

17. Doherty M, Dieppe PA. The 'placebo' response in osteoarthritis and its implications for clinical practice. *Osteoarthritis Cartilage* 2009; 17:1255–62.

18. Uthman OA, van der Windt DA, Jordan JL, et al. Exercise for lower limb osteoarthritis: systematic review incorporating trial sequential analysis and network meta-analysis. *BMJ* 2013; 347:f5555.

19. Fransen M, McConnell S, Harmer AR, et al. Exercise for osteoarthritis of the knee (Review). *Cochrane Library* 2015; 1:CD004376.

20. Thomas K, Muir K, Doherty M, et al. Home based exercise programme for knee pain and osteoarthritis: randomised controlled trial. *BMJ* 2002; 325:752–5.

21. O'Reilly SC, Muir KR, Doherty M. Effectiveness of home exercise on pain and disability from osteoarthritis of the knee: a randomised controlled trial. *Ann Rheum Dis* 1999; 58:15–19.

22. American Geriatrics Society Panel on Exercise and Osteoarthritis. Exercise Prescription for older adults with osteoarthritis pain: consensus practice recommendations. *J Am Geriat Soc* 2001; 49:808–23.

23. Hurley MV, Scott DL. Improvements in sensorimotor function and disability of patients with knee osteoarthritis following a clinically practicable exercise regime. *Br J Rheumatol* 1998; 37:1181–7.

24. Messier SP, Royer TD, Craven TE, et al. Long-term exercise and its effect on balance in older, osteoarthritic adults: results from the Fitness, Arthritis, and Seniors Trial (FAST). *J Am Geriat Soc* 2000; 48:131–8.

25. Messier SP, Thompson CD, Ettinger WH. Effects of long-term aerobic or weight training regimens on gait in an older osteoarthritic population. *J Appl Biomech* 1997; 13:205–25.

26. McWilliams DF, Leeb BF, Muthuri SG, Doherty M, Zhang W. Occupational risk factors for osteoarthritis of the knee: a meta-analysis. *Osteoarthritis Cartilage* 2011; 19:829–39.

27. Muthuri SG, McWilliams D, Doherty M, Zhang W. History of knee injuries and knee osteoarthritis: a meta-analysis of observational studies. *Osteoarthritis Cartilage* 2013; 19:1286–93.

28. Bliddal H, Leeds AR, Christensen R. Osteoarthritis, obesity and weight loss: evidence, hypotheses and horizons—a scoping review. *Obes Rev* 2014; 15(7):578–86.

29. Christensen R, Henriksen M, Leeds AR, et al. Effect of weight maintenance on symptoms of knee osteoarthritis in obese patients: a twelve-month randomized controlled trial. *Arthritis Care Res* 2015; 67(5): 640–50.

30. Blount WP. Don't throw away the cane. *J Bone Joint Surg* 1956; 38(A):695–8.

31. Doherty M, Hawkey C, Goulder M, et al. A randomized controlled trial comparing oral ibuprofen, paracetamol and two doses of a fixed-dose combination tablet of ibuprofen/paracetamol in community-derived people with knee pain. *Ann Rheum Dis* 2011; 70:1534–41.

32. Hinz B, Brune K. Paracetamol and cyclooxygenase inhibition: is there a cause for concern? *Ann Rheum Dis* 71:20–25.

33. Roberts E, Nunes VD, Buckner S, et al. Paracetamol: not as safe as we thought? a systematic literature review of observational studies. *Ann Rheum Dis* 2016; 75(3):552–9.

34. Machado GC, Maher CG, Ferreira PH, et al. Efficacy and safety of paracetamol for spinal pain and osteoarthritis: systematic review and meta-analysis of randomised placebo controlled trials. *BMJ* 2015; 350:h1225.

35. Underwood M, Ashby D, Cross P, et al. Advice to use topical or oral ibuprofen for chronic knee pain in older people: randomised controlled trial and patient preference study. *BMJ* 2008; 336:138–42.

36. Zhang W, Robertson J, Jones A, Dieppe PA, Doherty M. The placebo response and its determinants in osteoarthritis—meta-analysis of randomised controlled trials. *Ann Rheum Dis* 2008; 67:1716–23.

37. Wylde V, Hewlett S, Learmonth ID, Dieppe P. Persistent pain after joint replacement: prevalence, sensory qualities, and postoperative determinants. *Pain* 2011; 152(3):566–72.

38. Kehlet H, Jensen TS, Woolf CJ Persistent postsurgical pain: risk factors and prevention. *Lancet* 2006; 367:1618–25.

39. Brandt KD, Bradley JD. Should the initial drug used to treat osteoarthritis pain be a nonsteroidal anti-inflammatory drug? *J Rheumatol* 2001; 28:467–73.

40. Bradley JD, Brandt KD, Katz BP, Kalasinski LA, Ryan SI. Comparison of an anti-inflammatory dose of ibuprofen, an analgesic dose of ibuprofen, and acetaminophen in the treatment of patients with osteoarthritis of the knee. *N Engl J Med* 1991; 325:87–91.

41. Jones A, Doherty M. Intra-articular corticosteroids are effective in osteoarthritis but there are no clinical predictors of response. *Ann Rheum Dis* 1996; 55:829–32.

42. Hirsch G, Kitas G, Klocke R. Intra-articular corticosteroid injection in osteoarthritis of the knee and hip: factors predicting pain relief—a systematic review. *Seminars in Arthritis Rheum* 2013; 42(5):451–73.

43. Williams HJ, Ward JR, Egger MJ, et al. Comparison of naproxen and acetaminophen in a two-year study of treatment of osteoarthritis of the knee. *Arthritis Rheum* 1993; 36:1196–206.

44. Dieppe PA, Cushnaghan J, Jasani MK, McCrae F, Watt I. A two-year, placebo-controlled trial of non-steroidal anti-inflammatory therapy in osteoarthritis of the knee joint. *Br J Rheumatol* 1993; 32:595–600.

45. Shekelle PG, Woolf SH, Eccles M, Grimshaw J. Clinical guidelines: developing guidelines. *BMJ* 1999; 318(7183):593–6.

46. Walach H. The efficacy paradox in randomized controlled trials of CAM and elsewhere: beware of the placebo trap. *J Altern Complement Med* 2001; 7(3):213–8.

47. Zhang W, Zou K, Doherty M. Placebos in knee osteoarthritis—reaffirmation that 'needle is better than pill'. *Ann Intern Med* 2015; 163(5):392–3.

48. Moerman DE, Jonas WB. Deconstructing the placebo effect and finding the meaning response. *Ann Intern Med* 2002; 136:471–6.

49. Abhishek A, Doherty M. Mechanisms of the placebo response in pain in osteoarthritis. *OA Cart* 2013; 21:1229–35.

50. OANation. OANation. 2012. http://www.arthritiscare.org.uk

51. Di Blasi Z, Harkness E, Ernst E, Georgiou A, Kleijnen J. Influence of context effects on health outcomes: a systematic review. *Lancet* 2001; 357:757–62.

CHAPTER 21

Patient information strategies for decision-making and management of osteoarthritis

Gillian Hawker, Anne Lyddiatt, Linda Li, Dawn Stacey, Susan Jaglal, Sarah Munce, and Esther Waugh

Introduction

Osteoarthritis (OA) is a chronic, progressive, and debilitating disease. Thus care that aligns with the principles of 'chronic disease management' [1,2] is indicated (Figure 21.1). Consistent with the tenets of chronic disease management, research conducted worldwide has consistently found that multidisciplinary team-based care is beneficial for people with OA [3,4]. Patients gain one-stop access to the expertise of different health professional specialties, each of which addresses an important aspect of OA management, including importantly engagement in OA self-management activities.

Self-management has been described as integral to quality chronic disease care [5]. Self-management has been defined by Lorig et al. [6] as 'learning and practicing skills necessary to carry on an active and emotionally satisfying life in the face of a chronic condition'; self-management is 'aimed at helping the participant

become an active, not adversarial, partner with healthcare providers'. Studies have shown that patients who are actively engaged in their care are more likely to be adherent to treatment recommendations, have enhanced self-efficacy, and, ultimately, experience better health outcomes [7,8]. Thus, motivating patients to be actively engaged in self-management, including pain management, weight control, physical activity, psychosocial health strategies [9], informed shared decision-making and goal setting is central to the success of chronic disease management.

In this chapter, we will review programmes that have been developed to enable people with or at risk for OA to achieve these goals, and summarize the evidence on their efficacy and effectiveness. Specifically, we will provide an overview of the following: strategies to enhance chronic disease and OA-specific self-management; the role of shared decision-making between the patient/family and

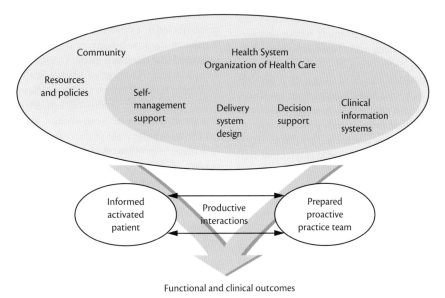

Figure 21.1 Model for improvement of chronic illness care.
Wagner EH. Chronic Disease Management: What Will It Take To Improve Care for Chronic Illness? *Effective Clinical Practice*, August/September 1998; 1:2–4.

healthcare providers; the use of patient decision aids to facilitate shared decision-making; advances in the use of information technologies to enhance patient education and self-management; and public health approaches to prevention of OA at a population level.

Chronic disease and osteoarthritis-specific self-management programmes

Traditional *patient education programmes* are intended to impart disease-specific *information and technical skills* designed to promote behaviour change (enhanced self-management of the condition or conditions) and, in turn, improve clinical outcomes [10]. They are often led by a healthcare professional. In comparison, *support groups* comprise a group of people with common experiences and concerns who provide emotional and moral support for one another. *Self-management programmes* typically combine aspects of both of these programmes; they may be led by a combination of a health professional, peer leader, or other patients, and generally take place in group settings. While self-management programmes provide some information and technical skills, the focus is principally on the development of patients' *problem-solving skills* or 'self-efficacy' (one's belief in one's ability to succeed in specific situations) [11] based on studies that show that greater patient self-efficacy, to make life-improving changes, yields better clinical outcomes.

Self-management programmes are multifaceted behavioural interventions that include both education and behaviour modification. Programmes vary in the content used to educate patients about their condition and to explain how they can best manage their symptoms. Some programmes specifically focus on managing the chronic condition itself, whereas others may take a more holistic approach to managing the overall general well-being of the individual. Substantial variation exists in the delivery of self-management programmes, such as the mode (face-to-face, Internet, telephone), the audience (group, individual), the duration (single session, several months, ongoing), the frequency (once a week, once every 2 months), and the personnel involved (healthcare professionals, lay leaders) [12].

Several models of self-management are known [13]; however, the core elements of all models involve building the patient's competency in (1) engaging in activities that promote health and prevent adverse sequelae; (2) interacting with healthcare providers; (3) performing improved self-monitoring of physical and emotional status; and (4) managing the effects of illness on a person's ability to function in important roles and the impact on emotions, self-esteem, and relationships with others [14]. As suggested above, the competencies required for these tasks include problem-solving, decision-making, finding and utilizing resources, forming partnerships with healthcare workers, and taking action to implement self-management activities [15].

The Stanford Arthritis Self-Management Program (ASMP) is one of the most well-known programmes [16]. It is a community-based programme for individuals with mild to moderate disease and is delivered by pairs of lay leaders, most of whom have arthritis. Caregivers or other support people are also encouraged to attend. The programme uses the principles of self-efficacy theory [11] aiming to enhance perceived ability to control various aspects of arthritis through mastery of skills, modelling, reinterpretation of symptoms, and persuasion. Overall, the programme aims to help individuals understand their arthritis, learn ways to cope with chronic pain, and take a more active role in managing their arthritis. Specific content of the programme includes exercising and healthy eating, managing pain, preventing fatigue and protecting joints, dealing with stress and depression, taking medications as prescribed and working with healthcare providers, and evaluating alternative treatments [17].

Evidence for efficacy and effectiveness of self-management programmes in osteoarthritis

A number of low-to-moderate-quality randomized clinical trials have evaluated the impact of self-management programmes on patient outcomes. In a systematic review by Kroon and colleagues [12], 29 studies (6753 participants) were included that compared self-management education programmes for OA to attention control (five studies), usual care (17 studies), information alone (four studies), or another intervention (seven studies). Most interventions included elements of skill and technique acquisition (94%), health-directed activity (85%), and self-monitoring and insight (79%). Social integration and support were addressed in only 12%. Eight studies included predominantly Caucasian, educated female participants, and only four provided any information on participants' health literacy. All studies were at high risk of performance and detection bias for self-reported outcomes; 20 studies were at high risk of selection bias, 16 were at high risk of attrition bias, two were at high risk of reporting bias and 12 were at risk of other biases. The attention control group was considered the most appropriate and thus the main comparator.

Self-management programme versus attention control in osteoarthritis

Compared with attention control groups, these studies showed that, on average, self-management programmes did not result in significant benefits, as they were defined, at 12 months. Low-quality evidence from one study (344 people) indicated that self-management skills were similar in active and control groups. Low-quality evidence from four studies (575 people) indicated that self-management programmes led to a small but clinically unimportant reduction in pain. Furthermore, low-quality evidence from one study (251 people) indicated that the mean global OA score was 4.2 on a 0- to 10-point symptom scale (lower score = better health) in the control group, and treatment reduced symptoms by a mean of 0.14 points. Low-quality evidence from three studies (574 people) showed no significant difference in function between groups; mean function was 1.29 points on a 0- to 3-point scale in the control group, and treatment resulted in a mean improvement of 0.04 points with self-management. Low-quality evidence from one study (165 people) showed no between-group difference in quality of life from a control group mean of 0.57 units on a 0–1 well-being scale. Moderate-quality evidence from five studies (937 people) indicated similar withdrawal rates between self-management (13%) and control groups (12%). Positive and active engagement in life was not measured.

Self-management programme versus usual care in osteoarthritis

Compared with usual care, the same review reported moderate-quality evidence from 11 studies (up to 1706 participants) that self-management programmes provided small benefits up to 21 months, in terms of self-management skills, pain, and OA symptoms and function. However, the authors concluded that these results were likely not clinically important, and no improvement in positive and active engagement in life or quality of life was observed. Withdrawal rates were similar between groups.

Self-management programme versus information alone or other interventions

Low-to-moderate-quality evidence indicated no important differences in self-management, pain, symptoms, function, quality of life, or withdrawal rates between self-management programmes and information alone or other interventions (exercise, physiotherapy, social support, or acupuncture).

Conclusions of systematic review and next steps

Based on this recent systematic review, there is currently only low-to-moderate-quality evidence that self-management programmes provide meaningful benefits in people with OA compared to any of attention controls or usual care. However, there are a number of limitations to self-management trials to date that may explain the absence of clinically meaningful impacts on patient outcomes. First, variation in the measures used to evaluate the success of self-management programmes has undoubtedly contributed to inconsistency in the reported efficacy and effectiveness of self-management programmes in OA. The Arthritis Self-Efficacy Scale (ASES) was the first arthritis-specific instrument developed to measure the effects of arthritis self-management programmes [18]. It consists of three subscales (pain, function, and other symptoms) and includes self-efficacy expectation items that ask individuals how certain they are that they can perform a specific activity (e.g. walking 100 feet on flat ground in 7 seconds); as well as performance attainment items (e.g. how certain they are that they can control their fatigue or deal with the frustration of arthritis). Although these items capture an individual's ability to self-manage, and are therefore useful in measuring outcomes of self-management programmes, the validity of the ASES as a true self-efficacy measure has been questioned [19,20]. For example, the ASES does not ask about an individual's confidence that different behaviours will produce the desired outcome (outcome expectations)—a key component of Bandura's theory of self-efficacy [21]. In addition, the function subscale items appear to capture *perceived* physical function rather than self-efficacy belief.

As outlined by Nolte and Osborne [22], while the Stanford ASMP includes content on communication with the physician, emotions and self-efficacy, it is questionable whether self-management programmes are able to have a significant effect on outcomes such as disability and physical functioning, as these outcomes are not specifically targeted by the programme. Given these limitations, research is ongoing to identify key indicators of effective self-management interventions from the patient perspective [23]. One such development has been the Health Education Impact Questionnaire (heiQ). This has involved extensive engagement and consultation with consumers and healthcare professionals regarding the outcomes they consider to be valuable and the direct benefits of self-management programmes. Eight independent domains were described and form the basis of the constructs of the questionnaire. Domains identified as key indicators of effective self-management programmes include health-directed behaviour; positive and active engagement in life; emotional well-being; self-monitoring and insight; constructive attitudes and approaches; skill and technique acquisition; social integration and support; and health service navigation. The constructs used in the heiQ have been determined to be robust across a range of settings [24,25].

As in other chronic disease self-management programmes, a further challenge in interpreting outcomes of self-management programmes concerns the time frame in which outcomes can be expected to occur. A programme logic model of impacts of self-management education could serve as a guide to categorize outcomes into short-, medium-, and long-term effects [22].

Finally, the impact of self-management programmes on patient outcomes may differ based on mode of delivery, for example, in person versus by telephone, and patient characteristics. For example, a study by Sperber and colleagues [26] explored whether the effects of a telephone-based OA self-management support intervention differed by race and health literacy. They determined that the Arthritis Impact Measurement Scales-2 (AIMS-2) mobility improved more among non-white than white people in the self-management programme compared with the health education and usual care groups. Furthermore, the AIMS-2 pain improved more among participants with low versus high literacy in the self-management group compared to the health education group. They also determined that non-white people with low literacy in the intervention group had the greatest improvement in pain. The authors concluded that this telephone intervention may be particularly beneficial for patients with OA who are racial/ethnic minorities and have low health literacy. Ackerman et al. [27] conducted a secondary analysis of data from their randomized controlled trial (RCT) of the Stanford ASMP in patients with hip/knee OA. In the trial, participation in the Stanford ASMP among those assigned to the intervention was only 30–53%, despite the absence of financial barriers and provision of flexible times. Review of the reasons for non-participation in the trial included disinterest, mobility challenges (pain, fear of falling, difficulty getting to programme), concurrent illness (a focus on arthritis versus living with more than one chronic condition), and lack of endorsement for the programme by the primary care physician. They additionally found that within those who agreed to participate, the baseline level of self-efficacy was high, indicating less potential for improvement with the intervention. Based on their findings, the authors made the following recommendations: targeting self-management programmes to individuals with low self-efficacy, who have the greatest potential for benefit; and provision of multiple options for delivery of self-management programmes (e.g. online, mail, telephone, and mobile devices).

Tailoring self-management/OA education programmes based on participant characteristics may be a necessary consideration in producing effective outcomes in OA self-management. As noted by Ackerman et al., programme delivery should capitalize on the rapidly growing use of online and mobile technologies. For example, in 2012, 83% of all Canadians and over 73% of rural residents had online access at home [28]. Of those, 67% used the Internet for medical/health-related activities [28]. Seniors are the fastest growing group of Internet users; two-thirds of people who are 65 or older use the Internet at least once a day [29]. Ownership of mobile devices is also growing rapidly, with over one-quarter of mobile phone users accessing health and wellness, fitness, or nutritional applications through their devices [30]. Given the increasing reach of communication technologies, initiatives that aim to integrate online tools in OA care are both relevant and timely.

Online and mobile tools use a variety of behavioural change techniques to increase physical activity participation [31]. Ensuring adherence to using technologies, however, can be a challenge. Approximately one-third of people in the United States who have owned a wearable product stopped using it within 6 months [32]. Furthermore, while one in ten people owned a physical activity tracker, half would use them on an ongoing basis [32]. While there is limited knowledge on strategies to improve adherence, emerging evidence suggests that a user friendly design for the tools, as well as the support and periodic review on their activity performance by health professionals, are facilitators for patients with arthritis to sustain the use of these tools [33].

Interactive health communication applications

Interactive health communication applications are computer-based information programs that aim to provide health information plus social support, decision support, and/or behaviour change support [34,35]. Users of these applications may also interact with clinical experts and other users. A Cochrane systematic review of 24 RCTs examining the effectiveness of these applications for people with chronic disease concluded that they had a moderately positive effect on the patient's knowledge and modest effect on the perceived social support, clinical outcomes, and behavioural outcomes, for example, being physically active and decreasing caloric intake [34]. Furthermore, there was a positive trend for self-efficacy.

One of the most successful online self-management interventions is the *Internet Chronic Disease Self-Management Program*. This 6-week online programme was a replicate of the original face-to-face programme [37,38]. Patients participated in weekly online workshops moderated by two trained peer moderators. In addition, they were required to log on at least three times a week to read the online content and join the bulletin board discussion. In a 12-month RCT (n = 958; 24.9% had arthritis), Lorig et al. [39] found significant improvement in participants' health distress, fatigue, pain, and participation in stretching and strengthening exercises, compared to the usual care group. In a subsequent RCT of the *Internet Arthritis Self-Management Program*, the authors found significant improvement in health distress, activity limitation, self-reported global health, and pain over the 12-month period for patients with OA [40].

Smartphones and mobile devices

Research on the use of smartphones and mobile devices in patients with OA is still at an early stage. A number of studies have examined the potential for using smartphones in delivering behaviour change interventions in other chronic diseases. For example, Fjeldsoe et al. [41] examined the use of a short message service (SMS) for supporting healthy behaviours, including smoking cessation, increased physical activity, and participation in chronic disease self-management. They concluded that tailored content and interactivity were important features of successful SMS interventions. A second narrative review by Wei et al. [42] concurred that the use of SMS could improve individuals' self-management behaviours, including adherence to medication and medical monitoring. In a review of RCTs on the use of smartphone messaging by

people with chronic diseases, de Jongh and associates [43] found moderate-quality evidence that smartphone messaging improved self-efficacy in patients with diabetes, and medication adherence in those with hypertension.

Role of shared decision-making in osteoarthritis care

As noted earlier, shared decision-making is a key skill necessary for patients to effectively self-manage chronic conditions, including OA. Shared decision-making is a process in which the patient and clinician jointly reach an informed decision about the plan of care on the basis of the patient's clinical needs, priorities, and values [44]. The clinician's expertise lies in diagnosing and identifying treatment options according to clinical priorities and evidence; the patient's role is to identify and communicate their informed values and personal priorities as shaped by their social circumstances, including culture and beliefs. Studies have consistently shown that patients that are involved in making decisions have improved quality of life, sense of control over their illness, fewer illness concerns and improved symptom relief [45]. Despite this, providers' engagement of patients in shared decision-making is suboptimal [45]. A systematic review of 33 studies using observers to evaluate current practice revealed that few practitioners engage their patients in shared decision-making [46]. In a study using standardized knee OA patients to evaluate gender bias in physicians' recommendations for knee replacement surgery, Borkhoff et al. [47] documented low levels of informed decision-making, using the Informed Decision-Making (IDM) checklist [48]. Fewer than 10% of all patient–physician discussions about knee replacement included all seven IDM elements; only 15% of the physicians elicited the patients' preference. Thus, there is room for improvement.

Patients with OA have multiple treatment options for managing their chronic illness, including choosing to do nothing. When treatments have risks of harm (e.g. non-steroidal anti-inflammatory drugs, surgery), patients' values concerning potential benefits and harms need to be considered. However, patients often have unrealistic expectations and clinicians are poor judges of patients' values [49]. The use of tools, such as patient decision aids, has been shown to be helpful in increasing the adoption of shared decision-making into clinical practice [50] and thus improving the quality of patient decisions.

Patient decision aids

Patient decision aids are tools that prepare patients for consultations by presenting evidence in user-friendly formats to help patients understand their options and consider what benefits and harms are most important to them [50,51]. They are typically used for decisions with multiple options (including the status quo) and where there are competing benefits and harms that patients may value differently. In these 'toss-up' decisions, the best option is one in which the expected outcomes are consistent with the patient's values and preferences. For example, one patient with OA may prefer a treatment option with a lower risk of side effects and not necessarily one that will result in better pain control. Another OA patient may prioritize avoiding surgery so s/he can continue to play a recreational sport.

At a minimum, patient decision aids make explicit the decision to be made, explain options, present evidence on benefits and harms of options, and help patients consider what is most important to them [49]. They may also: (1) provide additional information on the condition; (2) communicate probabilities of benefits and harms; (3) help patients better understand how much they value features of options and use their values to inform the decision (e.g. values clarification exercises, worksheets); (4) share patients' experiences; and (5) provide a structured process to guide patients in the steps of deliberation and communication. These tools may be used in preparation for or during the consultation with a clinician.

A number of patient decision aids have been developed for managing OA, including patient decision aids that focus on surgery (e.g. hip, knee, or shoulder replacement) and non-surgery OA treatment options (e.g. medicines, acupuncture, physical therapy). Common formats are paper-based booklets, DVDs, and Internet-based materials. A comprehensive inventory of patient decision aids may be found online at http://www.ohri.ca/decisionaid. For each patient decision aid inventoried, a summary is provided, including a link to obtain the patient decision aid and assessment of its quality using results from the International Patient Decision Aid Standards (IPDAS) [52]. The A to Z inventory of publicly available patient decision aids is a subset from the full Decision Aid Library Inventory (DALI); this inventory includes patient decision aids in development and indicates those no longer available. A second inventory provides links to patient decision aids in a number of different languages (http://www.med-decs.org/nl).

Evidence for efficacy and effectiveness of patient decision aids in osteoarthritis

There are over 115 RCTs evaluating the effectiveness of patient decision aids [49]; of these, 86 trials evaluated patient decision aids compared to usual practice (two of the trials were in patients with OA) [53,54]. In brief, these 86 trials have found that patients who use a patient decision aid as an adjunct to practitioner counselling experience improved decision quality and better outcomes: 13% higher knowledge, 82% more accurate perception of the chances of benefits and harms, and 51% better match between patient values and the option chosen [49]. Compared to usual practices, patient decision aids improve the decision-making process by reducing decisional conflict (i.e. uncertainty about choosing a course of action), decreasing the proportion of patients who are passive in decision-making, having a lower proportion of patients remaining undecided, enhancing patient involvement in decision-making (less practitioner controlled), and improving patient–practitioner communication [49].

Importantly, patient decision aids have not been found to adversely impact patient health outcomes, including overall and condition-specific quality of life, anxiety, and depression [49]. This is not surprising given that decision aids typically target decisions where there is no clear right choice and options may have different impacts on health outcomes. The change in uptake of options depends on whether they are over-used or under-used. For surgery decisions (e.g. herniated disc, benign uterine bleeding), 21% of patients given patient decision aids chose conservative surgery or medical options instead of more invasive surgical options. Patient decision aids have had more variable effect on the uptake of other treatment options; a recent systematic review found no impact of patient decision aids on costs, cost-effectiveness, or patient adherence to treatment [55].

Table 21.1 Key education/information strategies to enhance OA patient self-management and decision-making and their possible outcomes

Educational strategy	Outcomes
Multidisciplinary care	Increased provision of evidence-based OA care
	Appropriate use of each health discipline, e.g. orthopaedic surgeon only once non-surgical therapies tried and failed
Self-management programmes	Improved knowledge about OA pathogenesis and treatment
	Increased self-efficacy to participate in self-management activities (impact greater if baseline self-efficacy low and delivery tailored to patient circumstances)
	Better adherence to self-management activities, e.g. physical activity, healthy diet
Shared decision-making	Better quality of life
	More sense of control over illness
	Fewer illness concerns
	Improved symptom relief
Patient decision aids	Improved knowledge
	More realistic expectations of benefits and harms
	Better match between chosen option and patients' preferences
	Improved decision-making process (e.g. less decisional conflict, better engagement in decision-making)

Three RCTs have evaluated patient decision aids focused on hip and/or knee arthroplasty for OA [54,56,57]. All trials used the same patient decision aid (e.g. DVD and booklet) produced by the Informed Medical Decisions Foundation and one trial included a health coach to help patients navigate the decision-making process [56]. These studies demonstrated that, compared to controls, patients in the patient decision aid group experienced less decisional conflict, felt more knowledgeable, were better prepared for the surgical consultation, and a higher proportion achieved good decision quality. In addition, in the trial using health coaches, orthopaedic surgeons reported greater satisfaction and consultation efficiency, and indicated that patients asked more appropriate questions [56]. Given their demonstrated effectiveness, more concerted efforts are required to ensure that decision aids are effectively implemented into OA patient care.

Educational strategies and expected outcomes are summarized in Table 21.1.

Public health strategies to prevent osteoarthritis

While much attention and effort has been directed towards patient information strategies for decision-making and management of OA, relatively less has been paid to population-based public health strategies to reduce the incidence of OA. Education at a population level (e.g. schools, work place, recreational and competitive sport) regarding risk factors for development of OA is also important. Public health interventions aim to promote health and prevent disease and disability at the population level rather than the individual level. A comprehensive public health approach to promote primary prevention of OA is needed to stem the expected dramatic increase in the incidence of this condition and its consequent significant health and socioeconomic impact.

Recently, detailed recommendations regarding a public health agenda for OA have been developed [58,59]. First and foremost, there is a need to change societal beliefs about OA and challenge the widespread perception that it is an inevitable consequence of ageing as this belief may discourage people from taking preventative action [60–62]. As well, emphasizing the long-term and significant impact of OA on quality of life may spur behavioural change.

Public health interventions focus on addressing modifiable risk factors for OA including increasing physical activity, decreasing obesity, and minimizing musculoskeletal injuries. Promotion of physical activity and a healthy diet throughout life is important for both primary and secondary prevention of OA; these strategies are integral to weight management and maintenance of muscle strength and joint flexibility. As obesity and physical inactivity are risk factors shared by other higher-profile diseases such as diabetes and cardiovascular disease, integrating mutually beneficial health promotion strategies could broaden the dissemination of the information to a larger audience.

Given the strong evidence for a relationship between joint injuries and OA [63,64], interventions aimed at reducing injury risk have the potential to be an important public health approach to decreasing the incidence of OA. Injury prevention programmes such as those developed to prevent anterior cruciate ligament injuries in adolescents [65–67] or the prevention programme developed by FIFA (the Fédération Internationale de Football Association) [68] have been shown to significantly decrease knee and ankle injuries. Such programmes should be widely promoted to adolescents and young adults through physical health and education curricula and sports associations [65]. Repetitive micro-trauma from occupational activities, such as frequent kneeling or heavy lifting, may also increase the risk for OA, thus, promoting work-related modifications in high-risk industries is another important strategy.

Health communication and education approaches as outlined above are only one part of an overall public health approach that requires a broad strategy including policy initiatives at all levels of government and strategic alliances among all stakeholders who have the common goal of preventing chronic disease. This broad population-based approach is necessary to substantially reduce the burden of OA on individuals, healthcare services, and society at large.

Key contextual factors to consider in osteoarthritis patient education

In the design and implementation of educational strategies to enhance OA prevention and care, potential barriers and facilitators must be recognized. Research has consistently found that the adoption of recommended preventive measures, such as weight loss and physical activity, as well as the impact of therapies on OA outcomes, are influenced by myriad contextual factors (Figure 21.2).

These include the effects of patients' psychological and physical health [69,70], social support [71], gender [72], coping behaviours [73–75], and level of self-efficacy [76]. Specifically, female gender,

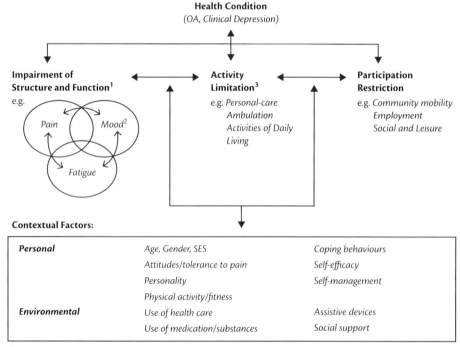

Figure 21.2 Key contextual factors influencing OA care and outcomes.

greater motivation [77], self-efficacy [10,78–81], perception of symptoms as more serious or bothersome [82], and access to allied health professionals (e.g. dietitian for dietary recommendations) [77] have been linked to greater engagement of patients in chronic disease self-care and improved health outcomes. Identified barriers to self-care include lower education and financial constraints, depressed mood [77], lack of social support [83], lack of time and caregiving duties [84], lack of continuity of care, logistical obstacles to being seen by their physician, for example, transportation, prioritization of another health problem by the patient, and competing demands resulting from comorbid health conditions, which are common among people with OA [85].

Conclusion

Information strategies are essential to enabling self-management and informed, shared decision-making in patients with OA, and thus optimizing patient outcomes. Such strategies are best delivered by a multidisciplinary team of health providers, taking into consideration the characteristics, preferences, and values of the individual OA patient. The use of tools, specifically patient decision aids, in clinical practice has the potential to improve shared decision-making in patients with OA, who face multiple, complex, healthcare decisions in the course of their illness. More participatory decision-making has the potential to improve OA patient satisfaction, adherence to treatment recommendations, appropriate use of healthcare resources, and health outcomes [86–89].

References

1. Wagner EH, Austin BT, Von Korff M. Improving outcomes in chronic illness. *Manag Care Q* 1996; 4(2):12–25.
2. Wagner EH. Chronic disease management: what will it take to improve care for chronic illness? *Eff Clin Pract* 1998; 1(1):2–4.
3. Lineker SC, Bell MJ, Badley EM. Evaluation of an inter-professional educational intervention to improve the use of arthritis best practices in primary care. *J Rheumatol* 2011; 38(5):931–7.
4. Schofield D, Fuller J, Wagner S, Friis L, Tyrell B. Multidisciplinary management of complex care. *Aust J Rural Health* 2009; 17(1):45–8.
5. Committee on Quality of Health Care in America and Institute of Medicine. *Crossing the Quality Chasm: A New Health System for the 21st Century*. Washington, DC: The National Academies Press; 2001.
6. Lorig K. Self-management of chronic illness: a model for the future. *Generations XVII* 1993(3):11–14.
7. Hibbard JH, Greenlick M, Jimison H, Capizzi J, Kunkel L. The impact of a community-wide self-care information project on self-care and medical care utilization. *Eval Health Prof* 2001; 24(4):404–23.
8. Brousseau L, Egan M, Wells G, et al. Ottawa panel evidence-based clinical practice guidelines for patient education programmes in the management of osteoarthritis. *Health Educ J* 2010; 70(3):318–58.
9. March L, Amatya B, Osborne RH, Brand C. Developing a minimum standard of care for treating people with osteoarthritis of the hip and knee. *Best Pract Res Clin Rheumatol* 2010; 24(1):121–45.
10. Bodenheimer T, Lorig K, Holman H, Grumbach K. Patient self-management of chronic disease in primary care. *JAMA* 2002; 288(19):2469–75.
11. Bandura A. Self-efficacy mechanism in human agency. *Am Psychol* 1982; 37:122–47.
12. Kroon FP, van der Burg LR, Buchbinder R, Osborne RH, Johnston RV, Pitt V. Self-management education programmes for osteoarthritis. *Cochrane Database Syst Rev* 2014; 1:CD008963.
13. Osborne RH, Spinks JM, Wicks IP. Patient education and self-management programs in arthritis. *Med J Aust* 2004; 180(5 Suppl):S23–26.
14. Von Korff M, Gruman J, Schaefer J, Curry SJ, Wagner EH. Collaborative management of chronic illness. *Ann Intern Med* 1997; 127(12):1097–102.
15. Lorig KR, Holman H. Self-management education: history, definition, outcomes, and mechanisms. *Ann Behav Med* 2003; 26(1):1–7.
16. Lorig K, Holman H. Arthritis self-management studies: a twelve-year review. *Health Educ Q* 1993; 20(1):17–28.
17. The Arthritis Society of Canada. *Arthritis Self-Management Program.* 2015. http://www.arthritis.ca/asmp
18. Lorig K, Chastain RL, Ung E, Shoor S, Holman HR. Development and evaluation of a scale to measure perceived self-efficacy in people with arthritis. *Arthritis Rheum* 1989; 32(1):37–44.
19. Brady TJ. Do common arthritis self-efficacy measures really measure self-efficacy? *Arthritis Care Res* 1997; 10(1):1–8.
20. Brady TJ. Measures of self-efficacy: Arthritis Self-Efficacy Scale (ASES), Arthritis Self-Efficacy Scale-8 Item (ASES-8), Children's Arthritis Self-Efficacy Scale (CASE), Chronic Disease Self-Efficacy Scale (CDSES), Parent's Arthritis Self-Efficacy Scale (PASE), and Rheumatoid Arthritis Self-Efficacy Scale (RASE). *Arthritis Care Res (Hoboken)* 2011; 63(Suppl 11):S473–85.
21. Bandura A. Self-efficacy: toward a unifying theory of behavioral change. *Psychol Rev* 1977; 84(2):191–215.
22. Nolte S, Osborne RH. A systematic review of outcomes of chronic disease self-management interventions. *Qual Life Res* 2013; 22(7):1805–16.
23. Osborne RH, Elsworth GR, Whitfield K. The Health Education Impact Questionnaire (heiQ): an outcomes and evaluation measure for patient education and self-management interventions for people with chronic conditions. *Patient Educ Couns* 2007; 66(2):192–201.
24. Nolte S, Elsworth GR, Sinclair AJ, Osborne RH. The extent and breadth of benefits from participating in chronic disease self-management courses: a national patient-reported outcomes survey. *Patient Educ Couns* 2007; 65(3):351–60.
25. Nolte S, Elsworth GR, Sinclair AJ, Osborne RH. Tests of measurement invariance failed to support the application of the 'then-test'. *J Clin Epidemiol* 2009; 62(11):1173–80.
26. Sperber NR, Bosworth HB, Coffman CJ, et al. Differences in osteoarthritis self-management support intervention outcomes according to race and health literacy. *Health Educ Res* 2013; 28(3):502–11.
27. Ackerman IN, Buchbinder R, Osborne RH. Factors limiting participation in arthritis self-management programmes: an exploration of barriers and patient preferences within a randomized controlled trial. *Rheumatology (Oxford)* 2013; 52(3):472–9.
28. Statistics Canada. *The Daily. Individual Internet Use and e-Commerce, 2012.* Catalogue no. 11-001-X. Ottawa; 2013. http://www.statcan.gc.ca/daily-quotidien/131028/dq131028a-eng.htm
29. Statistics Canada. *Internet Use by Individuals, by Selected Frequency of Use and Age (at Least Once a Day).* CANDSIM table 358-0129. Ottawa; 2010. http://www.statcan.gc.ca/tables-tableaux/sum-som/l01/cst01/comm32a-eng.htm
30. Statistics Canada and Organisation for Economic Co-operation and Development (OECD). *Learning a Living: First Results of the Adult Literacy and Life Skills Survey.* Ottawa and Paris; 2005. http://www.statcan.gc.ca/pub/89-603-x/2005001/4071714-eng.htm
31. Lyons EJ, Lewis ZH, Mayrsohn BG, Rowland JL. Behavior change techniques implemented in electronic lifestyle activity monitors: a systematic content analysis. *J Med Internet Res* 2014; 16(8):e192.
32. Ledger D. *Inside Wearables—Part 2: A Look at the Uncertain Future of Smart Wearable Devices, and Five Industry Developments that will be Necessary for Meaningful Mass Market Adoption and Sustained Engagement.* Cambridge, MA: Endeavour Partners; 2014. http://endeavourpartners.net/assets/Endeavour-Partners-Inside-Wearables-Part-2-July-2014.pdf
33. Leese J, Tran B, Backman C, et al. *A Qualitative Study of Barriers and Facilitators to Arthritis Patients' Use of Physical Activity Monitoring Tools.* Submitted abstract to 2016 American College of Rheumatology/Association of Rheumatology Health Professionals Annual Meeting.

http://rheum.ca/images/documents/2016_Abstracts_Selected_for_
Poster_Session_(updated_Feb_16).pdf

34. Murray E, Burns J, See TS, Lai R, Nazareth I. Interactive Health Communication Applications for people with chronic disease. *Cochrane Database Syst Rev* 2005(4):CD004274.

35. Leese J, Tran BC, Backman C, et al. A qualitative study of barriers and facilitators to arthritis patients' use of physical activity monitoring tools. *Arthritis Rheum* 2015; 66(10 (Suppl)):2879.

36. Macdonal GG, Leese J, Backman CL, et al. Integrating wearable physical activity monitoring tools into rehabilitation practice for patients with arthritis: the healthcare professional perspective. Arthritis & Rheum 2015; 66(10(Suppl)):2883.

37. Lorig KR, Sobel DS, Stewart AL, et al. Evidence suggesting that a chronic disease self-management program can improve health status while reducing hospitalization: a randomized trial. *Med Care* 1999; 37(1):5–14.

38. Lorig KR, Ritter P, Stewart AL, et al. Chronic disease self-management program: 2-year health status and health care utilization outcomes. *Med Care* 2001; 39(11):1217–23.

39. Lorig KR, Ritter PL, Laurent DD, Plant K. Internet-based chronic disease self-management: a randomized trial. *Med Care* 2006; 44(11):964–71.

40. Lorig KR, Ritter PL, Laurent DD, Plant K. The internet-based arthritis self-management program: a one-year randomized trial for patients with arthritis or fibromyalgia. *Arthritis Rheum* 2008; 59(7):1009–17.

41. Fjeldsoe BS, Marshall AL, Miller YD. Behavior change interventions delivered by mobile telephone short-message service. *Am J Prev Med* 2009; 36(2):165–73.

42. Wei J, Hollin I, Kachnowski S. A review of the use of mobile phone text messaging in clinical and healthy behaviour interventions. *J Telemed Telecare* 2011; 17(1):41–8.

43. de Jongh T, Gurol-Urganci I, Vodopivec-Jamsek V, Car J, Atun R. Mobile phone messaging for facilitating self-management of long-term illnesses. *Cochrane Database Syst Rev* 2012; 12:Cd007459.

44. Makoul G, Clayman ML. An integrative model of shared decision making in medical encounters. *Patient Educ Couns* 2006; 60(3):301–12.

45. Kiesler DJ, Auerbach SM. Optimal matches of patient preferences for information, decision-making and interpersonal behavior: evidence, models and interventions. *Patient Educ Couns* 2006; 61(3):319–41.

46. Couet N, Desroches S, Robitaille H, et al. Assessments of the extent to which health-care providers involve patients in decision making: a systematic review of studies using the OPTION instrument. *Health Expect* 2015; 18(4):542–61.

47. Borkhoff CM, Hawker GA, Kreder HJ, et al. Influence of patients' gender on informed decision making regarding total knee arthroplasty. *Arthritis Care Res (Hoboken)* 2013; 65(8):1281–90.

48. Braddock CH, 3rd, Edwards KA, Hasenberg NM, Laidley TL, Levinson W. Informed decision making in outpatient practice: time to get back to basics. *JAMA* 1999; 282(24):2313–20.

49. Stacey D, Legare F, Col NF, et al. Decision aids for people facing health treatment or screening decisions. *Cochrane Database Syst Rev* 2014; 1:CD001431.

50. Legare F, Stacey D, Turcotte S, et al. Interventions for improving the adoption of shared decision making by healthcare professionals. *Cochrane Database Syst Rev* 2014; 9:CD006732.

51. Brouwers M, Stacey D, O'Connor A. Knowledge creation: synthesis, tools and products. *CMAJ* 2010; 182(2):E68–72.

52. Elwyn G, O'Connor A, Stacey D, et al. Developing a quality criteria framework for patient decision aids: online international Delphi consensus process. *BMJ* 2006; 333(7565):417.

53. Fraenkel L, Rabidou N, Wittink D, Fried T. Improving informed decision-making for patients with knee pain. *J Rheumatol* 2007; 34(9):1894–8.

54. de Achaval S, Fraenkel L, Volk RJ, Cox V, Suarez-Almazor ME. Impact of educational and patient decision aids on decisional conflict associated with total knee arthroplasty. *Arthritis Care Res (Hoboken)* 2012; 64(2):229–37.

55. Trenaman L, Stirling B, Bansback N. The cost-effectiveness of patient decision aids: a systematic review. *Healthcare* 2014; 2(4):251–7.

56. Bozic KJ, Belkora J, Chan V, et al. Shared decision making in patients with osteoarthritis of the hip and knee: results of a randomized controlled trial. *J Bone Joint Surg Am* 2013; 95(18):1633–9.

57. Stacey D, Hawker G, Dervin G, et al. Decision aid for patients considering total knee arthroplasty with preference report for surgeons: a pilot randomized controlled trial. *BMC Musculoskelet Disord* 2014; 15:54.

58. Centers for Disease Control and Prevention and The Arthritis Foundation. *A National Public Health Agenda for Osteoarthritis*. CDC; 2010. http://www.cdc.gov/arthritis/docs/OAagenda.pdf

59. Arthritis Research UK. *Musculoskeletal Health: A Public Health Approach*. Arthritis Research UK; 2014. http://www.arthritisresearchuk.org/policy-and-public-affairs/public-health.aspx

60. Ali F, Jinks C, Ong BN. '…Keep mobile, I think that's half the battle.' A qualitative study of prevention of knee pain in symptomless older adults. *BMC Public Health* 2012; 12:753.

61. Turner AP, Barlow JH, Buszewicz M, Atkinson A, Rait G. Beliefs about the causes of osteoarthritis among primary care patients. *Arthritis Rheum* 2007; 57(2):267–71.

62. Hurley MV, Walsh N, Bhavnani V, Britten N, Stevenson F. Health beliefs before and after participation on an exercised-based rehabilitation programme for chronic knee pain: doing is believing. *BMC Musculoskelet Disord* 2010; 11:31.

63. Lohmander LS, Englund PM, Dahl LL, Roos EM. The long-term consequence of anterior cruciate ligament and meniscus injuries: osteoarthritis. *Am J Sports Med* 2007; 35(10):1756–69.

64. Amin S, Guermazi A, Lavalley MP, et al. Complete anterior cruciate ligament tear and the risk for cartilage loss and progression of symptoms in men and women with knee osteoarthritis. *Osteoarthritis Cartilage* 2008; 16(8):897–902.

65. Ratzlaff CR, Liang MH. New developments in osteoarthritis. Prevention of injury-related knee osteoarthritis: opportunities for the primary and secondary prevention of knee osteoarthritis. *Arthritis Res Ther* 2010; 12(4):215.

66. Gilchrist J, Mandelbaum BR, Melancon H, et al. A randomized controlled trial to prevent noncontact anterior cruciate ligament injury in female collegiate soccer players. *Am J Sports Med* 2008; 36(8):1476–83.

67. Pasanen K, Parkkari J, Pasanen M, et al. Neuromuscular training and the risk of leg injuries in female floorball players: cluster randomised controlled study. *BMJ* 2008; 337:a295.

68. FIFA Medical Assessment and Research Centre. *Prevention of Injuries 11+ Programme*. 2014. http://f-marc.com/11plus/manual/

69. Seeman TE. Health promoting effects of friends and family on health outcomes in older adults. *Am J Health Promot* 2000; 14(6):362–70.

70. Rowe J, Kahn R. *Successful Aging*. New York: Pantheon; 1998.

71. George L. Social factors and illness. In Binstock H, George K (eds) *Handbook of Aging and the Social Sciences*, 4th ed. San Diego, CA: Academic Press; 1996:229–52.

72. Walen H, Lachman M. Social support and strain from partner, family, and friends: costs and benefits for men and women in adulthood. *J Soc Pers Relat* 2000; 17:5–30.

73. Keefe FJ, Lefebvre JC, Egert JR, et al. The relationship of gender to pain, pain behavior, and disability in osteoarthritis patients: the role of catastrophizing. *Pain* 2000; 87(3):325–34.

74. Lorig K, Gonzalez VM, Laurent DD, Morgan L, Laris BA. Arthritis self-management program variations: three studies. *Arthritis Care Res* 1998; 11(6):448–54.

75. Klinger L, Spaulding SJ, Polatajko HJ, MacKinnon JR, Miller L. Chronic pain in the elderly: occupational adaptation as a means of coping with osteoarthritis of the hip and/or knee. *Clin J Pain* 1999; 15(4):275–83.

76. Keefe FJ, Lefebvre JC, Maixner W, Salley AN, Jr, Caldwell DS. Self-efficacy for arthritis pain: relationship to perception of thermal laboratory pain stimuli. *Arthritis Care Res* 1997; 10(3):177–84.

77. Ali HI, Baynouna LM, Bernsen RM. Barriers and facilitators of weight management: perspectives of Arab women at risk for type 2 diabetes. *Health Soc Care Community* 2010; 18(2):219–28.

78. Lorig KR, Sobel DS, Ritter PL, Laurent D, Hobbs M. Effect of a self-management program on patients with chronic disease. *Eff Clin Pract* 2001; 4(6):256–62.

79. Hurley AC, Shea CA. Self-efficacy: strategy for enhancing diabetes self-care. *Diabetes Educ* 1992; 18(2):146–50.

80. Glasgow RE, Toobert DJ, Hampson SE, et al. Improving self-care among older patients with type II diabetes: the 'Sixty Something …' Study. *Patient Educ Couns* 1992; 19(1):61–74.

81. Clark NM, Dodge JA. Exploring self-efficacy as a predictor of disease management. *Health Educ Behav* 1999; 26(1):72–89.

82. Kart CS, Engler CA. Predisposition to self-health care: who does what for themselves and why? *J Gerontol* 1994; 49(6):S301–8.

83. Lukkarinen H, Hentinen M. Self-care agency and factors related to this agency among patients with coronary heart disease. *Int J Nurs Stud* 1997; 34(4):295–304.

84. King AC, Castro C, Wilcox S, et al. Personal and environmental factors associated with physical inactivity among different racial-ethnic groups of U.S. middle-aged and older-aged women. *Health Psychol* 2000; 19(4):354–64.

85. Bayliss EA, Steiner JF, Fernald DH, Crane LA, Main DS. Descriptions of barriers to self-care by persons with comorbid chronic diseases. *Ann Fam Med* 2003; 1(1):15–21.

86. Hall JA, Roter DL, Katz NR. Meta-analysis of correlates of provider behavior in medical encounters. *Med Care* 1988; 26(7):657–75.

87. Kaplan SH, Gandek B, Greenfield S, Rogers W, Ware JE. Patient and visit characteristics related to physicians' participatory decision-making style. Results from the Medical Outcomes Study. *Med Care* 1995; 33(12):1176–87.

88. Bertakis KD, Roter D, Putnam SM. The relationship of physician medical interview style to patient satisfaction. *J Fam Pract* 1991; 32(2):175–81.

89. Roter D. The medical visit context of treatment decision-making and the therapeutic relationship. *Health Expect* 2000; 3(1):17–25.

CHAPTER 22

Exercise for the person with osteoarthritis

Kim L. Bennell, Ans Van Ginckel, Fiona Dobson, and Rana S. Hinman

Introduction

Osteoarthritis (OA) is a prevalent chronic musculoskeletal condition that commonly affects the joints of the knee, hip, hand, and spine. Societal burden and healthcare costs aside, affected individuals suffer from considerable pain, experience difficulty performing activities of daily living, sleep problems, and fatigue. Specifically, OA patients present with a range of physical impairments such as joint stiffness, muscle weakness, altered proprioceptive acuity, or balance and gait abnormalities. Psychological disabilities such as depression and anxiety are also known to contribute to the burden of the disease as it is experienced by the patients themselves [1].

Since no effective cure exists, contemporary management primarily aims to relieve pain, improve function, and, as such, enhance quality of life. Ultimately, these strategies should assist in preventing or postponing the need for costly joint arthroplasty surgery. Clinical guidelines recommend exercise as a vital component of conservative management [2–6], irrespective of patient age, joint involved, radiographic disease severity, pain intensity, functional levels, and comorbidities.

This chapter summarizes the role of exercise in the management of OA based on evidence from systematic reviews and key randomized controlled trials (RCTs). The first section synthesizes the evidence to support the efficacy of exercise in alleviating symptoms of OA. Following this, practical recommendations are presented regarding exercise prescription modalities such as exercise type or dosage, as well as delivery methods and assessment methods of individual outcomes following an exercise treatment programme. A separate section will address how to maximize these outcomes and how to preserve exercise benefits in the longer term. This chapter focuses on knee, hip, and hand joints as common OA sites but will not address evidence related to spinal OA. The current body of evidence is presented and directions for future research avenues are made.

Does exercise alleviate symptoms of osteoarthritis?

Recommendations to prescribe exercise in OA are largely directed to people with hand, hip, and knee OA. The evidence informing these guidelines is primarily based on trials comparing exercise to no exercise, as few placebo-controlled trials are available. Thus, the majority of evidence as described in this section is based on studies involving participants who were aware of their treatment, which may have overestimated treatment outcomes [7]. While most of the clinical trials have addressed knee OA, however, at present there is a paucity of literature to conclusively inform clinical guidelines of OA at other joints such as the hip and hand.

Systematic reviews and meta-analyses consistently conclude that exercise is a beneficial strategy to improve pain and physical function in the short term for people diagnosed with knee OA [8–10]. Amongst these, one recent review performed a trial sequential analysis and network meta-analysis of 60 trials for lower limb OA (44 knee, 2 hip, and 14 mixed) that covered 12 different types of exercise interventions [9]. The authors concluded that as of 2002, sufficient evidence had accumulated to confirm the significant benefit of exercise interventions over no exercise as a control, for a range of exercise types. These benefits also seem to apply to patients with severe disease such as those awaiting total joint replacement [8,11]. A recent update of a Cochrane review of the evidence for exercise in knee OA agreed with this contemporary point of view [10]. By pooling outcomes from up to 3913 participants, the authors compared treatment responses of land-based exercise programmes to non-exercise or non-treatment control groups and presented moderate- to high-quality evidence for benefits of exercise for knee pain reduction or improved physical function. As short-term benefits were sustained for 2–6 months after cessation of formal treatment, effect sizes were generally small to moderate, albeit comparable to those of simple analgesics and oral non-steroidal anti-inflammatory drugs [12]. Importantly, as opposed to conservative drug treatments, those undergoing exercise therapies seemed to experience relatively fewer side effects [12]. While effective in the short term, any longer-term benefits of exercise, however, are largely dependent upon patients' adherence to the programme, which is known to decline over time [13]. Reasons for this and strategies to maximize any (long-term) effects of exercise are discussed in a later section.

Whilst an abundance of studies focused on treatment responses to exercise in knee OA, much less research specifically involved patients with hip OA. One of the few high-quality placebo-controlled RCTs evaluated the efficacy of a multimodal physical therapy programme including home exercise and manual therapy in this patient group [14]. It found that the physical therapy programme did not confer clinically relevant benefits in terms of pain reduction or functional improvement when compared to placebo [14]. An updated Cochrane review including 10 trials (594 participants) conversely found that in hip OA patients, land-based exercise alleviated pain and improved physical function, yet with small to moderate effect sizes, immediately after treatment compared to no exercise control which suggests that part of the benefits with exercise may be due to non-specific effects [15]. Similar to knee OA, exercise programmes elicited few side effects with improvements sustained for up to 3–6 months following cessation of treatment [10]. One long-term follow-up of an RCT involving 109 participants with hip OA found that a combined programme of exercise therapy plus education exerted more beneficial effects on the 6-year cumulative survival of the native hip shown by an increased median time to joint replacement surgery as opposed to those patients undertaking education alone [16]. In summary, the relatively limited research investigating hip OA treatments shows that current non-surgical and exercise treatments are only modestly effective, or even ineffective, for improving pain and function. However, current clinical exercise guidelines in hip OA are based on research from people with knee OA, which may be erroneous because of differences in biomechanics, risk factors, and clinical presentation between the two joints. More insight is needed into the determinants of clinical presentation in people with hip OA in order to optimize clinical recommendations and reconcile differing conclusions drawn from the currently available evidence.

Exercise recommendations from current clinical guidelines for hand OA [5] are largely based on expert consensus due to a lack of adequately powered studies and conflicting results in available trials at the time the guidelines were developed. More recently, two larger exercise RCTs have been published. One trial in 80 women reported that compared with information alone, home-based range of motion and strengthening exercises three times per week over a 3-month time frame in addition to information improved activity performance measured by the Patient-Specific Functional Scale [17]. Although the adjusted mean difference between treatment groups was below the threshold of the minimal clinically important difference for this performance outcome measure [17], more women in the exercise group achieved clinically important improvements when compared to the control group whereas none versus two in the exercise and control group respectively exhibited a negative change. Additionally, a larger proportion of participants in the exercise group as opposed to the control group fulfilled the Outcome Measures in Rheumatology–Osteoarthritis Research Society International (OMERACT–OARSI) response criteria. While these results are promising, the largest RCT of exercise for hand OA published to date (n = 257) conversely showed that hand exercises were not effective for improving outcomes at 6 months when OMERACT–OARSI responder criteria were appraised [18]. The home programme included daily stretching and strengthening exercises of hand and thumb. Clearly, further research is warranted to underpin the benefit and most optimal modalities of dedicated and efficacious exercise for hand OA.

What type of exercise should be prescribed for patients with osteoarthritis?

Despite few studies directly comparing the effects of different types of exercise, systematic reviews support clinical benefits from a

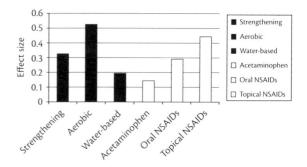

Figure 22.1 Effect sizes of different types of exercise (black bars) for pain compared with those for common drug therapies (white bars) in knee osteoarthritis.

Reprinted from *Osteoarthritis Cartilage*, 18/4, Zhang W, Nuki G, Moskowitz RW, Abramson S, Altman RD, Arden NK, et al, OARSI recommendations for the management of hip and knee osteoarthritis: Part III: Changes in evidence following systematic cumulative update of research published through January 2009 476–99. Copyright (2010) with permission from Elsevier.

range of exercise types in people with OA [9,10,12] (Figure 22.1). Exercise types include muscle strengthening/resistance training, stretching/range of motion, cardiovascular/aerobic conditioning (such as cycling and walking), neuromuscular exercise, balance training, and Tai Chi.

Clinical guidelines [4] confirm that people with knee and hip OA should be recommended to participate in aerobic and/or resistance land-based exercise, as well as aquatic exercise. Despite similar effects on pain relief following cardiovascular, strengthening, and performance exercise [19], uncertainty remains as to whether exercise programmes should contain specific single-type components or whether combinations of exercises should be implemented that address different impairments. Whilst a recent meta-analysis of RCTs including patients with lower limb OA supports the combination of strengthening, flexibility, and aerobic exercise as opposed to no exercise as most efficacious in achieving pain relief and functional improvement [9], in another meta-analysis Juhl et al. [19] conversely concluded that single-type exercise programmes appeared more effective than programmes comprising a combination of different exercise types [19]. While this evidence is predominantly summarized from RCTs in knee OA, for hand OA both strengthening and range of motion exercises have been recommended. Yet, the limited number of RCTs in hand OA highlights the need for more and adequately powered trials to inform evidence-based guidelines for this patient group [5].

Although strengthening exercise is recommended, there is no evidence to suggest that a specific type of strengthening is superior over another in terms of beneficial effects on pain or function in people with OA. Isotonic (through range), isometric (without movement), and isokinetic (performed on specific machines) strengthening exercise [8] as well as strengthening exercise performed in weight-bearing or non-weight-bearing positions, all have similar benefits on symptom relief [5,20]. In addition, strengthening programmes for knee OA have either focused on the quadriceps muscle as a single target or included strengthening of other lower limb muscles in addition to the quadriceps. A 2015 systematic review revealed moderate to large effect sizes for quadriceps strengthening for both pain and physical function while effect sizes were slightly smaller for muscle strengthening that included several lower limb muscles [10]. This suggests that it is preferable to include strengthening exercises for the major lower limb muscles and confirms a previous recommendation by Juhl et al. [19] who showed that greater pain reduction and functional improvements were observed with quadriceps-specific exercise compared with exercise aiming to improve overall lower limb strength.

Aerobic exercise (e.g. walking or cycling) is a popular choice for the management of lower limb OA. Although this has not been specifically investigated in people with hip OA, aerobic exercise is beneficial for improving pain and physical function. A recent 2014 meta-analysis revealed small to moderate effects of walking exercise on pain relief at short-term (≤2 months) and mid-term (>2 months–12 months) follow-up in patient groups suffering chronic musculoskeletal pain such as low back pain, OA, or fibromyalgia. Functional improvements were similarly seen at short- and mid-term as well as long-term (>12 months) follow-ups [21]. Additionally, aerobic exercise also has several other potential benefits. Combined with dietary restriction, aerobic exercise can facilitate weight loss in patients who are overweight or obese. An 18-month RCT compared the efficacy of exercise, intensive diet, and their combination in 454 overweight and obese people with knee OA [22]. Results revealed that combining intensive dieting with exercise resulted in greater pain reduction and better function compared with either treatment options alone. Given the intensive nature of the intervention and the considerable support provided for participants in this efficacy trial, future research needs to confirm whether similar results can be obtained in 'real-life' conditions. Aerobic exercise has also been shown to have positive effects on psychological impairments in a range of rheumatic conditions such as depressive symptoms [23,24], which constitute a common comorbidity in people with OA.

Since reduced joint range of motion is a common observation in the clinical assessment of OA patients, stretching or flexibility exercises comprise a logical component of any exercise programme to maintain periarticular soft tissue flexibility and extensibility of nearby muscles. However, these exercises generally form part of an overall exercise programme for OA and as such, their effects in isolation have not yet been studied.

Limited evidence is available concerning the usefulness of specific balance exercises for people with OA hampering formulation of any clinical recommendation as of yet [25]. However, given that people with lower limb OA may have poor balance, increasing their risk of falling [26], clinicians should assess balance impairments and incorporate specific and dedicated exercises in the exercise programme whenever appropriate and whenever safety can be guaranteed.

Because of its potential to improve muscle strength, balance as well as anxiety and stress, Tai Chi is conditionally recommended for people with knee OA according to the latest American College of Rheumatology guidelines [4,27–29]. Tai Chi involves gentle, low-impact exercise with slow, controlled movements. Although Tai Chi is gaining popularity among people with OA, there are few well-designed clinical trials of Tai Chi. The most recent systematic review published to date concluded Tai Chi as an effective way of relieving pain and improving physical function for people with knee OA. Nonetheless, the authors highlighted the need for further dedicated larger-scaled RCTs that should incorporate longer follow-up periods [30].

When compared to non-treatment controls or land-based exercise programmes, aquatic exercise appears to have significant, yet small, effects on pain, self-reported and performance-based physical functioning, joint stiffness, as well as quality of life in people with lower limb OA [6,31,32]. While relatively few aquatic exercise RCTs have been conducted, studies evaluated a heterogeneous set of outcome measures in relatively small samples implying that at this point any conclusions should be drawn cautiously. Aquatic exercise, however, may be particularly useful in overweight/obese patients or in those who have severe joint-related symptoms. The resilience and agreeable temperature of the water can assist in improving the range of motion and pain with reduced loading to joints. Additionally, if performed at a level of at least 50% of the patient's heart reserve, aquatic exercise can also improve aerobic capacity.

More recently, the efficacy of neuromuscular exercise to relieve symptoms has been described for people with lower limb OA. Neuromuscular training covers a broad range of exercises that are typically performed in functional weight-bearing positions and emphasize quality and efficiency of movement, which also includes alignment of the trunk and lower limb joints [33]. Neuromuscular exercise proved to be able to improve pain and function in people with knee OA, even in those with more advanced disease [33–35]. However, the addition of such exercise to a general strengthening programme does not appear to enhance any of these benefits, even in those patients with self-reported and/or biomechanically assessed knee joint instability [34,36]. Findings of a recent RCT concur that no significant between-group differences in pain or function could be attained at the end of a 12-week programme of either neuromuscular exercise or quadriceps strengthening exercises in people with medial knee OA and moderate varus malalignment [37].

Since people with OA are not meeting public health physical activity guidelines [38], increasing overall physical activity levels in addition to therapeutic exercise is also important, especially since physical activity levels also predict functional performance levels in knee OA [39]. The use of a pedometer or accelerometer as simple and relatively inexpensive tools can facilitate this by providing additional motivation. Worn at the waist, leg, or arm, pedometers assess the number of steps taken while accelerometers assess the amount of overall movement. These devices can thus provide patients with feedback regarding the amount of daily physical activity performed and can facilitate motivating them to reach set goals.

How can the response to exercise be maximized?

Although most forms of therapeutic exercise proved effective in managing symptoms, especially in patients with knee OA, effect sizes of exercise therapy are modest at best. It is possible that different subgroups of people with OA respond differently to different therapy modalities. Previous RCTs have applied a 'one-size-fits-all' approach to exercise prescription, which may have attenuated treatment effects in clinical trials because treatments were evaluated in heterogeneous groups. This general approach may also have hampered drawing sound conclusions as to what exercise type is superior in eliciting desirable or optimal treatment responses. There is increasing international recognition that OA manifests differently across individuals, and that specific characteristics or 'phenotypes' may influence exercise treatment outcomes.

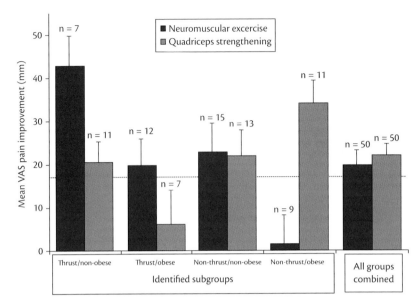

Figure 22.2 Mean (standard error, SE) change in pain with the neuromuscular and strengthening exercise programmes in each of the mutually exclusive subgroups based on characteristics of obesity and varus thrust. The mean (SE) change in pain when all participants are analysed as per randomized exercise intervention without consideration of these characteristics is shown in the right-hand columns. The minimal clinically important change in pain of 18 mm [42] is indicated by the dashed horizontal line.

Reprinted from *Arthritis Care Res*, 10, Bennell KL, Dobson F, Roos EM, Skou SR, Hodges P, Wrigley TV, et al, The influence of biomechanical characteristics on pain and function outcomes from exercise in medial knee osteoarthritis and varus malalignment: exploratory analyses from a randomised controlled trial, Copyright (2015) with permission from Elsevier.

New avenues to maximize the benefits of exercise according to clinical phenotype for people with knee OA has been the focus of more recent international work. Sub-group analyses from an RCT comparing neuromuscular exercise versus strengthening in people medial knee OA and varus malalignment [37] showed that clinically measurable, biomechanical subgroups responded differently to these two types of exercise. Specifically, people with a visually observable varus thrust (a dynamic outward bowing of the knee during walking) experienced significantly more pain relief with neuromuscular exercise, whereas non-thrusters had greater pain reduction with strengthening. Additionally, obese people without a varus thrust, experienced more pain relief following quadriceps strengthening, whilst non-obese, non-thrusters did equally well in both the neuromuscular or strengthening programme. (Figure 22.2) [40,41]. A further recent subgroup analysis of another RCT in The Netherlands [36] observed that patients with greater baseline lower-limb muscle strength had a greater functional benefit from knee stabilization exercises whereas patients with weaker muscles experienced more benefits from traditional strengthening exercises. These findings support the contention that not all patients respond equally well to different exercise regimens and that baseline clinical assessment of the patient should be interpreted as to how optimal adjustment of individual treatment plans can be obtained. Nevertheless, conclusive evidence for this premise is required [42,43].

Next to tailoring programme components to clinical phenotypes, long-term patient adherence to a regular exercise programme is critical in order to achieve and, most importantly, maintain optimal clinical outcomes. Dose–response relationships seem to exist between adherence and exercise effects, with increasing adherence found to associate with decreased pain, ameliorated walking ability, and reduced self-reported disability [44]. A study by van Baar et al. [45] showed that the beneficial effects of exercise last only as long as the patient with OA continues to participate in exercise. In these patients, the beneficial effects of exercise on symptoms were lost 6 months after the 12-week exercise programme under study had been completed [45]. It appears that once people commence an exercise programme, adherence is often high in the early stages but can diminish relatively quickly as time passes [46]

Whether one adheres to regular exercise depends upon interactions amongst the individual and his/her social and physical environment [47]. The effectiveness of this dynamic process relies on a complex array of both intrinsic factors (e.g. a person's beliefs, attitudes, personal experiences, perceptions, and knowledge about OA and exercise, severity of symptoms, personality and self-image, motivation) and extrinsic factors (e.g. transportation, proximity and availability of adequate facilities, weather or social support, and/or care from a (exercise) partner or healthcare professional) [48–59]. These factors may either be general or disease-specific in nature and may constitute barriers or facilitators to exercise adherence. Given that the barriers to exercise adherence are complex, changeable over time, and variable across individuals, an individualized and proactive approach to exercise prescription by health professionals is required. Strategies as to how to improve or optimize adherence in people with knee OA are discussed elsewhere in this textbook.

Should exercise be delivered in individual treatments, or class-based or home-based programmes?

Due to the growing burden of OA worldwide and rising associated healthcare costs, exercise therapy should be delivered in the most efficacious but also cost-effective way. Exercise can be broadly categorized into three different delivery modes including individual

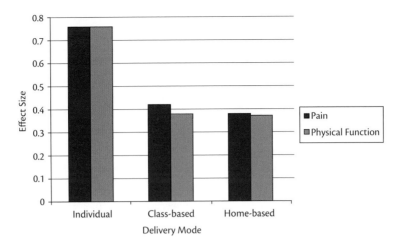

Figure 22.3 Mean effect size for different modes of exercise delivery including individual treatments, class-based programmes, and home based programmes on self-reported pain (black bars) and physical function (grey bars). Note: effect sizes were derived from the pooled data including extreme outliers. After removal of outliers from the respective meta-analyses, for both pain and physical dysfunction differences amongst the three modes of delivery no longer reached statistical significance. Data from Fransen M, McConnell S, Harmer AR, van der Esch M, Simic M, Bennell KL. Exercise for osteoarthritis of the knee. Cochrane, 2015, Wiley.

(one-on-one) treatments, class-based (group) programmes, and home-based programmes. Other common mixed-mode alternatives comprise individual treatment sessions combined with home-based exercise or home exercise supplemented with either a class-based programme or supervised home visits by a trained healthcare professional.

A recently updated meta-analysis [10] showed that individual, class-based, and home-based programmes all achieved beneficial small to large treatment effects in terms of reduced self-reported pain and improved self- reported physical function. Treatment effects for pain and function were greatest for individual programmes followed by class-based and home-based programmes (Figure 22.3). After exclusion of extreme outliers in the individual treatment category, significant differences across delivery modes were no longer evident. Thus, to establish clear superiority of one mode over the other additional factors should be considered, such as cost and the patient's clinical presentation and preferences [60,61]. These factors are further explored below.

A dearth of studies has evaluated different exercise delivery modes for people with hip OA [62–65]. While most of these studies incorporated mixed modes of delivery, using individual treatments combined with either home-based exercise [63,66] or a gym-based programme [62], one study investigated a class-based programme specifically designed for hip OA [65] and found non-significant and small treatment effects for both pain and function. These findings may have been due to the small sample size and relatively few treatment sessions (eight sessions in total) incorporated in this class-based programme.

Even less evidence is available on the effects of exercise delivery modes for hand OA. In a recent RCT, where exercise was delivered using a class-based programme supplemented by a daily home programme, hand exercises to improve grip strength and dexterity were not effective for improving pain and function [67], nor was a 6-month, daily home programme of strengthening and stretching exercise when the OMERACT–OARSI responder criteria were appraised [18]. Further evaluation of exercise delivery in hand OA is required. These studies should include individualized treatments targeted to patient-specific impairments.

In clinical practice, patients are often prescribed a supplementary home exercise programme despite participation in regular supervised individual or class-based exercise sessions. Home-based programmes can be either supervised or unsupervised by a qualified health professional. The decision as to how exercise delivery is best organized should take into account the variable clinical presentation of patients with OA (i.e. pain severity, joints affected, functional ability, and comorbidities). In this respect, outcomes following exercise treatment are most likely optimized to meet individual goals, needs, and interests of the patient when they are initially supervised by an appropriately qualified health professional (such as a physiotherapist) [68]. Trained health professionals should ensure supervision to promote the safe and correct execution of the exercise programme either in class or at home, especially during the initial phase of the programme. These measures will facilitate reducing the risk of adverse events. Although not consistently studied, the risk of adverse events for group and home programmes is considered low once individuals have been appropriately assessed for the suitability of the exercises by a qualified health professional at the start of the programme [2,68,69].

While class-based and home-based programmes appear to have somewhat smaller, yet not significantly different, treatment effects compared to those established for individual programmes [10], supervised programmes are potentially more cost-effective than unsupervised strategies despite initial direct costs. Economic analyses indicated that additional costs associated with a supervised classed-based exercise to supplement a home-based programme were attenuated by reduced use of other healthcare services [69]. Thus, supervised exercise class supplementation is a relatively cost-effective approach to maximize the relatively smaller benefits of home exercise.

Nevertheless, evidence shows that taking a 'recipe-based' or 'general-purpose' approach to exercise intervention is ineffective in patients with hip and knee OA [70]. Such an approach will be less likely to achieve meaningful benefits as there is less opportunity for variation, progression or optimization of programme parameters. As a result, patients may be less likely to maintain adherent to the programme or may perform the exercises incorrectly, further reducing the effectiveness of the programme.

In summary, conclusive superiority of one delivery mode over the other remains to be clearly established. Therefore, the choice between individual, class-based, or home-based programmes should ultimately also be informed by patient preference as part of the shared decision-making process [71].

What exercise dosage should be implemented?

Exercise dosage encompasses the number of sessions within a programme, the frequency (number of sessions per week), duration (time length of session) or volume (the amount such as number of repetitions/sets), and the intensity (amount of muscular effort or exertion, typically expressed as a percentage of the individual's maximal capacity). Variations in any of these parameters may affect the outcome and, thus, efficacy of the exercise programme [72].

Due to a lack of studies directly comparing dosage parameters between exercise programmes and the noticeable variation in dosage applied amongst available studies, the optimal dosage of exercise in OA remains unclear. Furthermore, appropriate indirect comparisons between studies are hampered by insufficient detail of exercise dosage provided.

The number of sessions incorporated in exercise programmes for lower limb OA was evaluated in an updated meta-analysis on exercise for knee OA [10]. While studies were divided into those having either 12 or more or less than 12 occasions of directly supervised sessions, beneficial moderate treatment effects for self-reported pain and physical function were found for those evaluating programmes providing at least 12 directly supervised occasions. In contrast, the studies evaluating programmes providing less than 12 directly supervised sessions showed only small effect sizes for physical function and moderate effect sizes for pain [10]. Although this meta-analysis failed to establish significant differences for both pain and physical function between the two categories of contact occasions, this tendency of more benefit with increased frequency was also supported by Juhl et al. [19] who revealed a positive dose–response effect between the number of supervised sessions of aerobic exercise and corresponding extent of pain relief [19]. Greater improvements became also apparent when single type exercise programmes were performed at least three times per week compared to those performed less than two sessions per week.

The American Geriatric Society has advised specific guidelines for flexibility, strengthening, and aerobic exercise in people with OA. These guidelines are based on the literature and consensus reached by a multidisciplinary panel of experts [72] (Table 22.1). Other guidelines for physical activity in older adults are provided by the World Health Organization [73]. The World Health Organization recommends 150 minutes of moderate-intensity aerobic activity to be performed each week, with additional health benefits to be gained when training is increased up to 300 minutes per week. In case of chronic conditions such as OA, it is recommended to be as physically active as possible within the limits of the condition. Greater training volumes are desirable in individuals with coexisting obesity who make a considerable proportion of people with OA [74].

Although Juhl et al. [19] did not discern any impact of exercise intensity or duration of individual sessions on treatment effects, moderate-quality evidence described greater strength gains in people with OA with higher-intensity training programmes.

Table 22.1 General guidelines for training parameters in people with OA, as developed by the American Geriatrics Society

Exercise type	Intensity	Volume	Frequency
Flexibility: static stretching initially	Stretch to subjective sensation of resistance	1 stretch/muscle group; hold 5–15 seconds	Once daily
Flexibility: longer-term goal	Stretch to full range of motion	3–5 stretches/muscle group; hold 20–30 seconds	3–5/week
Strengthening: isometric	Low-moderate: 40–60% MVC	1–10 submax contractions/muscle group; hold 1–6 seconds	Daily
Strengthening: isotonic	Low: 40% 1 RM	10–15 reps	2–3/week
	Mod: 40–60% 1 RM	8–10 reps	
	High: >60% 1 RM	6–8 reps	
Endurance: aerobic	Low–mod: 40–60% of VO_2 max/ HR max RPE: 12–14 = 60–65% VO_2 max	Accumulation of 20–30 min/day	2–5/week

1 RM, one repetition maximum; MVC, maximal voluntary contraction; reps, repetitions; RPE, rating of perceived exertion; HR max = age-predicted heart rate maximum; VO_2 max = maximal aerobic capacity.

American Geriatrics Society Panel on Exercise and Osteoarthritis, *Exercise Prescription for Older Adults with Osteoarthritis Pain: Consensus Practice Recommendations*, 2001, Wiley.

A meta-analysis by Zacharias et al. published in 2014 [75] appraised 40 RCTs of which all but one comprised patients with knee OA. Where the majority of studies (77%) involved resistance exercise programmes to enhance lower limb muscle strength, the authors presented high-quality evidence for increased knee extension and flexion strength at short-term follow-up following low-intensity resistance programmes. Although high-intensity resistance programmes were able to generate larger treatment responses that were sustained up to intermediate follow-up time points when compared to a control, quality of this evidence was rated as moderate only. One recent RCT in 46 women with hip OA compared daily high-velocity to low-velocity home-based resistance training in terms of its effect on muscle properties and physical performance. At completion of the 8-week programme, high-velocity resistance training induced partially greater beneficial changes in muscle properties and physical performance than low-velocity training ([76]. However, there have been concerns that higher intensity programmes could potentially overload the joint [77] and, thus, exacerbate symptoms [78,79]. Even though adverse events were reported to be no more likely in these programmes as compared to lower-intensity schemes, larger scaled direct comparisons of exercise intensity in view of adverse events and sustainability of treatment responses in the longer term are required before strong recommendations about intensity can be made [75].

Nevertheless, experiences of pain during exercise may assist decisions about exercise dosage and may co-determine the patient's willingness to continue complying with the programme. Therefore, patients should be advised that they may feel some discomfort or pain while exercising and that this does not necessarily means the joint is deteriorating. If necessary, pain medication can be taken prior to commencing exercise bouts and/or ice packs applied to the joint following exercise. However, increased or unsettling pain and/or swelling following exercise sessions may be signs that the exercise programme is too intensive and that changes to the type or dosage may be required [1].

How can clinicians monitor the effects of exercise?

Clinicians are encouraged to use validated outcome measures to assess the effectiveness or progress of an exercise programme and/or to promote adherence to the programme by providing the patients with potential positive outcome experiences (strategies on how to promote adherence are discussed elsewhere in this textbook). These outcome measures can include simple and reliable patient self-report measures of pain via a 10 cm visual analogue scale or a 0–10 numeric rating scale. For knee or hip OA, a variety of other self-report measures of pain and physical function are available including the Western Ontario and McMaster Universities Osteoarthritis Index (WOMAC), the Lower Extremity Functional Scale, or the Hip (HOOS) and Knee (KOOS) Osteoarthritis Outcome Scales [80]. Although the latter are mostly indicated in clinical research settings because of the required administration and processing time, these outcome measures should be administered prior to commencing the exercise programme to gain a measure at baseline, re-administered at regular intervals, such as monthly, as well as at completion of the programme. Patients can also rate the overall change they feel once they have completed a programme using a global rating of change scale.

In addition to self-report measures, physical performance measures evaluate what a patient actually is able to achieve physically rather than what they perceive or think they can do. These measures may also assist in monitoring patient progress as to the extent programme objectives are being achieved such as increases in strength, joint mobility or other functional goals. These performance measures usually consist of functional tasks or movements based on common activities of daily living and provide separate yet complementary information about patient status. Based on an international modified Delphi exercise rating the relevant evidence, OARSI has recommended a core set of physical performance measures for use in patients with hip and knee OA including those with OA and those following joint replacement [81]. The set comprises the 30-second chair stand test, 40-minute fast-paced walk test, and a stair climb test with additional tests including the timed up and go test and the 6-minute walk test. These are summarized in Table 22.2 with further information available from the OARSI website (http://www.oarsi.org).

For hand OA, several self-reported questionnaires have been described to rate the severity of symptoms such as the Australian/Canadian (AUSCAN) hand index, the Functional Index of Hand OsteoArthritis (FIHOA), Cochin Hand Function Scale, the Score for Assessment and Quantification of Chronic Rheumatic Affections of the Hand (SACRAH), the Arthritis Impact Measurement Scales 2 (AIMS 2), the Health Assessment Questionnaire, and the Michigan Hand Outcomes Questionnaire (MHQ). Objective measurements including the Arthritis Hand Function Test or evaluation of grip

Table 22.2 Description of the core set of physical performance measures for hip and knee osteoarthritis as recommended by the Osteoarthritis Research Society International

Test	Equipment needed	Description
30-second chair stand test	◆ Timer/stop watch ◆ Straight back chair with a 44 cm (17 inch) seat height, preferably without arms	Maximum number of chair stand repetitions possible in 30 seconds
40 m fast-paced walk test	◆ Timer/stop watch ◆ 10 m marked walkway with space to safely turn around at each end ◆ 2 cones placed approximately 2 m beyond each end of the walkway ◆ Calculator to convert time to speed	A fast paced walking test that is timed over 4 × 10 m for a total of 40 m performed in comfortable footwear
Stair climb test	◆ Timer/stop watch ◆ Set of stairs	Time in seconds it takes to ascend and descend a flight of stairs. The number of stairs will depend on individual availability

Reprinted from *Osteoarthritis Cartilage*, 21,8, Dobson F, Hinman RS, Roos EM, Abbott JH, Stratford P, Davis AM, et al., OARSI recommended performance-based tests to assess physical function in people diagnosed with hip or knee osteoarthritis, 1042–52, Copyright (2013) with permission from Elsevier.

strength constitute site-specific physical performance measures [82]. The OMERACT Hand Osteoarthritis Special Interest group acknowledges the availability of several instruments to assess symptom severity and physical dysfunction in people with hand OA, but highlights that at the present time it is impossible to recommend the use of one instrument over another [83].

Box 22.1 Practice points

◆ Exercise should be recommended for all patients with OA as part of the conservative management of their condition regardless of age, disease severity, levels of pain and physical dysfunction, and/or presence of co-morbidities.

◆ Exercise modalities such as type or dosage should be targeted to the patient's clinical characteristics, and should consider the patient's wishes and preferences.

◆ Patients and allied healthcare professionals should be educated about benefits of exercise. Patients should be informed it is normal to experience some discomfort/pain during exercise. While settling in the few hours after exercise completion, discomfort does not necessarily indicate worsening of structural damage to the joint.

◆ Referral to an exercise specialist such as a physical therapist is recommended.

◆ Barriers and facilitators to exercise should be identified and flexible, proactive strategies implemented to optimize adherence to exercise.

Conclusion

The take home messages of this chapter are summarized in Box 22.1. Non-surgical, non-drug treatments are considered important in the management of symptomatic OA. Exercise is universally recommended by OA clinical guidelines as an integral component of such a conservative approach. While considerable research has investigated the effects of exercise for knee OA, there is much less evidence to underpin its benefits for other joints such as the hip and hand. As the optimal dosage of exercise and particular choice of exercise type or delivery mode for people with OA remain unclear, treatment benefits of exercise of all types may be considered small to moderate. Importantly, these effects are comparable to those of drug treatments but are associated with relatively fewer side effects. In order to achieve optimal clinical outcomes with exercise, programme parameters and modalities should be individualized according to clinical phenotype, patient symptomatic status, and/or preferences of delivery mode. Additionally, adherence to exercise in the longer term should be encouraged in order to sustain longer-term clinical outcomes. Whilst the value of exercise for OA at other joint sites warrants further investigation, future trials should also continue to determine the ability of exercise in delaying the need for joint replacement. In this respect, when designing dedicated RCTs, placebo comparisons should be preferred to minimize the risk of bias in appraising the true effects of exercise on symptoms of OA.

References

1. Bennell KL, Dobson F, Hinman RS. Exercise in osteoarthritis: moving from prescription to adherence. *Best Pract Res Clin Rheumatol* 2014; 28(1):93–117.
2. Conaghan PG, Dickson J, Grant RL. Care and management of osteoarthritis in adults: summary of NICE guidance. *BMJ* 2008; 336(7642):502–3.
3. Fernandes L, Hagen KB, Bijlsma JW, et al. EULAR recommendations for the non-pharmacological core management of hip and knee osteoarthritis. *Ann Rheum Dis* 2013; 72(7):1125–35.
4. Hochberg MC, Altman RD, Toupin April K, et al. American College of Rheumatology 2012 recommendations for the use of nonpharmacologic and pharmacologic therapies in osteoarthritis of the hand, hip, and knee. *Arthritis Care Res* 2012; 64(4):465–74.
5. Zhang W, Doherty M, Leeb BF, et al. EULAR evidence based recommendations for the management of hand osteoarthritis: report of a Task Force of the EULAR Standing Committee for International Clinical Studies Including Therapeutics (ESCISIT). *Ann Rheum Dis* 2007; 66(3):377–88.
6. Zhang W, Moskowitz RW, Nuki G, et al. OARSI recommendations for the management of hip and knee osteoarthritis, Part II: OARSI evidence-based, expert consensus guidelines. *Osteoarthritis Cartilage* 2008; 16(2):137–62.
7. Savovic J, Jones H, Altman D, et al. Influence of reported study design characteristics on intervention effect estimates from randomised controlled trials: combined analysis of meta-epidemiological studies. *Health Technol Assess* 2012; 16(35):1–82.
8. Pelland L, Brosseau L, Wells G, et al. Efficacy of strengthening exercises for osteoarthritis (Part I): A meta-analysis. *Phys Ther Rev* 2004; 9(2):77–108.
9. Uthman OA, van der Windt DA, Jordan JL, et al. Exercise for lower limb osteoarthritis: systematic review incorporating trial sequential analysis and network meta-analysis. *BMJ* 2013; 347:f5555.
10. Fransen M, McConnell S, Harmer AR, et al. Exercise for osteoarthritis of the knee. *Cochrane Database Syst Rev* 2015; 1:CD004376.
11. Wallis JA, Taylor NF. Pre-operative interventions (non-surgical and non-pharmacological) for patients with hip or knee osteoarthritis awaiting joint replacement surgery—a systematic review and meta-analysis. *Osteoarthritis Cartilage* 2011; 19(12):1381–95.
12. Zhang W, Nuki G, Moskowitz RW, et al. OARSI recommendations for the management of hip and knee osteoarthritis: Part III: Changes in evidence following systematic cumulative update of research published through January 2009. *Osteoarthritis Cartilage* 2010; 18(4):476–99.
13. Pisters MF, Veenhof C, van Meeteren NL, et al. Long-term effectiveness of exercise therapy in patients with osteoarthritis of the hip or knee: a systematic review. *Arthritis Rheum* 2007; 57(7):1245–53.
14. Bennell KL, Egerton T, Martin J, et al. Effect of physical therapy on pain and function in patients with hip osteoarthritis. A randomised clinical trial. *JAMA* 2014; 311(19):1987–97.
15. Fransen M, McConnell S, Hernandez-Molina G, Reichenbach S. Exercise for osteoarthritis of the hip. *Cochrane Database Syst Rev* 2014; 4:CD007912.
16. Svege I, Nordsletten L, Fernandes L, Risberg MA. Exercise therapy may postpone total hip replacement surgery in patients with hip osteoarthritis: a long-term follow-up of a randomised trial. *Ann Rheum Dis* 2015; 74(1):164–9.
17. Hennig T, Haehre L, Hornburg VT, et al. Effect of home-based hand exercises in women with hand osteoarthritis: a randomised controlled trial. *Ann Rheum Dis* 2015; 74(8):1501–8.
18. Dziedzic K, Nicholls E, Hill S, et al. Self-management approaches for osteoarthritis in the hand: a 2x2 factorial randomised trial. *Ann Rheum Dis* 2015; 74(1):108–18.
19. Juhl C, Christensen R, Roos EM, Zhang W, Lund H. Impact of exercise type and dose on pain and disability in knee osteoarthritis: a systematic review and meta-regression analysis of randomized controlled trials. *Arthritis Rheum* 2014; 66(3):622–36.
20. Tanaka R, Ozawa J, Kito N, Moriyama H. Efficacy of strengthening or aerobic exercise on pain relief in people with knee osteoarthritis: a systematic review and meta-analysis of randomized controlled trials. *Clin Rehabil* 2013; 27(12):1059–71.
21. O'Connor SR, Tully MA, Ryan B, et al. Walking exercise for chronic musculoskeletal pain: systematic review and meta-analysis. *Arch Phys Med Rehabil* 2015; 96(4):724–734.e3.
22. Messier SP, Mihalko SL, Legault C, et al. Effects of intensive diet and exercise on knee joint loads, inflammation, and clinical outcomes among overweight and obese adults with knee osteoarthritis: the IDEA randomized clinical trial. *JAMA* 2013; 310(12):1263–73.
23. Bridle C, Spanjers K, Patel S, Atherton NM, Lamb SE. Effect of exercise on depression severity in older people: systematic review and meta-analysis of randomised controlled trials. *Br J Psychiatry* 2012; 201(3):180–5.
24. Kelley GA, Kelley KS, Hootman JM. Effects of exercise on depression in adults with arthritis: a systematic review with meta-analysis of randomized controlled trials. *Arthritis Res Ther* 2015; 17(1):21.
25. Chaipinyo K, Karoonsupcharoen O. No difference between home-based strength training and home-based balance training on pain in patients with knee osteoarthritis: a randomised trial. *Aust J Physiother* 2009; 55(1):25–30.
26. Arnold CM, Gyurcsik NC. Risk factors for falls in older adults with lower extremity arthritis: a conceptual framework of current knowledge and future directions. *Physiother Can* 2012; 64(3):302–14.
27. Escalante Y, Saavedra JM, Garcia-Hermoso A, Silva AJ, Barbosa TM. Physical exercise and reduction of pain in adults with lower limb osteoarthritis: a systematic review. *J Back Musculoskelet Rehabil* 2010; 23(4):175–86.
28. Wang C. Role of Tai Chi in the treatment of rheumatologic diseases. *Curr Rheumatol Rep* 2012; 14:598–603.
29. Wang C, Schmid CH, Hibberd PL, et al. Tai Chi is effective in treating knee osteoarthritis: a randomized controlled trial. *Arthritis Rheum* 2009; 61(11):1545–53.
30. Ye J, Cai S, Zhong W, Cai S, Zheng Q. Effects of tai chi for patients with knee osteoarthritis: a systematic review. *J Phys Ther Sci* 2014; 26(7):1133–7.

31. Bartels E, Lund H, Hagen K, et al. Aquatic exercise for the treatment of knee and hip osteoarthritis. *Cochrane Database Syst Rev* 2007; 4:CD005523.

32. Barker AL, Talevski J, Morello RT, et al. Effectiveness of aquatic exercise for musculoskeletal conditions: a meta-analysis. *Arch Phys Med Rehabil* 2014; 95(9):1776–86.

33. Ageberg E, Link A, Roos EM. Feasibility of neuromuscular training in patients with severe hip or knee OA: the individualized goal-based NEMEX-TJR training program. *BMC Musculoskelet Disord* 2010; 11:126.

34. Skou ST, Odgaard A, Rasmussen JO, Roos EM. Group education and exercise is feasible in knee and hip osteoarthritis. *Dan Med J* 2012; 59(12):A4554.

35. Thorstensson CA, Henriksson M, von Porat A, Sjodahl C, Roos EM. The effect of eight weeks of exercise on knee adduction moment in early knee osteoarthritis—a pilot study. *Osteoarthritis Cartilage* 2007; 15(10):1163–70.

36. Knoop J, van der Leeden M, Roorda LD, et al. Knee joint stabilization therapy in patients with osteoarthritis of the knee and knee instability: subgroup analyses in a randomized, controlled trial. *J Rehabil Med* 2014; 46(7):703–7.

37. Bennell KL, Kyriakides M, Metcalf B, et al. Neuromuscular versus quadriceps strengthening exercise in people with medial knee osteoarthritis and varus malalignment: a randomised controlled trial. *Arthritis Rheum* 2014; 66:950–9.

38. Dunlop DD, Song J, Semanik PA, et al. Objective physical activity measurement in the osteoarthritis initiative: are guidelines being met? *Arthritis Rheum* 2011; 63(11):3372–82.

39. Dunlop DD, Semanik P, Song J, et al. Moving to maintain function in knee osteoarthritis: evidence from the osteoarthritis initiative. *Arch Phys Med Rehabil* 2010; 91(5):714–21.

40. Bellamy N, Carette S, Ford PM, et al. Osteoarthritis antirheumatic drug trials. III. Setting the delta for clinical trials—results of a consensus development (Delphi) exercise. *J Rheumatol* 1992; 19(3):451–7.

41. Bennell KL, Dobson F, Roos EM, et al. The influence of biomechanical characteristics on pain and function outcomes from exercise in medial knee osteoarthritis and varus malalignment: exploratory analyses from a randomised controlled trial. *Arthritis Care Res* 2015; 67(9):1281–8.

42. Hancock MJ, Kjaer P, Korsholm L, Kent P. Interpretation of subgroup effects in published trials. *Phys Ther* 2013; 93:852–9.

43. Hancock MJ, Herbert R, Maher CG. A guide to interpretation of studies investigating subgroups of responders to physical therapy interventions. *Phys Ther* 2009; 89:698–704.

44. Ettinger WH, Jr., Burns R, Messier SP, et al. A randomized trial comparing aerobic exercise and resistance exercise with a health education program in older adults with knee osteoarthritis. The Fitness Arthritis and Seniors Trial (FAST). *JAMA* 1997; 277(1):25–31.

45. van Baar M, Dekker J, Oostendorp R, et al. Effectiveness of exercise in patients with osteoarthritis of the hip or knee: nine months follow up. *Ann Rheum Dis* 2001; 60(12):1123–30.

46. Campbell R, Evans M, Tucker M, et al. Why don't patients do their exercises? Understanding non-compliance with physiotherapy in patients with osteoarthritis of the knee. *J Epidemiol Community Health* 2001; 55:132–8.

47. Mihalko SL, Brenes GA, Farmer DF, et al. Challenges and innovations in enhancing adherence. *Control Clin Trials* 2004; 25(5):447–57.

48. Brittain DR, Gyurcsik NC, McElroy M, Hillard SA. General and arthritis-specific barriers to moderate physical activity in women with arthritis. *Womens Health Issues* 2011; 21(1):57–63.

49. Gyurcsik NC, Brawley LR, Spink KS, Sessford JD. Meeting physical activity recommendations: self-regulatory efficacy characterizes differential adherence during arthritis flares. *Rehabil Pychol* 2013; 58(1):43–50.

50. Marks R. Knee osteoarthritis and exercise adherence: a review. *Curr Aging Sci* 2012; 5(1):72–83.

51. Mazieres B, Thevenon A, Coudeyre E, et al. Adherence to, and results of, physical therapy programs in patients with hip or knee

52. McAuley E, Lox C, Duncan TE. Long-term maintenance of exercise, self-efficacy, and physiological change in older adults. *J Gerontol* 1993; 48(4):P218–24.

53. Minor MA, Brown JD. Exercise maintenance of persons with arthritis after participation in a class experience. *Health Educ Q* 1993; 20(1):83–95.

54. Petursdottir U, Arnadottir S, Halldorsdottir S. Facilitators and barriers to exercising among people with osteoarthritis: a phenomenological study. *Phys Ther* 2010; 90(7):1014–25.

55. Resnick B, Spellbring AM. Understanding what motivates older adults to exercise. *J Gerontol Nurs* 2000; 26(3):34–42.

56. Rhodes RE, Martin AD, Taunton JE, et al. Factors associated with exercise adherence among older adults. An individual perspective. *Sports Med* 1999; 28(6):397–411.

57. Schutzer KA, Graves BS. Barriers and motivations to exercise in older adults. *Prev Med* 2004; 39(5):1056–61.

58. U Seçkin, Gunduz S, Borman P, Akyuz M. Evaluation of the compliance to exercise therapy in patients with knee osteoarthritis. *J Back Musculoskelet* 2000; 14:133–7.

59. Wilcox S, Der Ananian C, Abbott J, et al. Perceived exercise barriers, enablers, and benefits among exercising and nonexercising adults with arthritis: results from a qualitative study. *Arthritis Rheumatism* 2006; 55(4):616–27.

60. Baker K, Nelson M, Felson D, et al. The efficacy of home-based progressive strength training in older adults with knee osteoarthritis: a randomized controlled trial. *J Rheumatol* 2001; 28:1655–65.

61. O'Reilly SC, Muir KR, Doherty M. Effectiveness of home exercise on pain and disability from osteoarthritis of the knee: a randomised controlled trial. *Ann Rheum Dis* 1999; 58(1):15–9.

62. Fernandes L, Storheim K, Sandvik L, Nordsletten L, Risberg MA. Efficacy of patient education and supervised exercise vs patient education alone in patients with hip osteoarthritis: a single blind randomized clinical trial. *Osteoarthritis Cartilage* 2010; 18(10):1237–43.

63. French HP, Cusack T, Brennan A, et al. Exercise and Manual Physiotherapy Arthritis Research Trial (EMPART) for osteoarthritis of the hip: a multicenter randomized controlled trial. *Arch Phys Med Rehabil* 2013; 94(2):302–14.

64. Juhakoski R, Tenhonen S, Malmivaara A, et al. A pragmatic randomized controlled study of the effectiveness and cost consequences of exercise therapy in hip osteoarthritis. *Clin Rehabil* 2011; 25(4):370–83.

65. Tak E, Staats P, Van Hespen A, Hopman-Rock M. The effects of an exercise program for older adults with osteoarthritis of the hip. *J Rheumatol* 2005; 32:1106–13.

66. Juhakoski R, Tenhonen S, Anttonen T, Kauppinen T, Arokoski JP. Factors affecting self-reported pain and physical function in patients with hip osteoarthritis. *Arch Phys Med Rehabil* 2008; 89(6):1066–73.

67. Osteras N, Hagen KB, Grotle M, et al. Limited effects of exercises in people with hand osteoarthritis: results from a randomized controlled trial. *Osteoarthritis Cartilage* 2014; 22(9):1224–33.

68. Bennell KL, Hinman RS. A review of the clinical evidence for exercise in osteoarthritis of the hip and knee. *J Sci Med Sport* 2011; 14(1):4–9.

69. McCarthy C, Mills P, Pullen R, et al. Supplementation of a home-based exercise programme with a class-based programme for people with osteoarthritis of the knees: a randomised controlled trial and health economic analysis. *Health Technol Assess* 2004; 8(46):1–61.

70. Ravaud P, Giraudeau B, Logeart I, et al. Management of osteoarthritis (OA) with an unsupervised home based exercise programme and/or patient administered assessment tools. A cluster randomised controlled trial with a 2x2 factorial design. *Ann Rheum Dis* 2004; 63(6):703–8.

71. Roddy E, Zhang W, Doherty M, et al. Evidence-based recommendations for the role of exercise in the management of osteoarthritis of

osteoarthritis. Development of French clinical practice guidelines. *Joint Bone Spine* 2008; 75(5):589–96.

the hip or knee—the MOVE consensus. *Rheumatology (Oxford)* 2005; 44(1):67–73.

72. American Geriatrics Society Panel on Exercise and Osteoarthritis. Exercise prescription for older adults with osteoarthritis pain: consensus practice recommendations. *J Am Geriatr Soc* 2001; 49:808–23.

73. World Health Organization. *Global Recommendations on Physical Activity for Health*. Geneva: World Health Organization; 2010.

74. World Health Organization. Obesity: preventing and managing the global epidemic. Report of a WHO consultation. *World Health Organ Tech Rep Ser* 2000; 894:i–xii, 1–253.

75. Zacharias A, Green RA, Semciw AI, Kingsley MI, Pizzari T. Efficacy of rehabilitation programs for improving muscle strength in people with hip or knee osteoarthritis: a systematic review with meta-analysis. *Osteoarthritis Cartilage* 2014; 22(11):1752–73.

76. Fukumoto Y, Tateuchi H, Ikezoe T, et al. Effects of high-velocity resistance training on muscle function, muscle properties, and physical performance in individuals with hip osteoarthritis: a randomized controlled trial. *Clin Rehabil* 2014; 28(1):48–58.

77. van Baar ME, Dekker J, Lemmens JA, Oostendorp RA, Bijlsma JW. Pain and disability in patients with osteoarthritis of hip or knee: the relationship with articular, kinesiological, and psychological characteristics. *J Rheumatol* 1998; 25(1):125–33.

78. Baliunas AJ, Hurwitz DE, Ryals AB, et al. Increased knee joint loads during walking are present in subjects with knee osteoarthritis. *Osteoarthritis Cartilage* 2002; 10(7):573–9.

79. Lucchinetti E, Adams CS, Horton WE, Jr, Torzilli PA. Cartilage viability after repetitive loading: a preliminary report. *Osteoarthritis Cartilage* 2002; 10(1):71–81.

80. Collins NJ, Misra D, Felson DT, Crossley KM, Roos EM. Measures of knee function: International Knee Documentation Committee (IKDC) Subjective Knee Evaluation Form, Knee Injury and Osteoarthritis Outcome Score (KOOS), Knee Injury and Osteoarthritis Outcome Score Physical Function Short Form (KOOS-PS), Knee Outcome Survey Activities of Daily Living Scale (KOS-ADL), Lysholm Knee Scoring Scale, Oxford Knee Score (OKS), Western Ontario and McMaster Universities Osteoarthritis Index (WOMAC), Activity Rating Scale (ARS), and Tegner Activity Score (TAS). *Arthritis Care Res* 2011; 63(Suppl 11):S208–28.

81. Dobson F, Hinman RS, Roos EM, et al. OARSI recommended performance-based tests to assess physical function in people diagnosed with hip or knee osteoarthritis. *Osteoarthritis Cartilage* 2013; 21(8):1042–52.

82. Poole JL. Measures of hand function: Arthritis Hand Function Test (AHFT), Australian Canadian Osteoarthritis Hand Index (AUSCAN), Cochin Hand Function Scale, Functional Index for Hand Osteoarthritis (FIHOA), Grip Ability Test (GAT), Jebsen Hand Function Test (JHFT), and Michigan Hand Outcomes Questionnaire (MHQ). *Arthritis Care Res* 2011; 63(Suppl 11):S189–99.

83. Kloppenburg M, Boyesen P, Smeets W, et al. Report from the OMERACT Hand Osteoarthritis Special Interest Group: advances and future research priorities. *J Rheumatol* 2014; 41(4):810–8.

CHAPTER 23

Weight loss

Marius Henriksen, Robin Christensen,
Berit L. Heitmann, and Henning Bliddal

Obesity and osteoarthritis

The global prevalence of osteoarthritis (OA) continues to escalate, both due to an ageing population [1] and as a result of the current obesity epidemic, with obesity among the elderly becoming an increasing problem [2]. In the year 2000, 600 million people worldwide were aged 60 years or older, representing a threefold increase compared with the 1950 population [1]. This trend is a cause for concern given that, as evidenced by data from the United States, the prevalence of OA rises steeply in older people, with approximately 34% of those aged 65 years or older estimated to have OA, compared with 14% of adults aged 25 years or older [3]. OA is a leading cause of disability and has a significant impact on health-related quality of life [3,4]. Approximately 80% of affected individuals have some degree of movement limitation, while 25% are unable to perform major activities of daily living [3]. Knee OA is of particular importance, as the knee is pivotal for ambulation and therefore social participation [5]. In a survey looking at the changing profile of joint disorders with age, knee and back problems were most frequently reported (approximately10%), with knee problems having the greatest increase in prevalence with age compared with other joints [6]. Knee pain is present in a large proportion of the elderly, with 25% of people aged over 55 years experiencing a persistent episode of knee pain and around 10% experiencing painful disabling knee OA [7]. OA is also costly, accounting for more than a $10 billion per year healthcare spend in the United States [8], much of this attributable to loss of working days and the cost of knee and hip replacements [9].

The global epidemic of obesity is also well recognized with the worldwide prevalence of obesity being nearly doubled between 1980 and 2014. It has been estimated in 2014 that about 40% of adults worldwide were overweight and 11% of men and 15% of women were obese. Thus, more than half a billion adults worldwide are classed as obese [10]. Obesity has wide-ranging implications on many aspects of health, including musculoskeletal health. Similar to many musculoskeletal conditions, obesity affects mobility and physical function leading to disability and loss of independent lifestyle.

Obesity and knee OA share pathogenetic phenotypes and the development of one disease increases the risk of the other and may trigger the onset of a vicious circle [5]. Obesity has long been recognized as a risk factor for knee OA and the relationship was documented for the first time in the middle of last century [11]. Now, more than 60 years later, we are facing immense and increasing socioeconomic costs due to the complications associated with OA and the obesity pandemic. The increasing prevalence of these two interlinked conditions and the associated health, social, and economic consequences, make it imperative to advance our knowledge of the interrelation between OA and obesity, and apply this to improve care for these patients.

Obesity is widely acknowledged as a risk factor for OA, with every 5 kg of weight gain conferring a 36% increase in the risk of knee OA incidence [12]. There is evidence that the risk accumulates with increased exposure to high body mass index (BMI) throughout adulthood, with an association between BMI and later knee OA starting as early as from age 20 years in men and 15 years in women [13]. In addition, body weight influences the severity of OA; obese individuals have significantly more severe joint damage in the knees compared with normal weight or underweight individuals [14]. Data from a case–control study have also indicated a strong association between high BMI and surgical replacement of hip and knee joints [15]. Of note, obesity and OA collectively reduce mobility, which can initiate a vicious cycle of events: reduced activity, further weight gain, and decreased muscle strength, leading to increased joint problems and disease progression [5]. Hence, weight loss is a primary goal in obese individuals with OA [16–18].

Aetiologically, two main pathways are suggested to lead to knee OA: a biochemical pathway and a biomechanical pathway. The two pathways may interlink or alternate in the individual, and both mechanisms seem to be significantly influenced by heritage [19,20], with definite indications of overlapping syndromes [21,22]. In particular, the pathomechanical effects of abnormal knee joint loadings during walking have been in focus in knee OA because of the repetitive high joint loadings that walking creates daily. Obesity and knee OA are traditionally thought to be associated due to excess joint loads that are thought to be pathogenic and lead to knee OA [23,24] and OA may lead to an increase in body weight [25]. Yet, not all obese individuals develop knee OA, nor are all knee OA patients obese; some obese people may adapt functionally and/or biologically and avoid development of OA, and overweight and joint loads are not by themselves a sufficient explanation for osteoarthritic degeneration of the knee [26]. Thus, the relationships between knee OA, obesity, and biomechanical factors are complex. Longitudinal studies that relate knee OA development and progression to mechanical loading (including those of overweight and obesity) are sparse and it is not possible to confidently link OA to mechanical overload [27].

Intriguingly, obesity is also associated with hand OA in spite of the lack of an intuitive link between excess joint loads and OA in non-weight bearing joints, such as those in the hand [28,29]. This suggests that non-mechanical mechanisms must also play important roles [30]. In particular, there is interest in the potential role of adipokines (cytokines secreted by adipose tissue). For example, leptin has long been considered to be implicated in the pathogenesis of OA, independent of the mechanical effect of obesity [31] and recent data indicate that a significant part of the obesity–OA association may be due to excess levels of leptin [32]. Of note, the infrapatellar fat pad, an adipose tissue depot located in the knee joint, may contribute to the pathophysiological changes which occur in the OA joint via local production of cytokines and adipokines [33]. Indeed, definite signs of increased perfusion (a possible marker of inflammation) of the infrapatellar fat pad have been demonstrated in obese patients with knee OA, indicating a local inflammatory active fatty tissue [34]. Relative loss of muscle mass and strength over time may also contribute to the onset of OA in obese individuals. Although both muscle and fat mass increase with weight gain, overall, the volume of muscle mass remains relatively low and inadequate to match the demands placed upon it [35].

There is also evidence that OA is associated with release of a range of pro-inflammatory mediators from joint tissues, including interleukin (IL)-1 beta, IL6, IL8, cyclooxygenase 2, prostaglandin E2, matrix metalloproteinase (MMP)-2, MMP3, MMP9, MMP13, receptor activator of nuclear factor kappa B ligand, fibroblast growth factor 2 [36–39], and adipokines [33]. Of note, proinflammatory cytokines such as IL6 and C-reactive protein (CRP) have been shown to predict both the incidence [40] and progression of arthritis [41,42]. Furthermore, recent evidence from the Intensive Diet and Exercise for Arthritis (IDEA) study illustrates the association between weight and inflammation [43]. Indeed, leptin may exert its effect via upregulation of IL6 expression in synovial fibroblasts [44]. Levels of CRP are only to a very limited extent elevated in OA, which may be interpreted as a sign of OA being a localized inflammatory process involving mostly the joint rather than a systemic disease, such as rheumatoid arthritis, as influenced by IL6 in the circulation.

Also worthy of note is the association of obesity and OA with metabolic abnormalities, such as hyperinsulinaemia and other cardiometabolic defects. OA of the knee is associated with hyperinsulinaemia, which may play a role in OA in overweight patients, possibly via changes in insulin-like growth factor 1 [45]. Furthermore, an increased risk of OA has been observed in obese women with cardiometabolic clustering versus those without [46]. Notably, obesity was found to be significantly associated with pain measures or many of the physical functioning performance measures only when it was accompanied by cardiometabolic clustering [46]. This observation may have significance in terms of optimizing treatment for knee OA. Vincent et al. published a review of the potential complex and multifactorial mechanisms linking obesity and OA [35].

Weight loss in osteoarthritis

There is evidence that weight loss as a primary treatment of patients with knee OA and concomitant obesity improves both pain and functional status dramatically [5,43,47–49]. As a consequence, current international recommendations for treatment of knee OA highlight weight loss as a core management strategy in concomitant knee OA and overweight/obesity [16–18,50].

Weight loss relieves symptoms in obese patients with OA including, importantly, pain. Significantly, decreasing body fat and increasing physical activity are particularly important in producing symptomatic relief of knee OA [51]. Data from a cohort study of 1410 individuals with symptomatic knee OA suggest that a significant dose–response relationship exists between changes in body weight and corresponding changes in self-reported pain and physical function scores [52]. While loss of approximately 5% of body weight has been shown to provide some symptomatic relief in obese patients with OA [53], several studies have indicated that the ultimate goal should be an initial decrease in body weight of at least 10%, in order to provide significant reductions in pain [52,54]. This is supported by clinical guidelines on the identification, evaluation, and treatment of overweight and obesity in adults from the Obesity Education Initiative of the National Institutes of Health (NIH) in the United States, which recommend an initial goal for weight loss of 10% from baseline in obese individuals [55]. If successful, maintenance of the weight loss is important and further weight loss may be attempted if required. Importantly, in parallel with OA pain reduction, mobility and physical function improve [52,54,56]. Quality of life is also improved following weight loss in patients with OA, as evidenced by improvements in the composite physical health score of the SF-36 Health Survey, as well as improvements in satisfaction with body function and appearance [57].

Further insight comes from the Influence of Weight Loss or Exercise on Cartilage in Obese Knee OA Patients (CAROT) study, which evaluated the effects of an intensive weight-loss programme over 16 weeks in obese patients with knee OA. This low-energy, formula-diet, weight-loss programme was shown to reduce OA symptoms [48], although no changes were demonstrated in bone marrow lesions in response to weight loss [58]. The IDEA study suggests that besides symptomatic effects, weight loss through diet and combined diet and exercise may have anti-inflammatory benefits in obese subjects with concomitant knee OA, as evidenced by reduced levels of IL6 following a weight loss [43].

Guidelines from the American College of Rheumatology (ACR) (17) and European League Against Rheumatism (EULAR) [16] recommend the need for weight loss as well as exercise in the management of overweight or obese patients with OA. Several studies support the combination of exercise and weight loss, together with appropriate analgesia, as a cornerstone for these patients [56,59]. These studies have highlighted important benefits of combined exercise and diet therapy compared with either exercise or diet alone, including greater improvements in gait, knee pain, and physical function [59]. Although long-term weight loss can be achieved through calorie restriction alone, the addition of exercise is also required in order to significantly improve mobility (an important determinant of disability), self-reported function, and pain [56]. In addition, the CAROT study indicated a decrease in lower extremity muscle mass and muscle strength following weight loss in obese patients with knee OA, suggesting that significant weight loss should be followed by an exercise regimen to restore or increase muscle mass in this patient population [60].

Theoretically weight loss could improve dysfunction of the knee related to OA by virtue of the pain reduction reported as a concomitant result of weight loss [54]. Recent studies of weight loss show that the peak knee compressive force can be reduced more than what can be accounted for by the weight loss alone [61,62]. The Arthritis Diet and Activity Promotion Trial (ADAPT) study

[62] showed a 1:4 association between weight loss and reduction in peak knee joint load during walking even though the weight loss was moderate in magnitude (<5%). In the CAROT study [61], these results were confirmed reporting a larger weight loss (>10%) and a 1:2 association between weight loss and peak knee joint load reduction during walking. Thus, biomechanical adaptations that 'off-load' the knee occur to a higher extent than what can be accounted for by the mere weight loss, indicating changes in the neuromuscular coordination strategies used during walking. From the CAROT study Aaboe et al. [61] also reported that the axial knee load impulse was significantly reduced by 13% after weight loss. The axial impulse represents the total or cumulative mechanical load on the knee during one step cycle. These results may have important implications in that not only the peak knee loading but also the total cumulative amount of joint loading exposed to the knee is reduced. The clinical relevance however, of a reduced peak knee joint load and axial impulse currently is unknown as no studies have addressed the long-term consequences of weight loss on knee OA progression. On the other hand, one-third of the participants in the CAROT study surprisingly increased their peak knee joint loads after the significant weight loss [26]. The presumably unfavourable increase in knee joint loading was due to improved ambulatory function and walking speed following weight loss, yet no acceleration of symptomatic and structural disease progression was observed in these patients with increased joint loads relative to those with reduced joint loads 1 year later [26]. The solution to the paradox lies in the interaction between pain and knee joint loading/usage. Weight loss significantly reduces knee OA pain [48,54,61] but conversely, pain relief has been shown to increase knee joint loading during walking and stair climbing [63–66]. Given adequate time, musculoskeletal tissues including cartilage and bone, adapt their properties to gradual changes in loads; bone mineral density in the proximal tibia varies as a function of joint loading [67,68], and bone marrow lesions appear frequently in areas of increased bone mass density in support of the hypothesis that the local density of bone reflects historical loading of a joint [69].

Does weight loss have an impact on development and progression of osteoarthritis?

Results from the Framingham study have demonstrated that weight loss reduces the risk for developing knee OA in women [70]. In this study, a 5.1 kg reduction in weight over a 10-year period decreased the likelihood of women developing symptomatic knee OA by 50% [70]. In a subgroup analysis, weight loss was associated with a significant reduction in OA risk in individuals with high baseline BMI (≥ 25 kg/m^2), but not in those with BMI less than 25 kg/m^2 [70].

While the short-term benefits of weight loss in obese patients with OA are undisputed, the effect of weight loss on the progression of OA remains a topic for debate. Some results have suggested a positive effect of weight loss on cartilage in non-OA subjects. For example, in a prospective study of obese adults recruited from gastric banding or diet and exercise programmes, weight loss was found to be associated with improvements in both the quality and quantity of knee articular cartilage [71].

However, other studies have indicated that weight loss does not alter the course of OA, and an association between symptom relief and altered course of structural damage remains to be shown. In the ADAPT study, no difference in joint space width (a measure of disease progression) was seen between patients treated with diet, exercise, diet plus exercise, or healthy lifestyle (the control group) [56]. However, the authors noted that the relatively short duration of the intervention (18 months) coupled with the number of subjects per group (approximately 80) probably prevented the detection of meaningful differences in radiographic disease progression. The ADAPT study results were later confirmed in the IDEA trial on both X-ray and magnetic resonance imaging with considerably more participants, but the same duration [72]. Hence, more research on possible long-term associations between weight loss and alterations in the course of OA is required.

Weight loss management

In contrast to weight loss among the general population, where rapid initial weight loss can indicate a poorer long-term prognosis in terms of regaining weight [55,56], greater initial weight loss in obese people with OA is associated with better long-term prognosis of weight maintenance, and can be associated with better compliance with weight management [73]. However, this is in contrast with clinical opinion recommending a slower rate of weight loss [73]. The NIH guidelines recommend that, in order to achieve a 10% weight loss over 6 months, overweight patients (BMI 27–35 kg/m^2) should aim for a decrease of 300–500 kcal/day (1300–2100 kJ/day), resulting in weight loss of about 250–500 g/week. For more severely obese patients (BMI > 35 kg/m^2), deficits of up to 500–1000 kcal/day (2100–4200 kJ/day) are required for weight loss of about 500–1000 g/week [55]. For obese people with established OA, who may have relatively low activity levels and inactivity-induced lean mass atrophy [74], weight loss tends to be less than expected [75] and the energy deficit of an effective diet has to be greater to compensate for this.

Opinions on the optimal method for weight loss are varied. While evidence supports a calorie-restricted diet, the evidence to support differences in diet composition is limited and inconclusive. Although it is critical—especially in elderly OA patients—to introduce a low-calorie diet that still provides all the essential nutrients, maintenance of recommended daily calcium intake is particularly important for elderly women who may be at risk of osteoporosis [55]. For some obese patients, compliance with long-term lifestyle changes is low and other approaches, such as bariatric surgery (e.g. laparoscopic adjustable gastric banding or sleeve gastrectomy) [35,76] or pharmacotherapy, may be the best way to achieving weight loss. A hierarchy of approaches for weight loss is illustrated in Figure 23.1.

It has been postulated that exercise may cause further joint damage in obese patients with OA due to the increased strain and load on the joints. This leads to the hypothesis that weight loss should be achieved prior to commencing exercise. This theory is supported by evidence from an 8-week study assessing the effect of rapid diet-induced weight loss on physical function in 80 obese knee OA patients [54]. In this study, implementation of a low-energy diet (3.4 MJ/day) led to a weight loss of 11.1%, compared with 4.3% in individuals on a control diet (5 MJ/day). In the group on the low-energy diet, physical function—as assessed by the Western Ontario and McMaster Universities Osteoarthritis Index function score—was significantly improved; there was no significant change in the control group [54]. This finding suggests that rapid weight loss

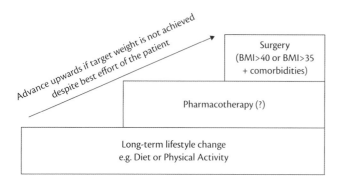

Figure 23.1 A hierarchy of approaches for weight loss.

enabled obese OA patients to subsequently obtain a higher degree of physical activity compared with the control group.

The CAROT study applied a well-documented weight loss programme consisting of full meal replacement for 8 weeks and a graduate return to 'normal food' and dietary consultancy over the subsequent 8 weeks [48,54,77]. However, although the applied intensive dietary intervention resulted in major weight losses and symptomatic and functional improvements, the majority of the participants were still categorized as obese (BMI > 30 kg/m²) at the end of the intervention. Further, only participants subsequently randomized to continuous weekly counselling sessions with a dietician over 1 year were able to maintain the weight loss; participants allocated to exercise or control groups regressed towards baseline body weight during the weight maintenance period (1 year) [47]. Importantly, the initial (16-week) symptomatic and functional improvements obtained by all participants dissipated in all groups during the 1-year weight maintenance period [47]—independently of the weight change during maintenance. Despite evidence of its benefits, these results support the general notion that weight loss is notoriously difficult to sustain in the long term. Of note, while the general advice is to exercise to maintain weight loss, this may not be possible in obese knee OA patients due to activity-induced knee pain—despite current recommendations advocating exercise as a core treatment of knee OA [16,17]. This was highlighted in the CAROT study, in which adherence to exercise as a weight loss maintenance strategy was extremely poor [47]. Altogether, this highlights the need for additional strategies to support knee OA patients in maintaining or enhancing weight loss.

Pharmacological and surgical approaches to weight loss/maintenance

With continued lifestyle treatment, weight regain can be ameliorated but not eliminated. Originally medications for the treatment of obesity were proposed as short-term adjuncts for patients, who would presumably then acquire the skills necessary to continue to lose weight, reach 'ideal body weight', and maintain a reduced weight indefinitely. The need for constant vigilance to sustain behavioural changes in the face of pressures to regain weight emphasizes the challenges faced by even the most motivated patients. Currently among 'obesiologists' it is generally accepted that there is a need for adjunctive therapies that can help patients who are not able to lose or sustain sufficient weight loss to improve health with lifestyle interventions alone. Pharmacological therapy is considered

appropriate for patients as an adjunct to lifestyle interventions to facilitate weight loss and prevent weight regain.

Surprisingly the scientific literature on drug treatment for obesity is limited, particularly for studies conducted before the requirement for registration of all clinical trials, by short intervention periods, high attrition, inadequate description of methods, and data analyses that used biased approaches such as inferring from those completing the trial rather than the rigorous intention-to-treat approach [78]. However, according to meta-analyses of weight loss compounds [79], drugs like orlistat, lorcaserin, and phentermine, when used as an adjunct to lifestyle intervention, all increase the likelihood that a patient will achieve a clinically meaningful (>5%) 1-year weight loss. Thus, although there are no 'wonder drugs' available, medications approved for long-term obesity treatment, when used as an adjunct to lifestyle intervention, lead to greater mean weight loss and an increased likelihood of achieving clinically meaningful 1-year weight loss relative to placebo [80].

Although bariatric surgery is commonly performed, it is not universally accepted as an obesity treatment. The reason for this might very well be that most published studies of bariatric surgery are retrospective, short-term studies with insufficient follow-up. Methodological issues in these studies typically preclude definitive conclusions about the outcomes of procedures. There is ample short-term evidence about the benefits and risks of bariatric surgery up to 1 year after surgery, few data are available about long-term outcomes or groups [81]. Based on a systematic review, the quality of evidence and treatment effectiveness 2 years after bariatric procedures for weight loss for type 2 diabetes, hypertension, and hyperlipidaemia in severely obese adults was assessed [81]. It was concluded that gastric bypass has better outcomes than gastric banding procedures for long-term weight loss, type 2 diabetes control and remission, hypertension, and hyperlipidaemia [81].

Strategies to enhance behavioural change and adherence

Weight loss is clearly important in managing the obese OA patient, but once it has been achieved, how difficult is it to maintain this weight loss? In a prospective study assessing the effects of physical activity on weight maintenance in 32 women who had recently (within 3 months) achieved their target for weight loss, the amount of physical activity required to minimize weight gain for 1 year after weight loss was estimated [82]. It was apparent that active women maintained their weight loss better than inactive women, although the relationship was found to be non-linear. Instead, a threshold-like relationship was observed between physical activity and weight control, with the threshold corresponding to a physical activity level of 80 minutes of moderate exercise or 35 minutes of vigorous exercise per day in order to prevent weight regain following weight loss [82].

Despite evidence of its benefits, weight loss maintenance through diet and exercise is notoriously difficult in the long term, with non-compliance being a key problem. Factors that appear to pose a particular risk for weight regain include a history of weight cycling, disinhibited eating, binge eating, more hunger, eating in response to negative emotions and stress, and more passive reactions to problems [73]. In the Look AHEAD trial, which evaluated the cardiovascular effects of intensive lifestyle intervention in type 2 diabetes patients, initial mean weight loss was 8.6%, declining to an average weight loss of 6.0% after 10 years [83]. Although modest weight loss was sustained over the length of the trial, patients were specifically recruited if they were motivated to lose weight through a lifestyle intervention and were only included in the study if they could complete a maximal-fitness test at baseline [83]. Maintenance of weight loss in non-motivated individuals is likely to be even more difficult over time, with particular difficulties encountered in maintaining standard diet and exercise programmes in previously sedentary, overweight adults with OA and its associated mobility disability [47,56]. This highlights the need for strategies to increase motivation and improve patient adherence to diet and exercise programmes, as well as additional ways to support patients in achieving sustainable weight loss.

In fact, there are a number of approaches aimed at improving compliance and supporting long-term weight control. A review of factors associated with weight loss maintenance by Elfhag and Rössner proposes that contributors to successful long-term weight loss include achieving initial weight loss, reaching a self-determined goal weight, having a physically active lifestyle, maintaining a regular meal rhythm including breakfast and healthier eating, exerting control of overeating, and instigating self-monitoring of behaviours [73]. In addition to an internal motivation to lose weight, other important factors include social support, better coping strategies and ability to handle life stress, self-efficacy, autonomy, assuming responsibility in life, and overall more psychological strength and stability [73]. Patient–therapist contact appears to be a key factor in achieving weight loss of approximately 10% over a period of 16–26 weeks. Continued contact appears to be effective whether it occurs in person (e.g. by attending weight maintenance classes) or through telephone, post, or email-based communications.

Strategies for weight loss maintenance

The vast majority of overweight and obese adults have endured several weight loss attempts and struggle lifelong against the scales. In agreement, the real challenge is not to lose weight but to keep the lost weight off in the long term. Thus, studies show that only 5–10% of persons are successful in keeping weight off for more than 5 years [84]. However, there is still a lack of knowledge about the strategies for a permanent weight loss beyond 5 years. A recent review [85] concluded that interventions that target both diet and activity seem superior to diet or activity alone, in weight loss maintenance. Addition of pharmacological treatment further added to the effect. Similarly, a report from the NIH on the problem of weight regain after weight loss likewise specified that 'Specific barriers to successful weight loss maintenance include poor adherence to behavioural regimens and physiological adaptations that promote weight regain' and concluded that physiologists and behavioural researchers need to collaborate for weight loss maintenance to be successful [86]. Finally, The US National Weight Control Registry that has followed successful weight losers for more than 10 years, recently emphasized that sustained behaviour change and a large initial weight loss are important strategies for long-term weight maintenance, whereas decreased leisure-time physical activity, dietary restraint, and frequency of self-weighing and increased dietary energy intake from fat and disinhibition, will increase the risk of weight regain [87].

Conclusion and perspectives

It is imperative to diagnose OA as early as possible—in particular among overweight and obese individuals. Because obese patients have a greater risk of developing OA, they should be monitored for signs of the disease. In the future, earlier diagnosis of OA may be aided by the identification of effective biomarkers. For all obese patients with OA, weight loss should be advocated as a first-line management approach, with a goal of rapid initial weight loss of at least 10% of body weight. The challenge of how to maintain weight loss, and the question of whether or not weight loss can alter progression of OA, remain key areas of ongoing research.

Another area for focus is advancing our knowledge of the pathophysiology that underpins both OA and obesity. This, in turn, may facilitate the identification of alternative therapeutic approaches. In particular, any approach that tackles both OA and obesity would be a major step forward in stemming the global epidemic of these two interlinked conditions.

References

1. United Nations. *World Population Aging*. New York: United Nations; 2009.
2. Mathus-Vliegen EM. Prevalence, pathophysiology, health consequences and treatment options of obesity in the elderly: a guideline. *Obes Facts* 2012; 5(3):460–83.
3. Centers for Disease Control. *Osteoarthritis*. Atlanta, GA: Centers for Disease Control; 2011.
4. Lementowski P, Zelicof S. Obesity and osteoarthritis. *Am J Orthop* 2008; 37:148–51.
5. Bliddal H, Christensen R. The management of osteoarthritis in the obese patient: practical considerations and guidelines for therapy. *Obes Rev* 2006; 7(4):323–31.
6. Badley EM, Tennant A. Changing profile of joint disorders with age: findings from a postal survey of the population of Calderdale, West Yorkshire, United Kingdom. *Ann Rheum Dis* 1992; 51(3):366–71.
7. Peat G, McCarney R, Croft P. Knee pain and osteoarthritis in older adults: a review of community burden and current use of primary health care. *Ann Rheum Dis* 2001; 60(2):91–7.
8. Bliddal H. Guidelines for the use of nonsurgical interventions in osteoarthritis management. *Expert Rev Clin Immunol* 2008; 4(5):583–90.
9. Lethbridge-Cejku M, Helmick C, Popovic J. Hospitalizations for arthritis and other rheumatic conditions: data from the 1997 National Hospital Discharge Survey. *Med Care* 2003; 41(12):1367–73.
10. World Health Organization. *Global Status Report on Noncommunicable Diseases 2014*. Geneva: World Health Organization; 2014.
11. Fletcher E, Lewis-Fanning E. Chronic rheumatic diseases – part IV: a statistical study of 1,000 cases of chronic rheumatism. *Postgrad Med J* 1945; 21(235):176–85.
12. Lementowski PW, Zelicof SB. Obesity and osteoarthritis. *Am J Orthop (Belle Mead NJ)* 2008; 37(3):148–51.
13. Wills AK, Black S, Cooper R, et al. Life course body mass index and risk of knee osteoarthritis at the age of 53 years: evidence from the 1946 British birth cohort study. *Ann Rheum Dis* 2012; 71(5):655–60.
14. Muehleman C, Margulis A, Bae W, Masuda K. Relationship between knee and ankle degeneration in a population of organ donors. *BMC Med* 2010; 28(8):48.
15. Wendelboe AM, Hegmann KT, Biggs JJ, et al. Relationships between body mass indices and surgical replacements of knee and hip joints. *Am J Prev Med* 2003; 25(4):290–5.
16. Fernandes L, Hagen KB, Bijlsma JW, et al. EULAR recommendations for the non-pharmacological core management of hip and knee osteoarthritis. *Ann Rheum Dis* 2013; 72(7):1125–35.
17. Hochberg MC, Altman RD, April KT, et al. American College of Rheumatology 2012 recommendations for the use of

nonpharmacologic and pharmacologic therapies in osteoarthritis of the hand, hip, and knee. *Arthritis Care Res (Hoboken)* 2012; 64(4):465–74.

18. McAlindon TE, Bannuru RR, Sullivan MC, et al. OARSI guidelines for the non-surgical management of knee osteoarthritis. *Osteoarthritis Cartilage* 2014; 22(3):363–88.

19. Waalen J. The genetics of human obesity. *Transl Res* 2014; 164(4):293–301.

20. Doherty M, Watt I, Dieppe P. Influence of primary generalised osteoarthritis on development of secondary osteoarthritis. *Lancet* 19832; 2(8340):8–11.

21. Yerges-Armstrong LM, Yau MS, Liu Y, et al. Association analysis of BMD-associated SNPs with knee osteoarthritis. *J Bone Miner Res* 2014; 29(6):1373–9.

22. Lim YZ, Wang Y, Wluka AE, et al. Association of obesity and systemic factors with bone marrow lesions at the knee: a systematic review. *Semin Arthritis Rheum* 2014; 43(5):600–12.

23. Andriacchi TP, Mündermann A. The role of ambulatory mechanics in the initiation and progression of knee osteoarthritis. *Curr Opin Rheumatol* 2006; 18(5):514–8.

24. Andriacchi TP. Dynamics of knee malalignment. *Orthop Clin North Am* 1994; 25(3):395–403.

25. Bucknor MD, Nardo L, Joseph GB, et al. Association of cartilage degeneration with four year weight gain—3T MRI data from the Osteoarthritis Initiative. *Osteoarthritis Cartilage* 2015; 23(4):525–31.

26. Henriksen M, Hunter DJ, Dam EB, et al. Is increased joint loading detrimental to obese patients with knee osteoarthritis? A secondary data analysis from a randomized trial. *Osteoarthritis Cartilage* 2013; 21(12):1865–75.

27. Henriksen M, Creaby MW, Lund H, Juhl C, Christensen R. Is there a causal link between knee loading and knee osteoarthritis progression? A systematic review and meta-analysis of cohort studies and randomised trials. *BMJ Open* 2014; 4(7):e005368.

28. Yusuf E, Nelissen RG, Ioan-Facsinay A, et al. Association between weight or body mass index and hand osteoarthritis: a systematic review. *Ann Rheum Dis* 2010; 69(4):761–5.

29. Carman WJ, Sowers M, Hawthorne VM, Weissfeld LA. Obesity as a risk factor for osteoarthritis of the hand and wrist: a prospective study. *Am J Epidemiol* 1994; 139(2):119–29.

30. Bliddal H, Leeds AR, Christensen R. Osteoarthritis, obesity and weight loss: evidence, hypotheses and horizons—a scoping review. *Obes Rev* 2014; 15(7):578–86.

31. Conde J, Scotece M, Gomez R, Lopez V, Gomez-Reino JJ, Gualillo O. Adipokines and osteoarthritis: novel molecules involved in the pathogenesis and progression of disease. *Arthritis* 2011; 2011:203901.

32. Fowler-Brown A, Kim DH, Shi L, et al. The mediating effect of leptin on the relationship between body weight and knee osteoarthritis in older adults. *Arthritis Rheumatol* 2015; 67(1):169–75.

33. Klein-Wieringa IR, Kloppenburg M, Bastiaansen-Jenniskens YM, et al. The infrapatellar fat pad of patients with osteoarthritis has an inflammatory phenotype. *Ann Rheum Dis* 2011; 70(5):851–7.

34. Ballegaard C, Riis RG, Bliddal H, et al. Knee pain and inflammation in the infrapatellar fat pad estimated by conventional and dynamic contrast-enhanced magnetic resonance imaging in obese patients with osteoarthritis: a cross-sectional study. *Osteoarthritis Cartilage* 2014; 22(7):933–40.

35. Vincent H, Heywood K, Connelly J, Hurley R. Obesity and weight loss in the treatment and prevention of osteoarthritis. *PMR* 2012; 4:S59–67.

36. Sanchez C, Gabay O, Salvat C, Henrotin YE, Berenbaum F. Mechanical loading highly increases IL-6 production and decreases OPG expression by osteoblasts. *Osteoarthritis Cartilage* 2009; 17(4):473–81.

37. Takao M, Okinaga T, Ariyoshi W, et al. Role of heme oxygenase-1 in inflammatory response induced by mechanical stretch in synovial cells. *Inflamm Res* 2011; 60(9):861–7.

38. Wang Y, Tang Z, Xue R, et al. Combined effects of TNF-alpha, IL-1beta, and HIF-1alpha on MMP-2 production in ACL fibroblasts under mechanical stretch: an in vitro study. *J Orthop Res* 2011; 29(7):1008–14.

39. Sanchez C, Pesesse L, Gabay O, et al. Regulation of subchondral bone osteoblast metabolism by cyclic compression. *Arthritis Rheum* 2012; 64(4):1193–203.

40. Livshits G, Zhai G, Hart DJ, et al. Interleukin-6 is a significant predictor of radiographic knee osteoarthritis: the Chingford Study. *Arthritis Rheum* 2009; 60(7):2037–45.

41. Sharif M, Shepstone L, Elson CJ, Dieppe PA, Kirwan JR. Increased serum C reactive protein may reflect events that precede radiographic progression in osteoarthritis of the knee. *Ann Rheum Dis* 2000; 59(1):71–4.

42. Spector TD, Hart DJ, Nandra D, et al. Low-level increases in serum C-reactive protein are present in early osteoarthritis of the knee and predict progressive disease. *Arthritis Rheum* 1997; 40(4):723–7.

43. Messier SP, Mihalko SL, Legault C, et al. Effects of intensive diet and exercise on knee joint loads, inflammation, and clinical outcomes among overweight and obese adults with knee osteoarthritis: the IDEA randomized clinical trial. *JAMA* 2013; 310(12):1263–73.

44. Yang WH, Liu SC, Tsai CH, et al. Leptin induces IL-6 expression through OBRl receptor signaling pathway in human synovial fibroblasts. *PLoS One* 2013; 8(9):e75551.

45. Silveri F, Brecciaroli D, Argentati F, Cervini C. Serum levels of insulin in overweight patients with osteoarthritis of the knee. *J Rheumatol* 1994; 21(10):1899–902.

46. Sowers M, Karvonen-Gutierrez CA, Palmieri-Smith R, et al. Knee osteoarthritis in obese women with cardiometabolic clustering. *Arthritis Rheum* 2009; 61(10):1328–36.

47. Christensen R, Henriksen M, Leeds AR, et al. The effect of weight maintenance on symptoms of knee osteoarthritis in obese patients: 12 month randomized controlled trial. *Arthritis Care Res (Hoboken)* 2015; 67(5):640–50.

48. Riecke BF, Christensen R, Christensen P, et al. Comparing two low-energy diets for the treatment of knee osteoarthritis symptoms in obese patients: a pragmatic randomized clinical trial. *Osteoarthritis Cartilage* 2010; 18(6):746–54.

49. Miller GD, Nicklas BJ, Davis C, et al. Intensive weight loss program improves physical function in older obese adults with knee osteoarthritis. *Obesity (Silver Spring)* 2006; 14(7):1219–30.

50. National Institute for Health and Clinical Excellence (NICE). *Osteoarthritis. The Care and Management of Osteoarthritis in Adults*. NICE Clinical Guideline 59. London: NICE; 2008.

51. Toda Y, Toda T, Takemura S, et al. Change in body fat, but not body weight or metabolic correlates of obesity, is related to symptomatic relief of obese patients with knee osteoarthritis after a weight control program. *J Rheumatol* 1998; 25(11):2181–6.

52. Riddle DL, Stratford PW. Body weight changes and corresponding changes in pain and function in persons with symptomatic knee osteoarthritis: a cohort study. *Arthritis Care Res (Hoboken)* 2013; 65(1):15–22.

53. Christensen R, Bartels EM, Astrup A, Bliddal H. Effect of weight reduction in obese patients diagnosed with knee osteoarthritis: a systematic review and meta-analysis. *Ann Rheum Dis* 2007; 66(4):433–9.

54. Christensen R, Astrup A, Bliddal H. Weight loss: the treatment of choice for knee osteoarthritis? A randomized trial. *Osteoarthritis Cartilage* 2005; 13(1):20–7.

55. NHLBI Obesity Education Initiative Expert Panel on the Identification, Evaluation, and Treatment of Obesity in Adults (US). *Clinical Guidelines on the Identification, Evaluation, and Treatment of Overweight and Obesity in Adults*. Bethesda, MD: National Heart, Lung, and Blood Institute; 1998.

56. Messier SP, Loeser RF, Miller GD, et al. Exercise and dietary weight loss in overweight and obese older adults with knee osteoarthritis: the Arthritis, Diet, and Activity Promotion Trial. *Arthritis Rheum* 2004; 50(5):1501–10.

57. Rejeski WJ, Focht BC, Messier SP, et al. Obese, older adults with knee osteoarthritis: weight loss, exercise, and quality of life. *Health Psychol* 2002; 21(5):419–26.

58. Gudbergsen H, Boesen M, Christensen R, et al. Changes in bone marrow lesions in response to weight-loss in obese knee osteoarthritis patients: a prospective cohort study. *BMC Musculoskelet Disord* 2013; 14:106.

59. Messier SP, Loeser RF, Mitchell MN, et al. Exercise and weight loss in obese older adults with knee osteoarthritis: a preliminary study. *J Am Geriatr Soc* 2000; 48(9):1062–72.

60. Henriksen M, Christensen R, Danneskiold-Samsoe B, Bliddal H. Changes in lower extremity muscle mass and muscle strength after weight loss in obese patients with knee osteoarthritis: a prospective cohort study. *Arthritis Rheum* 2012; 64(2):438–42.

61. Aaboe J, Bliddal H, Messier SP, Alkjaer T, Henriksen M. Effects of an intensive weight loss program on knee joint loading in obese adults with knee osteoarthritis. *Osteoarthritis Cartilage* 2011; 19(7):822–8.

62. Messier SP, Gutekunst DJ, Davis C, DeVita P. Weight loss reduces knee-joint loads in overweight and obese older adults with knee osteoarthritis. *Arthritis Rheum* 2005; 52(7):2026–32.

63. Henriksen M, Simonsen EB, Alkjaer T, et al. Increased joint loads during walking—a consequence of pain relief in knee osteoarthritis. *Knee* 2006; 13:445–50.

64. Hurwitz DE, Ryals AR, Block JA, et al. Knee pain and joint loading in subjects with osteoarthritis of the knee. *J Orthop Res* 2000; 18(4):572–9.

65. Schnitzer TJ, Popovich JM, Andersson GB, Andriacchi TP. Effect of piroxicam on gait in patients with osteoarthritis of the knee. *Arthritis Rheum* 1993; 36(9):1207–13.

66. Shrader MW, Draganich LF, Pottenger LA, Piotrowski GA. Effects of knee pain relief in osteoarthritis on gait and stair-stepping. *Clin Orthop* 2004; 421:188–93.

67. Hurwitz DE, Sumner DR, Andriacchi TP, Sugar DA. Dynamic knee loads during gait predict proximal tibial bone distribution. *J Biomech* 1998; 31(5):423–30.

68. Thorp LE, Wimmer MA, Block JA, et al. Bone mineral density in the proximal tibia varies as a function of static alignment and knee adduction angular momentum in individuals with medial knee osteoarthritis. *Bone* 2006; 39(5):1116–22.

69. Lo GH, Hunter DJ, Zhang Y, et al. Bone marrow lesions in the knee are associated with increased local bone density. *Arthritis Rheum* 2005; 52(9):2814–21.

70. Felson DT, Zhang Y, Anthony JM, Naimark A, Anderson JJ. Weight loss reduces the risk for symptomatic knee osteoarthritis in women. The Framingham Study. *Ann Intern Med* 1992; 116(7):535–9.

71. Anandacoomarasamy A, Leibman S, Smith G, et al. Weight loss in obese people has structure-modifying effects on medial but not on lateral knee articular cartilage. *Ann Rheum Dis* 2012; 71(1):26–32.

72. Hunter DJ, Beavers DP, Eckstein F, et al. The Intensive Diet and Exercise for Arthritis (IDEA) trial: 18-month radiographic and MRI outcomes. *Osteoarthritis Cartilage* 2015; 23(7):1090–8.

73. Elfhag K, Rössner S. Who succeeds in maintaining weight loss? A conceptual review of factors associated with weight loss maintenance and weight regain. *Obes Rev* 2005; 6(1):67–85.

74. Segal NA, Toda Y. Absolute reduction in lower limb lean body mass in Japanese women with knee osteoarthritis. *J Clin Rheumatol* 2005; 11(5):245–9.

75. Christensen P, Bartels EM, Riecke BF, et al. Improved nutritional status and bone health after diet-induced weight loss in sedentary osteoarthritis patients: a prospective cohort study. *Eur J Clin Nutr* 2012; 66(4):504–9.

76. Edwards C, Rogers A, Lynch S, et al. The effects of bariatric surgery weight loss on knee pain in patients with osteoarthritis of the knee. *Arthritis* 2012; 2012:504189.

77. Bliddal H, Leeds AR, Stigsgaard L, Astrup A, Christensen R. Weight loss as treatment for knee osteoarthritis symptoms in obese patients: 1-year results from a randomised controlled trial. *Ann Rheum Dis* 2011; 70(10):1798–803.

78. Simons-Morton DG, Obarzanek E, Cutler JA. Obesity research—limitations of methods, measurements, and medications. *JAMA* 2006; 295(7):826–8.

79. Christensen R, Kristensen PK, Bartels EM, Bliddal H, Astrup A. Efficacy and safety of the weight-loss drug rimonabant: a meta-analysis of randomised trials. *Lancet* 2007; 370(9600):1706–13.

80. Yanovski SZ, Yanovski JA. Long-term drug treatment for obesity: a systematic and clinical review. *JAMA* 2014; 311(1):74–86.

81. Puzziferri N, Roshek TB, III, Mayo HG, et al. Long-term follow-up after bariatric surgery: a systematic review. *JAMA* 2014; 312(9):934–42.

82. Schoeller DA, Shay K, Kushner RF. How much physical activity is needed to minimize weight gain in previously obese women? *Am J Clin Nutr* 1997; 66(3):551–6.

83. Wing RR, Bolin P, Brancati FL, et al. Cardiovascular effects of intensive lifestyle intervention in type 2 diabetes. *N Engl J Med* 2013; 369(2):145–54.

84. Sarlio-Lahteenkorva S, Rissanen A, Kaprio J. A descriptive study of weight loss maintenance: 6 and 15 year follow-up of initially overweight adults. *Int J Obes Relat Metab Disord* 2000; 24(1):116–25.

85. Dombrowski SU, Knittle K, Avenell A, Araujo-Soares V, Sniehotta FF. Long term maintenance of weight loss with non-surgical interventions in obese adults: systematic review and meta-analyses of randomised controlled trials. *BMJ* 2014; 348:g2646.

86. MacLean PS, Wing RR, Davidson T, et al. NIH working group report: Innovative research to improve maintenance of weight loss. *Obesity (Silver Spring)* 2015; 23(1):7–15.

87. Thomas JG, Bond DS, Phelan S, Hill JO, Wing RR. Weight-loss maintenance for 10 years in the National Weight Control Registry. *Am J Prev Med* 2014; 46(1):17–23.

CHAPTER 24

Addressing adverse mechanical factors

Christelle Nguyen and François Rannou

Introduction

Optimal treatment of osteoarthritis (OA) requires a combination of non-pharmacological and pharmacological strategies individualized to the patient's requirements. Non-pharmacological approaches include biomechanical interventions such as braces, orthoses, insoles, joint protection, joint-preserving surgical procedures, walking sticks, and other aids. Weight loss, specific and non-specific exercises, patient education, and self-care programmes are discussed in other chapters. Whereas pharmacological treatments are usually the same whatever the anatomical OA location, the non-pharmacological approach must be adjusted to the individual patient and to the biomechanical specificities of each affected joint [1].

Braces, orthoses, and insoles are prescribed to modulate mechanical stress on the symptomatic joint compartment. Besides this mechanical effect, they have effects on muscle contraction and proprioception [2,3]. Braces and orthoses are external devices used for knee and hand OA. For knee OA, orthoses are rest orthoses, knee sleeves, unloader knee braces, patella tape, and patellofemoral braces. There are no orthoses that have demonstrated efficacy in hip OA. Foot pronation and cushioning insoles are commonly prescribed for lower-limb OA. Information on the use of orthoses and insoles is elaborated by the physiotherapist, occupational therapist, podiatrist, prosthetist, and orthotist, depending on the use and professional legislation in each country. The aim and the way to use non-pharmacological treatments must be clearly explained to patients in order to improve their adherence to the treatment. Patient education involves various forms of vehicles for delivery and information.

Recommendations for the management of OA are numerous. They are mainly based on literature analyses to calculate the effect size of a treatment strategy, along with expert opinion. The most important information for the physician in daily practice is that effect sizes of non-pharmacological interventions are in the same range (0–1) as those of pharmacological interventions, which suggest the importance of the use of non-pharmacological approaches in treating OA. In addition, the absence of side effects of non-pharmacological interventions is a major point regarding their use in primary care practice. The main international recommendations are from the Osteoarthritis Research Society International (OARSI) [4,5], the European League Against Rheumatism (EULAR) [6,7], and the American College of Rheumatology (ACR) [8]. Besides

these international guidelines, national recommendations are usually adjusted to the domestic healthcare system.

Here, we use an evidence-based approach, including the most recent OARSI, EULAR, and ACR recommendations, to describe and review non-pharmacological strategies available in daily clinical practice, designed to modulate joint mechanical load, with a focus on the management of hand, hip, and knee OA.

Biomechanical interventions for the treatment of hand osteoarthritis

Hand OA must be divided into two distinct clinical and biomechanical entities, namely interphalangeal joint OA, and thumb base OA. These two hand OA subtypes have very different pathophysiological processes. Whereas finger OA pathogenesis involves mainly hormonal and metabolic factors [9], thumb base OA pathogenesis mainly involves local adverse mechanical factors [10].

International clinical recommendations for the management of hand OA have been developed by EULAR in 2007 [7], and ACR in 2012 [8]. However, as pointed out in Mahendira and Towheed's 2009 systematic review of non-surgical therapies for osteoarthritis of the hand, hand OA is a more heterogeneous disease than hip or knee OA, and high-quality randomized controlled trials (RCTs) are lacking in this condition [11]. Therefore, EULAR [7] and ACR [8] international recommendations are based solely on expert opinion, and do not result from an analysis of RCTs. At the time of EULAR recommendations no effect sizes were available to assess these biomechanical interventions.

Orthoses

EULAR recommendation #5 for orthoses is as follows: 'Splints for thumb base OA and orthoses to prevent/correct lateral angulation and flexion deformity are recommended' [7]. Consistently, ACR recommends providing splints for patients with trapeziometacarpal joint OA [8]. At the time of development of EULAR recommendations, no results from RCTs were available. Only two small head-to-head RCTs compared the treatment effects of a full splint versus a half splint. The results showed more pain relief from the full splint than from the half splint (effect size = 0.64, 95% confidence interval (CI) 0.02–1.26). In 2009, our group showed a significant reduction in pain and disability at 12 months, in a high-quality RCT assessing the efficacy of biomechanical intervention consisting of a rest splint in thumb base OA [10]. Our study confirmed the

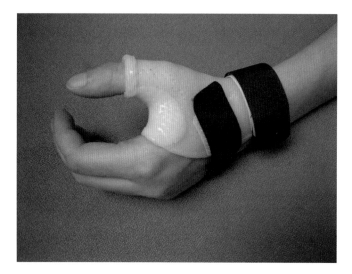

Figure 24.1 Opponens splint for base-of-thumb osteoarthritis (palmar view).

expert opinion and supported the use of rest splints for thumb base OA to reduce pain and to maintain hand function (Figure 24.1). In addition, the treatment was well tolerated. At 12 months, 86% of the patients in the intervention group, who wore the rest splint for more than 5 nights a week, did not show any adverse effects [10]. Lastly, even if in this RCT the health economic aspects were not addressed, the price of a rest splint seems to be largely cost-effective in a primary care setting.

For interphalangeal joint OA, stacked or static finger splints could be used to immobilize and correct distal and/or proximal finger joints (Figure 24.2). These splints can be used as a rest orthosis or just after a joint injection to immobilize the injected joint for a few days. Recently, night-time short-term splinting of distal interphalangeal OA joint has been shown to reduce pain at 6 months and improve digit extension at 3 months, in a small non-blinded controlled trial of 36 patients [12].

Overall, orthoses for hand OA are safe and effective biomechanical interventions, and there is some evidence of their efficacy in reducing pain and disability. However, to date, no study has assessed the efficacy of splinting in decreasing structural damage in hand OA.

Joint protection

EULAR recommendation #3 for joint protection is as follows: 'Education concerning joint protection (how to avoid adverse mechanical factors) together with an exercise regimen (involving both range of motion and strengthening exercises) are recommended for all patients with hand OA' [7], and ACR recommends instruction in joint protection techniques for the management of hand OA [8]. In a 3-month RCT, in combination with home exercises, joint protection has been shown to improve grip strength and global hand function [13]. However, joint protection advice delivered by the physician and the occupational and physical therapists is usually given as part of a broader multidisciplinary education intervention and whether any benefit is directly attributable to avoidance of adverse mechanical factors remains unproved.

Surgery

EULAR recommendation #3 for surgery is as follows: 'The potential benefits of surgery compared with conservative management, and the most appropriate surgical procedure for thumb base OA, remain to be determined'. Non-replacement surgery modalities can be considered as biomechanical interventions in that they will modify adverse mechanical factors affecting OA joints. Various surgical procedures have been assessed in the treatment for patients with severe thumb base OA refractory to conventional treatment, such as arthrodesis, trapeziectomy, or osteotomy [7]. Surgery can reduce pain and improve function. More adverse events were observed when two surgical procedures were combined and trapeziectomy seemed to be the procedure with fewer complications [14].

Biomechanical interventions for the treatment of hip osteoarthritis

As for other OA locations, the optimal management of hip OA requires a combination of non-pharmacological and pharmacological treatment modalities [15]. If non-pharmacological modalities for treatment of knee OA are widely described in the international literature, fewer studies are specifically devoted to hip OA. For this reason, EULAR [6, 15], OARSI [5], and ACR [8] international recommendations are more based on expert opinion than on literature analyses with effect size calculations. The other main difference with knee OA is the absence of possibilities for bracing.

Insoles and footwear

The aim of insoles in the treatment of hip OA is to decrease the load applied on the hip. No RCTs have investigated insoles in hip OA. The 2005 EULAR recommendations describe insoles for patients with hip OA solely on the basis of expert opinion [15]. The 2013 EULAR recommendations include the use of appropriate footwear

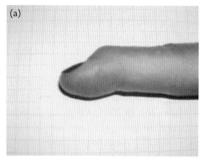
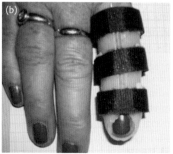
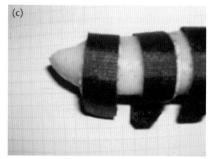

Figure 24.2 Distal interphalangeal OA (a). Finger splint, dorsal view (b) and lateral view (c).

in patients with hip OA, even though there is no evidence to support the effect of specific shoes or insoles on pain or function [6].

In contrast, no OARSI recommendation describes insoles for hip OA but OARSI does point out the importance of delivering advice concerning appropriate footwear for hip OA [5]. This last recommendation is based solely on expert opinion. Insoles and footwear are not included in ACR non-pharmacological recommendations for the management of hip OA [8]. The type of insole and precise footwear are not described in international recommendations. These recommendations can only be based on clinical experience. Specific RCTs are required to address the efficacy of cushioning insoles and footwear with shock absorbance for pain and disability reduction for hip OA.

Walking sticks and other walking aids

There is no research evidence for appliances such as a stick or walking aids for hip OA. They are assumed to help to reduce the adverse forces across the joint [15]. They are included in the 2005 EULAR recommendation #3 as follows 'Non-pharmacological treatment of hip OA should include regular education, exercise, appliances (stick, insoles) and weight reduction if obese or overweight' [15], and in 2013 #10 as follows 'Walking aids, assistive technology and adaptations at home and/or at work should be considered, to reduce pain and increase participation, for example: a walking stick used on the contralateral side, walking frames and wheeled walkers' [6]. ACR conditionally recommends that patients with hip OA should use walking aids, as needed [8].

Joint preserving surgery

2005 EULAR recommendation #9 for surgery is as follows: 'osteotomy and joint preserving surgical procedures should be considered in young adults with symptomatic hip OA, especially in the presence of dysplasia or varus/valgus deformity' [15]. This kind of surgical procedures should be considered as a biomechanical intervention as osteotomies of the pelvis and/or femoral osteotomies can alter force transmission through the hip joint and thus potentially influence clinical symptoms and the course of the OA process. Symptomatic and structural effects have been evaluated in retrospective and prospective cohort studies, showing significant improvement in clinical outcomes including pain, walking ability, and overall functional scores [15]. Data from observational studies also support more recently advocated joint-preserving surgical procedures such as arthroscopic debridement and surgical dislocation of the hip with offset reconstruction [15]. Altogether, joint-preserving surgery appears to be a useful procedure for younger patients with painful hip dysplasia or deformity. However, its effectiveness and cost effectiveness in patients with advanced age and/or OA stages have yet to be established [15].

Biomechanical interventions for the treatment of knee OA

Knee OA is the OA location for which the efficacy on pain and function of biomechanical interventions have been the most extensively assessed in RCTs. International recommendations have been published by OARSI [4,5], EULAR [6,16], and ACR [8]. The most recent guidelines were published by OARSI in 2014 [4].

Orthosis

For knee OA, orthosis consists of rest orthoses, knee sleeves, unloader knee brace, and patella tape and patellofemoral braces. Rest orthoses are used for joint immobilisation, which excludes any dynamic effect. Rest orthoses are created by a stiff composite, by casting or a line. The effectiveness of rest orthoses for lower-limb OA has not been studied in clinical trials. To date, they cannot be recommended [17]. Knee sleeves are elastic non-adhesive orthoses associated with various devices aimed at patellar alignment or frontal femorotibial stabilization. Unloader knee braces are, like knee sleeves, functional devices. They are composed of external stems, hinges and straps. Their purpose is to decrease compressive loads transmitted to the joint surfaces, either in the medial or lateral femorotibial compartment, depending on the *valgus* or *varus* position of the device (Figure 24.3).

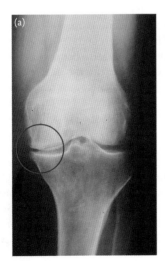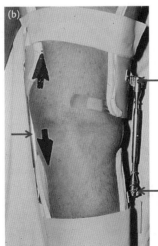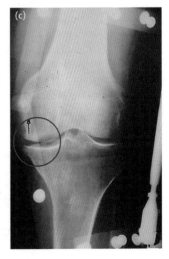

Figure 24.3 Schematic diagram illustrating how a valgus unloading knee brace theoretically counteracts the external adduction moment acting about the knee during walking. (a) X-ray of unbraced right knee with medial femorotibial OA (red circle). (b) The unloading brace applies points of force at three locations (arrows), which create two moment arms, and result in a valgus moment of the knee. (c) X-ray of braced right knee showing unloading of the medial femorotibial compartment (red circle).

The 2003 EULAR recommendation #3 is devoted to the non-pharmacological approach in the treatment of knee OA [16]. Orthotic devices are recommended but mainly on the basis of expert opinion. Only one RCT, comparing one group with knee sleeve, one group with a *valgus* brace and a control group without a knee sleeve or brace, was described [18]. This study showed a significant improvement in pain and function for the two intervention groups. In addition, *valgus* brace treatment is more effective than simple knee sleeve. Effect size could be calculated, but the strength of the recommendation was moderate (B), which points out the importance of expert opinion in this recommendation. Cochrane reviews and 2008 OARSI recommendations include one more study, but the device used was an unloader knee brace, not a knee sleeve [5,19,20]. The 2008 OARSI recommends a knee brace for patients with knee OA and mild or moderate *varus* or *valgus* instability so as to reduce pain, improve stability and diminish the risk of falling [5]. As part of available biomechanical interventions for knee OA, knee braces and sleeves are also recommended in the 2014 OARSI guidelines [4]. They are mainly based on Raja and colleagues systematic review suggesting that knee braces are effective in decreasing pain, joint stiffness, and drug dosage and in improving physical function, with insignificant adverse events [21]. Biomechanical effects of valgus knee brace were assessed by Moyer and colleagues in a meta-analysis of 17 studies. The authors found that knee braces could influence knee joint biomechanics though different mechanisms. The most frequently reported mechanism is that valgus knee brace directly opposes knee abduction moment during walking with a statistically significant decrease in the external knee adduction and a moderate to high effect size (standardized mean differences [SMD] = 0.61; 95% CI 0.39, 0.83; p < 0.001). Optimal dosage was unclear, and studies were heterogeneous in design, disease severity of patients, brace type and data collection and analysis procedures [22]. In another meta-analysis from the same group, clinical benefit of valgus knee brace was assessed in a meta-analysis of six RCTs [23]. When compared to a control group that did not use an orthosis, a significant difference favouring the valgus bracing group for improvement in pain and in function was found, with a moderate effect size for pain (SMD = 0.56; 95% CI, 0.03–1.09, p = 0.04) and function (SMD = 0.48; 95% CI, 0.02–0.95, p = 0.04) [23]. Regarding unloader knee braces, Beaudreuil and colleagues reviewed 16 studies [17]. Unfortunately, these studies were of poor quality, and the recommendation for using an unloader knee brace was again based on the Kirkley study [17,18]. Finally, Beaudreuil and colleagues pointed out the potential adverse effects of unloader knee braces, such as venous thromboembolic events [17]. This last point has to be considered in daily medical practice.

Patellar taping or patellofemoral bracing are not included in the most recent ACR, EULAR or OARSI recommendations for the non-pharmacological management of knee OA [4,6,8]. However patellofemoral joint OA should be considered as a distinct clinical entity that requires specific and targeted biomechanical interventions to alleviate joint stress [24]. Data regarding medially directed patellar taping on pain reduction are conflicting as one review reported no benefit [25], one reported conflicting evidence [26], and one reported positive effects [27]. Callaghan and Selfe included five small heterogeneous RCTs in their meta-analysis and found no significant difference between taping and non-taping in pain at the end of the treatment programmes with time points ranging from 1 week to 3 months and various taping methods (i.e. tailored

and untailored) [25]. Swart and colleagues included 8 studies in their analysis with a similar definition for short term (4–12 weeks), but did not to pool data [26]. These authors concluded that there was conflicting evidence for the additive effectiveness of tape to exercise therapy on pain and function [26]. In a systematic review of 16 studies, Warden and colleagues found that tape applied to exert a medially-directed force on the patella significantly decreased chronic knee pain compared with no tape or sham tape [27]. The effectiveness of patellar bracing is reported to be inconsistent [27], although data suggest that bracing can be effective at providing immediate pain reduction [28].

RCTs are needed to determine whether bracing can be effective to decrease structural damage in knee OA. In addition, instability, misalignment, and the main symptomatic knee compartment (medial, lateral, and patellar) must be evaluated for their importance in the response to bracing treatment. Biomechanical interventions such as knee braces or orthoses are no longer included in 2013 EULAR recommendations [6].

Insoles and footwear

Insoles can be neutral, lateral-wedged or cushioning. The biomechanical concept for the use of insoles for knee OA has not yet been clearly validated and has been described only for lateral-wedged insoles. Two different biomechanical theories have been elaborated: adduction moment theory and kinetic chain theory [29]. The adduction moment theory estimates the loading on the medial knee compartment by the product of the mechanical axis force and the distance between this axis and the knee joint centre. With a lateral-wedge insole, the mechanical axis might reach a more upright position and reduce the distance between the axis and the joint centre, thus decreasing the knee medial loading. For the kinetic chain theory, a lateral-wedge insole creates a *valgus* hind foot and then a *valgus* knee joint, as well as a decrease in medial compartment load. Whatever the theory, lateral-wedge insoles could decrease the load on the knee joint and probably more on the medial compartment.

The 2003 EULAR recommendation #9 describes insoles, without specification, with a strength of recommendation of B [16]. The calculation of the effect-size was not possible. In the latest 2013 EULAR recommendations, the use of insoles in knee OA was rejected for no clinical effects and the report of adverse effects [6]. The Cochrane review described a better pain effect with a strapped insole as compared with an inserted insole but with a poor long-term adherence [19,30–33]. However, strapped insoles are not disseminated in many countries. For the latest 2014 OARSI recommendations, the authors included Raja and colleagues 2011 systematic review and 3 RCTs [21,34–36], the effect size for pain and function was not available for the same reason, but quality of evidence for the use of foot orthoses in the non-pharmacological management of knee OA was considered as fair [4].

Finally, in light of the literature and recommendations, lateral-wedge insoles could be of interest to decrease pain and non-steroidal anti-inflammatory drugs consumption in patients with medial knee OA. To date, no evidence suggests a structural or functional impact of insoles [34,37,38]. ACR also recommends to wear medially wedged insoles if the lateral compartment is affected by OA [8], but no results from a RCT exist to comment on the other sites (lateral and patellar). No RCT has evaluated footwear and a cushioning insole. OARSI recommendations point out an interest to give advice to patients about appropriate footwear [4], consistently with EULAR latest recommendations [6]. The optimal shoes could have a flat or low heel, be flexible, and have lateral wedged soles [39]. From a practical point of view : lateral-wedge insole could reduce symptoms in medial knee OA and are recommended by OARSI and ACR, but its use was rejected in the latest EULAR recommendations, a strapped insole could have a good symptomatic effect, a neutral and cushioning insole could be of interest in knee OA, whatever the compartment affected.

Walking stick

Based on the results of a recent RCT [40], OARSI and EULAR also recommends the use of a walking stick [4,6], to decrease pain, improve function and some aspects of quality of life in patients with knee OA. However, the use of a walking stick was not recommended in individuals with multiple-joint type OA, as cane use to relieve knee pain may increase weight-bearing load on other affected joints. Finally, evidence was considered as insufficient in the absence of available trials to support the use of crutches as an appropriate alternative to cane use [4].

Joint-preserving surgery

The 2008 OARSI recommendation #23 for joint-preserving surgery is as follows: 'for the young and physically active patient with significant symptoms from unicompartmental knee OA, high tibial osteotomy may offer an alternative intervention that delays the need for joint replacement some 10 years' with a IIb level of evidence (at least one well-designed quasi-experimental study) [5]. This proposition was mainly supported by a 2004 review of the literature and meta-analysis of follow-up studies of 2406 osteotomies in 19 uncontrolled cohort studies [41]. Less pain and improved walking ability or improvement on the Hospital for Special Surgery score were achieved in 75% of patients at 60 months and 60% of patients at 100 months [41]. The average time between high tibial osteotomy and arthroplasty was 6 years [41]. A more recent meta-analysis included 46 studies of high tibial valgus osteotomy and consistently showed that after a 5- to 8-year follow-up, 91.0% of the patients did not need a total replacement, and 84.4% after a 9- to 12-year follow-up. Mean survival time to total knee replacement was 9.7 years [42].

Conclusion

Non-pharmacological management OA requires a combination of general non-pharmacological treatment and specific treatment for the affected OA joint. Whatever the localization of the OA (knee, hip, or hand), aerobic, strengthening, and range-of-motion exercise; diet; and patient education should be proposed. Besides these general recommendations, and depending on OA location, specific biomechanical interventions aiming to reduce adverse biomechanical factors on the joint should be considered. For hand OA, splinting and joint protection techniques are recommended. For lower-limb OA, cushioning insoles, braces, orthoses, walking sticks, and joint-preserving surgeries are of interest to reduce pain and improve function, when prescribed properly, after an accurate physical examination. Many recommendations are based solely on expert opinion, and therefore should be adjusted to each individual patient. RCTs with appropriate methodology adapted to non-pharmacological treatments are needed.

References

1. Rannou F, Poiraudeau S. Non-pharmacological approaches for the treatment of osteoarthritis. *Best Pract Res Clin Rheumatol* 2010; 24(1):93–106.
2. Birmingham TB, Kramer JF, Kirkley A, et al. Knee bracing for medial compartment osteoarthritis: effects on proprioception and postural control. *Rheumatology (Oxford)* 2001; 40(3):285–9.
3. Ramsey DK, Briem K, Axe MJ, Snyder-Mackler L. A mechanical theory for the effectiveness of bracing for medial compartment osteoarthritis of the knee. *J Bone Joint Surg Am* 2007; 89(11):2398–407.
4. McAlindon TE, Bannuru RR, Sullivan MC, et al. OARSI guidelines for the non-surgical management of knee osteoarthritis. *Osteoarthritis Cartilage* 2014; 22(3):363–88.
5. Zhang W, Moskowitz RW, Nuki G, et al. OARSI recommendations for the management of hip and knee osteoarthritis, Part II: OARSI evidence-based, expert consensus guidelines. *Osteoarthritis Cartilage* 2008; 16(2):137–62.
6. Fernandes L, Hagen KB, Bijlsma JW, et al. EULAR recommendations for the non-pharmacological core management of hip and knee osteoarthritis. *Ann Rheum Dis* 2013; 72(7):1125–35.
7. Zhang W, Doherty M, Leeb BF, et al. EULAR evidence based recommendations for the management of hand osteoarthritis: report of a Task Force of the EULAR Standing Committee for International Clinical Studies Including Therapeutics (ESCISIT). *Ann Rheum Dis* 2007; 66(3):377–88.
8. Hochberg MC, Altman RD, April KT, et al. American College of Rheumatology 2012 recommendations for the use of nonpharmacologic and pharmacologic therapies in osteoarthritis of the hand, hip, and knee. *Arthritis Care Res (Hoboken)* 2012; 64(4):465–74.
9. Berenbaum F, Eymard F, Houard X. Osteoarthritis, inflammation and obesity. *Curr Opin Rheumatol* 2013; 25(1):114–8.
10. Rannou F, Dimet J, Boutron I, et al. Splint for base-of-thumb osteoarthritis: a randomized trial. *Ann Intern Med* 2009; 150(10):661–9.
11. Mahendira D, Towheed TE. Systematic review of non-surgical therapies for osteoarthritis of the hand: an update. *Osteoarthritis Cartilage* 2009; 17(10):1263–8.
12. Watt FE, Kennedy DL, Carlisle KE, et al. Night-time immobilization of the distal interphalangeal joint reduces pain and extension deformity in hand osteoarthritis. *Rheumatology (Oxford)* 2014; 53(6):1142–9.
13. Stamm TA, Machold KP, Smolen JS, et al. Joint protection and home hand exercises improve hand function in patients with hand osteoarthritis: a randomized controlled trial. *Arthritis Rheum* 2002; 47(1):44–9.
14. Wajon A, Vinycomb T, Carr E, Edmunds I, Ada L. Surgery for thumb (trapeziometacarpal joint) osteoarthritis. *Cochrane Database Syst Rev* 2009; 4:CD004631.
15. Zhang W, Doherty M, Arden N, et al. EULAR evidence based recommendations for the management of hip osteoarthritis: report of a task force of the EULAR Standing Committee for International Clinical Studies Including Therapeutics (ESCISIT). *Ann Rheum Dis* 2005; 64(5):669–81.
16. Jordan KM, Arden NK, Doherty M, et al. EULAR Recommendations 2003: an evidence based approach to the management of knee osteoarthritis: Report of a Task Force of the Standing Committee for International Clinical Studies Including Therapeutic Trials (ESCISIT). *Ann Rheum Dis* 2003; 62(12):1145–55.
17. Beaudreuil J, Bendaya S, Faucher M, et al. Clinical practice guidelines for rest orthosis, knee sleeves, and unloading knee braces in knee osteoarthritis. *Joint Bone Spine* 2009; 76(6):629–36.
18. Kirkley A, Webster-Bogaert S, Litchfield R, et al. The effect of bracing on varus gonarthrosis. *J Bone Joint Surg Am* 1999; 81(4):539–48.
19. Brouwer RW, Jakma TS, Verhagen AP, Verhaar JA, Bierma-Zeinstra SM. Braces and orthoses for treating osteoarthritis of the knee. *Cochrane Database Syst Rev* 2005; 1:CD004020.
20. Brouwer RW, van Raaij TM, Verhaar JA, Coene LN, Bierma-Zeinstra SM. Brace treatment for osteoarthritis of the knee: a prospective

randomized multi-centre trial. *Osteoarthritis Cartilage* 2006; 14(8):777–83.

21. Raja K, Dewan N. Efficacy of knee braces and foot orthoses in conservative management of knee osteoarthritis: a systematic review. *Am J Phys Med Rehabil* 2011; 90(3):247–62.

22. Moyer RF, Birmingham TB, Bryant DM, et al. Biomechanical effects of valgus knee bracing: a systematic review and meta-analysis. *Osteoarthritis Cartilage* 2015; 23(2):178–88.

23. Moyer RF, Birmingham TB, Bryant DM, et al. Valgus bracing for knee osteoarthritis: a meta-analysis of randomized trials. *Arthritis Care Res (Hoboken)* 2015; 67(4):493–501.

24. Hinman RS, Crossley KM. Patellofemoral joint osteoarthritis: an important subgroup of knee osteoarthritis. *Rheumatology (Oxford)* 2007; 46(7):1057–62.

25. Callaghan MJ, Selfe J. Patellar taping for patellofemoral pain syndrome in adults. *Cochrane Database Syst Rev* 2012; 4:CD006717.

26. Swart NM, van Linschoten R, Bierma-Zeinstra SM, van Middelkoop M. The additional effect of orthotic devices on exercise therapy for patients with patellofemoral pain syndrome: a systematic review. *Br J Sports Med* 2012; 46(8):570–7.

27. Warden SJ, Hinman RS, Watson MAJr, et al. Patellar taping and bracing for the treatment of chronic knee pain: a systematic review and meta-analysis. *Arthritis Rheum* 2008; 59(1):73–83.

28. Barton CJ, Lack S, Hemmings S, Tufail S, Morrissey D. The 'Best Practice Guide to Conservative Management of Patellofemoral Pain': incorporating level 1 evidence with expert clinical reasoning. *Br J Sports Med* 2015; 49(14):923–34.

29. Gélis A, Coudeyre E, Hudry C, et al. Is there an evidence-based efficacy for the use of foot orthotics in knee and hip osteoarthritis? Elaboration of French clinical practice guidelines. *Joint Bone Spine* 2008; 75(6):714–20.

30. Toda Y, Segal N. Usefulness of an insole with subtalar strapping for analgesia in patients with medial compartment osteoarthritis of the knee. *Arthritis Rheum* 2002; 47(5):468–73.

31. Toda Y, Segal N, Kato A, Yamamoto S, Irie M. Effect of a novel insole on the subtalar joint of patients with medial compartment osteoarthritis of the knee. *J Rheumatol* 2001; 28(12):2705–10.

32. Toda Y, Tsukimura N. A six-month followup of a randomized trial comparing the efficacy of a lateral-wedge insole with subtalar strapping and an in-shoe lateral-wedge insole in patients with varus deformity osteoarthritis of the knee. *Arthritis Rheum* 2004; 50(10):3129–36.

33. Toda Y, Tsukimura N. A 2-year follow-up of a study to compare the efficacy of lateral wedged insoles with subtalar strapping and in-shoe lateral wedged insoles in patients with varus deformity osteoarthritis of the knee. *Osteoarthritis Cartilage* 2006; 14(3):231–7.

34. Bennell KL, Bowles KA, Payne C, et al. Lateral wedge insoles for medial knee osteoarthritis: 12 month randomised controlled trial. *BMJ* 2011; 342:d2912.

35. Erhart JC, Mündermann A, Elspas B, Giori NJ, Andriacchi TP. Changes in knee adduction moment, pain, and functionality with a variable-stiffness walking shoe after 6 months. *J Orthop Res* 2010; 28(7):873–9.

36. van Raaij TM, Reijman M, Brouwer RW, Bierma-Zeinstra SM, Verhaar JA. Medial knee osteoarthritis treated by insoles or braces: a randomized trial. *Clin Orthop Relat* Res 2010; 468(7):1926–32.

37. Maillefert JF, Hudry C, Baron G, et al. Laterally elevated wedged insoles in the treatment of medial knee osteoarthritis: a prospective randomized controlled study. *Osteoarthritis Cartilage* 2001; 9(8):738–45.

38. Pham T, Maillefert JF, Hudry C, et al. Laterally elevated wedged insoles in the treatment of medial knee osteoarthritis. A two-year prospective randomized controlled study. *Osteoarthritis Cartilage* 2004; 12(1):46–55.

39. Hinman RS, Bennell KL Advances in insoles and shoes for knee osteoarthritis. *Curr Opin Rheumatol* 2009; 21(2):164–70.

40. Jones A, Silva PG, Silva AC, et al. Impact of cane use on pain, function, general health and energy expenditure during gait in patients with knee osteoarthritis: a randomised controlled trial. *Ann Rheum Dis* 2012; 71(2):172–9.

41. Virolainen P, Aro HT. High tibial osteotomy for the treatment of osteoarthritis of the knee: a review of the literature and a meta-analysis of follow-up studies. *Arch Orthop Trauma Surg* 2004; 124(4):258–61.

42. Spahn G, Hofmann GO, von Engelhardt LV, et al. The impact of a high tibial valgus osteotomy and unicondylar medial arthroplasty on the treatment for knee osteoarthritis: a meta-analysis. *Knee Surg Sports Traumatol Arthrosc* 2013; 21(1):96–112.

CHAPTER 25

Psychological strategies in osteoarthritis of the knee or hip

Joost Dekker, Daniel Bossen, Jasmijn Holla,
Mariëtte de Rooij, Cindy Veenhof,
and Marike van der Leeden

Introduction

Characteristic clinical presentations of osteoarthritis (OA) include pain, activity limitations (e.g. problems in walking, stair climbing, and rising up), and restrictions in participation (e.g. loss of work opportunities). These presentations are dependent in part on psychological processes, including psychological distress, and specific personal and environmental factors. This is illustrated in Figure 25.1, which is derived from the International Classification of Functioning, Disability and Health (ICF) [1]. Psychological distress in OA comprises depression and anxiety, as well as fatigue. Personal factors include maladaptive cognitions (e.g. low self-efficacy), lack of physical exercise, and avoidance of activity. An environmental factor is lack of social support. Various interventions aim to regulate the OA patient's functioning. These interventions may contribute to amelioration of pain, activity limitations, and restrictions in participation (see Figure 25.1).

This chapter will first review studies on the prevalence of psychological distress, that is, depression, anxiety, and fatigue in osteoarthritis. Second, risk factors for an increase in pain and activity limitations will be reviewed. Specifically, the impact of psychological distress, personal factors, and environmental factors on pain and activity limitations will be addressed. A theoretical explanation about how psychological distress affects activity limitations (i.e. via avoidance of activity) will be provided, and evidence supporting

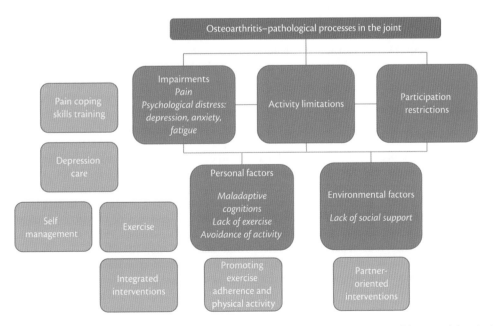

Figure 25.1 Interventions and patient functioning in osteoarthritis. Red: pathological processes in the joint. Blue: aspects of the patient's functioning. Green: interventions. Note: the interventions are located close to the impairments and factors, which the interventions are targeting.

this theory will be reviewed. Third, psychological interventions aiming to regulate the patient's functioning, as well as psychological strategies to improve exercise adherence and promote physical activity will be reviewed.

Psychological distress

Depression

Consistent evidence points to an elevated level of symptoms of depression in subjects with OA. Controlled studies have repeatedly shown higher rates of depression in subjects with OA than control subjects [2–4] (see Table 25.1). Prevalence rates in subjects with OA range from 5.0% to 28.7% (see Table 25.1). Prevalence rates seem to depend on how depression is assessed, with lower rates in studies using a psychiatric interview or a physician diagnosis of depression (range 5.0–12.4%) [2,3] than in studies using questionnaires or self-report (range 11.8–28.7%).

Anxiety

Symptoms of anxiety are more prevalent in subjects with OA than controls, as observed in several controlled studies [2,3] (see Table 25.1). Prevalence rates in subjects with OA vary from 2.9% to 6.6% (see Table 25.1). These rates are lower than for depression. It should be noted, however, that only studies using a psychiatric interview or a physician diagnosis of anxiety disorder are available.

Fatigue

The prevalence rate of fatigue is less clear, primarily because of the lack of consensus on diagnostic criteria or cut off values. In a study using a visual analogue scale (scores ranging from 0 to 10; fatigue defined as a score of 2.0 or more), the prevalence of fatigue in subjects with OA was 41% [5]. In two studies, fatigue on a continuous measure was higher in subjects with OA than controls [6,7]. In one of these studies [7], fatigue was assessed with questions from the PROMIS item bank, like 'How often do you feel tired?' and 'How often were you too tired to think clearly?' (http://www.assessmentcenter.net). Fatigue needs to be distinguished from depression, although unusual fatigue and a loss of energy are symptoms of depression. Studies in OA have shown that fatigue is to a large extent independent from symptoms of depression and anxiety [8,9].

Osteoarthritis clinical phenotype: depressive mood

OA is a heterogeneous disease. It has been hypothesized that knee OA actually consists of homogeneous subgroups or phenotypes [10]. Recently, clinical patient characteristics (i.e. upper leg muscle strength, body mass index, radiographic severity, and depressive mood) were used to identify homogeneous clinical phenotypes. Cluster analysis resulted in five clinical phenotypes, including the 'depressive mood phenotype': a distinct group of patients with knee OA with depressive mood as defining characteristic [11]. This finding has been replicated in a different sample of knee OA patients, using different measures of clinical patient characteristics [12]. Apparently, five clinical phenotypes including the 'depressive mood phenotype' is a robust finding. Patients of the 'depressive mood phenotype' may benefit from treatment for their depressive mood, alongside their OA specific management. Interventions aiming to ameliorate

depressive mood may need to target a specific subgroup of patients, that is, the 'depressive mood phenotype'.

Impact of psychological risk factors on pain and activity limitations

Psychological factors can negatively influence future pain and activity limitations. The evidence on psychological risk factors has been summarized in two systematic reviews, on knee OA [13] and on hip OA [14].

Psychological distress

The presence of depressive symptoms was found to be a consistent predictor of future pain [8,15–18] and activity limitations [8,17,19–21] in knee OA. The literature is less consistent with regard to anxiety; two studies found an association [20, 22], while one study failed to find an association [8]. Low vitality was found to be a predictor of future activity limitations in both knee and hip OA [23,24]. Thus, psychological distress has been shown to have prognostic value in OA.

Personal factors

Personal factors include exercise, physical activity, coping strategies, and self-efficacy. Aerobic exercises were found to protect against activity limitations in patients with knee OA [25]. Similar results were shown in patients with hip OA [26]. Physical activity can vary from light-intensity to high-intensity/high-impact activities. In a recent study using data from the Osteoarthritis Initiative, an association was shown between greater daily time spent in light-intensity physical activities (measured by accelerometer monitoring) and reduced risk of onset and progression of activity limitations in adults with (a risk of) knee OA [27]. In studies using questionnaires to record physical activity level, no association between physical activity and future activity limitations was found [19,23,28]; however, the validity of such questionnaires is questionable. High-impact physical activities, such as marathon running and occupational-related kneeling, may increase the risk of onset and progression of radiological progression [29], and may have a negative influence on physical functioning. Thus, exercise and physical activity seem to protect against activity limitations in knee and hip OA if executed at a light to moderate intensity.

In general, there is only weak or inconsistent evidence for coping strategies to predict future pain and activity limitations [13]. A specific pain coping strategy, however—avoidance of activity—seems to play a role in the course of activity limitations. In cross-sectional studies the relationship between avoidance of activities and activity limitations is firmly established [30]. Avoidance of activities was found to predict future activity limitations, in two longitudinal studies with 5 years of follow-up in people with early symptomatic knee OA [31] and in patients with established hip and/or knee OA [32]. Two other studies with a shorter follow-up period failed to find an association [23,33], possibly due to the short follow-up. Further information on the role of avoidance of activity is given in the next section.

Self-efficacy is defined as the conviction that one can successfully execute the behaviour required to complete a task or activity [34]. Lower self-efficacy was found to be a predictor for activity limitations in patients with knee OA [25,35]. In the absence of studies, no conclusions can be drawn on the impact of self-efficacy in hip OA.

Table 25.1 Prevalence of depression, anxiety, and fatigue in osteoarthritis

Authors, year of publication	Setting, total number of subjects	Target population	Reference population	Assessment of psychological distress	Results
Depression					
Gore et al., 2011 [2]	Database on medical and pharmacy claims, USA, n = 225 902	Subjects with a claim associated with a diagnosis of OA	Subjects without an OA-related claim	Diagnosis of depression	Prevalence of depression: 12.4% in OA, compared to 6.4% in controls
Patten et al., 2006 [3]	Canadian Community Health Survey, Canada, n = 36 984	Self-report on diagnosis by health professional of arthritis or rheumatism, excluding fibromyalgia	Self-report of no chronic condition	CIDI	Prevalence of major depression: 5.0 (95% CI: 4.3–5.7) in arthritis or rheumatism, compared to 2.4% (95% CI: 2.1–2.8) in no chronic condition
Kingsbury et al., 2014 [4]	Five European (5EU) National Health and Wellness Survey, Europe, n = 3750	Self-report on physician diagnosis of peripheral joint OA	Total population	Self-reported depression	Prevalence of depression: 21.5%, compared to 13.4% in total population
Riddle et al., 2011 [17]	Osteoarthritis Initiative (incidence and progression cohort), USA, n = 3407	Symptomatic knee OA or at risk of symptomatic knee OA, with knee pain	—	CES-D ≥16, indicating probable clinical depression	Prevalence of depression: 11.8%
Sale et al., 2008 [72]	Population cohort, Canada, n = 1227	Disabling hip or knee OA	—	CES-D ≥16, indicating probable clinical depression	Prevalence of depression: 21.3%
Gleicher et al., 2011 [73]	Population-based cohort, Canada, n = 2005	Moderate-to-severe hip or knee OA	—	SF-36, MH score <60/100, indicating probable depression	Prevalence of depression: 28.7%
Anxiety					
Gore et al., 2011 [2]	Database on medical and pharmacy claims, n = 225 902	Subjects with a claim associated with a diagnosis of OA	Subjects without an OA-related claim	Diagnosis of anxiety disorder	Anxiety prevalence of 6.6% in OA, compared to 3.5% in controls
Patten et al., 2006 [3]	Canadian Community Health Survey, Canada, n = 36 984	Self-report on diagnosis by health professional of arthritis or rheumatism, excluding fibromyalgia	Self-report of no chronic condition	CIDI	Prevalence of panic disorder 3.0% (95% CI: 2.5–3.6) in arthritis or rheumatism, compared to 1.0% (95% CI: 0.7–1.3) in no chronic condition. Prevalence of social phobia 2.9% % (95% CI: 2.4–3.4) in arthritis or rheumatism, compared to 2.2% (95% CI: 1.9–2.6) in no chronic condition
Depression or anxiety					
Stamm et al., 2014 [74]	Austrian Health Interview Survey, Austria, n = 3097	Self-reported osteoarthritis	No musculoskeletal disease	Self-reported depression or anxiety	Prevalence of depression or anxiety: 14.7%, compared to 8.8% in the subjects with no musculoskeletal disease
Fatigue					
Wolfe et al., 1996 [5]	Consecutive patients	Diagnosis of osteoarthritis	—	Fatigue of ≥2 on 10-point VAS	Prevalence of fatigue: 41%

CES-D, Centre for Epidemiological Studies Depression scale; CIDI, Composite International Diagnostic Interview; SF-36, MH score, Short Form 36, Mental Health score; VAS, Visual Analogue Scale.

Environmental factors

In knee OA, the literature is inconsistent with regard to the predictive value of social support. Some studies found less social support to be associated with future activity limitations [23,36], while other studies did not find an association [24,37]. In hip OA, evidence was found that social support is not associated with future activity limitations [23,24,37].

Avoidance of activity

The avoidance model aims to explain the impact of psychological distress (i.e. anxiety, depression, and fatigue) on activity limitations in people with knee or hip OA [38,39]. The model was introduced in 1992 [38], inspired by previous models in chronic pain, mainly low back pain [40,41]. According to the avoidance model, a person

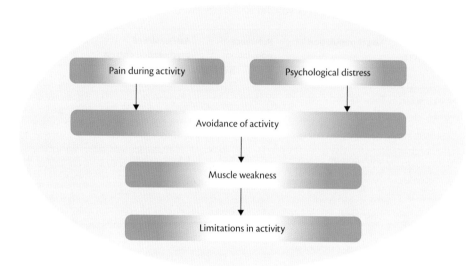

Figure 25.2 The avoidance model in people with knee or hip osteoarthritis, providing a behavioural explanation for the development of activity limitations. Dekker J., Exercise and Physical Functioning in Osteoarthritis. *Medical, Neuromuscular and Behavioral Perspectives,* 2014, Springer.

with OA experiences pain during physical activity (see Figure 25.2) [39]. This experience results in the expectation that renewed activity will again lead to pain. This expectation of pain induces the patient to avoid physical activity. In the short term, avoidance of activity leads to less pain due to the decreased load on the symptomatic joint. However, in the long term, avoidance of activity results in physical deconditioning, most notably a decrease in muscle strength. Decreased muscle strength leads to an increase in activity limitations. It is hypothesized that psychological distress enhances avoidance of activity.

The evidence for the validity of the avoidance model in people with knee and hip OA was summarized in a systematic literature of observational studies [30]. One cross-sectional study among people with early symptomatic knee OA examined the hypothesis that pain and psychological distress lead to avoidance of activity, which then results in muscle weakness (mediation by avoidance [42]). This hypothesis was confirmed.

Three studies examined the hypothesis that avoidance of activity leads to muscle weakness, which results in activity limitations (mediation by muscle weakness), in people with knee OA. All studies confirmed this hypothesis, including one longitudinal study [32] and two cross-sectional studies [43,44]. In the longitudinal study, the mediating role of muscle weakness was also found in people with hip OA [32].

Further support for the relationships hypothesized in the avoidance model was found in cross-sectional and longitudinal studies [30]. The avoidance model seems to provide a valid explanation for the impact of psychological distress on activity limitations in people with knee or hip OA. Further research is needed to confirm causal relationships.

Psychological interventions

Various interventions in OA have a psychological component. Some interventions (e.g. 'depression care', and pain coping skills training) use psychological or psychiatric treatments exclusively; in other cases, psychological interventions are embedded in other interventions (e.g. psychological interventions integrated into exercise therapy, or self-management). The various interventions with a psychological component are illustrated in Figure 25.1, and will be reviewed in the following subsections.

Depression care

In a pre-planned subgroup analysis of the IMPACT trial, Lin et al. [44] studied 1001 depressed older adults (a current diagnosis of major depression or dysthymia; ≥60 years) with coexisting arthritis; a diagnosis of OA was noted in 93.4% of medical records. In the 1-year long intervention, patients received improved depression care by a nurse or psychologist, working collaboratively with the patient and primary care physician. Treatment options included antidepressant medication, six to eight sessions of problem-solving therapy, and use of other mental health services. Compared to usual care, the intervention resulted in reduction of depressive symptoms, lower pain intensity, less interference with daily activities due to arthritis or pain, and improved general health. Although not designed to identify treatment mechanisms, the study shows that benefits of improved depression care extend beyond reduced depressive symptoms: improved depression care ameliorated pain and activity limitations.

Duloxetine is a selective serotonin and norepinephrine reuptake inhibitor, approved for the treatment of major depressive disorder, and also for use in OA. In a recent systematic review and meta-analysis, duloxetine was found to result in improved functioning, compared to placebo; however, the analysis suggested no difference in effect between duloxetine and non-steroidal anti-inflammatory drugs or opioids [45].

Pain coping skills training

Pain coping skills training aims to teach cognitive and behavioural techniques which enable patients to reduce the impact of pain on functioning. Common techniques include relaxation, attention diversion, activity pacing, and reducing pain-related cognitions and emotions [46]. Pain copings skills training in OA of the knee or hip has been shown to reduce symptoms of anxiety and depression, fatigue, catastrophizing, as well as pain and activity limitations—compared to usual care or education [46–48]. Interestingly, although the emphasis is on teaching techniques to deal with pain and although patients were not selected for symptoms of depression, pain coping skills training has been shown to also have an impact on depression, anxiety, and fatigue.

Behavioural strategies integrated into exercise therapy

Exercise therapy consists of supervised strengthening, aerobic, flexibility and/or functional exercises. The effectiveness of exercise therapy in knee and hip OA is well established; it has been found to reduce pain and activity limitations [49,50]. Since psychological factors have an impact on pain and activity limitations (see above), the integration of behavioural strategies into exercise therapy treatments seems a promising approach. Several integrated interventions have been developed and tested, among which behavioural graded activity (BGA) and cognitive behavioural therapy combined with exercise (ESCAPE-knee pain) [39].

BGA is an individually tailored exercise programme for patients with OA [51]. The intervention is directed at increasing the level of activities in a time-contingent way, with the goal to integrate these activities in the daily living of patients. Time-contingency management means that the amount of activities/exercises is based on preset quotas and is not based on pain or other tolerance factors. BGA is based on the concepts of operant conditioning. Essential features of the operant conditioning approach are positive reinforcement of healthy behaviour, and withdrawal of attention toward pain behaviour. BGA was compared with usual physiotherapy according to the Dutch OA guideline in 200 patients with OA of the hip and/or knee. Both groups showed beneficial within-group effects on the outcome measures pain and activity limitations, both in the short and long term. In patients with knee OA, no differences between treatments were found. In patients with hip OA, significant differences in favour of BGA were found in the outcome measures of pain and activity limitations, both after 3 and 9 months [51]. After 5 years, both interventions had similar beneficial effects on pain and activity limitations for both patients with hip and knee OA [52].

The ESCAPE-knee pain intervention aims to change the behaviour of participants by challenging inappropriate beliefs about their condition and physical activity, enabling self-management, and encouraging physical activity [53]. It is based on the principles of cognitive behavioural therapy, which can be delivered to either groups or individually. By the end of the programme, participants are supposed to have learnt how to utilize physical activity to self-manage their symptoms. The effectiveness of the ESCAPE-knee pain intervention was investigated among 418 patients with chronic knee pain. Six months after completing the ESCAPE-knee intervention, participants had significantly less limitations in activity, less pain, and more improvement in psychosocial outcomes compared to usual physiotherapy [53]. After 12 months, the beneficial effects of ESCAPE-knee pain and usual physiotherapy were similar. However, the healthcare costs of ESCAPE-knee pain were lower which made ESCAPE-knee pain more cost-effective [54].

It can be concluded that these integrated interventions reduce pain and activity limitations in patients with hip and knee OA. However, the added value of these interventions over exercise therapy alone, especially in the long term, is not firmly established yet and requires further study. It can be suggested to target integrated interventions to specific subgroups or phenotypes; in particular, patients with the depressive phenotype might benefit from these types of interventions.

Self-management

Self-management includes a wide range of activities, such as engaging in activities that promote health, interacting with healthcare providers, self-monitoring of physical and emotional status, and managing the effects of illness on a person's functioning [55,56]. Self-management interventions aim to support patients in these activities. In narrative reviews, beneficial outcomes of self-management interventions in OA were noted [57,58]. A recent systematic review provides a sobering perspective, however. No beneficial effects of self-management interventions were observed on self-management skills, pain, activity limitations (function), psychological distress, or quality of life, compared with an attention control intervention [55]. Compared with usual care, self-management interventions may slightly improve self-management skills, pain, and activity limitations (function), although these benefits were rather small [55]. In order to improve outcome, it can be suggested to tailor specific components of self-management to the specific needs of patients.

Partner-oriented interventions

Partners may play an important role in patients' adjustment to the disease and functioning. Outcomes of pain coping skills training in knee OA patients (see above) tended to be better if partners assisted in the training [47,48]. However, a study comparing a partner-oriented education and support intervention with a patient-oriented intervention found less reduction of pain and activity limitations in the partner-oriented condition [59]. Spouse support did increase in the couple-oriented intervention [60].

Improving exercise adherence

Adherence to exercise is crucial for the effectiveness of exercise therapy. In a narrative review, Marks [61] identified desirable attributes of programmes to promote exercise adherence. He concluded that psychological interventions are an important attribute of programmes to promote exercise adherence. In a systematic review, Jordan et al. [62] also pointed to the importance of psychological interventions. These authors concluded that therapeutic programmes that specifically address exercise adherence, self-management programmes, and the graded activity programme (see also [63]) are effective in improving several aspects of exercise adherence. The delivery mode was found to affect adherence as well: supervised exercise, supplementing home exercises with group exercise, and refresher sessions promote adherence.

Stronger input from evidence-based psychological theory into adherence programmes may lead to a significant advance in this field of research. Current approaches towards exercise adherence frequently lack a firm background in evidence-based psychological theory. The Health Action Process Approach (HAPA), developed by Schwarzer [64,65], has a firm basis in empirical evidence. The HAPA framework posits that patients pass through different phases on their way to being a regular exerciser. Programmes to promote exercise adherence may be most efficient when tailored to the individuals mind set. Schwarzer and colleagues [66] suggest that *pre-intenders*, who are deliberating whether or not to exercise,

Table 25.2 Integration of the HAPA framework and knowledge on desirable attributes of effective programmes to promote exercise adherence

Component in HAPA framework [65]	Desirable attributes according to Marks [61]	Integration of HAPA framework and Marks' attributes
Risk perception	Not among Marks' attributes	Address perception of being at risk of pain and activity limitations
Outcome expectancies	Comport with and correct beliefs, and perceptions about exercise and bodily states	Comport with and correct beliefs, and perceptions about exercise and bodily states
	Stress importance and benefits of exercise	Stress importance and benefits of exercise
Self-efficacy (action, maintenance, recovery)	Foster increased self-control, and efficacy expectations	Differentiate between action, maintenance, and recovery self-efficacy
		Foster increased self-control, and efficacy expectations—for action, maintenance, and recovery
Intention	Involve patient in goal setting	Involve patient in goal setting
	Set realistic goals	Set realistic goals
	Personal goals and interests	Personal goals and interests
Planning (action, coping)	Not among Marks' attributes	Formation of plans on when, where and how to exercise, and plans on how to cope with barriers and the design of alternative actions
Barriers and resources	Support services, reminders, follow-ups	Support services, reminders, follow-ups
	Peer and provider interaction, social support	Peer and provider interaction, social support
	Emotional, instrumental, and informational support	Emotional, instrumental, and informational support
Skills acquisition[a]	Simple and personalized programmes	Simple and personalized programmes
	Clear instructions	Clear instructions
	Modelling and mastery	Modelling and mastery
	Personalized feedback	Personalized feedback
	Encouragement, reassurance, advice, explanations	Encouragement, reassurance, advise, explanations
Identification of patient as pre-intender, intender, or actor	Not among Marks' attributes	Identification of patient as pre-intender, intender, or actor
Offer interventions tailored to pre-intenders, intenders, and actors		Offer interventions tailored to re-intenders, intenders, and actors

[a]Not in HAPA framework.

need information on the positive outcome of exercise (outcome expectation). They also need to develop an optimistic belief that they are capable of performing exercise (self-efficacy). *Intenders*, who are motivated to exercise but are not actually exercising, are supposed to benefit from interventions that help them to actually plan exercise and to plan strategies to cope with barriers and failures (planning). *Actors*, who are regularly doing exercise, may also benefit from interventions that bolster their beliefs in their capability to plan and maintain exercise and to recover from failure (self-efficacy).

Marks [61] has listed desirable attributes of programmes to promote exercise adherence. Table 25.2 lists these attributes, as well as the components suggested by the HAPA framework [65], and the integration of these two approaches. The HAPA framework points to essential attributes of effective adherence programmes, which Marks did not mention. Specifically, risk perception, planning, and tailoring of interventions to pre-intenders, intenders, and actors are not mentioned by Marks. It is suggested that effective adherence programmes need to incorporate these attributes. On the other hand, Marks points to skills acquisition: skilful instruction of exercise, modelling and shaping of exercise, and feedback on exercise performance are essential for the adoption and maintenance of exercise [67]. Marks also lists many specific attributes of effective

programmes. It seems that integration of the HAPA framework and available knowledge on effective programmes would result in improved adherence programmes. More generally, it is suggested that thoughtful integration of evidence-based psychological theory into research on exercise adherence programmes will significantly contribute to scientific progress in this field.

Promoting physical activity through web-based interventions

Regular physical activity, such as walking, cycling, or dancing, is proven to be beneficial in preserving physical function and improving pain in patients with knee OA [68]. Engagement in daily activity depends crucially on psychological factors. In particular, catastrophic thoughts and exaggerated anxiety of pain play a pivotal role in the performance of daily physical activity [69,70]. Furthermore, psychological distress enhances the tendency to avoid activity in response to pain, resulting in deterioration of physical functioning [30].

BGA is directed at increasing the level of activities in a time-contingent way, with the goal to integrate these activities in the daily living of patients (see above). A web-based version of the BGA intervention has been recently developed, entitled 'Join2move'

[71]. This programme was developed because of the high reach, low costs, and 24/7 accessibility of web-based interventions. The Join2move programme contains nine weekly modules in which users' favourite recreational activity is increased on fixed time points. In the first week, participants choose a central activity such as cycling, perform a 3-day self-test, and determine a short-term goal. Based on the results of the 3-day baseline test, eight modules are generated and weekly presented on the website. Users start with a low-intensity level which ensures success during the initial weeks.

The effectiveness of Join2move has been investigated in a randomized controlled trial [71]. Patients with knee and/or hip OA were assigned to Join2move or the waiting list control group. Primary outcome measures were physical activity levels, physical functioning, and self-perceived effect. At 3 months, patients in the intervention group reported a significantly improved physical function status and a positive self-perceived effect compared to the control group. However, no significant differences between the groups were found for physical activity. After 12 months, the intervention group reported higher levels of physical activity with respect to the control group. Non-significant differences were found for physical functioning and self-perceived effect.

Conclusion

The psychological approach towards OA is fruitful: the psychological approach has resulted in substantial contributions to the understanding and management of clinical presentations of OA, including pain and activity limitations. This chapter leads to a number of conclusions: (1) symptoms of depression, anxiety, and fatigue are more prevalent among patients with OA than among the general population. Recently, a depressive mood phenotype has been identified in knee OA. (2) Symptoms of depression, anxiety, and fatigue, as well as other psychological variables are established risk factors for future worsening of pain and activity limitations. (3) Psychological interventions such as depression care and pain coping skills training have been demonstrated to improve pain and activity limitations, as well as psychological outcomes. Self-management may have beneficial effects, although there is clearly room for improvement. Interventions combining psychological interventions with exercise therapy have been shown to be effective; improved outcome over exercise therapy alone stills needs to be demonstrated. (4) Psychological interventions are effective in improving exercise adherence and promoting physical activity.

With regard to future research, the following suggestions can be made: (1) further research on the impact of psychological risk factors on pain and activity limitations in OA; (2) further research on theoretical explanations on how psychological distress has impact on pain and activity limitations; (3) targeting psychological interventions on specific subgroups of patients, such as the 'depressive mood phenotype'; (4) tailoring specific components of psychological interventions to specific needs of patients; and (5) thoughtful integration of evidence-based psychological theory into research on psychological interventions and exercise adherence programmes.

References

1. World Health Organization. *International Classification of Functioning, Disability and Health.* Geneva: WHO; 2001.
2. Gore M, Tai KS, Sadosky A, Leslie D, Stacey BR. Clinical comorbidities, treatment patterns, and direct medical costs of patients with osteoarthritis in usual care: a retrospective claims database analysis. *J Med Econ* 2011; 14(4):497–507.
3. Patten SB, Williams JV, Wang J. Mental disorders in a population sample with musculoskeletal disorders. *BMC Musculoskelet Disord* 2006; 7:37.
4. Kingsbury SR, Gross HJ, Isherwood G, Conaghan PG. Osteoarthritis in Europe: impact on health status, work productivity and use of pharmacotherapies in five European countries. *Rheumatology (Oxford)* 2014; 53(5):937–47.
5. Wolfe F, Hawley DJ, Wilson K. The prevalence and meaning of fatigue in rheumatic disease. *J Rheumatol* 1996; 23(8):1407–17.
6. Grotle M, Hagen KB, Natvig B, Dahl FA, Kvien TK. Prevalence and burden of osteoarthritis: results from a population survey in Norway. *J Rheumatol* 2008; 35(4):677–84.
7. Christodoulou C, Schneider S, Junghaenel DU, Broderick JE, Stone AA. Measuring daily fatigue using a brief scale adapted from the Patient-Reported Outcomes Measurement Information System (PROMIS (R)). *Qual Life Res* 2014; 23(4):1245–53.
8. Parmelee PA, Harralson TL, McPherron JA, Schumacher HR. The structure of affective symptomatology in older adults with osteoarthritis. *Int J Geriatr Psychiatry* 2013; 28(4):393–401.
9. Stebbings S, Herbison P, Doyle TC, Treharne GJ, Highton J. A comparison of fatigue correlates in rheumatoid arthritis and osteoarthritis: disparity in associations with disability, anxiety and sleep disturbance. *Rheumatology (Oxford)* 2010; 49(2):361–7.
10. Bijlsma JW, Berenbaum F, Lafeber FP. Osteoarthritis: an update with relevance for clinical practice. *Lancet* 2011; 377(9783):2115–26.
11. Knoop J, van der LM, Thorstensson CA, et al. Identification of phenotypes with different clinical outcomes in knee osteoarthritis: data from the Osteoarthritis Initiative. *Arthritis Care Res (Hoboken)* 2011; 63(11):1535–42.
12. Van der Esch M, Knoop J, van der Leeden M, et al. Clinical phenotypes in patients with knee osteoarthritis: a study in the Amsterdam Osteoarthritis Cohort. *Osteoarthritis Cartilage* 2015; 23(4):544–9.
13. de Rooij M, van der Leeden M, Heymans M, et al. Prognosis of pain and physical functioning in patients with knee osteoarthritis: systematic review and meta-analysis. *Arthritis Care Res (Hoboken)* 2016; 68(4):481–92.
14. de Rooij M, van der Leeden M, Heymans MW, et al. Course and predictors of pain and physical functioning in patients with hip osteoarthritis: systematic review and meta-analysis. *J Rehabil Med* 2016; 48(3):245–52.
15. Blagojevic M, Jinks C, Jordan KP. The influence of consulting primary care on knee pain in older people: a prospective cohort study. *Ann Rheum Dis* 2008; 67(12):1702–9.
16. Jinks C, Jordan KP, Blagojevic M, Croft P. Predictors of onset and progression of knee pain in adults living in the community. A prospective study. *Rheumatology* 2008; 47(3):368–74.
17. Riddle DL, Kong X, Fitzgerald GK. Psychological health impact on 2-year changes in pain and function in persons with knee pain: data from the Osteoarthritis Initiative. *Osteoarthritis Cartilage* 2011; 19(9):1095–101.
18. Peat G, Thomas E. When knee pain becomes severe: a nested case-control analysis in community-dwelling older adults. *J Pain* 2009; 10(8):798–808.
19. Colbert CJ, Song J, Dunlop D, et al. Knee confidence as it relates to physical function outcome in persons with or at high risk of knee osteoarthritis in the osteoarthritis initiative. *Arthritis Rheum* 2012; 64(5):1437–46.
20. Mallen CD, Peat G, Thomas E, Lacey R, Croft P. Predicting poor functional outcome in community-dwelling older adults with knee pain: prognostic value of generic indicators. *Ann Rheum Dis* 2007; 66(11):1456–61.
21. Riddle DL, Stratford PW. Body weight changes and corresponding changes in pain and function in persons with symptomatic knee

osteoarthritis: a cohort study. *Arthritis Care Res (Hoboken)* 2013; 65(1):15–22.

22. Thomas E, Peat G, Mallen C, et al. Predicting the course of functional limitation among older adults with knee pain: do local signs, symptoms and radiographs add anything to general indicators? *Ann Rheum Dis* 2008; 67(10):1390–8.

23. Holla JF, Steultjens MP, Roorda LD, et al. Prognostic factors for the two-year course of activity limitations in early osteoarthritis of the hip and/or knee. *Arthritis Care Res (Hoboken)* 2010; 62(10):1415–25.

24. van Dijk GM, Veenhof C, van den Ende CHM, Lankhorst G, Dekker J. Vitality and the course of limitations in activities in osteoarthritis of the hip or knee. BMC *Musculoskelet Disord* 2011; 12:269.

25. Sharma L, Cahue S, Song J, et al. Physical functioning over three years in knee osteoarthritis: role of psychosocial, local mechanical and neuromuscular factors. *Arthritis Rheum* 2003; 48:3359–70.

26. Juhakoski R, Malmivaara A, Lakka TA, et al. Determinants of pain and functioning in hip osteoarthritis—a two-year prospective study. *Clin Rehabil* 2013; 27(3):281–7.

27. Dunlop DD, Song J, Semanik PA, et al. Relation of physical activity time to incident disability in community dwelling adults with or at risk of knee arthritis: prospective cohort study. *BMJ* 2014; 348:g2472.

28. Mansournia MA, Danaei G, Forouzanfar MH, et al. Effect of physical activity on functional performance and knee pain in patients with osteoarthritis: analysis with marginal structural models. *Epidemiology* 2012; 23(4):631–40.

29. Chapple CM, Nicholson H, Baxter GD, Abbott JH. Patient characteristics that predict progression of knee osteoarthritis: a systematic review of prognostic studies. *Arthritis Care Res (Hoboken)* 2011; 63(8):1115–25.

30. Holla JF, Sanchez-Ramirez DC, van der Leeden M, et al. The avoidance model in knee and hip osteoarthritis: a systematic review of the evidence. *J Behav Med* 2014; 37(6):1226–41.

31. Holla JF, van der Leeden M, Knol DL, et al. Predictors and outcome of pain-related avoidance of activities in persons with early symptomatic knee osteoarthritis: a 5-year follow-up study. *Arthritis Care Res (Hoboken)* 2015; 67(1):48–57.

32. Pisters MF, Veenhof C, van Dijk GM, Dekker J. Avoidance of activity and limitations in activities in patients with osteoarthritis of the hip or knee: a 5 year follow-up study on the mediating role of reduced muscle strength. *Osteoarthritis Cartilage* 2014; 22(2):171–7.

33. van Dijk GM, Veenhof C, Spreeuwenberg P, et al. Prognosis of limitations in activities in osteoarthritis of the hip or knee: a 3-year cohort study. *Arch Phys Med Rehabil* 2010; 91(1):58–66.

34. Harrison AL. The influence of pathology, pain, balance, and self-efficacy on function in women with osteoarthritis of the knee. *Phys Ther* 2004; 84(9):822–31.

35. Rejeski JW, Miller ME, Foy C, Messier SP, Rapp S. Self-efficacy and the progression of functional limitations and self-reported disability in older patients with knee pain. *J Gerontol Psychol Sci* 2001; 56(S261):S265.

36. Sharma L, Cahue S, Song J, et al. Physical functioning over three years in knee osteoarthritis: role of psychosocial, local mechanical, and neuromuscular factors. *Arthritis Rheum* 2003; 48(12):3359–70.

37. Pisters MF, Veenhof C, van Dijk GM, et al. The course of limitations in activities over 5 years in patients with knee and hip osteoarthritis with moderate functional limitations: risk factors for future functional decline. *Osteoarthritis Cartilage* 2012; 20(6):503–10.

38. Dekker J, Boot B, Woude LHV, Bijlsma JWJ. Pain and disability in osteoarthritis: a review of biobehavioral mechanisms. *J Behav Med* 1992; 15:189–214.

39. Dekker J (ed). *Exercise and Physical Functioning in Osteoarthritis. Medical, Neuromuscular and Behavioral Perspectives.* New York: Springer; 2014.

40. Lethem J, Slade PD, Troup JD, Bentley G. Outline of a fear-avoidance model of exaggerated pain perception—I. *Behav Res Ther* 1983; 21(4):401–8.

41. Turk DC, Flor H. Etiological theories and treatments for chronic back pain. II. Psychological models and interventions. *Pain* 1984; 19(3):209–33.

42. Holla JF, van der LM, Knol DL, et al. Avoidance of activities in early symptomatic knee osteoarthritis: results from the CHECK cohort. *Ann Behav Med* 2012; 44(1):33–42.

43. Steultjens MP, Dekker J, Bijlsma JW. Avoidance of activity and disability in patients with osteoarthritis of the knee: the mediating role of muscle strength. *Arthritis Rheum* 2002; 46(7):1784–8.

44. Lin EH, Katon W, Von KM, et al. Effect of improving depression care on pain and functional outcomes among older adults with arthritis: a randomized controlled trial. *JAMA* 2003; 290(18):2428–9.

45. Myers J, Wielage RC, Han B, et al. The efficacy of duloxetine, non-steroidal anti-inflammatory drugs, and opioids in osteoarthritis: a systematic literature review and meta-analysis. *BMC Musculoskelet Disord* 2014; 15:76.

46. Broderick JE, Keefe FJ, Bruckenthal P, et al. Nurse practitioners can effectively deliver pain coping skills training to osteoarthritis patients with chronic pain: a randomized, controlled trial. *Pain* 2014; 155(9):1743–54.

47. Keefe FJ, Caldwell DS, Williams DA, Gil KM, Mitchell D, Robertson C et al. Pain coping skills training in the management of osteoarthritic knee pain—II: Follow-up results. *Behav Ther* 1990; 21:435–47.

48. Keefe FJ, Caldwell DS, Baucom D, et al. Spouse-assisted coping skills training in the management of osteoarthritic knee pain. *Arthritis Care Res* 1996; 9(4):279–91.

49. Fransen M, McConnell S. Exercise for osteoarthritis of the knee. *Cochrane Database Syst Rev* 2008; 4:CD004376.

50. Fransen M, McConnell S, Hernandez-Molina G, Reichenbach S. Exercise for osteoarthritis of the hip. *Cochrane Database Syst Rev* 2014; 4:CD007912.

51. Veenhof C, Koke AJ, Dekker J, et al. Effectiveness of behavioral graded activity in patients with osteoarthritis of the hip and/or knee: a randomized clinical trial. *Arthritis Rheum* 2006; 55(6):925–34.

52. Pisters MF, Veenhof C, van Meeteren NL, et al. Long-term effectiveness of exercise therapy in patients with osteoarthritis of the hip or knee: a systematic review. *Arthritis Rheum* 2007; 57(7):1245–53.

53. Hurley MV, Walsh NE, Mitchell HL, et al. Clinical effectiveness of a rehabilitation program integrating exercise, self-management, and active coping strategies for chronic knee pain: a cluster randomized trial. *Arthritis Rheum* 2007; 57(7):1211–9.

54. Hurley MV, Walsh NE, Mitchell H, Nicholas J, Patel A. Long-term outcomes and costs of an integrated rehabilitation program for chronic knee pain: a pragmatic, cluster randomized, controlled trial. *Arthritis Care Res (Hoboken)* 2012; 64(2):238–47.

55. Kroon FP, van der Burg LR, Buchbinder R, et al. Self-management education programmes for osteoarthritis. *Cochrane Database Syst Rev* 2014; 1:CD008963.

56. Von Korff M, Gruman J, Schaefer J, Curry SJ, Wagner EH. Collaborative management of chronic illness. *Ann Intern Med* 1997; 127(12):1097–102.

57. Iversen MD, Hammond A, Betteridge N. Self-management of rheumatic diseases: state of the art and future perspectives. *Ann Rheum Dis* 2010; 69(6):955–63.

58. Fernandes L, Hagen KB, Bijlsma JW, et al. EULAR recommendations for the non-pharmacological core management of hip and knee osteoarthritis. *Ann Rheum Dis* 2013; 72(7):1125–35.

59. Martire LM, Keefe FJ, Rudy TE, Starz TW. Couple-oriented education and support intervention: effects on individuals with osteoarthritis and their spouses. *Rehabil Psychol* 2007; 52:121–32.

60. Martire LM, Schulz R, Keefe FJ, Rudy TE, Starz TW. Couple-oriented education and support intervention for osteoarthritis: effects on spouses' support and responses to patient pain. *Fam Syst Health* 2008; 26(2):185–95.

61. Marks R. Knee osteoarthritis and exercise adherence: a review. *Curr Aging Sci* 2012; 5(1):72–83.

62. Jordan JL, Holden MA, Mason EE, Foster NE. Interventions to improve adherence to exercise for chronic musculoskeletal pain in adults. *Cochrane Database Syst Rev* 2010; 1:CD005956.

63. Pisters MF, Veenhof C, de Bakker DH, Schellevis FG, Dekker J. Behavioural graded activity results in better exercise adherence and more physical activity than usual care in people with osteoarthritis: a cluster-randomised trial. *Aust J Physiother* 2010; 56(1):41–7.

64. Schwarzer R. Self-efficacy in the adoption and maintenance of health behaviors: theoretical approaches and a new model. In Schwarzer R (ed) *Self-efficacy: Thought Control of Action*. Washington, DC: Taylor & Francis; 1992:217–43.

65. Schwarzer R. Modeling health behavior change: how to predict and modify the adoption and maintenance of health behaviors. *Appl Psychol* 2008; 57:1–29.

66. Dekker J, Brosschot J, Schwarzer R, Tsutsumi A. Theory in behavioral medicine. In Fisher EB (ed) *Principles and Concepts of Behavioral Medicine: A Global Handbook*. Amsterdam: Springer; in press.

67. Dekker J. Osteoarthritis: promoting exercise for OA in ambivalent older adults. *Nat Rev Rheumatol* 2012; 8(8):442–4.

68. Fransen M, McConnell S. Land-based exercise for osteoarthritis of the knee: a metaanalysis of randomized controlled trials. *J Rheumatol* 2009; 36(6):1109–17.

69. Holden MA, Nicholls EE, Young J, Hay EM, Foster NE. Role of exercise for knee pain: what do older adults in the community think? *Arthritis Care Res (Hoboken)* 2012; 64(10):1554–64.

70. Somers TJ, Keefe FJ, Godiwala N, Hoyler GH. Psychosocial factors and the pain experience of osteoarthritis patients: new findings and new directions. *Curr Opin Rheumatol* 2009; 21(5):501–6.

71. Bossen D, Veenhof C, Van Beek KE, et al. Effectiveness of a web-based physical activity intervention in patients with knee and/or hip osteoarthritis: randomized controlled trial. *J Med Internet Res* 2013; 15(11):e257.

72. Sale JE, Gignac M, Hawker G. The relationship between disease symptoms, life events, coping and treatment, and depression among older adults with osteoarthritis. *J Rheumatol* 2008; 35(2):335–42.

73. Gleicher Y, Croxford R, Hochman J, Hawker G. A prospective study of mental health care for comorbid depressed mood in older adults with painful osteoarthritis. *BMC Psychiatry* 2011; 11:147.

74. Stamm TA, Pieber K, Blasche G, Dorner TE. Health care utilisation in subjects with osteoarthritis, chronic back pain and osteoporosis aged 65 years and more: mediating effects of limitations in activities of daily living, pain intensity and mental diseases. *Wien Med Wochenschr* 2014; 164(7–8):160–6.

CHAPTER 26

Miscellaneous physical therapies

Melanie A. Holden, Martin J. Thomas,
and Krysia S. Dziedzic

Introduction

This chapter reviews physical therapies for osteoarthritis (OA) that have not been covered elsewhere within the book (referred to as miscellaneous physical therapies), but feature within clinical guidelines for OA. These include assistive devices, thermotherapy, manual therapy, acupuncture, electrotherapy, and other miscellaneous physical therapies. Along with a brief description of each therapy, the recommendation within clinical guidelines for each therapy is summarized and an overview of the evidence base supporting guideline recommendations is provided.

To identify miscellaneous physical therapies that feature within clinical guidelines for OA, we made reference to three recent systematic reviews of guidelines for the management of OA that included literature searches up to 2013 [1–3]. We also completed an additional literature search of several electronic databases including Trip database, Physiotherapy Evidence Database (PEDro), National Guideline Clearing House, and NHS Evidence between January 2013 and July 2014, to identify more recently published clinical guidelines. The content of all identified guidelines was reviewed, and relevant data extracted (see Table 26.1) and summarized.

Overall aims and current use of miscellaneous physical approaches

Miscellaneous physical therapies predominantly aim to control pain, minimize joint stiffness, and limit joint damage with the minimum adverse treatment effects. They may also help to maximize function and health-related quality of life [4]. Conceptualized within the biopsychosocial model [5], outcome of treatment is related to more than the underlying pathology (see Chapter 3). Therefore, assessment and management of patients with OA should be holistic, considering the person with OA rather than the pathology of OA prior to selecting any therapy [4,6].

Miscellaneous physical therapies are commonly used to treat patients with OA, often as an adjunct to core treatment. A national survey of physiotherapists in the United Kingdom found that although exercise was the most commonly reported treatment approach for a patient with knee OA, 81% of physiotherapists (n = 538) would deliver one or more miscellaneous physical therapies in addition to exercise, including heat or ice (62%), manual therapy (36%), acupuncture (33%), and electrotherapy (33%) [7]. These findings have been mirrored elsewhere in Europe [8]. Walsh and Hurley [9] also found that physiotherapists used a median of four different treatment modalities with each patient with knee OA.

A recent international survey completed in the United Kingdom and Australia revealed that physiotherapists also utilize miscellaneous physical therapies, predominantly manual therapy (hip mobilizations/manipulations) in addition to exercise and advice for patients with hip OA. There were some differences in treatment approaches across the two countries, for example, Australian physiotherapists provided more treatment sessions than their United Kingdom colleagues (five or more treatment sessions reported by 75% and 40% of Australian and United Kingdom physiotherapists, respectively). Whether such differences or whether utilizing multi-modal miscellaneous therapies impacts on patient outcomes remains unknown [10].

Evidence and recommendations for miscellaneous physical approaches

Fifteen current clinical guidelines for OA were identified that addressed one or more miscellaneous physical therapies [6,11–24]. (Note: guidelines superseded by new editions were excluded, including the European League Against Rheumatism (EULAR) 2005 hip [25], 2003 knee [26], and 2000 knee [27] guidelines, as these have been superseded by the recently published EULAR hip and knee guidelines [19].) These were broadly grouped into assistive technology, thermotherapy, manual therapy, acupuncture, electrotherapy, and other miscellaneous physical therapies. Within the guidelines they were commonly seen as an adjunct to the core treatments of education, exercise, and weight loss if overweight or obese (see Chapters 22 and 23). Table 26.1 summarizes the recommendations for each miscellaneous physical therapy to accompany the detail provided in the following sections.

Assistive technology

Assistive technologies include a broad range of devices and appliances that are often designed as adjunctive interventions to facilitate both general mobility and activities of daily living (ADLs). The aim of these approaches is to support and correct biomechanical deficits in normal movement and to control joint instability.

Across the reviewed guidelines, 13 guidelines considered some form of assistive technology. For hand OA, three guidelines recommended joint protection [16,17,23], two recommended assistive devices for ADLs [6,23], and four advocated splinting [6,16,17,23]. Recommendations for most of these interventions are largely based on expert opinion due to a lack of evidence. However, evidence for the use of joint protection techniques for hand OA has recently been

Table 26.1 Miscellaneous physical therapies summary table

	Hip only			Knee only					Hip and knee			Hand, hip and knee		General	
	APTA-OS [12]	AAOS [11]	OARSI [13]	Philadelphia [14]	TLAR [15]	EULAR 2007 [16]	SIR [17]	DUTCH [18]	EULAR 2013 [19]	NHMRC [20]	OARSI 2008 (hip only+) [21]	SOFMER [22]	ACR [23]	NICE [6]	OTTAWA [24]
Assistive technology															
Joint protection					R	R	R						R hand		
ADL assistive devices									R				R hand	R	
Splinting					R	R	R						R hand	R	
Braces		?	R		R					NR			? knee	R	
Insoles/orthoses		NR	R		R				NR	NR		R knee ? hip	R knee	R	
Patella taping								R knee only		R knee only			R knee		
Walking aids	R		R knee* ? M-J		R				R		R hip		R hip R knee	R	
Footwear					R				R		R hip			R LL	
Thermotherapy															
Hot					R	R	R	?			R hip		R hand R hip R knee	R	
Cold				?	R			?		R knee only	R hip			R	
Manual therapy	R	?											? hip ? knee	R	
Manual therapy plus exercise								R		R			R hip R knee		R
Massage								NR		R knee only					
Acupuncture		NR	?							R knee			R knee	NR	
Electrotherapy		?	NR		R			NR							
TENS			? knee NR M-J	R	R			? knee only	R	R knee	R hip		R knee	R	
Ultrasound			? knee NR M-J	?	R	R	R	NR		NR					

Short-wave diathermy		R				
Laser				R	NR	R knee
Electromagnetic field					NR	
Magnetotherapy				R		
Electrical stimulation	?					NR
Other						
Balneotherapy	R M-J+ relevant co-morb. ?M-J +no relevant comorb. ?OA only	R		R	?	
Magnet therapy						R
Leech therapy						R

? = neither recommended or not recommended; AAOS, American Academy of Orthopaedic Surgeons; ACR, American College of Rheumatology; ADL, activities of daily living; APTA-OA, American Physical Therapy Association-Orthopaedic Section; co-morb, co-morbidity; EULAR, European League Against Rheumatism; LL, lower limb; NHMRC, National Health and Medical Research Council; NICE, National Institute for Health and Care Excellence; NR, not recommend; OARSI, Osteoarthritis Research Society International; R, recommended; SIR, Italian Society for Rheumatology; SOFMER, French Physical Medicine and Rehabilitation Society; TLAR, Turkish League Against Rheumatism.

+Hip only (knee recommendations superseded by [13]). *Cane (walking stick) is recommended, crutches are neither recommended nor not recommended.

strengthened, with patients more likely to be classed as responders at 6 months having received joint protection delivered by occupational therapists [28].

For hip and or knee OA, seven guidelines addressed and recommended the use of walking aids [6,12,13,15,19,21,23]. Theoretically, a walking aid such as a stick or cane should reduce impact loading through the joint, thus reduce pain, improve function, and may also reduce the rate of structural progression of OA [29]. However, there is only limited evidence to support this [30]. Four guidelines addressed and recommended appropriate footwear for patients with hip and/or knee OA [6,15,19,21]. Shoes with thick but soft soles and no raised heels minimize rebound upward force transmission and adverse knee, hip, and back alignment when walking [29]. Again, due to a lack of clinical evidence, this recommendation is primarily supported by expert opinion alone.

Many other forms of assistive technology were addressed within the guidelines for hip and knee OA including braces, insoles/orthoses, and joint protection. Recommendations for each were mixed, reflecting an overall lack of evidence in this area. For knee OA, braces are designed to offload increased focal stresses in the medial and lateral compartments of the knee, often associated with varus and valgus deformities. Braces were recommended by three guidelines [6,13,15], not recommended by one [20], and neither recommended nor not recommended by two others [11,23]. A recent meta-analysis suggested that valgus bracing may offer small-to-moderate benefits for knee OA-related pain and function [31]. The recommended use of insoles and orthoses to correct malalignment and help offload painful joints was also mixed, with five guidelines promoting their use as adjunctive treatments [6,13,15,22,23] and three not recommending their use [11,19,20]. A more recent meta-analysis of lateral wedge insoles concluded that there was insufficient evidence to substantiate the efficacy of orthoses for pain reduction associated with medial knee OA [32]. Patella taping used to correct abnormal patella tracking was recommended by three guidelines [18,20,23], and two guidelines advocated assistive devices for ADLs (e.g. increasing the height of chairs, beds, and toilet seats) [6,19].

Thermotherapy

Thermotherapy, involving the local application of heat or cold (cryotherapy) is commonly used to help manage symptomatic musculoskeletal problems in individuals with intact sensory perception [33]. Usually administered by patients themselves as part of self-management routines, heat treatments aim to reduce pain and stiffness and cold treatments aim to reduce pain and inflammation, with both approaches attempting to improve function and mobility [34]. Heat treatment includes applications such as hot packs, heating gels or sprays, warm water baths, and paraffin wax baths. Cold treatments can include the use of ice packs, ice baths, cooling gels or sprays, and local ice massage.

Of the 15 reviewed guidelines, seven recommended the use of thermotherapy for hand, hip, or knee OA [6,15,16,17,20,21,23] and two neither recommended nor discouraged its use [14,18]. The remainder did not consider their application.

To date, guideline recommendations are based predominantly on one Cochrane review of three randomized controlled trials (RCTs) for knee OA (179 patients) [34], with studies differing considerably

in terms of design and quality. The review found mixed results, with ice massage having statistically significant benefits for function, cold packs decreasing swelling but not reducing pain, and hot packs having no beneficial effect on oedema. Despite lacking evidence, these approaches are relatively safe and easily self-administered. In the clinical setting patients often report relief from heat or cold therapies and can be encouraged to trial both approaches for themselves at home.

Manual therapy

Manual therapy refers to the hands-on treatment of a trained musculoskeletal therapist (e.g. physiotherapist, occupational therapist, chiropractor, and osteopath), designed to reduce pain by passively facilitating normal functioning of bony articular surfaces and neural pathways, and surrounding soft tissue around restricted joints [33]. The hands-on physical contact provided by manual therapy can also have a positive psychological or placebo effect on patient perceived outcomes [35]. Techniques are commonly based on the following approaches: therapist-guided normal movements (physiological movements); therapist-performed movements within a joint's normal active range, but requiring external assistance to achieve (accessory movements); and small high-velocity therapist-performed movements at the limit of normal active range of motion (manipulation) [36]. Additional hands-on approaches can also include a range of soft tissue massage techniques.

Seven guidelines considered manual therapy. Of those, four recommended manual therapy in combination with exercise for hip and or knee OA [18,20,23,24]. Recommendations for the use of manual therapy alone were mixed, with two guidelines recommending it [6,12], and two neither recommending for or against its use [11,23]. In addition, one guideline recommended the use of massage for patients with knee OA [20], whereas one recommended against its use [18].

Guidelines recommending manual therapy for knee OA are generally based on a small number of RCTs offering support for this intervention in combination with other treatments including exercise [37,38], taping and exercise [39], and non-steroidal anti-inflammatory drugs [40]. In the short term, Swedish massage was shown to be beneficial compared to no intervention for knee OA [41], as was myofascial mobilization [42] and tibiofemoral joint mobilization [43]. A study of hip OA found manual therapy to be more favourable than exercise [44] and exercise combined with traction-mobilization was found to reduce hip disability in the short term [45]. Benefit among these studies was evaluated with a range of pain and function-related outcomes, and the quality of these studies was variable in terms of blinding, sample size, study length, and follow-up. One small pre- and post-test cohort study [46] has demonstrated improved pain and function outcomes for knee OA following hip mobilization. A small case series study also indicated that manual therapy and exercise reduced pain and increased function for hip OA [47].

More recently, two high-quality RCTs have strengthened the evidence base for manual therapy in OA. One trial including 206 patients with hip and knee OA found that manual physiotherapy provided benefits over usual care, and these were sustained over the long term. However, there was an antagonistic effect for usual care plus combined exercise therapy and manual therapy [48]. A second

RCT compared physiotherapy including manual therapy and exercise to a sham consisting of inactive ultrasound and inert gel in 102 patients with hip OA. The physiotherapy programme was not more effective than sham for pain and function [49]. This new evidence questions the usefulness of providing manual therapy alongside exercise for patients with OA, and as this reflects current guideline recommendations and typical clinical practice, further research in this field is required.

Acupuncture

Acupuncture is based on needle stimulation of points on the surface of the body (acupuncture points) and originates from Traditional Chinese Medicine. The mechanisms of traditional Chinese acupuncture cannot be explained by conventional physiology, but is the most common form of acupuncture practised throughout the world. In the United Kingdom, 'Western medical acupuncture' is used within the National Health Service. This is based upon neurophysiological mechanisms [6].

Acupuncture is most commonly used for pain relief [50]. It usually involves penetrating the skin at anatomical points on the body with thin, solid, metallic needles that are typically kept in place for 20–30 minutes. Whilst needles are *in situ* they are often manipulated manually or by electrical stimulation in order to achieve a 'needle sensation', or De Qi, usually described as a tingling, numbness, or dull ache sensation [50].

The role of acupuncture for OA is controversial, with two guidelines recommending that is should not be used [6,11], one neither recommending for or against it [13], and two advocating its use for knee OA [20,23]. One guideline that supports its use states that acupuncture should only be used for patients who meet a certain criteria: having knee OA; chronic moderate-to-severe pain; are a candidate for total knee arthroplasty but are either unwilling to undergo the procedure, have comorbid medical conditions, or are taking concomitant medications that lead to a relative or absolute contraindication to surgery; or the surgeon does not recommend the procedure [23].

Recommendations against the use of acupuncture are based on lack of evidence for its efficacy, rather than evidence of harm. Within RCTs, efficacy is often tested by comparing true acupuncture to a placebo 'sham acupuncture', involving inserting needles into the wrong place, not stimulating them, or by using blunt retractable needles that cause pressure but not skin penetration. However, there is concern over whether such sham controls are completely inactive [51]. Not surprisingly there is heterogeneity of results from RCTs and systematic reviews, contributing to the controversy around whether acupuncture should be recommended or not for patients with OA.

A Cochrane review by Manheimer et al. [50] included 16 RCTs (3498 people) comparing acupuncture to either a sham, waiting list control, or another active treatment in people with knee, hip, or hand OA. Compared to a sham, acupuncture showed a statistically significant short-term improvement in pain (standardized mean difference (SMD) 0.28, 95% confidence interval (CI) 0.11–0.45) and function (SMD 0.28, 95% CI 0.09–0.46), but did not reach pre-defined thresholds for clinical relevance. Compared to a waiting list control, acupuncture showed statistically significant, clinically relevant short-term improvements in pain (SMD 0.96, 95% CI 0.72–1.19) and function (SMD 0.89, 95% CI 0.60–1.18)

(four trials; 884 participants). In comparison to other active treatments acupuncture was associated with clinically relevant short- and long-term improvements in pain and function compared to 'supervised education' and 'physician consultation' control groups, and had similar treatment effects when compared with 'home exercises/advice leaflet' and 'supervised exercise'. The authors concluded that although sham-controlled trials show small and statistically significant benefits these are not of clinical relevance and are likely, in part, due to incomplete blinding. The statistically significant and clinically relevant benefits of acupuncture compared to a waiting list control suggest benefits are likely to be caused by expectation or placebo effects [50].

In addition to guideline evidence, two more recent meta-analyses concluded that acupuncture was effective for the treatment of chronic pain, including OA [51,52], suggesting that acupuncture was one of the more effective physical treatments for alleviating knee OA pain in the short term [51]. However, it was acknowledged that factors in addition to the specific effects of needling contributed to its therapeutic effects [51].

Electrotherapy

Electrotherapy involves the application of external energy into a tissue which stimulates physiological activity for therapeutic benefit [53]. Many different electrotherapy and electrophysical modalities exist and can be classified as either having 'thermal' or 'non-thermal' effects [54]. These include short-wave diathermy therapy, laser, transcutaneous electrical nerve stimulation (TENS), and ultrasound. All can be used to treat the signs and symptoms of OA such as pain, trigger point tenderness, and swelling [6], although their supporting evidence-base is generally limited. TENS and ultrasound are the forms of electrotherapy most commonly featured within non-pharmacological guidelines for OA and are described in more detail below.

Transcutaneous electrical nerve stimulation

TENS involves stimulation of cutaneous nerve fibres by a device worn and operated by the patient. It is based on the 'gate-control theory' of pain perception, providing pain relief by inhibiting the transmission of painful stimuli to the spinal cord and brain pain receptors [55]. The location of the stimulators, and the wave produced by the device (e.g. amplitude, rate, and width of pulse) all influence the quality of TENS administered to the patient and are generally adjusted depending on the patient's response [20]. It is recognized as a treatment modality with minimal contraindications [56].

TENS is recommended within six of the eight guidelines that consider its use, predominantly for patients with knee OA [6,14,15,20,21,23]. Two guidelines neither recommend for or against its use [13,18], and the Osteoarthritis Research Society International (OARSI) 2014 guidelines for knee OA recommend that it should not be used for patients with multi-joint OA [13]. This lack of consensus reflects inconclusive evidence regarding its clinical effectiveness. A 2009 Cochrane review included 18 small clinical trials (813 participants) comparing TENS with either a sham or no intervention in patients with knee OA [57]. Due to the poor quality and reporting of included studies, no firm conclusions could be drawn regarding the effectiveness of TENS for pain relief, although there was no evidence of it being unsafe [57].

Ultrasound

Therapeutic ultrasound consists of high-frequency vibrations that can be pulsed or continuous [58,59]. Pulsed ultrasound produces non-thermal effects (cavitation, acoustic streaming) that can alter the permeability of a cell membrane, thought to produce therapeutic benefits [60]. It is generally recommended for acute pain and inflammation. Continuous ultrasound generates thermal effects causing a rise in temperature within the tissue [61].

Therapeutic ultrasound is only recommended in three of the seven guidelines that consider its use, two of which are for hand OA [15,16,17]. These recommendations are based on expert opinion rather than RCT evidence. Other guidelines neither recommend for or against its use [13,14], or recommend that it should not be used in the management of patients with OA [13,18,20].

Two systematic reviews published in 2010 suggested a possible beneficial effect of ultrasound for knee OA, however the quality of the included evidence was low. No safety risks were reported to be associated with ultrasound [62,63]. One review included five small trials (341 patients with knee OA) that compared therapeutic ultrasound (including both pulsed and continuous ultrasound) with a sham or no intervention. For pain, there was an effect in favour of ultrasound and for function there was a trend in favour of ultrasound [62]. The other review included six trials and 378 patients with knee OA. They also found ultrasound improved pain and tended to improve self-reported physical function [63]. Within both reviews, as included studies were small, underpowered, and of low quality, no firm conclusions could be drawn.

Other miscellaneous physical therapies

Balneotherapy

Balneotherapy has been used since ancient times in the treatment of various illnesses, including OA. It is defined as the use of baths containing thermal mineral waters and involves various treatment methods, including Dead Sea salt or mineral baths, sulphur baths, and radon-carbon dioxide baths [64]. The temperature of the water (thermal water, seawater or tap water) is generally around 34°C. Common aims of balneotherapy are to relieve muscle spasm and reduce pain [65].

Four guidelines feature balneotherapy [13,15,17,18], with three recommending its use [13,15,17] and one neither recommending for or against it [18]. Although the OARSI guidelines for knee OA [13] recommend that it should be used for individuals with multi-joint OA and relevant co-morbidities (e.g. diabetes) they do not recommend either for or against its use for individuals without such co-morbidities or for people with knee OA alone [13].

A systematic review published in 2009 evaluated the effectiveness of natural thermal mineral waters in patients with knee OA [66]. Nine RCTs (493 participants) were included that were heterogeneous with regards to intervention, controls, samples and outcome measures, and were of varying quality. All interventions improved pain and functional capacity, and no serious adverse events were associated with balneotherapy. However, the authors concluded that additional higher quality RCTs were required to confirm these effects.

The effect of balneotherapy specifically for hand OA has also been investigated [67]. Sixty-three patients were randomized to bathe in thermal mineral water at either 36°C or 38°C five times a week for 3 weeks in addition to receiving magnetotherapy to their hands three times weekly. A third group received only magnetotherapy.

The combination of balneotherapy and magnetotherapy resulted in a greater improvement in pain severity and grip strength when compared to the magnetotherapy alone [67].

Magnet therapy

Magnet therapy involves the application of static magnetic fields to the body for purported health benefits, including pain relief [20]. Magnets are either worn directly over the affected area for a specified period each day, or on the wrist via a bracelet to provide an effect on the entire body [20]. There are many theories proposing why magnet therapy can influence pain, from magnets increasing blood flow through skin and muscles, to polarization influencing biological changes [68].

Only one guideline [20] addressed the use of magnetic therapy, and recommended the use of magnetic bracelets for patients with hip and knee OA. This was supported by one RCT including 194 patients with hip and knee OA [69]. Individuals were randomized to wear either a standard strength static bipolar magnetic bracelet, a weak magnetic bracelet, or a non-magnetic (dummy) bracelet for 12 weeks. There was a small but statistically significant difference in pain reduction in the standard magnet group compared to the dummy magnet group [69].

Leech therapy

Leech therapy has been proposed for the treatment of OA. It is suggested that leech saliva has analgesic effects, however early research failed to demonstrate either the ability of leech salivary secretions to reach the joint or the analgesic properties of leech saliva content [20].

Only one guideline addressed leech therapy, suggesting from weak evidence from one moderate quality RCT including 51 participants with knee OA that its use for treatment of knee and hip OA may be warranted [20]. Within the RCT individuals were randomized to receive a single treatment of four to six locally applied medicinal leeches, or diclofenac topical gel treatment for 28 days. There was reduced pain at 7 days in the leech therapy group compared to the control but this was not maintained at 4 weeks. However, differences in function, stiffness, total symptoms and quality of life remained significant in favour of leech therapy at 4 weeks [70].

Summary and conclusion

The main aims of miscellaneous physical therapies as adjuncts to written information and exercise are to control pain, minimize joint stiffness, and maximize function and health-related quality of life. Fifteen current clinical guidelines for OA address one or more miscellaneous physical therapies. The specific types of approaches addressed are variable, as are their recommendations. Differences in how guidelines are developed and consensus is reached are compounded by the overall quality of the evidence base. Small study sizes, heterogeneity in populations, study design, intervention delivery, and outcome measurement often make it difficult for guideline panels to effectively synthesis the available evidence. In light of the limited evidence base, this overview has not included detail of the strength of recommendation of evidence supporting each guideline, but rather included all levels of recommendation.

There appears to be greatest consensus for miscellaneous physical therapies in hand OA, with multiple guidelines addressing and consistently recommending joint protection, splinting and thermotherapy. However these recommendations are predominantly based on a small number of RCTs. Use of walking aids and footwear are commonly addressed and recommended for patients with hip and knee OA, although these recommendations are predominantly based on expert opinion. Other physical therapies that are addressed and recommended for hip and knee OA are variable, ranging from orthoses to less conventional leech therapy. When a recommendation for a miscellaneous physical therapy is not made, it is commonly due to limited clinical evidence, rather than evidence of harm. In light of this, and the lack of consensus between clinical guidelines, use of specific miscellaneous physical therapies in clinical practice should be based upon a holistic, individualized assessment of each patient with OA in addition to clinical guidelines and the underlying evidence base (Box 26.1).

The variability in clinical guideline recommendations for miscellaneous physical therapies, particularly for knee and hip OA, is also mirrored in clinical practice. A range of different therapies are currently utilized by healthcare professionals, but as adjuncts to core treatment rather than standalone interventions. A large number of interventions are used to treat individual patients, and there are some differences in the delivery of treatment internationally. As miscellaneous physical therapies are so commonly used as adjunctive approaches, further large-scale, high-quality RCTs would be useful to inform clinical guidelines and clinical practice as to which types of therapy are beneficial, which are not, and whether multiple miscellaneous physical therapies should be used simultaneously alongside core treatments for patients with OA.

Box 26.1 Summary of key messages regarding miscellaneous physical therapies for osteoarthritis

- Miscellaneous therapies aim to control pain, minimize joint stiffness, improve function, and maximize health-related quality of life

- Miscellaneous physical therapies are commonly used within clinical practice as adjuncts to core treatment

- The types of miscellaneous physical therapies used are wide ranging, and multiple therapies are often used for individual patients

- Fifteen current clinical guidelines for OA address one or more miscellaneous physical therapy. The specific types of approaches addressed are variable, as are recommendations

- For hand OA, multiple guidelines address and consistently recommend joint protection, splinting, and thermotherapy. These recommendations are based on a small number of RCTs

- Use of walking aids and appropriate footwear are commonly addressed and recommended for patients with hip and knee OA. These recommendations are predominantly based on expert opinion

- Variability in recommendations for other miscellaneous therapies reflects an overall limited evidence base

- Further large-scale, high-quality RCTs are required to strengthen the evidence base surrounding miscellaneous physical therapies for OA.

References

1. Brosseau L, Rahman P, Toupin-April K, et al. A systematic critical appraisal for non-pharmacological management of osteoarthritis using the appraisal of guidelines research and evaluation II instrument. *PLoS One* 2014; 9(1):e82986.
2. Larmer PJ, Reay ND, Aubert ER, et al. Systematic review of guidelines for the physical management of osteoarthritis. *Arch Phys Med Rehabil* 2014; 95(2):375–89.
3. Nelson AE, Allen KD, Golightly YM, et al. A systematic review of recommendations and guidelines for the management of osteoarthritis: the Chronic Osteoarthritis Management Initiative of the U.S. Bone and Joint Initiative. *Semin Arthritis Rheum* 2014; 43(6):701–12.
4. Bearne LM, Hurley MV. Physical therapies—treatment options in rheumatology. In Dziedzic K, Hammond A (eds) *Rheumatology: Evidence-Based Practice for Physiotherapists and Occupational Therapists.* New York: Churchill Livingstone; 2010: 111–22.
5. Main CJ, Spanswick CC, Watson P. The nature of disability. In Main CJ, Spanswick CC. *Pain Management: An Interdisciplinary Approach.* New York: Churchill Livingstone; Edinburgh, 2000:89–106.
6. National Institute for Health and Care Excellence. *Osteoarthritis: Care and Management in Adults.* NICE Clinical Guideline 177. London: Royal College of Physicians; 2014.
7. Holden MA, Nicholls EE, Hay EM, Foster NE. Physical therapists' use of therapeutic exercise for patients with clinical knee osteoarthritis in the United Kingdom: in line with current recommendations? *Phys Ther* 2008; 88(10):1109–21.
8. Jamtvedt G, Dahm KT, Holm I, Flottorp S. Measuring physiotherapy performance in patients with osteoarthritis of the knee: a prospective study. *BMC Health Serv Res* 2008; 8:145.
9. Walsh NE, Hurley MV. Evidence based guidelines and current practice for physiotherapy management of knee osteoarthritis. *Musculoskeletal Care* 2009; 7(1):45–56.
10. Holden MA, Foster NE, Mallen CD, et al. How do UK and Australian physiotherapists manage patients with hip osteoarthritis? Results of an international cross-sectional questionnaire. *Rheumatology* 2015; 54(Suppl 1):i112.
11. American Academy of Orthopaedic Surgeons. *Treatment of Osteoarthritis of the Knee*, 2nd ed. Rosemont, IL: American Academy of Orthopaedic Surgeons; 2013.
12. Cibulka MT, White DM, Woehrle J, et al. Hip pain and mobility deficits—hip osteoarthritis: clinical practice guidelines linked to the International Classification of Functioning, Disability, and Health from the Orthopaedic Section of the American Physical Therapy Association. *J Orthop Sports Phys Ther* 2009; 39(4):A1–25.
13. McAlindon TE, Bannuru RR, Sullivan MC, et al. OARSI guidelines for the non-surgical management of knee osteoarthritis. *Osteoarthritis Cartilage* 2014; 22(3):363–88.
14. Philadelphia Panel. Philadelphia Panel evidence-based clinical practice guidelines on selected rehabilitation interventions for knee pain. *Phys Ther* 2001; 81(10):1675–700.
15. Tuncer T, Çay HF, Kaçar C, et al. Evidence-based recommendations for the management of knee osteoarthritis: A consensus report of the Turkish League Against Rheumatism. *Turk J Rheumatol* 2012; 27(1):1–17.
16. Zhang W, Doherty M, Leeb BF, et al. EULAR evidence based recommendations for the management of hand osteoarthritis: report of a Task Force of the EULAR Standing Committee for International Clinical Studies Including Therapeutics (ESCISIT). *Ann Rheum Dis* 2007; 66(3):377–88.
17. Manara M, Bortoluzzi A, Favero M, et al. Italian Society for Rheumatology recommendations for the management of hand osteoarthritis. *Reumatismo* 2013; 65(4):167–85.
18. Peter WF, Jansen MJ, Hurkmans EJ, et al. Physiotherapy in hip and knee osteoarthritis: development of a practice guideline concerning initial assessment, treatment and evaluation. *Acta Reumatol Port* 2011; 36(3):268–81.

19. Fernandes L, Hagen KB, Bijlsma JW, et al. EULAR recommendations for the non-pharmacological core management of hip and knee osteoarthritis. *Ann Rheum Dis* 2013; 72(7):1125–35.

20. Brand C, Buchbinder R, Wluka A, et al. *Guideline for the Non-Surgical Management of Hip and Knee Osteoarthritis.* Melbourne: The Royal Australian College of General Practitioners; 2009.

21. Zhang W, Moskowitz RW, Nuki G, et al. OARSI recommendations for the management of hip and knee osteoarthritis, Part II: OARSI evidence-based, expert consensus guidelines. *Osteoarthritis Cartilage* 2008; 16(2):137–62.

22. Gélis A, Coudeyre E, Hudry C, et al. Is there an evidence-based efficacy for the use of foot orthotics in knee and hip osteoarthritis? Elaboration of French clinical practice guidelines. *Joint Bone Spine* 2008; 75(6):714–20.

23. Hochberg MC, Altman RD, April KT, et al. American College of Rheumatology 2012 recommendations for the use of nonpharmacologic and pharmacologic therapies in osteoarthritis of the hand, hip and knee. *Arthritis Care Res* 2012; 64(4):465–74.

24. Ottawa panel evidence-based clinical practice guidelines for therapeutic exercises and manual therapy in the management of osteoarthritis. *Phys Ther* 2005; 85(9):907–71.

25. Zhang W, Doherty M, Arden N, et al. EULAR evidence based recommendations for the management of hip osteoarthritis: report of a task force of the EULAR Standing Committee for International Clinical Studies Including Therapeutics (ESCISIT). *Ann Rheum Dis* 2005; 64(5):669–81.

26. Jordan KM, Arden NK, Doherty M, et al. EULAR Recommendations 2003: an evidence based approach to the management of knee osteoarthritis: Report of a Task Force of the Standing Committee for International Clinical Studies Including Therapeutic Trials (ESCISIT). *Ann Rheum Dis* 2003; 62(12):1145–55.

27. Pendleton A, Arden N, Dougados M, et al. EULAR recommendations for the management of knee osteoarthritis: report of a task force of the Standing Committee for International Clinical Studies Including Therapeutic Trials (ESCISIT). *Ann Rheum Dis* 2000; 59(12):936–44.

28. Dziedzic K, Nicholls E, Hill S, et al. Self-management approaches for osteoarthritis in the hand: a 2x2 factorial randomised trial. *Ann Rheum Dis* 2015; 74(1):108–18.

29. Paskins Z, Dziedzic K, Leeb B. *Osteoarthritis: Treatment.* [EULAR online course on rheumatic diseases] http://www.eular-onlinecourse.org/

30. Jones A, Silva PG, Silva AC, et al. Impact of cane use on pain, function, general health and energy expenditure during gait in patients with knee osteoarthritis: a randomised controlled trial. *Ann Rheum Dis* 2012; 71(2):172–9.

31. Moyer RF, Birmingham TB, Bryant DM, et al. Valgus bracing for knee osteoarthritis: a meta-analysis of randomised trials. *Arthritis Care Res* 2015; 67(4):493–501.

32. Parkes MJ, Maricar N, Lunt M, et al. Lateral wedge insoles as a conservative treatment for pain in patients with medial knee osteoarthritis: a meta-analysis. *JAMA* 2013; 310(7):722–30.

33. Hurley MV, Bearne LM. Non-exercise physical therapies for musculoskeletal conditions. *Best Pract Res Clin Rheumatol* 2008; 22(3):419–33.

34. Brosseau L, Younge KA, Robinson V, et al. Thermotherapy for treatment of osteoarthritis. *Cochrane Database Syst Rev* 2003; (4):CD004522.

35. Bialosky JE, Bishop MD, George SZ, Robinson ME. Placebo response to manual therapy: something or nothing? *J Man Manip Ther* 2011; 19(1):11–9.

36. Hengeveld E, Banks K. *Maitland's Peripheral Manipulation*, 4th ed. Edinburgh: Elsevier, Butterworth-Heinemann; 2005.

37. Deyle GD, Henderson NE, Matekel RL, et al. Effectiveness of manual physical therapy and exercise in osteoarthritis of the knee. A randomized, controlled trial. *Ann Intern Med* 2000; 132(3):173–81.

38. Deyle GD, Allison SC, Matekel RL, et al. Physical therapy treatment effectiveness for osteoarthritis of the knee: a randomized comparison of supervised clinical exercise and manual therapy procedures versus a home exercise program. *Phys Ther* 2005; 85(12):1301–17.

39. Bennell KL, Hinman RS, Metcalf BR, et al. Efficacy of physiotherapy management of knee joint osteoarthritis: a randomised, double blind, placebo controlled trial. *Ann Rheum Dis* 2005; 64(6):906–12.

40. Tucker M, Brantingham JW, Myburg C. The relative effectiveness of a non-steroidal anti-inflammatory medication (Meloxicam) versus manipulation in the treatment of osteo-arthritis of the knee. *Eur J Chiropr* 2003; 50(3):163–83.

41. Perlman AI, Sabina A, Williams AL, et al. Massage therapy for osteoarthritis of the knee: a randomized controlled trial. *Arch Intern Med* 2006; 166(22):2533–8.

42. Pollard H, Ward G, Hoskins W, Hardy K. The effect of a manual therapy knee protocol on osteoarthritic knee pain: a randomised controlled trial. *J Can Chiropr Assoc* 2008; 52(4):229–42.

43. Moss P, Sluka K, Wright A. The initial effects of knee joint mobilization on osteoarthritic hyperalgesia. *Man Ther* 2007; 12(2):109–18.

44. Hoeksma HL, Dekker J, Ronday HK, et al. Comparison of manual therapy and exercise therapy in osteoarthritis of the hip: a randomized clinical trial. *Arthritis Rheum* 2004; 51(5):722–9.

45. Vaarbakken K, Ljunggren AE. Superior effect of forceful compared with standard traction mobilizations in hip disability? *Adv Physiother* 2007; 9(3):117–28.

46. Cliborne AV, Wainner RS, Rhon DI, et al. Clinical hip tests and a functional squat test in patients with knee osteoarthritis: reliability, prevalence of positive test findings, and short-term response to hip mobilization. *J Orthop Sports Phys Ther* 2004; 34(11):676–85.

47. MacDonald CW, Whitman JM, Cleland JA, et al. Clinical outcomes following manual physical therapy and exercise for hip osteoarthritis: a case series. *J Orthop Sports Phys Ther* 2006; 36(8):588–99.

48. Abbott JH, Robertson MC, Chapple C, et al. Manual therapy, exercise therapy, or both, in addition to usual care, for osteoarthritis of the hip or knee: a randomized controlled trial. 1: clinical effectiveness. *Osteoarthritis Cartilage* 2013; 21(4):525–34.

49. Bennell KL, Egerton T, Martin J, et al. Effect of physical therapy on pain and function in patients with hip osteoarthritis: a randomized clinical trial. *JAMA* 2014; 311(19):1987–97.

50. Manheimer E, Cheng K, Linde K, et al. Acupuncture for peripheral joint osteoarthritis. *Cochrane Database Syst Rev* 2010; 1:CD001977.

51. Vickers AJ, Cronin AM, Maschino AC, et al. Acupuncture for chronic pain: individual patient data meta-analysis. *Arch Intern Med* 2012; 172(19):1444–53.

52. Corbett MS, Rice SJ, Madurasinghe V, et al. Acupuncture and other physical treatments for the relief of pain due to osteoarthritis of the knee: network meta-analysis. *Osteoarthritis Cartilage* 2013; 21(9):1290–8.

53. Watson T. Current concepts in electrotherapy. *Haemophilia* 2002; 8(3):413–8.

54. Low J, Reed A. *Electrotherapy Explained: Principles and Practice.* Oxford: Butterworth-Heinemann; 2000.

55. Melzack R, Wall PD. Pain mechanisms: a new theory. *Science* 1965; 150(3699):971–9.

56. Walsh D. *TENS Clinical Applications and Related Theory.* New York: Churchill Livingstone; 1997.

57. Rutjes AW, Nüesch E, Sterchi R, et al. Transcutaneous electrostimulation for osteoarthritis of the knee. *Cochrane Database Syst Rev* 2009; 4:CD002823.

58. Hartley A. *Therapeutic Ultrasound*, 2nd ed. Etobicoke, ON: Anne Hartley Agency; 1993.

59. Nelson RM, Hayes KW, Currier DP. *Clinical Electrotherapy*, 3rd ed. Stamford, CT: Appleton & Lange; 1999.

60. Baker KG, Robertson VJ, Duck FA. A review of therapeutic ultrasound: biophysical effects. *Phys Ther* 2001; 81(7):1351–8.

61. Rand SE, Goerlich C, Marchand K, Jablecki N. The physical therapy prescription. *Am Fam Physician* 2007; 76(11):1661–6.

62. Rutjes AW, Nüesch E, Sterchi R, Jüni P. Therapeutic ultrasound for osteoarthritis of the knee or hip. *Cochrane Database Syst Rev* 2010; 1:CD003132.

63. Loyola-Sánchez A, Richardson J, MacIntyre NJ. Efficacy of ultrasound therapy for the management of knee osteoarthritis: a systematic review with meta-analysis. *Osteoarthritis Cartilage* 2010; 18(9):1117–26.

64. Falagas ME, Zarkadoulia E, Rafailidis PI. The therapeutic effect of balneotherapy: evaluation of the evidence from randomised controlled trials. *Int J Clin Pract* 2009; 63(7):1068–84.

65. Verhagen AP, Bierma-Zeinstra SMA, Cardoso JR, et al. Balneotherapy for rheumatoid arthritis. *Cochrane Database Syst Rev* 2003; 4:CD000518.

66. Harzy T, Ghani N, Akasbi N, et al. Short- and long-term therapeutic effects of thermal mineral waters in knee osteoarthritis: a systematic review of randomized controlled trials. *Clin Rheumatol* 2009; 28(5):501–7.

67. Horváth K, Kulisch Á, Németh A, Bender T. Evaluation of the effect of balneotherapy in patients with osteoarthritis of the hands: a randomized controlled single-blind follow-up study. *Clin Rehabil* 2012; 26(5):431–41.

68. Brown CS, Ling FW, Wan JY, Pilla AA. Efficacy of static magnetic field therapy in chronic pelvic pain: a double-blind pilot study. *Am J Obstet Gynecol* 2002; 187(6):1581–7.

69. Harlow T, Greaves C, White A, et al. Randomised controlled trial of magnetic bracelets for relieving pain in osteoarthritis of the hip and knee. *BMJ* 2004; 329(7480):1450–4.

70. Michalsen A, Klotz S, Lüdtke R, et al. Effectiveness of leech therapy in osteoarthritis of the knee: a randomized, controlled trial. *Ann Intern Med* 2003; 139(9):724–30.

CHAPTER 27

Placebo, nocebo, and contextual effects

Abhishek Abhishek and Michael Doherty

Introduction

Placebo effect has been a topic of scientific and clinical interest for many decades. However, the use of placebos to treat patients antedates the development of modern medicine. In the Middle Ages and later years, placebo (Latin: 'I shall please') was regarded as anything given to make people believe that they were being treated, and to induce a sense of reassurance and well-being [1,2]. For example, the revised Quincy's *Lexicon Medicum* (*c*.early 1800s) defined placebo as 'an epithet given to any medicine adapted more to please than to benefit the patient' [2]. When effective drugs and other treatments began to be developed in the first half of the twentieth century, recognition of the benefits that patients receive from placebo led to inclusion of placebo arms in randomized controlled trials (RCTs) to account for non-specific contextual responses and to determine the specific 'true' effect of the treatment under study. Another reason to include a placebo in RCTs is to account for other factors such as natural fluctuation in disease severity, regression to the mean, and spontaneous disease remission. However, it was Beecher in 1955 who first drew attention to the magnitude of improvement seen with placebo treatment in clinical trials. In a landmark paper entitled 'The powerful placebo' [4] he reviewed 15 RCTs and concluded that 35% of patients in the placebo arm of these studies had significant clinical improvements in their symptoms. This and other observations subsequently catalysed research into placebo and its biological effects.

In the current biomedical model, placebo is regarded as any inert substance or sham procedure that does not have a direct effect on the disease process and therefore is not expected to directly influence its manifestations. The placebo response can be defined as the improvement in symptoms on unknowingly receiving an inert and non-therapeutic intervention in the place of an active treatment. It can be observed in placebo-controlled RCTs as the improvement in symptoms from baseline in the control arm of the trial [3] (Figure 27.1), and results from both non-specific effects, such as the Hawthorne effect (behaviour change while being observed) [5], and from more specific effects related to the treatment, such as the mode of delivery. Some factors that influence placebo response are person-specific, such as conditioning from previous experiences, illness perceptions, and expectation of improvement, whereas others are more dependent on the context in which the treatment is received, such as the therapeutic ritual, the setting (a positive or negative environment), and the patient–practitioner interaction. Confirmation that improvements on placebo are a true placebo response can be obtained by comparing the difference in outcome

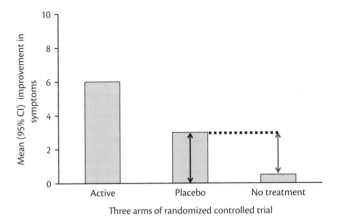

Figure 27.1 Placebo response and placebo effect. Placebo response (black line with arrowheads) is the improvement in symptoms in those treated surreptitiously with placebo in a blinded randomized controlled trial (RCT). Placebo effect (red line with arrowheads) is the difference in improvement in those treated with placebo and those who have had no treatment, and cannot be measured in traditional two-arm RCTs.

with a no-treatment (observation only) group in a three-arm RCT (Figure 27.1), and in some other study designs (see later).

Nocebo (Latin: 'I shall harm') is the opposite of placebo, and was introduced in the 1960s to distinguish the noxious from the pleasing effect of placebo [6]. Therefore, nocebo response can be regarded as the beginning of new symptoms or worsening of pre-existing symptoms caused by negative expectations on the part of the patient and/or negative verbal and non-verbal communications on the part of the treating person without any sham treatment [7]. In clinical practice, this most commonly refers to adverse effects generated by negative expectations that medical treatment will likely cause harm instead of healing [8]. Similarly, patients' expectation that symptoms will worsen, or affect other organ systems is also a form of nocebo response. Nocebo effect is similar to nocebo response but occurs during sham treatment or as a result of deliberate suggestion and/or negative expectations [7].

Study designs used to examine placebo and nocebo responses

The magnitude of placebo and nocebo responses can be examined in traditional RCTs that assume an additive model, that is, the

Box 27.1 Experimental study designs designed to investigate the placebo response

Balanced placebo design

Half the study participants receive active drug, while the other half receive a placebo.[1] Half of the participants in each group are given the correct information while the other half are given incorrect information about the intervention received. This allows the researchers to measure true drug response (measured in those who received a drug but were told that they received placebo), and true placebo response (measured in those who received a placebo but were told they received a drug) [3].

Half-balanced placebo design

All study participants receive a placebo.[1] Half told that they received an active drug while the other half told that they received a placebo. This design allows the researchers to measure the true placebo response [3].

Balanced cross-over design

All study participants are divided into four groups and told that they will receive active drug and placebo at different time points in a study without knowing the sequence. However, group 1 receives active drug at both time points, group 2 receives active drug and placebo, group 3 receives placebo and active drug, and group 4 receives placebo at both time points. The lowest mean improvement in group 1 reflects true drug response while the highest mean improvement in group 4 reflects the true placebo response.

[1]These study designs require deception of the subjects, and of the researchers in the half-balanced placebo design. For details please see the review by Enck et al. [3].

Box 27.2 Key facts: placebo response in OA

Placebo response in OA:

◆ Improves subjective outcomes such as pain and stiffness
◆ Improves function and mobility
◆ Does not affect objective outcomes such as range of movement or structural progression.

The ES of placebo analgesia is greater than that due to the specific effect of most treatments, including NSAIDs

The ES of placebo analgesia is highest in hand OA, then knee OA, and lowest in hip OA.

overall beneficial effect is equal to the specific treatment response plus the placebo response, though this may not always hold true. Non-additive models of placebo and drug response can be assessed in deception studies, for example, using a balanced placebo design, half-balanced placebo design, and balanced crossover design (Box 27.1) [3]. However, these are difficult to perform on patients due to ethical reasons, require blinding of the observer, and are incompatible with rules of informed consent unless the patient authorizes deception, that is, agrees to be deceived in some part of the study. Placebo response can also be studied in hidden treatment designs in patients with acute pain, or Parkinsonism when the timing of administration of the treatment is not disclosed [3]. To the best of our knowledge, neither a deception study nor a hidden treatment study has been carried out in patients with osteoarthritis (OA).

Evidence for the existence of placebo response in osteoarthritis

The occurrence and magnitude of placebo response in patients with OA was convincingly demonstrated in a systematic review of RCTs by Zhang et al., published in 2008 [5]. This review included 198 OA RCTs, and synthesized data from 193 placebo (16 364 patients) and 14 untreated groups (1167 patients).

This study demonstrated that pain is the most placebo responsive of all the symptoms in OA (Box 27.2) with an overall effect size (95% confidence interval) (ES (95% CI)) of 0.51 (0.46–0.55) [5]. In the three trials where active treatment, placebo, and no-treatment arms were all present, the ES of placebo analgesia was significantly greater than that of no treatment (ES (95% CI) 0.77 (0.65–0.89) vs −0.08 (−0.65–0.48)). This confirms that placebo analgesia in OA occurs due to placebo effect and is not merely explained by other factors such as natural variation in disease severity and regression to the mean.

In this study [5], placebo response was also observed for other subjective outcomes such as joint stiffness (ES (95% CI) 0.43 (0.38–0.49)), self-reported function (0.49 (0.44–0.54)), and physician's global assessment (0.66 (0.53–0.78)). However, there was no evidence of placebo response for certain objective clinical measures of OA such as quadriceps strength, range of motion, and knee circumference and placebo was unable to slow down radiographic progression in terms of joint space narrowing. However, for some objective measures such as timed walking distance that need both analgesia and patients' cooperation, placebo had an intermediate ES (95% CI) of 0.22 (0.08–0.35) compared to that for pain relief in the same studies ES (95% CI) 0.51 (0.36–0.65). This suggests that the contextual factors associated with any treatment for OA have an effect that improves symptoms of OA and can enhance physical performance, but do not influence objective markers of structural change and disease progression.

This systematic review also reported factors that influence the magnitude of placebo response. For example, a greater degree of placebo analgesia is reported in studies that induce a higher degree of expectancy of improvement, for example, by not allowing the use of a rescue medication (implying the study drug is a strong treatment) and when a treatment is being used for the first time ('new is better than old'). Similarly, the mode of delivery makes a difference, the ES being highest for injections, particularly serial injections (ES 0.63 (0.15–1.12)), then topical applications, and lowest for oral systemic medications. Greater placebo response also occurs when the patient has a higher degree of baseline pain [5]. Furthermore, OA at different sites appears to show different responsiveness, the mean ES for placebo pain reduction being 0.8 (95% CI 0.65–0.96) for hand OA, 0.54 (0.49–0.60), for knee OA and 0.37 (0.21–0.53) for hip OA [5].

Placebo analgesia is not restricted to OA. Three systematic reviews and meta-analyses that included RCTs of a variety of diseases confirmed that placebo analgesia occurs in other conditions as well, although the ES was lower in these studies (−0.27 to −0.28) than in OA, suggesting that the magnitude of placebo response to pain varies from condition to condition [9–11]. Another systematic review that synthesized data from three-arm RCTs included in a previous Cochrane review reported that placebo effect (ES (95% CI) −0.59 (−0.90 to −0.27)) was not significantly different from treatment effect (−1.47 (−2.34 to −0.61)) in providing pain relief in a variety of conditions [12]. Thus, placebo response should be optimized when treating patients with chronic painful conditions like OA. The strategies to enhance placebo response are discussed later in this chapter.

Although placebo response due to prior conditioning with a drug may induce immunosuppression and influence hormone secretion [13–17], most of the evidence suggests that placebo effect does not affect laboratory parameters or objective markers of disease activity [9–11]. This is especially true for placebo response induced by verbal suggestion. Overall, these studies suggest that the context in which a treatment is given does not generally affect the pathophysiology of the disease, but has a significant effect on its symptoms, especially when the main symptom is pain. However, such improvement in symptoms is of great utility in the management of chronic painful conditions like OA, where most treatments only have a mild to moderate effect [18].

Evidence for nocebo response

Clinical experience suggests that nocebo response is common in patients with OA. However, this has not been examined formally in a systematic review of the published literature. Nevertheless, illness perceptions of OA are often negative due to its recognized chronic persistent nature, multiple unsatisfactory healthcare consultations, and the absence of an effective disease-modifying drug [19]. Consequently, patients with OA often have low expectancy of improvement and commonly do not adhere to modestly effective analgesics, and may not have a high incentive to exercise or lose weight. As a result, both the patient and the healthcare practitioner may adopt a pessimistic view of OA ('Nothing can be done', 'What do you expect anyway when you get older?'), and believe that gradual worsening of symptoms will be the norm. Therefore, any consultation adopts negative connotations, and the patient disengages from their family doctor, and also from other services like physiotherapy, occupational therapy, pain management, and weight loss programmes, which have the ability of making a meaningful difference to their long-term health outcome and quality of life. This is a typical self-perpetuating state which is common in patients with OA, where negative belief about OA is perpetuated by patients' own experiences, and also by their interaction with healthcare professionals. Such low expectancy may reduce their response to treatments, including total joint replacement [20].

Certainly, most guidelines on OA management reinforce the negative treatment expectancy. As in RCT reporting, the main focus is on the separation of active treatment from placebo (this is the basis of the ES calculation) and only those treatments that separate by a minimum clinically important difference are recommended by bodies such as the National Institute for Health and Care Excellence (NICE). Such a perspective, however, removes attention from the fact that the placebo group in RCTs usually do very well, and that the overall treatment effect (specific plus placebo) is often in the strong effect range of ES. This gives rise to the

'efficacy paradox' where clinicians are requested not to use certain treatments, such as acupuncture, because they hardly separate from sham acupuncture in RCTs and are deemed to have only 'weak treatment effects', whereas in clinical practice patients often derive great benefit. A shift in emphasis in RCT reports towards the overall treatment effect, and then explaining how much of that may be explained by placebo/contextual response (the 'proportional contextual response or') would help lessen the paradox [21], lead to a different hierarchy of 'strong treatments' for OA, and might lead to alterations in guideline recommendations (see Chapter 37 for further discussion of this).

Nocebo response is primarily driven by expectation of harm. In a systematic review that included 16 RCTs of pharmacological agents for fibromyalgia, nocebo response (adverse effects in placebo arm) was common, occurring in over two-thirds of the patients, and was responsible for approximately 10% of the patients dropping out from the study in the placebo arm [8]. The frequency of adverse events and dropouts because of intolerance in placebo arms correlated strongly with the corresponding frequencies in the active arms (weighted Pearson correlation 0.88, 0.92 respectively), suggesting that nocebo response was driven by expectation of harm which in turn was derived from pre-trial suggestion. This view is further supported by the fact that the five most common adverse events reported by placebo-treated patients in each study were comparable with the five most often adverse events reported by active drug-treated patients, and most of them were related to the specific drug under trial [8]. Further analysis carried out by the authors suggests that younger people, and those with depression, are more likely to have a nocebo response in fibromyalgia. It is possible that the nocebo response rates observed in patients with fibromyalgia may be higher than in patients with OA due to a higher prevalence of anxiety, depression, and other somatoform disorders but certainly this merits formal study in OA.

Mechanism of placebo and nocebo effects

Placebo and nocebo effects are learned cognitive responses. Placebo analgesia and painful nocebo responses are the best studied placebo and nocebo effects. Placebo effects are induced by a combination of verbal suggestion, conditioned response, prior experiences, observational and social learning, and expectation of improvement [22]. For instance, positive verbal suggestion about the treatment received reduced the need for buprenorphine in postoperative thoracotomy patients, and improved visceral pain in irritable bowel syndrome [22]. Conversely verbal suggestion can also induce a nocebo response. For example, healthy volunteers experience more pain when they are told that they are receiving a hyperalgesic medicine [22]. Pavlovian conditioned responses, where an innocuous stimulus is presented with an active intervention, and then the innocuous stimulus is presented alone, result in an improvement in pain perception in animal studies, and with immunosuppression treatment, and humoral changes in human studies [22]. Previous experience of efficacy also determines the magnitude of the placebo response. Participants made to believe that they have received a strong pain killer for an experimental pain stimulus (by reducing the intensity of the painful stimulus), show a greater placebo response, while those made to believe that they have received a weak pain killer (by increasing the intensity of the painful stimulus) show a very weak placebo response [22]. Similarly, observing pain relief in others in a social context also provides placebo analgesia. Expectation of improvement which is a summary of all the effects described above is responsible for placebo response. Finally, reward mechanisms are also activated during placebo response [23].

Neuroanatomical basis

Areas of the brain involved in short-term memory (hippocampus, parahippocampal gyrus), long-term memory (superior temporal gyrus), and in semantics/linguistic processing (angular gyrus) are activated in verbal suggestion mediated placebo response [24]. Verbally-induced placebo response also requires activation of the frontal lobe. For example, both experimentally induced frontal lobe disconnection (by transcranial magnetic stimulation), or that due to Alzheimer's disease results in loss of verbally induced placebo responses [25,26]. Regions of the frontal lobe such as the rostral anterior cingulate cortex (RACC—a cognitive emotional integrative region), dorsolateral prefrontal cortex, and orbitofrontal cortex are activated during the anticipatory phases of placebo response [27–30]. This cortical activation stimulates subcortical anti-nociceptive networks such as the periaqueductal grey (PAG) and amygdala [31–33], which in turn increase the activity within the descending pain modulatory pathway [27,31] and reduce activity in the nociceptive pain processing pathways in the dorsal horn of the spinal cord [34]. Neural activity in parts of the brain involved in pain transmission (e.g. thalamus, anterior insula, and caudal RACC) are decreased during placebo analgesia [30]. Deeper parts of the cortex, such as the nucleus accumbens (involved in the reward mechanism) and parts of the insula are also activated during placebo analgesia [29]. These findings were recently confirmed for the first time in patients with OA, showing that placebo reduces brain activation in three core regions of the pain-processing network (supramarginal gyrus, frontal lateral region, thalamus) and extended its effects towards the medial frontal region, the hippocampus, and the cerebellum [35].

Nocebo response occurs due to activation of an affective cognitive pain pathway [36]. Parts of the brain involved in memory, affect, and emotional cognition processing are activated as in states of placebo analgesia. The ACC, insula, left orbital frontal cortex, and right lateral prefrontal cortex, which form the medial system of the pain matrix, are activated during nocebo states. Apart from this, the left hippocampus which encodes relation between various learning context cues and mediates the affective characteristics of pain is also activated in nocebo states [36].

Neurochemical mechanisms

The neurochemical basis of placebo and nocebo response has been elucidated over the last 40 years. Several studies suggest that endogenous opioids (predominantly acting via their μ-receptors) play a key role in placebo analgesia. For example, the synapses between RACC, and the subcortical anti-nociceptive network comprised of PAG, amygdala, and rostral ventromedial medulla, and that between the subcortical anti-nociceptive network and the dorsal horn in the spinal cord are rich in opiate receptors [31–33]. Moreover, the administration of placebo reduces the binding of a μ-opioid receptor selective radiotracer [11C] carfentalin to the available μ-opioid receptors in an in vivo PET study (suggesting endogenous opioid release in response to placebo presented as active treatment), and this reduction in binding correlated with placebo analgesia [27]. Additionally, an opiate antagonist naloxone completely blocks the

placebo response induced by verbal suggestion with or without an additional conditioning procedure in tooth extraction and ischaemic arm models of pain [37,38]. Similarly, placebo-induced reduction in minute respiratory volume, and heart rate is also blocked by naloxone [39,40]. However, not all placebo analgesia is mediated by opiates. For example, placebo analgesia produced by prior conditioning with ketorolac, a non-steroidal anti-inflammatory drug (NSAID), is not blocked by naloxone, suggesting that placebo response is not exclusively mediated by opiates [38].

Dopamine is the other recognized mediator of placebo analgesia. Increased dopaminergic and opiate activity occurs simultaneously during states of heightened placebo analgesia [29]. Dopamine release also mediates the motor placebo response in Parkinson's disease, and is implicated in reward mechanisms [23]. The fact that dopamine plays a key role in mediating placebo analgesia is supported by the fact that people who metabolize dopamine slowly have a greater susceptibility to placebo response. For example, irritable bowel syndrome patients with Met/Met polymorphism in the catechol-O-methyl-transferase gene which results in slow dopamine breakdown have a greater placebo response than those with Val/Val polymorphism, whereas those with Val/Met polymorphism have an intermediate placebo response to augmented sham acupuncture [41]. This suggests that constitutional interpersonal variation in pain physiology, influenced in part by genetic factors, may influence placebo analgesia.

It is possible that placebo may also have a peripheral anti-inflammatory effect in joints with OA [42]. In a small cross-over pilot study where patients with knee OA were randomized to receive intra-articular injection of corticosteroid or saline in a sequential manner, the administration of placebo (saline injection) associated with a reduction in maximal synovial hypertrophy on ultrasound imaging. This could result from involvement of the hypothalamic–pituitary axis in descending pain inhibition and be analogous to the peripheral leucocyte effects demonstrated by placebo following conditioning with cyclophosphamide and ciclosporin [14,15,17]. Certainly this interesting finding merits further study.

Nocebo response occurs due to a reduction in opiate and dopaminergic activity [29], but also due to an increase in cholecystokinin-mediated neural activity [43]. This is supported by the observation that proglumide, a cholecystokinin antagonist, enhances placebo analgesia and blocks the hyperalgesic nocebo response [43,44]. In summary, neural pathways with opiates, dopamine, and cholecystokinin are involved in the generation of placebo and nocebo responses.

Evidence for placebo effects in other conditions

Placebo response also occurs in fibromyalgia, a common condition and co-morbidity especially in older women [45]. In a meta-analysis that synthesized data from 72 placebo-controlled RCTs in 9827 patients with fibromyalgia, the pooled ES (95% CI) on pain in the placebo group was 0.42 (0.35–0.49), while that in the treatment group was 0.82 (0.72–0.92) [46]. Based on this, the authors suggest that the 45% improvement in the active drug group could be attributed to placebo response based on the assumption that active drug effect and placebo response summate to give the total improvement in symptoms [46]. Just as has been observed in OA, the magnitude of placebo analgesia was greater in trials with higher baseline pain and in those with higher treatment ES, supporting the view that placebo response occurs at least in part due to expectancy [46]. Similarly, although the evidence is not as strong as that in the case of OA and fibromyalgia, placebo response also occurs in the treatment of chronic low back pain [47].

Conditioned immunosuppression

Placebo response due to Pavlovian conditioning but not due to verbal suggestion affects hormone secretion. For example, prior conditioning with sumatriptan (a 5-HT1B/1D agonist) but not prior verbal suggestion resulted in secretion of growth hormone and reduced secretion of cortisol in response to placebo [13]. Moreover, the placebo response was unaffected by verbal suggestion [13]. In classic conditioning studies, with simultaneous administration of flavoured syrup and immunosuppressants such as cyclophosphamide [15] or ciclosporin [14,17], the subsequent administration of the syrup alone produced immunosuppressive effects such as reduced leucocyte count [15], reduced cytokine secretion and proliferation [14], and impaired T-lymphocyte function [17].

Predictors of placebo and nocebo contextual response

In order to use contextual response in clinical practice it is important to understand its predictors. These have been reviewed previously [48], and are outlined in the following subsections.

Consultation/physician factors

The patient–practitioner interaction is an important determinant of patient-centred outcomes. A warm and attentive consultation where the physician undertakes a thorough assessment, appears confident and certain about the treatment, and suggests a good prognosis enhances patient improvement. Conversely, a negative interaction with the practitioner can worsen pain. It is interesting that the clinician's subconscious pessimism or optimism about the treatment can influence outcome even when not explicitly stated. As expected, a physician perceived as being an experienced practitioner, and one who wishes to see the patient again to monitor progress enhances contextual response.

Patient factors

The patient's expectation of improvement from a treatment is an important determinant of response. Expectancy is influenced by constitutional features of the patient but also by information given by the healthcare professional, and the patient's perception from observing others, including in a social context. For example, news items in the popular media may influence the patient's expectation of improvement. Similarly, mere knowledge of being treated can improve outcomes. Such a response usually has an earlier onset of action, and may be the reason why some patients with arthritis report an almost immediate improvement in symptoms on receiving joint injections, just as the rapid analgesia with parenteral opioid is largely contextual [49].

Personality traits such as optimism, pessimism (catastrophizing), anxiety, and neuroticism also influence the placebo response [50]. Those with state anxiety ('situational anxiety') are more likely to have placebo response, but not those with trait anxiety ('habitually anxious') [50]. This is because state anxiety reflects responsiveness to the context, and therefore may be easily affected, whereas trait anxiety, an intrinsic personality trait, may be more difficult to affect by changes in the context [50]. As expected, optimists are more likely to be placebo responsive while pessimists are more likely to be influenced by negative expectations.

Treatment factors

In general, the more invasive and frequently administered an intervention, the higher is the placebo effect. For example, sham arthroscopy in the context of OA is associated with the same high rate of symptom improvement as with actual treatments [51]. Indeed a recent systematic review of RCTs of various surgical procedures that included sham showed that in half of these sham was as good as the actual procedure [52]. Placebo response is also enhanced by treatment with medicine from a reputable brand. Similarly, knowledge that the treatment is expensive or new also enhances the placebo response. Treatment that involves administration of a greater number of tablets associates with a greater placebo response. The colour of tablets may also have additional effects. For example, blue or green placebo pills believed to be sedatives have a greater sedative effect than red pills, conversely red or orange placebo pills believed to be stimulants generally have a greater stimulant effect than blue pills [49]. The pharmaceutical industry are aware of these influences and often specifically select colour and packaging to complement the action of the medication.

Predictors of nocebo response

Just as with placebo response, nocebo response is driven by patients' beliefs, expectations, their psychological make-up, and by any external influences [53]. For example, patients who expect side effects, or have been conditioned by side effects from previous drugs are more likely to report nocebo responses. Similarly, certain psychological characteristics such as anxiety, depression, tendency to somatize and to amplify symptoms associate with nocebo response [53]. Negative patient–practitioner interaction, and a nihilistic consultation, (e.g. 'Nothing can be done', 'The pain will get worse slowly') can further enhance the nocebo response. Such negative information also may be derived from observing others in society or from the media [53].

Implications for clinical practice

Healthcare professionals managing patients with OA should try to optimize contextual effects to enhance positive outcomes and minimize unduly negative responses, whilst maintaining professional standards and honesty (Box 27.3). This is particularly important in OA since the contextual response to a treatment is usually greater than the additional specific effect of the treatment. For example, the ES of placebo analgesia in OA RCTs (0.5–0.7) is far greater than that of oral analgesics and NSAIDs (0.2–0.3) and even intra-articular steroid injection has a significant proportion (c.50%) of contextual effect [5].

Clearly it is unethical to intentionally deceive any patient by giving them an inert placebo with no expected specific effect. Equally it is unethical and inappropriate to select invasive or expensive treatments purely because of their high contextual effects in patients with OA. However, several simple steps, which reflect recommended best practice, can be taken to optimize the contextual response when an appropriate treatment that is recommended for OA is being administered [18]. To begin with, the consultation

---

Box 27.3 Top tips to enhance placebo response in OA

- Positive, professional, unhurried consultation
- A full, holistic patient assessment (both history and examination)
- Enquire about illness perceptions and discuss patient concerns
- Individualized education concerning OA (nature, outcome, treatment options)
- Involve patient in management decisions
- Realistic optimism about treatment benefits
- State the wish to see the patient again—arrange specific follow-up.

---

should be conducted in a professional, reassuring, and unhurried manner. The patient should be assessed thoroughly, by interview and examination. The patient's perceptions about their condition should be explored and any negative attitudes or concerns discussed and addressed in a positive manner. Similarly, psychological predictors of nocebo response such as depression, anxiety, and somatization, should be specifically elicited and addressed appropriately. The patient should be fully educated about OA in an individualized manner, and then involved in management decisions. The healthcare professional should show confidence in the treatment they are giving and emphasize the positive effects that these interventions can have on current symptoms of OA and, if appropriate, on longer-term outcomes. For example, when managing an overweight patient with knee OA the short- and long-term beneficial effects of weight loss, exercise, and safe analgesics such as topical NSAIDs should be emphasized. In summary, the healthcare professional should provide a positive consultation, assess the patient in a thorough and holistic way, provide full information and involve the patient in management decisions, and show realistic confidence in the management plan. In addition, follow-up should be arranged, ideally but not necessarily with the same health professional, to monitor the patient's progress and to adjust the management plan if required. Thus, contextual response in OA should be recognized and optimized to improve patient-centred outcomes such as pain, function, participation, and quality of life.

Some professionals do all of this intuitively or because they received an enlightened education or learnt this practice from observing role models. Unfortunately, however, when audited it appears that many aspects of the patient–practitioner encounter in clinical practice are often suboptimal, especially with respect to doctors [54]. Common complaints from patients are that the doctor was too busy to fully explain things or to address their concerns; the doctor did not examine them very thoroughly, or did not examine them at all; and the doctor did not want to see them again. Of course, most doctors do feel pressured with respect to time and would often wish to have longer with the patient and to offer personalized follow-up. Time, however, is money. Nevertheless, although there are no data on this for OA, it seems likely that investing more time with patients to assess and support them more thoroughly, especially in the first few consultations for OA, may prove cost-effective in the long term if it leads to better understanding of OA, better motivation and adherence to self-management

(e.g. exercise, weight loss if overweight), and subsequently improved patient-centred outcomes.

In conclusion, just as placebo and nocebo responses occur in RCTs, contextual response is an integral part of any treatment for OA and occurs with every patient–practitioner encounter. A significant proportion of any treatment is due to contextual response and health professionals need to be aware that their approach to the patient that they are treating can improve or worsen the patient's symptoms and outcomes. In a chronic condition such as OA for which there are no 'cures', optimizing the contextual response is key to any successful management plan. Many aspects of recommended best practice will enhance a positive contextual response. Although this may require more time form the practitioner, the subsequent increased improvement in patient outcomes should be the overriding consideration.

References

1. Finniss DG, Benedetti F. Mechanisms of the placebo response and their impact on clinical trials and clinical practice. *Pain* 2005; 114(1–2):3–6.
2. de Craen AJ, Kaptchuk TJ, Tijssen JG, Kleijnen J. Placebos and placebo effects in medicine: historical overview. *J R Soc Med* 1999; 92(10):511–5.
3. Enck P, Klosterhalfen S, Zipfel S. Novel study designs to investigate the placebo response. *BMC Med Res Methodol* 2011; 11:90.
4. Beecher HK. The powerful placebo. *JAMA* 1955; 159(17):1602–6.
5. Zhang W, Robertson J, Jones AC, Dieppe PA, Doherty M. The placebo effect and its determinants in osteoarthritis: meta-analysis of randomised controlled trials. *Ann Rheum Dis* 2008; 67(12):1716–23.
6. Kennedy WP. The nocebo reaction. *Med World* 1961; 95:203–5.
7. Hauser W, Hansen E, Enck P. Nocebo phenomena in medicine: their relevance in everyday clinical practice. *Dtsch Arztebl Int* 2012; 109(26):459–65.
8. Mitsikostas DD, Chalarakis NG, Mantonakis LI, Delicha EM, Sfikakis PP. Nocebo in fibromyalgia: meta-analysis of placebo-controlled clinical trials and implications for practice. *Eur J Neurol* 2012; 19(5):672–80.
9. Hrobjartsson A, Gotzsche PC. Is the placebo powerless? An analysis of clinical trials comparing placebo with no treatment. *N Engl J Med* 2001; 344(21):1594–602.
10. Hrobjartsson A, Gotzsche PC. Placebo interventions for all clinical conditions. *Cochrane Database Syst Rev* 2010; 1:CD003974.
11. Hrobjartsson A, Gotzsche PC. Is the placebo powerless? Update of a systematic review with 52 new randomized trials comparing placebo with no treatment. *J Intern Med* 2004; 256(2):91–100.
12. Howick J, Friedemann C, Tsakok M, et al. Are treatments more effective than placebos? A systematic review and meta-analysis. *PloS One* 2013; 8(5):e62599.
13. Benedetti F, Pollo A, Lopiano L, et al. Conscious expectation and unconscious conditioning in analgesic, motor, and hormonal placebo/nocebo responses. *J Neurosci* 2003; 23(10):4315–23.
14. Goebel MU, Trebst AE, Steiner J, et al. Behavioral conditioning of immunosuppression is possible in humans. *FASEB J* 2002; 16(14):1869–73.
15. Giang DW, Goodman AD, Schiffer RB, et al. Conditioning of cyclophosphamide-induced leukopenia in humans. *J Neuropsychiatry Clin Neurosci* 1996; 8(2):194–201.
16. Meissner K, Distel H, Mitzdorf U. Evidence for placebo effects on physical but not on biochemical outcome parameters: a review of clinical trials. *BMC Med* 2007; 5:3.
17. Albring A, Wendt L, Benson S, et al. Preserving learned immunosuppressive placebo response: perspectives for clinical application. *Clin Pharmacol Ther* 2014; 96(2):247–55.
18. NICE, Royal College of Physicians Guidelines on Osteoarthritis. *Osteoarthritis—National Clinical Guideline for Care and Management in Adults.* London: NICE, 2008.

19. Bijsterbosch J, Scharloo M, Visser AW, et al. Illness perceptions in patients with osteoarthritis: change over time and association with disability. *Arthritis Rheum* 2009; 61(8):1054–61.

20. Judge A, Cooper C, Arden NK, et al. Pre-operative expectation predicts 12-month post-operative outcome among patients undergoing primary total hip replacement in European orthopaedic centres. *Osteoarthritis Cartilage* 2011; 19(6):659–67.

21. Zou K. *The Proportion of Contextual Effect of Treatments in Osteoarthritis: Systematic Reviews and Meta-analyses of Randomised Controlled Trials.* PhD thesis, University of Nottingham. 2015.

22. Colloca L, Miller FG. How placebo responses are formed: a learning perspective. *Philos Trans R Soc Lond B Biol Sci* 2011; 366(1572):1859–69.

23. Scott DJ, Stohler CS, Egnatuk CM, et al. Individual differences in reward responding explain placebo-induced expectations and effects. *Neuron* 2007; 55(2):325–36.

24. Craggs JG, Price DD, Robinson ME. Enhancing the placebo response: functional magnetic resonance imaging evidence of memory and semantic processing in placebo analgesia. *J Pain* 2014; 15(4):435–46.

25. Krummenacher P, Candia V, Folkers G, Schedlowski M, Schonbachler G. Prefrontal cortex modulates placebo analgesia. *Pain* 2010; 148(3):368–74.

26. Benedetti F, Arduino C, Costa S, et al. Loss of expectation-related mechanisms in Alzheimer's disease makes analgesic therapies less effective. *Pain* 2006; 121(1–2):133–44.

27. Zubieta JK, Bueller JA, Jackson LR, et al. Placebo effects mediated by endogenous opioid activity on mu-opioid receptors. *J Neurosci* 2005; 25(34):7754–62.

28. Petrovic P, Kalso E, Petersson KM, Ingvar M. Placebo and opioid analgesia–imaging a shared neuronal network. *Science* 2002; 295(5560):1737–40.

29. Scott DJ, Stohler CS, Egnatuk CM, et al. Placebo and nocebo effects are defined by opposite opioid and dopaminergic responses. *Arch Gen Psychiatry* 2008; 65(2):220–31.

30. Wager TD, Rilling JK, Smith EE, et al. Placebo-induced changes in FMRI in the anticipation and experience of pain. *Science* 2004; 303(5661):1162–7.

31. Eippert F, Bingel U, Schoell ED, et al. Activation of the opioidergic descending pain control system underlies placebo analgesia. *Neuron* 2009; 63(4):533–43.

32. Wager TD, Scott DJ, Zubieta JK. Placebo effects on human mu-opioid activity during pain. *Proc Natl Acad Sci U S A* 2007; 104(26):11056–61.

33. Bingel U, Lorenz J, Schoell E, Weiller C, Buchel C. Mechanisms of placebo analgesia: rACC recruitment of a subcortical antinociceptive network. *Pain* 2006; 120(1–2):8–15.

34. Eippert F, Finsterbusch J, Bingel U, Buchel C. Direct evidence for spinal cord involvement in placebo analgesia. *Science* 2009; 326(5951):404.

35. Gimenez M, Pujol J, Ali Z, et al. Naproxen effects on brain response to painful pressure stimulation in patients with knee osteoarthritis: a double-blind, randomized, placebo-controlled, single-dose study. *J Rheumatol* 2014; 41(11):2240–8.

36. Kong J, Gollub RL, Polich G, et al. A functional magnetic resonance imaging study on the neural mechanisms of hyperalgesic nocebo effect. *J Neurosci* 2008; 28(49):13354–62.

37. Levine JD, Gordon NC, Fields HL. The mechanism of placebo analgesia. *Lancet* 1978; 2(8091):654–7.

38. Amanzio M, Benedetti F. Neuropharmacological dissection of placebo analgesia: expectation-activated opioid systems versus conditioning-activated specific subsystems. *J Neurosci* 1999; 19(1):484–94.

39. Benedetti F, Amanzio M, Baldi S, Casadio C, Maggi G. Inducing placebo respiratory depressant responses in humans via opioid receptors. *Eur J Neurosci* 1999; 11(2):625–31.

40. Pollo A, Vighetti S, Rainero I, Benedetti F. Placebo analgesia and the heart. *Pain* 2003; 102(1–2):125–33.

41. Hall KT, Lembo AJ, Kirsch I, et al. Catechol-O-methyltransferase val158met polymorphism predicts placebo effect in irritable bowel syndrome. *PLoS One* 2012; 7(10):e48135.

42. Hall M, Doherty S, Courtney P, et al. Ultrasound detected synovial change and pain response following intra-articular injection of corticosteroid and a placebo in symptomatic osteoarthritic knees: a pilot study. *Ann Rheum Dis* 2014; 73(8):1590–1.

43. Benedetti F, Amanzio M, Maggi G. Potentiation of placebo analgesia by proglumide. *Lancet* 1995; 346(8984):1231.

44. Benedetti F, Amanzio M, Casadio C, Oliaro A, Maggi G. Blockade of nocebo hyperalgesia by the cholecystokinin antagonist proglumide. *Pain* 1997; 71(2):135–40.

45. Jones GT, Atzeni F, Beasley M, Fluss E, Sarzi-Puttini P, Macfarlane GJ. The prevalence of fibromyalgia in the general population: a comparison of the American College of Rheumatology 1990, 2010, and modified 2010 classification criteria. *Arthritis Rheumatol* 2015; 67(2):568–75.

46. Hauser W, Bartram-Wunn E, Bartram C, Reinecke H, Tolle T. Systematic review: Placebo response in drug trials of fibromyalgia syndrome and painful peripheral diabetic neuropathy-magnitude and patient-related predictors. *Pain* 2011; 152(8):1709–17.

47. Puhl AA, Reinhart CJ, Rok ER, Injeyan HS. An examination of the observed placebo effect associated with the treatment of low back pain—a systematic review. *Pain Res Manag* 2011; 16(1):45–52.

48. Abhishek A, Doherty M. Mechanisms of the placebo response in pain in osteoarthritis. *Osteoarthritis Cartilage* 2013; 21(9):1229–35.

49. Blackwell B, Bloomfield SS, Buncher CR. Demonstration to medical students of placebo responses and non-drug factors. *Lancet* 1972; 1(7763):1279–82.

50. Watson A, Power A, Brown C, El-Deredy W, Jones A. Placebo analgesia: cognitive influences on therapeutic outcome. *Arthritis Res Ther* 2012; 14(2):206.

51. Moseley JB, O'Malley K, Petersen NJ, et al. A controlled trial of arthroscopic surgery for osteoarthritis of the knee. *N Engl J Med* 2002; 347(2):81–8.

52. Wartolowska K, Judge A, Hopewell S, et al. Use of placebo controls in the evaluation of surgery: systematic review. *BMJ* 2014; 348:g3253.

53. Barsky AJ, Saintfort R, Rogers MP, Borus JF. Nonspecific medication side effects and the nocebo phenomenon. *JAMA* 2002; 287(5):622–7.

54. Arthritis Care. *OA Nation 2012.* 2012. http://wwwarthritiscareorguk

SECTION 8

Pharmacological therapies

CHAPTER 28

Topical pharmacological treatments

Abhishek Abhishek, Adrian Jones, and Michael Doherty

Introduction

Topical pharmacological agents are safe, effective, and well tolerated in controlling pain due to osteoarthritis (OA) of hands and knees [1,2]. This has resulted in topical treatments being recommended as the first-line analgesic in OA [3–6]. However, many physicians remain sceptical of their efficacy due to the paucity of published controlled trials, the marked placebo response associated with topical applications, and their perceived high cost [7–9]. Nevertheless, despite the reservations of many physicians and government licensing agencies, increasing number of topical non-steroidal anti-inflammatory drugs (NSAIDs) have been marketed, and are often obtained 'over the counter' without a prescription. Available topical NSAIDs include diclofenac, felbinac (active form of the prodrug fenbufen), flurbiprofen, ibuprofen, indomethacin, ketoprofen, and piroxicam. As with oral NSAIDs, the major market for topical NSAIDs is for regional soft tissue pain. Although topical delivery of NSAIDs and salicylates has been investigated for over 80 years [10], only a minority of topical NSAIDs are specifically licensed for use in OA. However, once topical NSAIDs are available their usage is often extended to OA and to other forms of arthritis. In this chapter we review the potential advantages and disadvantages of topical treatments such as NSAIDs and capsaicin, and examine data relating to their use in OA.

Topical NSAIDs

At first sight, there seems several potential advantages to topical compared to oral NSAIDs (Table 28.1). For patients with only one, or a few painful joints—the usual situation with OA—it seems appropriate to target the site where analgesia is required, thereby avoiding unnecessary systemic exposure. Topical products are generally well tolerated and from a patient perspective it makes intuitive sense to apply a treatment where it is needed so adherence is usually high. Such popularity may partly relate to self-efficacy— the patient participating in, and controlling their own treatment. Importantly, compared to oral delivery, topical NSAIDs result in lower blood levels. Since the risk of major adverse events, especially gastrointestinal (GI), is dose- and blood-level related, topical NSAIDs should be safer.

Local application, however, may also have its problems. It may be less suitable than oral delivery for multiple regional pain, for relatively inaccessible sites such as the spine, or for pain arising from deep structures such as the hip or glenohumeral joints. Patients

Table 28.1 Theoretical advantages and disadvantages of topical application of NSAIDs

Advantages	Disadvantages
Makes sense for single regional pain syndromes	Inappropriate for multiple regional pain syndromes
Very popular with patients	May be difficult or messy to apply
Well tolerated	Possible local skin reactions
Good adherence	Systemic (especially hypersensitivity) reactions may still occur despite low serum levels
Self-efficacy—shift of locus of control to patient	
Possible concomitant benefit from massage	May not achieve adequate tissue (especially deep tissue) levels for therapeutic effect
Lower serum levels—therefore safer (especially with respect to gastrointestinal and renal/cardiovascular side effects)	Cost
	May be no better than cheaper rubefacients

with compromised hand function may have difficulty applying topical agents, and some products are messy and discolour clothing. Side effects may still occur, especially local reactions to the NSAIDs or carrier (reddening, itching, photosensitivity). More widespread hypersensitivity reactions (bronchoconstriction, extensive skin and mucous membrane reactions) and even severe renal adverse reactions such as interstitial nephritis and renal failure following excessive [11] or normal [12] application are reported. Whether topical agents penetrate locally and achieve adequate periarticular and joint tissue levels has also been questioned. Furthermore, many topical NSAIDs cost more per day than the equivalent oral drug. Whether they are better or safer than cheaper 'over the counter' rubefacients or embrocations (themselves not formally tested in OA) remains unknown. Given these various considerations, what is the evidence for their efficacy and safety?

Pharmacokinetics and mode of action

The skin presents a barrier through which only a limited amount of active substance from a given preparation will penetrate, for example, approximately 25% for ibuprofen. Several factors, such as dose, fat solubility, and ionized state of the drug determine penetration into the stratum corneum, with lipid-soluble, unionized drugs penetrating best. Diffusion through skin is accelerated by occlusive dressings and local hyperaemia. Some additives induce hyperaemia and thus influence absorption as well as exerting possible effects from hyperaemia per se. Topical NSAIDs come in a variety of delivery systems including creams, gels, foams, patches, and sprays. Pre-medicated patches offer better standardization of the dose of NSAID delivered, but all other modalities give variable self-administered dosing. This itself presents special problems for efficacy and costing studies.

For many drugs that penetrate the skin, rapid clearance via the skin capillaries prevents local drug accumulation. Such rapid clearance explains the systemic efficacy of transdermal nitrates and oestrogen. However, rapid clearance may not be inevitable and there are limited data from animal and human studies to support high local tissue levels of salicylate and certain NSAIDs, with only minor uptake into the systemic circulation, after topical delivery. In one study of felbinac applied to human knees 6 hours prior to orthopaedic surgery [13] the relative drug concentrations in different tissues were skin 750, subcutaneous fat 230, muscle 220, synovium 100, synovial fluid 3, and serum 1. Similarly, topical ibuprofen and piroxicam may reach several hundred-fold higher concentrations in periarticular tissues compared to plasma [14–16]. However, not all data support such high tissue concentrations from topical delivery. Another study that involved pre-dosing of orthopaedic patients with felbinac or oral fenbufen prior to knee surgery [17] found that oral fenbufen gave higher concentrations in periarticular tissues and synovial fluid than topical felbinac; all tissue concentrations were lower than those reported in the previous study [13]. It is clear that meticulous technique is required to avoid contamination during sampling of contiguous periarticular/articular tissues, and methodological differences may account for the disparity between these studies [17].

All studies concur in showing low plasma levels after topical salicylate or NSAIDs. Such levels are in the order of 20–100 times lower than those following oral administration of the identical or equivalent drug at recommended doses [13–19]. With few exceptions [18], drug concentrations in synovial fluid after topical application are significantly lower than those following oral administration [13,16,17,19]. When it has been examined, for example, for diclofenac [20], fenbufen [21], and piroxicam [16], similar synovial fluid concentrations are found in both the topically treated knee and the contralateral untreated knee of the same patient, suggesting that synovial fluid NSAID concentrations, rather than resulting from direct penetration down from skin, primarily result from secondary reperfusion into synovium after absorption into the bloodstream. However, in one study of topical salicylate, synovial fluid levels were achieved that were 60% of those following oral aspirin even though plasma levels were several hundred-fold lower [19], supporting local penetration as well as blood-borne delivery.

The balance of evidence, therefore, confirms low plasma concentrations following topical delivery, but questions whether adequate levels are achieved in target tissues. Such inconclusive pharmacokinetic evidence of efficacy, fuels the scepticism about topical NSAIDs [7–9]. However, the issue of tissue drug levels is clouded since:

- ‘adequate’ therapeutic levels of NSAIDs in periarticular and joint tissue sites are not established
- much pharmacokinetic data on topical NSAIDs is unpublished and remains ‘data on file’ in pharmaceutical houses
- synovial fluid data are only available for the knee and extrapolation to smaller, more superficial joints such as finger interphalangeal joints is problematic.

Of course, ‘adequate’ synovial fluid levels may not be required for symptom relief in OA. Mechanisms of pain production in OA are complex. Much of the pain that associates with OA may originate in periarticular rather than intracapsular structures [22]. Furthermore, it is possible that drug-induced effects on afferent nociceptor fibres in the skin might influence spinal cord handling of afferent impulses from adjacent joints [23]. Neurovascular interactions between skin and underlying deep structures might also modulate pain [24]. The relevance of synovial fluid drug concentrations to the clinical efficacy of topical NSAIDs has not been formally examined, though it is apparent that serum levels of NSAID following topical delivery do not correlate with clinical efficacy [25]. The relevance of serum and synovial fluid concentrations to the clinical efficacy of topical NSAIDs is therefore open to question and should not be a major reason for denying their use.

Data on clinical efficacy in osteoarthritis

Most clinical data on topical NSAIDs relate to studies of soft tissue lesions. A number of problems exist for most such studies, including:

- poor definition of acute regional pain syndrome, often with pooling of different conditions
- short observation periods, mainly 7–14 days
- the self-limiting nature of many lesions
- questionable assessments of pain, function, or clinical signs
- a marked placebo response in all studies (up to 40–70%).

Few such studies appear in peer-reviewed journals. Nevertheless, despite these caveats there are randomized placebo-controlled studies that attest to the efficacy of topical NSAIDs in acute and chronic soft tissue injury. Relatively fewer, particularly placebo-controlled, studies relate to OA. Again, there are problems common to many of these studies including:

- variable definitions of OA
- short observation periods, usually 14 days and a maximum of 12 weeks
- a very high placebo response
- often inappropriate primary and secondary outcome measures
- inadequate power to determine a good estimate of efficacy.

Placebo-controlled studies in osteoarthritis

Hand osteoarthritis

In a placebo-controlled, randomized, double-blind trial, men and women aged 40 years and older meeting the American College of Rheumatology (ACR) classification criteria for OA of the dominant hand were randomized to self-apply topical 1% diclofenac sodium gel (n = 198) or vehicle (n = 187) to both hands four times daily for 8 weeks [26]. In this study, significant differences favouring diclofenac sodium gel over vehicle were observed at week 4 for pain intensity and AUSCAN, with a trend for global rating of disease activity. At week 6, diclofenac sodium gel treatment significantly improved each primary outcome measure compared with vehicle [26].

An earlier double-blind, cross-over study of 50 patients with hand OA, reported greater pain relief and improvement in stiffness with topical trolamine salicylate than placebo cream, but the benefit largely went within 2 hours of application. The placebo in this study had no counterirritant action, and benefit from massage alone probably lasted for approximately 30 minutes [27].

Knee osteoarthritis

Several placebo-controlled RCTs have examined the efficacy of topical NSAID gels in knee OA [25,28–43], and most published studies report encouraging results. Recently published studies suggest that topical NSAIDs may be more effective than placebo for up to 12 weeks [33]. Apart from this, TDT 064, which contains ultra-deformable phospholipid (Sequessome™) vesicles, and was first developed as a novel drug-delivery system, can penetrate into the joint cavity, reduce friction, and has been proposed as a 'drug-free' treatment for OA pain [28,29].

A randomized, double-blind study of piroxicam versus placebo gel, applied three or four times daily to the most symptomatic knee of 246 OA patients, demonstrated greater efficacy with piroxicam gel at 2 weeks [44]. Global patient opinion showed improvement in 80 versus 68% of patients, with marked to moderate improvement in 51 versus 33%. Interestingly, improvement in the contralateral OA knee occurred to a lesser but equal extent in piroxicam (31%) and placebo (36%) patients, suggesting no clinical benefit at distant sites following single joint treatment.

A randomized, double-blind, parallel-group study of topical 2% diclofenac gel conducted in 70 patients with symptomatic knee OA and only modest radiographic change, showed clinical superiority over the placebo gel at the end of the 2-week study period, significant differences being observed for the aggregated and individual subscale (pain, stiffness, function) scores of the Western Ontario and McMaster Universities Arthritis Index (WOMAC) [41].

A 15-day randomized, placebo-controlled study of diclofenac plasters (180 mg active drug) applied twice daily in 155 patients with knee OA also showed superiority of the treatment plaster over placebo at all three assessments (days 4, 7, and 15), significant differences being observed for the primary outcomes of pain visual analogue scale (VAS) and the Lequesne Index [43].

However, two randomized placebo-controlled multicentre studies of eltenac, an NSAID showing structural similarity to diclofenac but with one benzene ring being substituted by a thiophen ring (a modification that improves absorption following topical application) did not report a significant improvement compared to placebo [25,42]. The first study compared eltenac gel (1%) to oral diclofenac (50 mg twice a day) and placebo over a 4-week period in 290 patients with knee OA using a three-arm double-dummy design [42]. No significant differences were observed between groups in terms of the Lequesne Index and pain VAS, though post hoc subgroup analysis showed significant, similar clinical benefit for both active agents compared to placebo (Lesquesne Index) in those with moderate to severe baseline pain. The second study compared three strengths of eltenac gel (0.1%, 0.3%, and 1%) to placebo gel over a 4-week period in 237 patients with knee OA [25]. Again, sub-analysis of those with highest baseline pain showed significantly better efficacy for the 1% gel compared to placebo. Several problems inherent in topical NSAID studies are well illustrated by this study. For example, almost half the patients (102/234) were protocol violators through use of too little or too much of the un-metered gel as judged by the weight of returned tubes (an intention-to-treat analysis was appropriately used); the standardized effect size of

0.5 used in the power calculation was not achieved; up to 2 g of paracetamol was permitted daily in all groups, perhaps masking the independent effect size of the gel; the ability to fully explore predictors of response was not incorporated into the design; and the pre-study notion that better efficacy might be seen in those with milder pain was not realized.

A multicentre, randomized, double-blind, placebo-controlled trial of diclofenac gel 1% (4 g/day applied four times a day) in patients with mild to moderate knee OA of at least 6 months' duration (n = 492) reported a statistically significant improvement in WOMAC pain, WOMAC global function, and global rating of disease by week 1, and this improvement was maintained up to week 12 [31]. Patients recruited in this study were required to have moderate to severe symptoms (WOMAC pain of ≥9/20) and have a baseline pain on movement score of 50 or higher on a 100-point VAS scale. Effect sizes for WOMAC pain, WOMAC function, global rating of disease, and pain on movement at 12 weeks were 0.23, 0.30, 0.31, and 0.34 respectively.

In contrast, a randomized controlled, double-blind trial with 1395 participants meeting the ACR clinical classification for knee OA failed to show any improvement in WOMAC pain, stiffness and function nor in joint stiffness and patient global assessment of efficacy with ketoprofen gel administered as a transfersome [29]. This may be because only patients with milder pain were recruited in this study—the patients were required to have a total average WOMAC pain subscale score of less than 7 at the first and second baseline visits (separated by 2–5 days) [29]. However, a previous study which demonstrated improvement with the same drug formulation over a 6-week period in patients with flare of knee OA (n = 397) could be confounded by pre-selection of patients who are likely to respond to NSAIDs [30]. Some other studies that pre-selected patients for severity of knee pain and/or a flare of knee pain on withdrawing treatment also report improvement with topical NSAIDs [33,34,36–38]. Although the transfersome TDT 064 in its own right has been suggested as an effective 'drug-free' treatment for OA based on its non-inferiority to oral celecoxib, superiority over oral placebo and effect size greater than topical NSAIDs or placebo in other studies, its efficacy has not been directly compared against other conventional topical NSAIDs or topical placebo cream [45]. Therefore at present TDT 064 cannot be recommended as a treatment for OA pain.

Comparative studies in osteoarthritis

Several studies report similar efficacy when the topical NSAID is compared to the parent or alternative oral NSAID. For example, in a double-blind, double-dummy study of 275 patients with mild–moderate knee OA, felbinac was as effective over a 2-week period as oral fenbufen, with a similar low incidence of side effects [46]. Parity was also demonstrated in a similarly designed study of 235 patients with mild knee OA, comparing piroxicam gel and oral ibuprofen (1200 mg per day) thrice daily over a 4-week period [47]. Both active agents appeared comparable in the study of 290 patients comparing oral diclofenac (100 mg daily) and 1% eltenac gel to placebo [39]. In three smaller (40–50 patients) double-blind, double-dummy studies of patients with various diagnoses, including OA, equal efficacy after 1 week was found with salicylate cream or oral aspirin (2600 mg daily) at various peripheral and axial sites [48,49]. Topical salicylate, however, had advantages of faster pain relief and fewer side effects.

The ability to substitute topical for oral NSAID has been demonstrated in one open UK study [50]. One hundred and ninety-one elderly subjects on oral NSAID for OA (mainly knee) were randomized to continue their NSAID for 4 weeks, or to use piroxicam gel plus half their oral NSAID dose for 2 weeks, and then gel alone for a further 2 weeks. Both groups improved from baseline, but the gel group showed greater improvements in joint tenderness and movement, and in AIMS (Arthritis Impact Measurement Scale) scores. When topical NSAIDs have been directly compared in OA or chronic musculoskeletal pain there are little or no differences in efficacy between products [51–53]. The design of such studies, however, is often questionable with a strong likelihood of type II error. Possible differences between various topical agents that are in current use, therefore, have yet to be adequately examined.

Systematic review

The Cochrane review of topical NSAIDs was updated by Moore et al. in 2012 [54]. Thirty-four studies were included in this comprehensive review. Most included studies were carried out on patients with knee or hand OA, and the mean age of the participants in the included studies ranged between 59 and 65 years. They defined primary outcome as 'clinical success', defined as a 50% reduction in pain, or an equivalent measure such as a 'very good' or 'excellent' global assessment of treatment, or 'none' or 'slight' pain on rest or movement, measured on a categorical scale as defined in their previous review [55]. The overall relative benefit (RB) for successful treatment compared to placebo was 1.29 (95% confidence interval (CI) 1.21–1.38). However, when data were stratified according to the duration of trial, there was a significant decline in RB. The RB for successful treatment with topical NSAID gel for trials lasting 2 weeks, 4–6 weeks, and 8–12 weeks were 2.0 (95% CI 1.5–2.6), 1.7 95% CI (1.3–2.2), and 1.2 (95% CI 1.1–1.3) respectively. Apart from this, there was no difference in efficacy between gel and solution formulations of topical NSAIDs. However, of interest there was no difference between topical and oral NSAIDs in providing successful treatment (RB 1.02 (95% CI 0.94–1.1), and topical NSAIDs carried a significantly lower risk of systemic adverse effects (0.66, 95% CI 0.56–0.77). These findings are also supported by the results of an equivalence study designed to compare the effect of advice to use preferentially oral or topical NSAID) on knee pain and disability using a randomized controlled trial and a patient preference study [56].

Safety and economic considerations

Local adverse reactions to topical NSAIDs include skin irritation, dry skin, redness/erythema, and pruritus. These are generally regarded as mild and transient by patients. However, they can result in treatment discontinuation. The relative risk of local adverse effects seems to be slightly higher for diclofenac gel (RR 1.8, 95% CI 1.5–2.2) compared to other topical NSAIDs (RR 1.3, 95% CI 0.96–1.8) [54].

Although anecdotal reports of systemic harm due to topical NSAIDs exist, they do not result in systemic adverse effects. Data from over 1800 study participants suggests that overall there was no significant difference in the number of participants experiencing systemic adverse events with topical NSAIDs than with controls, either for topical diclofenac (RR 0.89, 95% CI 0.57–1.4) or for all other topical NSAIDs combined (RR 1.2, 95% CI 0.72–1.7) [54]. There was no difference in GI adverse events in the two groups.

A large case–control study evaluated the risk of a major upper GI event associated with topical NSAID use [57]. Using a record-linkage database, 1103 patients, hospitalized for upper GI bleeding or perforation, were each compared to matched community and hospital controls (eight controls per case) for prior drug exposures. After adjusting for the confounding effect of concomitant exposure to oral NSAIDs and ulcer-healing drugs, no association between topical NSAIDs and upper GI events was discerned.

A number of studies have estimated the economic benefits of topical versus oral NSAIDs, using various models of comparative efficacy, GI ulcer rates, and clinical decision-making. Two studies, suggest that topical piroxicam should be more cost-effective than oral ibuprofen for the treatment of mild OA [47,51], as would felbinac compared to oral fenbufen [46].

Capsaicin

Capsaicin (trans-8-methyl-n-vanillyl-6-nonenamide) (Figure 28.1), an alkaloid derived from the Nightshade family of plants, was first isolated in 1816 in partially purified crystalline form by Bucholz and in pure crystalline form in 1876 by Thresh [58]. It is also the active ingredient in Tabasco sauce (Figure 28.2) and is present in several over-the-counter preparations. Capsaicin has been used in the treatment of a variety of painful disorders, including post-herpetic neuralgia, cluster headaches, diabetic neuropathy, phantom limb pain, and post-mastectomy pain.

Mode of action

Initially, it was believed that capsaicin worked by a 'counterirritant' mechanism, and subsequently, it was shown that capsaicin, when applied topically, stimulates the release of the neuropeptide, substance P, from the peripheral nerves and prevents its re-accumulation from cell bodies and nerve terminals in both the central and peripheral nervous system, thus, reducing neural transmission [59]. This is because substance P is an important chemical mediator responsible for the transmission of pain from the periphery to the central nervous system.

Recently, capsaicin has been shown to act also by stimulation of the transient receptor potential channel of the vanilloid receptor family subtype 1 (TRPV1) receptor [60,61]. TRPV1 is a non-selective cation channel, and once activated by capsaicin, allows influx of calcium which results in sensory neuronal depolarization which can induce local sensitization and lead to the sensations of heat, burning, stinging, or itching [62]. Inactivation of voltage-gated Na^+ channels soon after activation of calcium channels and direct pharmacological desensitization of plasma membrane TRPV1 receptors may contribute to an immediate reduction in neuronal excitability and responsiveness [62]. Repeated applications can

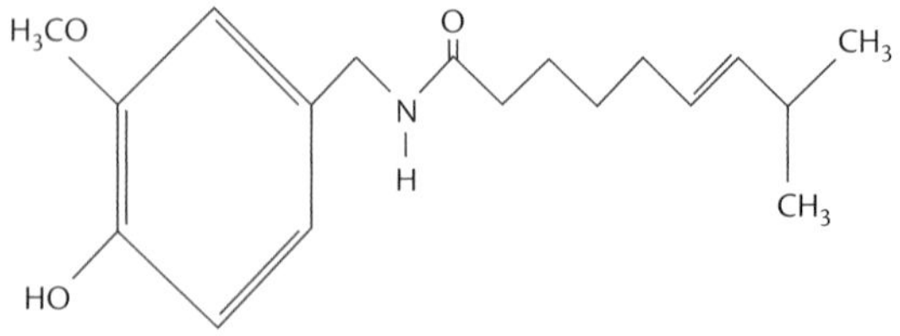

(trans-8-methyl-n-vanillyl-6-nonenamide)

Figure 28.1 Chemical structure of capsaicin.

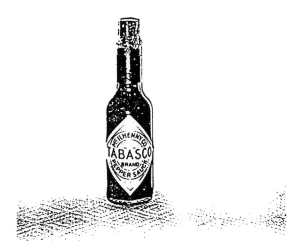

Figure 28.2 Capsaicin is derived from the pepper plant and is the active ingredient in Tabasco sauce.
Photo by Kathie Lane.

produce a persistent local effect on cutaneous nociceptors, which is best described as 'defunctionalization' and is constituted by reduced spontaneous activity and a loss of responsiveness to a wide range of sensory stimuli [62]. This may be due to overwhelming of intracellular Ca^{2+} buffering capacity by extracellular Ca^{2+} entering through TRPV1 and being released from intracellular stores, with subsequent activation of calcium-dependent proteases and cytoskeleton breakdown [62]. Microtubule depolymerisation may interrupt fast axonal transport [62].

TRPV1 activation may result in the depletion of substance P from the entire neuron, so that branches from the peripheral nerves to deeper structures such as the joint are effectively depleted. Although normal articular cartilage has no nerve supply and therefore cannot be a source of pain, histological studies of joint innervation have shown that the joint capsule, tendons, ligaments, subchondral bone, and periosteum are extensively innervated [63–65].

Furthermore, as the pathological changes of OA progress, capillaries originating in the medullary spaces of the subchondral bone and carrying nerve endings within their walls invade the normally avascular articular cartilage [24]. Small diameter nerve fibres in the synovium and subchondral plate have been shown to stain

immunohistochemically for substance P, as has sclerotic bone and areas of bony eburnation and of fibrillated cartilage in OA joints [66–69]. Synovial concentrations of substance P are increased in patients with OA [69,70].

Placebo-controlled studies in osteoarthritis

In 1991, Deal et al. reported the results of a randomized, double-blind, placebo-controlled multicentre trial involving patients with moderate to very severe pain due to knee OA [71]. Patients in the active treatment group applied 0.025% capsaicin cream, or the vehicle, four times daily to anterior, posterior, and lateral aspects of the most severely affected knee. The results are shown in Table 28.2. Improvement in joint pain was significantly greater (p = 0.02) in subjects who received capsaicin than in the placebo group. After 4 weeks of treatment, the evaluation of the physician and the pain score of the patient both showed a mean reduction of 22% (p = 0.05) for those using the active cream, but of only 14% (p = 0.05) and 10% (p = 0.06), respectively, for those using the placebo cream.

A local burning sensation was noted by 44% of patients using the capsaicin preparation and by one patient in the placebo group. However, burning diminished with continuation of treatment, and 94% of patients in the active treatment group and 88% of those in the placebo group completed the study. Although the burning at the site of application obviously affected blinding of the study and may have favoured a positive response to the capsaicin, the authors attempted to take this into account by comparing the results in patients treated with capsaicin who experienced burning, with those in capsaicin-treated patients who did not have this side effect. No difference in drug response was apparent between the two groups.

In 1992, McCarthy and McCarty reported a more potent formulation of capsaicin (0.075%) in a placebo-controlled, 4-week, double-blind randomized trial involving 14 subjects with painful OA of the distal or proximal interphalangeal joints or first carpometacarpal joint (Table 28.2) [72]. By week 4, the topical application of capsaicin had reduced joint pain by nearly 60% and joint tenderness by approximately 40% in comparison with the baseline values, while improvement in these parameters in patients treated with topical application of the vehicle alone was only about 20% and 10%, respectively. No changes were noted, however, with respect to grip strength, joint swelling, duration of morning stiffness or joint

Table 28.2 Results of placebo-controlled trials of capsaicin cream in patients with OA

Study	OA joint site	Capsaicin strength (%)	Duration of study (weeks)	Number of subjects treated	Decrease in joint pain at end of study (%)	
					Capsaicin 0.25%	Capsaicin 0.025%
Deal et al. [71]	Knee	0.025	4	36 capsaicin 34 placebo	22	14
McCarthy and McCarty [72]	DIP, PIP, MCP	0.075	4	7 capsaicin 7 placebo	60	20
Altman et al. [26]	Various (70% knee)	0.025	12	57 capsaicin 56 placebo	53	27
Schnitzer et al. [76]	Various (approx. 80% knee)	0.25 vs 0.025	4	31 capsaicin 29 placebo	74	66

DIP, distal interphalangeal joints; PIP, proximal interphalangeal joints; MCP, metacarpophalangeal joints.

function. As in the study by Deal et al., all patients who received capsaicin reported a burning sensation in the skin. However, none discontinued treatment because of this side effect, and the local discomfort diminished over the first week and became increasingly tolerable with continued treatment.

In both of the above-mentioned studies, patients were permitted to continue their usual treatment with NSAIDs or analgesics so capsaicin was used as an adjunct to their usual therapy. In contrast, Altman et al. reported a clinical trial of 0.025% capsaicin cream as monotherapy for OA (Table 28.2) [71]. In this double-blind study, NSAIDs and other medications that the patients were receiving for the treatment of OA were discontinued before entry into the study. Use of acetaminophen was permitted during the study but was restricted to 3 days per month, and patients were given only 12 tablets of acetaminophen per month, to be used for non-arthritic pain or fever. Patients were evaluated for 12 weeks which is considerably longer than in either of the two trials cited earlier. Although subjects had OA at a variety of joint sites, 70% of those treated with capsaicin and 79% of those treated with the vehicle had knee OA. Among the 113 patients in the study, 57 received capsaicin and 56 were treated with the vehicle.

Baseline pain scores in the two groups, measured on a VAS, were comparable (57 mm for capsaicin, 56 mm for vehicle). Based on global evaluation of the patients, those who received capsaicin reported significantly greater reduction of pain at weeks 4, 8, and 12, than did the controls. At week 12 the mean improvement in pain in the capsaicin group was 53% while that in the placebo group was 27.4% (p = 0.02) (Figure 28.3) (Table 28.2). This study is important insofar as it shows that improvement in joint pain can occur with use of capsaicin as the sole analgesic and that pain relief can be sustained. Indeed, pain relief was as great after 12 weeks of treatment as after only 4 weeks. Furthermore, the magnitude of improvement in joint pain was as great as that seen with oral NSAIDs.

In a single-blind study of patients with OA at a variety of joint sites, a high-strength (0.25%) capsaicin cream (not currently available in

the United States) applied just twice a day provided greater pain relief, with a considerably more rapid onset of action, than 0.025% capsaicin cream applied four times daily [73]. It is unclear, however, whether the fact that the dosing regimens were not comparable may have affected outcomes in the two treatment groups. As in the study by Altman et al., medications that might have interfered with efficacy evaluation (e.g. NSAIDs, systemic analgesics) were withdrawn prior to randomization so capsaicin was studied as the sole analgesic agent. Furthermore, only one patient in the high-strength capsaicin treatment group discontinued therapy because of a sensation of burning at the site of application. Although the incidence of burning was initially greater with the high-strength formulation, by day 7 and subsequently for the remainder of this 28-day study the number of patients who reported burning was no greater in the high-strength capsaicin group than in the 0.025% capsaicin group.

In 2010, Kosuwon et al. [74] reported the results of a cross-over, double blinded, randomized controlled trial of 100 participants with mild to moderate symptomatic radiographic knee OA (K&L knee OA score < 4) in which a weaker topical capsaicin preparation (0.0125%) was used. All participants received either capsaicin or placebo gel applied to the affected knee, three times daily for 4 weeks, then had a 1-week washout period after which the treatment switched to either capsaicin gel or placebo gel for the next 4 weeks. In this study, the mean difference of VAS, total WOMAC score, WOMAC pain, stiffness, and functional subscales in the capsaicin group versus the placebo group was statistically significant. Burning sensation still occurred in approximately 67% of patients, but none withdrew for this reason.

There are no comparative studies of the efficacy of capsaicin and another drug in osteoarthritis.

Systematic reviews

A systematic review of randomized controlled trials of topical capsaicin in OA catalogued in PubMed, EMBASE, and ISI Web of Knowledge identified five double-blind, placebo-controlled RCTs and one case–cross-over study [75].

Capsaicin treatment efficacy (versus placebo) for change in VAS pain score was moderate, at 0.44 (95% CI 0.25–0.62) over 4 weeks of treatment [75]. Two studies reported treatment beyond 4 weeks, with contradictory results. One study reported maximal between-group differences at 4 weeks, while the second study reported that between-group differences increase over time up to 20 weeks. Capsaicin was safe with no systemic toxicity. Application site burning affected 35–100% of capsaicin treated patients, with a risk ratio of 4.22 (3.25–5.48), the incidence peaking in week 1 and

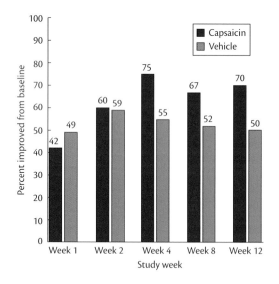

Figure 28.3 Mean percentage change in pain intensity over 12 weeks of therapy with capsaicin, 0.025%, or vehicle in 89 evaluable patients with OA. VAS, visual analogue scale; p < 0.05 vs vehicle.

Taken from Altman R.D., Avon A., Holmburg C.E., et al. 1994. *Sem Arthritis Rheum* 23(Suppl. 3):25–33.

Box 28.1 Use of topical capsaicin for treatment of OA pain

1. Is safe

2. May be employed as an adjunct to systemic analgesic/NSAID treatment

3. May be effective as monotherapy

4. The magnitude of response may be as great as with NSAIDs or acetaminophen

5. Somewhat inconvenient: irritating to eyes and mouth, requires three or four applications per day, and improvement may not occur until 3–4 weeks after regular use.

Table 28.3 Mean daily analgesic use at week 6, number of tablets taken per day[a]

Treatment group	Mean daily analgesic use	Standard error
Placebo	4.00	0.20
GTN	3.52[b]	0.16
Capsaicin	3.72[c]	0.16
Capsaicin/GTN	3.25[b]	0.18

GTN, glyceryl trinitrate.

[a]Pretreatment mean analgesic consumption was 4 tablets per day.

[b]p = 0.01.

[c]p = 0.05.

declining subsequently. Topical capsaicin therapy appears to be safe and effective, and warrants consideration in the management of OA pain (Box 28.1). A 6-week study of patients with radiographically confirmed OA of the hip, knee, shoulder, or hand indicated that the addition of glyceryl trinitrate to capsaicin (0.025%) resulted in less local discomfort than capsaicin alone and a greater decrease in the use of concurrent analgesic than either agent alone (Table 28.3) [76].

The place of topical treatments in management guidelines

Several publications have provided guidelines on the management of OA. The EULAR hand OA guidelines [3] recommend using topical treatments before systemic treatments, including paracetamol, in patients with mild to moderate pain especially when only a few joints are affected. The earlier EULAR knee OA guideline [6] also recommended topical treatments for managing pain due to OA. In keeping with these, the ACR recommendations support the use of both capsaicin and topical NSAIDs in the treatment of hand OA, and that of topical NSAIDs alone in the treatment of knee OA [4].

Other pharmacological topical treatments

Topical application of 5% lignocaine patches to the knees of people with knee OA (maximum four patches applied to cover the most painful areas changed daily) have been evaluated in two prospective, open-label pilot studies enrolling 237 patients between them [77,78]. The topical lignocaine patches were offered predominantly as an add-on treatment to those on stable analgesia (n = 225) but also on their own (n = 12). There was a statistically significant improvement in pain at the end of 2 weeks compared to baseline, but these studies were not placebo controlled.

Conclusion

Although topical treatments have gained acceptability in the treatment of OA pain, there are still relatively few published studies in this area and a number of outstanding issues such as cost-effectiveness of topical NSAIDs at common OA sites, and clarification of the site of action via this route of delivery need to be clarified.

References

1. Peniston JH, Gold MS, Wieman MS, Alwine LK. Long-term tolerability of topical diclofenac sodium 1% gel for osteoarthritis in seniors and patients with comorbidities. *Clin Interv Aging* 2012; 7:517–23.
2. Peniston JH, Gold MS, Alwine LK. An open-label, long-term safety and tolerability trial of diclofenac sodium 1% gel in patients with knee osteoarthritis. *Phys Sportsmed* 2011; 39(3):31–8.
3. Zhang W, Doherty M, Leeb BF, et al. EULAR evidence based recommendations for the management of hand osteoarthritis: report of a Task Force of the EULAR Standing Committee for International Clinical Studies Including Therapeutics (ESCISIT). *Ann Rheum Dis* 2007; 66(3):377–88.
4. Hochberg MC, Altman RD, April KT, et al. American College of Rheumatology 2012 recommendations for the use of nonpharmacologic and pharmacologic therapies in osteoarthritis of the hand, hip, and knee. *Arthritis Care Res* 2012; 64(4):465–74.
5. National Clinical Guideline Centre. *Osteoarthritis: Care and Management in Adults.* London: National Institute for Health and Care Excellence; 2014.
6. Jordan KM, Arden NK, Doherty M, et al. EULAR Recommendations 2003: an evidence based approach to the management of knee osteoarthritis: Report of a Task Force of the Standing Committee for International Clinical Studies Including Therapeutic Trials (ESCISIT). *Ann Rheum Dis* 2003; 62(12):1145–55.
7. Topical NSAIDs: a gimmick or a godsend? *Lancet* 1989; 2(8666):779–80.
8. Anonymous. Topical NSAIDs for joint disease. *Drug Therapeut Bull* 1997; 37:87–8.
9. Abhishek A, Doherty M. Mechanisms of the placebo response in pain in osteoarthritis. *Osteoarthritis Cartilage* 2013; 21(9):1229–35.
10. Nothmann M, Wolff, M. The absorption of salicylic acid by human skin. *Klin Wochscht* 1933; 12(345–6)
11. O'Callaghan CA, Andrews PA, Ogg CS. Renal disease and use of topical non-steroidal anti-inflammatory drugs. *BMJ (Clin Res Ed)* 1994; 308(6921):110–1.
12. Fernando AH, Thomas S, Temple RM, Lee HA. Renal failure after topical use of NSAIDs. *BMJ (Clin Res Ed)* 1994; 308(6927):533.
13. Sugawara Y. Percutaneous absorption and tissue absorption of L-141 topical agent. *Jpn Med Pharmacol* 1985; 13:183–94.
14. Peters H, Chlud K, Berner G, et al. Percutaneous kinetics of ibuprofen. *Akt Rheumatol* 1987; 12:208–11.
15. Kanazawa M, Ito H, Shimooka K, Mase K. The pharmaco- kinetics of 0.5 per cent piroxicam gel in humans. *Eur J Rheumatol Inflamm* 1987; 8:117.
16. Sugawara S, Ohno H, Ueda R, et al. Studies of percutaneous absorption and tissue distribution of piroxicam gel. *Jpn Med Pharmacol Sci* 1984; 12:1233–8.
17. Bolten W, Salzmann G, Goldmann R, Miehlke K. [Plasma and tissue concentrations of biphenylacetic acid following 1 week oral fenbufen medication and topical administration of Felbinac gel on the knee joint]. *Z Rheumatol* 1989; 48(6):317–22.
18. Riess W, Schmid K, Botta L, et al. Percutaneous absorption of diclofenac. *Arzneimittel Forschung Drug Res* 1986; 36:1092–6.
19. Rabinowitz JL, Feldman ES, Weinberger A, Schumacher HR. Comparative tissue absorption of oral 14C-aspirin and topical triethanolamine 14C-salicylate in human and canine knee joints. *J Clin Pharmacol* 1982; 22(1):42–8.
20. Radermacher J, Jentsch D, Scholl MA, Lustinetz T, Frolich JC. Diclofenac concentrations in synovial fluid and plasma after cutaneous application in inflammatory and degenerative joint disease. *Br J Clin Pharmacol* 1991; 31(5):537–41.
21. Dawson M, McGee CM, Vine JH, et al. The disposition of biphenylacetic acid following topical application. *Eur J Clin Pharmacol* 1988; 33(6):639–42.
22. Creamer P, Lethbridge-Cejku M, Hochberg MC. Where does it hurt? Pain localization in osteoarthritis of the knee. *Osteoarthritis Cartilage* 1998; 6(5):318–23.
23. Woolf CJ, Wall PD. Relative effectiveness of C primary afferent fibers of different origins in evoking a prolonged facilitation of the flexor reflex in the rat. *J Neurosci* 1986; 6(5):1433–42.
24. Kidd BL, Mapp PI, Blake DR, Gibson SJ, Polak JM. Neurogenic influences in arthritis. *Ann Rheum Dis* 1990; 49(8):649–52.

25. Ottillinger B, Gomor B, Michel BA, et al. Efficacy and safety of eltenac gel in the treatment of knee osteoarthritis. *Osteoarthritis Cartilage* 2001; 9(3):273–80.

26. Altman RD, Dreiser RL, Fisher CL, et al. Diclofenac sodium gel in patients with primary hand osteoarthritis: a randomized, double-blind, placebo-controlled trial. *J Rheumatol* 2009; 36(9):1991–9.

27. Rothacker D, Difigilo C, Lee I. A clinical trial of topical 10% trolamine salicylate in osteoarthritis. *Curr Ther Res* 1994; 55:584–97.

28. Rother M, Conaghan PG. A randomized, double-blind, phase III trial in moderate osteoarthritis knee pain comparing topical ketoprofen gel with ketoprofen-free gel. *J Rheumatol* 2013; 40(10):1742–8.

29. Conaghan PG, Dickson J, Bolten W, Cevc G, Rother M. A multicen-tre, randomized, placebo- and active-controlled trial comparing the efficacy and safety of topical ketoprofen in Transfersome gel (IDEA-033) with ketoprofen-free vehicle (TDT 064) and oral celecoxib for knee pain associated with osteoarthritis. *Rheumatology (Oxford)* 2013; 52(7):1303–12.

30. Rother M, Lavins BJ, Kneer W, et al. Efficacy and safety of epicutaneous ketoprofen in Transfersome (IDEA-033) versus oral celecoxib and pla-cebo in osteoarthritis of the knee: multicentre randomised controlled trial. *Ann Rheum Dis* 2007; 66(9):1178–83.

31. Barthel HR, Haselwood D, Longley S, 3rd, Gold MS, Altman RD. Randomized controlled trial of diclofenac sodium gel in knee osteo-arthritis. *Semin Arthritis Rheum* 2009; 39(3):203–12.

32. Ergun H, Kulcu D, Kutlay S, Bodur H, Tulunay FC. Efficacy and safety of topical nimesulide in the treatment of knee osteoarthritis. *J Clin Rheumatol* 2007; 13(5):251–5.

33. Niethard FU, Gold MS, Solomon GS, et al. Efficacy of topical diclofenac diethylamine gel in osteoarthritis of the knee. *J Rheumatol* 2005; 32(12):2384–92.

34. Baer PA, Thomas LM, Shainhouse Z. Treatment of osteoarthritis of the knee with a topical diclofenac solution: a randomised controlled, 6-week trial [ISRCTN53366886]. *BMC Musculoskelet Disord* 2005; 6:44.

35. Tugwell PS, Wells GA, Shainhouse JZ. Equivalence study of a topi-cal diclofenac solution (pennsaid) compared with oral diclofenac in symptomatic treatment of osteoarthritis of the knee: a randomized controlled trial. *J Rheumatol* 2004; 31(10):2002–12.

36. Trnavsky K, Fischer M, Vogtle-Junkert U, Schreyger F. Efficacy and safety of 5% ibuprofen cream treatment in knee osteoarthritis. Results of a randomized, double-blind, placebo-controlled study. *J Rheumatol* 2004; 31(3):565–72.

37. Roth SH, Shainhouse JZ. Efficacy and safety of a topical diclofenac solution (pennsaid) in the treatment of primary osteoarthritis of the knee: a randomized, double-blind, vehicle-controlled clinical trial. *Arch Intern Med* 2004; 164(18):2017–23.

38. Bookman AA, Williams KS, Shainhouse JZ. Effect of a topical diclofenac solution for relieving symptoms of primary osteoar-thritis of the knee: a randomized controlled trial. *CMAJ* 2004; 171(4):333–8.

39. Bruhlmann P, Michel BA. Topical diclofenac patch in patients with knee osteoarthritis: a randomized, double-blind, controlled clinical trial. *Clin Exp Rheumatol* 2003; 21(2):193–8.

40. Rovensky J, Micekova D, Gubzova Z, et al. Treatment of knee osteo-arthritis with a topical non-steroidal antiinflammatory drug. Results of a randomized, double-blind, placebo-controlled study on the efficacy and safety of a 5% ibuprofen cream. *Drugs Exp Clin Res* 2001; 27(5–6):209–21.

41. Grace D, Rogers J, Skeith K, Anderson K. Topical diclofenac versus placebo: a double blind, randomized clinical trial in patients with osteoarthritis of the knee. *J Rheumatol* 1999; 26(12):2659–63.

42. Sandelin J, Harilainen A, Crone H, et al. Local NSAID gel (eltenac) in the treatment of osteoarthritis of the knee. A double blind study com-paring eltenac with oral diclofenac and placebo gel. *Scand J Rheumatol* 1997; 26(4):287–92.

43. Dreiser RL, Tisne-Camus M. DHEP plasters as a topical treatment of knee osteoarthritis—a double-blind placebo-controlled study. *Drugs Exp Clin Res* 1993; 19(3):117–23.

44. Kageyama T. A double blind placebo controlled multicenter study of piroxicam 0.5% gel in osteoarthritis of the knee. *Eur J Rheumatol Inflamm* 1987; 8:114–5.

45. Conaghan PG, Bijlsma JW, Kneer W, et al. Drug-free gel containing ultra-deformable phospholipid vesicles (TDT 064) as topical therapy for the treatment of pain associated with osteoarthritis: a review of clinical efficacy and safety. *Curr Med Res Opin* 2014; 30(4):599–611.

46. Tsuyama N, Kurokawa T, Nihei T, et al. Clinical evaluation of L-141 topical agent on osteoarthrosis deformans of the knees. *Clin Med* 1985; 1:697–729.

47. Dickson DJ. A double-blind evaluation of topical piroxicam gel with oral ibuprofen in osteoarthritis of the knee. *Curr Ther Res Clin Exp* 1991; 49:199–207.

48. Shamszad M, Perkal M, Golden EL, Marlin R. Two double- blind comparisons of a topically applied salicylate cream and orally ingested aspirin in the relief of chronic musculoskeletal pain. *Curr Ther Res* 1986; 39:470–9.

49. Golden EL. A double-blind comparison of orally ingested aspirin and a topically applied salicylate cream in the relief of rheumatic pain. *Curr Ther Res* 1978; 24:524–9.

50. Browning RC, Johson K. Reducing the dose of oral NSAIDs by use of Feldene Gel: an open study in elderly patients with osteoarthritis. *Adv Ther* 1994; 11(4):198–207.

51. Rau R, Hockel S. [Piroxicam gel versus diclofenac gel in active gonar-throses]. *Fortschr Med* 1989; 107(22):485–8.

52. Balthazar-Letawe D. [Voltaren Emugel in clinical rheumatology. Comparative trial with Indocid gel]. *Acta Belg Med Phys* 1987; 10(3):109–10.

53. Burgos A, Pérez Busquier M, Reino JG, et al. Double-blind, double-dummy comparative study of local action transcutaneous flurbiprofen (flurbiprofen LAT) versus piketoprofen cream in the treatment of extra-articular rheumatism. *Clin Drug Invest* 2001; 21:95–102.

54. Derry S, Moore RA, Rabbie R. Topical NSAIDs for chronic musculo-skeletal pain in adults. *Cochrane Database Syst Rev* 2012; 9:CD007400.

55. Mason L, Moore RA, Edwards JE, Derry S, McQuay HJ. Topical NSAIDs for chronic musculoskeletal pain: systematic review and meta-analysis. *BMC Musculoskelet Disord* 2004; 5:28.

56. Underwood M, Ashby D, Carnes D, et al. Topical or oral ibuprofen for chronic knee pain in older people. The TOIB study. *Health Technol Assess (Winchester)* 2008; 12(22):iii–iv, ix–155.

57. Evans JM, McMahon AD, McGilchrist MM, et al. Topical non-steroidal anti-inflammatory drugs and admission to hospital for upper gastroin-testinal bleeding and perforation: a record linkage case-control study. *BMJ* 1995; 311(6996):22–6.

58. Bode AM, Dong Z. The two faces of capsaicin. *Cancer Res* 2011; 71(8):2809–14.

59. Virus RM, Gebhart GF. Pharmacologic actions of capsaicin: appar-ent involvement of substance P and serotonin. *Life Sci* 1979; 25(15):1273–83.

60. Caterina MJ, Schumacher MA, Tominaga M, et al. The capsaicin recep-tor: a heat-activated ion channel in the pain pathway. *Nature* 1997; 389(6653):816–24.

61. Haanpää M, Treede RD. Capsaicin for neuropathic pain: linking tradi-tional medicine and molecular biology. *Eur Neurol* 2012; 68(5):264–75.

62. Anand P, Bley K. Topical capsaicin for pain management: therapeutic potential and mechanisms of action of the new high-concentration capsaicin 8% patch. *Br J Anaesth* 2011; 107(4):490–502.

63. Samuel EP. The autonomic and somatic innervation of the articular capsule. *Anat Rec* 1952; 113(1):53–70.

64. Ralston HJ, 3rd, Miller MR, Kasahara M. Nerve endings in human fasciae, tendons, ligaments, periosteum, and joint synovial membrane. *Anat Rec* 1960; 136:137–47.

65. Cooper RR. Nerves in cortical bone. *Science (New York)* 1968; 160(3825):327–8.

66. Badalamente MA, Cherney SB. Periosteal and vascular innervation of the human patella in degenerative joint disease. *Semin Arthritis Rheum* 1989; 18(4 Suppl 2):61–6.

67. Nixon AJ, Cummings JF. Substance P immunohistochemical study of the sensory innervation of normal subchondral bone in the equine metacarpophalangeal joint. *Am J Vet Res* 1994; 55(1):28–33.

68. Wojtys EM, Beaman DN, Glover RA, Janda D. Innervation of the human knee joint by substance-P fibers. *Arthroscopy* 1990; 6(4):254–63.

69. Marshall KW, Chiu B, Inman RD. Substance P and arthritis: analysis of plasma and synovial fluid levels. *Arthritis Rheum* 1990; 33(1):87–90.

70. Menkes CJ, Mauborgne A, Loussadi S, et al. Substance P (SP) levels in synovial tissue and synovial fluid from rheumatoid arthritis (RA) and osteoarthritis (OA) patients. In *Scientific Abstracts of the 54th Annual Meeting of the American College of Rheumatology*, Seattle, WA, 27 October–1 November, 1991.

71. Deal CL, Schnitzer TJ, Lipstein E, et al. Treatment of arthritis with topical capsaicin: a double-blind trial. *Clin Ther* 1991; 13(3):383–95.

72. McCarthy GM, McCarty DJ. Effect of topical capsaicin in the therapy of painful osteoarthritis of the hands. *J Rheumatol* 1992; 19(4):604–7.

73. Schnitzer TJ, Posner M, Lawrence ID. High strength capsaicin cream for osteoarthritis pain: rapid onset of action and improved efficacy with twice daily dosing. *J Clin Rheumatol* 1995; 1(5):268–73.

74. Kosuwon W, Sirichatiwapee W, Wisanuyotin T, Jeeravipoolvarn P, Laupattarakasem W. Efficacy of symptomatic control of knee osteoarthritis with 0.0125% of capsaicin versus placebo. *J Med Assoc Thai* 2010; 93(10):1188–95.

75. Laslett LL, Jones G. Capsaicin for osteoarthritis pain. *Prog Drug Res* 2014; 68:277–91.

76. McCleane G. The analgesic efficacy of topical capsaicin is enhanced by glyceryl trinitrate in painful osteoarthritis: a randomized, double blind, placebo controlled study. *Eur J Pain* 2000; 4(4):355–60.

77. Burch F, Codding C, Patel N, Sheldon E. Lidocaine patch 5% improves pain, stiffness, and physical function in osteoarthritis pain patients. A prospective, multicenter, open-label effectiveness trial. *Osteoarthritis Cartilage* 2004; 12(3):253–5.

78. Gammaitoni AR, Galer BS, Onawola R, Jensen MP, Argoff CE. Lidocaine patch 5% and its positive impact on pain qualities in osteoarthritis: results of a pilot 2-week, open-label study using the Neuropathic Pain Scale. *Curr Med Res Opin* 2004; 20(Suppl 2):S13–9.

CHAPTER 29

Systemic analgesics (including paracetamol and opioids)

Bernard Bannwarth and Francis Berenbaum

Introduction

Pain, stiffness, and the resultant impaired functional capacities are the main clinical features of symptomatic osteoarthritis (OA). Current evidence indicates that pain related to OA is primarily nociceptive in nature [1]. Although cartilage degradation is a hallmark imaging sign of OA, cartilage which is aneural, does not directly generate pain. On the other hand, pathological changes in subchondral bone, synovium, ligaments, and joint capsule which are richly innervated, may be the source of nociceptive stimuli in OA [1,2]. Thus, while acknowledging that central pain sensitization may occur in OA, and keeping in mind that the experience of pain may be modulated by social, psychological, and other contextual factors, peripheral pain sensitization is a major feature of the OA joint [1]. Accordingly, analgesics might have a major role in the pharmacological management of symptomatic OA.

Apart from non-steroidal anti-inflammatory drugs (NSAIDs), two categories of systemic analgesics, namely paracetamol (acetaminophen) and opioids, are currently available worldwide for clinical use. It is worthy of note that analgesics form a therapeutic class which comprises old drugs only. Since no novel broadly acting painkillers have been approved over the past decades, special attention is being paid to drugs under development as potential innovative analgesics [3]. These include biological drugs, particularly nerve growth factor (NGF) antagonists [3].

Paracetamol

Paracetamol is the active metabolite of phenacetin which was withdrawn from the market of Western countries in the 1970s–1980s, especially because its long-term use was linked to kidney damage, known as analgesic nephropathy. Both compounds exhibit similar antipyretic and analgesic properties, while being virtually devoid of any anti-inflammatory activities in humans [4].

Mechanism of action

Although paracetamol has been in clinical use for over a century, its mechanism of action is still unclear. It was shown to be a weak inhibitor of the synthesis of prostaglandins [4]. However, the capacity of paracetamol to inhibit the cyclooxygenase (COX) enzymes varies dramatically between tissues and cell types. In this respect, there are several lines of evidence that the antipyretic and analgesic properties of paracetamol result primarily from its biological activity within the central nervous system (CNS)—where the drug exerts its most potent inhibitory effects on prostaglandin

production [4]. Conversely, inflammatory cells are much less susceptible to the action of paracetamol [4].

Pharmacokinetics

Paracetamol is generally administered by oral route that allows rapid absorption of the drug, peak plasma concentrations being achieved within 0.5–1.5 hours [5]. At usually recommended doses ($\leq$4 g/day), paracetamol is largely catabolized in the liver before being excreted via the kidneys [5]. More than 80% is thus transformed into glucuronide or sulphate-conjugated derivatives. A small proportion (<10%) is oxidized by the cytochrome P450 mixed function oxidase system, producing a reactive intermediate, N-acetyl-p-benzoquinone imine, that is immediately neutralized by reduced glutathione. Less than 10% of the dose administered is found unchanged in the urine [5]. Finally, the plasma elimination half-life of paracetamol is about 2–2.5 hours, and its effects generally last 4–6 hours [5].

Several pathophysiological factors may alter the pharmacokinetics of paracetamol [5]. Its plasma clearance is decreased in elderly subjects, particularly in frail individuals, and in patients with severe renal impairment, thereby requiring dose adjustments in these patients. Furthermore, paracetamol is contraindicated in patients with advanced hepatic insufficiency [5].

Drug interactions

There are few pharmacokinetic drug–drug interactions with paracetamol, partly because of its negligible binding to plasma proteins [5]. Furthermore, cytochrome P450-inducers (e.g. rifampicin, barbiturates, phenytoin, and carbamazepine) or inhibitors (e.g. cimetidine) did not appear to produce clinically significant changes in paracetamol clearance [5].

Conversely, paracetamol was shown to induce a statistically significant and possible clinical relevant increase in the international normalized ratio (INR), with a dose-dependent relationship in patients receiving vitamin K antagonists [6]. The mean increase of the INR was 0.17 (95% confidence interval (CI): 0.004 to 0.33) per each daily gram of paracetamol [6]. Therefore, patients treated concomitantly with vitamin K antagonists and paracetamol should be monitored more regularly for possible dosage adjustment of the anticoagulant agent [6].

Clinical efficacy in osteoarthritis

Meta-analyses of randomized, placebo-controlled trials showed that paracetamol displayed statistically significant efficacy in symptomatic OA [7–9]. However, the effect size (ES) was small and even of questionable clinical relevance [7–9]. A 2010 systematic review identified ten placebo-controlled trials (published between 1983 and 2007) which enrolled 3004 patients with OA of the knee and/or hip [8]. Trial duration ranged from 1 to 24 weeks. Meta-analysis of the data showed a pooled ES of 0.18 (95% CI 0.11–0.25) for pain, 0.16 (95% CI 0.01–0.31) for physical function, and 0.20 (95% CI 0.09–0.32) for stiffness, all favouring paracetamol [8]. According to a network meta-analysis, the corresponding median ES with 95% central credible intervals (CCIs) were 0.18 (95% CCI 0.04–0.33), 0.15 (95% CCI 0.02–0.29), and 0.10 (95% CCI −0.05 to 0.26), respectively, in patients with knee OA [9]. Of note, paracetamol was the least efficacious treatment for knee OA-related pain among the four pharmacological interventions studied [9]. In this respect, unlike systemic NSAIDs, intra-articular corticosteroids, and intra-articular hyaluronic acid, paracetamol did not produce clinically significant improvement in pain at 3 months [9]. Incidentally, oral NSAIDs were slightly, but statistically significantly, superior to paracetamol, with an ES of 0.26 (95% CCI 0.10–0.42) [9].

Prior meta-analyses of randomized clinical trials that provided a head-to-head comparison between paracetamol and NSAIDs already showed better efficacy and patient preference for NSAIDs, although side effects were greater [7,10–12]. In patients with symptomatic OA of the knee and/or hip (five trials) or multiple joints (one trial), NSAIDs outperformed paracetamol for pain relief (ES = 0.20, 95% CI 0.10–0.30) [10]. The number of patients who preferred NSAIDs was 2.46 times (95% CI 1.51–4.12) the number of those preferring paracetamol [10]. A further meta-analysis of 14 randomized controlled trials comparing NSAIDs (2991 patients) versus paracetamol (1561 patients) confirmed that the former are superior to the latter for improving pain due to knee and hip OA (ES = 0.29, 95% CI 0.22–0.35) [12].

Adverse effects of paracetamol

Paracetamol at therapeutic dosage is classically considered to have an excellent safety record. However, this traditional view has been questioned in recent years [8].

Paracetamol poisoning is a leading cause of acute liver failure as a result of overproduction of N-acetyl-p-benzoquinone imine relative to glutathione stores [13]. Indeed, this metabolite derivative binds covalently to cellular proteins thereby inducing cell death [13]. Serious liver damage after a single 75 mg/kg body weight dose of paracetamol is rare, even in patients with predisposing risk factors such as excessive alcohol consumption, prior abnormal renal or hepatic function, malnutrition, or cachexia [13]. There were, however, case reports of clinically evident liver injury associated with chronic paracetamol administration at therapeutic doses, some of them being suggestive of an idiosyncratic-allergic drug reaction [14]. Furthermore, a high incidence (>30%) of serum alanine aminotransferase elevations was observed after initiation of recurrent daily intake of 4 g of paracetamol in healthy volunteers [15]. Finally, there is controversy about whether the highest safe daily dose of paracetamol is 3–3.25 g or 4 g [16]. See Box 29.1.

Peripheral COX inhibition, albeit weak, might account for possible adverse effects of the drug. Firstly, while retrospective epidemiological studies generated conflicting results regarding the gastrointestinal (GI) toxicity of paracetamol [17], a 13-week randomized clinical trial showed that paracetamol 3 g/day caused similar

---

Box 29.1 Adverse effects of paracetamol

Hepatogastrointestinal:

- Liver toxicity (usually from overdosage)
- Dyspepsia symptoms, occult GI bleeding (to be confirmed), potentiation of the GI toxicity of NSAIDs.

Cardiovascular:

- Hypertension
- Myocardial infarction (chronic/frequent use) (to be confirmed)
- Dose-related increased activity of vitamin K antagonists.

Allergic or pseudo-allergic:

- Hypersensitivity reaction (rare)
- Cross-reactivity in patients with aspirin/NSAID intolerance.

(See [13,14,17–25].)

---

degrees of blood loss (as documented by a decrease in haemoglobin level ≥ 1 g/dL) as ibuprofen 1200 mg/day [18]. Moreover, the combination of the two appeared to be additive, or even synergistic in terms of the number of patients with a greater than 2 g/dL decrease in haemoglobin [18]. These findings lend support to the hypothesis that paracetamol not only might induce occult GI bleeding, but might also potentiate the GI toxicity of NSAIDs [18]. Secondly, observational studies linked long-term or regular use of paracetamol to the development of hypertension [19]. However, due to possible biases and confounding factors, they did not allow any definitive conclusions to be drawn [19]. A small randomized clinical trial showed that treatment with paracetamol (3 g/day) resulted in a statistically significant increase in blood pressure from baseline compared to placebo in patients with coronary artery disease [20]. This increase (2–3 mm) was within the range of the hypertensive effects of NSAIDs [21]. Accordingly, it might have a significant impact on the incidence of cardiovascular thrombotic events [20]. Interestingly, a prospective cohort study reported that women who frequently (≥22 days/month) used paracetamol or NSAIDs had a relative risk for a major cardiovascular event of 1.35 (95% CI 1.14–1.59) and 1.44 (95% CI 1.27–1.65), respectively, compared with non-users [22]. On the other hand, moderate use (≤21 days/month) did not confer a significant cardiovascular risk [22]. It is noteworthy that a recent systematic literature review, based on eight cohort studies fulfilling the inclusion criteria, highlighted a dose–response significant increase of the cardiovascular risk [23]. Furthermore, paracetamol (2 g/day) was shown to destabilize blood pressure control in OA patients with stable treated hypertension [23]. In summary, regular monitoring of blood pressure may be recommended for patients taking long-term paracetamol. Thirdly, paracetamol may precipitate or aggravate asthma, rhinitis, urticaria, and/or angio-oedema in patients with aspirin/NSAIDs intolerance [24]. These reactions are elicited by non-allergic mechanisms via inhibition of COX-1 and subsequent alteration in eicosanoid biosynthesis, most prominently leukotriene overproduction [24]. Patients with aspirin-induced asthma displayed the highest rates of cross reactivity to paracetamol [24]. In these patients, the incidence of cross sensitivity to paracetamol was estimated at 7% (95% CI 0–16%) while cross sensitivity to non-selective NSAIDs occurred in almost all of them [25]. Although most reactions to paracetamol were mild compared with those induced by NSAIDs, patients diagnosed with asthma or chronic urticaria should be aware of the increased risk of experiencing a hypersensitivity reaction to paracetamol [24,25]. On the other hand, there is no sound evidence that frequent paracetamol use may be associated with an increased risk of asthma in both children and adults [26]. Similarly, despite numerous epidemiological studies on the subject, current data are inconsistent regarding an association between either renal function decline or end-stage renal failure and long-term use of paracetamol [27]. However, chronic exposure to paracetamol might favour the progression of renal disease in patients with pre-existing chronic kidney disease [27].

Role for paracetamol in the management of osteoarthritis

Taken together, available data indicate that paracetamol would offer little advantage over placebo in relieving pain and improving physical function in patients with OA of the lower limb joints. For OA of other joints, especially the hand, the efficacy of paracetamol remains unclear, since there have been no placebo-controlled trials [28]. Nevertheless, paracetamol has been almost consistently recommended as the oral analgesic of first choice by expert guidelines [29]. Conversely, the 2013 American Academy of Orthopaedic Surgeons (AAOS) guidelines for knee OA did not recommend for or against the use of paracetamol because of inconclusive evidence for efficacy [29]. It was, however, specified that 'practitioners should feel little constraint in following a recommendation labelled as inconclusive', more especially as individual patient preference has to play a role in treatment decision making [29]. The 2014 Osteoarthritis Research Society International (OARSI) guidance on non-surgical management of knee OA considered paracetamol as an appropriate analgesia option for those patients without relevant co-morbidities because of safety concerns, particularly when the drug is used for extended durations [30]. Finally, the National Institute for Health and Care Excellence kept paracetamol as first-line treatment in the most recent UK guidelines despite the draft guidelines having said that it should be avoided [31].

To justify the place of paracetamol as first-line systemic analgesic for OA, it may be argued that many treated patients do experience satisfactory improvement in symptoms even if the actual 'treatment effect' (i.e. difference between the paracetamol group and the placebo group) is of minimal value. In fact, there is clear evidence for positive benefits from placebo, referred to as the 'placebo effect' (i.e. difference between baseline and endpoint). For pain relief, the ES was 0.47 (95% CI 0.17–0.78) for placebo in randomized clinical trials of paracetamol [32]. Placebo is also effective for other subjective outcomes such as stiffness and self-reported function [32]. Furthermore, paracetamol poses a lower risk of severe adverse drug reactions and has fewer contraindications and drug interactions than NSAIDs. It is also better tolerated than opioids while being devoid of any abuse potential.

Opioids

Mechanism of action

The biological effects of opioids are mediated by receptors that are mainly expressed in the CNS [33]. There are three main types of opioid receptors, namely μ (mu), κ (kappa), and δ (delta), each of them being associated with a range of psychological and physiological responses to endogenous or exogenous ligands [33].

Commonly prescribed opioid compounds are primarily μ agonists, and hence they produce similar desirable (analgesia) and untoward effects [33,34]. Tramadol, unlike other opioids, also inhibits the reuptake of noradrenaline and serotonin, thereby enhancing inhibitory effects on pain transmission in the spinal cord [33]. Despite this unique mechanism of action, the adverse effect profile of tramadol is typical of an opioid analgesic [33].

Although opioid analgesics share a similar pharmacodynamic profile, they differ from each other in some respects, probably because they interact with opioid receptor types with variable affinity and intrinsic activity [33]. Indeed, individual opioids do differ in their analgesic efficacy [33]. Thus, opioid analgesics can be classified according to the pain intensity for which they are conventionally used for relieving cancer pain [33]. As such, they are usually divided into 'weak opioids' (e.g. codeine, and tramadol) and 'strong opioids' (e.g. morphine, oxycodone, hydrocodone, hydromorphone, fentanyl, and tapentadol) [33]. Although weak opioids and strong opioids are primarily intended for moderate and severe pain, respectively, an alternative approach for patients with moderate pain incorporates the use of a low dose of a strong opioid [33].

Opioid equianalgesic dose ratios have been proposed to help clinicians estimate daily morphine equivalent dose taken by a patient [35]. In this respect, codeine 200 mg, tramadol 120 mg, hydrocodone 30 mg, and oxycodone 20 mg were reported to be equianalgesic to oral morphine 30 mg [33,35]. However, these are approximates only [33,35]. Furthermore, there is great variability of patient response to individual opioids. Therefore, equianalgesic dose ratios should not be used for conversion from one opioid to another [35]. When switching from an opioid to another, the second opioid should generally be started at half the dose equivalent of the first in order to prevent overdose [36].

Pharmacological features of commonly used opioids

Opioid analgesics are characterized by a short plasma elimination half-life in patients with normal renal function [33]. Since their mean duration of action ranges from 2 to 6 hours, standard oral formulations require frequent dosing in patients with chronic pain [33]. To improve the convenience of therapy in these patients, controlled-release preparations were developed for once- or twice-daily administration [33]. Many opioids are also marketed as fixed-dose combination products with paracetamol or an NSAID [33].

As already mentioned, there are significant interindividual variations in the response to opioids. Several factors may contribute to this variability, including genetic factors [37]. Codeine (methylmorphine) is a prodrug that is converted to its active moiety (morphine) by the cytochrome P450 CYP2D6 enzyme. Thus, patients who are deficient in that enzyme (6% of the Caucasian population) are unlikely to get analgesia from codeine [37]. Similarly, patients with low CYP2D6 activity may be less responsive to tramadol as compared to those with normal CYP2D6 activity [37]. Factors affecting drug bioavailability have also to be considered. Intersubject differences in first-pass metabolism of orally administered opioids, particularly morphine and oxycodone may result in significant interindividual variability in their bioavailability [33]. Furthermore, caution is required in the setting of impaired renal function because these patients may accumulate both the parent opioid compounds and their active and/or toxic metabolites [33].

Clinical efficacy in osteoarthritis

A 2007 published meta-analysis of six placebo-controlled trials found that opioids as a class produced analgesic effects similar to oral NSAIDs in patients with knee OA associated with moderate to severe pain [38]. The maximum efficacy of opioids relative to placebo appeared at 2–4 weeks and corresponded to 10.5 mm (95% CI 7.4–13.7) on a 100-mm visual analogue scale (VAS) [38]. This effect, while just exceeding the minimal perceptible clinical improvement threshold (i.e. 9.7 mm), may be inflated by high withdrawal rates (24–50%) and 'best-case' scenarios reported in intention-to-treat analyses [38]. Further meta-analyses were performed separately for tramadol and non-tramadol opioids.

A meta-analysis of 11 randomized clinical trials with a mean duration of 35 days (7–91 days) showed that mean daily doses of 200 mg of tramadol, given either alone (nine studies) or in combination with paracetamol (two studies), decreased pain intensity and improved function in patients with knee and/or hip OA [39]. Compared to placebo, the benefits were, however, small. They represented 8.5 units (95% CI 4.9–12.1) on a 0–100 scale for pain, and 0.34 (95% CI 0.19–0.49) on a 0–10 scale for the total WOMAC score [39]. Finally, tramadol increased by 37% the likelihood of a moderate global improvement compared to placebo (69% vs 50% of the patients, respectively) [39].

A recently updated Cochrane review identified 22 randomized or quasi-randomized controlled trials of non-tramadol opioids involving 8275 patients with knee or hip OA [40]. Oral oxycodone was studied in ten trials, transdermal buprenorphine and oral tapentadol in four, oral codeine in three, oral morphine and oxymorphone in two, and transdermal fentanyl and oral hydromorphone in one trial each [40]. The median follow-up for pain and function was 4 and 5 weeks, respectively [40]. Analyses of pain relief found a mean ES of 0.28 (95% CI 0.20–0.38) for these drugs over placebo. This corresponds to a difference in pain score of 7 mm on 100-mm VAS or a difference in improvement of 12% (95% CI 9–15%) between opioids and placebo. Regarding function, the improvement was of similar small magnitude with an ES of 0.26 (95% CI 0.17–0.35), corresponding to a difference in improvement of 11% (95% CI 7–14%) between opioids and placebo [40]. There were no substantial differences in effects according to type of opioid, analgesic potency, daily dose, or route of administration, whereas trials with shorter treatment durations (≤4 weeks) showed larger pain relief than trials with longer treatment duration [40].

In summary, short-term clinical trials provided evidence that patients with knee or hip OA may derive some clinical benefit from using opioids. However, the average benefit is modest and may even decline over time [40]. Unfortunately, no placebo-controlled or active-controlled studies evaluated long-term (>1 year) outcomes related to pain, function, or quality of life [41]. Finally, it is unknown how strong opioids compare with NSAIDs in patients with an inadequate response to paracetamol and/or weak opioids.

Adverse effects and safety issues

By activating opioid receptors, opioid analgesics have the potential to produce a broad range of adverse events (Box 29.2) that would make patients stop taking the medication. Data from clinical trials of opioids in OA indicated that 7% of the patients given placebo dropped out from the study due to side effects and that this risk was about fourfold (3.96, 95% CI 3.43–4.56) higher among participants

---

Box 29.2 Adverse effects of opioid analgesics

Gastrointestinal:
- Nausea, vomiting, constipation
- GI or biliary spasm.

Neurological and psychiatric:
- Sedation, dizziness, hyperalgesia, seizures, or myoclonus (high doses)
- Cognitive impairment, mental clouding, confusion, sleep disorders, nightmare, hallucinations, euphoria
- Behavioural disorders, including misuse, abuse, and addiction.

Cardiopulmonary:
- Respiratory depression, bronchoconstriction (high doses)
- Orthostatic hypotension, bradycardia (high doses).

Urinary:
- Urinary retention.

Endocrine:
- Androgen deficiency, reduced testosterone production
- Menstrual irregularities.

Allergic or immunological:
- Pruritus
- Immunosuppression (not clearly established).

(See [32,33,39–41].)

---

who received opioids [40]. Studies with strong opioids resulted in a significantly higher risk of dropouts compared to weak opioids, with odds ratios of 6.37 (95% CI 5.03–8.05) and 3.01 (95% CI 2.52–3.60), respectively [42]. These findings are in agreement with those reported in meta-analyses of clinical trials of tramadol and non-tramadol opioids [39,40]. The overall dropout rate due to adverse events was 21% in tramadol-treated patients compared to 9% in placebo-treated patients [39]. Similarly, dropouts were more frequent in patients receiving non-tramadol opioids compared to controls (pooled risk ratio 3.76, 95% CI 2.93–4.82) [40].

The overall incidence of adverse events seems to be similar for different opioids at the same level of analgesia, even though there are interindividual differences in the tolerability to a specific agent [33,36,40]. Furthermore, older people are more susceptible to these adverse effects because of altered opioid pharmacokinetics and/or increased sensitivity to CNS acting drugs associated with ageing [33].

The most frequent side effects include gastrointestinal (nausea, vomiting, constipation), neurological and psychiatric (sedation, cognitive impairment, dizziness,) and skin (itching) disorders [33–35,39,40]. CNS adverse effects, including dizziness and altered state of consciousness, may explain why opioids, as a class, appeared to be associated with an increased risk of fractures and motor vehicles accidents [41]. Furthermore, epidemiological studies suggested that opioids may increase the risk of myocardial infarction [41].

Although respiratory depression is potentially the most serious untoward effect, clinically significant respiratory depression rarely occurs when the opioid dose is carefully titrated [33]. Of note, both sedative and respiratory depressant effects of opioids may be potentiated by concomitant use of other sedating drugs such as benzodiazepines [33].

Except for constipation, tolerance to opioid-induced adverse effects usually develops rapidly so that symptoms resolve in most patients within the first several days of stable opioid therapy [33]. Accordingly, the risk of an adverse event is usually greater shortly after the initial opioid prescription or after dose escalation [33,41]. Since constipation is, in addition, the most common adverse effect occurring with chronic opioid use, prophylactic treatments are essential to minimize this complication [33]. Tolerance may also develop to opioid-induced analgesia, thereby bringing about the need for dose escalation to maintain equipotent analgesic effects [34,36]. However, the need for dose escalation may also be related to the development of a paradoxical increase in pain sensitivity, also known as 'opioid-induced hyperalgesia' [34,36]. This pronociceptive process which is characterized by both an increase in pain perception and lower nociceptive threshold, is more likely to occur in patients treated with higher doses of opioids [34].

Most importantly, along with the dramatic increase in the use of opioids for chronic non-cancer pain, including OA pain, during the past decade [43], there has been a steep increase in abuse, misuse, and both fatal and non-fatal overdoses involving prescription opioids, particularly strong opioids [34,35,41]. Moreover, opioid therapy poses a risk of addiction, that is, a psychological and behavioural syndrome characterized by a continued craving for an opioid drug to achieve a psychic effect, and associated aberrant drug-related behaviours, including compulsive use and continued use despite harm to self or others [33]. Psychiatric illness, history of substance abuse, and younger age may predispose to problem use of opioid medications [33,34].

Role for opioids in the management of osteoarthritis

Meta-analyses of short-term clinical trials showed that, on average, the small clinical benefits of opioids did not outweigh the side effects in patients with symptomatic OA [42]. Indeed, the small mean benefits of non-tramadol opioids were contrasted by a significant increase in the risk of adverse events [40], and tramadol exhibited similar number needed to treat (NNT) for pain relief (NNT = 6, 95% CI 4–9) and for a major adverse event leading to study withdrawal (NNT = 8, 95% CI 7–12) [39]. Furthermore, it appeared that patients preferred to stop opioids more often than placebo, regardless of the reason for treatment discontinuation [42]. Regarding long-term opioid therapy, there is still uncertainty about its effectiveness whereas there is evidence of serious adverse events and potential harms [40,42]. However, there are few other analgesics, and none of them have proven particularly effective and safe. Thus, there is general agreement that opioid use may be warranted in selected OA patients [2,29,39,40,42].

Indeed, most current guidelines support the use of opioids for refractory pain related to hip and knee OA, but not to hand OA [28,29]. Nevertheless, the American College of Rheumatology guidelines conditionally recommend the use of tramadol (to the exclusion of all other opioids) in patients with hand OA [44]. For knee or hip OA, these guidelines conditionally recommend tramadol as an initial pharmacological therapy, and strongly recommend opioid analgesics for patients who have not had an adequate response to both pharmacological and nonpharmacological modalities and are either unwilling to undergo or are not candidates for total joint arthroplasty [44]. The European League Against Rheumatism recommendations for the management of knee and hip OA stated that 'opioid analgesics, with or without paracetamol, are useful alternatives in patients in whom NSAIDs are contraindicated, ineffective, and/or poorly tolerated' [45,46]. On the other hand, the updated OARSI guidelines consider opioids (oral or transdermal) as treatments of uncertain appropriateness for any patients with knee OA [29]. While the guidelines did not differentiate between weak and strong opioids, some experts proposed to reserve strong opioids for special situations, such as for short-term treatment of later stage OA awaiting surgery [2,39].

Nerve growth factor antagonists

In view of the limited efficacy and/or potential harms of available drugs, there is an obvious unmet need for new effective and safe analgesics for OA. Unfortunately, new chemical molecules targeting novel neurotransmitters or receptors involved in pain processing produced disappointing results, and none has yet been approved for clinical use [3].

Since NGF was shown to function as a key mediator in both nociceptive and neuropathic pain, special attention has been paid to humanized monoclonal antibodies (mAbs) that operate as NGF-capturing agents [3] (Figure 29.1). Among these, tanezumab is at an advanced stage of clinical development while fulranumab and fasinumab are in early phases of development [3]. All three were investigated in patients with symptomatic OA of the knee and/or hip [47]. Compared to placebo, tanezumab 5 mg and 10 mg administered intravenously at 8-week intervals provided similar clinically meaningful and statistically significant improvements in pain and physical function [47]. Moreover, tanezumab appeared to be clearly superior to oxycodone, and it was shown to be more efficacious than celecoxib and naproxen in patients who experienced partial symptomatic relief with an NSAID [47]. Phase II placebo-controlled trials of fulranumab and fasinumab also generated positive results [47].

Treatment-emergent adverse events were similar across anti-NGF mAbs, thus being suggestive of 'class-specific effects' [47]. These consisted mainly of peripheral oedema, arthralgia, pain in the extremities, and neurosensory symptoms such as paraesthesia, hypoesthesia, or allodynia [47]. Most peripheral sensory symptoms resolved without sequelae within 1 month [47]. However, there were reported cases with long-lasting, persistent symptoms [47]. Moreover, some patients developed peripheral neuropathies, including focal mononeuropathy (predominantly carpal tunnel syndrome) and, more rarely, radiculopathy or peripheral polyneuropathy [47]. Thus, given the possible role of NGF for the maintenance of adult neurons, there may be fears that NGF inhibition might be associated with irreversible structural neurotoxic effects [3]. But the most problematic issue was joint failure requiring total joint arthroplasty, an unpredicted safety signal that led the US Food and Drug Administration to place the non-cancer related trials of NGF antagonists on clinical hold in 2010 [47]. Indeed, patients given NGF mAbs had a dose-dependent increased risk for developing rapidly destructive arthropathies [47]. This risk was greater with longer duration of anti-NGF exposure and even greater when NSAIDs were used concurrently [47]. Of note, both weight-bearing and non-weight-bearing joints were affected as were joints with

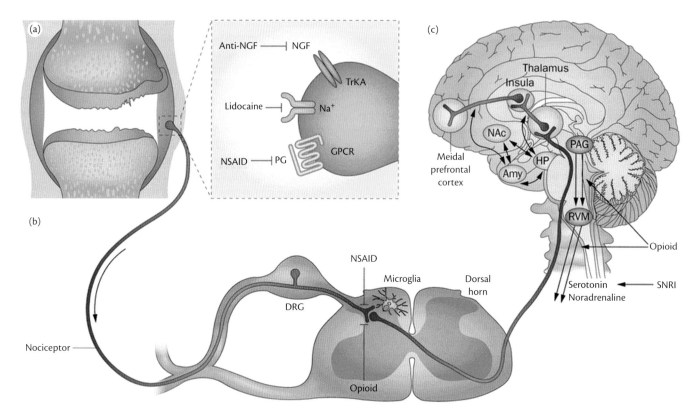

Figure 29.1 Neuroanatomy of the pain pathway and analgesic targets in OA. (a) Pain signals are detected by nociceptors in the periphery and carried to the dorsal horn of the spinal cord. Various analgesics that are efficacious against joint pain act in the periphery by targeting receptors expressed at nociceptor peripheral terminals. (b) The central terminals of the afferent nociceptors synapse with second-order neurons in the dorsal horn, in a stratified pattern that is anatomically very precisely organized. Second-order neurons are either interneurons (not shown) or projection neurons that cross to the contralateral side and carry the signal up the spinal cord. Central sensitization can occur through the strengthening of synapses and through the loss of inhibitory mechanisms. In addition, the activation of microglia contributes to enhanced pain sensitivity. Prostaglandins can also have a sensitizing effect in the dorsal horn, and NSAIDs can thus exert central analgesic actions, in addition to their peripheral actions. Opioids can inhibit incoming pain signals in the dorsal horn. (c) Projection neurons relay pain signals along the spinothalamic tract to the thalamus, and along the spinoreticulothalamic tract to the brainstem. From there, the signals can be propagated to different areas of the brain, including the cortex. Descending pathways (black arrows), both facilitating and inhibitory, modulate pain transmission; descending inhibitory pathways release noradrenaline and serotonin onto the spinal circuits. SNRIs engage these descending inhibitory pathways. RVM neurons are opioid sensitive, and morphine has an analgesic effect through engaging descending inhibition. Amy, amygdala; DRG, dorsal root ganglion; GPCR, G-protein-coupled receptor; HP, hippocampus; NAc, nucleus accumbens; NGF, nerve growth factor; PAG, periaqueductal grey; PG, prostaglandin; RVM, rostral ventromedial medulla; SNRI, serotonin–noradrenaline reuptake inhibitor.
From Malfait AM, Schnitzer TJ. Towards a mechanism-based approach to pain management in osteoarthritis. *Nature Rev Rheum* 2013; 9:654–64.

no-to-minimal OA [47]. The underlying pathophysiological mechanism is unknown. However, it must be kept in mind that NGF was reported to contribute to processes involved in tissue homeostasis and repair [3]. Whereas some experts consider that the dramatic analgesia induced by anti-NGF could accelerate the OA process by overutilization of the damaged joint, others suggest that NGF inhibition itself might thereby impair bone remodelling and compromise joint integrity [3].

Notwithstanding that pharmaceutical companies may have been allowed to resume clinical trials of NGF mAbs under the conditions of implementing adequate risk minimization measures, it may be *anticipated* that these drugs, if approved for marketing, will be reserved for selected and well-defined patients with OA.

Conclusion

Due to the limited efficacy along with safety issues of drug therapy, it is unquestionable that optimal management of OA requires a combination of non-pharmacological and pharmacological treatment modalities, as already stressed by current guidelines [28,29,30,44,45,47].

References

1. Dieppe PA, Lohmander LS. Pathogenesis and management of pain in osteoarthritis. *Lancet* 2005; 365:965–73.
2. Bijlsma JW, Berenbaum F, Lafeber FP. Osteoarthritis: an update with relevance for clinical practice. *Lancet* 2011; 377:2115–26.
3. Bannwarth B, Kostine M. Biologics in the treatment of chronic pain: a new era of therapy? *Clin Pharmacol Ther* 2015; 97:122–4.
4. Graham GG, Scott KF. Mechanism of action of paracetamol. *Am J Ther* 2005; 12:46–55.
5. Bannwarth B, Péhourcq F. Pharmacological rationale for the clinical use of paracetamol: pharmacokinetic and pharmacodynamic issues. *Drugs* 2003; 63(Special Issue 2):5–13.
6. Caldeira D, Costa J, Barra M, et al. How safe is acetaminophen use in patients treated with vitamin K antagonists? A systematic reviewed meta-analysis. *Thromb Res* 2015; 135:58–61.
7. Towheed T, Maxwell L, Judd M, et al. Acetaminophen for osteoarthritis. *Cochrane Database Syst Rev* 2006:CD004257.

8. Bannuru RR, Dasi UR, McAlindon TE. Reassessing the role of acetaminophen in osteoarthritis. Systematic review and meta-analysis. *Osteoarthritis Cartilage* 2010; 18(Suppl 2):S250 [abstract 558].

9. Bannuru RR, Schmid CH, Kent DM, et al. Comparative effectiveness of pharmacologic interventions for knee osteoarthritis. *Ann Intern Med* 2015; 162:46–54.

10. Zhang W, Jones A, Doherty M. Does paracetamol (acetaminophen) reduce the pain of osteoarthritis? A meta-analysis of randomised controlled trials. *Ann Rheum Dis* 2004; 63:901–7.

11. Lee C, Straus WL, Balshaw R, et al. A comparison of the efficacy and safety of nonsteroidal antiinflammatory agents versus acetaminophen in the treatment of osteoarthritis: a meta-analysis. *Arthritis Rheum* 2004; 51:746–54.

12. Verkleij SP, Luijsterburg PA, Bohnen AM, et al. NSAIDs vs acetaminophen in knee and hip osteoarthritis: a systematic review regarding heterogeneity influencing the outcomes. *Osteoarthritis Cartilage* 2011; 19:921–9.

13. Ferner RE, Dear JW, Bateman DN. Management of paracetamol poisoning. *BMJ* 2011; 342:d2218.

14. Vitols S. Paracetamol hepatotoxicity at therapeutic doses. *J Intern Med* 2003; 253:95–8.

15. Watkins PB, Kaplowitz N, Slattery JT, et al. Aminotransferase elevations in healthy adults receiving 4 grams of acetaminophen daily. A randomized controlled trial. *JAMA* 2006; 296:87–93.

16. Krenzelok EP, Royal MA. Confusion: acetaminophen dosing changes based on no evidence in adults. *Drugs R D* 2012; 12:45–8.

17. Bannwarth B. Gastrointestinal safety of paracetamol: is there any cause for concern? *Expert Opin Drug Saf* 2004; 3:269–72.

18. Doherty M, Hawkey C, Goulder M, et al. A randomised controlled trial of ibuprofen, paracetamol or a combination tablet of ibuprofen/paracetamol in community-derived people with knee pain. *Ann Rheum Dis* 2011; 70:1534–41.

19. Montgomery B. Does paracetamol cause hypertension? *BMJ* 2008; 336:1190–1.

20. Sudano I, Flammer AJ, Périat D, et al. Acetaminophen increases blood pressure in patients with coronary artery disease. *Circulation* 2010; 122:1789–96.

21. Chan AT, Manson JE, Albert CM, et al. Nonsteroidal antiinflammatory drugs, acetaminophen, and the risk of cardiovascular events. *Circulation* 2006; 113:1578–87.

22. Roberts E, Delgado Nunes V, Buckner S, et al. Paracetamol: not as safe as we thought? A systematic literature review of observational studies. *Ann Rheum Dis* 2016; 75(3):552–9.

23. Gualtierotti R, Zoppi A, Mugellini A, et al. Effect of naproxen and acetaminophen on blood pressure lowering by ramipril, valsartan and aliskiren in hypertensive patients. *Expert Opin Pharmacother* 2013; 14:1875–84.

24. Kim YJ, Lim KH, Kim MY, et al. Cross-reactivity to acetaminophen and celecoxib according to the type of nonsteroidal anti-inflammatory drug hypersensitivity. *Allergy Asthma Immunol Res* 2014; 6:156–62.

25. Jenkins C, Costello J, Hodge L. Systematic review of prevalence of aspirin induced asthma and its implications for clinical practice. *BMJ* 2004; 328:434–7.

26. Dharmage SC, Allen KJ. Does regular paracetamol ingestion increase the risk of developing asthma? *Clin Exp Allergy* 2011; 41:459–60.

27. Kuo HW, Tsai SS, Tiao MM, et al. Analgesic use and the risk for progression of chronic kidney disease. *Pharmacoepidemiol Drug Saf* 2010; 19:745–51.

28. Zhang W, Doherty M, Leeb BF, et al. EULAR evidence based recommendations for the management of hand osteoarthritis: report of a Task Force of the EULAR Standing Committee for International Clinical Studies Including Therapeutics (ESCISIT). *Ann Rheum Dis* 2007; 66:377–88.

29. Nelson AE, Allen KD, Golightly YM, et al. A systematic review of recommendations and guidelines for the management of osteoarthritis: The chronic osteoarthritis management initiative of the U.S. bone and joint initiative. *Semin Arthritis Rheum* 2014; 43:701–12.

30. McAlindon TE, Bannuru RR, Sullivan MC, et al. OARSI guidelines for the non-surgical management of knee osteoarthritis. *Osteoarthritis Cartilage* 2014; 22:363–88.

31. Zhang W, Robertson J, Jones AC, et al. The placebo effect and its determinants in osteoarthritis: meta-analysis of randomised controlled trials. *Ann Rheum Dis* 2008; 67:1716–23.

32. Wise J. NICE keeps paracetamol in UK guidelines on osteoarthritis. *BMJ*. 2014; 348:g1545.

33. Cherny NI. Opioid analgesics. Comparative features and prescribing guidelines. *Drugs* 1996; 51:713–37.

34. Crofford LJ. Adverse effects of chronic opioid therapy for chronic musculoskeletal pain. *Nat Rev Rheumatol* 2010; 6:191–7.

35. Franklin GM. Opioids for chronic noncancer pain. A position paper of the American Academy of Neurology. *Neurology* 2014; 83:1277–84.

36. Ballantyne JC, Mao J. Opioid therapy for chronic pain. *N Engl J Med* 2003; 349:1943–53.

37. Zahari Z, Ismail R. Influence of cytochrome P450, subfamily D, polypeptide 6 (CYP2D6) polymorphisms on pain sensitivity and clinical response to weak opioid analgesics. *Drug Metab Pharmacokinet* 2014; 29:29–43.

38. Bjordal JM, Klovning A, Ljunggren AE, et al. Short-term efficacy of pharmacotherapeutic interventions in osteoarthritic knee pain: a meta-analysis of randomised placebo-controlled trials. *Eur J Pain* 2007; 11:125–38.

39. Cepeda MS, Camargo F, Zea C, et al. Tramadol for osteoarthritis. *Cochrane Database Syst Rev* 2006; (3):CD005522.

40. Da Costa BR, Nüesch E, Kasteler R, et al. Oral or transdermal opioids for osteoarthritis of the knee or hip. *Cochrane Database Syst Rev* 2014; 9:CD003115.

41. Chou R, Turner JA, devine EB, et al. The effectiveness and risks of long-term opioid therapy for chronic pain: a systematic review for a National Institutes of Health Pathways to Prevention Workshop. *Ann Intern Med* 2015; 162(4):276–86.

42. Gehling M, Hermann B, Tryba M. Meta-analysis of dropout rates in randomized controlled clinical trials: opioid analgesia for osteoarthritis pain. *Schmerz* 2011; 25:296–305.

43. Wright EA, Katz JN, Abrams S, et al. Trends in prescription of opioids from 2003-2009 in persons with knee osteoarthritis. *Arthritis Care Res* 2014; 66:1489–95.

44. Hochberg MC, Altman RD, April KT, et al. American College of Rheumatology 2012 recommendations for the use of nonpharmacologic and pharmacologic therapies in osteoarthritis of the hand, hip, and knee. *Arthritis Care Res* 2012; 64:465–74.

45. Jordan KM, Arden NK, Doherty M, et al. EULAR recommendations 2003: an evidence based approach to the management of knee osteoarthritis: report of a Task Force of the Standing Committee for International Clinical Studies Including Therapeutic Trials (ESCISIT). *Ann Rheum Dis* 2003; 62:1145–55.

46. Zhang W, Doherty M, Arden N, et al. EULAR evidence based recommendations for the management of hip osteoarthritis: report of a task force of the EULAR Standing Committee for International Clinical Studies Including Therapeutics (ESCISIT). *Ann Rheum Dis* 2005; 64:669–81.

47. Bannwarth B, Kostine M. Targeting nerve growth factor for pain management: what does the future hold for NGF antagonists? *Drugs* 2014; 74:619–26.

48. Malfait AM, Schnitzer TJ. Towards a mechanism-based approach to pain management in osteoarthritis. *Nature Rev Rheum* 2013; 9:654–64.

CHAPTER 30

Non-steroidal anti-inflammatory drugs

Lee S. Simon and Marc C. Hochberg

Introduction

Non-steroidal anti-inflammatory drugs (NSAIDs) are a chemically diverse group of compounds that share three cardinal characteristics: they are anti-inflammatory, analgesic, and antipyretic [1,2]. They are approved by regulatory authorities for the treatment of patients with osteoarthritis (OA), rheumatoid arthritis, ankylosing spondylitis, acute gout, and some forms of juvenile idiopathic arthritis. They are also used for the treatment of acute pain, dysmenorrhea, chronic low back pain, and postoperative pain, especially after dental extraction. There are at least 20 chemically different NSAIDs currently available in Europe and the United States (Table 30.1). These include not only the 'traditional' non-selective cyclooxygenase (COX) inhibitors that inhibit both the COX1 and COX2 enzymes but also the COX2 selective inhibitors (coxibs, e.g. celecoxib and etoricoxib), which have similar efficacy in the treatment of patients with OA but significantly decreased gastrointestinal (GI) adverse effects and antiplatelet effects (see later in chapter).

NSAIDs are one of the most commonly used classes of drugs in developed countries. It has been reported that more than 17 million Americans use these agents on a daily basis for the relief of pain and, at times, swelling related to inflammation [3]. With the ageing of the US population, the Centers for Disease Control and Prevention predicted a significant increase in the prevalence of painful arthritis and rheumatic conditions and thus an increased use of NSAIDs [3]. Approximately 60 million NSAID prescriptions are written each year in the United States; the number for elderly patients exceeds those for younger patients by approximately 3.6-fold. Based on calendar year 2013 data for the United States, the five most commonly prescribed NSAIDs were ibuprofen followed by meloxicam, naproxen, diclofenac, and celecoxib [4].

Mechanism of action

The primary mechanism of action of NSAIDs is inhibition of prostaglandin biosynthesis.

Prostaglandins of the E series are pro-inflammatory, and increase vascular permeability and sensitivity to the release of bradykinins. Decreasing the synthesis of these mediators leads to reduced pain, swelling, and oedema in the peripheral tissues. In addition, there is accumulating evidence that central effects of pain modulation may be as important as the effects on the peripheral tissues. The hypothesis is that prostaglandin synthesis is upregulated in the brain with peripheral stimulation of pain particularly associated with inflammation, and those NSAIDs that are more lipophilic penetrate better into the central nervous system and inhibit synthesis of both peripheral and central prostaglandins [5].

Prostaglandins are derived from polyunsaturated fatty acids, such as arachidonic acid, that are constituents of all cell membranes. These molecules exist in ester linkage in the glycerols of phospholipids and are converted through multiple enzymatic steps to prostaglandins or leukotrienes first through the action of phospholipase A2. Free arachidonic acid, released by the phospholipase from the fatty acids, acts as a substrate for the prostaglandin (PG) H synthase complex, which includes both COX and peroxidase. These enzymes catalyse the conversion of arachidonic acid to the unstable cyclic-endoperoxide intermediates, PGG2 and PGH2, which are then converted to the more stable PGE2 and PGF2 compounds by specific tissue prostaglandin syntheses. NSAIDs specifically inhibit COX and thereby reduce the conversion of arachidonic acid to PGG2 (Figure 30.1).

At least two isoforms of the COX enzymes have now been identified. They are products of two different genes yet share approximately 60% homology in the amino acid sequences considered important for catalysis of arachidonic acid. The differences are primarily in their regulation and expression [6,7]. COX1, or prostaglandin synthase H1 (PGHS1), regulates normal cellular physiologic processes and is stimulated by hormones or growth factors. It is constitutively expressed in most tissues, and is inhibited by all non-selective NSAIDs to varying degrees depending on the applied experimental model system used to measure drug effects [8–11]. It has an important role in maintaining the integrity of the mucosa of the GI tract, and many of the adverse effects of the NSAIDs on the GI tract are attributed to its inhibition [12–17]. It has been described as a 'housekeeping enzyme'.

The other isoform, prostaglandin synthase H2 (PGHS2 or COX2) is an inducible enzyme and is usually undetectable in most tissues. Its expression is increased during states of inflammation or experimentally in response to mitogenic stimuli. In monocyte/macrophage systems, endotoxin stimulates COX2 expression; in fibroblasts various growth factors, phorbol esters, and interleukin 1 do so [2,6]. This isoform is also constitutively expressed in the brain, specifically the cortex and hippocampus, in the female reproductive tract, the male vas deferens, in bone, and in human kidney [6,7]. In the brain it appears that COX2 is upregulated with increased inflammation-induced pain impulses; thus, the inhibition of COX2 in the brain is thought to be an important modulator of pain in

Table 30.1 Non-steroidal anti-inflammatory drugs

Medication	Proprietary (trade) name	Usual daily dose (adults)	Serum half-life hours
Non-selective NSAIDS			
Carboxylic acid derivatives			
Aspirin (acetylsalicylic acid)	Multiple	2.4–6 g/24 h in four divided doses	4–15
Salsalate	Disalcid	1.5–3.0 g/24 h bid	Same
Diflunisal	Dolobid	0.5–1.5 g/24 h bid	7–15
Choline magnesium trisalicylate[†]	Trilisate	1.5–3 g/24 h bid–tid	
Proponic acid derivatives			
Ibuprofen[†]	Motrin, Rufen, OTC	OTC: 200–400 mg qid	2
		Rx: 400, 600, 800, maximum: 3200 mg	
Naproxen[†]	Naprolan, Anaprox, Naprosyn EC	250, 375, 500 mg bid	13
Fenoprofen	Nalfon	300–600 mg qid	3
Ketoprofen	Orudis	75 mg tid	2
Flurbiprofen	Ansaid	100 mg bid–tid	3–9
Oxaprozin	Daypro	600–1800 mg/24h	40–50
Tolmetin	Tolectin	400, 600, 800 mg; 800–2400 mg	1
Acetic acid derivatives			
Indomethacin[†]	Indocin, Indocin SR	25–50 mg tid or qid	3–11
	Indocin SR	SR: 75 mg bid; rarely > 150 mg/24h	
Tolmetin	See above		1
Sulindac	Clinoril	150, 200 mg bid–tid	16
Diclofenac	Voltaren, Arthrotec	50 tid, 75 mg bid	1–2
Etodolac	Lodine	200–300 mg bid–tid–qid	2–4
		maximum: 1200 mg	
Ketorolac	Toradol	20–40 mg	2
Fenamates			
Meclofenamate	Meclomen	50–100 mg tid–qid	2–3
Mefenamic acid	Ponstel	250 mg qid	2
Enolic acid derivatives			
Piroxicam	Feldene	10, 20 mg once a day	30–86
Meloxicam	Mobic	7.5–15 mg	20
Naphthylkanones			
Nabumetone	Relafen	500 mg bid up to 1500 mg/24 h	19–30
COX-2 selective NSAIDS			
Celecoxib	Celebrex	100, 200 mg bid, 200 mg once day	11
Etoricoxib*	Arcoxia	30, 60, or 90 mg once a day	15–22

*Not approved by the Food and Drug Administration for use in United States.

[†]Available in liquid form.

bid, twice a day; tid, three times a day; qid, four times a day.

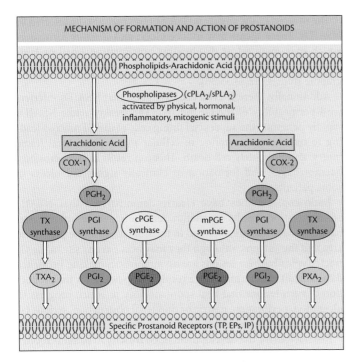

Figure 30.1 Mechanism of formation and action of prostanoids.
Patrono C. Non-steroidal anti-inflammatory drugs. Chapter 53 in Hochberg MC, Silman JA, Smolen JS, Weinblatt ME, Weisman MH, eds. *Rheumatology*, 6th ed. Mosby/Elsevier, 2015, 415–22.

states of inflammation [5]. COX2 is also inhibited by all of the currently available NSAIDs to a greater or lesser degree, and its inhibition leads to a decrease in those prostanoid products associated with increased pain and swelling [7–10]. Therefore, we have observed the effects of prolonged inhibition of COX2 for more than 50 years since the introduction of 'traditional' non-selective NSAIDs.

The *in vitro* systems used to define the actions of the available NSAIDs are based on using cell-free systems, pure enzyme, or whole-cells systems [8]. Each drug studied to date has demonstrated different measurable effects within each system. As an example, it appears that non-acetylated salicylates inhibit the activity of COX1 and COX2 in whole-cell systems but are not active against either COX1 or COX2 in recombinant enzyme or cell membrane systems. This suggests that non-acetylated salicylates act early in the arachidonic acid cascade similar to glucocorticoids, perhaps by inhibiting enzyme expression rather than direct inhibition of cyclooxygenase.

Several NSAIDs are selective and inhibit the COX2 enzyme more so than the COX1 enzyme. For example, *in vitro* effects of low doses of both etodolac and meloxicam demonstrate primary inhibition of COX2 compared with COX1 [18,19]. However, at higher approved doses, this effect appears to be mitigated, as both COX1 and COX2 are inhibited to variable degrees. Very potent, COX2 selective inhibitors have no measurable effect on COX1 mediated events at therapeutic doses; these agents include celecoxib, which is available in both Europe and the United States, and etoricoxib which is available in Europe but not the United States. Three other COX2 selective inhibitors, rofecoxib, valdecoxib, and lumericoxib, were removed from the market either voluntarily by the sponsor or at the request of regulatory authorities throughout the world because of adverse effects.

Other potential mechanisms of action that may explain the clinical effects of the NSAIDs include interruption of protein–protein interactions important for signal transduction, inhibition of activation, adherence and chemotaxis of neutrophils, as well as reduction in toxic oxygen radical production in stimulated neutrophils, inhibition of nuclear factor kappa B, inhibition of inducible nitric oxide synthase, and increased generation of lipoxins [20–27].

Pharmacology

NSAIDs are efficiently absorbed after oral administration, but absorption rates may vary in patients with altered GI blood flow or motility, as well as when the agents are taken with food in the stomach as opposed to on an empty stomach. Furthermore, enteric coating or over-encapsulation of pills may also reduce the rate of absorption.

Most non-selective NSAIDs are weak organic acids; once absorbed they are more than 95% bound to serum albumin. This is a saturable process. Clinically significant decreases in serum albumin levels or institution of other highly protein-bound medications may lead to an increase in the free concentration of NSAID in serum. This may be important in patients who are elderly or chronically ill, especially those with associated hypoalbuminaemic states. Importantly, as a result of increased vascular permeability in localized sites of inflammation, this high degree of protein binding may result in delivery of higher levels of NSAIDs.

NSAIDs are metabolized predominantly in the liver by the cytochrome P450 (CYP) system and the CYP2C9 isoform, and are excreted by the kidney in the urine. This must be taken into consideration when prescribing NSAIDs for patients with hepatic or renal dysfunction. NSAIDs should be used with caution, if at all, and at lowest possible doses in patients with clinically significant liver disease, including patients with cirrhosis with or without ascites, prolonged prothrombin times, low serum albumin levels, or important elevations in liver transaminases. Similarly, NSAIDs should be used with caution and at lowest possible doses in patients with mildly impaired renal function (chronic kidney disease stage 2 and 3A [estimated glomerular filtration rate (eGFR) of 60–80 and 45–60 mL/min], respectively), and not at all in patients with chronic kidney disease stage 3B, 4 and 5, corresponding to an eGFR below 45 mL/min. In addition, some NSAIDs (e.g. indomethacin, sulindac, and piroxicam) have a prominent enterohepatic circulation, resulting in a prolonged half-life, and should be used with caution, if at all, in the elderly. Significant differences in plasma half-lives of the NSAIDs may be important in explaining their diverse clinical effects. NSAIDs with long half-lives typically do not attain maximum plasma concentrations quickly and important clinical responses may be delayed. In most chronic conditions that are appropriate for the use of these drugs, the acute effects are not as important as in the treatment of acute gout or other forms of acute pain. Plasma concentrations can vary widely because of differences in renal clearance and metabolism. Piroxicam has the longest serum half-life of currently marketed NSAIDs: 57 ± 22 hours. In comparison, diclofenac has one of the shortest: 1.1 ± 0.2 hours (see Table 30.1). Although drugs have been developed with very long half-lives to improve patient adherence with therapy, in the older patient it is sometimes preferable to use drugs of shorter half-life so that, when the drug is discontinued, any unwanted effects may more rapidly disappear.

Sulindac and nabumetone are 'pro-drugs' in which the active compound is produced after first-pass metabolism through the liver. Theoretically, pro-drugs were developed to decrease the exposure of the GI mucosa to the local effects of the NSAIDs. Unfortunately, as was noted, the patient is placed at substantial risk of an NSAID-induced GI adverse event as long as COX1 activity is inhibited. This is true for drugs such as ketorolac given as an injection or by these pro-drugs when given at adequate therapeutic doses.

Adverse effects

Side effects attributed to NSAIDs are listed in Box 30.1. Many of these adverse effects are mechanism based due to inhibition of prostaglandin synthesis in local tissues, while others are idiosyncratic. The common adverse effects will be described in the following subsections.

Gastrointestinal events

The most common adverse effects associated with NSAIDs occur in the GI tract, affecting the GI mucosa [28–33]. NSAIDs cause a wide range of GI problems including symptoms of intolerance, often referred to as 'nuisance' symptoms, such as abdominal pain, dyspepsia, nausea, vomiting, and diarrhoea, as well as serious problems including esophagitis, oesophageal ulcers and strictures, gastritis, erosions, gastric, duodenal and small bowel ulceration resulting in haemorrhage, perforation, and obstruction, lower GI bleeding, and, rarely, death. The 'nuisance' symptoms may be observed in about 40–60% of patients but are not related to COX1 inhibition in the GI mucosa [14–16,34]. The exact cause of these symptoms remains unknown; however, use of H2-receptor antagonists and proton pump inhibitors typically alleviates these unpleasant symptoms and allows continued therapy if the NSAID is effective in relieving painful symptoms of OA. Upper GI erosions and ulcers as well as ulcer complications are predominantly due to the effects of NSAID-induced inhibition of COX1, resulting in a reduction of those prostaglandins that serve to protect the stomach mucosa from toxins. This protection consists of a mucous layer serving as a barrier, a bicarbonate gradient serving to buffer the mucous layer from the effects of the extremely acidic lumen, developing glutathione to serve as a scavenger of superoxides, prostaglandin-mediated inhibition of gastric acid production, and prostaglandin-mediated increases in mucosal blood flow. All of these effects are inhibited by the NSAIDs which inhibit COX1 activity.

The mucosa of the small and large bowel may also be affected by NSAIDs. These agents may induce ulcers and stricture formation, which may manifest as diaphragms precipitating small or large bowel obstruction, and can be hard to detect on contrast radiographic studies [32,33,35,36].

Additionally, there is evidence to suggest that NSAIDs interfere with permeability of the GI mucosa. The weakly acidic NSAIDs rapidly penetrate the superficial lining cells of the GI mucosa leading to oxidative uncoupling of cellular metabolism, local tissue injury, and ultimately cell death. This can result in local erosions, haemorrhages, and formation of clinically significant ulcers in some patients.

Endoscopic studies have clearly demonstrated that NSAID administration results in shallow erosions and/or submucosal haemorrhages that are observed in the stomach near the prepyloric area and the antrum, although they may occur at any site in the GI tract. Typically, these lesions are asymptomatic, making incidence data difficult to determine. As a result, we do not know the proportion of such lesions that heal spontaneously or which progress to ulceration, perforation, gastric or duodenal obstruction, serious GI haemorrhage, or subsequent death.

Risk factors for the development of GI toxicity in patients receiving NSAIDs include age above 60 years, prior history of peptic ulcer disease, prior use of antiulcer therapies for any reason, concomitant use of glucocorticoids and Helicobacter pylori infection, comorbidities such as significant cardiovascular disease, and use in patients with severe rheumatoid arthritis (Box 30.2). Additional risk factors for GI bleeding include concomitant administration of anticoagulants, often given to older patients for treatment of atrial fibrillation or recurrent deep venous thrombosis, and antiplatelet agents, often given to older patients for secondary prevention of cardiovascular thrombotic events such as myocardial infarction and stroke as well as for primary prevention of thrombosis in patients at increased risk for myocardial infarction or who have received a drug-eluting stent during a percutaneous transluminal angioplasty for treatment of either coronary artery or peripheral arterial disease. Furthermore, there are differences in risk between individual NSAIDs as well as dose-related effects for each individual NSAID. Data from a systematic review and meta-analysis of 28 observational studies, conducted under the auspices of the Safety of Nonsteroidal Anti-inflammatory Drugs (SOS) Project, estimated the pooled relative risk (RR) for serious GI complications of 16 different NSAIDs and

---

Box 30.1 Adverse reactions of the NSAIDs

Common:
- Gastrointestinal
- Cardiovascular
- Renal
- Hypersensitivity.

Uncommon:
- Hepatic
- Skin
- Central nervous system
- Pregnancy related.

Box 30.2 Risk factors for NSAID-induced upper GI toxicity

1. Age 60 and above
2. History of previous GI bleed, peptic ulcer disease, perforation, or obstruction
3. History of previous NSAID-induced GI toxicity
4. Concomitant illnesses such as cardiovascular disease leading to increased disability
5. Higher dose of a traditional non-selective NSAID
6. Combinations of traditional non-selective NSAIDs
7. Concomitant use of glucocorticoids
8. Infection with Helicobacter pylori.

Table 30.2 Relative risks of serious upper GI events with coxibs and non-selective NSAIDs

Regimen	NSAID vs placebo (95% CI)	Coxib vs non-selective NSAID (95% CI)
Coxibs	1.81 (1.17–2.81)	NA
Naproxen	4.22 (2.71–6.56)	0.37 (0.28–0.49)
Diclofenac	1.89 (1.16–3.09)	0.94 (0.72–1.24)
Ibuprofen	3.97 (2.22–7.10)	0.40 (0.25–0.64)

CI, confidence interval.

Data derived from [38], supplemental material webtable 3.

Table 30.3 Estimated relative risks for myocardial infarction by use of individual NSAIDs compared to non-use

NSAID	Number of studies	Relative risk (95% CI)
Naproxen	17	1.06 (0.94–1.20)
Ibuprofen	13	1.14 (0.98–1.31)
Meloxicam	3	1.25 (1.04–1.49)
Diclofenac	11	1.38 (1.26–1.52)
Indomethacin	4	1.40 (1.21–1.62)
Etodolac	3	1.55 (1.16–2.06)
Celecoxib	18	1.12 (1.00–1.24)
Rofecoxib	17	1.34 (1.22–1.48)
Etoricoxib	3	1.97 (1.35–2.89)

CI, confidence interval.

Data derived from [42], supplemental material eFigure 1.

divided them into three groups: aceclofenac, celecoxib, and ibuprofen had an estimated RR of less than 2.0; diclofenac, ketoprofen, meloxicam, nimesulide, rofecoxib, and sulindac had an estimated RR of between 2.0 and 3.9; and azapropazone, diflunisal, indomethacin, ketorolac, naproxen, piroxicam, and tenoxicam had an estimated RR of 4.0 or above [37]. Finally, for all NSAIDs except celecoxib, there was a two- to threefold higher estimated RR for higher compared to lower doses of individual NSAIDs.

Recent data on the GI adverse effects of both non-selective and COX2 selective NSAIDs was developed by the Coxib and NSAID Trialists Collaboration [38]. This group performed an individual patient data meta-analysis that included 124 513 participants of 280 trials of NSAID versus placebo and 229 296 participants from 474 comparative trials of NSAIDs. Compared with placebo, there was an increased risk of serious upper GI complications, most of which were bleeds, in association with the use of non-selective NSAIDs ibuprofen, naproxen, and diclofenac and coxibs including celecoxib, etoricoxib, lumiracoxib, rofecoxib, and valdecoxib (Table 30.2). The relative risk for celecoxib, based on data from 16 trials, was not significantly greater than placebo and there was no evidence of a dose–response relationship for increased GI risk with increasing doses of celecoxib. This is in contrast to a significantly increased relative risk for rofecoxib compared to placebo, based on data from 18 trials. The rate of events in participants receiving celecoxib was significantly lower than that for participants receiving either ibuprofen or naproxen. Thus, these data support the relative GI safety of celecoxib as compared to these non-selective NSAIDs.

Cardiovascular thrombotic events

The cardiovascular thrombotic adverse effects of NSAIDs were not identified until the large randomized clinical trials of coxibs were conducted in the late 1990s and early part of the twenty-first century [39–41]. Since then, a large number of observational pharmacoepidemiological studies have been published focusing on the association of use of coxibs and non-selective NSAIDs and the risk of myocardial infarction and other cardiovascular and cerebrovascular thrombotic events. The SOS Project conducted a systematic review of 31 observational studies published from 1990 to 2011 that reported on the association of NSAID use with myocardial infarction; data from 18 independent study populations were used for the meta-analysis [42]. In general, use of all NSAIDs, except naproxen, was associated with a significantly increased risk of myocardial infarction compared to non-use with etoricoxib having the highest estimated RR = 1.97 (95% confidence interval (CI) 1.35–2.89)

(Table 30.3). In general, there was a dose–response relationship for all NSAIDs, except for naproxen, such that higher risk was associated with higher average daily dose. The estimated risks did not differ between subjects with a history of prior myocardial infarction or coronary heart disease and those at risk for their first event.

Recent data on the cardiovascular thrombotic adverse effects of both non-selective and COX2 selective NSAIDs was developed by the Coxib and NSAID Trialists Collaboration [38]. The primary outcome in this analysis was major vascular events, defined as non-fatal myocardial infarction, non-fatal stroke, or death from a vascular cause; secondary outcomes included major coronary events, stroke, and hospitalization for heart failure. Compared with placebo, there was an increased risk of major vascular events, most of which were major coronary events, in association with the use of non-selective NSAIDs ibuprofen and diclofenac, but not naproxen, and coxibs including celecoxib, etoricoxib, lumiracoxib, rofecoxib, and valdecoxib (Table 30.4). There was no evidence to support an increased risk of stroke, either fatal or non-fatal, with any of the three non-selective NSAIDs or coxibs as a group. The relative risk for major vascular events for celecoxib, based on data from 41 trials, was significantly greater than placebo (RR = 1.36, 95% CI 1.00–1.84) and there was a significant dose–response relationship for increased risk for major vascular events with increasing doses of celecoxib: the RR for the recommended dose for OA of 200 mg daily was 0.95 (95% CI 0.30–3.00) while that for the dose of 800 mg daily was 2.96 (95% CI 1.21–7.25). Thus, these data support the relative safety of not only naproxen, when used at a dose of 500 mg twice daily, but also celecoxib, when used at a dose of 200 mg once daily, with respect to the outcome of major vascular and major coronary events.

The physiological mechanisms for the increased risk of cardiovascular thrombotic events with NSAIDs appear to be related to relative inhibition of COX1-mediated synthesis of thromboxane A2 by the platelet versus COX2-mediated synthesis of prostacyclin by the vascular endothelial cell as well as the pharmacodynamic half-lives of the individual compounds [43]. The greater the COX2 selectivity and the higher the dose and longer the half-life of the COX2 selective inhibitor, the more sustained the inhibition of prostacyclin synthesis and inhibition of vasodilatation. Similarly,

Table 30.4 Relative risks of major vascular events with coxibs and non-selective NSAIDs compared to placebo

Regimen	Major vascular events (95% CI)	Major coronary events (95% CI)	Stroke (95% CI)	Hospitalization for heart failure (95% CI)
Coxibs	1.37 (1.14–1.66)	1.76 (1.31–2.37)	1.09 (0.78–1.52)	2.28 (1.62–3.20)
Naproxen	0.93 (0.69–1.27)	0.84 (0.52–1.35)	0.97 (0.59–1.60)	1.87 (1.10–3.16)
Diclofenac	1.41 (1.12–1.78)	1.70 (1.19–2.41)	1.18 (0.79–1.78)	1.85 (1.17–2.94)
Ibuprofen	1.44 (0.89–2.33)	2.22 (1.10–4.48)	0.97 (0.42–2.24)	2.49 (1.19–5.20)

CI, confidence interval.

Data derived from [38], Figures 1–4.

the lower the COX2 selectivity and the higher the dose and longer half-life of the non-selective NSAID, the more sustained the inhibition of platelet-derived thromboxane and inhibition of thrombosis. Hence, this would explain the apparent lack of an adverse cardiovascular thrombotic effect of high-dose naproxen taken at a regular twice-daily dosing interval since it suppresses platelet-derived COX1 activity to the same extent as low-dose aspirin.

Renal adverse effects

The effects of the NSAIDs on renal function include changes in the excretion of sodium, changes in tubular function, the potential for interstitial nephritis, and reversible renal failure due to alterations in glomerulofiltration rate and renal plasma flow [44–46]. Prostaglandins and prostacyclins are important for maintenance of intrarenal blood flow and tubular transport. All NSAIDs, except non-acetylated salicylates, have the potential to induce reversible impairment of glomerular filtration rate; this effect occurs more frequently in patients with established renal disease with altered intrarenal plasma flow including diabetes, hypertension, or atherosclerosis; and with induced hypovolaemia, salt depletion, or significant hypoalbuminemia. Potassium-sparing diuretics and angiotensin-converting enzyme (ACE) inhibitors, especially when used in patients with congestive heart failure, may predispose those taking NSAIDs to acute kidney injury.

NSAID-associated interstitial nephritis is typically manifested as nephrotic syndrome, characterized by oedema or anasarca, proteinuria, haematuria, and pyuria. The usual stigmata of drug-induced allergic nephritis such as eosinophilia, eosinophiluria, and fever may not be present. Interstitial infiltrates of mononuclear cells are seen histologically with relative sparing of the glomeruli. The phenylpropionic acid derivative, fenoprofen, is most commonly associated with the development of interstitial nephritis.

All NSAIDs, including the COX2 inhibitors, have been associated with increases in mean arterial blood pressure in hypertensive patients but not in patients with normal blood pressure [47–49]. Patients receiving antihypertensive agents including beta blockers, ACE inhibitors, and thiazide and loop diuretics, must be checked regularly when initiating therapy with a new NSAID to ensure that there are no significant continued and sustained rises in blood pressure.

Hypersensitivity

Patients with allergic rhinitis, nasal polyposis, and/or a history of asthma, in whom all non-selective NSAIDs effectively inhibit prostaglandin synthesis, are at increased risk for anaphylaxis. In high doses, even non-acetylated salicylates may sufficiently decrease prostaglandin synthesis to induce an anaphylactic reaction in sensitive patients [50]. Although the exact mechanism for this effect remains unclear, it is known that prostaglandins serve as bronchodilators. When COX1 activity is inhibited in patients at risk, a decrease in synthesis of prostaglandins that contribute to bronchodilation results. Another explanation implicates other enzymatic pathways that utilize the arachidonate pool after it is converted from phospholipase, whereby shunting of arachidonate into the leukotriene pathway occurs when cyclooxygenase is inhibited [51]. The leukotriene pathway converts arachidonic acid by 5-lipoxygenase, leading to products such as leukotriene B4 as well as others clearly associated with anaphylaxis. This explanation implies that large stores of arachidonate released in certain inflammatory situations lead to excess substrate for leukotriene metabolism. This process results in release of products that are highly reactive, leading to increased bronchoconstriction and the risk for anaphylaxis in the right patient. Whether the main mechanism of effect is inhibition of prostaglandin synthesis or shunting of arachidonate into conversion by 5-lipoxygenase or a combination of the two, it is clear that patients who are sensitive are at great risk when NSAIDs are used. A recent meta-analysis of clinical trials showed that COX2 selective inhibitors are safe in these patients: no significant differences were found in respiratory symptoms, decrease in forced expiratory volume in 1 second of 20% or greater, or nasal symptoms during treatment [52]. Hence, if NSAIDs need to be used in patients with OA and a history of nasal polyposis or aspirin sensitivity, then COX2 selective inhibitors should be chosen.

Use in patients with osteoarthritis

Several professional societies have published evidence-based recommendations for the management of patients with OA [53–58]. All of these recommend the use of oral NSAIDs in patients with persistent symptoms that have not responded adequately to acetaminophen (paracetamol) with or without concomitant use of topical NSAIDs or, in the European Society for Clinical and Economic Aspects of Osteoporosis and Osteoarthritis recommendations [58], the use of the slow-acting symptomatic drugs glucosamine sulphate and chondroitin sulphate. There is no convincing evidence that the efficacy of any one NSAID is superior to that of another [59].

The choice of the individual NSAID by the individual practitioner is usually based on a combination of relative safety, frequency of administration, and cost, as there is no convincing evidence of superior efficacy for one drug versus another within the class. Since use of NSAIDs is associated with an increased risk for serious upper GI side effects, it is recommended that concomitant therapy be given with a proton pump inhibitor even in patients who are at low risk for these events (see Table 30.3). In patients at high risk for serious upper GI side effects, the best option would be the combination of a COX2 selective inhibitor with a proton pump inhibitor. For patients at low risk of a cardiovascular thrombotic event, the decision regarding choice of NSAID depends on the GI risk. For patients at moderate risk of a cardiovascular thrombotic event, one would consider using naproxen with a proton pump inhibitor. For patients at high risk of a cardiovascular thrombotic event, especially those with a prior history of a myocardial infarction or known coronary heart disease, oral NSAIDs should be avoided and alternative analgesic agents should be used to manage the patient's pain. As noted above, oral NSAIDs should be avoided in patients with established moderate-to-severe chronic kidney disease and moderate-to-severe congestive heart failure (New York Heart Association class III and IV).

Summary

NSAIDs are known to be analgesic, anti-inflammatory, and antipyretic, and are efficacious for the management of pain and other symptoms in patients with OA. Their role in management of patients continues to be controversial, however, largely because of common and potentially severe adverse effects. Numerous clinical practice guidelines and recommendations provide help to the practising clinician in their decision about their use in the treatment of the individual patient with OA.

References

1. Day RO, Graham GG. Non-steroidal antiinflammatory drugs. *BMJ* 2013; 346:f3195.
2. Patrono C. Non-steroidal anti-inflammatory drugs. In Hochberg MC, Silman JA, Smolen JS, Weinblatt ME, Weisman MH (eds) *Rheumatology*, 6th ed. Philadelphia, PA: Mosby/Elsevier; 2015:415–22.
3. Baum C, Kennedy DL, Forbes MB. Utilization of nonsteroidal anti-inflammatory drugs. *Arthritis Rheum* 1985; 28:686–91.
4. Aitken M, Kleinrock M, Lyle J, Caskey L. *Medicine Use and Shifting Costs of Healthcare: A Review of the Use of Medicines in the United States in 2013*. Parsinnapany, NJ: IMS Institute for Healthcare Informatics; 2014.
5. Samad TA, Moore KA, Sapirstein A, et al. Interleukin-1beta-mediated induction of COX-2 in the CNS contributes to inflammatory pain hypersensitivity. *Nature* 2001; 410:471–5.
6. Crofford LJ, Lipsky PE, Brooks P, et al. Basic biology and clinical application of cyclooxygenase-2. *Arthritis Rheum* 2000; 43(1):4–13.
7. Dubois RN, Abramson SB, Corfford L, et al. Cyclooxygenase in biology and disease. *FASEB J* 1998; 12:1063–73.
8. Mitchell JA, Akarasereenont P, Thiemermann C, et al. Selectivity of nonsteroidal antiinflammatory drugs as inhibitors of constitutive and inducible cyclooxygenase. *Proc Natl Acad Sci U S A* 1994; 90:11693–7.
9. Patrignani P, Panara MR, Greco A, et al. Biochemical and pharmacological characterization of the cyclooxygenase activity of human blood prostaglandin endoperoxide synthases. *J Pharmacol Exp Ther* 1994; 271:1705–12.
10. Meade EA, Smith WL, Dewitt DL. Differential inhibition of prostaglandin endoperoxide synthase (cyclooxygenase) isoenzymes by aspirin and other non-steroidal anti-inflammatory drugs. *J Biol Chem* 1993; 268(9):6610–4.
11. Laneuville O, Breuer DK, DeWitt DL, et al. Differential inhibition of human prostaglandin endoperoxide H synthases-1 and -2 by nonsteroidal antiinflammatory drugs. *J Pharmacol Exp Ther* 1994; 271: 927–39.
12. Fries JP, Miller SR, Spitz PW. Toward an epidemiology of gastropathy associated with nonsteroidal antiinflammatory drug use. *Gastroenterology* 1989; 96:647–55.
13. Gabriel SE, Jaaklimainen L, Bombadier C. Risk for serious gastrointestinal complications related to use of nonsteroidal antiinflammatory drugs: a meta-analysis. *Ann Intern Med* 1991; 115:787–96.
14. Wolfe MM, Lichtenstein DR, Singh G. Gastrointestinal toxicity of the nonsteroidal antiinflammatory drugs. *N Engl J Med* 1999; 340:1888–99.
15. Scheiman JM. NSAIDs, gastrointestinal injury, and cytoprotection. *Gastroenterol Clin North Am* 1996; 25:279–98.
16. Laine L. Nonsteroidal antiinflammatory drug gastropathy. *Gastrointest Endosc Clin North Am* 1996; 6:489–504.
17. Hollander D. Gastrointestinal complications of nonsteroidal anti-inflammatory drugs: prophylactic and therapeutic strategies. *Am J Med* 1994; 96:274–81.
18. DeWitt DL, Meade EA, Smith WL. PGH synthase isoenzyme selectivity: the potential for safer nonsteroidal antiinflammatory drugs. *Am J Med* 1993; 95(Suppl 2A):40S–44S.
19. Glaser K, Sung M-L, O'Neill K, et al. Etodolac selectively inhibits human prostaglandin G/H synthase 2 (PGHS-2) versus human PGHS-1. *Eur J Pharmacol* 1995; 281:107–11.
20. Mahmud T, Rafi SS, Scott DL, et al. Nonsteroidal antiinflammatory drugs and uncoupling of mitochondrial oxidative phosphorylation. *Arthritis Rheum* 1996; 39:1998–2003.
21. Abramson SB, Leszczynska-Piziak J, Clancy RM, et al. Inhibition of neutrophil function by aspirin-like drugs (NSAIDs): requirement for assembly of heterotrimeric G proteins in bilayer phospholipid. *Biochem Pharmacol* 1994; 47:563–72.
22. Amin AR, Vyas P, Attur M, et al. The mode of action of aspirin-like drugs: effect on inducible nitric oxide synthase. *Proc Natl Acad Sci U S A* 1995; 92:7926–30.
23. Díaz-González F, González-Alvero I, Companero MR, et al. Prevention of *in vitro* neutrophil-endothelial attachment through shedding of L-selectin by nonsteroidal antiinflammatory drugs. *J Clin Invest* 1995; 95:1756–65.
24. Friman C, Johnston C, Chew C, Davis P. Effect of diclofenac sodium, tolfenamic acid and indomethacin on the production of superoxide induced by N-fromyl-methionyl-leucyl-phenylalanine in normal human polymorphonuclear leukocytes. *Scand J Rheumatol* 1986; 15:41–6.
25. Gay JC, Lukens JN, English DK. Differential inhibition of neutrophil superoxide generation by nonsteroidal antiinflammatory drugs. *Inflammation* 1984; 8:209–22.
26. Eisen DP. Manifold beneficial effects of acetyl salicylic acid and nonsteroidal anti-inflammatory drugs on sepsis. *Intensive Care Med* 2012; 38(8):1249–57.
27. Scher JU, Pillinger MH. The anti-inflammatory effects of prostaglandins. *J Invest Med* 2009; 57:703–8.
28. Garcia Rodriguez LA, Walker AM, Perez Gutthann S. Nonsteroidal antiinflammatory drugs and gastrointestinal hospitalizations in Saskatchewan: a cohort study. *Epidemiology* 1992; 3:337–42.
29. Griffin MR, Piper JM, Daugherty JR, et al. Nonsteroidal antiinflammatory drug use and increased risk for peptic ulcer disease in elderly persons. *Ann Intern Med* 1991; 114:257–63.
30. Garcia Rodriguez LA. Nonsteroidal antiinflammatory drugs, ulcers and risk: a collaborative meta-analysis. *Semin Arthritis Rheum* 1997; 26(Suppl):16–20.
31. Bjarnason I, Thjodleifsson B. Gastrointestinal toxicity of non-steroidal anti-inflammatory drugs: the effect of numesulide compared with naproxen on the human gastrointestinal tract. *Rheumatology* 1999; 38 (Suppl):24–32.
32. Holt S, Rigoglioso V, Sidhu M, et al. Nonsteroidal antiinflammatory drugs and lower gastrointestinal bleeding. *Dig Dis Sci* 1993; 38:1619–23.
33. Wilcox CM, Alexander LN, Cotsonis GA, Clark WS. Nonsteroidal antiinflammatory drugs are associated with both upper and lower gastrointestinal bleeding. *Dig Dis Sci* 1997; 42:990–7.

34. Larkai EN, Smith JL, Lidsky MD, Graham DY. Gastroduodenal mucosa and dyspeptic symptoms in arthritic patients during chronic nonsteroidal anti-inflammatory drug use. *Am J Gastroenterol* 1987; 82:1153.

35. Allison MC, Howatson AG, Torance CJ. Gastrointestinal damage associated with the use of nonsteroidal antiinflammatory drugs. *N Engl J Med* 1992; 327:749–54.

36. Reuter BK, Asfaha S, Buret A, et al. Exacerbation of inflammation-associated colonic injury in rat through inhibition of cyclooxygenase-2. *J Clin Invest* 1996; 98:2076–85.

37. Castellsague J, Riera-Guardia N, Calingaert B, et al. Individual NSAIDs and upper gastrointestinal complicatiions: a systematic review and meta-analysis of observational studies (the SOS project). *Drug Saf* 2012; 35:1127–46.

38. Coxib and traditional NSAID Trialists' (CNT) Collaboration. Vascular and upper gastrointestinal effects of nonsteroidal anti-inflammatory drugs: meta-analyses of individual participant data from randomized trials. *Lancet* 2013; 382:769–79.

39. Bombardier C, Laine L, Reicin A, et al. Comparison of upper gastrointestinal toxicity of rofecoxib and naproxen in patients with rheumatoid arthritis. VIGOR Study Group. *N Engl J Med* 2000; 343:1520–8.

40. Bresalier RS, Sandler Rs, Quan H, et al. Cardiovascular events associated with rofecoxib in a colorectal adenoma chemoprevention trial. *N Engl J Med* 2005; 352:1092–102.

41. Solomon SD, McMurray JJ, Pfeffer MA, et al. Cardiovascular risk associated with celecoxib in a clinical trial for colorectal adenoma prevention. *N Engl J Med* 2005; 352:1071–80.

42. Varas-Lorenzo C, Riera-Guardia N, Calingaert B, et al. Myocardial infarction and individual nonsteroidal anti-inflammatory drugs meta-analysis of observation studies. *Pharmacoepidemiol Drug Saf* 2013; 22 (6):559–70.

43. Patrono C, Baigent C. Nonsteroidal anti-inflammatory drugs and the heart. *Circulation* 2014; 129(8):907–16.

44. Schlondorff D. Renal complications of nonsteroidal anti-inflammatory drugs. *Kidney Int* 1993; 44:643–53.

45. Whelton A. Renal and related cardiovascular effects of conventional and COX-2 specific NSAIDs and non-NSAID analgesics. *Am J Ther* 2000; 7:63–74.

46. Murray MD, Brater DC: Renal toxicity of the nonsteroidal anti-inflammatory drugs. *Annu Rev Pharmacol Toxicol* 1993; 33:435–65.

47. Pope JE, Anderson JJ, Felson DT. A meta-analysis of the effects of nonsteroidal anti-inflammatory drugs on blood pressure. *Arch Intern Med* 1993; 153:477–84.

48. Friedewald VE, Ram CV, Wesson DE, et al. The editor's roundtable: effect of nonsteroidal anti-inflammatory drugs on blood pressure. *Am J Cardiol* 2010; 105(12):1759–67.

49. Zhao SZ, Burge TA, Whelton A, von Allmen H, Henderson SC. Blood pressure destabilization and related healthcare utilization among hypertensive patients using nonspecific NSAIDs and COX-2 specific inhibitors. *Am J Manag Care* 2002; 8(15 Suppl):S401–13.

50. Stevenson DD, Hougha m, Schrank PJ, et al. Salsalate cross-sensitivity in aspirin-sensitive patients with asthma. *J Allergy Clin Immunol* 1990; 86:749–58.

51. Robinson DR, Skosliewicz M, Bloch KJ, et al. Cyclooxygenase blockade elevates leukotriene E4 production during acute anaphylaxis in sheep. *J Exp Med* 1986; 163:1509–17.

52. Morales DR, Lipworth BJ, Guthrie B, et al. Safety risks for patients with aspirin-exacerbated respiratory disease after acute exposure to selective nonsteroidal anti-inflammatory drugs and COX-2 inhibitors: meta-analysis of controlled clinical trials. *J Allergy Clin Immunol* 2014;134(1):40–5.

53. Jordan KM, Arden NK, Doherty M, et al. EULAR recommendations 2003; an evidence based approach to the management of knee osteoarthritis. *Ann Rheum Dis* 2003; 62:1145–55.

54. Zhang W, Doherty M, Arden N, et al. EULAR evidence based recommendations for the management of hip osteoarthritis. *Ann Rheum Dis* 2005; 64(5):669–81.

55. Hochberg MC, Altman RD, April KT, et al. American College of Rheumatology 2012 recommendations for the use of nonpharmacologic and pharmacologic therapies in osteoarthritis of the hand, hip, and knee. *Arthritis Care Res (Hoboken)* 2012; 64:465–74.

56. McAlindon TE, Bannuru RR, Sullivan MC, et al. OARSI guidelines for the non-surgical management of knee osteoarthritis. *Osteoarthritis Cartilage* 2014; 22:363–88.

57. National Clinical Guideline Centre (UK). *Osteoarthritis: Care and management in Adults*. London: National Institute for Health and Care Excellence; 2014.

58. Bruyere O, Cooper C, Pelletier JP, et al. An algorithm recommendation for the management of knee osteoarthritis in Europe and internationally: a report from a task force of the European Society for Clinical and Economic Aspects of Osteoporosis and Osteoarthritis (ESCEO). *Semin Arthritis Rheum* 2014; 44(3):253–63.

59. Burmester G, Lanas A, Biasucci L, et al. The appropriate use of nonsteroidal anti-inflammatory drugs in rheumatic disease: opinions of a multidisciplinary European expert panel. *Ann Rheum Dis* 2011; 70(5):818–22.

CHAPTER 31

Supplements for the treatment of osteoarthritis

Allen D. Sawitzke and Daniel O. Clegg

Introduction

Osteoarthritis (OA; degenerative joint disease, DJD) is the one form of arthritis for which effective therapies have been especially difficult to elucidate. While it has long been fashionable to consider modification of what we eat as an effective approach to modifying our health, current therapies demonstrate that any benefits of dietary modification are likely to be small as is readily evident by studying any of the OA therapy reviews [1–6]. There is a clear nexus between our environment and our own bodies through what we eat and, further, it is one of the few environmental factors over which an individual can exert their influence. To this end, most cultures from ancient to modern have proscriptions and prescriptions related to dietary intake, seen in the Hebrew Bible as kosher practices [7], or in current Western trends such as gluten sensitivity [8]. Further, these principles may be more easily embraced at a lay level than are treatments with which the untrained person has little common experience such as the use of chemical-based medications. It is well appreciated that food can be both beneficial and toxic as anyone who has experienced food poisoning can attest. This connection between diet and health makes understanding, or at least accepting, potential toxicity easier for us.

While several terms are used to describe these food-based therapies, we will use the general term 'dietary supplement' throughout this chapter. A number of helpful reviews of dietary supplements for arthritis can also be recommended including these noted references [9–11]. Dietary supplement use is also a point of intersection between the concepts of Eastern medicine that aim to adjust the balance of various life forces, and those of Western medicine, where prevention of illness is thought to be achievable through modification of risk factors such as smoking, diet, inactivity and so forth. Individuals typically consider dietary additions as therapy, but frequently neglect to consider omission of nutritional items as therapy as well. Particularly relevant to the treatment of OA are the well-demonstrated weight loss benefits for OA of the knee. As such, caloric restriction is likely one of the most effective 'supplements' for the treatment of OA that can be prescribed [12,13].

Before we begin the review of specific data related to many, but certainly not all, dietary supplement approaches to the treatment of OA, a few cautions are worth special consideration. First, we have very little ability to compare products from different manufacturers, sources, or formulations. Typically, no information on bioavailability, stability, drug interactions, or toxicity have been gathered or at least published. The indications promoting the use of a supplement are typically painted very broadly, such as 'it helps digestion'. Dietary supplement manufacturers typically reference internally funded studies adding at least the potential for additional bias. Despite these issues, dietary supplements are a very popular adjunct to health. Another measure of the human interest in this topic is the complementary and alternative medicine (CAM) registry at the Cochrane Library, which demonstrates a fivefold increase in CAM citations from 2006 to 2010 [14]. While the most comprehensive data are available for knee OA, additional data exist for DJD of the spine, hand, and hip [15]. This chapter will recognize many, but definitely not all of the dietary supplements putatively ascribed with benefit in the treatment of OA. In an effort to provide some organization, much like the hit 1950s American TV show, the dietary supplement categories have been classified as animal, vegetable, or mineral with one additional category for synthetic or chemical-based therapies.

Data review

For each category, a general discussion of the mechanisms shown to be associated with each dietary supplement (Table 31.1) will be followed by discussions of efficacy, safety and practical issues. Then, systematic reviews or meta-analysis data will be summarized to highlight the best understanding of their efficacy and safety. Finally, a focus on combination products, as they are commonly seen in the dietary supplement industry, will include some additional points.

Animal

A significant number of animal-derived dietary supplements have been suggested as having potential benefit in the treatment of OA. These include, among many others, antler velvet [16], collagen (intact and fragments), chondroitin sulphate (CS), eggshell membrane, fish oils, glucosamine, hyaluronic acid, and even the lips of an aquatic mussel [17]. Reviews have detailed some of these agents extensively and are referenced for more information [9,18–21]. The purported active ingredients often include a mix of proteins, carbohydrates, and oils. In some cases, minimal purification is necessary to prepare the dietary supplement for use and in others, such as for CS, a thorough chemical extraction technique is required.

Glucosamine is likely the most extensively studied dietary supplement for the treatment of OA as it has been the focus of more than 20 randomized controlled trials [22], several meta-analyses [23,24], and several iterations of Cochrane review [20,25]. Trials of glucosamine sulphate and glucosamine hydrochloride have been described

Table 31.1 Target mechanisms of supplements used to treat OA

Supplements	Target mechanisms	Dosage	Adverse drug reactions	References
ASU	Inhibit IL1B	300 mg/day	None	[9,68]
Cat's claw	Inhibit COX1 Inhibit LOX Increase IGF1	1800 mg/day	Diarrhoea, abdominal pain, rash	[11]
Chondroitin sulphate	Inhibit PLA2 Inhibit COX2 Stimulate matrix	1200 mg/day	Diarrhoea, abdominal pain, dyspepsia	[41,42]
Collagen hydrolysates	Stimulate matrix	10 g/day	Nausea, diarrhoea, dyspepsia	[46]
Devil's claw	Antioxidant Decrease NFkB Increase SOD	2–3 g powder	Diarrhoea, abdominal pain, rash	[22]
Frankincense	Inhibit LOX Inhibit COX Inhibit Complement	600–3000 g/day	Weakness, diarrhoea, abdominal pain, nausea,	[64,88,89]
Ginger	Inhibit COX Inhibit LOX	500–1000 mg/day	Bad taste, dyspepsia	[62,72,90]
Glucosamine	Decrease NFkB Stimulate matrix	1500 mg/day	Gastrointestinal	[31,32]
Omega-3 PUFA Fish oil GLM	Decrease COX2 Decrease LOX Change microbiome Inhibit COX2 Decrease catabolism	1.2 g/day 1150 mg/day powder or 210 mg lipid extract	Bad breath, dyspepsia, nausea, diarrhoea Increased stiffness, flatulence, epigastric discomfort, nausea, exacerbation of symptoms and fluid retention	[10,54] [17,60,91]
Pineapple	Decrease PGE2, TBX -A2	100–150 mg/day	None	[92]
Rose hips	Antioxidant	2–3 g/day	Mild gastrointestinal	[93,94]
SAMe	Stimulate matrix	400–1200 mg/day	Dyspepsia, diarrhoea, anxiety, rash	[63]
Strontium	Increase OPG Increase IGF1	1–2 g/day	Diarrhoea, thromboembolic events, rash	[69,71,95]

COX, cyclooxygenase; GLM, green-lipped mussels; IGF1, insulin like growth factor; iNOS, inducible nitric oxide synthase; LOX, lipoxygenase; NFkB, nuclear factor kappa B; OPG, osteoprotegerin; PGE2, prostaglandin E2; PLA2, phospholipase A2; PUFA, polyunsaturated fatty acids; SAMe, S-adenosylmethionine; TBX-A2 thromboxane A2.

in OA of the knees, hips, hands, and back [15,26]. Glucosamine can be administered either as a sulphate or hydrochloride salt and substantial debate surrounds the asserted differences [27–29]. Recent reviews segregate the data for the two salts [4,20,30]. Glucosamine has been examined when administered alone and in combination with other supplements. Glucosamine can be purified from shellfish or produced chemically. Two major mechanisms of action have been suggested: (1) inhibition of the transcriptional regulator nuclear factor kappa-light-chain-enhancer of activated B cells and thereby downstream cytokines [31], and (2) by supplying the 'building blocks' for *de novo* proteoglycan synthesis [32]. The typical recommended dosage is 1500 mg of glucosamine daily (Table 31.2). Glucosamine is well tolerated with minimal adverse drug reactions (ADRs) primarily including gastrointestinal symptoms such as dyspepsia, nausea, diarrhoea, and constipation [33–35]. No studies of ADRs longer than 2–3 years have been reported [36–38]. While concerns have been expressed over potential shellfish allergies or increasing a patient's likelihood of developing diabetes, neither

have been seen in studies of 2 years' duration [22,37]. Efficacy is extensively reviewed in the most recent Cochrane review [20] and the Osteoarthritis Research Society International (OARSI) review of 19 randomized controlled trials using glucosamine which found moderate effect sizes (ES) for pain with an ES = 0.46 (95% confidence interval (CI) 0.23–0.69) (Table 31.2). The data has been analysed many different ways in order to isolate different effects such as which salt was used, who funded the study, trial size, the year the study was performed, and so on. These analyses showed the estimated benefit to be smaller for studies of high quality, that is, Jadad score = 5 (ES = 0.29, 95% CI 0.003–0.57) and no benefit was seen with trials using glucosamine hydrochloride [4]. The results for structural joint space narrowing (JSN) showed a smaller yet significant ES = 0.24 (95% CI 0.04–0.43) [4]. The use of glucosamine in combination with CS will be discussed below.

CS has also been studied extensively. CS varies considerably in quality manufacturer to manufacturer [39,40] complicating direct comparisons of different products. CS is harvested through

Table 31.2 Systematic reviews and meta-analyses

Agent	Design	Efficacy (ES) when available	References
ASU	Meta	0.38 (0.01–0.76)	[4]
		0.22 (−0.06 to 0.51) for high-quality trials	
CH	Systematic	Insufficient to recommend	[48]
Chondroitin sulphate	Meta	0.78 (0.60–0.75): pain	[23]
	Meta	Superior to placebo: pain	[101]
	Meta	Structural efficacy: pain	[24]
	Meta	Minimal or no symptom benefit	[44]
	Meta	0.75 (0.50–1.01): pain	[4]
		0.005 (−0.11 to 0.12) for high-quality trials	
		0.26 (0.16–0.36): JSN	
	Cochrane	10% Better than placebo: pain	[45]
		Better than placebo: JSN	
Frankincense	Systematic	Suggestive: pain	[89]
Ginger	Meta	Modest efficacy: pain	[90]
GLM	Systematic	May be effective: pain	[59]
Glucosamine salt	Meta	0.44 (0.24–0.64): pain	[23]
	Cochrane	Superior to placebo: pain	[26]
	Cochrane	Superior to placebo: pain	[20]
	Systematic	For GS	[30]
		For GH	
	Meta	0.46 (0.23–0.69) all	[4]
		0.58 (0.30–0.87) for GS	
		0.02 (−0.15 to 0.11) for GH	
		0.29 (0.003–0.57) for high-quality trials	
MSM	Systematic	No conclusion	[79]
	Meta	Not effective	[80]
Rose hips	Systematic	Moderate effect	[102]
	Meta	0.37 (0.13–0.60)	[4]
SAMe	Meta	No efficacy	[103]
	Meta	0.22 (−0.25 to 0.69)	[4]

ASU, avocado soybean unsaponifiables; CH, collagen hydrolysates; GH, glucosamine hydrochloride; GS, glucosamine sulphate; JSN, joint space narrowing; MSM, methylsulfonylmethane; SAMe, S-adenosylmethionine.

purification from animal sources including fish, beef, chicken, or pig cartilage [41]. Proposed mechanisms of action include diminishing phospholipase A2, cyclooxygenase 2, and inflammatory cytokines [42]. The usual dosage is 1200 mg daily. Serious ADRs following exposure to CS are not associated with its use, while mild gastrointestinal symptoms are the most commonly observed adverse events. Evidence for efficacy for treatment of pain associated with knee OA using CS was estimated in the OARSI guideline at an ES = 0.75 (95% CI 0.50–1.01) (Table 31.2) [4] although this might have been skewed by one trial. Increasing evidence for a benefit in slowing JSN is also suggested [43] and the OARSI review showed an ES = 0.26 (95% CI 0.16–0.36) for structural change [4].

In contrast, Reichenbach et al. found that high-quality studies found essentially no benefit for CS [44]. Some concerns about confounding due to including combination therapies in this review and also non-oral use may limit its conclusions. Recently, a Cochrane review has been published in the Cochrane Library [45] that describes analysis of trial information including 4962 subjects treated with CS. A small yet statistically significant benefit for pain relief (about 10%) was also shown with CS compared to placebo in studies of less than 6 months' duration. The benefit persisted with most sensitivity analysis. No statistical difference in ADRs was found between the CS and placebo groups.

Dietary supplements of collagen have been administered both as intact type II collagen, and as processed fragments usually referred to as collagen hydrolysates (CH) [46]. Oral administration of CH has demonstrated increase of proteoglycan levels in animal cartilage [47]. A recent systematic review provides an excellent summary of these data. The usual dose of CH is 10 g daily and the most common ADRs are nausea, diarrhoea, and dyspepsia (Table 31.1). In conclusion, existing studies 'found insufficient evidence to recommend generalized use in OA' without further supportive high-quality trial data [48] (Table 31.2).

Fish oil has been used for a number of different ailments including inflammatory vascular disease and it has been suggested as a treatment for OA since as early as 1989 [49]. More recent studies support a modest symptom benefit in dogs and cats with experimental OA [50–52] although this benefit is not supported by all studies [53]. It is thought that the omega-3 unsaturated fatty acids are the active component. Fish oil is typically given as a mix of eicosapentaenoic acid and docosahexaenoic acid [54] and both of these agents are well tolerated with halitosis, dyspepsia and diarrhoea as the most common ADRs.

In similar fashion, *Perna canaliculus*, green-lipped mussels (GLM) have been shown to be effective in reducing pain associated with OA in dogs and horses [55–57]. In addition, GLM has been examined in human trials for hand, knee, and hip OA. Once again, omega-3 fatty acids are believed to be the active component. The dosage is 1150 mg powder daily or 210 mg of lipid extract. No serious ADRs have been associated with its use [58] and non-serious adverse effects include increased stiffness, flatulence, epigastric discomfort, nausea, and fluid retention [59]. In one study, GLM powder was thought to help prevent non-steroidal anti-inflammatory drug (NSAID)-associated gastrointestinal symptoms as well [60]. There have been four single-centre trials of this agent in humans and one systematic review (Table 31.2) [59]. Overall, just over 100 patients have been reported in trials and the results appear to show only a small pain benefit over placebo [59]. Clearly, a larger well-performed trial is needed [10,61].

Vegetable

In general, vegetable products seem more commonly available and are more familiar to most users as many of them have culinary uses as well as therapeutic applications. Agents with proposed therapeutic applications comprise a very extensive list. The most clinically studied in regard to OA would be avocado soybean unsaponifiables (ASU), frankincense, and devil's claw. Excellent reviews of these agents have been published by Akhtar and Haqqi [11] and Henrotin and colleagues [10].

Dietary supplements derived from plant roots include ginger, devil's claw, and turmeric among others. Ginger has been used medicinally for millennia for headaches, nausea and vascular conditions among other uses [11]. It has been shown to limit inducible nitric oxide synthase expression as well as having beneficial effects on prostaglandins, tumour necrosis factor and cyclooxygenase 2 expression [11]. No ADRs are reported in the British Herbal Compendium, although some studies report gastrointestinal adverse effects. Efficacy of ginger in treating the pain of OA, however, is limited [62].

Devil's claw is used extensively in Europe as an analgesic. It has potent antioxidant properties and potentially multiple active components. The primary active agent seems to be harpagoside. The recommended dose is 2–3 g of powder or 50–100 mg of harpagoside daily. Extracts are well tolerated with only minor ADRs including diarrhoea, abdominal pain, loss of taste, and skin reactions [22]. Devil's claw components appear to be effective in reducing pain [11,63] and more definitive studies would be of benefit.

The stems of plants have contributed to several dietary supplements, including the pine bark extracts: cat's claw, and frankincense. Cat's claw is harvested from *Uncaria tomentosa*. The bark has antioxidant and anti-inflammatory effects, but the dosage is not well established. It can cause mild nausea and/or diarrhoea and may reduce pain. Frankincense is from the *Boswellia serrata* plant. Its use results in inhibition of lipoxygenase and metalloproteinase activity [11]. Associated ADRs include weakness, diarrhoea, abdominal pain and nausea (Table 31.1). Studies have reported benefit in reducing the pain of OA [64], but again, more research is needed (Table 31.2).

Many fruits have also been used in the treatment of OA, including tart cherries, grapes, olives, pineapple, pomegranate, rose hips, seeds, nuts, and soybeans. However, in most cases very few clinical trial data have been documented. Strong support has not been published for any of this group of agents [11]. The best supported of the vegetable group is the avocado soybean unsaponifiables. These are the portion of the two plant oils that do not form soaps and generally are mixed 1/3 avocado to 2/3 soybean oil [65]. It is given in a dosage of 300 mg daily and has no reported ADRs. It has been reviewed by Henrotin and colleagues [10] and more recently by Ragle and Sawitzke [9] as well as by a meta-analysis [66]. All analyses suggest a benefit likely exists, but that further study is needed. The OARSI summary estimate when used to treat pain was an ES = 0.38 (95% CI 0.01–0.76) (Table 31.2) [4].

Rose hips are thought to work through antioxidant mechanisms. They are used in a dosage of 2–3 g powder daily and ADRs include dyspepsia. Only minimal data is available, but the OARSI estimate of ES for treatment of the pain of OA was 0.37 (95% CI 0 0.13–0.60) [4], again suggesting a need for more study (Table 31.2).

Plant leaves contribute derivatives of green tea as common dietary supplements for many and varied uses, including the treatment of OA. The proposed mechanisms are protean [11], but those likely most relevant to the treatment of OA are the antioxidant and anti-inflammatory mechanisms. No significant clinical efficacy data exists.

Mineral

Trace elements, minerals, and vitamins have long been used as dietary supplements and they have broad appeal to the general public as a 2013 Gallop poll found that 50% of Americans are thought to use them on a daily basis [67]. Many were recommended for bone health, but some have been studied in relationship to the treatment of OA. Chief among these are calcium, selenium, strontium, and

boron. A number of theoretical reasons exist for why minerals could be important to the treatment of OA. In particular, several enzymes of collagen metabolism including lysine oxidase, metalloproteinases, and others require mineral/metal co-factors such as magnesium, copper, zinc, or selenium. Of course, calcium is critical to bone health. Clinical trials have used mineral supplementation with mixtures containing amounts of calcium, magnesium, selenium, strontium, and others. Evidence from one small, double-blind, randomized, placebo-controlled trial suggests that boron supplementation may benefit patients with OA [68].

Strontium is sold as citrate and as ranelate salts. The Strontium ranelate Efficacy in Knee OsteoarthrItis trial (SEKOIA) was a 3- year, international, multicentre, randomized, placebo-controlled, double blind trial of two dosages of strontium versus placebo assessed for effect on JSN and pain [69]. Remarkably, the study met the structural endpoints more robustly than it did for those that were symptom related. Statistically smaller loss of joint space width was observed in both the 1 g and 2 g/day strontium groups. In fact a 27% reduction in JSN was observed in the 2 g/day arm. A statistical improvement in Western Ontario and McMaster Universities Osteoarthritis Index (WOMAC) pain was seen in the 2 g/day group. Subsequently, an analysis using magnetic resonance imaging (MRI) on a subset of patients from this trial has shown decreased bone marrow lesion progression and decreased cartilage volume loss [70]. Thus far, only one large clinical trial using strontium has been reported. Therefor a confirmatory trial is critical before clear recommendations for its use can be made. Furthermore, concern over thrombotic complications has been raised when it has been used to treat osteoporosis and more data regarding ADRs are needed [71]. Although strontium ranelate is not strictly a diet supplement, strontium citrate is available as one. The SEKOIA trial suggests that strontium citrate should be investigated for similar effects.

Synthetics

Synthetics are the agents most closely related to traditional pharmaceutical agents. These include S-adenosylmethionine (SAMe), the sweetener aspartame, methylsulfonylmethane (MSM) and several of the vitamins, including vitamins C, D and niacinamide [72–75]. Others, including vitamin E, have been shown not to be of benefit to symptoms of OA [76]. Of these, only DMSO/MSM and SAMe have enough data to consider in significant detail.

Dimethyl sulfoxide (DMSO) has been studied in many different ways for the treatment of OA along with its protean uses in *in vitro* assays [77,78]. It is a pro-drug in that *in vivo* is converted to MSM and that is the oral agent most often used by the dietary supplement industry. It is typically given in dosages of 4–6 g/day. It has been studied in a number of small trials, perhaps best reviewed in the systematic reviews by Ameye and Chee [61] and Brien [79]. Small benefits for pain are suggested, but many methodological weaknesses preclude a strong endorsement. A recent meta-analysis found 'no definite conclusion' could be drawn (Table 31.2) [80].

A number of studies have found SAMe to be more effective than placebo in improving pain and stiffness related to OA. However, many of these studies were non-randomized, and people find SAMe to have a prohibitively high cost [72]. Reported dosage ranges vary from 400 to 1200 mg per day [68]. A meta-analysis found SAMe to be of value similar to an NSAID (Table 31.2) [63]. The small summary ES for treatment of pain from OARSI was 0.22 (95% CI −0.025 to 0.69 [4].

Combination products

Using dietary supplements in combination adds another level of complexity to our obtaining of acceptable data as the composition of each product is not standardized nor found in peer-reviewed publications. A list of some examples of the common pairings in this category is shown (Table 31.3). Readily apparent is the pairing of dietary supplements from many of our categories without any logical rationale being provided. For example, is there 'synergy' gained by adding MSM to glucosamine as manufacturers purport? Robust clinical data exists for a very small number of combination products and summary data for combinations of pharmacological therapies were not examined by the OARSI group [4].

Probably most extensively studied is the combination of glucosamine with CS, which will be discussed in detail later, but further combinations of glucosamine and CS and additional ingredients such as 'selected minerals 'or MSM are common. While the best evidence seems to be for the GS salt alone, the best combination data is for GH and CS. As was first suggested in Glucosamine/chondroitin Arthritis Intervention Trial (GAIT) [34], patients with moderate to severe pain appeared to have symptomatic benefit while taking the combination as compared to placebo. The most recent randomized control trial to examine this is the Multicenter Osteoarthritis interVEntion trial with SYSADOA (MOVES) trial which examined 605 subjects in two arms: (1) celecoxib 200 mg daily and (2) glucosamine hydrochloride 1500 mg plus CS 1200 mg daily. The study was a 6-month international, double-blind multicentre randomized controlled trial. Improvement in WOMAC pain was the primary outcome. MOVES was designed as a non-inferiority trial, in which a study agent is compared to a well-established therapy. Fundamental to non-inferiority trials is the choice of a pre-defined interval that would be considered 'close enough' to the benefit of standard therapy to be considered non-inferior. In MOVES at 6 months, the combination of GH and CS was found to be non-inferior for pain and well tolerated as an equal number of subjects discontinued treatment for ADRs in each treatment group [81]. The combination of GH + CS is suggesting evidence for a structural benefit in MRI outcomes [43,82] as the paper by Martel-Pelletier et al. demonstrated benefit at 24 months by quantitative MRI. However, not all MRI studies agree as the Long-term Evaluation of Glucosamine Sulfate (LEGS) study failed to show benefit at 24 weeks [83].

Table 31.3 Selected example combination products

Product	Main ingredients
AR7 Joint Complex	Collagen II and MSM [96]
Articulin-F	*Withania somnifera*, frankincense, turmeric, zinc [97]
CS & G	GS + CS GH + CS [34,43,81,82,98]
Move Free Advanced	Chondroitin, glucosamine, hyaluronic acid, proprietary extract
Phytalgic	Fish oils, *Urtica dioica*, zinc, and vitamin E [99]
RA-11	*Withania somnifera*, frankincense, ginger, and turmeric [100]

CS, chondroitin sulphate; GH, glucosamine hydrochloride; GS, glucosamine sulphate; MSM, methylsulfonylmethane.

Supplements in the future

The process of matching dietary supplements to individuals and how best to recognize individuals whose OA is caused or worsened by vitamin D, borate, copper, calcium, or other nutritional deficiency(ies) remains our challenge. While blood tests may be one approach, the circulating pool may not be representative of the functional location. It may be that measurement of transporter systems or genes associated with systemic absorption might provide a better way for us to enrich the treatment population for individuals at highest potential benefit from dietary supplementation [84]. This would allow the targeting of 'specific' dietary supplements to those most likely to gain from their use, much like that done with iron, vitamin B12 and other nutrition related molecules in current practice. Providing nutrients to populations genetically at risk could limit disease onset similar to studies that are being undertaken for the onset of type 1 diabetes [85]. It is also likely that absorption of the entire range of foodstuffs may further be affected by the microbiome [86] and the concurrent use of the many potent medications such as proton pump inhibitors that potentially change the absorption chemistry of many molecules. Further sophisticated pharmacokinetic studies need to be conducted so as to determine how to appropriately 'prescribe' dietary supplements in the future. Benefit could also be achieved if regulatory agencies treated supplements like other pharmacologic compounds as is currently done in Europe. This way, the specifics of the dietary supplement preparation could be standardized from dose-to-dose and manufacturer-to-manufacturer and interpretation of the clinical trials might be more objective.

Conclusions

Even though there has been great hope that foods and dietary supplements may provide significant relief to patients with OA, the supportive evidence has been quite modest. How to best explain to lay people the interpretation of traditional superiority trials and the newer non-inferiority designs remains a major unmet need. A paper by Tsui and colleagues has compared two models of information transfer and found that although scientific evidence was an important factor in decision-making by patients, it was not as important as was advice from providers, family, and friends [87]. This is likely particularly true when the data are sparse, the methods flawed, the outcomes somewhat subjective, or when the standards are not clearly defined. Undoubtedly, there is more work to do. Among the dietary supplements, supportive evidence for reducing pain in OA is suggested for treatment with GS, CS, and G + CS combinations, while structural benefit appear best supported for the use of CS, and combined G and CS. Others like ASU and strontium have enough suggestive evidence to support additional study.

References

1. Bannuru RR, Schmid CH, Kent DM, et al. Comparative effectiveness of pharmacologic interventions for knee osteoarthritis: a systematic review and network meta-analysis. *Ann Intern Med* 2015; 162(1):46–54.
2. Pendleton A, Arden N, Dougados M, et al. EULAR recommendations for the management of knee osteoarthritis: report of a task force of the Standing Committee for International Clinical Studies Including Therapeutic Trials (ESCISIT). *Ann Rheum Dis* 2000; 59(12):936–44.
3. Jordan KM, Arden NK, Doherty M, et al. EULAR Recommendations 2003: an evidence based approach to the management of knee

osteoarthritis: Report of a Task Force of the Standing Committee for International Clinical Studies Including Therapeutic Trials (ESCISIT). *Ann Rheum Dis* 2003; 62(12):1145–55.

4. Zhang W, Nuki G, Moskowitz RW, et al. OARSI recommendations for the management of hip and knee osteoarthritis: part III: Changes in evidence following systematic cumulative update of research published through January 2009. *Osteoarthritis Cartilage* 2010; 18(4):476–99.

5. Bruyere O, Cooper C, Pelletier JP, et al. An algorithm recommendation for the management of knee osteoarthritis in Europe and internationally: a report from a task force of the European Society for Clinical and Economic Aspects of Osteoporosis and Osteoarthritis (ESCEO). *Semin Arthritis Rheum* 2014; 44(3):253–63.

6. McAlindon TE, Bannuru RR, Sullivan MC, et al. OARSI guidelines for the non-surgical management of knee osteoarthritis. *Osteoarthritis Cartilage* 2014; 22(3):363–88.

7. Deuteronomy 14. *The Holy Bible*.

8. Khamsi R. The trouble with gluten. *Sci Am* 2014; 310(2):30, 31A.

9. Ragle RL, Sawitzke AD. Nutraceuticals in the management of osteoarthritis: a critical review. *Drugs Aging* 2012; 29(9):717–31.

10. Henrotin Y, Lambert C, Couchourel D, et al. Nutraceuticals: do they represent a new era in the management of osteoarthritis?—a narrative review from the lessons taken with five products. *Osteoarthritis Cartilage* 2011; 19(1):1–21.

11. Akhtar N, Haqqi TM. Current nutraceuticals in the management of osteoarthritis: a review. *Ther Adv Musculoskelet Dis* 2012; 4(3):181–207.

12. Hochberg MC, Altman RD, April KT, et al. American College of Rheumatology 2012 recommendations for the use of nonpharmacologic and pharmacologic therapies in osteoarthritis of the hand, hip, and knee. *Arthritis Care Res (Hoboken)* 2012; 64(4):465–74.

13. Messier SP, Gutekunst DJ, Davis C, DeVita P. Weight loss reduces knee-joint loads in overweight and obese older adults with knee osteoarthritis. *Arthritis Rheum* 2005; 52(7):2026–32.

14. Wieland LS, Manheimer E, Sampson M, et al. Bibliometric and content analysis of the Cochrane Complementary Medicine Field specialized register of controlled trials. *Syst Rev* 2013; 2:51.

15. Rozendaal RM, Koes BW, van Osch GJ, et al. Effect of glucosamine sulfate on hip osteoarthritis: a randomized trial. *Ann Intern Med* 2008; 148(4):268–77.

16. Gilbey A, Perezgonzalez JD. Health benefits of deer and elk velvet antler supplements: a systematic review of randomised controlled studies. *N Z Med J* 2012; 125(1367):80–6.

17. Cho SH, Jung YB, Seong SC, et al. Clinical efficacy and safety of Lyprinol, a patented extract from New Zealand green-lipped mussel (Perna Canaliculus) in patients with osteoarthritis of the hip and knee: a multicenter 2-month clinical trial. *Eur Ann Allergy Clin Immunol* 2003; 35(6):212–6.

18. Deal CL, Moskowitz RW. Nutraceuticals as therapeutic agents in osteoarthritis. The role of glucosamine, chondroitin sulfate, and collagen hydrolysate. *Rheum Dis Clin North Am* 1999; 25(2):379–95.

19. Fillmore CM, Bartoli L, Bach R, Park Y. Nutrition and dietary supplements. *Phys Med Rehabil Clin N Am* 1999; 10(3):673–703.

20. Towheed TE, Maxwell L, Anastassiades TP, et al. Glucosamine therapy for treating osteoarthritis. *Cochrane Database Syst Rev* 2005; 2:CD002946.

21. McAlindon TE. Nutraceuticals: do they work and when should we use them? *Best Pract Res Clin Rheumatol* 2006; 20(1):99–115.

22. Gregory PJ, Sperry M, Wilson AF. Dietary supplements for osteoarthritis. *Am Fam Physician* 2008; 77(2):177–84.

23. McAlindon TE, LaValley MP, Gulin JP, Felson DT. Glucosamine and chondroitin for treatment of osteoarthritis: a systematic quality assessment and meta-analysis. *JAMA* 2000; 283(11):1469–75.

24. Richy F, Bruyere O, Ethgen O, et al. Structural and symptomatic efficacy of glucosamine and chondroitin in knee osteoarthritis: a comprehensive meta-analysis. *Arch Intern Med* 2003; 163(13):1514–22.

25. Bliddal H, Christensen RD, Kristensen PK, Astrup AV. [Glucosamine effectiveness in the treatment of knee osteoarthritis. Presentation of a Cochrane analysis with the perspective on the GAIT trial]. *Ugeskr Laeger* 2006; 168(50):4405–9.

26. Towheed TE, Anastassiades TP, Shea B, et al. Glucosamine therapy for treating osteoarthritis. *Cochrane Database Syst Rev* 2001; 1:CD002946.

27. Barnhill JG, Fye CL, Williams DW, et al. Chondroitin product selection for the glucosamine/chondroitin arthritis intervention trial. *J Am Pharm Assoc (2003)* 2006; 46(1):14–24.

28. Block JA, Oegema TR, Sandy JD, Plaas A. The effects of oral glucosamine on joint health: is a change in research approach needed? *Osteoarthritis Cartilage* 2010; 18(1):5–11.

29. Aghazadeh-Habashi A, Jamali F. The glucosamine controversy; a pharmacokinetic issue. *J Pharm Pharm Sci* 2011; 14(2):264–73.

30. Vlad SC, LaValley MP, McAlindon TE, Felson DT. Glucosamine for pain in osteoarthritis: why do trial results differ? *Arthritis Rheum* 2007; 56(7):2267–77.

31. Gouze JN, Bianchi A, Bécuwe P, et al. Glucosamine modulates IL-1-induced activation of rat chondrocytes at a receptor level, and by inhibiting the NF-kappa B pathway. *FEBS Lett* 2002; 510(3):166–70.

32. Dodge GR, Jimenez SA. Glucosamine sulfate modulates the levels of aggrecan and matrix metalloproteinase-3 synthesized by cultured human osteoarthritis articular chondrocytes. *Osteoarthritis Cartilage* 2003; 11(6):424–32.

33. Herrero-Beaumont G, Ivorra JA, Del Carmen Trabado M, et al. Glucosamine sulfate in the treatment of knee osteoarthritis symptoms: a randomized, double-blind, placebo-controlled study using acetaminophen as a side comparator. *Arthritis Rheum* 2007; 56(2):555–67.

34. Clegg DO, Reda DJ, Harris CL, et al. Glucosamine, chondroitin sulfate, and the two in combination for painful knee osteoarthritis. *N Engl J Med* 2006; 354(8):795–808.

35. Fox BA, Stephens MM. Glucosamine hydrochloride for the treatment of osteoarthritis symptoms. *Clin Interv Aging* 2007; 2(4):599–604.

36. Pavelka K, Gatterová J, Olejarová M, et al. Glucosamine sulfate use and delay of progression of knee osteoarthritis: a 3-year, randomized, placebo-controlled, double-blind study. *Arch Intern Med* 2002; 162(18):2113–23.

37. Reginster JY, Deroisy R, Rovati LC, et al. Long-term effects of glucosamine sulphate on osteoarthritis progression: a randomised, placebo-controlled clinical trial. *Lancet* 2001; 357(9252):251–6.

38. Sawitzke AD, Shi H, Finco MF, et al. Clinical efficacy and safety of glucosamine, chondroitin sulphate, their combination, celecoxib or placebo taken to treat osteoarthritis of the knee: 2-year results from GAIT. *Ann Rheum Dis* 2010; 69(8):1459–64.

39. Volpi, N. Quality of different chondroitin sulfate preparations in relation to their therapeutic activity. *J Pharm Pharmacol* 2009; 61(10):1271–80.

40. Calamia V, Fernández-Puente P, Mateos J, et al. Pharmacoproteomic study of three different chondroitin sulfate compounds on intracellular and extracellular human chondrocyte proteomes. *Mol Cell Proteomics* 2012; 11(6):M111 013417.

41. Hochberg M, Chevalier X, Henrotin Y, Hunter DJ, Uebelhart D. Symptom and structure modification in osteoarthritis with pharmaceutical-grade chondroitin sulfate: what's the evidence? *Curr Med Res Opin* 2013; 29(3):259–67.

42. Iovu M, Dumais G, du Souich P. Anti-inflammatory activity of chondroitin sulfate. *Osteoarthritis Cartilage* 2008; 16(Suppl 3):S14–8.

43. Martel-Pelletier J, Roubille C, Abram F, et al. First-line analysis of the effects of treatment on progression of structural changes in knee osteoarthritis over 24 months: data from the osteoarthritis initiative progression cohort. *Ann Rheum Dis* 2015; 74(3):547–56.

44. Reichenbach S, Sterchi R, Scherer M, et al. Meta-analysis: chondroitin for osteoarthritis of the knee or hip. *Ann Intern Med* 2007; 146(8):580–90.

45. Singh JA, Noorbaloochi S, MacDonald R, Maxwell LJ. Chondroitin for osteoarthritis. *Cochrane Database Syst Rev* 2015; 1:CD005614.

46. Clark KL, Sebastianelli W, Flechsenhar KR, et al. 24-Week study on the use of collagen hydrolysate as a dietary supplement in athletes with activity-related joint pain. *Curr Med Res Opin* 2008; 24(5):1485–96.

47. Ohara H, Iida H, Ito K, Takeuchi Y, Nomura Y. Effects of Pro-Hyp, a collagen hydrolysate-derived peptide, on hyaluronic acid synthesis using in vitro cultured synovium cells and oral ingestion of collagen hydrolysates in a guinea pig model of osteoarthritis. *Biosci Biotechnol Biochem* 2010; 74(10):2096–9.

48. Van Vijven JP, Luijsterburg PA, Verhagen AP, et al. Symptomatic and chondroprotective treatment with collagen derivatives in osteoarthritis: a systematic review. *Osteoarthritis Cartilage* 2012; 20(8):809–21.

49. Stammers T, Sibbald B, Freeling P. Fish oil in osteoarthritis. *Lancet* 1989; 2(8661):503.

50. Fritsch D, Allen TA, Dodd CE, et al. Dose-titration effects of fish oil in osteoarthritic dogs. *J Vet Intern Med* 2010; 24(5):1020–6.

51. Roush JK, Cross AR, Renberg WC, et al. Evaluation of the effects of dietary supplementation with fish oil omega-3 fatty acids on weight bearing in dogs with osteoarthritis. *J Am Vet Med Assoc* 2010; 236(1):67–73.

52. Corbee RJ, Barnier MM, van de Lest CH, Hazewinkel HA. The effect of dietary long-chain omega-3 fatty acid supplementation on owner's perception of behaviour and locomotion in cats with naturally occurring osteoarthritis. *J Anim Physiol Anim Nutr (Berl)* 2013; 97:846–53.

53. Hielm-Bjorkman A, Roine J, Elo K, et al. An un-commissioned randomized, placebo-controlled double-blind study to test the effect of deep sea fish oil as a pain reliever for dogs suffering from canine OA. *BMC Vet Res* 2012; 8:157.

54. Hutchins-Wiese HL, Kleppinger A, Annis K, et al. The impact of supplemental n-3 long chain polyunsaturated fatty acids and dietary antioxidants on physical performance in postmenopausal women. *J Nutr Health Aging* 2013; 17(1):76–80.

55. Bui LM, Bierer TL. Influence of green lipped mussels (Perna canaliculus) in alleviating signs of arthritis in dogs. *Vet Ther* 2003; 4(4):397–407.

56. Pollard B, Guilford WG, Ankenbauer-Perkins KL, Hedderley D. Clinical efficacy and tolerance of an extract of green-lipped mussel (Perna canaliculus) in dogs presumptively diagnosed with degenerative joint disease. *N Z Vet J* 2006; 54(3):114–8.

57. Cayzer J, Hedderley D, Gray S. A randomised, double-blinded, placebo-controlled study on the efficacy of a unique extract of green-lipped mussel (Perna canaliculus) in horses with chronic fetlock lameness attributed to osteoarthritis. *Equine Vet J* 2012; 44(4):393–8.

58. Zawadzki M, Janosch C, Szechinski J. Perna canaliculus lipid complex PCSO-524 demonstrated pain relief for osteoarthritis patients benchmarked against fish oil, a randomized trial, without placebo control. *Mar Drugs* 2013; 11(6):1920–35.

59. Brien S, Prescott P, Coghlan B, Bashir N, Lewith G. Systematic review of the nutritional supplement Perna Canaliculus (green-lipped mussel) in the treatment of osteoarthritis. *QJM* 2008; 101(3):167–79.

60. Coulson S, Vecchio P, Gramotnev H, Vitetta L. Green-lipped mussel (Perna canaliculus) extract efficacy in knee osteoarthritis and improvement in gastrointestinal dysfunction: a pilot study. *Inflammopharmacology* 2012; 20(2):71–6.

61. Ameye LG, Chee WS. Osteoarthritis and nutrition. From nutraceuticals to functional foods: a systematic review of the scientific evidence. *Arthritis Res Ther* 2006; 8(4):R127.

62. Altman RD, Marcussen KC. Effects of a ginger extract on knee pain in patients with osteoarthritis. *Arthritis Rheum* 2001; 44(11):2531–8.

63. Soeken KL. Selected CAM therapies for arthritis-related pain: the evidence from systematic reviews. *Clin J Pain* 2004; 20(1):13–8.

64. Kimmatkar N, Thawani V, Hingorani L, Khiyani R. Efficacy and tolerability of Boswellia serrata extract in treatment of osteoarthritis of knee—a randomized double blind placebo controlled trial. *Phytomedicine* 2003; 10(1):3–7.

65. Ernst E. Avocado-soybean unsaponifiables (ASU) for osteoarthritis—a systematic review. *Clin Rheumatol* 2003; 22(4–5):285–8.

66. Christensen R, Bartels EM, Astrup A, Bliddal H. Symptomatic efficacy of avocado-soybean unsaponifiables (ASU) in osteoarthritis (OA) patients: a meta-analysis of randomized controlled trials. *Osteoarthritis Cartilage* 2008; 16(4):399–408.

67. GALLUP. *Half of Americans Take Vitamins Regularly*. 2013, December 19. http://www.gallup.com/poll/166541/half-americans-vitamins-regularly.aspx

68. Morelli V, Naquin C, Weaver V. Alternative therapies for traditional disease states: osteoarthritis. *Am Fam Physician* 2003; 67(2):339–44.

69. Reginster JY, Badurski J, Bellamy N, et al. Efficacy and safety of strontium ranelate in the treatment of knee osteoarthritis: results of a double-blind, randomised placebo-controlled trial. *Ann Rheum Dis* 2013; 72(2):179–86.

70. Pelletier JP, Roubille C, Raynauld JP, et al. Disease-modifying effect of strontium ranelate in a subset of patients from the Phase III knee osteoarthritis study SEKOIA using quantitative MRI: reduction in bone marrow lesions protects against cartilage loss. *Ann Rheum Dis* 2015; 74(2):422–9.

71. Donneau AF, Reginster JY. Cardiovascular safety of strontium ranelate: real-life assessment in clinical practice. *Osteoporos Int* 2014; 25(2):397–8.

72. McCarty MF, Russell AL. Niacinamide therapy for osteoarthritis—does it inhibit nitric oxide synthase induction by interleukin 1 in chondrocytes? *Med Hypotheses* 1999; 53(4):350–60.

73. Ringdahl E, Pandit S. Treatment of knee osteoarthritis. *Am Fam Physician* 2011; 83(11):1287–92.

74. Edmundson AB, Manion CV. Treatment of osteoarthritis with aspartame. *Clin Pharmacol Ther* 1998; 63(5):580–93.

75. Manion CV, Hochgeschwender U, Edmundson AB, Hugli TE, Gabaglia CR. Dietary aspartyl-phenylalanine-1-methyl ester delays osteoarthritis and prevents associated bone loss in STR/ORT mice. *Rheumatology (Oxford)* 2011; 50(7):1244–9.

76. Brand C, Snaddon J, Bailey M, Cicuttini F. Vitamin E is ineffective for symptomatic relief of knee osteoarthritis: a six month double blind, randomised, placebo controlled study. *Ann Rheum Dis* 2001; 60(10):946–9.

77. Rosenbaum EE, Jacob SW. Dimethyl Sulfoxide (DMSO) in musculoskeletal injuries and Inflammations. Ii. Dimethyl sulfoxide in rheumatoid arthritis, degenerative arthritis and gouty arthritis. *Northwest Med* 1964; 63:227–9.

78. Aliabeva AP, Akimova TF, Trusova TM. [Treatment of joint diseases with dimethyl sulfoxide (DMSO) applications]. *Ter Arkh* 1979; 51(7):52–5.

79. Brien S, Prescott P, Bashir N, Lewith H, Lewith G. Systematic review of the nutritional supplements dimethyl sulfoxide (DMSO) and methylsulfonylmethane (MSM) in the treatment of osteoarthritis. *Osteoarthritis Cartilage* 2008; 16(11):1277–88.

80. Brien S, Prescott P, Lewith G. Meta-analysis of the related nutritional supplements dimethyl sulfoxide and methylsulfonylmethane in the treatment of osteoarthritis of the knee. *Evid Based Complement Alternat Med* 2011; 2011:528403.

81. Hochberg MC, Martel-Pelletier J, Monfort J, et al. Combined chondroitin sulfate and glucosamine for painful knee osteoarthritis: a multicentre, randomised, double-blind, non-inferiority trial versus celecoxib. *Ann Rheum Dis* 2016; 75(1):37–44.

82. Fransen M, Agaliotis M, Nairn L, et al. Glucosamine and chondroitin for knee osteoarthritis: a double-blind randomised placebo-controlled clinical trial evaluating single and combination regimens. *Ann Rheum Dis* 2015; 74(5):851–8.

83. Kwoh CK, Roemer FW, Hannon MJ, et al. Effect of oral glucosamine on joint structure in individuals with chronic knee pain: a randomized, placebo-controlled clinical trial. *Arthritis Rheumatol* 2014; 66(4):930–9.

84. Morgan K. Food as medicine. *Genome* 2014; Winter:34–41.

85. Franciscus M, Nucci A, Bradley B, et al. Recruitment and retention of participants for an international type 1 diabetes prevention trial: a coordinators' perspective. *Clin Trials* 2014; 11(2):150–8.

86. Zhao L, Shen J. Whole-body systems approaches for gut microbiota-targeted, preventive healthcare. *J Biotechnol* 2010; 149(3):183–90.

87. Tsui T, Boon H, Boecker A, Kachan N, Krahn M. Understanding the role of scientific evidence in consumer evaluation of natural health products for osteoarthritis an application of the means end chain approach. *BMC Complement Altern Med* 2012; 12:198.

88. Sengupta K, Alluri KV, Satish AR, et al. A double blind, randomized, placebo controlled study of the efficacy and safety of 5-Loxin for treatment of osteoarthritis of the knee. *Arthritis Res Ther* 2008; 10(4):R85.

89. Ernst E. Frankincense: systematic review. *BMJ* 2008; 337:a2813.

90. Bartels EM, Folmer VN, Bliddal H, et al. Efficacy and safety of ginger in osteoarthritis patients: a meta-analysis of randomized placebo-controlled trials. *Osteoarthritis Cartilage* 2015; 23(1):13–21.

91. Coulson S, Butt H, Vecchio P, Gramotnev H, Vitetta L. Green-lipped mussel extract (Perna canaliculus) and glucosamine sulphate in patients with knee osteoarthritis: therapeutic efficacy and effects on gastrointestinal microbiota profiles. *Inflammopharmacology* 2013; 21(1):79–90.

92. Dave M, Attur M, Palmer G, et al. The antioxidant resveratrol protects against chondrocyte apoptosis via effects on mitochondrial polarization and ATP production. *Arthritis Rheum* 2008; 58(9):2786–97.

93. Warholm O, Skaar S, Hedman E, Mølmen HM, Eik L. The effects of a standardized herbal remedy made from a subtype of Rosa canina in patients with osteoarthritis: a double-blind, randomized, placebo-controlled clinical trial. *Curr Ther Res Clin Exp* 2003; 64(1):21–31.

94. Winther K, Rein E, Kharazmi A. The anti-inflammatory properties of rose-hip. *Inflammopharmacology* 1999; 7(1):63–8.

95. Reginster JY, Pelousse F, Bruyere O. Safety concerns with the long-term management of osteoporosis. *Expert Opin Drug Saf* 2013; 12(4):507–22.

96. Xie Q, Shi R, Xu G, et al. Effects of AR7 Joint Complex on arthralgia for patients with osteoarthritis: results of a three-month study in Shanghai, China. *Nutr J* 2008; 7:31.

97. Kulkarni RR, Patki PS, Jog VP, et al. Treatment of osteoarthritis with a herbomineral formulation: a double-blind, placebo-controlled, cross-over study. *J Ethnopharmacol* 1991; 33(1–2):91–5.

98. Sawitzke AD, Shi H, Finco MF, et al. The effect of glucosamine and/or chondroitin sulfate on the progression of knee osteoarthritis: a report from the glucosamine/chondroitin arthritis intervention trial. *Arthritis Rheum* 2008; 58(10):3183–91.

99. Jacquet A, Girodet PO, Pariente A, et al. Phytalgic, a food supplement, vs placebo in patients with osteoarthritis of the knee or hip: a randomised double-blind placebo-controlled clinical trial. *Arthritis Res Ther* 2009; 11(6):R192.

100. Chopra A, Lavin P, Patwardhan B, Chitre D. A 32-week randomized, placebo-controlled clinical evaluation of RA-11, an Ayurvedic drug, on osteoarthritis of the knees. *J Clin Rheumatol* 2004; 10(5):236–45.

101. Leeb BF, Schweitzer H, Montag K, Smolen JS. A metaanalysis of chondroitin sulfate in the treatment of osteoarthritis. *J Rheumatol* 2000; 27(1):205–11.

102. Chrubasik C, Duke RK, Chrubasik S. The evidence for clinical efficacy of rose hip and seed: a systematic review. *Phytother Res* 2006; 20(1):1–3.

103. Soeken KL, Lee WL, Bausell RB, Agelli M, Berman BM. Safety and efficacy of S-adenosylmethionine (SAMe) for osteoarthritis. *J Fam Pract* 2002; 51(5):425–30.

CHAPTER 32

Intra-articular injection therapy

Nigel Arden and Terence O'Neill

Introduction

Intra-articular injection therapy is widely used in the management of osteoarthritis (OA). In this chapter, the rationale for intra-articular therapy and practical considerations relating to administration of therapy are discussed. The evidence for efficacy and safety of two commonly used intra-articular injection therapies, corticosteroids (CS) and hyaluronic acid (HA), is reviewed and other intra-articular therapies that have been used in the management of OA are briefly considered.

Rationale

Management of OA focuses on reducing symptoms and functional impairment. Current oral therapies used in the management of symptomatic OA are often limited by their relatively short duration of action, efficacy, and also adverse effects. For patients who fail to gain relief from oral therapy and other non-pharmacological therapies, intra-articular injection therapy offers significant potential benefits including targeted and relatively long-lasting therapy to the affected joint combined with the ability to achieve relatively high local drug concentrations and a lower risk of systemic adverse effects.

Intra-articular therapy: practical considerations

Intra-articular therapy can be administered in both primary and secondary care settings. It is an invasive procedure and an aseptic technique is therefore required. Gloves may be worn though need not necessarily be sterile provided a no-touch technique is used. During the procedure the patient should be seated comfortably with the injection area clearly exposed. Following preparation the skin should be cleaned with antiseptic solution. Local anaesthesia, either topical or subcutaneous infiltration prior to injection, may be used though is not required unless the procedure is being undertaken in children. For large joints a green (21-gauge) needle should be used though a larger needle may be needed if purulent material is present. Smaller-gauge needles can be used for smaller joints. Depending on the joint there may be a number of possible injection sites. Injections undertaken 'blind' without imaging are, depending on the joint site, often inaccurate [1]. Image guidance (e.g. using ultrasound) may help in localization of the joint and is recommended for some joints such as the hip and spine where there is difficulty in clinical localization of the joint. Aspiration of the joint should be attempted as the presence of fluid confirms localization of the needle within the joint; also the appearance of synovial fluid (SF) can help provide clues about any coexisting pathology. Following aspiration of fluid, the joint should then be injected using either the same, or an accompanying syringe, using the same needle portal. The injection should flow smoothly and if there is resistance the needle should be withdrawn slightly, though taking care not to displace it. Following the injection, on withdrawal of the needle, gentle pressure should be applied to the injection site with use of a small adhesive strip to cover the site. If there is any concern about underlying joint infection or the presence of coexisting pathology (e.g. crystal arthropathy), the SF withdrawn should be retained for cytological and/or microbiological analysis. Following the procedure, patients are typically advised to rest during the subsequent 24 hours, however, the evidence base for this is not strong. One study in a group of hospitalized patients with rheumatoid arthritis found no benefit associated with resting joints for 48 hours following steroid injection. In another study, however, of patients with inflammatory arthritis, intra-articular steroid injection of the knee followed by 24 hours of observed bed rest (in hospital) was associated with greater symptom and functional improvement at 6 months compared with no rest [2,3].

Intra-articular steroid therapy

Following the identification of steroids as an effective therapy for use in the relief of symptoms in patients with rheumatoid arthritis in the 1940s, intra-articular steroid injections have become widely used in the management of inflammatory and non-inflammatory arthritis. Their use in large series of OA patients was popularized by Hollander in 1951; since then they have become widely used in the management of patients with OA [4]. A survey among rheumatologists in the United States found intra-articular steroid injections to be popular, with over 95% of them using them at least 'sometimes' and more than 50% using them 'frequently' [5]. Intra-articular steroids are currently recommended for the clinical management of OA as part of European League Against Rheumatism (EULAR), National Institute for Health and Care Excellence (NICE), Osteoarthritis Research Society International (OARSI) and American College of Rheumatology (ACR) guidelines [6–12].

Pharmacology

Following injection, the intra-articular steroid is taken up by synovial lining cells and then gradually diffuses into the blood and is cleared. The magnitude and duration of any effect is related to the dose and potency of the steroid and its solubility. Synthetic steroids used in clinical practice today are derivatives of prednisolone. Methyl prednisolone is the methyl derivative of prednisolone whereas betamethasone, dexamethasone, and triamcinolone are all fluorinated derivatives of prednisolone; the inclusion of fluorine augmenting the pharmacological properties. Most steroid preparations contain steroid esters which are highly insoluble in water (hydrophobic) and thus form a microcrystalline suspension. Dexamethasone is not an ester and is freely soluble in water (hydrophilic), and so preparations are clear and non-particulate [13]. Steroid esters require hydrolysis by cellular esterases to release the active moiety. Water-soluble preparations such as dexamethasone and betamethasone are taken up rapidly by cells and thus have a quicker onset of effect though with a concomitant reduced duration of action. Given the fact that ester preparations require metabolism within the joint it might be expected that they would have a longer half-life than non-ester preparations though this is not always observed in clinical practice; in a recent trial comparing triamcinolone hexacetonide, a compound with poor solubility with methylprednisolone acetate, a compound with intermediate solubility, it was the methylprednisolone acetate which had a more sustained clinical effect on pain [14]. Steroid preparations may be combined also with local anaesthetic preparations (e.g. lignocaine).

Mechanism of action

Glucocorticoids have potent anti-inflammatory effects and immunosuppressive effects. They act through a combination of genomic and non-genomic mechanisms. It is thought though that their effect on reducing symptoms in OA is through their anti-inflammatory effect and this is consistent with their relatively rapid onset of effect. Synovial inflammation (synovitis) is a well-recognized feature of OA; histological studies in patients with knee OA show evidence of inflammatory change ranging from mild to severe almost rheumatoid like. On arthroscopy, synovitis is seen in approximately 50% of the knees of patients with painful OA and in an even higher percentage using MRI [15, 16]. Loeuille et al. [17] compared magnetic resonance imaging (MRI), histological, and arthroscopic appearance of synovium in persons with symptomatic knee OA and reported a high correlation between the degree of synovial thickening on MRI and macroscopic scoring of synovitis by an arthroscopist (r = 0.58). Thickness was also correlated with infiltration of inflammatory cells into the subsurface layers of synovium (r = 0.46). Data from observational studies suggest an association between synovitis as assessed by MRI and knee pain in both cross-sectional and prospective studies [18–20]. The cause of synovial inflammation is unknown though may be related to the release of cartilage degradation products into the joint and triggering of the inflammatory cascade within the synovial lining layer. Recent data suggest evidence of synovial shrinkage following intra-articular steroid therapy and also an increase in synovial thickening on relapse (recurrence of pain) suggesting that the synovium is a target tissue [21].

Adverse effects

Intra-articular CS injections have an excellent safety record over many years. The most serious and feared complication of CS and other intra-articular therapies is the risk of joint infection (septic arthritis). The risk is very small and it is difficult therefore to obtain accurate estimates. In a retrospective survey of 69 rheumatologists in France, the overall risk was estimated at just under 1 in 80 000 injections [22], while in a case-note survey undertaken in Nottingham only eight cases of infection, possibly related to steroid injection, were seen over a 10-year period in two large teaching hospitals serving a catchment area of 632 000 people [23].

In neither study was it possible to determine the level of risk by underlying disease type. Apart from local discomfort during the time of the injection, one of the most frequent adverse effects is a post-injection flare, a local increase in inflammation that develops within hours and can last a couple of days. The cause is unknown but may be due to microcrystalline steroid esters inducing a crystal-induced arthritis, though a post-injection flare may occur also following placebo injection suggesting other mechanisms [24,25]. Other adverse effects are less common. There is a small risk of skin atrophy or subcutaneous atrophy/skin depigmentation at the injection site; however, this is more frequently seen with use of extra-articular injections. It may be due to inaccurate localization of the injection outside the joint or steroid leaking from the joint. Systemic absorption of steroids can occur following steroid injections though systemic side effects are uncommon and include facial flushing which was reported, in a series of mixed inflammatory and non-inflammatory arthritides, as being unpleasant in up to 15% of patients [26,27]. In diabetic patients, glucose control can be affected with a transient increase in blood glucose levels over a few days [27] and diabetic patients should be warned to look for changes in their blood glucose. Suppression of the hypothalamic–pituitary–adrenal axis may occur with reduction in the level of cortisol within hours and which can last for several days with the degree dependent on the dose and type of intra-articular steroid and also the number of joints injected [27]. Bone turnover markers may be affected—with osteocalcin level falling within a day after injection and returning to pre-treatment levels after 2 weeks [28]. Anaphylaxis following intra-articular injection in knee OA is rare though has been reported [29, 30]. Tendon weakening or rupture after injection of an arthritic joint has also been described [31]. Systemic infection is very rare.

There are few data concerning potential long-term adverse effects. There are theoretical concerns about damage to the joint following injection. Animal studies have, however, been somewhat inconsistent with studies in rabbits suggesting evidence of cartilage damage following steroid injection; this was not supported by studies in other animals [32,33], while other studies suggest there may be a protective effect [34]. In the longest human study to date—a randomized trial of repeated intra-articular steroid injections given every 3 months for 2 years—there was no change in joint space narrowing when compared with intraarticular saline [35]. A number of observational studies suggest that following steroid injection at the hip, patients with hip OA who go on to have hip surgery may have an increased risk of infection following surgery and subsequent revision arthroplasty [36]. In a recent systematic review of safety of intra-articular CS injection prior to total knee arthroplasty, three of four observational studies suggested no increased risk of post-arthroplasty infection though one suggested an increased risk of deep infection post arthroplasty. Further studies are thus required to evaluate the safety of steroid injection in this setting [37].

Indications and contraindications

The main indication for intraarticular steroid therapy is joint pain or discomfort. There are relatively few contraindications; the main one being suspected joint sepsis or bacteraemia. There is some evidence that steroids inhibit bone healing in intra-articular fracture and so should be avoided in this setting and in the presence also of markedly unstable joints. A relative contraindication is the presence of a prosthetic joint, and injection should only be performed after discussion with orthopaedic surgeons. Caution is required in patients taking anticoagulant therapy and it is prudent to check anticoagulant control prior to any injection because of concern about bleeding. A recent study, however, reported no clinical haemarthroses or complications in 21 patients taking warfarin with an international normalized ratio less than 3 [38].

Efficacy

Knee

There have been a number of trials performed looking at the effect of intra-articular steroid injections in patients with symptomatic knee OA. They vary significantly in terms of design, setting, the dose and type of steroid used, and also comparator intervention. In a meta-analysis of randomized trials comparing CS with placebo injections, Arroll and Goodyear-Smith [39] reported the superiority of CS injections in reducing symptoms in the short term. The treatment effect was large, with the number needed to treat ranging from 1.3 to 3.5. Less is known about longer-term efficacy, primarily because of the paucity of long-term trials [40]. Two meta-analyses have looked at long-term efficacy of intra-articular steroid injection [39,40] and included two high-quality trials, [41,42] though in one the steroid injection was given at the time of arthroscopy [42]. Bellamy et al. [40] reported no compelling evidence of benefit from 4–24 weeks post injection though Arroll and Goodyear-Smith [39] suggested improvement among methodologically sound studies at 16–24 weeks (relative risk 2.09, 95% confidence interval 1.20–3.65) with a number needed to treat of 4.4.

The effect of steroid injection on physical function is less well established, primarily because few randomized controlled trials (RCTs) included validated, joint-specific functional scores for assessment of function [35,42–44]. Meta-analyses, however, do not support evidence for either short-term or long-term effects on function [40]. A more recent study reported no additional improvement, compared to controls, in short- or medium-term outcomes (including pain and function) when steroid injection was given prior to an exercise programme [45].

Effect of dose and type of steroid on response

There are few studies which allow comparison of either the dose or type of steroid used in management of knee OA. Arroll and Goodyear-Smith [39] reported that higher doses of steroid (equivalent to 50 mg prednisolone) may be required to show benefit in the longer term (16–24 weeks). Valtonen [46] in a study of 42 patients with OA, reported that the duration of effect of triamcinolone hexacetonide (THA) (20 mg) was longer than a combination of betamethasone acetate and betamethasone disodium-phosphate (6 mg). In another study which compared THA 20 mg and methylprednisolone acetate (MPA) 40 mg, THA was more effective than MPA in terms of pain reduction at 3 weeks though its effect was lost by week 8 while MPA continued to show benefit at week 8 [14].

Site and accuracy of injection

In a systematic review of knee joint injections, Maricar et al. [47] reported that overall about 80% of blinded injections were accurate in terms of localization within the joint. There was variation though in the degree of accuracy by site of injection with the superolateral approach being the most accurate (87%) and also some evidence that greater clinical experience was linked with improved accuracy. Use of image guidance also increased accuracy of the injection. Based on a small number of studies there was some evidence of improved short-, but not longer-term, outcomes when injections were administered using image guidance (compared to non-image-guided injections); to date though there are no studies which have looked at accuracy of knee injection (with confirmation of localization) and subsequent outcome [48].

Predictors of response

Evidence from meta-analyses suggest that not all patients respond to steroids and among those who respond, the duration of response varies [21,39,40]. An understanding of the person-, disease-, and treatment-related factors that influence response to steroid injection would be of potential help in clinical practice in guiding or targeting therapy. Evidence from two recent systematic reviews, however, suggest no factor which has been consistently linked with response; data from single studies suggest individual disease factors which are linked with response though these are either not confirmed, or contradicted in other studies [48,49]. There was relatively little evidence also to support the impression that the presence of knee effusion was associated with response; with only two of six studies suggesting that response was better in those with effusion [14,25,43,50–52]. In one study, the absence of synovitis, as assessed using ultrasound, was linked with a better response [43]. However, the numbers of patients in these studies was relatively small and further larger studies are needed to better define the disease- and non-disease-related factors which are linked to response.

Hip

Clinical localization of the hip joint is difficult and use of imaging is recommended for aspiration and/or injection; in a study of cadaver specimens using dye to help determine accuracy, injection without image guidance using the anterior approach was successful in only 60% of injections and the lateral approach successful in 80% [53]. In contrast to knee OA there are relatively few randomized trials that have been performed looking at the effect of intra-articular steroids in patients with symptomatic hip OA. These do, however, suggest that steroid injection at the hip is efficacious in delivering short-term, but clinically significant, pain reduction in those with hip OA, and may also lead to transient improvement in function [54–58]. Treatment effect appears to be relatively quick with a large treatment effect size after 1 week post injection. The magnitude of pain reduction and functional improvement would appear to decrease thereafter, although two trials report clinically significant differences in both pain and function at 8 weeks post injection [57,58]. Caution though is needed in interpreting these data given the relatively small number of subjects; in addition, many of the trial subjects had severe OA and were awaiting hip surgery.

Effect of dose and type of steroid on response

In the randomized trials which have been performed, because each used a different preparation or dose of steroid it was not possible to determine the effect of any particular type or dose of steroid on outcome. In an open-label study of patients with symptomatic hip OA, injection of 40 mg of methylprednisolone resulted in a significant reduction in pain at 6 though not 12 weeks while injection of 80 mg was associated with reduction in both time points, providing some evidence for a dose–response effect [59].

Predictors of response

In a systematic review, Hirsch et al. [49] was unable to identify any disease or patient factors which were consistently associated with treatment response following hip injection. In one randomized study, in which patients were randomized to one of four interventions including 120 mg methylprednisolone acetate, the presence of synovitis assessed at baseline (determined by the presence of synovial tissue volume > 7 mm) was linked with responder status, however the number of people who received the intervention was relatively small [18] [58]. A further study, using a lower dose of steroids, did not find any association between semi-quantitative capsular thickness assessed on ultrasound and response [59]. Studies looking at the impact of disease severity as determined by radiographs and response are somewhat inconsistent with most suggesting no association while others either a better or worse response among those with more severe disease [49].

Hand

Most of the published trials of steroid injection therapy in hand OA have focused on the first carpometacarpal joint. All but one of these was undertaken using blinded imaging. This may have limited efficacy as up to 58% of such injections may be inaccurate [60]. The number of participants studied also was relatively small and studies used both different doses and types of steroids, precluding comparisons, and only a couple looked at the effect compared with saline placebo [61–64]. In all studies there was an improvement in pain in those who received the injection, however, none of the trials showed any between-group differences in pain or function. To date, there are no published trials of steroid injections in patients with OA at other hand joints including distal interphalangeal and proximal interphalangeal joints. The role of steroids therefore in the management of hand OA remains unclear. There are also few studies which have looked at factors which may predict response to therapy. In an open-label study of 30 patients with carpometacarpal OA injected with 40 mg methylprednisolone acetate (and local anaesthetic), followed by immobilization in a thumb spica spline for 3 weeks, those with mild disease as determined by the Eaton classification had better response in the short- and long-term than those with more severe disease [65,66]. However, in a separate study of 83 patients with thumb base OA injected with 40 mg triamcinolone and local anaesthetic, disease severity was not linked with response [67]. Synovitis as assessed using ultrasound (capsular thickness) did not predict treatment response in an open-label study of 31 patients with symptomatic thumb base OA treated with 40 mg triamcinolone acetonide and 1% lidocaine [68].

Other joints

Steroids have been widely used in the management of OA at other joint sites including the wrist/shoulder, elbows, and feet including metatarsophalangeal, subtalar and true ankle joint. There are, however, few trials which have looked at efficacy in these settings. Trials of steroid injection to the facet joints do not suggest any benefit over placebo [69,70].

Hyaluronic acid

HA is a naturally occurring glycosaminoglycan, which is present in a number of tissues throughout the body. It is present in large quantities in SF, and cartilage of articular joints where it enhances the viscoelastic properties of SF in terms of lubrication, shock absorption, and elasticity [71]. It has a strong affinity for water that increases with the molecular weight (MW) of HA, which is 4–5 MDa in normal SF [72]. In joints with OA, the concentration of HA is reduced and, as importantly, the MW is also reduced. These

two factors together lead to a reduction in the beneficial effects of HA [73–75].

HA was initially thought to exert its beneficial effects solely through restoration of HA concentration, which optimized the viscoelastic properties of SF. However a number of other properties of HA have since been discovered that may partially explain its clinical benefit. HA is thought to have chondroprotective actions, including a reduction of chondrocyte apoptosis and increase in proliferation, largely mediated through binding to the CD44 receptors [76,77]. Intra-articular HA administration has been demonstrated to increase the synthesis of endogenous HA by synoviocytes [78] in addition to proteoglycan (PG) and glycosaminoglycan (GAG) synthesis and these effects may be greater for higher MW HA [79]. They may have an anti-inflammatory effect through the suppression of interleukin 1 beta (IL1B)-mediated via binding to the CD44 receptor [80]. Finally, HA may have direct analgesic properties by blocking sensitized nociceptive nerve endings [81]. It is not currently clear, however, which of these mechanism(s) explain the beneficial effects of HA. Intra-articular injections of HA do appear to increase the endogenous production of native HA, which may explained the sustained benefit beyond the intra-articular half-life of the injected HA.

Initial HA products were derived from avian sources, predominantly from rooster combs. This may be an issue for use in patients who are vegetarians or vegans, but may also be the cause of some of the reported localized adverse reactions [82]. More recently, several HA products produced by bacterial formation have been marketed. These may potentially have less localized reactions, however more research is required before this is confirmed [82]. The available preparations also vary in their MW, varying from 0.5 to 7 MDa; however, for the cross-linked products, it is hard to define a true MW. There is considerable debate about the importance of MW of the injected product. There is some evidence that higher MW HA has superior binding to CD44, GAG, and PG production and blocking of nociceptors, but whether this is translated into better clinical response is uncertain (see below). What is clinically important, however, is the frequency of injection required per course. This can vary from one injection for some of the high MW and cross-linked products, to five weekly injections for lower MW products. This obviously has a large impact on patient time and the use of health facilities and professionals and hence costs.

In relation to safety, as with all intra-articular injections the risk of infection is the most feared though is rare. As with steroids, intra-articular HA injections are associated with an increased risk of minor post injection flares, although a small percentage of patients may develop an inflammatory effusion. Patients with allergies to eggs or chicken should ideally avoid products derived from rooster combs.

Efficacy

Intra-articular injections of HA have been used in a number of joints, however, the vast majority of trials have been performed in the knee and hip. The traditional trial is to compare the injection of HA to a placebo injection. The 'placebo arm', however, is often accompanied by aspiration of the joint, which is associated with its own clinical benefit. This arm of the trial should therefore be called a control arm, rather than a placebo arm. Furthermore, the clinical decision faced by the clinician and patient is whether to give an HA injection or not, as opposed to an HA injection or a 'placebo' injection. The 'placebo'-controlled RCT therefore does not answer this question and may provide spurious results when performing cost effectiveness analyses.

Knee

The response to intra-articular HA is different to that of intra-articular CS in that they have a gradual and delayed onset of pain reduction, but a more prolonged effect when compared to intra-articular CS as demonstrated in a 26-week trial comparing intra-articular methyl prednisolone and NASHA (Non-animal stabilised Hyaluronic acid) (Figure 32.1). There is some early evidence that repeated courses of injections may lead to cumulative benefit. A number of international guidelines have assessed the role of HA injections for knee OA. The OARSI analysed the literature and performed an expert consensus meeting and published guidance in 2014 [82]. They concluded that intra-articular HA had benefit over placebo, but that the effect size was variable, between small and moderate [83,84], and that it was inferior to intra-articular CS at 2 weeks, but superior at 12 and 26 weeks [84]. HA was not recommended for multi-joint OA, but for single-joint OA the recommendation was 'uncertain', in part due to the discrepancy of effect sizes. The ACR published guidelines in 2012 and conditionally recommended using intra-articular HA in patients over the age of 75 who did not respond to conservative therapies [10]. The American Society of Orthopaedic Surgeons' guidelines issued in 2013 changed the previous recommendation of 'inconclusive' to 'not recommended', although they did note that some studies of high MW HA were positive [85].

The discrepancy in the guidelines reflects the difficulty in assessing the published data for the use of intra-articular HA in the treatment of knee OA. Many of the issues are shared with the assessment of other treatment modalities. These include the inclusion of a number of different compounds in the same statistical analysis; the use of different outcomes; and more importantly that the time of outcome differs, which is critically important when comparing to intra-articular CS that have a very different time course of benefit. The most important issue, however, is the lack of allowance for the phenotype of the patients. This limits analyses in two ways: the first is that studies will often have different inclusion and exclusion criteria, making comparisons difficult, but more importantly, they do not allow the assessment of personalized medicine, that is, targeting the treatment to an individual patient rather than expecting all patients to have the same response. Overall, the evidence for the use of intra-articular HA in knee OA is still unclear. Whilst it is not the panacea for knee OA it is likely that it is of benefit in subsets of patients.

Hip and other joints

As outlined earlier, injections of the hip OA joint are constrained by the need for either fluoroscopy or ultrasound to confirm intra-articular placement, adding to the complexity and costs of the treatment. Although a number of trials of intra-articular HA have been performed, there is still considerable heterogeneity; however, there does appear to be a small improvement over a 'control arm', but no benefit over intra-articular CS [86]. There is less evidence for its use in other joints. There are only a limited numbers of trials for shoulder, ankle, and thumb base OA that are often underpowered and results are both heterogeneous and inconclusive, making firm conclusions difficult.

In summary, HAs are not a first-line treatment for patients with OA, but may be useful in small subsets of patients in whom other treatments are either ineffective or contraindicated for example, patients with risk factors for non-steroidal anti-inflammatory drug-induced gastrointestinal bleeds and cardiovascular system disease. We need to know more also about the predictors of response to treatment for HAs, and all drugs, to allow targeted treatments of patients with OA.

Other intra-articular therapies

A number of other intra-articular therapies have been used in the management of OA though the evidence base to support their use is generally either limited or poor, often with data from small-scale or pilot studies only; some of these are outlined below.

Biological therapy

Biological therapy including anti-tumour necrosis factor blockade has revolutionized the management of many inflammatory disorders. It has also been used in some patients with symptomatic OA. In a randomized trial of 170 patients with symptomatic knee OA, intra-articular injection of anakinra, a recombinant IL1 receptor antagonist, at doses of either 50 mg or 150 mg was well tolerated though not linked with any improvement in OA symptoms compared to placebo [87]. In contrast, in a small pilot study of intra-articular infliximab, there was some evidence suggesting benefit in women with hand OA [88]. Ten women with bilateral erosive hand OA, received treatment with monthly intra-articular injections of 0.2 mL infliximab (0.1 mg/mL) in each affected proximal and distal interphalangeal joint of the most involved hand with the other hand treated with physiological saline. The patients were blinded to the hand which was treated with infliximab. After 12 months there was a significant within group reduction in pain in the hand treated with infliximab [88].

Analgesic therapy

Many clinicians include local anaesthetic in combination with steroids; however, evidence to support the efficacy of this in terms of pain reduction is relatively weak. Local anaesthetic agents have been used

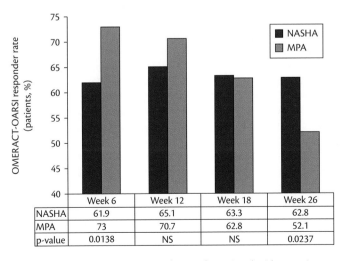

	Week 6	Week 12	Week 18	Week 26
NASHA	61.9	65.1	63.3	62.8
MPA	73	70.7	62.8	52.1
p-value	0.0138	NS	NS	0.0237

Figure 32.1 OMERACT-OARSI responder rates for a 26 week trial comparing methylprednisolone (MPA) and NASHA (non-animal stabilised hyaluronic acid). Data from National Institute for Health and Care Excellence. *Osteoarthritis: Care and Management in Adults*. NICE Clinical Guideline 177. February 2014 http://www.nice.org.uk/guidance/CG177

alone; in one study patients were randomized to receive either small volume (5 mL) of bupivacaine or saline [89]. There was a significant improvement in pain (assessed using a visual analogue pain score) within the bupivacaine group though this did not persist beyond 1 hour, though there were prolonged changes in the McGill pain questionnaire observed up to 7 days. In a cross-over randomized trial of 23 patients with knee OA, patients received either intra-articular morphine (1 mg) and intravenous saline or an intra-articular injection of saline and intravenous morphine [90]. Intra-articular morphine was linked with significantly greater pain relief than intra-articular saline. Another randomized trial looked at the efficacy of intra-articular morphine and bupivacaine in a group of 39 patients with knee OA; mean joint range of movement and also pain improved in both groups though there were no between group differences [91].

Oral non-steroidal anti-inflammatory drugs are effective in management of pain however their use is often limited by adverse effects or concerns about adverse effects. Intraarticular therapy with phenyl-butazone was linked with improvement in pain in one uncontrolled study of 15 patients with painful knees who had had previous unsuccessful intra-articular steroid therapy [92]. In a randomized trial, 30 patients with an acute knee effusion and grade 2–3 OA were assigned to intra-articular tenoxicam or oral therapy. The intra-articular group had more rapid pain relief than the oral group and at the end of 1 year the number of effusions was lower in the intra-articular group [93].

Radio-synovectomy

Intra-articular injection of yttrium and other chemical toxins such as osmium have been used in the management of patients with predominantly inflammatory arthritis though have been used also in some patients with OA. In a small trial of 15 patients with chronic pyrophosphate arthropathy of the knee, one knee was randomly assigned to receive yttrium-90 injection + 20 mg triamcinolone hexacetonide and the other knee triamcinolone and saline. After 6 months there was significantly less pain and stiffness in the yttrium-90 injected knees with no changes in joint deformity or instability [94]. Edmonds et al. [95] in a trial which included patients with rheumatoid arthritis [51] and knee OA [14] and given either yttrium-90 or dysprosium-165 found no difference in the proportion of patients reporting a subsequent reduction in knee pain on use, pain at rest, or stiffness. Long-term response appeared less good for the OA group compared to the inflammatory group. This impression was confirmed in a retrospective review of patients with both inflammatory and non-inflammatory arthritis treated during 1981–1995 in Wellington, New Zealand, which suggested that patients with OA tended to fare worse than others with only 10% (vs 51%) having improved at 12 months [96].

Platelet-rich plasma

Platelet-rich plasma (PRP) is a concentrate derived from peripheral blood and hypothesized to have anti-inflammatory and analgesic effects. However, qualitative reviews and meta-analyses, while promising, have to date failed to provide conclusive evidence of the efficacy of PRP in part due to methodological limitations of the trials which have been performed [97–100].

Other therapies

Data from several studies suggest intra-articular therapy with autologous or allogenic mesenchymal stem cells is linked with beneficial effects including reduction in pain and improvement in function

in patients with OA without significant adverse effects; however, further studies are needed to confirm these findings [101–105].

In a small trial of 53 patients with knee OA, treatment with polymerized type 1 collagen, given as 12 intra-articular injections over a 6-month period was linked with some improvement in symptoms compared to placebo injections [106].

Oral bisphosphonates have both bone and may also have chondroprotective effects; however, the results of clinical trials with oral bisphosphonates in knee OA have been disappointing. In a randomized trial of 150 men and women with symptomatic knee OA and using different doses of an intra-articular bisphosphonate, clodronate, given up to weekly for 4 weeks or hyaluron there was improvement in pain and function in all treatment groups though no between group differences [107].

Orgotein, the pharmaceutical form of the bovine Cu-Zn superoxide dismutase, has anti-inflammatory effects. A randomized double-blind study of 36 patients with knee OA comparing orgotein injections (8 mg or 16 mg) with intra-articular methylprednisolone (40 mg) injection suggested that those who received higher-dose orgotein had improved pain compared to those who received steroids [108].

Botulinum toxin has been used in the past for its muscle paralysing effects though there is some evidence to support a role in pain modulation. In a pilot study, 60 patients with painful knee OA were randomized to either 40 mg methylprednisolone acetate or one of two doses (100 units/200 units) of botulinum toxin type A. All three groups showed significant improvements in WOMAC scores at 8 weeks though there was no significant between-group difference [109].

Lastly, in a small randomized trial of joint distension (vs placebo) among patients with unilateral hip pain and OA there was no significant difference in outcome between groups [110].

Summary

Intra-articular therapy has significant advantages over oral therapy in the management of OA in that it can provide targeted therapy to individual joint sites and at higher dose than could be achieved through oral administration and with fewer adverse effects. Intra-articular steroid therapy, the most widely used intra-articular therapy, is safe and effective in the short term particularly at the knee; though more studies are needed to better characterize the longer-term benefit. The role of intra-articular hyaluronic acid in clinical management of OA is less clear though it may have a role in selected patients in whom other therapies are contraindicated. Currently there are no factors which have been identified which consistently predict response to intra-articular therapy. Other intra-articular agents have been used in the management of OA, however, because of the limited evidence base relating to efficacy and safety they cannot currently be recommended for use in routine clinical practice.

References

1. Jones A, Regan M, Ledingham J, et al. Importance of placement of intra-articular steroid injections. *BMJ* 1993; 307(6915):1329–30.
2. Chatham W, Williams G, Moreland L, et al. Intraarticular corticosteroid injections: should we rest the joints? *Arthritis Care Res* 1989; 2(2):70–4.
3. Chakravarty K, Pharoah PD, Scott DG. A randomized controlled study of post-injection rest following intra-articular steroid therapy for knee synovitis. *Br J Rheumatol* 1994; 33(5):464–8.

4. Hollander JL, Brown EM, Jr, Jessar RA, Brown CY. Hydrocortisone and cortisone injected into arthritic joints; comparative effects of and use of hydrocortisone as a local antiarthritic agent. *JAMA* 1951; 147(17):1629–35.

5. Hochberg MC, Perlmutter DL, Hudson JI, Altman RD. Preferences in the management of osteoarthritis of the hip and knee: results of a survey of community-based rheumatologists in the United States. *Arthritis Care Res* 1996; 9(3):170–6.

6. Zhang W, Doherty M, Arden N, et al. EULAR evidence based recommendations for the management of hip osteoarthritis: report of a task force of the EULAR Standing Committee for International Clinical Studies Including Therapeutics (ESCISIT). *Ann Rheum Dis* 2005; 64(5):669–81.

7. Zhang W, Moskowitz RW, Nuki G, et al. OARSI recommendations for the management of hip and knee osteoarthritis, part I: critical appraisal of existing treatment guidelines and systematic review of current research evidence. *Osteoarthritis Cartilage* 2007; 15(9):981–1000.

8. Zhang W, Moskowitz RW, Nuki G, et al. OARSI recommendations for the management of hip and knee osteoarthritis, Part II: OARSI evidence-based, expert consensus guidelines. *Osteoarthritis Cartilage* 2008; 16(2):137–62.

9. Zhang Y, Niu J, Felson DT, et al. Methodologic challenges in studying risk factors for progression of knee osteoarthritis. *Arthritis Care Res (Hoboken)* 2010; 62(11):1527–32.

10. Hochberg MC, Altman RD, April KT, et al. American College of Rheumatology 2012 recommendations for the use of nonpharmacologic and pharmacologic therapies in osteoarthritis of the hand, hip, and knee. *Arthritis Care Res (Hoboken)* 2012; 64(4):465–74.

11. McAlindon TE, Bannuru RR, Sullivan MC, et al. OARSI guidelines for the non-surgical management of knee osteoarthritis. *Osteoarthritis Cartilage* 2014; 22(3):363–88.

12. National Institute for Health and Care Excellence. *Osteoarthritis: Care and Management* (Clinical Guideline 177). February 2014. http://www.nice.org.uk/guidance/CG177

13. MacMahon PJ, Eustace SJ, Kavanagh EC. Injectable corticosteroid and local anesthetic preparations: a review for radiologists. *Radiology* 2009; 252(3):647–61.

14. Pyne D, Ioannou Y, Mootoo R, Bhanji A. Intra-articular steroids in knee osteoarthritis: a comparative study of triamcinolone hexacetonide and methylprednisolone acetate. *Clin Rheumatol* 2004; 23(2):116–20.

15. Ayral X, Pickering EH, Woodworth TG, Mackillop N, Dougados M. Synovitis: a potential predictive factor of structural progression of medial tibiofemoral knee osteoarthritis—results of a 1 year longitudinal arthroscopic study in 422 patients. *Osteoarthritis Cartilage* 2005; 13(5):361–7.

16. Roemer FW, Kassim Javaid M, Guermazi A, et al. Anatomical distribution of synovitis in knee osteoarthritis and its association with joint effusion assessed on non-enhanced and contrast-enhanced MRI. *Osteoarthritis Cartilage* 2010; 18(10):1269–74.

17. Loeuille D, Chary-Valckenaere I, Champigneulle J, et al. Macroscopic and microscopic features of synovial membrane inflammation in the osteoarthritic knee: correlating magnetic resonance imaging findings with disease severity. *Arthritis Rheum* 2005; 52(11):3492–501.

18. Hill CL, Gale DG, Chaisson CE, et al. Knee effusions, popliteal cysts, and synovial thickening: association with knee pain in osteoarthritis. *J Rheumatol* 2001; 28(6):1330–7.

19. Hill CL, Hunter DJ, Niu J, et al. Synovitis detected on magnetic resonance imaging and its relation to pain and cartilage loss in knee osteoarthritis. *Ann Rheum Dis* 2007; 66(12):1599–603.

20. Zhang W, McWilliams DF, Ingham SL, et al. Nottingham knee osteoarthritis risk prediction models. *Ann Rheum Dis* 2011; 70(9):1599–604.

21. O'Neill TW, Parkes MJ, Maricar N, et al. Synovial tissue volume: a treatment target in knee osteoarthritis (OA). *Ann Rheum Dis* 2016; 75(1):84–90.

22. Seror P, Pluvinage P, d'Andre FL, Benamou P, Attuil G. Frequency of sepsis after local corticosteroid injection (an inquiry on 1160000

injections in rheumatological private practice in France). *Rheumatology (Oxford)* 1999; 38(12):1272–4.

23. Weston VC, Jones AC, Bradbury N, Fawthrop F, Doherty M. Clinical features and outcome of septic arthritis in a single UK Health District 1982–1991. *Ann Rheum Dis* 1999; 58(4):214–9.

24. Berger RG, Yount WJ. Immediate 'steroid flare' from intraarticular triamcinolone hexacetonide injection: case report and review of the literature. *Arthritis Rheum* 1990; 33(8):1284–6.

25. Gaffney K, Ledingham J, Perry JD. Intra-articular triamcinolone hexacetonide in knee osteoarthritis: factors influencing the clinical response. *Ann Rheum Dis* 1995; 54(5):379–81.

26. Pattrick M, Doherty M. Facial flushing after intra-articular injection of steroid. *Br Med J (Clin Res Ed)* 1987; 295(6610):1380.

27. Habib GS. Systemic effects of intra-articular corticosteroids. *Clin Rheumatol* 2009; 28(7):749–56.

28. Emkey RD, Lindsay R, Lyssy J, et al. The systemic effect of intraarticular administration of corticosteroid on markers of bone formation and bone resorption in patients with rheumatoid arthritis. *Arthritis Rheum* 1996; 39(2):277–82.

29. Karsh J, Yang WH. An anaphylactic reaction to intra-articular triamcinolone: a case report and review of the literature. *Ann Allergy Asthma Immunol* 2003; 90(2):254–8.

30. Mace S, Vadas P, Pruzanski W. Anaphylactic shock induced by intraarticular injection of methylprednisolone acetate. *J Rheumatol* 1997; 24(6):1191–4.

31. Tonkin MA, Stern HS. Spontaneous rupture of the flexor carpi radialis tendon. *J Hand Surg Br* 1991; 16(1):72–4.

32. Gibson T, Burry HC, Poswillo D, Glass J. Effect of intra-articular corticosteroid injections on primate cartilage. *Ann Rheum Dis* 1977; 36(1):74–9.

33. Papacrhistou G, Anagnostou S, Katsorhis T. The effect of intraarticular hydrocortisone injection on the articular cartilage of rabbits. *Acta Orthop Scand Suppl* 1997; 275:132–4.

34. Vandeweerd JM, Zhao Y, Nisolle JF, et al. Effect of corticosteroids on articular cartilage: have animal studies said everything? *Fundam Clin Pharmacol* 2015; 29(5):427–38.

35. Raynauld JP, Buckland-Wright C, Ward R, et al. Safety and efficacy of long-term intraarticular steroid injections in osteoarthritis of the knee: a randomized, double-blind, placebo-controlled trial. *Arthritis Rheum* 2003; 48(2):370–7.

36. Ravi B, Escott BG, Wasserstein D, et al. Intraarticular hip injection and early revision surgery following total hip arthroplasty: a retrospective cohort study. *Arthritis Rheumatol* 2015; 67(1):162–8.

37. Marsland D, Mumith A, Barlow IW. Systematic review: the safety of intra-articular corticosteroid injection prior to total knee arthroplasty. *Knee* 2014; 21(1):6–11.

38. Conway R, O'Shea FD, Cunnane G, Doran MF. Safety of joint and soft tissue injections in patients on warfarin anticoagulation. *Clin Rheumatol* 2013; 32(12):1811–4.

39. Arroll B, Goodyear-Smith F. Corticosteroid injections for osteoarthritis of the knee: meta-analysis. *BMJ* 2004; 328(7444):869.

40. Bellamy N, Campbell J, Robinson V, et al. Intraarticular corticosteroid for treatment of osteoarthritis of the knee. *Cochrane Database Syst Rev* 2006(2):Cd005328.

41. Ravaud P, Moulinier L, Giraudeau B, et al. Effects of joint lavage and steroid injection in patients with osteoarthritis of the knee: results of a multicenter, randomized, controlled trial. *Arthritis Rheum* 1999; 42(3):475–82.

42. Smith MD, Wetherall M, Darby T, et al. A randomized placebo-controlled trial of arthroscopic lavage versus lavage plus intra-articular corticosteroids in the management of symptomatic osteoarthritis of the knee. *Rheumatology (Oxford)* 2003; 42(12):1477–85.

43. Chao J, Wu C, Sun B, et al. Inflammatory characteristics on ultrasound predict poorer longterm response to intraarticular corticosteroid injections in knee osteoarthritis. *J Rheumatol* 2010; 37(3):650–5.

44. Young L, Katrib A, Cuello C, et al. Effects of intraarticular glucocorticoids on macrophage infiltration and mediators of joint damage in

osteoarthritis synovial membranes: findings in a double-blind, placebo-controlled study. *Arthritis Rheum* 2001; 44(2):343–50.

45. Henriksen M, Christensen R, Klokker L, et al. Evaluation of the benefit of corticosteroid injection before exercise therapy in patients with osteoarthritis of the knee: a randomized clinical trial. *JAMA Intern Med* 2015; 175(6):923–30.

46. Valtonen EJ. Clinical comparison of triamcinolonehexacetonide and betamethasone in the treatment of osteoarthrosis of the knee-joint. *Scand J Rheumatol Suppl* 1981; 41:1–7.

47. Maricar N, Parkes MJ, Callaghan MJ, Felson DT, O'Neill TW. Where and how to inject the knee—a systematic review. *Semin Arthritis Rheum* 2013; 43(2):195–203.

48. Maricar N, Callaghan MJ, Felson DT, O'Neill TW. Predictors of response to intra-articular steroid injections in knee osteoarthritis—a systematic review. *Rheumatology (Oxford)* 2013; 52(6):1022–32.

49. Hirsch G, Kitas G, Klocke R. Intra-articular corticosteroid injection in osteoarthritis of the knee and hip: factors predicting pain relief—a systematic review. *Semin Arthritis Rheum* 2013; 42(5):451–73.

50. Jones A, Doherty M. Intra-articular corticosteroids are effective in osteoarthritis but there are no clinical predictors of response. *Ann Rheum Dis* 1996; 55(11):829–32.

51. Pendleton A, Millar A, O'Kane D, Wright GD, Taggart AJ. Can sonography be used to predict the response to intra-articular corticosteroid injection in primary osteoarthritis of the knee? *Scand J Rheumatol* 2008; 37(5):395–7.

52. Arden NK, Reading IC, Jordan KM, et al. A randomised controlled trial of tidal irrigation vs corticosteroid injection in knee osteoarthritis: the KIVIS Study. *Osteoarthritis Cartilage* 2008; 16(6):733–9.

53. Leopold SS, Battista V, Oliverio JA. Safety and efficacy of intraarticular hip injection using anatomic landmarks. *Clin Orthop Relat Res* 2001(391):192–7.

54. Flanagan J, Casale FF, Thomas TL, Desai KB. Intra-articular injection for pain relief in patients awaiting hip replacement. *Ann R Coll Surg Engl* 1988; 70(3):156–7.

55. Kullenberg B, Runesson R, Tuvhag R, Olsson C, Resch S. Intraarticular corticosteroid injection: pain relief in osteoarthritis of the hip? *J Rheumatol* 2004; 31(11):2265–8.

56. Qvistgaard E, Christensen R, Torp-Pedersen S, Bliddal H. Intra-articular treatment of hip osteoarthritis: a randomized trial of hyaluronic acid, corticosteroid, and isotonic saline. *Osteoarthritis Cartilage* 2006; 14(2):163–70.

57. Lambert RG, Hutchings EJ, Grace MG, et al. Steroid injection for osteoarthritis of the hip: a randomized, double-blind, placebo-controlled trial. *Arthritis Rheum* 2007; 56(7):2278–87.

58. Atchia I, Kane D, Reed MR, Isaacs JD, Birrell F. Efficacy of a single ultrasound-guided injection for the treatment of hip osteoarthritis. *Ann Rheum Dis* 2011; 70(1):110–6.

59. Robinson P, Keenan AM, Conaghan PG. Clinical effectiveness and dose response of image-guided intra-articular corticosteroid injection for hip osteoarthritis. *Rheumatology (Oxford)* 2007; 46(2):285–91.

60. Helm AT, Higgins G, Rajkumar P, Redfern DR. Accuracy of intra-articular injections for osteoarthritis of the trapeziometacarpal joint. *Int J Clin Pract* 2003; 57(4):265–6.

61. Meenagh GK, Patton J, Kynes C, Wright GD. A randomised controlled trial of intra-articular corticosteroid injection of the carpometacarpal joint of the thumb in osteoarthritis. *Ann Rheum Dis* 2004; 63(10):1260–3.

62. Stahl S, Karsh-Zafrir I, Ratzon N, Rosenberg N. Comparison of intraarticular injection of depot corticosteroid and hyaluronic acid for treatment of degenerative trapeziometacarpal joints. *J Clin Rheumatol* 2005; 11(6):299–302.

63. Fuchs S, Monikes R, Wohlmeiner A, Heyse T. Intra-articular hyaluronic acid compared with corticoid injections for the treatment of rhizarthrosis. *Osteoarthritis Cartilage* 2006; 14(1):82–8.

64. Heyworth BE, Lee JH, Kim PD, et al. Hylan versus corticosteroid versus placebo for treatment of basal joint arthritis: a prospective, randomized, double-blinded clinical trial. *J Hand Surg* 2008; 33(1):40–8.

65. Eaton RG, Lane LB, Littler JW, Keyser JJ. Ligament reconstruction for the painful thumb carpometacarpal joint: a long-term assessment. *J Hand Surg* 1984; 9(5):692–99.

66. Day CS, Gelberman R, Patel AA, et al. Basal joint osteoarthritis of the thumb: a prospective trial of steroid injection and splinting. *J Hand Surg* 2004; 29(2):247–51.

67. Swindells MG, Logan AJ, Armstrong DJ, et al. The benefit of radiologically-guided steroid injections for trapeziometacarpal osteoarthritis. *Ann R Coll Surg Engl* 2010; 92(8):680–4.

68. Mallinson PI, Tun JK, Farnell RD, Campbell DA, Robinson P. Osteoarthritis of the thumb carpometacarpal joint: correlation of ultrasound appearances to disability and treatment response. *Clin Radiol* 2013; 68(5):461–5.

69. Lilius G, Laasonen EM, Myllynen P, Harilainen A, Gronlund G. Lumbar facet joint syndrome. A randomised clinical trial. *J Bone Joint Surg Br* 1989; 71(4):681–4.

70. Carette S, Marcoux S, Truchon R, et al. A controlled trial of corticosteroid injections into facet joints for chronic low back pain. *N Engl J Med* 1991; 325(14):1002–7.

71. Elmorsy S, Funakoshi T, Sasazawa F, et al. Chondroprotective effects of high-molecular-weight cross-linked hyaluronic acid in a rabbit knee osteoarthritis model. *Osteoarthritis Cartilage* 2014; 22(1):121–7.

72. van den Bekerom MP, Lamme B, Sermon A, Mulier M. What is the evidence for viscosupplementation in the treatment of patients with hip osteoarthritis? Systematic review of the literature. *Arch Orthop Trauma Surg* 2008; 128(8):815–23.

73. Moreland LW. Intra-articular hyaluronan (hyaluronic acid) and hylans for the treatment of osteoarthritis: mechanisms of action. *Arthritis Res Ther* 2003; 5(2):54–67.

74. Kosinska MK, Ludwig TE, Liebisch G, et al. Articular joint lubricants during osteoarthritis and rheumatoid arthritis display altered levels and molecular species. *PLoS One* 2015; 10(5):e0125192.

75. Band PA, Heeter J, Wisniewski HG, et al. Hyaluronan molecular weight distribution is associated with the risk of knee osteoarthritis progression. *Osteoarthritis Cartilage* 2015; 23(1):70–6.

76. Brun P, Zavan B, Vindigni V, et al. In vitro response of osteoarthritic chondrocytes and fibroblast-like synoviocytes to a 500-730 kDa hyaluronan amide derivative. *J Biomed Mater Res B Appl Biomater* 2012; 100(8):2073–81.

77. Karna E, Miltyk W, Surazynski A, Palka JA. Protective effect of hyaluronic acid on interleukin-1-induced deregulation of beta1-integrin and insulin-like growth factor-I receptor signaling and collagen biosynthesis in cultured human chondrocytes. *Mol Cell Biochem* 2008; 308(1–2):57–64.

78. Greenberg DD, Stoker A, Kane S, Cockrell M, Cook JL. Biochemical effects of two different hyaluronic acid products in a co-culture model of osteoarthritis. *Osteoarthritis Cartilage* 2006; 14(8):814–22.

79. Homandberg GA, Ummadi V, Kang H. The role of insulin-like growth factor-I in hyaluronan mediated repair of cultured cartilage explants. *Inflamm Res* 2004; 53(8):396–404.

80. Sasaki A, Sasaki K, Konttinen YT, et al. Hyaluronate inhibits the interleukin-1beta-induced expression of matrix metalloproteinase (MMP)-1 and MMP-3 in human synovial cells. *Tohoku J Exp Med* 2004; 204(2):99–107.

81. Gomis A, Miralles A, Schmidt RF, Belmonte C. Intra-articular injections of hyaluronan solutions of different elastoviscosity reduce nociceptive nerve activity in a model of osteoarthritic knee joint of the guinea pig. *Osteoarthritis Cartilage* 2009; 17(6):798–804.

82. Kirchner M, Marshall D. A double-blind randomized controlled trial comparing alternate forms of high molecular weight hyaluronan for the treatment of osteoarthritis of the knee. *Osteoarthritis Cartilage* 2006; 14(2):154–62.

83. Bannuru RR, Natov NS, Dasi UR, Schmid CH, McAlindon TE. Therapeutic trajectory following intra-articular hyaluronic acid injection in knee osteoarthritis—meta-analysis. *Osteoarthritis Cartilage* 2011; 19(6):611–9.

84. Rutjes AW, Juni P, da Costa BR, et al. Viscosupplementation for osteoarthritis of the knee: a systematic review and meta-analysis. *Ann Intern Med* 2012; 157(3):180–91.

85. Jevsevar DS, Brown GA, Jones DL, et al. The American Academy of Orthopaedic Surgeons evidence-based guideline on: treatment of osteoarthritis of the knee, 2nd edition. *J Bone Joint Surg Am* 2013; 95(20):1885–6.

86. Colen S, Haverkamp D, Mulier M, van den Bekerom MP. Hyaluronic acid for the treatment of osteoarthritis in all joints except the knee: what is the current evidence? *BioDrugs* 2012; 26(2):101–12.

87. Chevalier X, Goupille P, Beaulieu AD, et al. Intraarticular injection of anakinra in osteoarthritis of the knee: a multicenter, randomized, double-blind, placebo-controlled study. *Arthritis Rheum* 2009; 61(3):344–52.

88. Fioravanti A, Fabbroni M, Cerase A, Galeazzi M. Treatment of erosive osteoarthritis of the hands by intra-articular infliximab injections: a pilot study. *Rheumatol Int.* 2009; 29(8):961–5.

89. Creamer P, Hunt M, Dieppe P. Pain mechanisms in osteoarthritis of the knee: effect of intraarticular anesthetic. *J Rheumatol* 1996; 23(6):1031–6.

90. Likar R, Schafer M, Paulak F, et al. Intraarticular morphine analgesia in chronic pain patients with osteoarthritis. *Anesth Analg* 1997; 84(6):1313–7.

91. Gazi MB, Sakata RK, Issy AM. Intra-articular morphine versus bupivacaine for knee motion among patients with osteoarthritis: randomized double-blind clinical trial. *Sao Paulo Med J* 2008; 126(6):309–13.

92. Moens B, Moens CH. Intra-articular injection of phenylbutazone in gonarthrosis. *Ann Rheum Dis* 1986; 45(9):788.

93. Oztuna V, Eskandari M, Bugdayci R, Kuyurtar F. Intra-articular injection of tenoxicam in osteoarthritic knee joints with effusion. *Orthopedics* 2007; 30(12):1039–42.

94. Doherty M, Dieppe PA. Effect of intra-articular yttrium-90 on chronic pyrophosphate arthropathy of the knee. *Lancet* 1981; 2(8258):1243–6.

95. Edmonds J, Smart R, Laurent R, et al. A comparative study of the safety and efficacy of dysprosium-165 hydroxide macro-aggregate and yttrium-90 silicate colloid in radiation synovectomy—a multicentre double blind clinical trial. Australian Dysprosium Trial Group. *Br J Rheumatol* 1994; 33(10):947–53.

96. Taylor WJ, Corkhill MM, Rajapaske C. A retrospective review of yttrium-90 synovectomy in the treatment of knee arthritis. *Br J Rheumatol* 1997; 36:1100–5.

97. Hsu WK, Mishra A, Rodeo SR, et al. Platelet-rich plasma in orthopaedic applications: evidence-based recommendations for treatment. *J Am Acad Orthop Surg* 2013; 21(12):739–48.

98. Khoshbin A, Leroux T, Wasserstein D, et al. The efficacy of platelet-rich plasma in the treatment of symptomatic knee osteoarthritis: a systematic review with quantitative synthesis. *Arthroscopy* 2013; 29(12):2037–48.

99. Chang KV, Hung CY, Aliwarga F, et al. Comparative effectiveness of platelet-rich plasma injections for treating knee joint cartilage degenerative pathology: a systematic review and meta-analysis. *Arch Phys Med Rehabil* 2014; 95(3):562–75.

100. Laudy AB, Bakker EW, Rekers M, Moen M. Efficacy of platelet rich plasma injections in osteoarthritis of the knee: a systematic review. *Br J Sports Med* 2015; 49:657–72.

101. Centeno CJ, Schultz JR, Cheever M, et al. Safety and complications reporting update on the re-implantation of culture-expanded mesenchymal stem cells using autologous platelet lysate technique. *Curr Stem Cell Res Ther* 2011; 6(4):368–78.

102. Jo CH, Lee YG, Shin WH, et al. Intra-articular injection of mesenchymal stem cells for the treatment of osteoarthritis of the knee: a proof-of-concept clinical trial. *Stem Cells (Dayton, Ohio)* 2014; 32(5):1254–66.

103. Rodriguez-Merchan EC. Intra-articular injections of mesenchymal stem cells for knee osteoarthritis. *Am J Orthop (Belle Mead, NJ)* 2014; 43(12):E282–91.

104. Emadedin M, Ghorbani Liastani M, Fazeli R, et al. Long-term follow-up of intra-articular injection of autologous mesenchymal stem cells in patients with knee, ankle, or hip osteoarthritis. *Arch Iran Med* 2015; 18(6):336–44.

105. Vega A, Martin-Ferrero MA, Del Canto F, et al. Treatment of knee osteoarthritis with allogeneic bone marrow mesenchymal stem cells: a randomized controlled trial. *Transplantation* 2015; 99(8):1681–90.

106. Furuzawa-Carballeda J, Munoz-Chable OA, Macias-Hernandez SI, Agualimpia-Janning A. Effect of polymerized-type I collagen in knee osteoarthritis. II. In vivo study. *Eur J Clin Invest* 2009; 39(7):598–606.

107. Rossini M, Viapiana O, Ramonda R, et al. Intra-articular clodronate for the treatment of knee osteoarthritis: dose ranging study vs hyaluronic acid. *Rheumatology (Oxford)* 2009; 48(7):773–8.

108. Gammer W, Broback LG. Clinical comparison of orgotein and methylprednisolone acetate in the treatment of osteoarthrosis of the knee joint. *Scand J Rheumatol* 1984; 13(2):108–12.

109. Boon AJ, Smith J, Dahm DL, et al. Efficacy of intra-articular botulinum toxin type A in painful knee osteoarthritis: a pilot study. *PM R* 2010; 2(4):268–76.

110. Hoilund-Carlsen PF, Meinicke J, Christiansen B, et al. Joint distension arthrography for disabling hip pain. A controlled clinical trial. *Scand J Rheumatol* 1985; 14(2):179–83.

SECTION 9

Surgery

CHAPTER 33

Arthroplasty and its complications

Andrew Price, Paul Monk, and David Beard

Introduction

Hip and knee replacement surgery is one of the most commonly performed orthopaedic procedures in the world. Within the United States approximately 1 000 000 arthroplasty surgeries are performed a year [1]. Within the United Kingdom around 200 000 hip and knee replacements are performed annually [2]. There is considerable evidence to show the clinical and cost-effectiveness of these interventions. Many patients will get very effective relief of the pain and immobility resulting in a general improvement in the quality of life. However, there can be complications from the surgery and approximately 10–15% of patients may not do well after joint replacement. This chapter outlines the key points of arthroplasty practice including indications for surgery, the type of surgery performed, and review of the benefits and risks of the procedure.

Who should be treated by arthroplasty?

Osteoarthritis of the synovial joints is a common and disabling condition that creates a very large global healthcare problem [3]. Its incidence is age related and patients present with pain, poor mobility and a decrease in their quality of life. When pain becomes severe and resistant to non-operative measures then joint replacement should be considered. The decision to undergo hip or knee replacement is based around balancing the potential advantages and disadvantages of undergoing the treatment [4]. The treatments have a large effect size with approximately 90% of patients recognizing improvement in their symptoms, some undergoing very dramatic improvement. However, for the remaining 10% of patients symptoms do not improve. This means that before proceeding to surgery patients must have an accurate expectation of the potential outcome and an understanding that in up to 1% of patients medical complications can occur. Attempts have been made to identify the optimum time for patients with arthritis to undergo hip and knee replacement, but this still remains unclear [5]. Balancing these issues is a complicated process and recent developments in decision support have attempted to aid the process. Such developments help to obtain a well-informed shared decision made by both clinician and patient together.

Hip and knee replacement epidemiology

Arthroplasty is the standard treatment for end-stage osteoarthritis when conservative measures have failed. Using large datasets it has been established that the lifetime risk of requiring hip or knee replacement is approximately 10% [6]. Data from joint registries demonstrate increasing demand for these procedures. In 2004, Dixon et al. reviewed the United Kingdom Department of Health statistics between 1991 and 2000 for primary and revision total knee replacement (TKR) and total hip replacement (THR) [7]. The research showed that the incidence of primary TKR doubled, with revision TKR increasing by 300%; primary THR increased by 18% whilst revision THR doubled. Based on these trends, the authors predicted a 63% rise in TKR to 54 000 primary TKR procedures and 47 000 primary THR by 2010. There has been a progressive increase in the numbers of primary TKR operations performed between 2005 and 2010, increasing from 62 217 cases to 79 263 cases, showing earlier predictions of 54 000 procedures to be conservative [2]. The Swedish Knee Arthroplasty Register (SKAR) initiated in 1975 has 100% compliance by all Swedish institutions performing arthroplasty, and shows a similar trend to the United Kingdom data. Most notable are the statistics regarding younger patients [8]. In Sweden, knee surgery for osteoarthritis in patients less than 55 years of age has doubled during the past 10 years, with the use of TKR increasing significantly. This trend is predicted to continue to increase in the future, with recent studies predicting the demand for primary TKR to increase by more than 670% by 2030 in the United States alone, with the revision rate predicted to increase by 600% [1,9]. In comparison, the projected demand for primary THR is less acute, reflecting more closely the predicted change in demographics over time. Primary hip replacement is predicted to rise 174% by 2030 in line with ageing trends.

History

The earliest recorded attempts of hip replacement are from Professor Gluck in Germany in 1891, using ivory in tuberculosis patients. At a similar time, Pierre Delbet (1861–1925) at La Fert´e Gaucher, Departement Seine-et-Marne, France was the first to use a rubber femoral prosthesis to replace one-half of the hip joint in 1919. Simultaneously, the American surgeon Marius Smith-Peterson created a smooth, glass, biocompatible acetabular socket which failed to withstand the compressive forces across the hip joint and later shattered. Ernest W. Hey-Groves (1872–1944) used ivory in the same manner in 1927, but later described what, in his opinion, was a preferable method to treat hip arthritis.

The first attempt at replacing both sides of the joint (THR) was made in 1938 by Philip Wiles with Smith-Peterson (1899–1966) at the Middlesex Hospital in London, United Kingdom, using precisely fitted stainless steel components which were fixed to the bone with screws and bolts. The Judet brothers (Robert and Jean) in 1948 used an acrylic femoral prosthesis again to replace one-half of the hip joint which was exceptionally susceptible to wear. This design was refined upon by Frederick Reck Thompson (1907–1983) and Harold R. Bohlman (1893–1979) with Austin Moore (1899–1963). Both the Thompson and Bohlman–Moore prostheses went on to be the first hip arthroplasty products that were widely distributed and were until recently still widely used for replacement of the femoral head and neck following intracapsular femoral neck fractures in the elderly. Kenneth McKee (1905–1991) experimented with dental acrylic cement for fixation in the late 1940s and later used the Thompson prosthesis on the femoral side that articulated with a three claw-type cup that was screwed into the acetabulum. Peter Ring (b. 1922), in 1964 using cementless components with a metal-on-metal articulation achieved good results. Both the McKee–Farrar and the Ring models were abandoned in the 1970s due to unfavourable local effects of metal particles seen at revision.

In the early 1960s, Sir John Charnley (1911–1982) from Manchester, United Kingdom, pioneered a low-friction arthroplasty cemented total hip joint replacement which remains similar in principle to many prostheses available today [10]. The technique combines a high-density polyethylene cup with a metal stem, held in place with polymethylmethacrylate bone cement. The use of a small femoral head size is believed to reduce wear due to low surface area creating a low friction environment.

Professor Gluck is again credited with the implantation of the earliest total knee joint replacement in 1890. The ivory, hinged design failed due to high infection rate and inadequate fixation. Until the early 1970s, the Waldius hinge was popularized, first manufactured from acrylic, followed by cobalt chrome. Similar European designs of the hinged knee prosthesis were evident around this time, but due to the extreme constraint applied to the joint, they were coupled with the emergence of the early condylar knee designs. The Freeman Swanson/ICLH invention provided a landmark design with a single radius femoral component and a 'roller in trough' articulation of the tibia. Goodfellow and O'Connor introduced the idea that prosthesis design should use articular surfaces and retention of ligament function that allowed freedom for the knee to move whilst remaining stable [11]. They introduced the concept of a mobile bearing design. A landmark change occurred with the development of the IB-2 total-condylar knee replacement by Insall, where the bony surfaces of the knee are replaced with metal shaped more anatomically and the stability of the reconstruction relying on the collateral ligaments of the knee [12]. Insertion of the femoral component required removal of the cruciate ligaments, followed by medial and lateral collateral ligament balancing, a technique that has remained largely unchanged to this day.

General principles of modern use

Fixation of prostheses

All hip and knee prostheses are implanted into bony surfaces and implant fixation can be broadly classified into those that are *cemented* using polymethylmethacrylate (PMMA), and those employing *cementless* fixation [13]. Cement fixation is achieved with a micro-interlock with endosteal bone. PMMA bone cement has excellent tissue compatibility and was first introduced into

clinical surgery in the 1940s to close gaps in the scalp. Modern bone cements are provided as two component materials: powder (prepolymerized PMMA, an initiator, and a radio-opacifier) and liquid (containing methylmethacrylate monomer, stabilization, and an inhibitor). When mixed together, the two components undergo free radical polymerization forming bone cement. Over approximately 10 minutes, bone cement viscosity increases from a runny liquid to a solid material. During this setting time the cement is inserted under pressure into the introductory canal, and the prosthetic device inserted.

Contemporary cementing techniques have evolved in response to early failures. Cement will fatigue under cyclical loading and failure has been shown to start at stress points within the cement mantle. Any defects in the cement mantle where the prosthesis touches bone create an area of significant stress concentration which can rapidly lead to loosening, failure of fixation, and consequent revision. Current fourth-generation cementing techniques include vacuum mixing to reduce cement porosity, pressurization to enhance into interdigitization with bone, pulsed lavage to provide clean, dry bone, and in hip replacement stem centralization to promote a uniform cement mantle.

Cementless fixation involves bone growth into the prosthesis to secure the implant. This can be achieved using porous coating, where the prosthesis surface is fabricated with tiny pores (50–150 micrometres) incorporated into the metal alloy provides bone *in-growth* whilst hydroxy-appetite coating provides bone *on-growth*. Successful biological fixation of uncemented prostheses is influenced by both manufacturing tolerances and implantation considerations. Optimal porosity (40–50%), pore size, and depth, are all directly related to fixation strength. Surgical factors that enhance fixation include ensuring there is cortical contact with bone at implantation. This enables internal rigid fixation to exclude minimal implant micromotion. Furthermore, cortical contact with allows load transfer to the weight-bearing regions of bone. This is the theoretical foundation of the *line-to-line* and *press fit* techniques, the latter requiring the bone to be prepared to receive a slightly oversized implant.

Computer-assisted radiostereometric analysis (RSA) of tibial component migration can detect very small changes in the prosthetic position over time [14]. Recent literature suggests that most implants migrate for up to 1 year after insertion, but then stabilize. Cases that were eventually revised for loosening all belonged to the continuously migrating group. Thus, the loosening process was gradual and started shortly after implantation. The pattern was the same, whether the interface material was bone cement, polyethylene, or metal. Of note, less migration was seen when a water-cooled saw-blade was used to cut bone, and following optimal alignment of the leg.

RSA has also been used to record the inducible displacement of the tibial component when the replaced knee is physiologically loaded. The observed micromotion occurs at a level that inhibits bone ingrowth in porous surfaces. However, stems and screws have a stabilizing effect, which reduces interfacial motion.

RSA indicates that the early findings govern the final outcome of the arthroplasty, influenced by prosthetic design, surgical technique, fixation and position of implants, alignment, and bone quality. The interface in stable implants has been shown to be mainly dense fibrocartilage. Unstable implants have a softer, fibrous tissue encapsulation permeable to polyethylene wear particles. These, and other wear particles, induce an inflammatory reaction capable of inducing bone resorption (osteolysis), making failure more likely.

Bearing surfaces of hip and knee prostheses

To allow joint movement, all hip and knee replacements have a bearing surface. Tribology is the science and engineering of interacting surfaces and involves the application of friction, lubrication, and wear principles. The definitive choice of bearing couple is based on patient factors, wear properties of the material, and manufacturing techniques. Both hard (metals and ceramics) and soft (polyethylene) bearings are available and can be used either together or in combination [15]. The classical combination is for a metal stem (stainless steel/cobalt–chromium–molybdenum) to be used with a high-molecular-weight polyethylene (HMWPE) acetabular component, a *hard-on-soft* bearing. The rate of wear of the bearing couple is related to surface roughness of the head (carbide asperities can cause scratching), the sphericity of the head, and the quality of manufacture, sterilization, and irradiation of the polyethylene. Whilst a hard-on-hard bearing combination has benefits in terms of its wear profile, the metal-on-metal and ceramic-on-ceramic options are not without problems. Metal wear is characterized by very small particles (0.015 micrometres). Whilst the volumetric wear is minimal the absolute number of particles generated is significantly greater than for metal–polyethylene bearings. The particles have an ability to generate metal ions which can be detected in the urine and blood. Similarly, metal debris has been associated with T-cell lymphocyte hypersensitivity reactions and pseudotumour or aseptic lymphocyte-dominated vasculitis-associated lesion formation. The ceramic–ceramic pairing couple has the lowest wear profile with bioinert debris, but is restricted in terms of the head size allowed, and is prone to squeaking and fracture of the material due to its low toughness.

Contemporary hip arthroplasty

Modern THR has not changed in principle from the Charnley concept. The implants combine an acetabular (cup) component and a femoral component (stem). The stem component is designed to incorporate a head, on the neck of the stem, which can be of variable head size. The choice of head size is determined by the requirements for the patient and the interaction of stability and range of motion, with increasing use of a larger head seen over the last 10 years. The metal components are commonly made of steel, cobalt chrome alloy, or titanium (acetabular side). The final reconstruction attempts to recreate the normal biomechanics of the joint by restoring the correct hip offset and leg length. Resurfacing hip arthroplasty, using a metal cap on the femoral head (no stem) and an acetabular cup, did enjoy increasing popularity over the last 10 years but has subsequently declined in use due to problems related to the bearing surface.

There are many different types of THR used in modern practice [16]. The United Kingdom National Joint Registry data reveals that over 140 different brands are available. In terms of fixation, cementless fixation predominates at 43%, all cemented THA at 33%, and hybrid fixation at 20%. In the United States, the majority of implantations performed are with cementless prostheses. However, in Scandinavian registries, the usual procedure is a cemented THR using modern cementing techniques including a cement-restricting plug, lavage, cleaning of the bone bed, and cement pressurization

of vacuum-mixed cement with a gun. The technique has become standard practice and does improve revision rate, according to the Swedish Total Hip Arthroplasty Register [17]. Head sizes used on the whole vary between 22 and 28 mm diameter in the majority of cases. Metal-on-polyethylene remains the most popular bearing choice, although ceramic on ceramic is a popular choice in the younger patient.

Contemporary knee arthroplasty

The majority of contemporary knee replacement designs maintain the use of the total condylar design [8], in effect, a resurfacing of the femur and tibia largely recreating anatomical shapes of the native knee, using cobalt–chrome metal alloy as the primary material. The patellar can be resurfaced with a polyethylene insert but debate remains as to the need for this part of the procedure and many surgeons choose not to do this. The goals of total knee arthroplasty (TKA) are to restore the neutral mechanical alignment of the limb, to restore the joint line, and to balance the ligaments and patella tracking. Intraoperative resection of the distal femur and proximal tibia are guided by preoperative analysis of radiographs (full-length standing bilateral anteroposterior knee, flexion and extension lateral and patella views). A range of instrumentation is available to the surgeon and includes intra- and extramedullary guides to aid measured resection. Coronal (mediolateral) plane balancing, when necessary, is performed by sequential release of soft tissue structures as required. Optimum survival following TKA has been shown in older patients (70 years or older), rheumatoid arthritis patients, and when using cemented fixation.

Generalized osteoarthritis can be treated with tri-compartmental TKA [18]. TKA designs can be described relative to the level of mechanical constraint they provide to the knee joint. The highest constraint is provided by a hinged knee joint, which is largely reserved for complex primary (e.g. massive infection, after complex fracture, or following resection of pathological lesion within the knee joint) and complex revision procedures. The vast majority of primary TKA is performed using the least constraint, employing designs that either retain (cruciate retaining) or require excision ('cruciate sacrificing') of the posterior cruciate ligament (PCL). The PCL helps regulate flexion stability by influencing femoral rollback, defined as the progressive change in the tibia femoral contact point throughout flexion. In cruciate-sacrificing TKA designs, a spine and cam mechanism control rollback. A cam on the femoral component engages a vertical tibial post during flexion. In general, cruciate-retaining tibial designs are flatter to accommodate rollback. A rotating (tibial) platform knee is thought to provide intermediate constraint by allowing better articular conformity throughout the entire knee range. However, equivalent survivorship has been shown when compared to the fixed-bearing knee designs.

Single compartment arthritis of the knee can be treated with partial or uni-compartmental knee arthroplasty. First described by MacIntosh (1954) and McKeever (1960) for the medial and lateral compartments, these designs are in widespread use today. Most designs incorporate a metal femoral component (either polycentric or spherical in design) and a polyethylene bearing (fixed or mobile). In comparison to contemporary TKA surgery, more non diseased native structures are preserved and the postoperative rehabilitation is more rapid. Furthermore, there appears to be a more physiological postoperative gait and an improved range of movement. Isolated patellofemoral joint osteoarthritis can also be treated with partial knee replacement; however, patellofemoral joint arthroplasty is not performed in very large numbers and its role in treating knee arthritis is still evolving.

Contemporary knee arthroplasty practice shows that most implantations are performed as cemented total condylar knee replacements, with very few cementless prostheses used. A much smaller number of partial implants are used as demonstrated in the National Joint Registry in the United Kingdom where 91% of TKAs are cemented, 8% being unicompartmental replacement (medial or lateral) and 1% isolated patellofemoral joint replacement [2].

Development of methods to implant joint replacements

The surgical approach used when implanting joint replacements is an important contributing factor to the procedure and the final outcome. The approach is adapted to the requirements of the planned procedure but must give adequate exposure to allow the surgeon to perform the implantation. In recent years, a drive to perform minimally invasive incisions has been observed based around reducing morbidity for patients and increasing their ability to mobilize quickly after surgery.

For the hip, the anterolateral and posterior approaches are the most widely used. The posterior approach is associated with a higher revision rate but better functional recovery compared to the anterolateral approach. In more recent years, the direct anterior approach has become more popular, particularly in association with a minimally invasive approach.

In the knee, the midline approach is the most widely used skin incision with a medial approach though the joint capsule running alongside the patella and quadriceps tendons. A number of modifications of this technique have been developed including the sub-vastus and mid-vastus approaches to preserve the quadriceps tendon. Minimally invasive approaches have been adopted particularly for unicompartmental knee replacement.

Successful outcome of both hip and knee arthroplasty is dependent on correct alignment of prosthetic components at implantation and malalignment of the components, in any anatomical plane, can cause major complications. As a result, significant advances have been made in the development of instruments to implant prostheses in an accurate manner. For the hip, this involves making sure the orientation of the acetabular component (cup) is precisely placed in relation to the bony acetabulum, that the alignment of the femoral component follows the line of the femur and the reconstruction does not lengthen the leg. In the knee, instruments allow the predetermined position of femoral and tibial components to be achieved, producing in most cases a limb with neutral mechanical alignment, as the weight-bearing axis of the leg passes from the head of the femur though the centre of the knee to the ankle.

A number of different systems have been developed to assist the precision of implantation. Computer navigation systems for use in joint arthroplasty involve the combination of markers attached to the bony skeleton and a motion capture system. Alternatively, patient-specific instrumentation (PSI) jigs can be prepared from a surgical reconstruction plan created from preoperative imaging. The PSI jigs are then used in theatre to guide the bony cuts that determine the component position. Robots have also been developed to assist implantation, being employed to create very accurate bony cuts based on a preoperative plan. The current literature offers some evidence that these technologies may prevent major errors in implantation (outliers) but it remains to be seen if their use, if widely adopted, will improve outcome for patients in the longer term.

Development of enhanced recovery for patients

One of the most important aspects of arthroplasty care is the perioperative management of the patient. This includes the preoperative assessment of patients, the intraoperative management, and the postoperative treatment of patients as they recover from surgery [19].

Preoperative assessment is used to identify if a patient's health can be optimized prior to surgery to reduce risk of complications (e.g. identifying treatable high blood pressure that may predispose a patient to postoperative stroke). In some patients, a detailed assessment of the risk of morbidity or mortality after surgery may be pivotal in the shared decision to go ahead with surgery or not.

The intraoperative management of each patient centres on the anaesthetic techniques employed. Significant advances have been made over the last 20 years in this area with the use of general or spinal anaesthesia being the mainstay of care. These are augmented by local anaesthetic blocks and the use of multimodal medication to reduce intraoperative and immediate postoperative pain. Surgical techniques have also advanced to decrease the risk of bleeding and the requirement for postoperative blood transfusion. Pharmacological and physical treatments have been developed to reduce the risk of thrombosis. Routine use of intraoperative intravenous antibiotics and the introduction of clean air laminar flow operating theatres have reduced the incidence of infection.

In the postoperative phase of treatment, advances have been made in the pain relief techniques, which allows for early mobilization of patients after surgery. A multidisciplinary approach involving nursing staff, physiotherapists, occupational therapists, and the surgical team is now commonplace.

Over the last 10 years, the optimization of all three phases of the patient's perioperative care has led to the development of enhanced recovery protocols to reduce variation in practice and deliver evidence-based rehabilitation. This has brought about a significant reduction in the time spent in hospital by patients after surgery and is likely to improve morbidity and even mortality rates after arthroplasty surgery.

Complications and outcome after hip and knee arthroplasty

The outcome of joint replacement for an individual patient can be assessed in a number of different ways; the occurrence of serious medical complications including death, intraoperative surgical complications, the requirement for early reoperation, the rate of deep infection, the rate of failure of the replacement leading to revision, and the restoration of a patient's quality of life through reduction of pain and improved mobility.

Analysis of population data reveals that death (within 90 days) after hip or knee replacement occurs in approximately 1 in 200 patients [20]. The risk is higher in patients with greater preoperative co-morbidity and higher American Society of Anesthesiologists (ASA) grade.

Subclinical lower limb thrombosis is very common after hip and knee surgery. With the use of modern antithrombotic treatment, the risk of major lower limb thrombosis requiring treatment is 2.7%, with a smaller proportion of patients suffering pulmonary embolism which is fatal in 0.02% of cases [21,22].

Intraoperative complications do occur at a low rate. Significant intraoperative haemorrhage with damage to large arteries and periprosthetic fracture during implantation can occur but are rare occurrences, especially with contemporary surgical techniques. They are best treated with early recognition and appropriate immediate vascular control/reconstruction and bony stabilization.

Reoperation within the first 12 months following surgery can be required following a number of different complications. Significant haematoma with or without wound breakdown may require washing out and re-suturing. Following hip replacement, early dislocation requiring a closed or open reduction of the prosthesis occurs at a rate of 1–2% [2]. After TKR some patients do not regain an adequate range of motion and a manipulation under general anaesthetic is required in an attempt to improve movement.

Infection is one of the most serious and difficult complications of prosthetic joint infection that required reoperation. The rate of infection in large data series is approximately 1% [23]. It can occur in the early postoperative phase (within 6 weeks) due to contamination during the primary surgery or much later secondary to seeding of infection from other sites in the body (e.g. a tooth abscess). Treatment depends on whether the implant remains well fixed or is loose and deemed to have failed. In the first case, open surgical debridement of the joint, retention of implants, and antibiotic therapy can be an effective treatment that salvages the patient's joint replacement. However, if this fails to control the infection or the components are loose then revision of the prosthesis will be required. This involves removal of the primary implant and implantation of a second new revision joint replacement. The surgery is completed in one or two stages and debate remains as to the most effective mode of treatment. In the two-stage strategy a gap of 3–4 months occurs after primary implant removal before the second stage implantation with revision prosthesis is performed. In some cases the infection is not controlled after surgery and recurrence occurs. Salvage surgery may save the limb with implantation of an endoprosthesis but in a minority of cases amputation is required.

Failure of a prosthesis requiring revision surgery is one of the most widely used measures of the outcome of joint arthroplasty [2]. The most common reason for revision is loosening of prostheses secondary to polyethylene wear and subsequent loosening of the components. This mode of failure is often associated with significant osteolysis (loss of bone). The revision procedure usually requires implantation of a stemmed prosthesis with augmentation to replace lost bone stock. Revision for instability is sometimes required where the bony and ligamentous structures around a joint replacement may fail to provide adequate support. In the hip, this usually manifests itself as dislocation and revision to a more constrained device may be required. In knee replacement, a true dislocation of the joint is rare but patients develop a progressive instability of the joint and, as with the hip, revision to a more constrained device may be required. In a small number of cases, mal-positioning of prostheses at the primary surgery may result in early failure and revision.

Over the last 20 years, a number of National Joint Registries have offered great insight into the true rate of revision in large populations of patients [2]. They calculate survival rates of different prostheses using survival analysis with revision as a very hard endpoint. For total hip and knee replacement, 95% survival at 10 years post implantation is normally achieved. For most patients over the age of 70 years revision of their primary implantation revision will not be required in their remaining lifetime. Unfortunately much higher rates of revision are seen in the patients under the age of 60.

Over the last 10 years there has been increasing focus on the outcome of arthroplasty as reported by patients themselves. Patient-reported outcome measures (PROMs) are now widely used to determine the success of the intervention in restoring a patient's quality of life. This is achieved by reduction in their pain and restoration of their functional ability. The United Kingdom has been at the forefront of PROM development and use in joint replacement surgery, where collection of the Oxford Hip or Knee score has been mandatory for the last 8 years [24,25]. Following knee replacement this resource has identified that approximately 85% of patients have a very good outcome after surgery, with the treatment registering a very high effect size. However, 15% of patients still have pain after surgery with some patients reporting no improvement or a worsening of pain [26]. Many of these patients are dissatisfied with their final outcome. A similar pattern is seen after THR but a higher proportion of patients achieve a good outcome (approximately 90%).

The collection of large data sets of PROMs of patients undergoing hip and knee replacement has also facilitated the calculation of the cost-effectiveness of the procedure. Numerous studies have now identified both hip and knee replacement as one of the most cost-effective surgical interventions performed.

Future developments in hip and knee replacement

The application of new technology drives the continued efforts to develop and improve all aspects of joint replacement [18]. Implant design remains a major focus for development including the use of novel new materials and nanotechnology to improve fixation and reduce infection. Attempts continue to develop better bearing surfaces to reduce failure due to wear and loosening. In the knee, implants that preserve rather than sacrifice ligaments are being developed and may improve patient outcome. In the hip, novel designs of femoral stem that preserve normal bone are being assessed. In parallel with these developments a greater emphasis is being placed on developing the regulatory framework that surrounds the introduction of new implants to protect patients. This new approach is driven by the need to identify early and new modes of joint failure with new devices, as seen with the widespread use and then failure of metal-on-metal hip replacement.

Major advances have been made in the methods for reproducibly implanting both hip and knee prostheses. The influence of the surgical approach to the joint has been recognized and the sophistication of instruments used for implanting devices will continue to be improved. The use of computer-assisted methods and robotic surgery are likely to become more commonly used [27].

Increasingly, similar technology is being used to help train surgeons in joint replacement techniques. The development of virtual reality technology to assist in training is a very exciting new use of technology.

The perioperative management of patients is also advancing with new methods employed to reduce complications and enhance recovery after surgery. Day-case hip and knee replacement can now be safely performed in a subset of patients and overall length of hospital stay for joint replacement has been reduced.

The advances in prostheses design and implantation methods have also driven the need to gain a better understanding of the outcome of surgery. New outcome measures and novel ways to collect data, such as mobile phone applications, are being developed and tested. The importance of following long-term outcome is also increasingly recognized and has driven the increasing importance of National Joint Registries to track outcome.

Arthroplasty in other joints of the body

Arthroplasty in the other joints of the body are performed but not as commonly as hip and knee replacement. However, the same considerations occur in terms of design, materials, bearing surfaces, fixation, and implantation methods.

Shoulder replacement has been performed for over 20 years, albeit in relatively small numbers. The surgery is performed for patients with either inflammatory joint disease or osteoarthritis of the shoulder [28]. The critical importance of preserving the rotator cuff muscles in achieving good functional outcome has been recognized. The major design issue in this area has been whether hemiarthroplasty or total joint replacement is most effective, and both types are still widely used.

Elbow replacement has been more commonly used to treat patients with end-stage inflammatory arthropathy. The first elbow replacements employed a constrained hinge type of prostheses but this predetermines a significant failure rate due to prosthesis loosening. The second generation of elbow replacement designs introduced a constrained surface replacement, such as the Kudo [29]. As with shoulder replacement, very good pain relief can be achieved with this surgery, but functional outcome can be more limited.

Ankle replacement has only really been used in significant numbers over the last 10 years, although designs have been around for much longer [30]. Ankle fusion is the operation of choice for many patients with ankle arthritis with successful outcomes. However, the indications for ankle replacement have grown with increasing confidence in the design of implants available. Where patients have arthrosis of the ankle, without deformity, instability, or neuropathic disorder, an ankle joint replacement can be considered.

Key points

- Joint replacement is most commonly performed for patients who have end-stage osteoarthritis of the large joints, with smaller numbers of patients undergoing surgery for inflammatory conditions.

- Throughout the world several million joint replacement procedures are undertaken each year, with hip and knee arthroplasty most commonly performed.

- THR remains the commonest method for replacing the hip joint, with both cementless and cemented types used widely.

- Cemented TKR remains the commonest type of arthroplasty operation performed in the knee, with partial or unicompartmental implants used in approximately 10% of cases.

- Technological advances are being made in all aspects of joint replacement including bearing surfaces, fixation methods, implant designs, and implantation methods.

- Modern joint replacement practice puts greater emphasis on the optimization of the perioperative treatment of patients, as evidenced by the development of Enhanced Recovery Programmes.

- The rate of postoperative complication following joint replacement has reduced over the last 20 years but acute medical problems (including myocardial infarction, stroke, and pulmonary embolus) and infection still occur in up to 1% of patients.

- Revision of joint replacement may be required if the prosthesis fails, with the commonest causes of failure being implant loosening with polyethylene wear, infection, implant instability, periprosthetic fracture, and increasing pain in the replaced joint.

- The use of PROMs has given a new level of insight into the outcome of joint replacement, demonstrating a very large positive treatment effect for approximately 85% of patients but highlighting that 15% of patient do less well and can be dissatisfied with the outcome of surgery.

- Joint replacement remains one of the most cost-effective surgical interventions that has ever been performed.

References

1. Kurtz S, Ong K, Lau E, Mowat F, Halpern M. Projections of primary and revision hip and knee arthroplasty in the United States from 2005 to 2030. *J Bone Joint Surg Am* 2007; 89(4):780–5.
2. National Joint Registry. *12th Annual Report of the UK NJR*. 2015. http://www.njrcentre.org.uk/njrcentre/Reports,PublicationsandMinutes/Annualreports/tabid/86/Default.aspx
3. Cross M, Smith E, Hoy D, et al. The global burden of hip and knee osteoarthritis: estimates from the global burden of disease 2010 study. *Ann Rheum Dis* 2014; 73(7):1323–30.
4. Dieppe P, Lim K, Lohmander S. Who should have knee joint replacement surgery for osteoarthritis? *Int J Rheum Dis* 2011; 14(2):175–80.
5. Riddle DL, Jiranek WA, Hayes CW. Use of a validated algorithm to judge the appropriateness of total knee arthroplasty in the United States: a multicenter longitudinal cohort study. *Arthritis Rheumatol* 2014; 66(8):2134–43.
6. Mukherjee S, Culliford D, Arden N, Edwards C. What is the risk of having a total hip or knee replacement for patients with lupus? *Lupus* 2015; 24(2):198–202.
7. Dixon T, Shaw M, Ebrahim S, Dieppe P. Trends in hip and knee joint replacement: socioeconomic inequalities and projections of need. *Ann Rheum Dis* 2004; 63(7):825–30.
8. Nemes S, Rolfson O, W-Dahl A, et al. Historical view and future demand for knee arthroplasty in Sweden. *Acta Orthop* 2015; 86(4):426–31.
9. Culliford D, Maskell J, Judge A, et al. Future projections of total hip and knee arthroplasty in the UK: results from the UK Clinical Practice Research Datalink. *Osteoarthritis Cartilage* 2015; 23(4):594–600.
10. Wroblewski BM, Siney PD, Fleming PA. Charnley low-frictional torque arthroplasty: follow-up for 30 to 40 years. *J Bone Joint Surg Br* 2009; 91(4):447–50.

11. O'Connor JJ, Goodfellow JW. Theory and practice of meniscal knee replacement: designing against wear. *Proc Inst Mech Eng H* 1996; 210(3):217–22.

12. Insall J, Ranawat CS, Scott WN, Walker P. Total condylar knee replacement: preliminary report. *Clin Orthop Relat Res* 1976(120):149–54.

13. Friedman RJ, Black J, Galante JO, Jacobs JJ, Skinner HB. Current concepts in orthopaedic biomaterials and implant fixation. *Instr Course Lect* 1994; 43:233–55.

14. Pijls BG, Valstar ER, Nouta KA, et al. Early migration of tibial components is associated with late revision: a systematic review and meta-analysis of 21,000 knee arthroplasties. *Acta Orthop* 2012; 83(6):614–24.

15. Berry DJ, Abdel MP, Callaghan JJ, Members of the Clinical Research Group. What are the current clinical issues in wear and tribocorrosion? *Clin Orthop Relat Res* 2014; 472(12):3659–64.

16. Kynaston-Pearson F, Ashmore AM, Malak TT, et al. Primary hip replacement prostheses and their evidence base: systematic review of literature. *BMJ* 2013; 347:f6956.

17. Hailer NP, Garellick G, Karrholm J. Uncemented and cemented primary total hip arthroplasty in the Swedish Hip Arthroplasty Register. *Acta Orthop* 2010; 81(1):34–41.

18. Carr AJ, Robertsson O, Graves S, et al. Knee replacement. *Lancet* 2012; 379(9823):1331–40.

19. Christelis N, Wallace S, Sage CE, et al. An enhanced recovery after surgery program for hip and knee arthroplasty. *Med J Aust* 2015; 202(7):363–8.

20. Liddle AD, Judge A, Pandit H, Murray DW. Adverse outcomes after total and unicompartmental knee replacement in 101,330 matched patients: a study of data from the National Joint Registry for England and Wales. *Lancet* 2014; 384(9952):1437–45.

21. Parvizi J, Huang R, Raphael IJ, Arnold WV, Rothman RH. Symptomatic pulmonary embolus after joint arthroplasty: stratification of risk factors. *Clin Orthop Relat Res* 2014; 472(3):903–12.

22. Bjornara BT, Gudmundsen TE, Dahl OE. Frequency and timing of clinical venous thromboembolism after major joint surgery. *J Bone Joint Surg Br* 2006 Mar; 88(3):386–91.

23. Kapadia BH, Berg RA, Daley JA, et al. Periprosthetic joint infection. *Lancet* 2016; 387(10016):386–94.

24. Dawson J, Fitzpatrick R, Carr A, Murray D. Questionnaire on the perceptions of patients about total hip replacement. *J Bone Joint Surg Br* 1996; 78(2):185–90.

25. Dawson J, Fitzpatrick R, Murray D, Carr A. Questionnaire on the perceptions of patients about total knee replacement. *J Bone Joint Surg Br* 1998; 80(1):63–9.

26. Noble PC, Conditt MA, Cook KF, Mathis KB. The John Insall Award: patient expectations affect satisfaction with total knee arthroplasty. *Clin Orthop Relat Res* 2006; 452:35–43.

27. Lang JE, Mannava S, Floyd AJ, et al. Robotic systems in orthopaedic surgery. *J Bone Joint Surg Br* 2011; 93(10):1296–9.

28. Wiater JM, Fabing MH. Shoulder arthroplasty: prosthetic options and indications. *J Am Acad Orthop Surg* 2009; 17(7):415–25.

29. Qureshi F, Draviaraj KP, Stanley D. The Kudo 5 total elbow replacement in the treatment of the rheumatoid elbow: results at a minimum of ten years. *J Bone Joint Surg Br* 2010; 92(10):1416–21.

30. Bartel AF, Roukis TS. Total ankle replacement survival rates based on Kaplan-Meier survival analysis of national joint registry data. *Clin Podiatr Med Surg* 2015; 32(4):483–94.

CHAPTER 34

Other surgical approaches in the management of osteoarthritis

Jonas Bloch Thorlund and L. Stefan Lohmander

Arthroscopy

Arthroscopic interventions have been used for many years to treat osteoarthritic joints. Most commonly the procedures have been carried out on the knee but are also used for the ankle, elbow, shoulder, and hip. Arthroscopic procedures for the knee are particularly frequent [1,2] with yearly incidences of meniscal procedures close to 200 per 100 000 in patients aged 60–74 in 2010–2012 in the United Kingdom [3]. Even higher yearly incidences of more than 300 meniscal procedures per 100 000 have been reported in Danish patients aged 55 or older in 2010 and 2011 [4]. However, procedures for the hip and shoulder are also increasing [5–7]. For example, the number of subacromial decompressions has been reported to have increased in the United Kingdom from 5.2 to 40.2 yearly procedures per 100 000 from 2000/2001 to 2009/2010 [7]. The rationale for these treatments is that degenerated or damaged parts of the different joint structures, or fragments thereof, are the cause of pain, symptoms, and joint dysfunction, and that their removal will relieve pain and improve joint function. Debridement, or in lay terms 'house-cleaning', of the joint may involve resection of cartilage flaps, meniscectomy, synovectomy and removal of loose cartilage, osteochondral and meniscal fragments, and in some cases removal of osteophytes. Debridement was previously carried out by arthrotomy [8,9] but nowadays the procedure is arthroscopic. Joint irrigation (i.e. lavage) is part of the debridement procedure but can also be carried out as an isolated arthroscopic or non-arthroscopic procedure. The aim of lavage is to wash out loose tissue and debris from the joint space. This has typically been performed as tidal irrigation lavage using one entry point to alternately inject and draw out fluid or non-arthroscopic lavage with two entry points (i.e. one to inject fluid and one for withdrawal) but without visual inspection of the joint or by arthroscopy.

Knee arthroscopy

Debridement and lavage has for many years been recommended for patients with knee pain and degenerative knee disease. However, several studies questioned the effect of arthroscopic lavage for patients with knee osteoarthritis in the late 1990s and early 2000s [10]. In 2010, Reisenbach et al. [10] synthesized the evidence from available studies on all types of lavage (i.e. arthroscopic and non-arthroscopic lavage and tidal irrigation) as treatment for knee pain in patients with knee osteoarthritis. The authors concluded that overall methodological study quality and the quality of reporting was poor and showed no relevant benefit in terms of pain reduction

or improvement in function compared to control interventions (including sham interventions).

Debridement for degenerative knee disease often involves resection or shaving of cartilage, synovium, meniscus, and bone, making it hard to assign any benefit to a specific intervention. The effect of debridement has been challenged since Chang et al. [11] showed no difference in improvement in pain in a randomized study comparing the effect of debridement with that of closed-needle lavage. Expanding on these findings, the landmark study by Moseley and co-workers in 2002 [12] showed no difference between debridement and lavage for patients with established knee osteoarthritis. More importantly, this randomized controlled trial found no difference between either debridement or lavage compared to the treatment arm receiving sham surgery only (i.e. skin incisions only) (Figure 34.1). Despite the strong study design the Moseley study was heavily criticized for looking at a specific subgroup of patients [13] and for using a non-validated pain measure as primary outcome [14]. The evidence for the effectiveness of arthroscopic debridement for knee osteoarthritis was summarized in a systematic review in 2008 [15], concluding that there

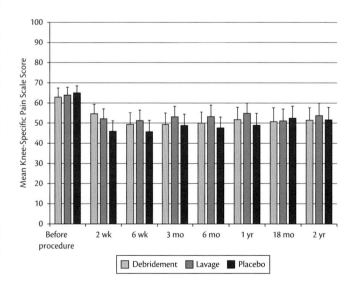

Figure 34.1 Mean values (with 95% confidence intervals) on the Knee-Specific Pain Scale between interventions at the different study time points.
Moseley JB, O'Malley K, Petersen NJ, Menke TJ, Brody BA, Kuykendall DH, Hollingsworth JC, Ashton CM, Wray NP. A controlled trial of arthroscopic surgery for osteoarthritis of the knee. *N Engl J Med* 2002; 347(2):81–8.

was 'gold level' evidence that arthroscopic debridement provided no relevant benefit for knee osteoarthritis of indeterminate cause. However, the review also stated that there might be subgroups of patients or levels of disease severity where the intervention may be effective.

Meniscal tears are often stated as a main indication for debridement. In particular, the treatment of these tears in patients with degenerative knee disease (osteoarthritis) has been debated [16,17]. Following the study by Moseley et al. [12], seven randomized controlled trials [18–24] have investigated the benefit of arthroscopic partial meniscectomy with or without concomitant additional debridement in comparison to sham surgery [23] or exercise therapy [22], or in addition to exercise therapy compared to exercise therapy alone [18,19,20,21,24]. The mean age of patients in these studies ranged between 50 and 63 years and the degree of degenerative knee disease (osteoarthritis) in the included patients ranged from degenerative meniscal tears without radiographic signs of knee osteoarthritis [23,24], over studies including both patients with and without radiographic knee osteoarthritis [18,19,20,22], to studies also including patients with severe radiographic knee (i.e. Kellgren and Lawrence grade 4 [25]) [21]. A recent systematic review and meta-analysis including all randomized trials up to August 2014 summarized the most current evidence [26]. The results showed that there was a minimal short-term (3–6 months) pain benefit, corresponding to 3–5 mm on a 0–100 mm VAS scale, of surgery compared to control interventions (Table 34.1). However, this effect is comparable to the benefit provided by paracetamol for knee osteoarthritis, and no difference was observed between surgery and non-operative interventions after 6 months. There was no benefit found for function. Importantly, these findings were consistent for studies across the entire spectrum of patients from those with degenerative meniscal tears to those with established radiographic knee osteoarthritis [26]. Of note is that no studies including a sham surgery control intervention showed a benefit of the arthroscopic intervention compared with the sham treatment.

Adverse events

Like other surgical procedures, arthroscopic meniscal surgery (with or without debridement) is associated with risk of adverse events such as deep venous thrombosis, pulmonary embolism, infection, and death [26]. The most frequent of the symptomatic adverse events is venous thromboembolism with an incidence of almost 6 per 1000 performed procedures [26].

Clinical practice

Despite this accumulating evidence of limited or no effect of debridement including meniscectomy for patients with knee pain and degenerative knee disease, and associated adverse events, these procedures are still widely and frequently practised [1,2,4]. Many orthopaedic surgeons maintain a strong belief in the treatment despite the published studies [16,17,27]. In particular, the presence of 'mechanical symptoms', such as a sensation of catching (pseudo-locking) or locking of the knee provides a strong rationale for the surgeon to offer the patient surgery. However, a benefit of partial meniscectomy for the subgroup of patients with mechanical symptoms remains to be documented, and it is often forgotten that 172/180 patients in the Moseley study had one or more mechanical symptoms [28].

The absence of benefit, or very limited benefit, observed in studies of debridement (including partial meniscectomy) for patients with early or established radiographic knee osteoarthritis may lie in the assumption that pain and diminished function can be 'cut' away. Challenging this perception, studies have shown that meniscal tears are very common in asymptomatic knees in individuals aged 50 years and older and that the prevalence of tears increases with age [29]. However, such asymptomatic tears are also common in younger subjects [30], questioning the direct link between pain and meniscal tears. Indeed, one study investigating the link between meniscal tears and pain, aching, and stiffness concluded that the presence of these symptoms was due to the presence of knee osteoarthritis rather than by a direct link between pain and meniscal tears [31].

Recommendations

The Osteoarthritis Research Society International (OARSI) recommendations for management of knee OA discourage the use of lavage and debridement for patients with knee OA [32]. Likewise, the guidelines from the American Academy of Orthopaedic Surgeons (AAOS) advise against the use of debridement and lavage for patients with a primary diagnosis of knee osteoarthritis [33]. However, the AAOS guidelines also state that the evidence for use of arthroscopic meniscectomy in patients with knee osteoarthritis is 'inconclusive' and do not advice against such a procedure [33]. There now seems to be a need to revisit these guidelines.

Hip arthroscopy

In recent years, the number of performed hip arthroscopies has increased dramatically (up to 600%) in the United States [5,6] and other countries. In particular, treatment for acetabular labral tears

Table 34.1 Difference in effect of interventions including arthroscopic knee surgery compared with control interventions (i.e. placebo surgery or exercise) at different follow-up time points after surgery

	3 months	6 months	12 months	18 months	24 months
Difference in pain, mm on 0–100 mm VAS scale (95% CI)	4.6 (2.3–6.9)	3.0 (0.9–5.1)	1.0 (−1.1–3.1)	0.0 (−5.5–5.5)	1.0 (−2.2–4.3)
No. trials	9	6	7	2	3
No. patients	1162	1002	1049	308	434
I² (%)	20.6	0.0	0.0	48.9	0.0

I² = estimate of heterogeneity.

Data from Thorlund JB, Juhl CB, Roos EM, Lohmander LS. Arthroscopic surgery for degenerative knee: systematic review and meta-analysis of benefits and harms. *BMJ* 2015; 350:h2747.

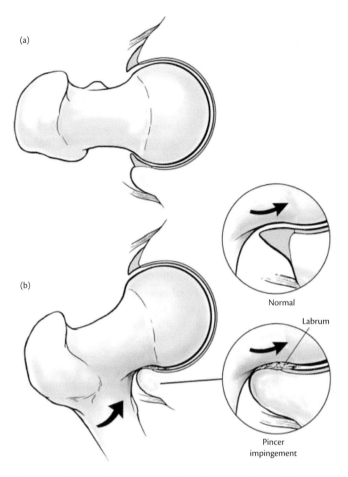

Figure 34.2 Pincer impingement occurs from a bony prominence of the anterior acetabulum crushing the labrum against the neck of the femur (a → b). Secondary articular failure occurs over time.

Reproduced with permission from Byrd, J.W.T., Femoroacetabular Impingement in Athletes, Part 1: Cause and Assessment, *Sports Health*, Vol. 2 No. 4, 2010, with permission from SAGE publications.

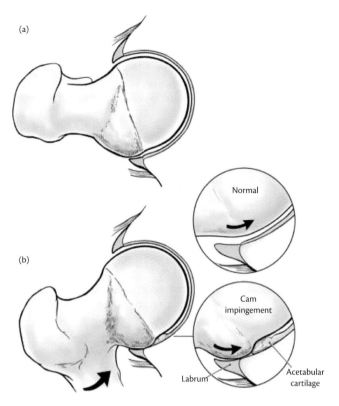

Figure 34.3 Cam impingement occurs with hip flexion as the bony prominence of the non-spherical portion of the femoral head (cam lesion) glides under the labrum, engaging the edge of the articular cartilage and resulting in progressive delamination (a → b). Initially, the labrum is relatively preserved, but secondary failure occurs over time.

Reproduced with permission from Byrd, J.W.T., Femoroacetabular Impingement in Athletes, Part 1: Cause and Assessment, *Sports Health*, Vol. 2 No. 4, 2010, with permission from SAGE publications.

has gained in popularity as these together with femoroacetabular impingement (FAI) are considered important risk factors for osteoarthritis [34]. *In vitro* and modelling studies have suggested that the function of the acetabular labrum is much like the meniscus in the knee to increase the joint surface area, distribute the forces transmitted to the cartilage, enhance joint stability, and provide proprioceptive feedback [35–37]. The major cause of acetabular labrum tears is considered to be FAI [38]. FAI is divided into two distinct pathomechanical types (which may be seen alone or in combination): pincer and cam. Pincer impingement results from local or global acetabular over-coverage, causing impact between the acetabular rim and the head–neck junction [39,40] (Figure 34.2). Cam impingement is caused by abnormal contact between the acetabular rim and the femoral head or the head-neck junction due to a dysmorphic shape of the femoral head [39,40] (Figure 34.3).

The surgical treatment of FAI and/or labral tears involves correction of deformities causing bony contact during hip motion as well as associated cartilage and labral tears and can be conducted as an open surgical treatment (also known as the surgical dislocation technique) [41,42], arthroscopic treatment, or a combination of the two [40]. In recent years the arthroscopic method has been increasingly used [40]. The optimal surgical techniques remain to

be determined [40,43]. A prospective study [44] making a head-to-head comparison of the surgical dislocation technique compared to hip arthroscopy for FAI and labral tears showed better outcome for those receiving hip arthroscopy as measured with the Hip Outcome Score—Sport-Specific Subscale (HOS-SSS) [45]. However, this finding needs to be confirmed in randomized and blinded trials. Labral tears are either treated by debridement or re-attachment.

Several systematic reviews have investigated the effectiveness of surgical treatment of FAI and labral tears. One systematic review [41] reported pain relief and improved function in 68–96% of patients undergoing surgery for FAI and another systematic review reported a mean rate of 'good' results in 82% of patients undergoing labral debridement [43]. A more recent systematic review investigating the effectiveness of hip arthroscopic surgery for patients with hip osteoarthritis reported improvement after the procedure but this improvement was less compared to patients without hip osteoarthritis [46]. Greater hip osteoarthritis severity and higher patient age were both predictors of a more rapid conversion to total hip arthroplasty [46]. Importantly, the authors of this systematic review noted that all included papers were level IV evidence (case series) with the exception of three studies, which were level III evidence (case–control studies). The authors further stated that the observed positive effects may be inflated as a result of methodological limitations of the included studies and that high-quality comparative studies are required to confirm the effects of hip arthroscopy.

Adverse events

Adverse events reporting following FAI and acetabulum labral surgery is very limited. Conversion rates to total hip arthroplasty to have been reported to range from 0% to 26% and major complications from 0% to 18% in studies on surgical treatment for FAI [41,43]. Large register studies are needed to fully appreciate the extent of adverse events.

Clinical practice

Current practice of surgical treatment for FAI and labral tears is thus based on insufficient evidence [40,41]. As noted, FAI and labral tears are considered a significant contributing factor in the aetiology of osteoarthritis [47]. However, it remains to be shown that surgical intervention to correct these features can postpone or prevent hip osteoarthritis development. Furthermore, as seen with meniscal tears, labral tears in a degenerated labrum may represent an early sign of osteoarthritis [48] and if this is so, then surgery is less likely to provide benefit [46]. A major limitation in evaluating the true efficacy of surgical treatments for FAI and/or labral tears is the lack of randomized trials comparing the benefit to that of non-surgical treatments such as exercise/physiotherapy, or to sham surgery [48,49].

Osteotomy

The osteotomy procedure involves cutting and re-fixing the bone to correct any malalignment and thereby redistribute mechanical loading of the joint surfaces. The intended redistribution of load to areas with less severe joint damage is considered to alleviate patient symptoms and postpone the need for joint replacement [50].

Osteotomies around the knee

Several procedures exist, with high tibial osteotomy for re-alignment of the knee being the most common and having been in use since the 1960s [51,52]. Osteotomies for unicompartmental knee OA are carried out to correct either varus or valgus malalignment, with osteotomies for varus alignment and medial compartment knee OA being most frequent owing to the higher prevalence of medial compartment knee osteoarthritis [53]. With increasing use of total knee replacements, high tibial osteotomies are now less frequently performed [54,55].

Early results after high tibial osteotomy are usually good, with patients reporting improved function and reduced pain [55–61] compared to baseline values. The deterioration in effect over time is likely caused by progression of knee osteoarthritis. Survival of the osteotomy (usually defined as not revised to total knee replacement) after 10 years has been reported to vary substantially [62]. A more recent national register study reporting on revision rates from more than 3000 osteotomies in Sweden reported cumulative revision rates to be 30% at 10 years [55]. However, revision rates seem to be highly dependent on patient age, with younger patients (<50 years) having increased life expectancy of the osteotomy [55,63,64]. This is in contrast to knee replacements where longevity of the implant is shorter in younger more active patients [65].

Correct patient selection and precise technique may be critical for the success of high tibial osteotomy. Knee replacement surgery is not ideal for active young patients with physically demanding work, making osteotomy a viable alternative. The main characteristics for the optimal candidate for high tibial osteotomy have been summarized to be younger than 50–60 years, isolated medial compartment pain/osteoarthritis, varus malalignment, and a good range of motion [50,62]. No decisive evidence seems to exist on any perioperative conditions improving/worsening the outcome of high tibial osteotomy [66].

Several high tibial osteotomy surgical techniques exist, with opening wedge and closing wedge osteotomies being the most frequently performed [50,62]. Lateral closing wedge osteotomy has typically been the treatment of choice providing a large bone contact area supporting postoperative bone healing but it requires a fibular osteotomy, two saw cuts, and extensor muscle detachment [50]. In later years, the opening wedge osteotomy has become increasingly used owing to the simple medial approach not requiring fibular osteotomy and potentially lower risk of neurovascular complications as well as easier conversion to total joint replacement [67]. A systematic review from 2007 [66] showed no evidence of better outcome of either of the two procedures. A more recent systematic review and meta-analysis showed no difference between an opening and a closing high tibial osteotomy with respect to pain and physical function as well as incidence of adverse events such as infection, deep vein thrombosis, personal nerve palsy, or conversion to knee replacement [67]. In contrast, the results of a 6-year follow-up from a trial randomizing patients to either closing or opening wedge high tibial osteotomy showed more complications in patients receiving an opening wedge osteotomy compared to closing wedge, whereas those receiving a closing wedge osteotomy had more early conversions to knee arthroplasty [68].

A systematic review and meta-analysis based on a of mix of retrospective, cohort, and randomized studies comparing high tibial osteotomy and unicompartmental knee joint replacement showed no difference in improvement in pain and function [66,69]. No differences were observed in either revision rate or amount of complications between treatments. Age seems to be the most important factor when deciding between unicompartmental knee replacement and high tibial osteotomy, recommending unicompartmental knee joint replacement to those above 65 years of age [70].

Adverse events

Information on adverse events associated with high tibial osteotomy surgery is sparse with only small cohort studies and no large register-based studies. The most common adverse events requiring additional non-operative treatment include delayed union, cellulitis, and limited hardware failure but also stiffness and deep venous thrombosis is observed [71]. More serious adverse events requiring additional surgery or long-term non-operative medical care are reported to be aseptic non-union, deep infection, complex regional pain syndrome, and hardware failure with loss of correction [71].

Recommendations

A major limitation in determining the 'true' effectiveness of high tibial osteotomy is the lack of randomized trials comparing with non-surgical treatments. Thus, there is no high-level evidence to suggest that osteotomies are superior to non-surgical treatment [66]. Nevertheless, the authors of the most recent systematic review concluded that there was 'silver' level evidence that high tibial osteotomy provides reduction in pain and improvement in function. The OARSI guidelines state that a high tibial osteotomy may be offered as an alternative treatment to delay the need for joint replacement [72], which is in line with the AAOS guidelines [33].

Osteotomies around the hip

Various corrective hip osteotomy techniques exist such as juxta-articular triple osteotomies [73], spherical osteotomies [74], and periacetabular osteotomies [75] for treatment of symptomatic dysplasia. Osteotomies of the hip are rarely carried out in older patients. Rather, these procedures are performed on children and young adults with anatomical deficiencies of the hip such as dysplasia, in order to prevent or postpone later development of hip osteoarthritis. The goal is to restore the hip anatomy as close to normal as possible in patients with acetabular structural abnormalities consistent with hip dysplasia. The preferred method in Northern America and Europe to achieve this is the periacetabular osteotomy owing to its minimal exposure and ability to provide optimal correction and least amount of complications [76].

A systematic review from 2009 on the effectiveness of periacetabular osteotomy reported that pain relief and improved hip function was observed in most patients at short- to midterm follow-up (average follow-up range: 2.9–12 years) [77]. A more recent retrospective study supports these findings by reporting decreased pain and increased physical activity level in young patients (mean age 27.3 years) 2 years after periacetabular osteotomy for hip dysplasia [78].

Conversion to total hip arthroplasty is reported to occur in 0–17% of patients 1–12 months after periacetabular osteotomy, mainly in those with moderate to severe hip osteoarthritis at the time of surgery [77]. The rate of major complications is reported to range between 6% and 37%, with the most common being symptomatic heterotopic ossification, wound haematomas, nerve palsies, loss of fixation, and malreductions [77]. Obesity (i.e. BMI over 30) is a major independent risk factor for complications following periacetabular osteotomy [79]. A more recent study [80] reporting on complications from experienced surgeons provides a major complication rate of 5.9%, suggesting that surgeon experience may be important for a low complication rate. However, precise estimates of complications rates are hampered by the large diversity in quality of reporting of adverse events. Main characteristics of the ideal patient for consideration for hip osteotomy were suggested to be young age (<40 years), Tönnis grade 0 or 1 [81], no or mild osteoarthritis, and not obese (BMI < 30 kg/m^2) [76,77].

Recommendations

The evidence level for hip osteotomy is low with no randomized trials investigating the effectiveness of the procedure compared to non-operative treatments. A systematic review reported that the literature almost exclusively consisted of retrospective case series of low-quality (level IV evidence) [77]. Nevertheless, the OARSI guidelines for management of hip osteoarthritis suggest that osteotomies for the hip should be considered in young adults with symptomatic hip osteoarthritis, especially in the presence of dysplasia [72].

Other treatments

Numerous other surgical interventions are used to manage osteoarthritis. Overall, these interventions are directed towards specific subgroups of patients and often lack high-level evidence to support their clinical efficacy.

Joint distraction

Joint distraction is a surgical procedure whereby the two sides of the joint are gradually separated by means of an external frame, creating 2–3 months of unloading of the osteoarthritic joint. The procedure has so far been practised mainly on the ankle and knee joints [82]. The majority of the published studies represent retrospective case reports, with some prospective observational studies, but only few and small controlled trials. Results of improved joint structure, tissue repair, and pain and function benefit have been reported [83,84], but need to be confirmed in low-risk-of-bias randomized trials with appropriate controls. There is insufficient evidence to either support or refute this procedure as a treatment for osteoarthritis.

Bone marrow stimulation techniques

These methods include abrasion chondroplasty, Pridie drilling, and microfracturing with the aim of exposing the bone marrow space underlying the subchondral bone plate. This may induce a spontaneous repair response based on bleeding, clot formation, and the presence of mesenchymal stem cells. Unfortunately, this response is variable and the 'cartilage' tissue formed is often fibrous with a limited durability as a bearing surface within the joint [85]. Based largely on observational studies, short-term positive clinical outcomes have been reported. The best results are suggested to be obtained in younger patients, possibly due to their larger numbers of precursor cell pools. On the basis of the published reports, there is insufficient evidence to either support or refute this procedure as a treatment for osteoarthritis.

Osteochondral autografting

This technique, sometimes termed mosaicplasty, is based on the harvesting of full-thickness cartilage–bone plugs from the unloaded, marginal areas of the joint, and inserting them into large, full-thickness joint surface lesions [85]. Concerns have been raised with regard to the viability and integration of the autografted plugs due to the traumatic procedures needed to both remove and insert them. This method was introduced primarily to deal with large joint defects resulting from, for example, osteonecrosis, and there is insufficient evidence to support its benefits as a treatment for osteoarthritis.

Autologous chondrocyte implantation

A pivotal report using this technique for treatment of joint cartilage defects in the human knee joint was published by Brittberg and co-workers in 1994, and was met with great enthusiasm and hope [86]. The technique is based on the arthroscopic harvesting of joint cartilage fragments from which chondrocytes are then isolated and expanded in culture. In a subsequent open surgery session, the chondrocyte suspension is deposited in the joint defect to be treated, and covered with a periosteal membrane harvested from the tibia. Later modifications of this technique have used chondrocytes embedded in a matrix of, for example, collagen or hyaluronan, and used an off-the-shelf collagen membrane to cover the implant instead of periosteum [85]. Autologous chondrocyte implantation is most commonly used to treat symptomatic cartilage defects of the knee. In spite of many years of practice, the published evidence is insufficient to prove the superiority of one variation of the technique over the other; the published reports suffer from small patient numbers, heterogeneous indications, loss to follow-up, and, importantly, lack of appropriate control treatments for comparison, such as sham surgery. Notably, the highest quality studies have failed to show a difference in long-term patient-reported outcome between chondrocyte implantation treatment and the considerably simpler method of microfracturing [87,88]. Published studies have included a variable proportion of patients that may fulfil criteria for having early-stage osteoarthritis, but there is insufficient evidence to either support or refute this procedure as a treatment for osteoarthritis.

Mesenchymal stem cell injections

Mesenchymal stem cells are now used in a variety of experimental and insufficiently documented and monitored procedures to treat symptomatic joints with osteoarthritis or injury. Mesenchymal stem cells are precursors of connective tissue cells and can be isolated from every tissue of the adult joint. The rationale of these procedures is based on the accessibility of mesenchymal stem cells in, for example, adipose tissue, where they can be harvested by liposuction, and the capacity of these cells for self-renewal [89–91]. There is a growing recognition that the critical property of these stem cells that provides them with a therapeutic potency may be their capacity to secrete in a paracrine manner potent growth and differentiation factors at the site of implantation, thereby stimulating a tissue repair or regeneration response of the host tissue. Several early-stage human clinical trials of stem cell therapy for joint injury or osteoarthritis can be found through searching clinical trials registries (e.g. http://www.clinicaltrials.gov). These are, in general, phase I trials targeting the knee and with a focus on safety evaluation, not clinical efficacy. Much further work remains to improve our mechanistic understanding of this therapy. There is insufficient evidence to support its safety or efficacy in treating osteoarthritis.

Conclusion

The surgical approaches to the management of osteoarthritis summarized in this chapter range from those that have been widely practised for many years, such as arthroscopic surgery and osteotomy, to those that have been more recently introduced, such as joint distraction, chondrocyte implantation, and mesenchymal stem cell injections. Arthroscopic surgery for the osteoarthritic knee continues to be widely practised in spite of high-level evidence against its benefit compared with sham surgery or with non-surgical interventions. The use of osteotomies around the knee has decreased in recent years, possibly due to the increasing commodification of total knee arthroplasty. More recent surgical techniques have been introduced based on, for example, implantation of chondrocytes or stem cells, but their utility for treating osteoarthritis has not yet been shown by low-risk-of bias clinical trials.

A systematic review of the evaluation of surgery found that half of the studies that used placebo controls provided evidence against the continued use of the investigated surgical procedures [92]. Trials without sham control may show benefit for the surgical procedure when compared with no treatment or ineffective non-operative treatment, or when compared with pre-treatment status. It is, however, difficult to justify invasive surgery with associated risks to obtain an effect similar to the placebo effect of sham surgery [27]. There is a great need for continued innovation and development of surgical techniques for managing in particular the earlier stages of osteoarthritis. To reduce the risk of future costly failures, a stepwise introduction of new surgical procedures and devices must be encouraged [93].

References

1. Bohensky MA, Sundararajan V, Andrianopoulos N, et al. Trends in elective knee arthroscopies in a population-based cohort, 2000–2009. *Med J Aust* 2012; 197(7):399–403.
2. Cullen K, Hall M, Golosinskiya A. Ambulatory surgery in the United States, 2006. *Natl Health Stat Report* 2009; 28(11):1–25.
3. Lazic S, Boughton O, Hing C, Bernard J. Arthroscopic washout of the knee: a procedure in decline. *Knee* 2014; 21(2):631–4.
4. Thorlund JB, Hare KB, Lohmander LS. Large increase in arthroscopic meniscus surgery in the middle-aged and older population in Denmark from 2000 to 2011. *Acta Orthop* 2014; 85(3):287–92.
5. Bozic KJ, Chan V, Valone FH, 3rd, Feeley BT, Vail TP. Trends in hip arthroscopy utilization in the United States. *J Arthroplasty* 2013; 28(8 Suppl):140–3.
6. Colvin AC, Harrast J, Harner C. Trends in hip arthroscopy. *J Bone Joint Surg Am* 2012; 94(4):e23.
7. Judge A, Murphy RJ, Maxwell R, Arden NK, Carr AJ. Temporal trends and geographical variation in the use of subacromial decompression and rotator cuff repair of the shoulder in England. *Bone Joint J* 2014; 96-B(1):70–4.
8. Haggart GE. The surgical treatment of degenerative arthritis of the knee joint. *J Bone Joint Surg* 1940; 2213.
9. Magnuson PB. Joint debridement: surgical treatment of degenerative arthritis. *Surg Gynecol Obstet* 1941; 739.
10. Reichenbach S, Rutjes AW, Nuesch E, Trelle S, Juni P. Joint lavage for osteoarthritis of the knee. *Cochrane Database Syst Rev* 2010; 5:CD007320.
11. Chang RW, Falconer J, Stulberg SD, et al. A randomized, controlled trial of arthroscopic surgery versus closed-needle joint lavage for patients with osteoarthritis of the knee. *Arthritis Rheum* 1993; 36(3):289–96.
12. Moseley JB, O'Malley K, Petersen NJ, et al. A controlled trial of arthroscopic surgery for osteoarthritis of the knee. *N Engl J Med* 2002; 347(2):81–8.
13. Jackson RW. Arthroscopic surgery for osteoarthritis of the knee. *N Engl J Med* 2002; 3471.
14. Chambers KG, Schulzer M. Arthroscopic surgery for osteoarthritis of the knee. *N Engl J Med* 2002; 3471.
15. Laupattarakasem W, Laopaiboon M, Laupattarakasem P, Sumananont C. Arthroscopic debridement for knee osteoarthritis. *Cochrane Database Syst Rev* 2008; 1:CD005118.
16. Lubowitz JH, Provencher MT, Rossi MJ. Could the New England Journal of Medicine be biased against arthroscopic knee surgery? Part 2. *Arthroscopy* 2014; 30(6):654–5.
17. Rossi MJ, D'Agostino RB, Jr, Provencher MT, Lubowitz JH. Could the New England Journal of Medicine be biased against arthroscopic knee surgery? *Arthroscopy* 2014; 30(5):536–7.
18. Gauffin H, Tagesson S, Meunier A, Magnusson H, Kvist J. Knee arthroscopic surgery is beneficial to middle-aged patients with meniscal symptoms: a prospective, randomised, single-blinded study. *Osteoarthritis Cartilage* 2014; 22(11):1808–16.
19. Herrlin S, Hallander M, Wange P, Weidenhielm L, Werner S. Arthroscopic or conservative treatment of degenerative medial meniscal tears: a prospective randomised trial. *Knee Surg Sports Traumatol Arthrosc* 2007; 15(4):393–401.
20. Katz JN, Brophy RH, Chaisson CE, et al. Surgery versus physical therapy for a meniscal tear and osteoarthritis. *N Engl J Med* 2013; 368(18):1675–84.
21. Kirkley A, Birmingham TB, Litchfield RB, et al. A randomized trial of arthroscopic surgery for osteoarthritis of the knee. *N Engl J Med* 2008; 359(11):1097–107.
22. Osteras H, Osteras B, Torstensen TA. Medical exercise therapy, and not arthroscopic surgery, resulted in decreased depression and anxiety in patients with degenerative meniscus injury. *J Bodyw Mov Ther* 2012; 16(4):456–63.

23. Sihvonen R, Paavola M, Malmivaara A, et al. Arthroscopic partial meniscectomy versus sham surgery for a degenerative meniscal tear. *N Engl J Med* 2013; 369(26):2515–24.

24. Yim JH, Seon JK, Song EK, et al. A comparative study of meniscectomy and nonoperative treatment for degenerative horizontal tears of the medial meniscus. *Am J Sports Med* 2013; 41(7):1565–70.

25. Kellgren JH, Lawrence JS. Radiological assessment of osteo-arthrosis. *Ann Rheum Dis* 1957; 16(4):494–502.

26. Thorlund JB, Juhl CB, Roos EM, Lohmander LS. Arthroscopic surgery for degenerative knee: systematic review and meta-analysis of benefits and harms. *BMJ* 2015; 350:h2747.

27. Lohmander LS, Roos EM. The evidence base for orthopaedics and sports medicine. *BMJ* 2015; 350g7835.

28. Wray NP, Moseley JB, O'Malley K. Arthroscopic surgery for osteoarthritis of the knee. *N Engl J Med* 2002; 3471719.

29. Englund M, Guermazi A, Gale D, et al. Incidental meniscal findings on knee MRI in middle-aged and elderly persons. *N Engl J Med* 2008; 359(11):1108–15.

30. Boks SS, Vroegindeweij D, Koes BW, Hunink MM, Bierma-Zeinstra SM. Magnetic resonance imaging abnormalities in symptomatic and contralateral knees: prevalence and associations with traumatic history in general practice. *Am J Sports Med* 2006; 34(12):1984–91.

31. Englund M, Niu J, Guermazi A, et al. Effect of meniscal damage on the development of frequent knee pain, aching, or stiffness. *Arthritis Rheum* 2007; 56(12):4048–54.

32. Zhang W, Nuki G, Moskowitz RW, et al. OARSI recommendations for the management of hip and knee osteoarthritis: part III: Changes in evidence following systematic cumulative update of research published through January 2009. *Osteoarthritis Cartilage* 2010; 18(4):476–99.

33. American Academy of Orthopaedic Surgeons. *Treatment of Osteoarthritis of the Knee*, 2nd ed. Rosemont, IL: American Academy of Orthopaedic Surgeons; 2013.

34. Pun S, Kumar D, Lane NE. Review: femoroacetabular impingement. *Arthritis Rheum* 2015; 67(1):17–27.

35. Ferguson SJ, Bryant JT, Ganz R, Ito K. The influence of the acetabular labrum on hip joint cartilage consolidation: a poroelastic finite element model. *J Biomech* 2000; 33(8):953–60.

36. Ferguson SJ, Bryant JT, Ganz R, Ito K. An in vitro investigation of the acetabular labral seal in hip joint mechanics. *J Biomech* 2003; 36(2):171–8.

37. Kim YT, Azuma H. The nerve endings of the acetabular labrum. *Clin Orthop Relat Res* 1995(320):176–81.

38. Ito K, Leunig M, Ganz R. Histopathologic features of the acetabular labrum in femoroacetabular impingement. *Clin Orthop Relat Res* 2004(429):262–71.

39. Leunig M, Ganz R. The evolution and concepts of joint-preserving surgery of the hip. *Bone Joint J* 2014; 96-B(1):5–18.

40. MacFarlane RJ, Konan S, El-Huseinny M, Haddad FS. A review of outcomes of the surgical management of femoroacetabular impingement. *Ann R Coll Surg Engl* 2014; 96(5):331–8.

41. Clohisy JC, St John LC, Schutz AL. Surgical treatment of femoroacetabular impingement: a systematic review of the literature. *Clin Orthop Relat Res* 2010; 468(2):555–64.

42. Ng VY, Arora N, Best TM, Pan X, Ellis TJ. Efficacy of surgery for femoroacetabular impingement: a systematic review. *Am J Sports Med* 2010; 38(11):2337–45.

43. Haddad B, Konan S, Haddad FS. Debridement versus re-attachment of acetabular labral tears: a review of the literature and quantitative analysis. *Bone Joint J* 2014; 96-B(1):24–30.

44. Domb BG, Stake CE, Botser IB, Jackson TJ. Surgical dislocation of the hip versus arthroscopic treatment of femoroacetabular impingement: a prospective matched-pair study with average 2-year follow-up. *Arthroscopy* 2013; 29(9):1506–13.

45. Martin RL, Philippon MJ. Evidence of validity for the hip outcome score in hip arthroscopy. *Arthroscopy* 2007; 23(8):822–6.

46. Kemp JL, MacDonald D, Collins NJ, Hatton AL, Crossley KM. Hip arthroscopy in the setting of hip osteoarthritis: systematic review of outcomes and progression to hip arthroplasty. *Clin Orthop Relat Res* 2015; 473(3):1055–73.

47. Ganz R, Parvizi J, Beck M, et al. Femoroacetabular impingement: a cause for osteoarthritis of the hip. *Clin Orthop Relat Res* 2003(417):112–20.

48. Kemp JL, Crossley KM, Roos EM, Ratzlaff C. What fooled us in the knee may trip us up in the hip: lessons from arthroscopy. *Br J Sports Med* 2014; 48(16):1200–1.

49. Clohisy JC, Kim YJ, Lurie J, et al. Clinical trials in orthopaedics and the future direction of clinical investigations for femoroacetabular impingement. *J Am Acad Orthop Surg* 2013; 21(Suppl 1):S47–52.

50. Lutzner J, Kasten P, Gunther KP, Kirschner S. Surgical options for patients with osteoarthritis of the knee. *Nat Rev Rheumatol* 2009; 5(6):309–16.

51. Coventry MB. Osteotomy of the upper portion of the tibia for degenerative arthritis of the knee. A preliminary report. *J Bone Joint Surg Am* 1965; 479:84–90.

52. Jackson JP, Waugh W. Tibial osteotomy for osteoarthritis of the knee. *J Bone Joint Surg Br* 1961; 43-B:746–51.

53. Felson DT, Nevitt MC, Zhang Y, et al. High prevalence of lateral knee osteoarthritis in Beijing Chinese compared with Framingham Caucasian subjects. *Arthritis Rheum* 2002; 46(5):1217–22.

54. Nwachukwu BU, McCormick FM, Schairer WW, et al. Unicompartmental knee arthroplasty versus high tibial osteotomy: United States practice patterns for the surgical treatment of unicompartmental arthritis. *J Arthroplasty* 2014; 29(8):1586–9.

55. W-Dahl A, Robertsson O, Lohmander LS. High tibial osteotomy in Sweden, 1998–2007: a population-based study of the use and rate of revision to knee arthroplasty. *Acta Orthop* 2012; 83(3):244–8.

56. Adili A, Bhandari M, Giffin R, Whately C, Kwok DC. Valgus high tibial osteotomy. Comparison between an Ilizarov and a Coventry wedge technique for the treatment of medial compartment osteoarthritis of the knee. *Knee Surg Sports Traumatol Arthrosc* 2002; 10(3):169–76.

57. Brouwer RW, Bierma-Zeinstra SM, van Raaij TM, Verhaar JA. Osteotomy for medial compartment arthritis of the knee using a closing wedge or an opening wedge controlled by a Puddu plate. A one-year randomised, controlled study. *J Bone Joint Surg Br* 2006; 88(11):1454–9.

58. Magyar G, Ahl TL, Vibe P, Toksvig-Larsen S, Lindstrand A. Open-wedge osteotomy by hemicallotasis or the closed-wedge technique for osteoarthritis of the knee. A randomised study of 50 operations. *J Bone Joint Surg Br* 1999; 81(3):444–8.

59. Myrnerts R. High tibial osteotomy with overcorrection of varus malalignment in medial gonarthrosis. *Acta Orthop Scand* 1980; 51(3):557–60.

60. Odenbring S, Lindstrand A, Egund N. Early knee mobilization after osteotomy for gonarthrosis. *Acta Orthop Scand* 1989; 60(6):699–702.

61. W-Dahl A, Toksvig-Larsen S, Roos EM. A 2-year prospective study of patient-relevant outcomes in patients operated on for knee osteoarthritis with tibial osteotomy. *BMC Musculoskelet Disord* 2005; 61:8.

62. Amendola A, Bonasia DE. Results of high tibial osteotomy: review of the literature. *Int Orthop* 2010; 34(2):155–60.

63. Flecher X, Parratte S, Aubaniac JM, Argenson JN. A 12–28-year followup study of closing wedge high tibial osteotomy. *Clin Orthop Relat Res* 2006; 452:91–6.

64. Naudie D, Bourne RB, Rorabeck CH, Bourne TJ. The Insall Award. Survivorship of the high tibial valgus osteotomy. A 10- to -22-year followup study. *Clin Orthop Relat Res* 1999(367):18–27.

65. Robertsson O, Knutson K, Lewold S, Lidgren L. The Swedish Knee Arthroplasty Register 1975-1997: an update with special emphasis on 41,223 knees operated on in 1988–1997. *Acta Orthop Scand* 2001; 72(5):503–13.

66. Brouwer RW, Raaij van TM, Bierma-Zeinstra SM, et al. Osteotomy for treating knee osteoarthritis. *Cochrane Database Syst Rev* 2007; 3:CD004019.

67. Smith TO, Sexton D, Mitchell P, Hing CB. Opening- or closing-wedged high tibial osteotomy: a meta-analysis of clinical and radiological outcomes. *Knee* 2011; 18(6):361–8.

68. Duivenvoorden T, Brouwer RW, Baan A, et al. Comparison of closing-wedge and opening-wedge high tibial osteotomy for medial compartment osteoarthritis of the knee: a randomized controlled trial with a six-year follow-up. *J Bone Joint Surg Am* 2014; 96(17):1425–32.

69. Fu D, Li G, Chen K, et al. Comparison of high tibial osteotomy and unicompartmental knee arthroplasty in the treatment of unicompartmental osteoarthritis: a meta-analysis. *J Arthroplasty* 2013; 28(5):759–65.

70. Trieb K, Grohs J, Hanslik-Schnabel B, et al. Age predicts outcome of high-tibial osteotomy. *Knee Surg Sports Traumatol Arthrosc* 2006; 14(2):149–52.

71. Martin R, Birmingham TB, Willits K, et al. Adverse event rates and classifications in medial opening wedge high tibial osteotomy. *Am J Sports Med* 2014; 42(5):1118–26.

72. Zhang W, Moskowitz RW, Nuki G, et al. OARSI recommendations for the management of hip and knee osteoarthritis, Part II: OARSI evidence-based, expert consensus guidelines. *Osteoarthritis Cartilage* 2008; 16(2):137–62.

73. Tonnis D, Behrens K, Tscharani F. A modified technique of the triple pelvic osteotomy: early results. *J Pediatr Orthop* 1981; 1(3):241–9.

74. Ninomiya S, Tagawa H. Rotational acetabular osteotomy for the dysplastic hip. *J Bone Joint Surg Am* 1984; 66(3):430–6.

75. Ganz R, Klaue K, Vinh TS, Mast JW. A new periacetabular osteotomy for the treatment of hip dysplasias. Technique and preliminary results. *Clin Orthop Relat Res* 1988(232):26–36.

76. Perry KI, Trousdale RT, Sierra RJ. Hip dysplasia in the young adult: an osteotomy solution. *Bone Joint J* 2013; 95-B(11 Suppl A):21–5.

77. Clohisy JC, Schutz AL, St John L, Schoenecker PL, Wright RW. Periacetabular osteotomy: a systematic literature review. *Clin Orthop Relat Res* 2009; 467(8):2041–52.

78. Novais EN, Heyworth B, Murray K, et al. Physical activity level improves after periacetabular osteotomy for the treatment of symptomatic hip dysplasia. *Clin Orthop Relat Res* 2013; 471(3):981–8.

79. Novais EN, Potter GD, Clohisy JC, et al. Obesity is a major risk factor for the development of complications after peri-acetabular osteotomy. *Bone Joint J* 2015; 97-B(1):29–34.

80. Zaltz I, Baca G, Kim YJ, et al. Complications associated with the periacetabular osteotomy: a prospective multicenter study. *J Bone Joint Surg Am* 2014; 96(23):1967–74.

81. Tonnis D. Normal values of the hip joint for the evaluation of X-rays in children and adults. *Clin Orthop Relat Res* 1976(119):39–47.

82. Mastbergen SC, Saris DB, Lafeber FP. Functional articular cartilage repair: here, near, or is the best approach not yet clear? *Nat Rev Rheumatol* 2013; 9(5):277–90.

83. Intema F, Thomas TP, Anderson DD, et al. Subchondral bone remodeling is related to clinical improvement after joint distraction in the treatment of ankle osteoarthritis. *Osteoarthritis Cartilage* 2011; 19(6):668–75.

84. Wiegant K, van Roermund PM, Intema F, et al. Sustained clinical and structural benefit after joint distraction in the treatment of severe knee osteoarthritis. *Osteoarthritis Cartilage* 2013; 21(11):1660–7.

85. Hunziker EB, Lippuner K, Keel MJ, Shintani N. An educational review of cartilage repair: precepts & practice—myths & misconceptions—progress & prospects. *Osteoarthritis Cartilage* 2015; 23(3):334–50.

86. Brittberg M, Lindahl A, Nilsson A, et al. Treatment of deep cartilage defects in the knee with autologous chondrocyte transplantation. *N Engl J Med* 1994; 331(14):889–95.

87. Knutsen G, Drogset JO, Engebretsen L, et al. A randomized trial comparing autologous chondrocyte implantation with microfracture. Findings at five years. *J Bone Joint Surg Am* 2007; 89(10):2105–12.

88. Vanlauwe J, Saris DB, Victor J, et al. Five-year outcome of characterized chondrocyte implantation versus microfracture for symptomatic cartilage defects of the knee: early treatment matters. *Am J Sports Med* 2011; 39(12):2566–74.

89. Barry F, Murphy M. Mesenchymal stem cells in joint disease and repair. *Nat Rev Rheumatol* 2013; 9(10):584–94.

90. Bornes TD, Adesida AB, Jomha NM. Mesenchymal stem cells in the treatment of traumatic articular cartilage defects: a comprehensive review. *Arthritis Res Ther* 2014; 16(5):432.

91. Murphy M, Barry F. Cellular chondroplasty: a new technology for joint regeneration. *J Knee Surg* 2015; 28(1):45–50.

92. Wartolowska K, Judge A, Hopewell S, et al. Use of placebo controls in the evaluation of surgery: systematic review. *BMJ* 2014; 348:g3253.

93. McCulloch P, Altman DG, Campbell WB, et al. No surgical innovation without evaluation: the IDEAL recommendations. *Lancet* 2009; 374(9695):1105–12.

SECTION 10

Prospects for disease modification

CHAPTER 35

Prospects for disease modification

Shirley P. Yu and David J. Hunter

Introduction

Osteoarthritis (OA) is a highly prevalent and disabling disease that consequently has a formidable individual and societal impact. The disease occurs when the dynamic equilibrium between the breakdown and repair of joint tissues becomes unbalanced, often in a situation where the mechanical loads applied exceed those that can be tolerated by the joint tissues [1,2]. OA is a heterogeneous disease that is characterized by progressive cartilage loss, subchondral bone remodelling, osteophyte formation, and synovial inflammation, with resultant joint pain and increasing disability [1,2]. Whilst the progressive joint failure may cause pain and disability [3], approximately 50% of people with structural changes consistent with OA are asymptomatic [4].

Although in most cases the pathological changes of OA are asymptomatic, because of the sheer prevalence of OA, the prevalence of significant joint pain and disability in even a minority of those with pathological changes results in enormous medicoeconomic and socioeconomic burdens [5]. Until recently, pharmacological therapy for OA was aimed exclusively at symptom relief and has been based mainly on the use of paracetamol and other analgesics and non-steroidal anti-inflammatory drugs (NSAIDs). However, as greater understanding of the pathogenetic mechanisms in OA has accrued, interest has burgeoned in the development of new classes of drugs that are not primarily analgesics or anti-inflammatory agents but whose mechanism of action is directed at the inhibition of catabolic processes or stimulation of anabolic processes in the OA joint. These agents were originally called 'chondroprotective drugs', but because of the recognition that the pathological changes of OA are much more extensive than those in cartilage alone, more recently they have been designated disease-modifying OA drugs (DMOADs) or structure-modifying OA drugs (SMOADs).

Rationale for disease modification

The currently available treatments for OA focus on decreasing pain and improving function, with varying degrees of success. When this fails, destroyed joints can be replaced by arthroplasty, often with good long-term outcome. However, we still lack an effective means of intervening in the disease process of OA in order to stop or slow down the gradual destruction of joint tissues, and associated functional decline. Instead, the 'watchful waiting' of steady decline to end-stage joint disease is a major cause of disablement and loss of quality of life [6].

Research into the pathogenesis of the disease is rapidly progressing, but drug development is filled with hurdles [7]. Development of symptoms and disease progression is highly variable between each individual. Typically the disease process of OA is characterized by one of slow and inexorable progression. For some the rapidity of progression is faster, however for the majority there is a substantial window of opportunity to intervene in the disease process. Left unchecked the inexorable decline of joint tissues and associated function may lead to requirements for surgical intervention. Given the extraordinary prevalence of this disease and the enormity of expense associated with surgical intervention, opportunities to intervene in this process are worthy of pursuit.

In addition, several studies have highlighted the high risk of severe OA at a young age following joint injuries [8]. These young patients with OA, often in their thirties and forties, present a significant challenge. They have high expectations of physical activity and ability to work, while the orthopaedic surgeon is often reluctant to replace their failed joint due to the significantly increased risk of implant wear, loosening, and reoperation in these young patients.

Challenges inherent in disease modification

Preclinical studies with varying levels of efficacy suggest that a wide array of agents including glucosamine sulphate, chondroitin sulphate, sodium hyaluronan, doxycycline, matrix metalloproteinase (MMP) inhibitors, bisphosphonates, calcitonin, diacerein, and avocado/soybean unsaponifiables can modify disease progression [9]. At this point, however, there is no pharmacological agent that has been approved by regulatory authorities for disease modification in OA. It may be a while before a disease-modifying drug is available as current trial strategies remain neglectful of some simple fundamentals and/or are hampered by outdated regulatory requirements

Therefore, despite the important advances in our understanding of the pathogenetic mechanisms underlying tissue damage in the OA joint and the availability of pharmacological agents that may modify those pathogenetic processes, our inability to use valid and responsive outcome measures in clinical trials of DMOADs that would involve a reasonable number of patients and/or reasonable duration of treatment continues to inhibit significantly progress in DMOAD development.

A major problem facing the evaluation of any disease-modifying OA therapy is our inability to use reliable and convenient outcome measures to document changes in joint structure, function, or metabolism resulting from the treatment. There are a number of good studies advocating for particular imaging modalities that support the responsiveness and validity of newer imaging techniques [10]. At this point in time, however, they suffer from not being recognized by regulatory authorities to have that ability [11]. It may even be argued that until such measures are able to be used in clinical trials, it will be difficult to prove the efficacy of even the most promising drug candidate [12].

A comparison with the development of new osteoporosis treatments is instructive. For this disease, a reliable and convenient outcome measure in the form of bone density was available and subsequently supplemented with systemic biomarkers of bone turnover measured in urine and blood. These measures could in turn be related to a clinically relevant and measurable outcome: fracture. Finally, agents were available early on that could be used to probe validity of these measures in animal models.

In OA, the indirect measurement of joint cartilage thickness by plain radiography is still advocated by the regulatory authorities as the structural endpoint of interest [11]. Utilizing radiography as a means of defining disease serves to limit itself to a disease window that evaluates only some of the synovial joint features affected by OA, and this evaluation may reflect only the later stages of disease evolution. Magnetic resonance imaging (MRI) shows improved responsiveness and validity as an alternative or complementary method to monitor the structure of cartilage and other joint tissues [10]. Biochemical markers for OA are being developed and show promise, but for lack of an agent with proven disease-modifying effect, it remains difficult to validate biochemical markers for OA as outcome measures.

If non-surgical interventions as a single therapy are to be trialled effectively, selecting those with earlier disease, prior to the development of marked aberrant mechanics, is a preferable solution. In the recent iNOS trial [13] there may have been an effect in Kellgren–Lawrence (KL) grade 2 knees, supporting the perspective about needing to intervene earlier when biomechanical effects may not be as difficult to overcome. The fact that the effects were lost over the longer term suggests that perhaps targeting a single pathway even in milder disease may be insufficient.

It is unclear whether slowing the rate of progression of joint structural damage in OA pharmacologically will be accompanied by clinically meaningful benefit. Given the bulk of the evidence supporting an important relation of synovitis/effusion and bone marrow lesions to pain in OA, these appear, at present, to be the most promising targets for symptom modification. It should not be assumed a priori, that a pharmacological agent exhibiting DMOAD activity in humans will have a favourable impact on *clinically important* outcomes, such as joint pain, function, disability, and the need for joint replacement surgery. Although it is possible that the poor correlation that has been noted between radiographic progression and clinical progression is due to the lack of precision of plain radiography in evaluating structural change, the origin of joint pain in patients with knee OA is multifactorial and may relate to factors such as anxiety, depression, quadriceps strength, and the patient's coping skills—changes that do not have radiographic correlates [14]. For a disease-modifying agent to be approved by regulatory agencies it would likely have to have concomitant symptomatic benefits. Pain trials generally use subjective patient-reported outcomes, and these are susceptible to a high degree of variability, with resultant consequences on their responsiveness and ability to disentangle therapeutic effects from placebo. Placebo effects in OA trials can be high and persist over several months [15].

There is no shortage of *in vitro* and *in vivo* models that can be used for eliminating candidates from consideration, but establishing the validity and utility of these models for this selection and facilitating ready translation into the human model in the face of a paucity of successful candidates is challenging [9]. The applicability of preclinical models of OA to the human model is fraught with challenges, with many potentially promising DMOADs terminated because of difficulty in demonstrating clinical activity [16].

There are additional challenges that relate to safety and cost. OA is a chronic but not life-threatening disease. The acceptance level for side effects of disease-modifying pharmacological treatment of OA will likely be low. Similarly because of the typically slow progression of the disease requiring long-term administration and the availability of a cost-effective surgical intervention at the expense of disease-modifying interventions will need to be constrained accordingly [17].

Once a popular area for drug development, with a multitude of discovery and preclinical programmes at major pharmaceutical and biotech companies, and dozens of compounds moving through pharmaceutical pipelines toward pivotal clinical trials, today research on slowing or stopping progression of cartilage loss and other structural changes in the joint has been significantly scaled back, largely due to the challenges with target identification and clinical development referred to earlier [9].

Biological and clinical basis for tissue-targeted treatments

SMOADs have been defined as agents that reverse, retard, or stabilize the underlying pathology of OA, thereby slowing its progression and possibly providing symptomatic relief in the long term. SMOADs are considered to fall broadly into two categories: (1) those agents which slowed, arrested, or reversed structural changes in OA joints while concomitantly relieving the symptoms of the disease, and (2) drugs that achieved the same as (1) but provided no improvement in symptoms in the short term. For SMOADs corresponding to (2), symptomatic improvement was expected to occur in the long term and it was considered that other drugs, such as analgesics or NSAIDs, would probably have to be used to supplement this class of SMOADs in the intervening period. When they modify not only the structure but also the symptoms associated with the 'disease' they would be termed DMOADs.

While the 'structures' considered in this definition include articular cartilage and subchondral bone, these tissues are not of uniform composition and undergo continuous adaptation and remodelling throughout the development of OA. These circumstances render the evaluation of putative DMOADs extremely difficult since loss of tissue integrity in one part of a joint may be accompanied by a compensatory biosynthetic response in another, resulting in overall structural changes, which may appear to be beneficial. This is particularly evident in the early stages of OA, which are probably the most amenable to therapeutic intervention.

In human subjects, unlike animal models, direct tissue analysis is not generally possible and imaging techniques or biochemical markers are used to assess changes in synovial joint tissues. Joint space narrowing, as determined radiographically, is currently advocated by the regulatory authorities to follow cartilage loss in OA and has been employed to assess the effects of drugs on OA progression [11]. However, this approach has been shown to be open to many systematic errors and stringent precautions must be employed to ensure reproducible and meaningful measurements. MRI allows joint soft tissues to be visualized and this technique holds great promise as a potential means of determining the efficacy of DMOADs.

Irrespective of the time course of action, we require structural biomarkers that faithfully represent the status of the disease at a particular phase of its development and which would be amenable to modification by a therapeutic agent. With these structural biomarkers it is then assumed that these would allow the relative effects of a drug or placebo treatment, which was administered to a suitable number of patients, to be evaluated over a period of time, which was long enough for the structural component to change sufficiently for it to be accurately measured and permit differentiation between the respective treatments.

Fundamental to this approach is the identification of those structural features of OA that are amenable to observation using currently available non-invasive methodologies and which were meaningful in terms of our understanding of the pathology of the disease. As described more fully elsewhere in this book, OA is a disorder of multifactorial aetiology that generally has a long and variable period of asymptomatic development that affects the composition and structure of all tissues of the joint including articular cartilage, bone, ligaments, synovium, and synovial fluid. In the late stages of OA, the pathology is characterized by substantial damage to articular cartilage accompanied by subchondral bone necrosis, remodelling, and synovial inflammation [1]. However, since the functions of the respective components of the joint are integrated

and failure of one will inevitably lead to molecular and cellular changes in the others, it is important to appreciate that a DMOAD that may appear to produce a measurable change at one site in an OA joint may in fact be exerting its pharmacological effects elsewhere. For example, a drug that has no direct effects on cartilage metabolism may still mitigate its loss by decreasing the levels of cytokines released by synoviocytes, which promote catabolic proteinase production by chondrocytes.

The biological changes that take place in all OA joint tissues are extremely diverse and vary with the cause and the phase of the disease. Structural changes in OA and its modification by drugs must take into consideration the adaptable nature of joint connective tissues and accommodate such dynamic complexities into methods of assessment.

Emerging drugs for disease modification in osteoarthritis

Having considered the multitude of tissues that potentially can be targeted in this heterogeneous disease of OA we now consider the agents that can modify these tissues. In the first instance we focus on molecules targeting inflammatory pathways and then break that down by particular tissue targeted: specifically and in particular synovium, cartilage, and bone (Table 35.1).

The strategy for structural modification is to inhibit the effects of major cytokines, not dissimilar to the strategy adopted for the treatment of rheumatoid arthritis. Many new, novel drugs are currently under trial, but multiple drugs have failed to achieve a

Table 35.1 Emerging drugs targeting structural modification for osteoarthritis

Compound	ClinialTrials.gov identifier/ISRCTN registry/ANZCTR registry	Company/sponsor	Structure/mechanism of action	Stage of development
Targeting inflammatory pathways				
Tumour necrosis factor alpha inhibitors				
Infliximab	Not available	Dutch college of Health Insurances/Schering-Plough/ Centocor Inc./B.V	Chimeric monoclonal antibody	Open label
Adalimumab	NCT00296894	University Hospital, Ghent	Humanized monoclonal antibody	Phase II
	NCT00597623	Assistance Publique–Hôpitaux de Paris		Phase III
	NCT02471118	Canadian Research & Education in Arthritis/AbbVie		Phase II
DLX-105	NCT00819572	ESBATech AG (Germany/Switzerland)	Humanized monoclonal antibody (single-chain (scFv) antibody fragment against TNFA)	Phase II
Interleukin 1 beta inhibitors				
Anakinra	NCT00110916	Amgen	Recombinant IL1RA	Phase II
AMG-108	NCT00110942	Amgen	Fully humanized monoclonal antibody that binds type 1 IL1R and non-selectively inhibit IL1A and IL1B	Phase II
Gevokizumab	NCT01683396	Xoma (USA) Servier (France)	Humanized IgG2 MAb that binds to IL1B	Phase II

(continued)

Table 35.1 Continued

Compound	ClinialTrials.gov identifier/ISRCTN registry/ANZCTR registry	Company/sponsor	Structure/mechanism of action	Stage of development
ABT-981	NCT02087904	AbbVie (USA)	Anti-IL1A/B dual variable domain immunoglobulin	Phase II
Matrix metalloproteinase inhibitor				
PG-530742/ PG-116800	NCT00041756	Procter and Gamble	Matrix metalloproteinase inhibitors	Phase II
Inducible nitric oxide synthase inhibitor				
Cindunistat	NCT00565812	Pfizer (USA)	Inducible nitric oxide synthase (iNOS) inhibitor	Phase III
Mitogen-activate protein kinase inhibitor				
FX005	NCT01291914	Flexion Therapeutics (USA)	P38 mitogen-activated protein kinase (MAPK) inhibitor	Phase II
Bradykinin B2 receptor antagonist				
Icatibant	NCT00303056	Sanofi	Peptidic B2 receptor antagonist	Phase II
Fasitibant	NCT02205814	Menarini (Italy)	Non-peptide bradykinin 2 antagonist	Phase II
Cartilage catabolism and anabolism				
Bone morphogenetic protein				
Eptoterminalfa	NCT01111045	Stryker Biotech (USA)	Humanized recombinant bone morphogenetic protein 7	Phase IIb/III is planned
Fibroblast growth factor				
AS902330 (Sprifermin)	NCT01919164	Merck Serono (Germany)	Recombinant fibroblast growth factor 18	Phase II
Bone remodelling				
Calcitonin	NCT00376311	Université Catholique de Louvain/ Novartis	Oral salmon calcitonin	Phase II
	NCT00486434	Novartis/Nordic Bioscience A/S	Oral salmon calcitonin formulated with a 5-CNAC carrier	Phase III
	NCT00704847	Novartis/Nordic Bioscience A/S	Oral salmon calcitonin formulated with a 5-CNAC carrier	Phase III
Bisphosphonates				
Risedronate	ISRCTN01928173 (BRISK trial)	Procter and Gamble	Risedronate sodium	Phase not specified
	KOSTAR trial	Not specified	Risedronate sodium	Phase not specified
Zoledronic acid	ACTRN12613000039785	National Health and Medical Research Council (NHMRC)	Zoledronic acid	Phase III
Strontium ranelate				
Strontium ranelate	ISRCTN41323372	Institut de Recherches Internationales Servier (France)	Strontium ranelate	Phase III

clinically relevant result or have been withdrawn due to associated side effects.

Targeting inflammatory pathways

Tumour necrosis factor alpha inhibitors

Tumour necrosis factor alpha (TNFA) is one of the major cytokines involved in the destruction of articular matrix [18] that is produced predominantly by activated synoviocytes, phagocytic mononuclear cells, and articular cartilage [19]. Together with interleukin 1 beta (IL1B), it activates inflammatory signalling pathways that end in the activation of nuclear factor kappa B (NFKB), a transcription factor that regulates the expression of chemokines, cytokines, adhesion molecules, and matrix-degrading enzymes.

In vitro, the blockage of TNF decreases the production of proinflammatory mediators and enzymes in OA cartilage explants [20]. Because of these inflammatory mediators, the application of TNFA inhibitors from rheumatoid and psoriatic arthritis trials has been adopted in this context.

Infliximab appears to have potential effect on disease progression. In an open-label pilot study in erosive hand OA patients, there was a reduction in anatomical lesion radiological score at 12 months of follow-up [21]. The structural effect was further evaluated in patients with rheumatoid arthritis—infliximab (3–10 mg/kg) reduced both the radiological progression of existing hand OA and the incidence of secondary hand OA after 3 years of follow-up, compared to patients not treated with infliximab (6% versus 13% respectively) [22].

A small, open-label trial of 12 patients that received six fortnightly adalimumab injections for 12 weeks failed to demonstrate any pain improvement [23]. Similar results were seen with the Dora Study, a phase III randomized, double-blinded, placebo controlled study with adalimumab 40 mg (two subcutaneous injections at a 15-day interval versus placebo) for hand OA was conducted. The primary outcome was the percentage of patients with an improvement of more than 50% in the visual analogue scale between weeks 0 and 6, and this was not achieved [24].

Another randomized controlled trial in 60 patients with erosive OA demonstrating ongoing progression of erosive change or new erosion formation, failed to demonstrate any clinically significant change in symptomatology [25]. However, the adalimumab-treated group (40 mg every 2 weeks for 1 year) showed a significant decrease in the number of new erosions, which is its main end point. This is especially in the patient subset with clinical interphalangeal joint swelling at baseline.

DLX-105 (ESBA105) is a fully human antibody fragment of VH/VL domains that inhibits TNFA. In pre-clinical studies; in vitro cell cultures and animal studies, ESBA105 demonstrated inhibitory activity on TNFA similar to Infliximab and has the ability to penetrate the cartilage, synovium and surrounding tissues [26]. The phase II trial of DLX-105 has been completed (clinicaltrials.gov: NCT00819572), however no results have been published to date.

The failure of TNFA blockade may indicate that it is not the appropriate agent in a condition that only exhibits low-level inflammation in comparison to rheumatoid arthritis. The timing of drug delivery in OA, a condition with fluctuating inflammation will impact on its overall effectiveness on symptomatology. It is important to note that despite limited effects on pain in OA patients, there may be a potential effect on disease progression and erosion development.

Interleukin 1 beta inhibitors

IL1 is capable of inducing expression of MMPs and other catabolic genes, which stimulate the turnover of extracellular matrix remodelling. IL1B antagonist therapies, directed towards receptor targets (IL1 receptor antagonist protein, IL1RA), prevent the interaction of IL1B with cell surface receptors. IL1B antagonist has been shown to prevent cartilage breakdown in a multitude of animal models [27,28].

A phase II clinical trial with intra-articular injection of recombinant IL1RA, anakinra, showed promise and safety [29]; however, a randomized, multicentre, double-blind, placebo-controlled trial in 170 patients with knee OA failed to yield any statistical differences. The 160 patients who completed the study were randomized in a 2:2:1 ratio of single intra-articular injections at 50 mg, 150 mg of

anakinra, or placebo respectively, with primary outcome being the Western Ontario and McMaster Universities Osteoarthritis Index (WOMAC) score [30].

AMG-108, a fully humanized monoclonal antibody that binds Typ1 IL1R, and non-selectively inhibits the activity of both interleukin 1 alpha (IL1A) and IL1B, also failed to elicit a significant difference in WOMAC pain score compared with placebo in 159 patients with knee OA after 3 months of treatment [31].

A phase II, proof of concept study with subcutaneous injection of gevokizumab (NCT01683396), has been completed with no results published to date. Phase II study of ABT-981, an anti-IL1A/B dual variable domain-immunoglobulin is under recruitment (NCT02087904), with phase I studies that whilst had good tolerability in healthy individuals, showed a trend towards decreased absolute neutrophil count [32].

Matrix metalloproteinase inhibitors

MMP genes are expressed in all aspects of the articular joint, and one of its main roles is the enzymatic collagen breakdown in articular cartilage. Over 27 MMPs have been identified, with MMP1, MMP8, MMP13, and MMP14, which are collagenases, being implicated in cartilage collagen destruction [33,34]. MMP13 seems to be the most important one expressed in OA cartilage [35]. The approach of MMP inhibition has to date been relatively unsuccessful due to intolerable musculoskeletal side effects, likely due to the inhibition of interstitial collagenase. These side effects include musculoskeletal pain, Dupuytren's contracture, and frozen shoulder [36,37]. However, even with MMP1-sparing compounds such as PG-116800, the side effects are still seen [36].

Mitogen-activated protein kinase inhibitor

Given the side effects of MMP inhibition, alternate signal transduction pathways, which regulate MMP, are being examined. Mitogen-activated protein kinases (MAPKs) are also central regulators of cell signalling pathways that control cell proliferation, survival, and matrix synthesis [38]. They also regulates MMP production by chondrocytes [39].

The MAPKs include p38 MAPK (p38), extracellular signal-regulated kinase (ERK), and c-Jun N-terminal kinase (JNK). These are constitutively expressed in chondrocytes as well as most cell types [40]. In animal models of rheumatoid arthritis, p38 inhibitors have been shown to maintain joint integrity with a reduction in loss of cartilage and bone [41,42]. Several p38 inhibitors have been investigated in clinical trials, with only a few (VX702, SCIO469 and BIRB796) progressing to phase II trials due to poor safety profile with associated liver and central nervous system adverse effects [43]. The phase II clinical trial of FX005 (NCT01291914) has been completed with no published results.

Inducible nitric oxide synthase inhibition

Nitric oxide is involved in cartilage inflammation, catabolism, and pain associated with OA [44]. One isoform of nitric oxide synthase, named inducible nitric oxide synthase (iNOS), is highly expressed in chondrocytes. It activates MMPs, inhibits collagen and proteoglycan synthesis, and induces chondrocyte cell death [45].

Phase II/III study of cindunistat hydrochloride maleate (SD-6010), an inhibitor of iNOS (NCT00565812), has been completed in patients with symptomatic knee OA. The study did not demonstrate reduction in the rate of joint space narrowing. Post hoc analysis showed a beneficial effect at 48 weeks with joint space narrowing in patients with KL grade 2 OA. This effect was not sustained at the 96-week follow-up [13].

Bradykinin B2 receptor antagonist

The synovium in an osteoarthritic joint generates bradykinin, a vasodilator and inflammatory peptide. Bradykinin, through the B2 receptor, induces the release of proinflammatory cytokines including interleukins, cyclooxygenase, lipoxygenase, and MMPs, via the activation of chondrocytes and transcription factor NFKB. Through the activation of endothelial cells, it induces angiogenesis, and promotes vessel permeability, growth, and remodelling.

Icatibant (HOE140), an intra-articular peptidic B2 receptor antagonist, showed some initial potential with analgesic effects with high dosages [46]. However, further development of the drug was suspended possibly due to lack of efficacy [47]. Fasitibant (NCT02205814) has completed a phase II trial (ALBATROSS-3), with no published results to date.

Cartilage catabolism and anabolism

Bone morphogenetic protein 7

Bone morphogenetic protein 7 (BMP7), previously termed osteogenic protein-1, is expressed by human chondrocytes. It is a member of the transforming growth factor beta superfamily, which contributes to the repair of mature tissues [48]. Cartilage repair is achieved through the stimulation of proteoglycan, collagen, and hyaluronic acid synthesis. BMP7 also suppresses catabolic activities of cytokines, including IL1, IL6, IL8, MMP1, and MMP13 [49].

Recombinant BMP7, eptotermin alfa (NCT01111045), is undergoing a phase II trial. The phase I trial showed promise with 33 participants receiving weekly intra-articular BMP7 injections with a treatment randomization allocation in a 3:1 ratio. At 12-week follow-up, there was a trend towards symptomatic improvement in those who received 0.1 mg and 0.3 mg doses compared with placebo. Similar trends were seen in secondary endpoints of WOMAC pain and function subscales with the treatment group [50].

Fibroblast growth factor

Fibroblast growth factor (FGF)-18 is thought to have anabolic effects on cartilage, stimulating proteoglycan synthesis and cartilage growth in animal models of injury-induced OA [51]. This is likely through the activation of FGF receptor 3, thus increasing matrix formation, and at the same time as inhibiting cell proliferation [52].

Two phase I trials of intra-articular recombinant human FGF18 for knee OA treatment, have demonstrated a statistically significant dose-dependent improvement in tibiofemoral cartilage volume and reduction in joint space narrowing at the 12-month interval [53]. Sprifermin (AS902330) is still in its phase II trial (NCT01919164), with recruitment being concluded. Its initial proof of concept, double-blinded study recruited 192 knee OA patients who were randomized to single-ascending doses of sprifermin or placebo. Cartilage thickness at 6 and 12 months were measured using magnetic resonance imaging, and joint space width was assessed with X-rays. No statistical dose response in central medial tibiofemoral compartment cartilage or volume was seen at 12 months. However, a statistically significant dose-dependent reduction in loss of total and lateral tibiofemoral cartilage thickness and volume, and joint space width was observed. There were no safety or injection site adverse events [54].

Bone remodelling

Calcitonin

The main role of calcitonin is to regulate calcium homeostasis. It is a 32-amino acid polypeptide hormone produced primarily by the parafollicular C cells in the thyroid gland. It binds to calcitonin receptors on osteoclasts and promotes the inhibition of bone resorption, and thus increases the activity of osteoblasts. Calcitonin has shown to induce inhibition of MMP activity and cartilage degradation in both *in vivo* and *ex vivo* studies with cartilage explants and beneficial activities are seen in bone and cartilage of animal models [55].

Whilst it can be extracted from the ultimobranchial glands of salmon, most trial compounds are synthetic or recombinant peptides. It is mainly administrated in a parenteral or intranasal route.

Calcitonin inhalation therapy can potentially relieve pain. A clinical study of 50 Turkish female patients receiving a dose of 200 IU nasal calcitonin produced significant improvements in WOMAC pain, function, and stiffness scores, as well as in visual analogue scale, and 20-metre walking time [56]. However, the nasal calcitonin treatment was combined with exercise therapy, thus rendering it impossible to separate the effects of the individual therapies.

Pilot studies of salmon calcitonin comparing two doses of salmon calcitonin formulated with a 5-CNAC carrier against placebo demonstrated no difference in the 0.5 mg group. The placebo group and the group receiving 1 mg of salmon calcitonin exhibited a similar decrease in pain score, but a considerable improvement was seen in the function score with the two treatment groups [57].

A phase III trial of oral salmon calcitonin was conducted. A total of 1169 participants received either 0.8 mg twice-daily oral salmon calcitonin or placebo. After 24 months, those in the calcitonin group did not achieve the co-primary endpoint, which was improvement in joint space width. There was an increase in the cartilage volume, perhaps suggesting potential structure-modifying effect. Significant improvements in the WOMAC pain, function, and stiffness scores were also seen [58]. Another phase III study of oral salmon calcitonin (NCT00704847) also failed to provide any clinical benefits in patients. The study terminated male subjects early due to an imbalance in prostate cancer events [59].

Bisphosphonates

The therapeutic basis of bisphosphonates is based on their direct inhibitory effect on the function of osteoclasts, thus they have the potential to retard subchondral bone remodelling. In a study of patients with progressive OA, they were found to have higher urinary levels of C-terminal telopeptide of type II collagen (CTX-II), a marker of cartilage degradation [60]. Bisphosphonates can also exert a slight immunomodulating effect via the inhibition of proinflammatory cytokines, with etidronate *in vitro*, showing some inhibitory effect on MMPs when it binds to human cartilage [61].

Clinical trials of risedronate to date have yielded conflicting results. The BRISK trial [62] was a 1-year, double-blinded, placebo-controlled trial of patients with mild to moderate OA of the medial compartment of the knee. Patients were randomized to once-daily risedronate (5 mg or 15 mg) or placebo. The intention-to-treat population consisted of 284 patients. Those who received 15 mg of risedronate showed improvement in the WOMAC index, significant improvement of the patient global assessment, and decreased used of walking aids.

The Knee OA Structural Arthritis (KOSTAR) study [60], comprised of 2483 patient with medial compartment knee OA and 2–4 mm of joint space width (determined by fluoroscopically position, semi-flexed view radiography). Participants were enrolled in two parallel studies in North America and the European Union over 2 years. In Europe, risedronate dosages of 5 mg/day, 15 mg/day, and 35 mg/week were given, and in North America, 50 mg/week. The groups were compared against placebo. No treatment effects of risedronate were demonstrated, with all groups reporting a reduction in signs and symptoms measured by WOMAC and patient global assessment scores. There was no significant reduction in radiographic progression.

A reduction in the level of CTX-II was observed not surprisingly in the risedronate-treated groups. The lack of proper stratification of cohort in this study may have affected the outcome, given the population studied had little disease progression during the study period.

In a recent subanalysis of the KOSTAR study, subjects with accelerated cartilage degradation at baseline, and whose CTX-II levels returned to low levels at 6 months had a significant reduction in radiological progression compared with subjects with elevated CTX-II levels both at baseline and at 6 months [63].

Zoledronic acid, a once-yearly bisphosphonate infusion, has shown promise with the initial trial of a single infusion of zoledronic acid compared with placebo, showing a significant reduction in areal bone marrow lesion size at 6 months with a trend after 12 months. Significant reduction in visual analogue scale pain score was also seen at 6 months, which was not sustained by 12 months [64]. There is a phase III trial with annual zoledronic acid infusion underway in Australia (ANZCTR registry: ACTRN12613000039785).

Strontium

Strontium ranelate, an authorized treatment for osteoporosis in postmenopausal women, is a strontium salt of ranelic acid, an organic acid that chelated metal cations. The drug is classified as a dual action bone agent, given its ability to both increase the deposition of new bone by osteoblasts, and reduce bone resorption by osteoclasts, thereby improving the overall architecture of the bone. It has shown to lessen the progression of radiographic features of spinal OA and back pain in females with concomitant osteoporosis and spinal OA [65].

The SEKOIA trial was a 3-year, phase III, double-blinded, randomized control trial of patients randomly allocated to strontium ranelate 1 g/day, 2 g/day, or placebo was recently conducted. Treatment with strontium ranelate was associated with smaller degradations in joint space width, with treatment–placebo differences of 0.14 (standard error (SE) 0.04; 95% confidence interval (CI) 0.05–0.23, p <0.001) for 1 g/day and 0.10 (SE 0.04; 95% CI 0.02–0.19, p = 0.018 for 2 g/day). Strontium ranelate at 2 g/day also improved WOMAC total score and pain subscores.

MRI assessing cartilage volume loss and bone marrow lesions was done in a subset of patients in the SEKOIA trial. Treatment at 2 g/day of strontium ranelate was associated with a significant reduction in the cartilage volume loss in the plateau and bone marrow lesion progression in the medial compartment at 36 months [66].

Conclusion

There is a strong rationale for the development of disease-modifying agents in the context of OA. Current approaches to managing the disease remain largely palliative and focused on symptoms. There is widespread demonstration of the ability to modify disease in the context of preclinical models; however, this has not been translated to the human disease to the satisfaction of regulatory bodies at this point in time. There are a number of products currently in testing that demonstrate great promise although there remain considerable challenges to the demonstration of disease modification.

Acknowledgements

David J. Hunter is supported by an NHMRC practitioner fellowship.

We appreciate the valuable contributions made by the authors of this chapter in the prior version of the textbook. Some of the text from the previous chapter has been included in this version.

References

1. Brandt KD, Dieppe P, Radin EL. Etiopathogenesis of osteoarthritis. *Rheum Dis Clin North Am* 2008; 34(3):531–59.
2. Eyre DR. Collagens and cartilage matrix homeostasis. *Clin Orthop Relat Res* 2004; 42(Suppl):S118–22.
3. Guccione AA, Felson DT, Anderson JJ, et al. The effects of specific medical conditions on the functional limitations of elders in the Framingham Study. *Am J Public Health* 1994; 84(3):351–8.
4. Hannan MT, Felson DT, Pincus T. Analysis of the discordance between radiographic changes and knee pain in osteoarthritis of the knee. *J Rheumatol* 2000; 27(6):1513–7.
5. Hunter DJ, Schofield D, Callander E. The individual and socioeconomic impact of osteoarthritis. *Nat Rev Rheumatol* 2014; 10(7):437–41.
6. Hunter DJ. Osteoarthritis. *Best Pract Res Clin Rheumatol* 2011; 25(6):801–14.
7. Yu SP, Hunter DJ. Emerging drugs for the treatment of knee osteoarthritis. *Expert Opin Emerg Drugs* 2015; 20(3):361–78.
8. Muthuri SG, McWilliams DF, Doherty M, Zhang W. History of knee injuries and knee osteoarthritis: a meta-analysis of observational studies. *Osteoarthritis Cartilage* 2011; 19(11):1286–93.
9. Matthews GL, Hunter DJ. Emerging drugs for osteoarthritis. *Expert Opin Emerg Drugs* 2011; 16 (3):479–91.
10. Hunter DJ, Altman RD, Cicuttini F, et al. OARSI Clinical Trials Recommendations: knee imaging in clinical trials in osteoarthritis. *Osteoarthritis Cartilage* 2015; 23(5):698–715.
11. Conaghan PG, Hunter DJ, Maillefert JF, Reichmann WM, Losina E. Summary and recommendations of the OARSI FDA osteoarthritis Assessment of Structural Change Working Group. *Osteoarthritis Cartilage* 2011; 19(5):606–10.
12. Hunter DJ, Losina E, Guermazi A, et al. A pathway and approach to biomarker validation and qualification for osteoarthritis clinical trials. *Curr Drug Targets* 2010; 11(5):536–45.
13. Hellio le Graverand MP, Clemmer RS, Redifer P, et al. A 2-year randomised, double-blind, placebo-controlled, multicentre study of oral selective iNOS inhibitor, cindunistat (SD-6010), in patients with symptomatic osteoarthritis of the knee. *Ann Rheum Dis* 2013; 72(2):187–95.
14. Hunter DJ, Guermazi A, Roemer F, Zhang Y, Neogi T. Structural correlates of pain in joints with osteoarthritis. *Osteoarthritis Cartilage* 2013; 21(9):1170–8.
15. Zhang W, Robertson J, Jones AC, Dieppe PA, Doherty M. The placebo effect and its determinants in osteoarthritis: meta-analysis of randomised controlled trials. *Ann Rheum Dis* 2008; 67(12):1716–23.
16. Little CB, Hunter DJ. Post-traumatic osteoarthritis: from mouse models to clinical trials. *Nat Rev Rheumatol* 2013; 9(8):485–97.
17. Losina E, Daigle ME, Suter LG, et al. Disease-modifying drugs for knee osteoarthritis: can they be cost-effective? *Osteoarthritis Cartilage* 2013; 21(5):655–67.
18. Stannus O, Jones G, Cicuttini F, et al. Circulating levels of IL-6 and TNF-alpha are associated with knee radiographic osteoarthritis and knee cartilage loss in older adults. *Osteoarthritis Cartilage* 2010; 18(11):1441–7.

19. Sellam J, Berenbaum F. The role of synovitis in pathophysiology and clinical symptoms of osteoarthritis. *Nat Rev Rheumatol* 2010; 6(11):625–35.

20. Kobayashi M, Squires GR, Mousa A, et al. Role of interleukin-1 and tumor necrosis factor alpha in matrix degradation of human osteoarthritic cartilage. *Arthritis Rheum* 2005; 52(1):128–35.

21. Fioravanti A, Fabbroni M, Cerase A, Galeazzi M. Treatment of erosive osteoarthritis of the hands by intra-articular infliximab injections: a pilot study. *Rheumatol Int* 2009; 29 (8):961–5.

22. Guler-Yuksel M, Allaart CF, Watt I, et al. Treatment with TNF-alpha inhibitor infliximab might reduce hand osteoarthritis in patients with rheumatoid arthritis. *Osteoarthritis Cartilage* 2010; 18(10):1256–62.

23. Magnano MD, Chakravarty EF, Broudy C, et al. A pilot study of tumor necrosis factor inhibition in erosive/inflammatory osteoarthritis of the hands. *J Rheumatol* 2007; 34(6):1323–7.

24. Chevalier X, Ravaud P, Maheu E, et al. Adalimumab in patients with hand osteoarthritis refractory to analgesics and NSAIDs: a randomised, multicentre, double-blind, placebo-controlled trial. *Ann Rheum Dis* 2015; 74(9):1697–705.

25. Verbruggen G, Wittoek R, Vander Cruyssen B, Elewaut D. Tumour necrosis factor blockade for the treatment of erosive osteoarthritis of the interphalangeal finger joints: a double blind, randomised trial on structure modification. *Ann Rheum Dis* 2012; 71(6):891–8.

26. Urech DM, Feige U, Ewert S, et al. Anti-inflammatory and cartilage-protecting effects of an intra-articularly injected anti-TNF{alpha} single-chain Fv antibody (ESBA105) designed for local therapeutic use. *Ann Rheum Dis* 2010; 69(2):443–9.

27. Pelletier JP, Caron JP, Evans C, et al. In vivo suppression of early experimental osteoarthritis by interleukin-1 receptor antagonist using gene therapy. *Arthritis Rheum* 1997; 40(6):1012–9.

28. Santangelo KS, Nuovo GJ, Bertone AL. In vivo reduction or blockade of interleukin-1beta in primary osteoarthritis influences expression of mediators implicated in pathogenesis. *Osteoarthritis Cartilage* 2012; 20(12):1610–8.

29. Chevalier X, Giraudeau B, Conrozier T, et al. Safety study of intraarticular injection of interleukin 1 receptor antagonist in patients with painful knee osteoarthritis: a multicenter study. *J Rheumatol* 2005; 32(7):1317–23.

30. Chevalier X, Goupille P, Beaulieu AD, et al. Intraarticular injection of anakinra in osteoarthritis of the knee: a multicenter, randomized, double-blind, placebo-controlled study. *Arthritis Rheum* 2009; 61(3):344–52.

31. Cohen SB, Proudman S, Kivitz AJ, et al. A randomized, double-blind study of AMG 108 (a fully human monoclonal antibody to IL-1R1) in patients with osteoarthritis of the knee. *Arthritis Res Ther* 2011; 13(4):R125.

32. Wang SX, Medema J, Kosloski M, et al. Interleukin-1 dual variable-domain immunoglobulin reduces multiple inflammatory markers in knee osteoarthritis patients. *Ann Rheum Dis* 2014; 73(Suppl 2):756.

33. Davidson RK, Waters JG, Kevorkian L, et al. Expression profiling of metalloproteinases and their inhibitors in synovium and cartilage. *Arthritis Res Ther* 2006; 8(4):R124.

34. Ohuchi E, Imai K, Fujii Y, et al. Membrane type 1 matrix metalloproteinase digests interstitial collagens and other extracellular matrix macromolecules. *J Biol Chem* 1997; 272(4):2446–51.

35. Baragi VM, Becher G, Bendele AM, et al. A new class of potent matrix metalloproteinase 13 inhibitors for potential treatment of osteoarthritis: evidence of histologic and clinical efficacy without musculoskeletal toxicity in rat models. *Arthritis Rheum* 2009; 60(7):2008–18.

36. Krzeski P, Buckland-Wright C, Balint G, et al. Development of musculoskeletal toxicity without clear benefit after administration of PG-116800, a matrix metalloproteinase inhibitor, to patients with knee osteoarthritis: a randomized, 12-month, double-blind, placebo-controlled study. *Arthritis Res Ther* 2007; 9(5):R109.

37. Tu G, Xu W, Huang H, Li S. Progress in the development of matrix metalloproteinase inhibitors. *Curr Med Chem* 2008; 15(14):1388–95.

38. Loeser RF, Erickson EA, Long DL. Mitogen-activated protein kinases as therapeutic targets in osteoarthritis. *Curr Opin Rheumatol* 2008; 20(5):581–6.

39. Starkman BG, Cravero JD, Delcarlo M, Loeser RF. IGF-I stimulation of proteoglycan synthesis by chondrocytes requires activation of the PI 3-kinase pathway but not ERK MAPK. *Biochem J* 2005; 389(Pt 3):723–9.

40. Chun JS. Expression, activity, and regulation of MAP kinases in cultured chondrocytes. *Methods Mol Med* 2004; 100:291–306.

41. Badger AM, Griswold DE, Kapadia R, et al. Disease-modifying activity of SB 242235, a selective inhibitor of p38 mitogen-activated protein kinase, in rat adjuvant-induced arthritis. *Arthritis Rheum* 2000; 43(1):175–83.

42. Medicherla S, Ma JY, Mangadu R, et al. A selective p38 alpha mitogen-activated protein kinase inhibitor reverses cartilage and bone destruction in mice with collagen-induced arthritis. *J Pharmacol Exp Ther* 2006; 318(1):132–41.

43. Zhang J, Shen B, Lin A. Novel strategies for inhibition of the p38 MAPK pathway. *Trends Pharmacol Sci* 2007; 28(6):286–95.

44. Abramson SB. Nitric oxide in inflammation and pain associated with osteoarthritis. *Arthritis Res Ther* 2008; 10(Suppl 2):S2.

45. Schnitzer TJ. New pharmacologic approaches in the management of osteoarthritis. *Arthritis Care Res (Hoboken)* 2010; 62(8):1174–80.

46. Song IH, Althoff CE, Hermann KG, et al. Contrast-enhanced ultrasound in monitoring the efficacy of a bradykinin receptor 2 antagonist in painful knee osteoarthritis compared with MRI. *Ann Rheum Dis* 2009; 68(1):75–83.

47. Meini S, Maggi CA. Knee osteoarthritis: a role for bradykinin? *Inflamm Res* 2008; 57(8):351–61.

48. Griffith DL, Keck PC, Sampath TK, Rueger DC, Carlson WD. Three-dimensional structure of recombinant human osteogenic protein 1: structural paradigm for the transforming growth factor beta superfamily. *Proc Natl Acad Sci U S A* 1996; 93(2):878–83.

49. Elshaier AM, Hakimiyan AA, Rappoport L, Rueger DC, Chubinskaya S. Effect of interleukin-1beta on osteogenic protein 1-induced signaling in adult human articular chondrocytes. *Arthritis Rheum* 2009; 60(1):143–54.

50. Hunter DJ, Pike MC, Jonas BL, et al. Phase 1 safety and tolerability study of BMP-7 in symptomatic knee osteoarthritis. *BMC Musculoskelet Disord* 2010; 11:232.

51. Moore EE, Bendele AM, Thompson DL, et al. Fibroblast growth factor-18 stimulates chondrogenesis and cartilage repair in a rat model of injury-induced osteoarthritis. *Osteoarthritis Cartilage* 2005; 13(7):623–31.

52. Ellman MB, An HS, Muddasani P, Im HJ. Biological impact of the fibroblast growth factor family on articular cartilage and intervertebral disc homeostasis. *Gene* 2008; 420(1):82–9.

53. Mastbergen SC, Saris DB, Lafeber FP. Functional articular cartilage repair: here, near, or is the best approach not yet clear? *Nat Rev Rheumatol* 2013; 9(5):277–90.

54. Lohmander LS, Hellot S, Dreher D, et al. Intraarticular sprifermin (recombinant human fibroblast growth factor 18) in knee osteoarthritis: a randomized, double-blind, placebo-controlled trial. *Arthritis Rheumatol* 2014; 66(7):1820–31.

55. Karsdal MA, Sondergaard BC, Arnold M, Christiansen C. Calcitonin affects both bone and cartilage: a dual action treatment for osteoarthritis? *Ann N Y Acad Sci* 2007; 1117:181–95.

56. Armagan O, Serin DK, Calisir C, et al. Inhalation therapy of calcitonin relieves osteoarthritis of the knee. *J Korean Med Sci* 2012; 27(11):1405–10.

57. Manicourt DH, Azria M, Mindeholm L, Thonar EJ, Devogelaer JP. Oral salmon calcitonin reduces Lequesne's algofunctional index scores and decreases urinary and serum levels of biomarkers of joint metabolism in knee osteoarthritis. *Arthritis Rheum* 2006; 54(10):3205–11.

58. Karsdal MA, Alexandersen P, John MR, et al. Oral calcitonin demonstrated symptom-modifying efficacy and increased cartilage volume: results from a 2-year phase 3 trial in patients with osteoarthritis of the knee. *Osteoarthritis Cartilage* 2011; 19(Suppl 1):S35.

59. Karsdal MA, Byrjalsen I, Alexandersen P, et al. Treatment of symptomatic knee osteoarthritis with oral salmon calcitonin: results from two phase 3 trials. *Osteoarthritis Cartilage* 2015; 23(4):532–43.

60. Bingham CO, 3rd, Buckland-Wright JC, Garnero P, et al. Risedronate decreases biochemical markers of cartilage degradation but does not decrease symptoms or slow radiographic progression in patients with medial compartment osteoarthritis of the knee: results of the two-year multinational knee osteoarthritis structural arthritis study. *Arthritis Rheum* 2006; 54(11):3494–507.

61. Saag KG. Bisphosphonates for osteoarthritis prevention: 'Holy Grail' or not? *Ann Rheum Dis* 2008; 67(10):1358–9.

62. Spector TD, Conaghan PG, Buckland-Wright JC, et al. Effect of risedronate on joint structure and symptoms of knee osteoarthritis: results of the BRISK randomized, controlled trial [ISRCTN01928173]. *Arthritis Res Ther* 2005; 7(3):R625–33.

63. Garnero P, Aronstein WS, Cohen SB, et al. Relationships between biochemical markers of bone and cartilage degradation with radiological progression in patients with knee osteoarthritis receiving risedronate: the Knee Osteoarthritis Structural Arthritis randomized clinical trial. *Osteoarthritis Cartilage* 2008; 16(6):660–6.

64. Laslett LL, Dore DA, Quinn SJ, et al. Zoledronic acid reduces knee pain and bone marrow lesions over 1 year: a randomised controlled trial. *Ann Rheum Dis* 2012; 71(8):1322–8.

65. Bruyere O, Delferriere D, Roux C, et al. Effects of strontium ranelate on spinal osteoarthritis progression. *Ann Rheum Dis* 2008; 67(3):335–9.

66. Pelletier JP, Roubille C, Raynauld JP, et al. Disease-modifying effect of strontium ranelate in a subset of patients from the Phase III knee osteoarthritis study SEKOIA using quantitative MRI: reduction in bone marrow lesions protects against cartilage loss. *Ann Rheum Dis* 2015; 74(2):422–9.

SECTION 11

Delivery of care

CHAPTER 36

Delivery (organization and outcome)

Caroline A. Brand and Ilana N. Ackerman

Introduction

The inclusion of this chapter about models of care (MOC) in a textbook on osteoarthritis (OA) reflects growth in the burden of chronic disease over time, as well as pharmacological, technological, and societal changes that have necessitated new ways of thinking about the design and delivery of healthcare services.

The aims of this chapter are to inform readers about:

◆ factors that have influenced healthcare reforms for people with chronic conditions

◆ the development and characteristics of MOC for people with chronic conditions

◆ the evolution of OA MOC and evidence for their effectiveness

◆ ways in which to improve the design, implementation, and evaluation of MOC for chronic conditions

◆ the design of future OA MOC.

Factors driving healthcare reform

Healthcare reform has been driven by a complex array of factors. These include not only a rise in the prevalence of chronic conditions but also other factors including sociodemographic changes associated with ageing populations; economic issues associated with advancing technology and expensive pharmaceutical agents necessitating greater health system fiscal constraint; changes in consumer needs, expectations, and demands; as well as a community demand for greater transparency and accountability of healthcare managers, healthcare providers, policymakers, and funding providers [1].

The rise of chronic conditions

The epidemiology and impact of chronic conditions, including OA, on health-related, economic, and social outcomes has been well documented. In 2002, the World Health Organization (WHO) reported that chronic conditions were responsible for 60% of the global health burden and this was projected to increase to 80% by the year 2020 [2]. Further, the WHO acknowledged that there was a global paucity of health plans for management of chronic conditions. According to the landmark 2010 Global Burden of Disease Study, musculoskeletal conditions such as low back pain and OA now represent the second greatest cause of disability worldwide

and are responsible for 21% of all years lived with disability globally [3].

Gaps in care for people with chronic conditions

There is evidence that management of chronic conditions is suboptimal, with an early study reporting that about half the adults in the United States received care that was not in accordance with clinical practice guideline recommendations [4,5]. Such discrepancies in documentation and/or receipt of guideline-recommended generic and condition-specific care continue to be reported [6], including for people with OA and other musculoskeletal disorders (7–13).

The issues facing people with chronic conditions are both generic and disease specific. Healthcare is frequently not timely, accessible, or continuous and at times exposes the individual to harm. There is also failure to provide care according to recommended disease-specific guidelines, including underuse of effective treatment, overuse or inappropriate care, and more rarely, deliberate misuse of care [1].

Based on the changing needs of people with chronic conditions and evidence about suboptimal care provision, international policymakers [1,2] identified the key deficiencies in management of people with chronic conditions related to the organization and design of care, in particular:

◆ lack of integration between healthcare sectors and healthcare providers

◆ failure to put the patient and their family at the centre of care, to provide them with care in their community where possible, and to adequately support them with effective self-management strategies

◆ inadequate development of effective healthcare teams to coordinate care and deliver effective treatment based on evidence and patient preferences

◆ inadequate information and communications systems that would allow identification of at risk populations, provide decision support for healthcare providers and patients, and collect data for monitoring and evaluation.

There is, therefore, a strong rationale for healthcare reform to ensure that people with chronic conditions (including OA) are provided with evidence-based care that optimizes health outcomes for the individual, for communities, and for populations.

Models of care: definitions and development

Terminology and definitions

Investigating MOC for chronic conditions such as OA presents researchers and clinicians with a new lexicon of terms and theories that derive from multiple areas other than clinical medicine, including the social sciences, economics, and industry. The term 'model' can itself be defined in various ways and frequently, terms such as 'model', 'theory', or 'conceptual framework' are used interchangeably [14]. Conceptual theories and models present systematic ways of understanding an event, a process, or human behaviour [15] but often require more strategic and operational frameworks to facilitate their implementation [16].

Models of care are constructions that reflect a specific purpose and may be constrained by the nature of their use [15] at different levels of the health system: for international or national purposes (macro level); for jurisdictional and organizational purposes (meso level); and at the level of the clinical team, patients, and their families (micro level). Differences in MOC therefore largely reflect the composition of the developers and are inherently politicized by the 'diverse values, interests and scope of influence' of stakeholders [2].

At higher levels of the health system, the development of MOC is likely to be more formal and explicitly documented. In contrast, at the level of clinical teams and individual clinicians, changes in service MOC often occur in informal, incremental ways. Ideally, MOC should be designed for integration across health sector boundaries.

For the purposes of this chapter, the term MOC will refer to the conceptual design of a healthcare system developed at any level of the health system, which may or may not be accompanied by operational frameworks that articulate recommendations about actions, implementation and sustainability methods, and evaluation (Figure 36.1).

General principles in developing models of care for chronic conditions

Shared aspirations and fundamental principles can be discerned amongst MOC. Aspirational outcomes are based on quality theory, namely that care should be [1]:

- equitable
- timely and accessible
- effective
- appropriate
- safe
- efficient
- acceptable.

In order to attain these outcomes, international policymakers have recommended key principles specifying that care should be [1]:

- designed to be patient-centred
- coordinated to provide continuous support with ongoing monitoring and ready access to care when needed [2]
- organized to provide multidisciplinary team-based input as required
- integrated across healthcare sectors and healthcare providers
- provided appropriately in order to avoid underuse, overuse, or misuse

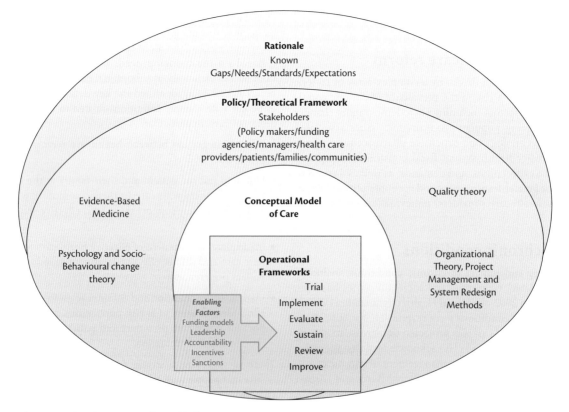

Figure 36.1 Development and implementation of a model of care.

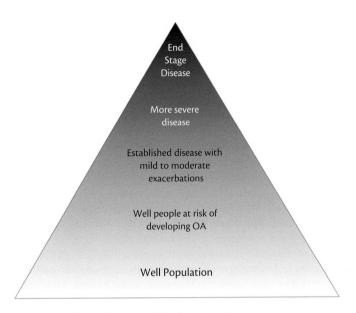

Figure 36.2 Chronic disease population hierarchy of risk.

♦ supported for healthcare providers and consumers by provision of healthcare information systems and decision support.

Further, there is a spectrum of populations that need to be considered within a hierarchical pyramid of risk (Figure 36.2), with the large base representing the population of well people and those at risk in the community and fewer people with established or more severe disease. The tip of the pyramid represents the small proportion of people with severe, end-stage disease.

National and international (macro-level) models of care for chronic conditions

The WHO Innovative Care for Chronic Conditions (ICCC) model [2] is an example of a macro healthcare model based on the

Chronic Care Model (CCM) [17,18]. The well-established CCM, a generic model for chronic condition management in primary care, includes the key domains of self-management support, delivery system design, decision support, clinical information systems, organization of care, and community linkages. It was designed in the mid 1990s and refined and expanded over the following decade [18–21]. As a macro model, the ICCC is strongly policy and advocacy oriented and has a public health focus on populations rather than individuals and on prevention to support risk reduction. As a high-level model, it does not provide detailed guidance about service components, service delivery methods, implementation, or evaluation but does provide a list of actions to be undertaken at each level of the health system (Table 36.1).

It is difficult to ascertain the effectiveness of a macro-level MOC. There is indirect evidence about the effectiveness of WHO ICCC policy from a recent WHO global survey of national capacity for the prevention and control of non-communicable diseases [22]. In 2010, in comparison to a previous survey, there had been a marked rise in the proportion of countries with chronic condition policies, plans, or strategies. However, only 79% of those with a policy indicated that it was operational and 71% had an operational policy with dedicated funding attached to it. Overall, the report identified ongoing major gaps in infrastructure, inadequate implementation and funding of policies, inadequate population surveillance, and insufficient funding for surveillance, particularly in lower-income countries. With regard to OA-specific macro MOC effectiveness, an Australian study also reported gaps in implementation of policy into practice for OA [23].

Meso and micro levels: service models of care

Early attempts to reduce the evidence gap and improve care for people with chronic conditions were focused at the micro level of the clinical team (including clinicians, patients, and their families) and involved implementation of evidence-based clinical practice guidelines (EB-CPG). However, the reported effectiveness of EB-CPG in changing practice and health outcomes has been varied [24,25], with multiple barriers identified that relate to EB-CPG

Table 36.1 WHO Innovative Care for Chronic Conditions[a] proposed actions for the healthcare system

Micro level	Meso level	Macro level
Patients and families are: ♦ Informed about their condition ♦ Motivated to change and sustain health behaviours and self-manage their condition ♦ Prepared with behavioural skills to self-manage their condition(s) ***Healthcare teams are:*** ♦ Informed about their roles and responsibilities ♦ Organized as teams ***Community partners are:*** ♦ Informed and skilled in management of chronic conditions ♦ Able to deliver services previously provided in the acute healthcare system	***Health care organizations*** create an environment to support chronic condition management through development of: ♦ Quality focus ♦ Leadership ♦ Workforce skills and mix ♦ Organization of healthcare teams ♦ Information systems ♦ Support for patient self-management ♦ Planning for continuity and coordination ♦ Community linkages and leadership development ♦ Incentives ♦ Coordination of resources to minimize redundancies	***Governments*** develop a positive policy environment through: ♦ Promoting leadership and advocacy ♦ Targeting policies at the population level ♦ Integrating policies to reduce redundancies ♦ Targeting policies to cross boundaries of specific chronic conditions ♦ Viewing policies and healthcare planning as a dynamic ongoing process, updated in accordance with changing needs, priorities and new information about effective treatments ♦ Promoting consistent financing based on principles of equity and effectiveness ♦ Integrating funding across chronic conditions and across divisions of the health system and sectors ♦ Developing and allocating resources (e.g. education curricula for clinicians, new types of healthcare workers) ♦ Strengthening partnerships among government sectors

[a]World Health Organization 2002; Innovative Care for Chronic Conditions: Building Blocks for Action.

factors (complexity, perceived utility, implementability), clinician factors (awareness, access, agreement with recommendations, prioritization, lack of incentives), and patient factors (awareness, understanding, support for behaviour change) [26]. Even when EB-CPG are effectively implemented in the short term, they may not be sustained [27].

These challenges may have reduced the enthusiasm of funding agencies to develop and sustain EB-CPG. A review of guidelines development in Canada between 1994 and 2005 found that over time, fewer guidelines were being released, fewer were based on literature reviews, and fewer strategies were being used to disseminate them [28].

The focus on meso/micro MOC design has shifted away from EB-CPG alone towards a broader systems focus, embedded in quality theory, that addresses not only evidence about therapeutic effectiveness but also outcomes across all quality domains [1]. Meso- and micro-level MOC are frequently overlapping and have an equal or greater focus on service design, service components, and delivery methods than macro models. They are therefore considered together as *service MOC* in this chapter.

There are many different service MOC that have been developed for chronic conditions in general and for specific musculoskeletal conditions such as OA [29,30]. With greater involvement of policy and funding providers in model development, there is a stronger focus on setting system-wide standards of care and accountability [30,31]. Also reflecting developer priorities, especially in acute care settings, service MOC frequently target specific high-risk or end-stage patient subpopulations (the 'tip' of the pyramid, as shown in Figure 36.2), such as patients waiting for joint replacement surgery.

Many chronic condition MOC have been based on the CCM. However, evaluation of the CCM remains challenging as it is a high-level conceptual model rather than a specific intervention and implementation can be difficult in the absence of clearly-defined methods [32]. However, there is evidence to support its effectiveness [17,33] and the CCM has now been widely implemented for a number of chronic conditions, particularly in primary care. A recent study of two large quality improvement collaboratives, one focusing on diabetes/heart failure and the other on depression/asthma, reported high levels of fidelity (congruence with CCM elements) and intensity (quantitative number of change activities) of CCM implementation but depth of implementation (qualitative assessment of likelihood of change making an impact) was less well rated [34]. There was variation in the degree to which the CCM and its specific components were implemented across different settings, and difficulty achieving change across all CCM elements within a 1-year study period. In an OA context, a large primary care study in Germany found that patients did not perceive their OA care to be well aligned with CCM elements, with greater alignment noted for patients who were younger, more educated, and less depressed [35].

Osteoarthritis models of care

A diverse range of OA MOC now exist internationally and these models span the spectrum of OA care from diagnosis, early intervention, education, and self-management support through to end-stage OA and timely provision of joint replacement surgery. OA MOC are commonly multidisciplinary in nature, with many having appropriate procedures in place to target the assessment, treatment, monitoring, referral, and communication aspects of care.

Changes in professional credentialing and greater willingness to redefine traditional work boundaries have also led to new advanced scope or extended practice roles for health professionals working in OA care, including nurses and physiotherapists. These roles have often been introduced with the overarching aims of reducing waiting times for specialist medical or surgical consultation, and minimizing inappropriate referral for joint replacement surgery. Advanced practice roles can include varied tasks such as ordering diagnostic and radiographic tests and postoperative follow-up of patients in joint replacement review clinics [36]. In some countries, nurse practitioners can administer joint injections and commence medications [37], while independent prescribing rights have now been afforded to appropriately-trained physiotherapists in the United Kingdom [38]. Physiotherapy-led musculoskeletal screening and assessment clinics have also been implemented in a number of hospital and community-based settings [39–41], and are designed to triage referrals to orthopaedic surgeons and optimize conservative (non-surgical) OA management. In some MOC, new musculoskeletal coordinator roles have been introduced for the purpose of assessing and monitoring patients, providing disease-relevant education, liaising with medical professionals and managing community referrals [42].

Evaluations of these advanced practice roles have demonstrated relatively short waiting times for assessment [39,43], high levels of satisfaction from patient and medical professional perspectives [36,39], and evidence of concordance with orthopaedic surgeons regarding diagnosis, imaging, and appropriateness for surgical referral (39,44,45]. Some discordance between advance practice physiotherapists and orthopaedic surgeons regarding conservative management options has been reported [44,45] and this may reflect differing professional backgrounds and treatment perspectives. A systematic review in this area found that advanced practice physiotherapists provided equally beneficial or better care than physicians for people with musculoskeletal conditions, with regard to diagnostic accuracy, patient satisfaction, resource use, and costs [46]. The review also reported equivalent clinical outcomes (using measures of pain, disability, quality of life, health status, and psychological well-being) for patients whose musculoskeletal problems were managed by advanced practice physiotherapists, compared to those who were managed by medical professionals.

Effectiveness of osteoarthritis models of care

To date, two systematic reviews have reported the effectiveness of integrated chronic condition management for OA, and both reviews classified the interventions tested with respect to the key elements of the CCM. The first review examined the outcomes of intervention programmes developed for a range of chronic conditions, and identified 12 studies relating to OA [47]. Of these studies, the majority (92%) focused on self-management support interventions such as educational sessions, motivational counselling, and provision of educational materials. Some positive outcomes of the interventions were noted, including improvements in health status and functional status. Only one study evaluated an intervention that was classified as 'health care organisation'; however, this was not further described and specific outcomes were not reported. None of the included studies incorporated clinical information systems, decision support for health professionals, delivery system design, or community resources as key operational design elements within their interventions.

A more recent review aimed to examine the effectiveness and cost-effectiveness of OA MOC [29]. This review included papers that addressed the organization or coordination of OA care between health professionals and/or across healthcare settings. Reflecting changing research priorities over the past decade, the review highlighted a shift in focus away from the evaluation of self-management support programmes to the evaluation of more comprehensive, multidisciplinary MOC. Several papers described complex interventions incorporating multiple operational elements such as delivery system design (or re-design), decision support mechanisms and clinical information systems. The studies reviewed were undertaken in a range of settings including primary care (general practice/primary care physician settings), hospitals, and community settings (allied health professional and pharmacy settings).

This review identified 13 studies that reported research involving coordinated care for lower limb or generalized OA. Of these, 9 papers incorporated an element of delivery system design (of which 7 additionally included other key operational elements). The delivery system design components were diverse, as demonstrated by the following examples:

◆ Provision of a collaborative pain intervention by primary care physicians, with regular telephone support from a psychologist care manager and liaison with relevant health professionals [48]

◆ Nurse care manager assessment, education and ongoing monitoring, liaison between the care manager and medical professionals, and referrals to other health professionals [49]

◆ Introduction of a musculoskeletal coordinator role, with a focus on patient assessment, coordination of community referrals, liaison with general practitioners, and provision of OA-related counselling and goal-setting plans [42]

◆ Introduction of a new clinical pathway for hip and knee replacement surgery that incorporated central intake clinics, care managers, targeted hospital resources, and standardized care guidelines [50]

◆ Introduction of a new clinical system for hip and knee arthritis that included standardized referral processes, a surgical prioritization instrument, dedicated orthopaedic-led and physiotherapy-led arthritis clinics, and provision of patient education [41]

◆ Introduction of a community pharmacy-based service that provided screening for knee OA, analgesia management, patient education, referral for physiotherapist-guided exercise, and communication with primary care physicians [51].

Eight studies evaluated the effectiveness of self-management support interventions, with or without the inclusion of other operational elements. Some of the self-management interventions that were evaluated included telephone-based or face-to-face monitoring, problem-solving, counselling or support sessions, provision of educational materials, group discussions, activity practice, and goal-setting or goal review activities. Three of the included studies incorporated decision support elements, such as standardized perioperative protocols [50], standardized joint replacement prioritization tools [41], and the drafting of treatment orders by care managers for the approval of primary care physicians [48]. Only two studies described the introduction or use of clinical information systems, such as an electronic system designed to capture care

pathway recommendations and produce summary reports regarding clinical outcomes and service utilization [42]. Two studies demonstrated linkage with community resources through referrals to physiotherapy exercise programmes, coordination of care between healthcare sectors (acute care, primary care, and community services) and coordination of community referrals [42,51]. None of the studies incorporated the element of healthcare organization.

Overall, these studies demonstrated only small to moderate effects on health outcomes (including reductions in pain and disability, changes in analgesia usage, and improvements in some dimensions of quality of life) and some improvements in process outcomes (including increased surgical throughput and reduced hospital length of stay), with varied impacts observed across the studies and across the range of outcome measures used [29]. These findings could relate to the heterogeneity of the interventions tested, the limited number of CCM elements included in the models, and the choice of outcome measures that focused predominantly on health outcomes. These limitations could potentially be addressed within the context of multicentre studies that utilize programme evaluation methods and consider broader quality of care outcomes. Table 36.2 summarizes the reported impacts for each of the included studies, and shows that few studies evaluated access or efficiency outcomes. Since publication of this review paper, an additional 'proof-of-concept' study has also been published. This study investigated the effect of multidisciplinary care for people with hip or knee OA referred to an outpatient orthopaedic clinic in the Netherlands [52]. During a single assessment visit, patients were reviewed by a multidisciplinary team (comprising a physical therapist, nurse practitioner, and junior orthopaedic surgeon), and personalized management advice was developed following team discussion. All patient management was undertaken in primary care, with relevant advice and patient education also provided. Assessment results and management advice were promptly communicated to the treating general practitioner. Significant improvements in OA pain and health-related quality of life scores were evident 10 weeks after the intervention; however, a control group was not included for comparison, and a future controlled trial is planned to further evaluate this MOC.

Most recently, a narrative review of musculoskeletal MOC was undertaken [30]. In their review, the authors summarized seven examples of models of OA care including hospital-based joint replacement MOC, self-management support programmes, and coordinated chronic care programmes delivered in hospital, primary care, and community care settings. Six of the seven examples were from Australia, with the remaining example from the United Kingdom. However, only limited outcomes data were available for the identified MOC; three of the seven implemented MOC had no data available, and an additional model was yet to be implemented. Consideration of the three literature reviews in this field shows that there is currently limited evidence for the effectiveness of OA MOC, particularly with regard to the assessment of healthcare access and efficiency outcomes. A major shortcoming in this field is the lack of empirical cost-effectiveness data to support new OA MOC [29]. These data are crucial for evaluating and justifying the value of integrated programmes to healthcare funders. While none of the papers described by Brand et al. [29] initially reported cost-effectiveness outcomes, the authors of one of the included studies have recently reported the results of their subsequent economic evaluation. Marra et al. [53] conducted a cost-utility analysis

Table 36.2 Summary of studies evaluating the impacts of multidisciplinary chronic disease management for osteoarthritis

Study, [reference], country and intervention elements[a] evaluated	Clinician process of care	Patient behaviour change	Health outcomes					
			Clinical	Psychological	Quality of Life	Access	Efficiency	Patient experience
Primary care models								
Dobscha et al. 2009 [48] USA DS, DSD, SMS	++		++	++	− −			− −
Rosemann et al. 2007 [130] Germany DSD, SMS	++		− −		+/−			
Unutzer et al. 2008 [49] USA DSD, SMS		+	+	+				+
Community care models								
Brosseau et al. 2012a [131] Brosseau et al. 2012b [132] Canada SMS		+/−	+/−		+/−			
Marra et al. 2012 [51] Marra et al. 2014[b] [53] Canada CR, DS, DSD	++		+/−		+/−		++	
Murphy et al. 2008 [133] USA SMS		+/−	+/−					
Secondary care models								
Brand et al. 2010 [42] Australia CIS, CR, DS, DSD, SMS	+	+	+					+
Doerr et al. 2013[c] [41] Australia CIS, DS, DSD		+				+	+	+
Gooch et al. 2012 [50] Frank et al 2011[c,d] [74] Canada DS, DSD	++				+/−	++	++	++
Hill et al. 2009 [134] UK DSD	++		− −					++
Hoogeboom et al. 2012 [135] Netherlands SMS		−	−					+/−
McKnight et al. 2010 [54] USA SMS			− −					

(continued)

Table 36.2 Continued

Study, [reference], country and intervention elements[a] evaluated	Clinician process of care	Patient behaviour change	Health outcomes					
			Clinical	Psychological	Quality of Life	Access	Efficiency	Patient experience
Oldmeadow et al. 2007 [39] Australia DSD	+							+

Adapted from Brand et al. 2014 [29].

The impacts are noted as: ++ if there was a reported improvement compared to a comparator group; + if there was a positive outcome in the absence of a comparison group (e.g. improvement over time or patient satisfaction data); – – if there was no difference in outcomes between comparison groups; – if there was no change over time for single-group studies; +/– if impacts varied across outcome measures; no symbol where the outcomes were not measured.

[a]Elements: CIS: Clinical Information Systems; CR: Community Resources; DS: Decision Support; DSD: Delivery System Design, SMS: Self-Management Support.

[b]Related paper reporting cost-utility outcomes.

[c]Statistical analyses not reported, only summary data presented.

[d]Related paper reporting access, efficiency and patient experience outcomes.

of their pharmacy-based multidisciplinary programme designed to screen for and manage knee OA in the community. Costs and incremental cost-effectiveness ratios (ICERs) were evaluated from both the Canadian healthcare system perspective (comprising direct healthcare costs including pharmacists' salaries) and the societal perspective (comprising out-of-pocket healthcare and medication costs, and lost productivity). While costs for the intervention group were higher than for usual care, ICERs indicated that the innovative MOC could be considered cost-effective from both the healthcare system and societal perspectives (Canadian $232 per quality-adjusted life year gained and $14 395 per quality-adjusted life year gained, respectively).

Barriers to osteoarthritis service models

A range of actual and potential barriers to the successful development, implementation, and sustainability of OA service MOC can be identified from the literature. At the patient level, clinical studies involving people with OA have demonstrated limited adherence to intervention programmes, suboptimal attendance, and limited uptake of recommended services [42,48,54]. Language barriers represent an important consideration when designing new MOC (particularly for multicultural settings) to ensure that programmes can be applied to broad patient populations [42]. Health literacy may limit an individual's understanding of their joint disease and impact on their ability to seek and use health information [55], although a recent systematic review reported that low health literacy was not consistently associated with worse functional outcomes for chronic musculoskeletal conditions [56]. Personal health beliefs (e.g. perceiving OA as a natural consequence of ageing) may affect concordance with healthcare recommendations and can lead to delays in seeking care [57–59]. Also, patients with multiple chronic conditions (multi-morbidity) can have competing self-management and treatment priorities, particularly where some medical conditions have a more obvious impact on health or mortality (e.g. diabetes or heart disease). Qualitative research has demonstrated that having multiple chronic conditions may affect patient engagement with self-management strategies, although individual priorities can change over time [60,61].

There are also a number of barriers at the health professional level, including the absence of an 'OA specialist' role, particularly in primary care settings [62]. While extended scope of practice roles are increasingly common in many countries, these can require legislative changes and professional body approval [39,43], and credentialing relies on the provision of appropriate training to ensure clinical competency. Developing and maintaining an appropriate skills mix within a healthcare team is also important, and may require role enhancement, role substitution, and/or the creation of new roles [63]. Workforce availability is also a potential barrier, particularly in view of future demand for primary care and surgery for OA [64–66]. In the United States, health workforce shortages have been forecast for rheumatology [67], physical therapy [68], and orthopaedic surgery [65] with demand for services predicted to outstrip supply. Additionally, improving the quality of care for OA is contingent on the uptake and implementation of published clinical guidelines and recommendations for evidence-based care by health professionals, to minimize evidence-practice gaps [11,69].

At the health system level, barriers to effective MOC are likely to include the current lack of evidence for cost-effectiveness in many settings [29], rising healthcare costs related to greater disease burden [70], and inadequate funding models for supporting longer-term integrated care in some jurisdictions. There are also pragmatic issues concerning the coordination of care within and across healthcare settings, and the need for adequate electronic systems to support effective patient management and clear communication between health professionals and between healthcare sectors. Many health systems currently provide OA services that are distinct to healthcare services provided for other coexistent medical conditions [71]; this approach is inefficient for health systems faced with a growing burden of multi-morbidity, impractical for patients, and unlikely to be sustainable.

Enabling factors

While these barriers warrant consideration, there are also a number of enablers that could facilitate the success of future OA MOC. Large-scale OA registries provide opportunities to monitor the development and progression of OA in populations over time, implement risk assessment and modification strategies, and evaluate the quality of care provided to people with OA. Some examples of these initiatives include the Better management of patients with OsteoArthritis (BOA) national quality register in Sweden [72] and the Osteoarthritis Initiative in the United States [73]. From a clinical perspective, successful examples of OA MOC exist in many countries and settings (e.g. the Alberta joint replacement MOC in Canada [74] and the Canadian community pharmacy MOC [51]), and these can be scrutinized and adapted for local requirements and capabilities.

Ongoing legislative changes enabling the growth of advanced practice roles will provide further opportunities for new career paths and career progression in fields such as physiotherapy and nursing. Shifts in traditional practice boundaries and the provision of more holistic patient management (considering both physical and mental well-being) also reflect a longer-term approach to OA care. This includes the delivery of pain coping skills training by physiotherapists [75] and nurse practitioners [76], and the provision of 'health coaching' to support behaviour change [77].

The availability of new technologies to support efficient assessment, monitoring, reporting, and interdisciplinary communication will also be an ongoing facilitator. Finally, changes to funding models and financial incentives to providing multidisciplinary OA management will be important for sustaining integrating MOC in the long term. For example, in Australia, access to multidisciplinary healthcare for chronic conditions exists via Medicare Australia Chronic Disease Management payment items that support team care arrangements and up to five allied health professional visits per calendar year for a chronic condition, if a management plan is developed by a general practitioner [78]. Funding for multidisciplinary case conferences is also available and can be used to plan and coordinate complex care needs for people with chronic conditions [79].

Improving the implementation and evaluation of models of care

Complex health service interventions

In the previous section, OA service MOC and factors associated with effective implementation were discussed. Many of the barriers described are common to other chronic condition MOC and to the implementation of complex health service interventions in general. In this section, these issues are further explored in relation to methods and tools that may assist researchers and clinicians working in this field.

A full discussion of the processes of implementing and evaluating MOC is beyond the scope of this chapter and readers are directed to other literature where appropriate, for additional information. Further, whilst the authors acknowledge the ongoing debate about the nature of 'knowledge' [80], the process of knowledge translation [81] and the plethora of terms used for reducing the evidence to practice gap (e.g. evidence into practice, knowledge translation, knowledge transfer, knowledge exchange, implementation science, diffusion, dissemination, and many others) [82], we have chosen to use terms about evidence and knowledge that are consistent with our cited references.

Classifying models of care: moving towards a consistent nomenclature

Lack of precision in defining elements of MOC and variation in the nomenclature of interventions and improvement methods and

strategies inhibits research [83–85]. It can reduce the efficiency of literature search methods and make it difficult to compare impacts across multiple studies and to generalize findings to other settings [33,86]. There are now a number of different generic tools available to guide classification of complex interventions and implementation strategies and the reporting of these [86–89]. Condition-specific taxonomies have also been developed, for instance, for chronic heart failure programmes [90]. A similar OA taxonomy has been developed based on this example, but has yet to be tested for its utility [29].

Planning the implementation and evaluation of models of care

Developing a program logic

In order to implement and evaluate the many components and impacts of a new MOC, it is essential to articulate, a priori, the 'inner workings' of the model and the likely short and intermediate impacts, as well as potential longer-term outcomes. This can be facilitated by development of a rationale or 'program logic', which is a conceptual diagram that links the primary aims of the MOC to the intervention components and implementation strategies/actions, and to the impacts and longer-term outcomes across care quality domains [91,92]. Ideally, researchers and end-users (clinicians, patients, carers, community groups) should be involved in this iterative process in order to capture the full range of stakeholder perspectives about outcomes and to ensure collective understanding and expectations of the planned service changes.

Using theory to support implementation and evaluation

The evolution of theory pertaining to improving dissemination and implementation and uptake of new knowledge is well summarized by Oborn et al. [93]. Traditionally, knowledge dissemination was perceived as being a largely technical and linear process, targeted to and premised on the professional motivation of (commonly medical) clinicians to provide optimal patient care. Evidence-based medicine, 'the conscientious, explicit and judicious use of current best evidence in making decisions about the care of individual patients', has drawn on this tradition and targets barriers to clinicians accessing and using evidence, but promotes a more interactive clinician–patient paradigm [94].

However, the process of disseminating and implementing evidence and complex health service interventions such as MOC usually involves multi-directional social processes operating within organizations and between groups and individuals [93]. As a result, collaborative research efforts between medical and other academic disciplines are increasing and psychological, sociobehavioural theories of change (e.g. specific theories of motivation, action, and organization) are being used to guide implementation and evaluation of innovative MOC [95–98]. The process of implementation can also be informed by the very many implementation/change theories now available [99]. Some of these are broad and abstract, such as the 'general theory of implementation', based on normalization process theory [100] whilst others are more specific and provide practical guidance with operational frameworks, such as the theoretical domains framework [101]. These theories and frameworks focus variably on context (e.g. organizational readiness, capacity, and capabilities) and interactions of groups or individuals [16]. In their review, Tabak et al. [16] summarized 61 theories and frameworks in relation to the major focus (dissemination, implementation, or both), the level of their application (broad or operational level) and the socioecological target (system, community organization, individual, or policy), allowing researchers to choose a theory or framework that best suits their needs.

Published systematic reviews also provide an overview of structural, organizational, provider, patient, and innovation factors and strategies that influence diffusion and implementation of innovations [102–106]. It is worth noting that strategy effectiveness may be context sensitive [107]. Grol [108] demonstrates the application of different theoretical perspectives to tailor implementation strategies. For instance, social interaction is informed by social learning, influence, and power theories that indicate the importance of social influence of significant peers and role models, thereby prompting inclusion of effective implementation strategies, such as peer review in local networks, outreach visits, and use of opinion leaders.

From a project management perspective, there is a need to identify and address not only general barriers to effective implementation, but also local contextual barriers and facilitators [82,108] and adapt a MOC to enable implementation without threatening the fidelity of key MOC principles and interventions. This often creates a tension, particularly in multicentre studies, where there may be a need to balance expectations of external academic researchers who seek to 'control' the research environment as tightly as possible and front-line staff who want to implement and refine processes to ensure greatest efficiency [109]. These issues are well discussed by Oborn et al. [110], who point out that 'high levels of external control negatively impacts on innovation outputs, as creativity and novelty are best supported by open processes and high levels of worker autonomy'. They suggest several ways in which organizations can design collaborations to bridge this divide.

Research designs for evaluating complex health service interventions

Even where new MOC include individual components associated with strong evidence of efficacy, a new MOC should be evaluated for its overall efficacy and effectiveness to justify future funding. A detailed analysis of disease management evaluation issues can be found in a recent RAND Europe report [111]. Use of randomized controlled trial (RCT) designs, including cluster RCTs may be limited by financial constraints, design issues, exposure of the control group to the intervention, ethical considerations, and lack of generalizability. Other research designs that can be considered include observational, interrupted time-series analyses, phased multisite/stepped-wedge implementation designs, and innovative designs such as a regression point displacement design (e.g. involving a single treated group and multiple control groups) [111]. Pragmatic trials, which are designed to include a broad range of patients from a variety of settings and which measure a range of outcomes of importance to different stakeholders can overcome issues of generalizability associated with RCTs but may be associated with bias [112].

Mixed-methods programme evaluation

The key questions when implementing complex MOC (particularly where the model already includes components of proven efficacy) relate largely to those of effectiveness, for instance:

◆ Was the MOC implemented as planned?

◆ If not, why not?

◆ What factors acted as barriers and enablers to effective MOC implementation and/or sustainability?

◆ How can the MOC be improved?

In a recent protocol publication, Manca et al. [92] demonstrate how researchers are now using planned mixed-methods evaluation and a variety of project evaluation management tools, such as the RE-AIM (Reach, Effectiveness, Adoption, Implementation, Maintenance) framework [113] to evaluate chronic condition programmes. Programme evaluation should be planned early and data collection should commence before implementation. For instance, quantitative and qualitative data about contextual factors that may influence implementation effectiveness, such as organizational/individual factors [114,115], organizational climate [116], leadership [117], and sustainability factors [118,119] can be used to inform choice of implementation strategies.

There is ongoing investigation of ways in which qualitative data, including patient views about effectiveness of programmes can be incorporated alongside quantitative data into systematic reviews [120,121]. Realist synthesis of evidence is also being used to 'unpack' the ways in which a complex intervention works or fails [122] and can augment quantitative evidence of effectiveness.

Future challenges for osteoarthritis models of care

A number of factors can influence the way in which principles for OA care are translated into practice, such as the unique needs of the population, funding models, incentives, and contextual constraints.

As alluded to earlier, a key challenge for future MOC will be to design services that best meet the needs of people with multimorbidity or multiple chronic conditions (defined as 'two or more concurrent chronic conditions that collectively have an adverse effect on health status, function, or quality of life and that require complex healthcare management, decision-making or coordination') [123]. In the United States, it is estimated that people with multiple chronic conditions comprise approximately one-quarter of the population [123]. The personal impacts have been well documented and include reduced functional status, reduced quality of life, and increased mortality risk as well as the need to see multiple health practitioners, the need to use multiple medications, and increased exposure to fragmented and inefficient healthcare [124,125].

Grembowski et al. [126] reviewed existing chronic care models relevant to people with multiple chronic conditions, including the CCM and concluded that there was a lack of alignment between patient needs and the capacity of the system to deliver this care.

Given the rising prevalence of people with multiple chronic conditions, it will not be practical to continue providing isolated OA-specific MOC. With this in mind, developers of future OA MOC need to explore ways in which to develop cross-condition research collaborations to build new service MOC that incorporate both generic and condition-specific elements. One option would be to focus on developing MOC for generic risk behaviour prevention or modification (e.g. for optimization of weight and physical activity). Such models could include shared components of self-management support and mental health management, as well as discretionary condition-specific modules that are tailored to individual needs (Figure 36.3).

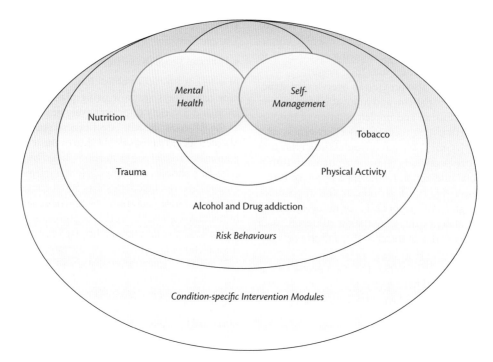

Figure 36.3 Redesigning care with a focus on preventing and managing multiple chronic conditions.

Future OA MOC also need to consider specific sub-populations such as the very old and also young people with OA who have been shown to have large reductions in quality of life, compared to age- and gender-matched norms [127]. Further research about key components of care for these groups and effective service delivery is required to inform tailored OA-specific module development.

Another ongoing challenge for new MOC research relates to the research and development process required to undertake such studies, such as the phased approach to developing and testing complex health service interventions described by Campbell et al. [128]. Using this approach, it is not until phase III that a definitive evaluation (RCT) is undertaken. However, preliminary phases (theory, modelling, and exploratory or pilot trials) require time and funding and it is difficult for researchers to access funding for such projects. Improved national funding schemes, such as those that fund strategic industry, clinical, and academic partnerships may assist in meeting this challenge.

Concluding comments

In this chapter we have considered the organization and delivery of OA care within the context of chronic condition management in general, and with specific regard to the current OA literature. Although there is a move towards OA MOC that incorporate design elements from comprehensive chronic condition MOC (such as the CCM), this is not yet as well-developed for OA as for some other chronic conditions. There remains limited evidence for the effectiveness and cost-effectiveness of MOC for OA, although evidence to support specific model components (particularly self-management support, delivery system design, and coordination of care) is increasing.

Implementing complex health service interventions is challenging but even small to moderate effects, as demonstrated in the studies presented in this chapter, can potentially translate to large population benefits, given the large numbers of people with OA

and in the absence of effective disease-modifying agents. Effective implementation of care models can be better supported by the use of theoretical models and frameworks and standardization of MOC taxonomy for planning programme implementation and evaluation. Evaluation of both programme efficacy and effectiveness, using mixed-methods research should be considered prior to, and alongside, programme implementation. There is a need to support researchers with appropriate knowledge translation training, delivered in a cost-efficient manner [129]. As impacts of programmes within one setting may not be transferable to other settings, research studies should include multiple sites, evaluated within cluster RCT or other innovative study designs.

Multidisciplinary arrangements and streamlined provision of OA care across different healthcare settings will become increasingly important given the prevalence of multi-morbidity among this patient group. This will likely require the design of specific OA modules, capable of integration with generic chronic condition MOC that focus on risk prevention and behaviour modification across the health spectrum from wellness to disease.

References

1. Institute of Medicine. *Crossing the Quality Chasm: A New Health System for the 21st Century*. Washington, DC: The National Academy of Sciences; 2001.
2. World Health Organization. *Innovative Care for Chronic Conditions: Building Blocks for Action*. Geneva: World Health Organization; 2002.
3. Vos T, Flaxman AD, Naghavi M, et al. Years lived with disability (YLDs) for 1160 sequelae of 289 diseases and injuries 1990-2010: a systematic analysis for the Global Burden of Disease Study 2010. *Lancet* 2012; 380:2163–96.
4. McGlynn EA, Asch SM, Adams J, et al. The quality of health care delivered to adults in the United States. *N Engl J Med* 2003; 348:2635–45.
5. Asch SM, Kerr EA, Keesey J, et al. Who is at greatest risk for receiving poor-quality health care? *N Engl J Med* 2006; 354:1147–56.

6. Runciman WB, Hunt TD, Hannaford NA, et al. CareTrack: assessing the appropriateness of health care delivery in Australia. *Med J Aust* 2012; 197:100–5.

7. Glazier RH, Badley EM, Wright JG, et al. Patient and provider factors related to comprehensive arthritis care in a community setting in Ontario, Canada. *J Rheumatol* 2003; 30:1846–50.

8. Ganz DA, Chang JT, Roth CP, et al. Quality of osteoarthritis care for community-dwelling older adults. *Arthritis Rheum* 2006; 55:241–7.

9. DeHaan MN, Guzman J, Bayley MT, et al. Knee osteoarthritis clinical practice guidelines—how are we doing? *J Rheumatol* 2007; 34:2099–105.

10. Curtis JR, Arora T, Narongroeknawin P, et al. The delivery of evidence-based preventive care for older Americans with arthritis. *Arthritis Res Ther* 2010; 12:R144.

11. Hunter DJ, Neogi T, Hochberg MC. Quality of osteoarthritis management and the need for reform in the US. *Arthritis Care Res* 2011; 63:31–8.

12. Li LC, Sayre EC, Kopec JA, et al. Quality of nonpharmacological care in the community for people with knee and hip osteoarthritis. *J Rheumatol* 2011; 38:2230–7.

13. McHugh GA, Campbell M, Luker KA. Quality of care for individuals with osteoarthritis: a longitudinal study. *J Eval Clin Pract* 2012; 18:534–41.

14. Kitson AL, Rycroft-Malone J, Harvey G, et al. Evaluating the successful implementation of evidence into practice using the PARiHS framework: theoretical and practical challenges. *Implement Sci* 2008; 3:1.

15. Green S. When one model is not enough: Combining epistemic tools in systems biology. *Stud Hist Philos Biol Biomed Sci* 2013; 44:170–80.

16. Tabak RG, Khoong EC, Chambers DA, et al. Bridging research and practice: Models for dissemination and implementation research. *Am J Prev Med* 2012; 43:337–50.

17. Bodenheimer T, Wagner EH, Grumbach K. Improving primary care for patients with chronic illness: the chronic care model, Part 2. *JAMA* 2002; 288:1909–14.

18. Von Korff M, Glasgow RE, Sharpe M. Organising care for chronic illness. *BMJ* 2002; 325:92–4.

19. Wagner EH. Chronic disease management: What will it take to improve care for chronic illness? *Effect Clin Pract* 1998; 1:2–4.

20. Bodenheimer T, Wagner EH, Grumbach K. Improving primary care for patients with chronic illness. *JAMA* 2002; 288:1775–9.

21. Barr VJ, Robinson S, Marin-Link B, et al. The expanded Chronic Care Model: an integration of concepts and strategies from population health promotion and the Chronic Care Model. *Hosp Q* 2003; 7:73–82.

22. World Health Organization. *Assessing National Capacity for the Prevention and Control of Noncommunicable Diseases: Report of the 2010 Global Survey.* Geneva: World Health Organization; 2012.

23. Brand C, Hunter D, Hinman R, et al. Improving care for people with osteoarthritis of the hip and knee: how has national policy for osteoarthritis been translated into service models in Australia? *Int J Rheum Dis* 2011; 14:181–90.

24. Woolf SH, Grol R, Hutchinson A, et al. Clinical guidelines: potential benefits, limitations, and harms of clinical guidelines. *Br Med J* 1999; 318:527–30.

25. Lugtenberg M, Burgers JS, Westert GP. Effects of evidence-based clinical practice guidelines on quality of care: a systematic review. *Qual Saf Health Care* 2009; 18:385–92.

26. Cabana MD, Rand CS, Powe NR, et al. Why don't physicians follow clinical practice guidelines? A framework for improvement. *JAMA* 1999; 282:1458–65.

27. Brand C, Landgren F, Hutchinson A, et al. Clinical practice guidelines: barriers to durability after effective early implementation. *Intern Med J* 2005; 35:162–9.

28. Kryworuchko J, Stacey D, Bai N, et al. Twelve years of clinical practice guideline development, dissemination and evaluation in Canada (1994 to 2005). *Implement Sci* 2009; 4:49.

29. Brand CA, Ackerman IN, Tropea J. Chronic disease management: improving care for people with osteoarthritis. *Best Pract Res Clin Rheumatol* 2014; 28:119–42.

30. Speerin R, Slater H, Li L, et al. Moving from evidence to practice: Models of care for the prevention and management of musculoskeletal conditions. *Best Pract Res Clin Rheumatol* 2014; 28:479–515.

31. NSW Agency for Clinical Innovation. *Musculoskeletal Network: Osteoarthritis Chronic Care Program Model of Care.* Chatswood, NSW: Agency for Clinical Innovation; 2012.

32. Hroscikoski MC, Solberg LI, Sperl-Hillen JM, et al. Challenges of change: a qualitative study of chronic care model implementation. *Ann Fam Med* 2006; 4:317–26.

33. Coleman K, Austin BT, Brach C, et al. Evidence on the Chronic Care Model in the new millennium. *Health Affairs* 2009; 28:75–85.

34. Pearson ML, Wu S, Schaefer J, et al. Assessing the implementation of the chronic care model in quality improvement collaboratives. *Health Serv Res* 2005; 40:978–96.

35. Rosemann T, Laux G, Szecsenyi J, et al. The Chronic Care Model: Congruency and predictors among primary care patients with osteoarthritis. *Qual Saf Health Care* 2008; 17:442–6.

36. Kennedy DM, Robarts S, Woodhouse L. Patients are satisfied with advanced practice physiotherapists in a role traditionally performed by orthopaedic surgeons. *Physiother Can* 2010; 62:298–305.

37. Solomon DH, Bitton A, Fraenkel L, et al. Roles of nurse practitioners and physician assistants in rheumatology practices in the US. *Arthritis Care Res* 2014; 66:1108–13.

38. Chartered Society of Physiotherapy. *Landmark Decision gives UK Physios a World First in Prescribing Rights.* 2012. http://www.csp.org.uk/news/2012/07/24/landmark-decision-gives-uk-physios-world-first-prescribing-rights

39. Oldmeadow LB, Bedi HS, Burch HT, et al. Experienced physiotherapists as gatekeepers to hospital orthopaedic outpatient care. *Med J Aust* 2007; 186:625–8.

40. Sephton R, Hough E, Roberts SA, et al. Evaluation of a primary care musculoskeletal clinical assessment service: a preliminary study. *Physiotherapy* 2010; 96:296–302.

41. Doerr CR, Graves SE, Mercer GE, et al. Implementation of a quality care management system for patients with arthritis of the hip and knee. *Aust Health Rev* 2013; 37:88–92.

42. Brand CA, Amatya B, Gordon B, et al. Redesigning care for chronic conditions: Improving hospital-based ambulatory care for people with osteoarthritis of the hip and knee. *Intern Med J* 2010; 40:427–36.

43. Passalent L, Kennedy C, Warmington K, et al. System integration and clinical utilization of the Advanced Clinician Practitioner in Arthritis Care (ACPAC) Program–Trained extended role practitioners in Ontario: a two-year, system-level evaluation. *Healthcare Policy* 2013; 8:56–70.

44. MacKay C, Davis AM, Mahomed N, et al. Expanding roles in orthopaedic care: a comparison of physiotherapist and orthopaedic surgeon recommendations for triage. *J Eval Clin Pract* 2009; 15:178–83.

45. Desmeules F, Toliopoulos P, Roy JS, et al. Validation of an advanced practice physiotherapy model of care in an orthopaedic outpatient clinic. *BMC Musculoskelet Disord* 2013; 14:162.

46. Desmeules F, Roy J-S, MacDermid J, et al. Advanced practice physiotherapy in patients with musculoskeletal disorders: a systematic review. *BMC Musculoskelet Disord* 2012; 13:107.

47. Zwar N, Harris M, Griffiths R, et al. *A Systematic Review of Chronic Disease Management.* Sydney: Australian Primary Health Care Research Institute; 2006.

48. Dobscha SK, Corson K, Perrin NA, et al. Collaborative care for chronic pain in primary care: a cluster randomized trial. *JAMA* 2009; 301:1242–52.

49. Unutzer J, Hantke M, Powers D, et al. Care management for depression and osteoarthritis pain in older primary care patients: a pilot study. *Int J Geriatr Psychiatry* 2008; 23:1166–71.

50. Gooch K, Marshall DA, Faris PD, et al. Comparative effectiveness of alternative clinical pathways for primary hip and knee joint

replacement patients: a pragmatic randomized, controlled trial. *Osteoarthritis Cartilage* 2012; 20:1086–94.

51. Marra CA, Cibere J, Grubisic M, et al. Pharmacist-initiated intervention trial in osteoarthritis: a multidisciplinary intervention for knee osteoarthritis. *Arthritis Care Res* 2012; 64:1837–45.

52. Voorn VM, Vermeulen HM, Nelissen RG, et al. An innovative care model coordinated by a physical therapist and nurse practitioner for osteoarthritis of the hip and knee in specialist care: a prospective study. *Rheumatol Int* 2013; 33:1821–8.

53. Marra CA, Grubisic M, Cibere J, et al. Cost-utility analysis of a multidisciplinary strategy to manage osteoarthritis of the knee: Economic evaluation of a cluster randomized controlled trial study. *Arthritis Care Res* 2014; 66:810–6.

54. McKnight PE, Kasle S, Going S, et al. A comparison of strength training, self-management, and the combination for early osteoarthritis of the knee. *Arthritis Care Res* 2010; 62:45–53.

55. Jordan JE, Buchbinder R, Osborne RH. Conceptualising health literacy from the patient perspective *Patient Educ Couns* 2010; 79:36–42.

56. Loke YK, Hinz I, Wang X, et al. Impact of health literacy in patients with chronic musculoskeletal disease—systematic review. *PLoS ONE* 2012; 7:e40210.

57. Sanders C, Donovan JL, Dieppe PA. Unmet need for joint replacement: a qualitative investigation of barriers to treatment among individuals with severe pain and disability of the hip and knee. *Rheumatology* 2004; 43:353–57.

58. Paskins Z, Sanders T, Hassell A. What influences patients with osteoarthritis to consult their GP about their symptoms? A narrative review. *BMC Fam Pract* 2013; 14:195.

59. Prasanna SS, Korner-Bitensky N, Ahmed S. Why do people delay accessing health care for knee osteoarthritis? Exploring beliefs of health professionals and lay people. *Physiother Can* 2013; 65:56–63.

60. Lindsay S. Prioritizing illness: Lessons in self-managing multiple chronic diseases. *Can J Sociol* 2009; 39:983–1002.

61. Morris RL, Sanders C, Kennedy AP, et al. Shifting priorities in multimorbidity: a longitudinal qualitative study of patient's prioritization of multiple conditions. *Chronic Illn* 2011; 7:147–61.

62. Mann C, Gooberman-Hill R. Health care provision for osteoarthritis: concordance between what patients would like and what health professionals think they should have. *Arthritis Care Res* 2011; 63:963–72.

63. Sibbald B, Shen J, McBride A. Changing the skill-mix of the health care workforce. *J Health Serv Res Policy* 2004; 9(Suppl 1):28–38.

64. Kurtz S, Ong K, Lau E, et al. Projections of primary and revision hip and knee arthroplasty in the United States from 2005 to 2030. *J Bone Joint Surg Am* 2007; 89A:780–85.

65. Fehring TK, Odum SM, Troyer JL, et al. Joint replacement access in 2016: a supply side crisis. *J Arthroplasty* 2010; 25:1175–81.

66. Turkiewicz A, Petersson IF, Bjork J, et al. Current and future impact of osteoarthritis on health care: a population-based study with projections to year 2032. *Osteoarthritis Cartilage* 2014; 22:1826–32.

67. Deal CL, Hooker R, Harrington T, et al. The United States rheumatology workforce: Supply and demand, 2005-2025. *Arthritis Rheum* 2007; 56:722–9.

68. Zimbelman JL, Juraschek SP, Zhang X, et al. Physical therapy workforce in the United States: forecasting nationwide shortages. *PM R* 2010; 2:1021–9.

69. Hunter DJ. Quality of osteoarthritis care for community-dwelling older adults. *Clin Geriatr Med* 2010; 26:401–17.

70. Murray CJL, Vos T, Lozano R, et al. Disability-adjusted life years (DALYs) for 291 diseases and injuries in 21 regions, 1990–2010: a systematic analysis for the Global Burden of Disease Study 2010. *Lancet* 2012; 380:2197–223.

71. Mallen CD. Osteoarthritis—the forgotten chronic disease. Time for a multimorbid approach? *Eur J Gen Pract* 2012; 18:131–2.

72. Thorstensson C, Dahlberg L, Garrelick G. *The BOA-Register Annual Report 2012. Better Management of Patients with OsteoArthritis.* 2012. http://utv.boaregistret.se/en/AnnualReport.aspx

73. University of California San Francisco Coordinating Center. *Osteoarthritis Initiative: A Knee Health Study.* https://oai.epi-ucsf.org/datarelease/About.asp

74. Frank C, Marshall D, Faris P, et al. Improving access to hip and knee replacement and its quality by adopting a new model of care in Alberta. *Can Med Assoc J* 2011; 183:E347–50.

75. Hunt MA, Keefe FJ, Bryant C, et al. A physiotherapist-delivered, combined exercise and pain coping skills training intervention for individuals with knee osteoarthritis: a pilot study. *Knee* 2013; 20:106–12.

76. Broderick JE, Keefe FJ, Bruckenthal P, et al. Nurse practitioners can effectively deliver pain coping skills training to osteoarthritis patients with chronic pain: a randomized, controlled trial. *Pain* 2014; 155:1743–54.

77. Bennell KL, Egerton T, Bills C, et al. Addition of telephone coaching to a physiotherapist-delivered physical activity program in people with knee osteoarthritis: a randomised controlled trial protocol. *BMC Musculoskelet Disord* 2012; 13:246.

78. Australian Government Department of Health. *Chronic Disease Management—Provider Information.* 2015. http://www.health.gov.au/internet/main/publishing.nsf/Content/mbsprimarycare-factsheet-chronicdisease.htm

79. Australian Government Department of Health. *Multidisciplinary Case Conferences.* 2015. http://www.health.gov.au/internet/main/publishing.nsf/Content/mbsprimarycare-caseconf-factsheet.htm

80. Greenhalgh T, Wieringa S. Is it time to drop the 'knowledge translation' metaphor? A critical literature review. *J R Soc Med* 2011; 104:501–9.

81. Trochim W, Kane C, Graham MJ, et al. Evaluating translational research: a process marker model. *Clin Transl Sci* 2011; 4:153–62.

82. Graham ID, Logan J, Harrison MB, et al. Lost in knowledge translation: Time for a map? *J Contin Educ Health Prof* 2006; 26:13–24.

83. Glasziou P, Meats E, Heneghan C, et al. What is missing from descriptions of treatment in trials and reviews? *BMJ* 2008; 336:1472–4.

84. Michie S, Abraham C. Advancing the science of behaviour change: a plea for scientific reporting. *Addiction* 2008; 103:1409–10.

85. Walshe K. Pseudoinnovation: the development and spread of healthcare quality improvement methodologies. *Int J Qual Health Care* 2009; 21:153–9.

86. Colquhoun HL, Levac D, O'Brien KK, et al. Scoping reviews: time for clarity in definition, methods, and reporting. *J Clin Epidemiol* 2014; 67:1291–4.

87. Leeman J, Baernholdt M, Sandelowski M. Developing a theory-based taxonomy of methods for implementing change in practice. *J Adv Nurs* 2007; 58:191–200.

88. Michie S, van Stralen MM, West R. The behaviour change wheel: a new method for characterising and designing behaviour change interventions. *Implement Sci* 2011; 6:42.

89. Michie S, Richardson M, Johnston M, et al. The behavior change technique taxonomy (v1) of 93 hierarchically clustered techniques: Building an international consensus for the reporting of behavior change interventions. *Ann Behav Med* 2013; 46:81–95.

90. Krumholz HM, Currie PM, Riegel B, et al. A taxonomy for disease management: a scientific statement from the American Heart Association Disease Management Taxonomy Writing Group. *Circulation* 2006; 114:1432–45.

91. Dwyer JJ, Makin S. Using a program logic model that focuses on performance measurement to develop a program. *Can J Public Health* 1997; 88:421–5.

92. Manca DP, Aubrey-Bassler K, Kandola K, et al. Implementing and evaluating a program to facilitate chronic disease prevention and screening in primary care: a mixed methods program evaluation. *Implement Sci* 2014; 9:135.

93. Oborn E, Barrett M, Racko G. Knowledge translation in healthcare: Incorporating theories of learning and knowledge from the management literature. *J Health Organ Manag* 2013; 27:412–31.

94. Sackett DL, Richardson WS, Rosenberg W, et al. *Evidence-Based Medicine: How to Practice and Teach EBM.* New York: Churchill Livingstone; 1997.

95. Sanson-Fisher RW, Grimshaw JM, Eccles MP. The science of changing providers' behaviour: the missing link in evidence-based practice. *Med J Aust* 2004; 180:205–6.

96. Lin MK, Marsteller JA, Shortell SM, et al. Motivation to change chronic illness care: results from a national evaluation of quality improvement collaboratives. *Health Care Manage Rev* 2005; 30:139–56.

97. Prochaska JJ, Spring B, Nigg CR. Multiple health behavior change research: an introduction and overview. *Prevent Med* 2008; 46:181–8.

98. Prochaska JO. Decision making in the transtheoretical model of behavior change. *Med Decis Making* 2008; 28:845–9.

99. Damschroder LJ, Aron DC, Keith RE, et al. Fostering implementation of health services research findings into practice: a consolidated framework for advancing implementation science. *Implement Sci* 2009; 4:50.

100. May C. Towards a general theory of implementation. *Implement Sci* 2013; 8:18.

101. Michie S, Johnston M, Abraham C, et al. Making psychological theory useful for implementing evidence based practice: a consensus approach. *Qual Saf Health Care* 2005; 14:26–33.

102. Bero LA, Grilli R, Grimshaw JM, et al. Closing the gap between research and practice: an overview of systematic reviews of interventions to promote the implementation of research findings. The Cochrane Effective Practice and Organization of Care Review Group. *Br Med J* 1998; 317:465–8.

103. Greenhalgh T, Robert G, Bate P, et al. *Diffusion of Innovations in Health Service Organisations: A Systematic Literature Review.* Oxford: Blackwell Publishing Ltd; 2005.

104. Grimshaw JM, Eccles MP, Lavis JN, et al. Knowledge translation of research findings. *Implement Sci* 2012; 7:50.

105. Chaudoir SR, Dugan AG, Barr CH. Measuring factors affecting implementation of health innovations: a systematic review of structural, organizational, provider, patient, and innovation level measures. *Implement Sci* 2013; 8:22.

106. Krause J, Van Lieshout J, Klomp R, et al. Identifying determinants of care for tailoring implementation in chronic diseases: an evaluation of different methods. *Implement Sci* 2014; 9:102.

107. Wensing M, van der Weijden T, Grol R. Implementing guidelines and innovations in general practice: which interventions are effective? *Br J Gen Pract* 1998; 48:991–7.

108. Grol R. Personal paper. Beliefs and evidence in changing clinical practice. *Br Med J* 1997; 315:418–21.

109. Jager C, Freund T, Steinhauser J, et al. Tailored Implementation for Chronic Diseases (TICD): a protocol for process evaluation in cluster randomized controlled trials in five European countries. *Trials* 2014; 15:87.

110. Oborn E, Barrett M, Prince K, et al. Balancing exploration and exploitation in transferring research into practice: a comparison of five knowledge translation entity archetypes. *Implement Sci* 2013; 8:104.

111. Conklin A, Nolte E. *Disease Management Evaluation: A Comprehensive Review of Current State of the Art.* Santa Monica, CA: RAND Corporation; 2010.

112. Ware JH, Hamel MB. Pragmatic trials—guides to better patient care? *N Engl J Med* 2011; 364:1685–7.

113. Glasgow RE, McKay HG, Piette JD, et al. The RE-AIM framework for evaluating interventions: what can it tell us about approaches to chronic illness management? *Patient Educ Couns* 2001; 44:119–27.

114. Holt DT, Helfrich CD, Hall CG, et al. Are you ready? How health professionals can comprehensively conceptualize readiness for change. *J Gen Intern Med* 2010; 25(Suppl 1):50–5.

115. Simpson KM, Porter K, McConnell ES, et al. Tool for evaluating research implementation challenges: a sense-making protocol for addressing implementation challenges in complex research settings. *Implement Sci* 2013; 8:2.

116. Ehrhart MG, Aarons GA, Farahnak LR. Assessing the organizational context for EBP implementation: The development and validity testing of the Implementation Climate Scale (ICS). *Implement Sci* 2014; 9:157.

117. Aarons GA, Ehrhart MG, Farahnak LR. The Implementation Leadership Scale (ILS): Development of a brief measure of unit level implementation leadership. *Implement Sci* 2014; 9:45.

118. Chambers DA, Glasgow RE, Stange KC. The dynamic sustainability framework: addressing the paradox of sustainment amid ongoing change. *Implement Sci* 2013; 8:117.

119. Doyle C, Howe C, Woodcock T, et al. Making change last: applying the NHS institute for innovation and improvement sustainability model to healthcare improvement. *Implement Sci* 2013; 8:127.

120. Thomas J, Harden A, Oakley A, et al. Integrating qualitative research with trials in systematic reviews. *BMJ* 2004; 328:1010–2.

121. Candy B, King M, Jones L, et al. Using qualitative evidence on patients' views to help understand variation in effectiveness of complex interventions: a qualitative comparative analysis. *Trials* 2013; 14:179.

122. Rycroft-Malone J, Seers K, Crichton N, et al. A pragmatic cluster randomised trial evaluating three implementation interventions. *Implement Sci* 2012; 7:80.

123. National Quality Forum. *Multiple Chronic Conditions Measurement Framework.* Washington, DC: National Quality Forum; 2012.

124. Fortin M, Dubois MF, Hudon C, et al. Multimorbidity and quality of life: a closer look. *Health Qual Life Outcomes* 2007; 5:52.

125. Fortin M, Soubhi H, Hudon C, et al. Multimorbidity's many challenges. *BMJ* 2007; 334:1016–7.

126. Grembowski D, Schaefer J, Johnson KE, et al. A conceptual model of the role of complexity in the care of patients with multiple chronic conditions. *Med Care* 2014; 52(Suppl 3):S7–S14.

127. Ackerman IN, Bucknill A, Page RS, et al. The substantial personal burden experienced by younger people with hip or knee osteoarthritis. *Osteoarthritis Cartilage* 2015; 23:1276–84.

128. Campbell M, Fitzpatrick R, Haines A, et al. Framework for design and evaluation of complex interventions to improve health. *BMJ* 2000; 321:694–6.

129. Holmes BJ, Schellenberg M, Schell K, et al. How funding agencies can support research use in healthcare: an online province-wide survey to determine knowledge translation training needs. *Implement Sci* 2014; 9:71.

130. Rosemann T, Joos S, Laux G, et al. Case management of arthritis patients in primary care: a cluster-randomized controlled trial. *Arthritis Rheum* 2007; 57:1390–7.

131. Brosseau L, Wells G, Kenny G, et al. The implementation of a community-based aerobic walking program for mild to moderate knee osteoarthritis (OA): a knowledge translation (KT) randomized controlled trial (RCT): Part I: The Uptake of the Ottawa Panel clinical practice guidelines (CPGs). *BMC Public Health* 2012; 12:871.

132. Brosseau L, Wells GA, Kenny GP, et al. The implementation of a community-based aerobic walking program for mild to moderate knee osteoarthritis: a knowledge translation randomized controlled trial: Part II: clinical outcomes. *BMC Public Health* 2012; 12:1073.

133. Murphy SL, Strasburg DM, Lyden AK, et al. Effects of activity strategy training on pain and physical activity in older adults with knee or hip osteoarthritis: a pilot study. *Arthritis Rheum* 2008; 59:1480–7.

134. Hill J, Lewis M, Bird H. Do OA patients gain additional benefit from care from a clinical nurse specialist? A randomized clinical trial. *Rheumatology* 2009; 48:658–64.

135. Hoogeboom TJ, Kwakkenbos L, Rietveld L, et al. Feasibility and potential effectiveness of a non-pharmacological multidisciplinary care programme for persons with generalised osteoarthritis: a randomised, multiple-baseline single-case study. *BMJ Open* 2012; 2:e001161.

SECTION 12

Guidelines

CHAPTER 37

Guidelines

Weiya Zhang and Michael Doherty

Introduction

Osteoarthritis (OA) is the most common form of arthritis and a major contributor to functional impairment and reduced independence in older adults [1]. The prevalence of symptomatic OA of the knee, hip, and hand is estimated to be 13%, 5%, and 3% of adults, whereas that of radiographic OA is 25%, 11%, and 41%, respectively [2]. Pain and functional restriction are the main presenting symptoms of OA and the main focus of treatment. Fifty-one non-pharmacological, pharmacological, and surgical treatments have been used to treat OA and more will continue to be added to the list [3]. However, not many of these treatments achieve the minimal clinically important difference (MCID), which is when the difference between active and placebo is at least half of the standard deviation of the difference, as recently recommended by the National Institute for Health and Care Excellence (NICE) [2]. According to this definition of MCID only two treatments for OA, specifically opioids and intra-articular steroid injection, are qualified. Clearly not all treatment guidelines require this MCID to recommend a treatment otherwise only these two would be recommended. The majority of OA treatment guidelines are based on the statistical difference between active treatment and placebo, including the recently updated American College of Rheumatology (ACR) guidelines, the NICE guidelines, the European League against Rheumatism (EULAR) evidence-based recommendations, and the Osteoarthritis Research Society International (OARSI) treatment guidelines. This chapter aims to summarize information from the currently published treatment guidelines or recommendations, compare the differences between them, and discuss the challenges in making guidelines relevant to everyday management of OA.

Definition

Clinical guidelines are frequently defined as 'systematically developed statements to assist practitioner and patient decisions about appropriate health care for specific clinical circumstances' [4]. Alternative or allied terms for guidelines include consensus statements, algorithms, standards of care, recommendations, and quality indicators [3]. Although there are differences between these terms, they all imply an attempt to improve the standard of care and therefore have been assessed together as a family [3]. According to the way they are developed, guidelines may be classified as opinion-based, evidence-based, or hybrid guidelines [3]. Opinion-based guidelines are developed mainly based on expert consensus, whereas evidence-based guidelines are developed solely according to the research evidence. The hybrid guidelines, however, combine both approaches, that is, research evidence and expert consensus to better translate research into clinical practice.

Development

It is generally agreed that modern guidelines should be evidence based, clinically driven, and patient-centred. Haynes et al. have proposed a model that takes into account *research evidence, clinical expertise, and patient preference* to guide the development of guidelines and other clinical decision-making processes [5] (Figure 37.1). In this model all three forms of evidence are equally weighted and it is only when all three concur that a true evidence-based decision is approached. As a result, the vast majority of guidelines combine a systematic literature review of research evidence together with an expert consensus approach to generate a guideline. Many organizations have also started to include patients in the guideline development team to take account of patient opinion and preferences. As well as patient opinion, NICE also includes the opinion of other stakeholders, including patient-carers and the pharmaceutical industry within the guideline development process [2].

Research evidence may be classified into different levels according to the quality of evidence. For therapeutic questions, the evidence hierarchy of Shekelle et al. (Table 37.1) has been well accepted and widely used [6]. For diagnostic questions, EULAR has suggested an evidence hierarchy for diagnostic test ranking in descending order from meta-analysis of multiple cohort or case–control studies, to single cohort or case–control studies, and finally expert opinion alone (Table 37.2) [7]. However, for prognosis questions there has been no agreed evidence hierarchy, although according to the nature of the studies assessing prognosis questions the hierarchy would be similar to that for diagnosis.

The expert consensus approach has also been evolving rapidly from non-anonymized (e.g. nominal voting) to anonymized

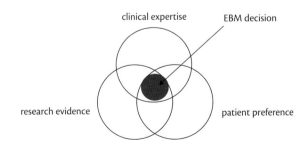

Figure 37.1 Evidence-based medicine (EBM) decision-making.
Adapted from Haynes B, Sackett DL, Cook J, Guyatt GH. Translating evidence from research into practice: 1. The role of clinical care research evidence in clinical decisions. *Evidence-Based Medicine* 1996; 1(7):196–198.

Table 37.1 Evidence hierarchy and traditional strength of recommendation

Category of evidence	Strength of recommendation
Ia—meta-analysis of randomized controlled trials	A—category 1 evidence
Ib—randomized controlled trial	
IIa—controlled study without randomization	B—category 2 evidence or extrapolated from category 1 evidence
IIb—quasi-experimental study	
III—non-experimental descriptive studies, such as comparative, correlation, and case-control studies	C—category 3 evidence or extrapolated from category 1 or 2 evidence
IV—expert committee reports or opinion or clinical experience of respected authorities, or both	D—category 4 evidence or extrapolated from category 2 or 3 evidence

Reproduced from *BMJ*, Shekelle PG, Woolf SH, Eccles M, Grimshaw J, 318, 593–596, copyright notice 1999 with permission from BMJ Publishing Group Ltd.

consensus (e.g. Delphi exercise) to avoid personal bias from more dominating experts [8]. This ensures that individual opinions can be fully expressed within the panel and are counted equally in the decision-making process. The most frequently used anonymized consensus is the Delphi exercise which has been used widely by many organizations including EULAR and OARSI [9–12].

One of the challenges for the development of guidelines is how to provide strength of recommendation (SOR). Shekelle et al. initially devised a scale to measure the SOR (Table 37.1) [6] which simply reflected the level of evidence for efficacy. However, clinical decisions are never based on treatment efficacy alone but also need to take account of other factors such as safety, availability, patient acceptability, cost, and so on. The scale was therefore replaced by the GRADE (Grading of recommendations Assessment, Development and Evaluation) system [13]. The GRADE system contains consensus statements gathered from a group of international experts in guideline development and recently has been updated [14]. The GRADE system aims to rank evidence according to (1) the level of evidence and (2) the quality of evidence at each level. To achieve simplicity and transparency the GRADE system classifies the quality of evidence into one of four levels:

◆ High quality—further research is very unlikely to change our confidence in the estimated effect

Table 37.2 EULAR level of evidence for diagnosis

Ia	Meta-analysis of cohort studies
Ib	Meta-analysis of case–control studies
IIa	Cohort studies
IIb	Case–control studies
III	Non-comparative descriptive studies
IV	Expert opinion

Reproduced from *Ann Rheum Dis*, Zhang W, Doherty M, Pascual E, Bardin T, Barskova V, Conaghan P et al., 6S, 1301–1311 copyright notice 2006 with permission from BMJ Publishing Group Ltd.

◆ Moderate quality—further research is likely to have an impact on our confidence in the estimate of effect and may change the estimate

◆ Low quality—further research is very likely to have an important impact on our confidence in the estimate of effect and is likely to change the estimate

◆ Very low—any estimate of effect is very uncertain [15].

Some organizations have chosen to combine the low and very low categories for decision-making purposes. Evidence based on randomized controlled trials (RCTs) begins as high-quality evidence, but it may be downgraded for several reasons including

◆ Study limitations (e.g. lack of allocation concealment, lack of blinding, large dropout rates, failure to undertake intention-to-treat analysis)

◆ Inconsistency of results

◆ Indirectness of evidence

◆ Imprecision

◆ Publication bias.

Although observational studies such as cohort and case–control studies start with a 'low-quality' rating, upgrading may be warranted if:

◆ the magnitude of the effect is very large (such as improvement following total joint replacement for severe hip OA)

◆ there is evidence of a dose–response relationship

◆ controlling all plausible biases would not decrease the magnitude of an apparent treatment effect [15].

The GRADE SOR is simply dichotomized as 'strong recommendation' or 'weak recommendation', although some guideline panels may prefer terms such as 'conditional' or 'discretionary' instead of weak [16]. Four key considerations should determine the SOR: (1) the balance between benefits and harms, (2) the quality of evidence as discussed above, (3) uncertainty or variability of evidence, and (4) cost-effectiveness.

As can be seen above, the GRADE system allows upgrading and downgrading of evidence according to its assessment and does not necessarily rely on RCTs. This is a significant advance in guideline development since RCTs have been used as the 'gold' standard since 1948 when the first RCT was introduced [17]. The arguments around what to do when faced with a bad RCT versus a good observational study for a therapeutic intervention were impossible to resolve until the GRADE system was established. However, whether an RCT is the 'gold' standard for all aspects of an intervention, for example, the safety of a treatment, remains a matter of debate. Nevertheless, what is clear from the GRADE system is that judgements on the quality of evidence should not be based purely on the type of the study but more on the quality of the study.

Although widely adopted, the GRADE system has also been criticized [18], especially since it has not been validated for use as an instrument but remains merely a group consensus. It is clearly subject to change between user groups in that different users may score the quality of evidence differently and hence give a different SOR for the same intervention in the same disease. It is apparent that the arbitrary classification may not readily reflect the complexity of clinical settings if just a 'strong' or a 'weak' recommendation to treat are the only options. In contrast, EULAR has proposed a simple visual analogue scale with 95% confidence interval for the SOR [10], taking into account the research evidence (efficacy, side effects, cost-effectiveness), clinical expertise, and perceived patient preference according to the evidence-based medicine decision model (Figure 37.1). The advantages of this method are twofold. Firstly, it is not dichotomous and therefore provides more leeway for individualized decision-making and for comparison between treatment options. Secondly, it gives a confidence estimate from experts for each recommendation, showing the variance of opinion within the panel and how uniform is the level of support for each recommendation. Such insight and transparency better informs the user about the true strength of the recommendation.

Multiple osteoarthritis guidelines

There are a number of clinical guidelines for both diagnosis and management of OA. A systematic review undertaken in 2006 identified 23 treatment guidelines on OA from the literature [3]. Six were based predominantly on opinion, five were based primarily on evidence, and twelve were based on both. Thirteen guidelines had been developed for specific care settings (five for primary care, three for rheumatology, three for physiotherapy, and two for orthopaedics), but ten did not specify the target users.

The quality of these guidelines was assessed using the AGREE (Appraisal of Guidelines for Research and Evaluation) instrument for scope and purpose, stakeholder participation, methodological rigour, clarity, applicability, editorial independence, and overall quality [19]. Overall quality was better in the evidence-based than opinion-based guidelines, and significantly better still in the hybrid guidelines that combined both research evidence and expert opinion (Figure 37.2). This was mainly attributed to better scores for scope and purpose (p = 0.007), rigour of development (p = 0.000), and editorial independence (p = 0.013) in the hybrid guidelines [3]. The tendency for evidence-based guidelines to have lower applicability may in part reflect the gap that exists between RCTs that demonstrate that an intervention works and how often and well that intervention works in clinical practice—the 'efficacy paradox'

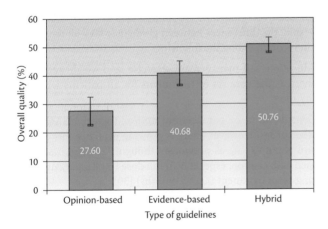

Figure 37.2 Quality of osteoarthritis guidelines.
Reprinted from *Osteoarthritis Cartilage*, 18/4, Zhang W, Nuki G, Moskowitz RW, Abramson S, Altman RD, Arden NK, et al, OARSI recommendations for the management of hip and knee osteoarthritis: Part III: Changes in evidence following systematic cumulative update of research published through January 2009 476–99. Copyright (2010) with permission from Elsevier.

that will be discussed later in this chapter. Hybrid guidelines can be expected to demonstrate improved applicability since clinical expertise can temper the rigidity of research data and close the gap between research and clinical practice.

In the development of hybrid guidelines by the EULAR OA Task Force, expert consensus on the most important propositions was followed by a systematic search for published supporting research evidence, prior to assigning a strength and confidence of recommendation for each treatment proposition. These were based on combined consideration of the research evidence and clinical expertise after also considering risks and benefits, including potential adverse effects and the cost of each treatment modality [10]. This method is clinically driven and evidence supported. The sequence of steps was modified slightly for the development of the OARSI Treatment Guidelines [3,12,20]. An initial systematic review of research evidence was undertaken prior to the development of expert consensus based on a combined consideration of the research evidence and the clinical expertise of the members of the committee. This was then followed by assignment of strength and confidence of recommendation for each proposition as before. It is evidence driven and clinically supported. Similar methods have been adapted by other organizations such as NICE [2,21] and the ACR [22].

Treatments recommended

Fifty-one treatments are available for OA, including 22 non-pharmacological treatments, 21 pharmacological treatments and 8 surgical treatments [3]. The recommendations for these treatments vary between guidelines depending on the research evidence examined and the consensus. In an attempt to summarize the 23 treatment guidelines reviewed by OARSI, treatments were classified according to the level of evidence and the level of recommendation (Table 37.3). The level of recommendation was defined as the percentage of guidelines which recommended the treatment when the treatment was addressed. Exercise, education, self-management, regular telephone contact, paracetamol, non-steroidal anti-inflammatory drugs (NSAIDs) plus a proton pump inhibitor (PPI), selective cyclooxygenase 2 (COX2) inhibitors, and opioids were fully recommended and supported by level Ia evidence. In contract to the individual guidelines, this classification system summarized commonality between the guidelines rather than individual recommendation hierarchy. The classification is therefore in line with but different to individual guidelines. In addition, this classification system found that the level of evidence did not necessarily reflect the level of recommendation (Table 37.3), reinforcing the need to improve on the SOR system of Shekelle et al. which reflects only the level of evidence [6]. For example, while walking canes/sticks, total joint replacement and osteotomy were not supported by RCTs, they were still universally recommended in the guidelines which addressed them. In contrast, despite evidence from systematic reviews of RCTs for the efficacy of chondroitin sulphate and ultrasound, they were recommended by less than 50% of the guidelines in which these modalities were considered (Table 37.3).

Several organizations have published updated OA guidelines or recommendations after 2006. NICE published its first clinical guidance for people with OA, containing its target diagram of core and option treatments that has been widely used in clinical practice

Table 37.3 Level of evidence and percentage of recommendation in existing guidelines¶

Level of evidence§	Percentage of recommendation (number of guidelines recommending the modality/total number of guidelines addressing the modality)				
	<25%	25%–	50%–	75%–	100%
Ia	Ultrasound (1/5)	Chondroitin sulphate (2/7)	Heat/ice (7/10) Glucosamine sulphate (6/10) NSAID + H2 blockers (5/8)	NSAIDs (15/16) Insole (12/13)* Braces (8/9)* Topical capsaicin (8/9)* IA HA (8/9)* IA steroid (11/13)* TENS (8/10) Topical NSAIDs (7/9)*	Aerobic exercise (21/21) Strengthening exercise (21/21) Acetaminophen (16/16) Education (15/15) COX-2 inhibitors (11/11) Opioid (9/9) Self-management (8/8) Water-based exercise (8/8) NSAID + PPI (8/8) NSAID + Misoprostol (8/8) Telephone (2/2)
Ib	Laser (1/6) Electrotherapy/ EMG (1/8)	Nutrients (1/3)	Acupuncture (5/8) Massage (1/2) Diacerhein (1/2)	Weight loss (13/14) Patellar tape (12/13)* Avocado soybean unsaponifiables (3/4)	Combination therapy (12/12) Joint lavage (3/3)* Herbs (2/2)
III					TJR (14/14) Osteotomy (10/10)
IV	Oral steroid (0/2)			Arthroscopic debridement (5/6)*	Cane/stick (11/11)* Referral (5/5) Knee fusion (2/2)* Knee aspiration (2/2)*

¶Modalities were grouped according to strength of agreement and level of evidence. Modalities addressed by only one guideline were not included, such as radiotherapy, sauna/spa, gait aid, topical rubefacients, oestrogen, patellar resurfacing, antidepressants. Modalities not directly related to the treatment such as consideration of risk factors, clinical features etc. were excluded.

§Level of evidence: Ia = systematic review of randomized controlled trials (RCTs); Ib = RCT, IIa = controlled trial; IIb = quasi-experiment; III = cohort/case-control study; IV = expert opinion. Only the highest level of evidence has been selected for each modality.

*Specific for knee OA.

Reprinted from *Osteoarthritis and Cartilage*, 15/9, Zhang W, Moskowitz RW, Nuki G, Abramson S, Altman RD, Arden N et al, OARSI recommendations for the management of hip and knee osteoarthritis, Part I: Critical appraisal of existing treatment guidelines and systematic review of current research evidence, 981–1000, Copyright (2007) with permission from Elsevier.

(Figure 37.3) in 2008 [21] and updated it in 2014 [2]. ACR updated its guidelines in 2012, expanding the joint coverage from just the hip and knee [23] to now also include the hand [22]. EULAR is unique in developing separate evidence-based recommendations for each of the hand [11], hip [10], and knee [24,25], both for diagnosis [26,27], and management [11,24]. EULAR also published in 2013 a more detailed guideline focused solely on non-pharmacological management of knee and hip OA to better guide practitioners in core elements of management [28]. In contrast, OARSI initially undertook a systematic review of all available treatments for knee and hip OA to produce a combined treatment guideline for both sites [7,12,20] but subsequently restricted its more recently updated guideline to non-surgical treatments for knee OA in recognition of the differences in aetiology, clinical presentation, progression, and management of OA at different joint sites [9]. In addition, in this update OARSI also provides further stratification according to number of affected joints and comorbidities in an attempt to optimize individual patient management. For example, topical NSAIDs are not recommended for people with multiple joint OA, selective COX2 inhibitors are not recommended in patients with cardiovascular comorbidity, etc. [9]. The differences between these major treatment guidelines are summarized in Table 37.4.

Despite the differences between guidelines they all tend to concur in recommending the following:

1. Education, self-management, exercise, and weight reduction if obese as the core set of treatments for all patients with OA at any site

2. Consideration of paracetamol and/or topical NSAID before other drugs. However, there is growing evidence that paracetamol is not as safe as previously thought [29] and it should be used with caution, especially in full dose (i.e. 4 g per day) and for long-term treatment (i.e. >3 months) [30]

3. Treatment may be stratified according to joint involvement, comorbidities, and clinical presentations such as severity of pain and functional limitation

4. An individualized package of care tailored to individual patient characteristics, rather than a uniform treatment algorithm, although evidence to support this is still sparse.

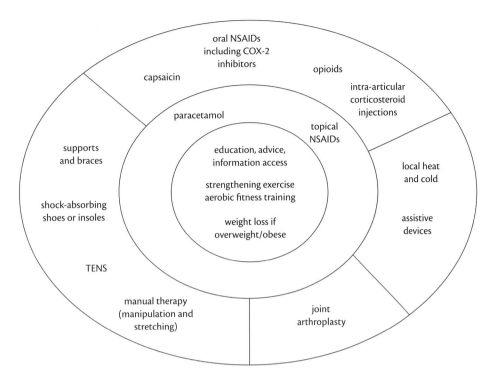

Figure 37.3 NICE overview figure showing core treatments at the centre, first-line analgesics in the middle ring, and other options to consider in the outer ring.
National Clinical Guideline Centre. *Osteoarthritis: Care and Management in Adults.* Clinical Guideline CG177. 2014. National Institute for Health and Care Excellence. 2014.

Challenges and changing perspectives

Stratified medicine

While we await new treatment developments, applying the right treatment for the right patient at the right time has been a research agenda for many organizations including Arthritis Research UK, EULAR, and more recently, OARSI. All guidelines recognize that guidance on treatment varies between joint sites because of differences in terms of aetiopathogenesis of OA, prognosis and suitability of certain treatments to only some sites (e.g. topical preparations). However, as discussed above, only EULAR has strategically produced separate recommendations for hand, hip and knee OA to better accommodate stratification by joint site [10,11,24] whereas other guidelines tend to give guidance for any joint site without specifying much difference between them. In practice, however, the vast majority of RCTs relate to knee OA, with fewer on hip OA and then hand OA, and very few indeed on OA at other joint sites. This means that advice on many treatments for joints other than the knee is often extrapolated and justified on the basis of knee OA research data with support from expert experience. Although always a caveat to such recommendations, such a pragmatic approach seems sensible since it is impractical to expect RCT data on all relevant treatments at all joint sites affected by OA.

In addition to joint site, OARSI recently has attempted to further stratify knee OA into four phenotypes according to joint involvement and comorbidities, specifically (1) isolated knee OA without comorbidities, (2) isolated knee OA with comorbidities, (3) multijoint OA without comorbidities, and (4) multijoint OA with comorbidities [9]. Treatments have been matched with each phenotype primarily according to the applicability and side effects of treatment. For example, topical NSAIDs are recommended for isolated knee OA with or without comorbidities, whereas oral NSAIDs are recommended for isolated knee OA or multijoint OA without comorbidities. However, although this stratification seems sensible in terms of adverse event consideration, it has no rationale in terms of improving treatment benefits which is the usual primary objective of stratified medicine.

Other stratifications have been proposed based on variables such as risk factors [31–33], pathology [34,35], clinical presentations [36,37], pain mechanisms [38,39], and inflammation [40,41]. For example, Knoop et al. [36] performed a cluster analysis of 842 participants with knee OA in the US Osteoarthritis Initiative (OAI) based on four clinically relevant and easily available variables—severity of radiographic OA, lower extremity muscle strength, body mass index, and depression. Five clinical phenotypes were identified, specifically (1) minimum joint disease phenotype, (2) strong muscle phenotype, (3) non-obese and weak muscle phenotype, (4) obese and weak muscle, and (5) depressive phenotype. The 'obese and weak muscle' and 'depressive' phenotypes showed higher pain levels and more severe activity limitation than the other three phenotypes. This stratification was subsequently replicated in the Netherlands [42]. Clearly three of the four features included in this stratification are potentially modifiable (muscle strength, body mass index, and depression) and there are RCT data to show that strengthening exercise, weight reduction, and antidepressants are statistically better than usual care or placebo controls for people with knee OA [9,20]. However, although such data support the already recommended full holistic assessment of people with OA to identify factors that then can be specifically targeted by available, often core treatments, such stratification adds nothing further to our current practice in terms of new strategies to guide selection of treatments to better optimize patient care.

Irrespective of whether inflammation is the primary or secondary feature of OA [40,43] selecting treatments according to the presence or absence of 'inflammation', detected predominantly by clinical assessment or imaging, remains a matter for frequent

Table 37.4 Comparison between NICE, OARSI, EULAR, ACR guidelines[a]

	NICE	OARSI	EULAR	ACR
Country	UK	Global	Europe	US
Target audience	All who manage OA	All who manage OA	Rheumatologists	Rheumatologists
Target joints	Knee, hip, and hand	Knee	Specific joint	Knee, hip, and hands
Stakeholders	All specialties plus patients	Rheumatologists, orthopaedics, and GPs	Rheumatologists, orthopaedics, and allied health professionals	Rheumatologists
Methods				
Systematic review	Yes	Yes	Yes	Yes
Delphi	No	Yes	Yes	No
Cost-effective assessment	Yes	Yes	No	No
Treatment algorithm	Yes	No	No	No
Stratification	Yes by joint	Yes by joint and co-morbidity	Yes by joint	Yes by joint
Exercise	Yes	Yes	Yes	Yes (knee and hip)
Education	Yes	Yes	Yes	Yes
Weight loss	Yes	Yes	Yes	Yes (knee and hip)
Acupuncture	No	Yes	?	?
Paracetamol	First-line drug	?	First-line drug	Yes
Topical NSAIDs	Yes (hand and knee)	Yes	Yes (hand and knee)	Yes
Oral NSAIDs	Yes	Yes	Yes	Yes
Opioids	Yes	?	Yes	Yes
Duloxetine	–	Yes	–	Yes
Glucosamine	No	?	?	?
Chondroitin	No	?	?	?
IA-steroid	Yes	Yes	Yes	Yes
IAHA	No	?	?	Yes
Lavage	No	No	?	?
TJR	Yes	–	Yes	–

[a]For guidelines with regular updates the latest version was used for the comparison.

– not covered; ? uncertain.

debate. For example, RCTS show superior pain relief from NSAIDs than paracetamol but whether this correlates to inflammation presence is unclear [44]. Intra-articular steroid is more effective in people with knee OA with more severe pain and possibly inflammation at baseline [45] and methotrexate, which is used successfully in rheumatoid arthritis and other inflammatory arthropathies, may relieve pain due to knee OA with clinical effusion [46]. However, the anti- tumour necrosis factor blocker adalimumab gives no benefit to people with hand OA that is insufficiently responsive to NSAIDs [47] or to those with erosive hand OA [48]. Therefore, whether inflammation should be a target of treatment and the utility of stratifying according to presence of inflammation remains an area of considerable interest and ongoing research.

Dissemination of guideline recommendations and influence on clinical practice

As OA is by far the commonest joint condition, it is predominantly managed in the community by general practitioners, allied health practitioners, and pharmacists. Only a very small proportion of people are seen by rheumatologists and in most countries secondary care referral predominantly is for late-stage OA and consideration of joint surgery. Paradoxically, however, the development of OA guidelines is led predominantly by doctors in secondary care. Furthermore, EULAR, ACR, and OARSI guidelines are published in specialist journals that will not reach the practitioners who manage the vast majority of patients with OA. These publications are also in a single format that is unsuitable for generalist and patient readers, and they are not readily available in open access format. A better model is that used by NICE in the United Kingdom which publishes multiple, freely available guidelines on their website, each in various formats to suit different readers (e.g. very brief summary, full guidelines for clinicians, expanded guidelines with all data, etc.). However, despite its better dissemination, NICE guidelines still have no power to influence the behaviour of general practitioners and health professionals within the National Health Service. This is because for OA, unlike certain other medical conditions, there is no agreed Quality and Outcomes Framework (QOF) that requires yearly audit of the standard of care for people with OA using approved quality indicators, with financial penalties if certain standards are not demonstrated. Without a QOF it is very hard to attract the attention of the general practice teams towards OA and independent audits continue to show more than just suboptimal care of people with OA [49]. Clearly the situation will vary from country to country. However, appropriate country-specific strategies to disseminate guidelines that can really effect change need to be developed if guidelines are to have an impact on improving standards of care.

Tackling the efficacy paradox

A further barrier to effective implementation of the guidelines is that there is frequent discordance between what the guidelines recommend and what clinicians have observed in clinical practice. For example, a practitioner may have used acupuncture for many years and seen it greatly help the majority of their patients with OA. However, the newly published NICE guideline on OA states that acupuncture gives no meaningful improvement in OA and therefore does not recommend its use. What should a doctor believe—his/her own experience or the evidence-based guideline recommendation? Only relatively recently has this 'efficacy paradox' been recognized—when the effect of a treatment that is tested in RCTs differs markedly from the effect observed in clinical practice [50].

How can this paradox happen? The effect of a treatment may result from two main components. Firstly, the specific treatment effect due to the active ingredients of the treatment itself and secondly, the non-specific (contextual) effects due to the context in which the treatment is being received. The latter is well known in RCTs as the 'placebo effect'. However, when a treatment is given to a patient in clinical practice, the outcome is always the overall treatment effect which is the sum of both the specific effects plus the contextual effects, and it is on this overall treatment effect that the worth of a treatment is judged. In contrast, in RCTs the whole focus is on the difference in the outcome between the treatment group and the placebo group. This between-group difference is used for calculation of the effect size of the treatment (how 'strong' it is) and only treatments that separate from placebo by a significant amount, or an MCID in the case of NICE, will be recommended.

This focus in RCTs on just the specific effect of the treatment distracts attention from the overall treatment effect even though this is often quite large and more akin to the effects seen in clinical practice. Furthermore it underemphasizes the large effect size of placebo/contextual response, even though this is often greater than the response due to the specific treatment effect [51]. Although the separation between specific and contextual effect of a treatment is essential for the establishment of a treatment, in clinical practice, patients receive benefit from both. The sole focus on the specific treatment effect reported from RCTs underestimates the overall benefit of treatment, therefore creates the 'efficacy paradox'. Guideline developers similarly ignore both the overall treatment effect and the magnitude of the contextual effect of a treatment and make recommendations based solely on specific treatment effects. As illustrated in Figure 37.4a, treatment A is not significantly better than placebo in one trial, whereas in another trial treatment B separates significantly from placebo. However, treatment A in fact is much better in terms of magnitude of benefit than treatment B if

we look at the overall treatment effects of the two. Unfortunately, if we look only at the evidence for the specific treatment effect from RCTs, we are likely to recommend treatment B but not treatment A.

A key question is whether the separation between specific and contextual effects matters to patients. Given the choice between treatments A and B most people will opt for A because that is likely to give them the largest overall treatment effect. Whether a higher or lower proportion of the treatment benefit results from specific treatment effects (Figure 37.4b) is not a big concern, as long as their patient-centred outcomes show a meaningful improvement. Very few people consult to hear just about specific treatment benefit, most want to know how much they may improve (overall) on any

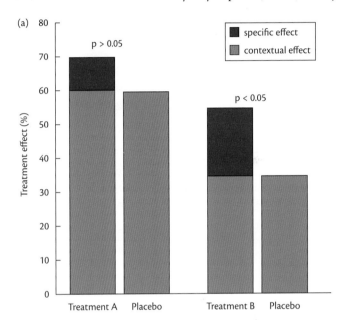

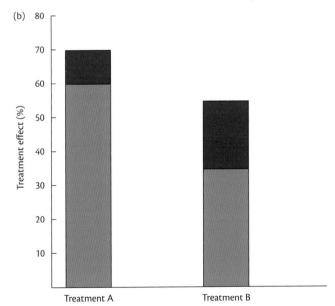

Figure 37.4 The efficacy paradox. In two RCTs, treatment A is not significantly better than placebo whereas treatment B is significantly better than placebo. However, the overall treatment effect of treatment A is in fact better than treatment B because treatment A associates with a much larger non-specific effect (or contextual effect) than treatment B. However, in most guidelines treatment B will be recommended whereas treatment A will not.

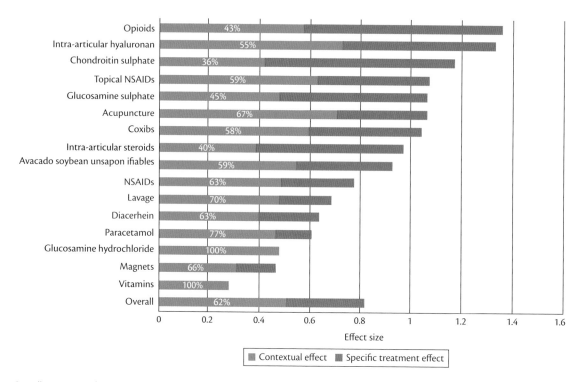

Figure 37.5 Overall treatment effect and contribution from specific and non-specific effects of treatment in OA. The data was estimated from the two systematic reviews of RCTs where both specific treatment effect and placebo effect were used to estimate the overall effect and proportion of contextual effect for each treatment [20,51].

Reprinted from Zhang W. Is placebo a possible therapy for osteoarthritis?—from placebo to obcalp. In: Lindgren KA, editor. Placebo—placebo effects in musculoskeletal disorders.Helsinki: Rehabilitation ORTON Foundation; 2013. p. 61–8.

particular treatment. Clearly it would be wrong to knowingly offer a treatment with no or very little specific effect purely to capitalize on contextual effects, but should we expect the magnitude of the specific effect on its own to be high enough to be 'clinically meaningful'? Perhaps the present bar is set too high. If we focus on the total treatment effect of various treatments in OA and show what proportion is explained by contextual factors in RCTs (Figure 37.5) this shows that (1) contrary to the widespread pessimism over treatments in OA, many of the treatments have a good to strong effect in terms of pain relief; and (2) the hierarchy of strength of treatment is re-ordered compared to one based just on specific treatment effects. Consideration of this approach may better explain the results of RCTs in terms that are relevant to clinical practice and better inform guideline developers, clinicians, and patients in making management decisions—in other words, better align with the stated philosophy of evidence-based medicine.

References

1. Peat G, McCarney R, Croft P. Knee pain and osteoarthritis in older adults: a review of community burden and current use of primary health care. *Ann Rheum Dis* 2001; 60(2):91–97.
2. National Clinical Guideline Centre. *Osteoarthritis: Care and Management in Adults*. Clinical Guideline CG177. London: National Institute for Health and Care Excellence; 2014.
3. Zhang W, Moskowitz RW, Nuki G, et al. OARSI recommendations for the management of hip and knee osteoarthritis, Part I: Critical appraisal of existing treatment guidelines and systematic review of current research evidence. *Osteoarthritis Cartilage* 2007; 15(9):981–1000.
4. Lohr KN, Field MJ. A provisional instrument for assessing clinical practice guidelines. In Field MJ, Lohr KN (eds) *Guidelines for Clinical Practice. From Development to Use*. Washington DC: National Academy Press; 1992.
5. Haynes B, Sackett DL, Cook J, Guyatt GH. Translating evidence from research into practice: 1. The role of clinical care research evidence in clinical decisions. *Evidence-Based Med* 1996; 1(7):196–8.
6. Shekelle PG, Woolf SH, Eccles M, Grimshaw J. Clinical guidelines: developing guidelines. *BMJ* 1999; 318(7183):593–6.
7. Zhang W, Doherty M, Pascual E, et al. EULAR evidence based recommendations for gout. Part I: Diagnosis. Report of a task force of the standing committee for international clinical studies including therapeutics (ESCISIT). *Ann Rheum Dis* 2006; 65(10):1301–11.
8. Jones J, Hunter D. Consensus methods for medical and health services research. *BMJ* 1995; 311(7001):376–80.
9. McAlindon TE, Bannuru RR, Sullivan MC, et al. OARSI guidelines for the non-surgical management of knee osteoarthritis. *Osteoarthritis Cartilage* 2014; 22(3):363–88.
10. Zhang W, Doherty M, Arden N, et al. EULAR evidence based recommendations for the management of hip osteoarthritis: report of a task force of the EULAR Standing Committee for International Clinical Studies Including Therapeutics (ESCISIT). *Ann Rheum Dis* 2005; 64(5):669–81.
11. Zhang W, Doherty M, Leeb BF, et al. EULAR evidence based recommendations for the management of hand osteoarthritis: Report of a Task Force of the EULAR Standing Committee for International Clinical Studies Including Therapeutics (ESCISIT). *Ann Rheum Dis* 2007; 66(3):377–88.
12. Zhang W, Moskowitz RW, Nuki G, et al. OARSI recommendations for the management of hip and knee osteoarthritis, Part II: OARSI evidence-based, expert consensus guidelines. *Osteoarthritis Cartilage* 2008; 16(2):137–62.

13. The GRADE Working Group. Grading quality of evidence and strength of recommendations. *BMJ* 2004; 328(7454):1490.

14. Guyatt GH, Oxman AD, Vist GE, et al. GRADE: an emerging consensus on rating quality of evidence and strength of recommendations. *BMJ* 2008; 336(7650):924–6.

15. Guyatt GH, Oxman AD, Kunz R, et al. What is 'quality of evidence' and why is it important to clinicians? *BMJ* 2008; 336(7651):995–8.

16. Guyatt GH, Oxman AD, Kunz R, et al. Going from evidence to recommendations. *BMJ* 2008; 336(7652):1049–51.

17. Marshall G, Blacklock JWS, Cameron C, et al. Streptomycin treatment of pulmonary tuberculosis. *BMJ* 1948; 2(4582):769–82.

18. Kavanagh BP. The GRADE system for rating clinical guidelines. *PLoS Med* 2009; 6(9):e1000094.

19. The AGREE Collaboration. *Appraisal of Guidelines for Research & Evaluation (AGREE) Instrument*. 2006. http://www.agreecollaboration.org

20. Zhang W, Nuki G, Moskowitz RW, et al. OARSI recommendations for the management of hip and knee osteoarthritis: part III: Changes in evidence following systematic cumulative update of research published through January 2009. *Osteoarthritis Cartilage* 2010; 18(4):476–99.

21. National Collaborating Centre for Chronic Conditions. *Osteoarthritis: National Clinical Guideline for Care and Management in Adults*. London: National Institute for Health and Care Excellence; 2008.

22. Hochberg MC, Altman RD, April KT, et al. American College of Rheumatology 2012 recommendations for the use of nonpharmacologic and pharmacologic therapies in osteoarthritis of the hand, hip, and knee. *Arthritis Care Res (Hoboken)* 2012; 64(4):465–74.

23. Recommendations for the medical management of osteoarthritis of the hip and knee: 2000 update. American College of Rheumatology Subcommittee on Osteoarthritis Guidelines. *Arthritis Rheum* 2000; 43(9):1905–15.

24. Jordan KM, Arden NK, Doherty M, et al. EULAR Recommendations 2003: an evidence based approach to the management of knee osteoarthritis: Report of a Task Force of the Standing Committee for International Clinical Studies Including Therapeutic Trials (ESCISIT). *Ann Rheum Dis* 2003; 62(12):1145–55.

25. Pendleton A, Arden N, Dougados M, et al. EULAR recommendations for the management of knee osteoarthritis: report of a task force of the Standing Committee for International Clinical Studies Including Therapeutic Trials (ESCISIT). *Ann Rheum Dis* 2000; 59(12):936–44.

26. Zhang W, Doherty M, Leeb BF, et al. EULAR evidence-based recommendations for the diagnosis of hand osteoarthritis: report of a task force of ESCISIT. *Ann Rheum Dis* 2009; 68(1):8–17.

27. Zhang W, Doherty M, Peat G, et al. EULAR evidence-based recommendations for the diagnosis of knee osteoarthritis. *Ann Rheum Dis* 2010; 69(3):483–9.

28. Fernandes L, Hagen KB, Bijlsma JW, et al. EULAR recommendations for the non-pharmacological core management of hip and knee osteoarthritis. *Ann Rheum Dis* 2013; 72(7):1125–35.

29. Roberts E, Delgado Nunes V, Buckner S, et al. Paracetamol: not as safe as we thought? A systematic literature review of observational studies. *Ann Rheum Dis* 2016; 75(3):552–9.

30. Doherty M, Hawkey C, Goulder M, et al. A randomised controlled trial of ibuprofen, paracetamol or a combination tablet of ibuprofen/paracetamol in community-derived people with knee pain. *Ann Rheum Dis* 2011; 70(9):1534–41.

31. Altman R, Asch E, Bloch D, et al. Development of criteria for the classification and reporting of osteoarthritis. Classification of osteoarthritis of the knee. Diagnostic and Therapeutic Criteria Committee of the American Rheumatism Association. *Arthritis Rheum* 1986; 29(8):1039–49.

32. Riordan EA, Little C, Hunter D. Pathogenesis of post-traumatic OA with a view to intervention. *Best Pract Res Clin Rheumatol* 2014; 28(1):17–30.

33. Herrero-Beaumont G, Roman-Blas JA, Castaneda S, Jimenez SA. Primary osteoarthritis no longer primary: three subsets with distinct etiological, clinical, and therapeutic characteristics. *Semin Arthritis Rheum* 2009; 39(2):71–80.

34. Roemer FW, Guermazi A, Niu J, et al. Prevalence of magnetic resonance imaging-defined atrophic and hypertrophic phenotypes of knee osteoarthritis in a population-based cohort. *Arthritis Rheum* 2012; 64(2):429–37.

35. Solomon L, Schnitzler CM. Pathogenetic types of coxarthrosis and implications for treatment. *Arch Orthop Trauma Surg* 1983; 101(4):259–61.

36. Knoop J, van der LM, Thorstensson CA, et al. Identification of phenotypes with different clinical outcomes in knee osteoarthritis: data from the Osteoarthritis Initiative. *Arthritis Care Res (Hoboken)* 2011; 63(11):1535–42.

37. Bijlsma JW, Berenbaum F, Lafeber FP. Osteoarthritis: an update with relevance for clinical practice. *Lancet* 2011; 377(9783):2115–26.

38. Murphy SL, Lyden AK, Phillips K, Clauw DJ, Williams DA. Association between pain, radiographic severity, and centrally-mediated symptoms in women with knee osteoarthritis. *Arthritis Care Res (Hoboken)* 2011; 63(11):1543–9.

39. Murphy SL, Phillips K, Williams DA, Clauw DJ. The role of the central nervous system in osteoarthritis pain and implications for rehabilitation. *Curr Rheumatol Rep* 2012; 14(6):576–82.

40. Berenbaum F. Osteoarthritis as an inflammatory disease (osteoarthritis is not osteoarthrosis!). *Osteoarthritis Cartilage* 2013; 21(1):16–21.

41. Siebuhr AS, Petersen KK, Arendt-Nielsen L, Egsgaard LL, Eskehave T, Christiansen C et al. Identification and characterisation of osteoarthritis patients with inflammation derived tissue turnover. *Osteoarthritis Cartilage* 2014; 22(1):44–50.

42. van der Esch M, Knoop J, van der Leeden M, et al. Clinical phenotypes in patients with knee osteoarthritis: a study in the Amsterdam osteoarthritis cohort. *Osteoarthritis Cartilage* 2015; 23(4):544–9.

43. Felson DT. Osteoarthritis as a disease of mechanics. *Osteoarthritis Cartilage* 2013; 21(1):10–15.

44. Zhang W, Jones A, Doherty M. Does paracetamol (acetaminophen) reduce the pain of osteoarthritis?: a meta-analysis of randomised controlled trials. *Ann Rheum Dis* 2004; 63(8):901–7.

45. van MM, Dziedzic KS, Doherty M, et al. Individual patient data meta-analysis of trials investigating the effectiveness of intra-articular glucocorticoid injections in patients with knee or hip osteoarthritis: an OA Trial Bank protocol for a systematic review. *Syst Rev* 2013; 2:54.

46. Abou-Raya A, Abou-Raya S, Khadrawe T. Methotrexate in the treatment of symptomatic knee osteoarthritis: randomised placebo-controlled trial. *Ann Rheum Dis* 2014; Mar 27. doi: 10.1136/annrheumdis-2013-204856. [Epub ahead of print]

47. Chevalier X, Ravaud P, Maheu E, et al. Adalimumab in patients with hand osteoarthritis refractory to analgesics and NSAIDs: a randomised, multicentre, double-blind, placebo-controlled trial. *Ann Rheum Dis* 2015; 74(9):1697–705.

48. Verbruggen G, Wittoek R, Vander CB, Elewaut D. Tumour necrosis factor blockade for the treatment of erosive osteoarthritis of the interphalangeal finger joints: a double blind, randomised trial on structure modification. *Ann Rheum Dis* 2012; 71(6):891–8.

49. Arthritis Care. *OA Nation 2012.* 2012. http://wwwarthritiscareorguk

50. Walach H. The efficacy paradox in randomized controlled trials of CAM and elsewhere: beware of the placebo trap. *J Altern Complement Med* 2001; 7(3):213–8.

51. Zhang W, Robertson J, Jones AC, Dieppe PA, Doherty M. The placebo effect and its determinants in osteoarthritis: meta-analysis of randomised controlled trials. *Ann Rheum Dis* 2008; 67(12):1716–23.

SECTION 13

Gout

CHAPTER 38

Epidemiology of gout

Samantha Hider and Edward Roddy

Introduction

Gout occurs when body tissues become super-saturated with urate, leading to the formation of monosodium urate (MSU) crystals in and around joints. The clinical features of gout are varied but include acutely painful attacks of peripheral joint synovitis, tophaceous deposition of MSU crystals in joints and other body tissues, chronic joint damage, renal stone formation, and renal insufficiency. It leads to impaired quality of life which arises from the excruciating pain of acute attacks, chronic arthropathy, associated co-morbidities, and frequent suboptimal management [1].

This chapter will review discuss evidence that the prevalence and incidence of gout are increasing, review epidemiological studies of risk factors for the development of gout (Table 38.1), and consider the evidence that gout is a risk factor for cardiovascular and renal disease. Data are presented from population-based prospective epidemiological studies where possible. Multivariate risk estimates are presented unless otherwise stated.

Prevalence and incidence of gout

Data from a number of countries across the globe suggest that the prevalence and incidence of gout are increasing. In the United Kingdom, the prevalence has increased steadily over a number of surveys from 0.26% in 1975 to a 1-year consultation prevalence of 2.49% in 2012 (Figure 38.1) [2,3]. Similarly, in the United States, the 1-year period prevalence of self-reported gout in the National Health Interview Surveys almost doubled from 0.48% in 1969 to 0.94% in 1996 [4,5]. In the National Health and Nutrition Examination Survey (NHANES), the lifetime prevalence of self-reported physician-diagnosed gout increased from 2.64% in NHANES-III (1988–1994) to 3.76% in NHANES 2007–2010 [6]. The prevalence of gout in New Zealand increased dramatically from 0.3% in European subjects and 2.7% in Maori subjects in 1958, to 2.9% and 6.4% respectively in 1992 but has remained stable since [7–10]. In the Health Search/Longitudinal Patient Primary Care database in Italy, the annual consultation prevalence of gout increased slightly from 0.67% in 2005 to 0.91% in 2009 [11].

There are fewer studies of gout incidence. In the Rochester Epidemiology Project, the annual incidence of primary gout (i.e. without diuretic exposure) doubled from 20.2/100 000 in 1977/1978 to 45.9/100 000 in 1995/1996, whereas diuretic-induced gout remained stable [12]. More recently, in the UK-Clinical Practice Research Datalink (UK-CPRD), the standardized incidence of gout increased from 1.36 per 1000 patient-years in 1997 to 1.77 per 1000 patient-years in 2012, although incidence reached a plateau from 2003 onwards (Figure 38.1) [3]. Gout incidence

Table 38.1 Risk factors for the development of gout

Increased risk	Reduced risk
Male gender	Dietary factors:
Age	◆ Low-fat dairy products
Socioeconomic deprivation	
Genetic factors (see Chapter 9)	◆ Coffee
Dietary factors:	◆ Vitamin C
◆ Animal purines (meat, seafood)	Diabetes mellitus
◆ Sugar-sweetened soft drinks, fructose	Medications:
◆ Alcoholic drinks (particularly beer)	◆ Fenofibrate
Metabolic syndrome	◆ Losartan
Obesity	◆ Calcium-channel blockers
Insulin resistance	
Hypertension	
Medications:	
◆ Loop and thiazide diuretics	
◆ Beta-blockers	
◆ Angiotensin-converting enzyme inhibitors	
◆ Non-losartan angiotensin II receptor blockers	
◆ Low-dose aspirin	
Chronic kidney disease	
Osteoarthritis	

was stable in UK primary care studies performed in The Health Improvement Network (UK-THIN) (2000–2007, 2.52 per 1000 patient-years) and Royal College of General Practitioners Weekly Returns Service (1994–2007, 12.4 per 10 000 patients per year) during this period [13,14]. Annual consultation rates for incident gout were also stable in Italy between 2005 and 2009, ranging from 0.93 to 0.95 per 1000 person-years [11].

Both the prevalence and incidence of gout are higher in men than women (Figure 38.1), and increase with age [3,9,11]. Whereas earlier studies reported that the greatest rise in prevalence and incidence was in primary gout in older men [12,15], the most recent study suggests slightly greater increases in gout prevalence and incidence in women than men [3].

Socioeconomic deprivation

Historically gout was considered to be the 'disease of kings' or a disease of affluence due in part to associations with alcohol and

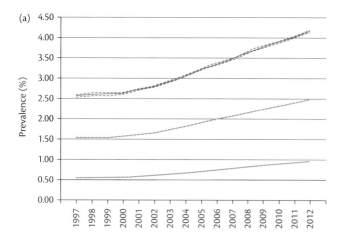

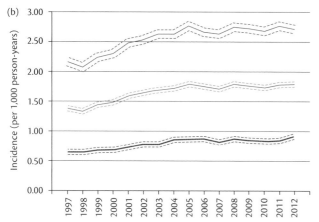

Figure 38.1 Gender differences in the trends of standardized prevalence (a) and incidence (b) of gout between 1997 and 2012 (blue: men; red: women; green: overall; dotted line: 95% confidence bounds).
Reproduced from *Annals of the Rheumatic Diseases*, Kuo CF et al., 2014 Jan 15. doi: 10.1136/annrheumdis-2013-204463, with permission from BMJ Publishing Group Ltd.

purine-rich food intake. However, the majority of studies to formally investigate this show an inverse correlation between gout and socioeconomic status. A study of 15 000 men aged 45–74 from three English towns with different socioeconomic backgrounds, found that people living in towns with a poorer economic status had higher prevalence of self-reported gout (proportion with gout: Preston 4.8%, Wakefield 4.5%, and Ipswich 3.9%) [16]. In New Zealand, the risk of gout was 41% higher in those living in the most socioeconomically deprived areas compared to those in the least deprived, even after adjustment for age, gender and ethnicity (relative risk (RR) 1.41, 95% confidence interval (CI) 1.31–1.52) [9]. A German health survey found an association between gout and lower socioeconomic class in women but not men [17]. A recent primary care cross-sectional study in the United Kingdom found that gout was associated with perceived inadequacy of income (odds ratio (OR) 1.44, 95% CI 1.13–1.84), although no association was seen with occupational class, education, or area-level socioeconomic status [18].

Dietary factors

Associations between gout and dietary factors, particularly excessive consumption of purine-rich foods and alcoholic drinks, have

been recognized since ancient times. Much of our current understanding of the role played by dietary factors in the aetiology of gout arises from the Health Professionals Follow-up Study (HPFS) which followed 51 529 male health professionals for a 12-year period, identifying 730 incident cases of gout [19] and the Nurses' Health Study which followed 89 433 female nurses for 26 years, during which 896 incident gout cases occurred [20]. High intake of total meat, seafood, sugar-sweetened soft drinks, and free and total fructose were associated with an increased risk of incident gout (Table 38.2) [21–23]. Consumption of low-fat dairy, coffee, decaffeinated coffee, and vitamin C protected against incident gout whereas purine-rich vegetables, high-fat dairy, tea, and diet-soft drinks did not appear to influence the risk of developing gout [19–24]. High total caffeine intake reduced the risk of incident gout in women but not in men [20,23].

A recent meta-analysis of alcohol intake and risk of gout identified 12 articles reporting a dose-dependent effect on alcohol consumption on the risk of gout [25]. Compared with those imbibing occasional or no alcohol, the RR of gout was 1.16 (95% CI 1.07–1.25) with light alcohol consumption (≤1 drink per day), 1.58 (1.50–1.66) with moderate consumption (1–3 drinks), and 2.64 (2.26–3.09) with heavy consumption (≥3 drinks per day), although there was significant heterogeneity. In the HPFS, the risk of incident gout in men drinking with 2 or more drinks per day compared to those drinking less than once per month was greatest for beer (RR 2.51, 95% CI 1.77–3.55), followed by spirits (1.60; 1.19–2.16) whereas wine consumption conferred little risk (1.05; 0.64–1.72) [26].

Whereas these studies have examined the role of dietary factors as risk factors for the development of gout, there has also been interest in their propensity to precipitate recurrent acute attacks of gout. An internet-based case–crossover study found that intake of purine-rich foods (OR 4.76, 95% CI 3.37–6.74; highest quintile consumed in preceding 48 hours versus lowest quintile) and alcoholic drinks (OR 1.51, 95% CI 1.09–2.09; >2–4 drinks in preceding 24 hours versus no drinks) triggered recurrent acute attacks whereas cherry consumption was associated with a lower risk of attacks (OR 0.65, 95% CI 0.50–0.85; any amount in preceding 48 hours versus none consumed) [27–29].

Comorbidities

The development of gout is commonly associated with a number of common comorbidities including the metabolic syndrome and its constituent conditions including obesity, hypertension, and insulin resistance or diabetes. In a cross-sectional study within NHANES-III, the prevalence of metabolic syndrome was higher in gout patients (62.8% vs 25.4%; OR 3.05, 95% CI 2.01–4.61) [30].

Obesity

A recent meta-analysis of ten studies (seven from the United States, two from Taiwan, and one from the United Kingdom) including 27 944 cases and 215 739 control subjects without gout, examined body mass index (BMI) and risk of incident gout and found an increased RR risk per 5-unit increase in BMI of 1.62 (95% CI 1.33–1.98) for males and 1.49 (95% CI 1.32,1.68) for females [31]. There was also evidence of a dose–response effect of BMI on gout risk, with an increased RR seen in those with a BMI of 25 (RR 1.78), 30 (RR 2.67), 35 (RR 3.62), and 40 (RR 4.64) compared to people

Table 38.2 Dietary factors and risk of incident gout

Dietary factor	Study	Exposure group	Comparator group	Multivariate relative risk (95% confidence interval)
Total meat	HPFS	Highest quintile	Lowest quintile	1.41 (1.07–1.86)
Seafood	HPFS	Highest quintile	Lowest quintile	1.51 (1.17–1.95)
Purine-rich vegetables	HPFS	Highest quintile	Lowest quintile	0.96 (0.79–1.19)
Dairy products	HPFS	Highest quintile	Lowest quintile	0.56 (0.42–0.74)
Low-fat dairy products	HPFS	Highest quintile	Lowest quintile	0.58 (0.45–0.76)
High-fat dairy products	HPFS	Highest quintile	Lowest quintile	1.00 (0.77–1.29)
Coffee	HPFS	≥6 cups/day	None	0.41 (0.19–0.88)
	Nurses' Health Study	≥4 cups/day	None	0.43 (0.30–0.61)
Decaffeinated coffee	HPFS	≥4 cups/day	None	0.73 (0.46–1.17)
	Nurses' Health Study	>1 cups/day	None	0.77 (0.63–0.95)
Tea	HPFS	≥4 cups/day	None	0.82 (0.38–1.75)
	Nurses' Health Study	≥4 cups/day	None	1.55 (0.98–2.47)
Total caffeine	HPFS	Highest quintile	Lowest quintile	0.83 (0.64–1.08)
	Nurses' Health Study	Highest quintile	Lowest quintile	0.52 (0.41–0.68)
Sugar-sweetened soft drinks	HPFS	≥2 servings/day	<1 serving/month	1.85 (1.08–3.16)
	Nurses' Health Study	≥2 servings/day	<1 serving/month	2.39 (1.34–4.26)
Diet soft drinks	HPFS	≥2 servings/day	<1 serving/month	1.12 (0.82–1.52)
	Nurses' Health Study	≥2 servings/day	<1 serving/month	1.18 (0.87–1.58)
Free fructose	HPFS	Highest quintile	Lowest quintile	2.02 (1.49–2.75)
	Nurses' Health Study	Highest quintile	Lowest quintile	1.62 (1.20–2.19)
Total fructose	HPFS	Highest quintile	Lowest quintile	1.81 (1.31–2.50)
	Nurses' Health Study	Highest quintile	Lowest quintile	1.44 (1.04–2.00)
Vitamin C	HPFS	≥1500 mg/day	<250 mg/day	0.55 (0.38–0.80)

HPFS, Health Professionals Follow-up Study.

with a BMI of 20. A similar dose–response relationship between BMI and incident gout was seen in a recent large UK-CPRD population study of 39 111 gout patients matched 1:1 with controls (BMI 25–29.9, OR 1.81, 95% CI 1.74–1.88; BMI ≥ 30, OR 3.15, 95% CI 3.01–3.30; compared with referent BMI 18.5–24.9) [32].

Fewer studies have assessed other measures of obesity such as waist/hip ratio or weight gain from young adulthood although pooled results from two studies [33,34] demonstrate an overall increase in the RR of gout per 0.1 unit change in the waist:hip ratio of 1.82 (95% CI 1.44–2.29) and similar overall risks from an increase in weight from young adulthood (1.82 per 5 kg increase; 1.44–2.29) [31].

Diabetes mellitus

The relationship between gout and hyperglycaemia and diabetes mellitus is complex. Hyperuricaemia is a risk factor for development of type 2 diabetes, with a recent review [35] suggesting that this is independent of other metabolic syndrome components.

However, once diabetes is present the risk of gout appears to lessen. In a case–control study nested in the UK-THIN database, the RR of incident gout was lower in those with diabetes compared

to age- and gender-matched controls (0.67, 95% CI 0.63–0.71). This effect was stronger for type 1 than type 2 diabetes (0.33 vs 0.69) and with increasing duration of diabetes (0–3 years 0.81, 95% CI 0.74–0.90 vs ≥10 years 0.52, 95% CI 0.46–0.58) [36].

A potential mechanism to explain this finding is via the relative effects of hyperinsulinaemia and glycosuria on serum urate levels. Hyperinsulinaemia and insulin resistance seen as part of the metabolic syndrome lead to an increase in serum urate levels, which is counteracted once frank diabetes develops by the uricosuric effect of glycosuria [37].

Hypertension and cardiovascular disease

The risk of incident gout in patients with hypertension has been investigated in several large-scale studies, although with differing magnitudes of risk. Within the UK-THIN database, the risk of incident gout in patients with hypertension was moderate (OR 1.18, 95% CI 1.13–1.23) [13], although, in the United States, the Atherosclerosis Risk in Communities (ARIC) study of 10 872 patients showed a higher risk of incident gout (hazard ratio (HR) 2.87, 95% CI 2.24–3.78) [38]. In NHANES-III, there was a small increased prevalence of gout in patients with uncontrolled hypertension alone, but an increasing magnitude of risk in in those with additional cardiovascular risk factors, with a prevalence ratio of 1.47 (95% CI 0.79–2.72) in those with uncontrolled hypertension alone, increasing to 2.41 (95% CI 1.52–3.85) in those with a second CVD risk factor and 4.45 (95% CI 3.13–6.32) in those with two additional risk factors [39].

In terms of other cardiovascular risk factors, within the UK-THIN dataset, hypertriglyceridaemia was associated with increased risk of incident gout (OR 1.45, 95% CI 1.18–1.79) but this effect was less clear for hypercholesterolaemia (OR 1.08, 95% CI 1.04–1.22) [13].

Furthermore, gout itself is associated with an increased risk of cardiovascular disease. Data from UK-CPRD, examining 8386 incident gout patients and 39 766 age- and gender-matched controls showed increased coronary heart disease risk in both men (HR 1.08, 95% CI 1.01–1.15) and women (HR 1.25, 95% CI 1.12–1.39) [40] whilst a meta-analysis of six studies showed an increased risk of cardiovascular mortality (HR 1.29, 95% CI 1.14–1.44) even after adjustment for traditional vascular risk factors [41].

Chronic kidney disease and nephrolithiasis

The association between gout and kidney disease is well recognized. It is thought that hyperuricaemia and gout occur as a consequence of impaired renal function, but then they lead to further impairment of renal function. Several epidemiological studies provide evidence that renal disease is an independent risk factor for the development of gout. In the HPFS, men with chronic renal failure had over three times the risk of incident gout compared to those without chronic renal failure (RR 3.61, 95% CI 1.60–8.14) [33]. In the UK-THIN database, incident gout was associated with a prior history of chronic renal failure (OR 2.48, 95% CI 2.19–2.81) [13]. These two studies defined renal disease using primary care diagnostic codes whereas two more recently published analyses used a more robust biochemical definition for chronic kidney disease. In the prospective ARIC cohort, those with an estimated glomerular filtration rate (eGFR) less than 60 mL/min had more than twice the odds of incident gout than those with normal renal function (eGFR >90 mL/min) (OR 2.43, 95% CI 1.50–3.94) [38]. Similarly, in the Multiple Risk Factor Intervention Trial, the HR for incident gout in those with eGFR less than 60mL/min compared to those with eGFR of 90 mL/min or higher was 2.8 (95% CI 1.3–6.0) [42].

A small number of studies have prospectively examined whether gout is a risk factor for renal disease. In a study from Canada, gout was an independent risk factor for decline in mean eGFR of at least 25% between 2001 and 2003 in adults aged 66 years or older (OR 1.5, 95% CI 1.1–2.1) [43]. A Taiwanese study found an increased risk of incident end-stage renal disease (ESRD) in people with gout compared with those without gout over an 8-year period (HR 1.57, 95% CI 1.38–1.79) [44] whereas there was no increased risk of ESRD over 25 years on multivariate analysis in a study undertaken in the United States [45].

A study undertaken in UK-CPRD has examined the risk of comorbidities prior to and after the diagnosis of incident gout [32]. People with gout were almost six times more likely to have a diagnosis of renal disease in the 10-year period prior to developing incident gout (OR 5.96, 95% CI 5.09–6.98) and had greater than three times the risk of developing incident renal disease after the diagnosis of gout (HR 3.18, 95% CI 2.88–3.50).

Although the association between gout and nephrolithiasis has been recognized for centuries, there is a paucity of prospective epidemiological studies. In the HPFS, men with gout had twice the risk of incident nephrolithiasis compared with men without gout (HR 2.12, 95% CI 1.22–3.68) [46]. In UK-CPRD, the HR for incident nephrolithiasis in people with gout was 1.26 (95% CI 1.02–1.55) [32].

Medications
Diuretics and antihypertensives

Several medications have been implicated in the development of gout. Loop and thiazide diuretics have been frequently implicated in gout pathogenesis via their effects on renal urate handling, including reduced uric acid excretion and direct effects on urate transporters at the renal proximal tubule. A recent systematic review (including two randomized controlled trials, six cohort, and five case–control studies) [47] showed an increased risk of gout in diuretic users but commented on the moderate quality of the included studies, with significant heterogeneity in study size, population, and adjustment for potential confounders, which is critical given that prescribing indications for diuretics (e.g. heart failure or hypertension) may themselves be associated with gout.

Data from the UK-THIN database of patients with hypertension, showed an increased risk of incident gout with current diuretic use (RR 2.36, 95% CI 2.21–2.52), beta blockers (RR 1.48, 95% CI 1.40–1.57), angiotensin-converting-enzyme inhibitors (RR 1.24, 95% CI 1.17–1.32), and non-losartan angiotensin II receptor blockers (RR 1.29, 95% CI 1.16–1.43). The risk was reduced in those taking calcium channel antagonists (RR 0.87, 95% CI 0.82–0.93) or losartan (RR 0.81, 95% CI 0.70–0.94) [48]. Similar increased risk of gout in diuretic users was observed in both men (RR 3.41, 95% CI 2.38–4.89) and women (RR 2.39, 95% CI 1.53–3.74) in the Framingham Heart Study [49].

Aspirin

Aspirin is known to have a bimodal effect on the handling of uric acid at the renal tubule. Classical studies by Yu and Gutman [50], established that lower doses (1–2 g/day) lead to uric acid retention, whilst very high doses (>3 g/day) are uricosuric. However, even the lowest doses of aspirin (75 mg/day), commonly used for its cardioprotective properties, have effects on uric acid transport. In a study of 49 older (61–94 years) hospital inpatients, 75 mg aspirin daily led to a 15% reduction in the rate of uric acid excretion, most marked in patients with hypoalbuminaemia, which returned to baseline levels within a week of stopping aspirin [51]. In an online case–crossover study of 724 gout patients, the use of low dose (≤325 mg/day) was associated with an increased risk of gout attacks (OR 1.81, 95% CI 1.30–2.51), the effect of which was strongest in lower doses (≤100 mg OR 1.91, 95% CI 1.32–2.85). However, concomitant use of allopurinol nullified this increased risk (OR 0.89, 95% CI 0.55–1.44) [52].

Osteoarthritis

Gout and osteoarthritis (OA) commonly coexist which can lead to diagnostic uncertainty. Clinical and radiographic studies show that acute attacks of gout commonly occur at joints already affected by OA, particularly at first metatarsophalangeal, midfoot, knee, and finger distal interphalangeal joints [53,54]. In a small UK cross-sectional study, nodal OA was no more common in 164 subjects with gout than in 656 control subjects without gout [55]. However, in the

UK-CPRD, people with incident gout were more likely to have been diagnosed with OA prior to the incidence of gout (OR 1.71, 95% CI 1.61–1.82), but also had greater risk of being diagnosed with incident OA subsequent to the diagnosis of gout (HR 1.45, 95% CI 1.35–1.54) [32]. This would appear to support the so-called amplification loop hypothesis whereby MSU crystals readily deposit in osteoarthritic cartilage and then initiate further cartilage damage [56].

Conclusion

Epidemiological data from several countries including the United Kingdom, United States, Italy, and New Zealand show that gout prevalence has markedly increased in recent decades. Whereas a similar pattern has been reported for incidence in the United Kingdom and United States, rising incidence may have stabilized more recently. Numerous dietary, comorbid, and pharmacological risk factors for gout have been described in prospective epidemiological studies. Excessive consumption of animal purines, alcohol, and fructose increase the risk if incident gout, in addition to obesity, metabolic syndrome, hypertension, chronic kidney disease, diuretics, aspirin, beta blockers, angiotensin-converting enzyme inhibitors, and non-losartan angiotensin II receptor blockers. In contrast, low-fat dairy products, coffee, vitamin C, calcium channel antagonists, and losartan appear to reduce the risk of developing gout. Gout itself is an important risk factor for both cardiovascular disease and chronic kidney disease, beyond the risk conferred by traditional comorbid risk factors for these conditions. These observations have increased our understanding of the aetiology and pathogenesis of hyperuricaemia and gout, and provided important insights into clinical complexity and key strategies for management.

References

1. Chandratre P, Roddy E, Clarson L, et al. Health-related quality of life in gout: a systematic review. *Rheumatology (Oxford)* 2013; 52(11):2031–40.
2. Currie WJ. Prevalence and incidence of the diagnosis of gout in Great Britain. *Ann Rheum Dis* 1979; 38(2):101–6.
3. Kuo C, Grainge MJ, Mallen C, Zhang W, Doherty M. Rising burden of gout in the UK but continuing suboptimal management: a nationwide population study. *Ann Rheum Dis* 2015; 74(4):661–7.
4. Lawrence RC, Hochberg MC, Kelsey JL, et al. Estimates of the prevalence of selected arthritic and musculoskeletal diseases in the United States. *J Rheumatol* 1989; 16(4):427–41.
5. Lawrence RC, Felson DT, Helmick CG, et al. Estimates of the prevalence of arthritis and other rheumatic conditions in the United States. Part II. *Arthritis Rheum* 2008; 58(1):26–35.
6. Juraschek SP, Miller ER 3rd, Gelber AC. Body mass index, obesity, and prevalent gout in the United States in 1988–1994 and 2007–2010. *Arthritis Care Res (Hoboken)* 2013; 65(1):127–32.
7. Lennane GA, Rose BS, Isdale IC. Gout in the Maori. *Ann Rheum Dis* 1960; 19:120–5.
8. Klemp P, Stansfield SA, Castle B, et al. Gout is on the increase in New Zealand. *Ann Rheum Dis* 1997; 56(1):22–6.
9. Winnard D, Wright C, Taylor WJ, et al. National prevalence of gout derived from administrative health data in Aotearoa New Zealand. *Rheumatology (Oxford)* 2012; 51(5):901–9.
10. Winnard D, Wright C, Jackson G, et al. Gout, diabetes and cardiovascular disease in the Aotearoa New Zealand adult population: co-prevalence and implications for clinical practice. *NZ Med J* 2013; 126(1368):53–64.
11. Trifirò G, Morabito P, Cavagna L, et al. Epidemiology of gout and hyperuricaemia in Italy during the years 2005-2009: a nationwide population-based study. *Ann Rheum Dis* 2013; 72(5):694–700.
12. Arromdee E, Michet CJ, Crowson CS, O'Fallon WM, Gabriel SE. Epidemiology of gout: is the incidence rising? *J Rheumatol* 2002; 29(11):2403–6.
13. Cea Soriano L, Rothenbacher D, Choi HK, Garcia-Rodriguez LA. Contemporary epidemiology of gout in the UK general population. *Arthritis Res Ther* 2011; 13(2):R39.
14. Elliot AJ, Cross KW, Fleming DM. Seasonality and trends in the incidence and of gout in England and Wales 1994–2007. *Ann Rheum Dis* 2009; 68(11):1728–33.
15. Wallace KL, Riedel AA, Joseph-Ridge N, Wortmann R. Increasing prevalence of gout and hyperuricemia over 10 years among older adults in a managed care population. *J Rheumatol* 2004; 31(8):1582–7.
16. Gardner MJ, Power C, Barker DJ, Padday R. The prevalence of gout in three English towns. *Int J Epidemiol* 1982; 11(1):71–5.
17. Helmert U, Shea S. Social inequalities and health status in western Germany. *Public Health* 1994; 108(5):341–56.
18. Hayward RA, Rathod T, Roddy E, et al. The association of gout with socioeconomic status in primary care: a cross-sectional observational study. *Rheumatology (Oxford)* 2013; 52(11):2004–8.
19. Choi HK, Atkinson K, Karlson EW, Willett W, Curhan G. Purine-rich foods, dairy and protein intake, and the risk of gout in men. *N Engl J Med* 2004; 350(11):1093–103.
20. Choi HK, Curhan G. Coffee consumption and risk of incident gout in women: the Nurses' Health Study. *Am J Clin Nutr* 2010; 92(4):922–7.
21. Choi HK, Curhan G. Soft drinks, fructose consumption and the risk of gout in men: a prospective cohort study. *BMJ* 2008; 336(7639):309–12.
22. Choi HK, Willett W, Curhan G. Fructose-rich beverages and risk of gout in women. *JAMA* 2010; 304(20):2270–8.
23. Choi HK, Willett W, Curhan G. Coffee consumption and risk of incident gout in men: a prospective study. *Arthritis Rheum* 2007; 56(6):2049–55.
24. Choi HK, Gao X, Curhan G. Vitamin C intake and the risk of gout in men: a prospective study. *Arch Intern Med* 2009; 169(5):502–7.
25. Wang M, Jiang X, Wu W, Zhang D. A meta-analysis of alcohol consumption and the risk of gout. *Clin Rheumatol* 2013; 32(11):1641–8.
26. Choi HK, Atkinson K, Karlson EW, Willett W, Curhan G. Alcohol intake and risk of incident gout in men: a prospective study. *Lancet* 2004; 363(9417):1277–81.
27. Neogi T, Chen C, Niu J, et al. Alcohol quantity and type on risk of recurrent gout attacks: an internet-based case-crossover study. *Am J Med* 2014; 127(4):311–8.
28. Zhang Y, Chen C, Choi H, et al. Purine-rich foods intake and recurrent gout attacks. *Ann Rheum Dis* 2012; 71(9):1448–53.
29. Zhang Y, Neogi T, Chen C, et al. Cherry consumption and decreased risk of recurrent gout attacks. *Arthritis Rheum* 2012; 64(12):4004–11.
30. Choi HK, Ford ES, Li C, Curhan G. Prevalence of the metabolic syndrome in patients with gout: the Third National Health and Nutrition Examination Survey. *Arthritis Rheum* 2007; 57(1):109–15.
31. Aune D1, Norat T, Vatten LJ. Body mass index and the risk of gout: a systematic review and dose-response meta-analysis of prospective studies. *Eur J Nutr* 2014; 53(8):1591–601.
32. Kuo CF, Grainge M, Mallen C, Zhang W, Doherty M. Comorbidities in patients with gout prior to and following diagnosis: case-control study. *Ann Rheum Dis* 2016; 75(1):210–7.
33. Choi HK, Atkinson K, Karlson EW, Curhan G. Obesity, weight change, hypertension, diuretic use, and risk of gout in men: the health professionals follow-up study. *Arch Intern Med* 2005; 165(7):742–8.
34. Maynard JW, McAdams DeMarco MA, et al. Incident gout in women and association with obesity in the Atherosclerosis Risk in Communities (ARIC) Study. *Am J Med* 2012; 125(7):717.e9–717.
35. Li C, Hsieh MC, Chang SJ. Metabolic syndrome, diabetes, and hyperuricemia. *Curr Opin Rheumatol* 2013; 25(2):210–6.

36. Rodríguez G, Soriano LC, Choi HK. Impact of diabetes against the future risk of developing gout. *Ann Rheum Dis* 2010; 69(12):2090–4.

37. Herman JB, Goldbourt U. Uric acid and diabetes: observations in a population study. *Lancet* 1982; 2(8292):240–3.

38. McAdams-DeMarco MA, Maynard JW, Baer AN, Coresh J. Hypertension and the risk of incident gout in a population-based study: the atherosclerosis risk in communities cohort. *J Clin Hypertens (Greenwich)* 2012; 14(10):675–9.

39. Juraschek SP, Kovell LC, Miller ER, Gelber AC. Dose-response association of uncontrolled blood pressure and cardiovascular disease risk factors with hyperuricemia and gout. *PLoS One* 2013; 8(2):e56546.

40. Clarson LE, Hider SL, Belcher J, et al. Increased risk of vascular disease associated with gout: a retrospective, matched cohort study in the UK Clinical Practice Research Datalink. *Ann Rheum Dis* 2015; 74(4):642–7.

41. Clarson L, Chandratre P, Hider S, et al. Increased cardiovascular mortality associated with gout: a systematic review and meta-analysis. *Eur J Prev Cardiol* 2015; 22(3):335–43.

42. Krishnan E. Chronic kidney disease and the risk of incident gout among middle-aged men: a seven-year prospective observational study. *Arthritis Rheum* 2013; 65(12):3271–8.

43. Hemmelgarn BR, Culleton BF, Ghali WA. Derivation and validation of a clinical index for prediction of rapid progression of kidney dysfunction. *QJM* 2007; 100(2):87–92.

44. Yu KH, Kuo CF, Luo SF, et al. Risk of end-stage renal disease associated with gout: a nationwide population study. *Arthritis Res Ther* 2012; 14(2):R83.

45. Hsu C, Iribarren C, McCulloch CE, Darbinian J, Go AS. Risk factors for end-stage renal disease—25-year follow-up. *Arch Intern Med* 2009; 169(4):342–50.

46. Kramer HJ, Choi HK, Atkinson K, Stampfer M, Curhan GC. The association between gout and nephrolithiasis in men: The Health Professionals' Follow-Up Study. *Kidney Int* 2003; 64(3):1022–6.

47. Hueskes BA, Roovers EA, Mantel-Teeuwisse AK, et al. Use of diuretics and the risk of gouty arthritis: a systematic review. *Semin Arthritis Rheum* 2012; 41(6):879–89.

48. Choi HK, Soriano LC, Zhang Y, Rodríguez LA. Antihypertensive drugs and risk of incident gout among patients with hypertension: population based case-control study. *BMJ* 2012; 344:d8190.

49. Bhole V1, de Vera M, Rahman MM, Krishnan E, Choi H. Epidemiology of gout in women: fifty-two-year followup of a prospective cohort. *Arthritis Rheum* 2010; 62(4):1069–76.

50. Yu TF, Gutman AB. Study of the paradoxical effects of salicylate in low, intermediate and high dosage on the renal mechanisms of excretion of urate in man. *J Clin Invest* 1959; 38:1298–313.

51. Caspi D, Lubart E, Graff E, et al. The effect of mini-dose aspirin on renal function and uric acid handling in elderly patients. *Arthritis Rheum* 2000; 43(1):103–8.

52. Zhang Y, Neogi T, Chen C, et al. Low-dose aspirin use and recurrent gout attacks. *Ann Rheum Dis* 2014; 73(2):385–90.

53. Roddy E, Zhang W, Doherty M. Are joints affected by gout also affected by osteoarthritis? *Ann Rheum Dis* 2007; 66(10):1374–7.

54. Kawenoki-Minc E, Eyman E, Leo W, Weryńska-Przybylska J. Osteoarthrosis and spondylosis in gouty patients. Analysis of 262 cases of gout. *Reumatologia* 1974; 12(3):267–77.

55. Roddy E, Zhang W, Doherty M. Gout and nodal osteoarthritis: a case-control study.*Rheumatology (Oxford)* 2008; 47(5):732–3.

56. Roddy E, Doherty M. Gout and osteoarthritis: a pathogenetic link? *Joint Bone Spine* 2012; 79(5):425–7.

CHAPTER 39

Pathophysiology of gout

Nicola Dalbeth

Introduction

Gout is a chronic disease of monosodium urate (MSU) crystal deposition. The clinical features of gout occur as a result of the individual's inflammatory response to these crystals. A number of pathophysiological checkpoints are required for the development of clinically apparent gout (Figure 39.1) [1]. The first is elevated urate concentrations at sites of deposition, usually mirrored by elevated serum urate concentrations (hyperuricaemia). Both overproduction and underexcretion of urate contribute to increased urate concentrations. The second checkpoint is formation of MSU crystals. The third checkpoint is the acute inflammatory response to these crystals, presenting as acute synovitis, which is typically self-limiting after 7–10 days. Finally, in those with severe persistent hyperuricaemia, advanced gout may develop, with tophi, chronic gouty arthropathy, and joint damage. This chapter details each of these checkpoints to describe the pathophysiology of gout.

Hyperuricaemia

The presence of hyperuricaemia is the major risk factor for development of gout, with concentration-dependent increased risk observed in those with serum urate concentrations above 7 mg/dL [2]. Serum urate concentrations represent the balance of urate production and excretion, with renal underexcretion of uric acid accounting for the major cause of hyperuricaemia and gout in the adult population [3]. Approximately two-thirds of urate is excreted in the urine and the remaining urate is excreted through the gut.

Purine metabolism and urate production

Urate is the end product of purine metabolism in humans. Purine compounds contain the nine-member purine nucleus, consisting of fused pyrimidine and imidazole rings [4]. Urate synthesis occurs primarily in the liver, with some contribution from the gut and other tissues. Purine nucleotides are essential compounds for

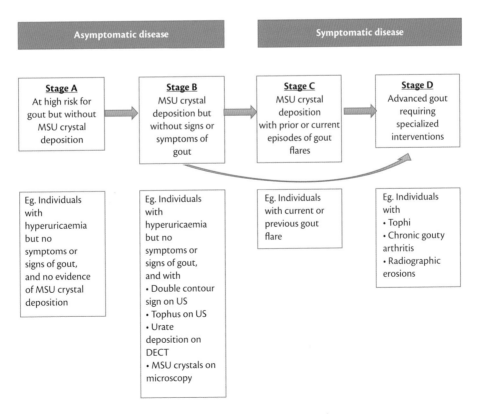

Figure 39.1 Key checkpoints in gout pathogenesis, representing the clinical stages of hyperuricaemia and gout.
Dalbeth N, Stamp L. Hyperuricaemia and gout: time for a new staging system? *Ann Rheum Dis* 2014; 73:1598–600.

nucleic acid synthesis and for many other cell functions including cell activation, energy metabolism, and other biosynthetic pathways. Purine metabolism involves a network of interacting pathways which includes purine synthesis, interconversion, and degradation (reviewed in detail in [5]) (Figure 39.2). This network is highly regulated and includes feedback inhibition at a number of steps.

Purine synthesis includes *de novo* synthesis pathways in which purine nucleotides are synthesized from non-purine precursors, and purine salvage pathways in which purine nucleotides are synthesized from dietary purines or products of endogenous purine interconversion pathways. *De novo* purine synthesis includes 11 enzymatic reactions to form the parent purine compound inosine monophosphate (IMP). Ribose-5′-phosphate and ATP are required to form phosphoribosylpyrophosphate (PRPP), the key substrate for *de novo* synthesis [6]; the initial step of this reaction is catalysed by the PRPP synthetase (PRS). Superactivity of PRS is a rare X-linked monogenic cause of hyperuricaemia, nephrolithiasis, and gout, which may be associated with neurodevelopmental disorders [7]. All newly synthesized purine compounds are formed from IMP which is converted to the two major purine nucleotides involved in DNA and RNA synthesis, adenosine monophosphate (AMP) and guanosine monophosphate (GMP), or is metabolized through the purine catabolic and degradation pathway, ultimately leading to irreversible production of urate.

De novo purine synthesis is a highly energy-demanding process. The purine salvage pathways allow efficient reutilization of preformed purines through salvage of nucleosides and interconversion of nucleotides. The purine nucleotides AMP and GMP formed during the salvage pathway regulate *de novo* purine synthesis through negative feedback inhibition mechanisms. Nucleoside salvage is mediated through the hypoxanthine-guanine phosphoribosyltransferase (HGPRT) and adenine phosphoribosyltransferase enzymes. HGPRT deficiency is a rare X-linked recessive disorder which in its most severe form leads to a condition with severe hyperuricaemia and gout, developmental delay, self-mutilation, and movement disorders (Lesch–Nyhan syndrome) [8]. Partial HGPRT deficiency leads to early-onset overproduction-type hyperuricaemia with nephrolithiasis and gout but without neurodevelopmental abnormalities (Kelley–Seegmiller syndrome) [9].

The purine pathways include interconversion pathways, in which purine nucleotides are interconverted to provide adequate supplies of adenylates and guanylates for nucleic acid synthesis and the essential purine compounds for cellular functions. Ultimately, purine nucleoside 5′-monophosphates (AMP, IMP, GMP) are dephosphorylated to their respective ribonucleosides (adenosine, inosine, and guanosine), which in turn are cleaved by purine nucleoside phosphorylase (PNP) to their respective purine bases, adenine, hypoxanthine, and guanine [10]. Adenine nucleotide catabolism occurs through conversion of AMP to IMP and of adenosine to inosine. Guanine is catalysed to xanthine by guanine deaminase.

Eventually, nucleosides are degraded to urate. Conversion of hypoxanthine to xanthine, and xanthine to urate is catalysed by xanthine oxidoreductase (XOR, xanthine oxidase). XOR exists in both oxidase and dehydrogenase forms [11], and in the oxidase form, generates both uric acid and the reactive oxygen species superoxide anion and H_2O_2. Inhibition of XOR is the most widely used method of reducing serum urate concentrations in gout therapy, with both allopurinol and febuxostat inhibiting this enzyme, and thus urate production [12,13].

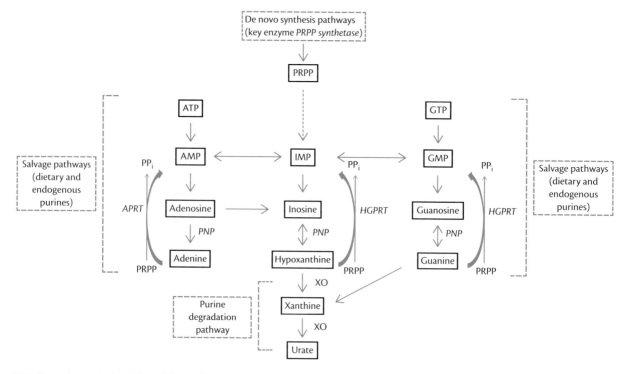

Figure 39.2 The purine synthesis and degradation pathways. AMP: adenosine monophosphate; APRT: adenine phosphoribosyltransferase; ATP: adenosine triphosphate; GMP: guanosine monophosphate; GTP: guanosine triphosphate; HGPRT: hypoxanthine-guanine phosphoribosyltransferase; IMP: inosine monophosphate; PNP: purine nucleoside phosphorylase; PRPP: phosphoribosylpyrophosphate; XO: xanthine oxidase.
Dalbeth N. The pathological basis of hyperuricemia and gout. In Dalbeth N, Perez Ruiz F, Schlesinger N (eds) *Gout*. London: Future Medicine; 2013:24–37.

Hyperuricaemia due to increased urate production can occur through rare inherited disorders of the purine pathways as described earlier, or potentially through genetic variants regulating glucose metabolism such as the glucokinase regulator GCKR or AMP-activated protein kinase (AMPK), both of which have been implicated in a recent, large genome-wide association study of hyperuricaemia [14]. These variants may increase levels of ribose-5′-phosphate which acts as a substrate for PRPP synthesis in the de novo synthesis pathway. Dietary risk factors for gout such as purine-rich foods, certain alcoholic beverages, and fructose intake also lead to hyperuricaemia through alteration in the purine synthesis pathways [15–17]. Purine-rich foods such as offal, seafood, meat, and beer provide high loads of dietary purine nucleotides that are salvaged and ultimately degraded to urate. Alcohol increases purine synthesis through direct ATP degradation via the salvage pathway [18]. Fructose phosphorylation leads to rapid ATP depletion, increased purine synthesis, and consequent increase in urate production [19]. Conditions such as haematological malignancies may lead to hyperuricaemia due to increased salvaged purines resulting from rapid cell turnover.

Renal uric acid excretion

Following synthesis primarily in the gut and liver, urate circulates in an unbound form, available for glomerular filtration [20]. Unionized uric acid predominates in normal acidic urine. Although urate is freely filtered at the glomerulus, the fractional excretion of uric acid (the uric acid clearance/creatinine clearance ratio) is typically 6–10% in healthy individuals, indicating that most filtered uric acid is reabsorbed. Uric acid interacts with a number of transporters within the proximal renal tubule (the renal urate transportasome) that lead to both reabsorption and secretion by the renal tubular cell (reviewed in [21]) (Figure 39.3). The importance of renal uric acid handling in the aetiology of hyperuricaemia was emphasized by the early genome-wide association studies which primarily identified variants in renal uric acid transporters as the major genetic risk factors for hyperuricaemia within the general population [22]. Furthermore, chronic kidney disease (due to many different aetiologies) is a major comorbid condition associated with development of hyperuricaemia and gout [23].

At the luminal surface of the renal proximal tubule cell, uric acid reabsorption is mediated by the anion transporters urate transporter 1 (URAT1) [24], organic anion transporter 10 (OAT10) [25], and OAT4 [26]. The sodium-dependent anion transporters SLC5A8 and SLC5A12 increase the intracellular concentrations of anions such as lactate and butyrate (and also salicylate, nicotinate, and pyrazinoate if present) which in turn promote reabsorption of uric acid through URAT1 and OAT10 [21]. The diuretic agent hydrochlorothiazide increases OAT4-mediated uric acid transport, which in turn may lead to hydrochlorothiazide-induced hyperuricaemia [27]. Inhibition of URAT1 by therapeutic agents such as probenecid, benzbromarone [28] and lesinurad prevents reabsorption of uric acid at the proximal tubule, leading to increased excretion of uric acid and subsequent reduction in serum urate concentrations.

At the basolateral surface of the proximal tubule cell, glucose transporter 9a (GLUT9a), the 540 residue N-terminal isoform of GLUT9, is the major transporter that mediates uric acid reabsorption [29]. This glucose (and possibly fructose) transporter is a high capacity urate transporter [30]. In genome wide association studies,

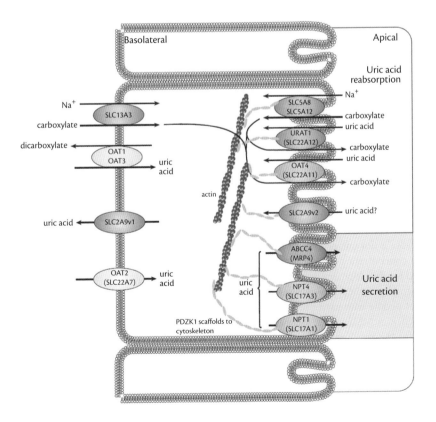

Figure 39.3 The proximal renal tubular uric acid transportasome.
Dalbeth N, Merriman T. Crystal ball gazing: new therapeutic targets for hyperuricaemia and gout. *Rheumatology (Oxford)* 2009; 48:222–6.

variants in the *SLC2A9* gene that encodes GLUT9 are highly and consistently associated with development of hyperuricaemia and gout [14] (see Chapter 40). Individuals with *SLC2A9* loss-of-function mutations have hypouricaemia due to complete absence of renal absorption of uric acid [31], with exercise-induced acute kidney injury and nephrolithiasis. In addition to its effects on URAT1, the uricosuric agent benzbromarone also inhibits GLUT9 [30].

At the basolateral surface of the proximal tubule cell, secretion of uric acid from the interstitium into the cell is mediated by the OAT1 and OAT3 transporters, which exchange urate with anions such as alpha-ketoglutarate [32], and OAT2 [33]. At the apical surface, uric acid is secreted into the lumen via multidrug resistance protein 4 (MRP4) [34], Na$^+$-phosphate transporter 1 (NPT1) [35], NPT4 [36], and also possibly ATP-binding cassette sub-family G member 2 (ABCG2) [37]. Loop and thiazide diuretic medications interact with NPT4, providing a further potential mechanism for diuretic-induced hyperuricaemia [36]. Although genetic variants in ABCG2, particularly the Q141K variant, are strongly associated with gout and hyperuricaemia [37], it is currently unclear whether ABCG2 variants increase serum urate through effects on renal uric acid excretion, or through extra-renal effects on gut excretion (see following subsection and see Chapter 40).

Gut uric acid excretion

The observation that *ABCG2* genetic variants were strongly associated with hyperuricaemia and gout has led to further examination of the role of this transporter in urate homeostasis. Surprisingly, given the postulated importance of ABCG2 in renal uric acid secretion, this work demonstrated that dysfunction in ABCG2 was actually associated with increased urinary uric acid excretion and overproduction-type hyperuricaemia [38]. Subsequent analysis of *Abcg2*-knockout mice demonstrated increased serum urate concentrations, increased renal uric acid excretion, and reduced intestinal urate excretion. These findings have led to the concept that 'overproduction-type hyperuricaemia' should be separated into two subtypes; 'extrarenal urate underexcretion', presumably due to gut underexcretion mediated by ABCG2, and true 'urate overproduction' due to disorders of purine pathway metabolism [38]. At present it is unclear what other transporters also contribute to uric acid excretion in the gut, and whether uric acid transport in the gut can be modified for therapeutic purposes.

Crystal deposition

MSU crystal deposition is the key pathogenic cause of gout. Although hyperuricaemia is the major risk factor for development of symptomatic gout, this disease is not universal in all people with even very high serum urate concentrations [2]. Therefore, other checkpoints must be required for development of clinically apparent disease. Recent ultrasonography studies have demonstrated that approximately one-quarter of people with asymptomatic hyperuricaemia have imaging evidence of MSU crystal deposition [39]. These data provide support for the concept that subclinical MSU crystal deposition is the next checkpoint for development of gout.

MSU crystals appear as negatively birefringent needle-shaped crystals under polarizing light microscopy, with a typical length of 10μm *in vivo*. These crystals can be observed within synovial fluid and tissue in those with gouty arthritis, and are also frequently detected in asymptomatic joints in those with previous gout flares [40].

Within synovial fluid, MSU crystals can exist as free crystals or within synovial fluid cells. Synovial fluid may also contain small cartilage fragments; microscopic analysis of these fragments shows MSU crystals lying in organized rows, following the direction of fibrillar matrix of the tissue fragments [41]. MSU crystals are present within the tophus in radiating aggregates. Consistent with well-described clinical observations, recent ultrasonography studies have highlighted the preferential sites of deposition of MSU crystals in people with gout; most commonly at sites such as the first metatarsophalangeal (MTP) joint, knee, and Achilles tendon [42].

Monosodium urate (NaC$_5$H$_3$N$_4$O$_3$·H$_2$O) exists as triclinic crystals, in which the urate molecules are linked by hydrogen bonds and stacked together leading to sheets of purine rings [43]. MSU crystallization includes a number of steps: saturation, MSU cluster formation, nucleation, and crystal growth (reviewed in [44]). Saturation is regulated by a number of factors including urate concentration, sodium concentration, pH, and temperature. At a temperature of 37°C and pH of 7.4, the saturation concentration for urate is 6.8 mg/dL (0.41 mmol/L) [45]). At concentrations below this level, dissolution occurs *in vitro* [46]. At pH 7.4, saturation occurs at lower concentrations if temperature is reduced; 6 mg/dL at 35°C and 4.5 mg/dL at 30°C [45]. Following MSU cluster formation, nucleation (the formation of new microcrystals) occurs. Factors that promote MSU crystal nucleation include calcium, low pH, mechanical shock, insoluble collagen, immunoglobulins, and proteoglycans [47–49]. In contrast to other tissues such as brain, liver, heart, and kidney, degraded cartilage strongly promotes MSU crystal formation [50]. Synovial fluid immunoglobulin G (IgG) from patients with gout, but not from patients with other forms of inflammatory arthritis, promotes MSU crystal nucleation [51]. In mice, IgM binds to MSU crystals by the Fab portion and facilitates MSU crystal formation and growth by stabilizing initial nucleating MSU monomers [52]. Under varying conditions, albumin may promote or inhibit crystallization [53]. Many factors that promote nucleation may also promote crystal growth. In particular, synovial and cartilage factors such as chondroitin sulphate and phosphatidylcholine may increase MSU crystal formation [48]. It has been postulated that the association between osteoarthritis and gout occurs through alteration or release of proteins of the joint cartilage surface, leading to a structure that can act as a template for crystal nucleation and growth [54].

The acute gout flare

The gout flare represents a sterile acute auto-inflammatory response to MSU crystals, characterized by heat, swelling, erythema, pain, and loss of joint movement. Histologically, the acute arthritis represents an intense inflammatory infiltration primarily of neutrophils, but also of mast cells, macrophages, and lymphocytes [55]. Other typical features include adherent fibrin on the synovial surface, synovial lining layer proliferation, and vascular congestion. MSU crystals are typically present in the inflamed synovial fluid, but may be absent from the acutely inflamed synovial tissue [55]. In the absence of treatment, the acute gout flare is self-limiting, typically resolving over a 7–10-day period [56]. In addition to neutrophils, many other cellular and soluble mediators have been implicated in the acute gout flare, including macrophages, mast cells, endothelial cells, complement, and arachidonic acid metabolites (reviewed in [57]) (Figure 39.4).

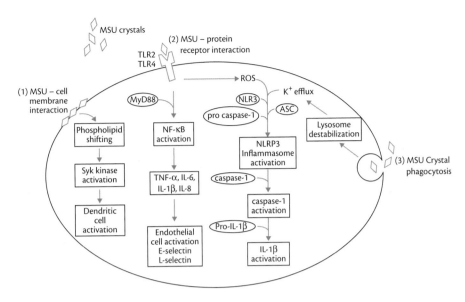

Figure 39.4 Summary of the acute inflammatory response to MSU crystals.
Dalbeth N, Lauterio TJ, Wolfe HR. Mechanism of action of colchicine in the treatment of gout. *Clin Ther* 2014; 36:1465–79.

Initiation

Initiation of the acute gout flare occurs when MSU crystals, acting as danger-associated molecular patterns (DAMPs), interact with cells of the innate immune system. Resident macrophages play a central role in this initiation process, and also in driving the early inflammatory response to MSU crystals [58]. Following internalization of crystals by phagocytosis, MSU crystals induce NACHT-LRR-PYD-containing protein 3 (NLRP3) inflammasome activation [59]. The NLRP3 inflammasome is a multimolecular complex present within the cytosol of the cell. This process requires reactive oxygen species, ASC, NALP3, and caspase 1, and leads to cleavage of pro-interleukin 1 beta (IL1B) to mature IL1B. Leukotriene B4 (LTB4) induces MSU crystal-induced production of reactive oxygen species and reactive oxygen species-dependent activation of the NLRP3 inflammasome [60]. Interactions between MSU crystals and Toll-like receptor (TLR)-2 and TLR4 on the cell surface in the presence of MyD88 also leads to nuclear factor kappa B activation, which in turn leads to transcription of pro-inflammatory cytokines such as tumour necrosis factor alpha (TNFA), IL6, IL8, and pro-IL1B [61]. In addition to NLRP3 inflammasome-dependent mechanisms described earlier, inflammasome-independent pathways also exist *in vivo*. Pro-IL1B can be cleaved to mature IL1B through a number of serine proteases present in neutrophils, mast cells, and monocytes [62]. The central role of IL1B in the pathogenesis of acute gouty arthritis has been confirmed by clinical trials demonstrating that anti-IL1B antibodies have potent anti-inflammatory effects in patients with established acute flares [63], and also prevent flares in those with recent flares and in those commencing urate-lowering therapy [64].

Amplification

Following initiation of acute gouty inflammation, an amplification phase occurs. Vascular endothelial cell activation occurs in response to pro-inflammatory cytokines such as IL1B and TNFA, leading to vasodilatation with increased blood flow, increased permeability to plasma proteins and the recruitment of leucocytes into the tissues, via the adhesion molecules E-selectin, intercellular adhesion molecule 1 (ICAM1) and vascular cell adhesion molecule 1 (VCAM1) [65]. Local generation of chemotactic factors such C5a, S100A8/A9 and IL8 contribute to leucocyte recruitment, leading to influx of neutrophils and immature monocytes into the joint [66–68]. Amplification of the inflammatory response occurs when neutrophils interact with MSU crystals both directly and through interactions with crystal bound iC3b and IgG [69]. These interactions lead to release of neutrophil-derived mediators including reactive oxygen species, prostaglandin (PG)-E2, antimicrobial peptides, lysosomal enzymes, pro-inflammatory cytokines including IL1B and chemokines [70–74]. Following recruitment into the joint, immature monocytes differentiate into an inflammatory M1 macrophage and interact with MSU crystals to produce pro-inflammatory cytokines such as TNFA, IL1B, and IL6, and the chemokines CCL2 and CXCL1 [75]. MSU crystals also induce cyclooxygenase (COX)-2 expression and PGE2 production in monocytes [76]. Mast cells are also present early in the inflammatory response to MSU crystals [77]. Mast cell-derived IL1B plays an important role in acute gouty arthritis [78], and release of preformed pro-inflammatory mediators from mast cells, including histamine, cytokines, and enzymes such as tryptase, mast cell chymase, and serine esterases may contribute to the promotion of downstream inflammatory cascades. Following phagocytosis of MSU crystals, synovial fibroblasts release arachidonic acid metabolites such as PGE2 [79]. Collectively these responses lead to amplification of the inflammatory response with further influx of leucocytes into the affected joint, leading to the vasodilatation, erythema, and pain observed during an acute gout flare.

Complement also contributes to both the initiation and amplification phases of the acute inflammatory response to MSU crystals. Complement activity is greatly increased in the synovial fluid in acute gout, and both the classical and alternative pathways are activated by MSU crystals [80]. In addition to the effects of iC3b on leucocyte-MSU crystal interactions, C3a and C5a act as leucocyte chemoattractants, and the membrane attack complex plays a key role in generation of the neutrophil chemokine IL8 into the inflamed joint in gout [81]. In monocytes, C5a acts as an endogenous priming signal in the initiation of uric acid crystal-induced IL1B production [82].

Pain is a central feature of the acute gout flare. The pattern of hypernociception in acute gout models closely mimics the pattern of IL1B release and is dependent on neutrophil influx into the joint, which requires NLRP3 activation [60]. Pain in acute gouty arthritis is further mediated by prostaglandins and bradykinin, sensitization of nociceptors and release of neuropeptides such as substance P [83].

Resolution

The characteristic of acute gouty arthritis is severe joint inflammation, which, even in the absence of therapy, self-resolves over 7–10 days. A number of factors have been implicated in the resolution phase of the acute gout attacks (reviewed in [84]). Apoptosis of neutrophils and subsequent non-inflammatory phagocytosis by differentiated macrophages and neutrophils represents an important pathway for resolution [85,86]. Following phagocytosis of apoptotic cells, TGFβ1 is produced; this cytokine is present at high concentrations in synovial fluid during the resolution phase [87]. TGFβ1 suppresses monocyte pro-inflammatory cytokine release in response to MSU crystals and endothelial cell activation in response to monocyte-derived cytokines [88].

In addition to TGFβ1, other anti-inflammatory soluble mediators and signalling pathways may also contribute to the resolution phase. IL1ra, IL10 and sTNFRI/II are present at high concentrations in the synovial fluid of patients with acute gouty arthritis [89]. Within acute gouty synovial fluid and tissue, gene expression of cytokine suppressors cytokine-inducible SH2-containing protein (CIS) and suppressor of cytokine signalling 3 (SOCS3) is up-regulated [89]. The transcription regulator peroxisome proliferator-activated receptor gamma (PPARG) is induced in monocytes by MSU crystals and a natural ligand of PPARG, 15-deoxy-PGJ2, can inhibit production of TNFA and IL1B by MSU-stimulated monocytes, and also early cellular infiltration in the air pouch model of acute gouty inflammation [90]. Anti-inflammatory hormones such as the melanocortins, adrenocorticotrophic hormone 1-39 and alpha-melanocyte-stimulating hormone, acting through the MC3-R may also contribute to the resolution phase [91,92].

Neutrophil extracellular traps (NETs) are formed by activated neutrophils as a mechanism for extracellular killing of pathogens [93]. NETosis (NET formation) is enhanced by reactive oxygen species and results in ejection of intracellular material such as chromatin, bactericidal molecules and enzymes into the extracellular space following rupture of the outer cell membrane. MSU crystals induce NET formation in vitro and in vivo [94]. At low neutrophil cell densities, MSU crystals induce pro-inflammatory NETosis with cytokine and chemokine release [95]. However, at high neutrophil density, NETs induced by MSU crystals form dense crystal aggregates that sequester and degrade pro-inflammatory cytokines including IL1B, IL6, and TNFA [95]. This degradation is mediated by NET-associated proteolytic activity. MSU crystal-induced aggregated NETosis is dependent on the presence of reactive oxygen species; lack of reactive oxygen species results in reduced aggregated NET formation and leads to persistent MSU crystal-induced arthritis. Collectively, these data indicate that reactive

oxygen species-dependent aggregated NET formation contributes to resolution of the acute gouty inflammation.

Maintenance of monosodium urate crystals in non-inflammatory state

As described above, both imaging and synovial fluid analysis studies have clearly demonstrated that MSU crystals are present within clinically uninflamed joints in most individuals with hyperuricaemia and previous gout attacks. Many of the mechanisms contributing to the resolution phase of the acute gout attack may also play a role in the maintenance of an anti-inflammatory state in intercritical gout despite presence of intra-articular MSU crystals. These observations also suggest that additional steps may be required to induce the acute inflammatory response to MSU crystals.

MSU crystals found in asymptomatic joints of patients with intercritical gout are usually present within macrophages and almost never within neutrophils [96], indicating that MSU crystals can interact with macrophages without inducing an inflammatory response. The differentiation stage of the resident macrophage may play a role in this non-inflammatory response, with differentiated macrophages responding to MSU crystal phagocytosis by production of TGFβ1, which in turn inhibits endothelial activation and production of pro-inflammatory cytokines [88]. Within the joint, MSU crystals may be also present within localized in tophus-like structures [97]. As with the resolution phase of gout described earlier, aggregated NETosis may play an important role in maintaining MSU crystals in an uninflamed state during intercritical gout [95]. Protein coating of crystals is a further important factor in regulation the inflammatory response to MSU crystals. In particular, IgG appears to have a pro-inflammatory effect [98], and apolipoprotein (APO)-B and APOE have a key anti-inflammatory effect [99, 100]. APOB and APOE coating of crystals suppress MSU crystal-induced neutrophil activation.

Induction of acute flares may occur due to de novo formation of new MSU crystals, but more likely results in changes in local factors that regulate the inflammatory response to preformed crystals; these factors include shedding of MSU crystals from contained tophus or aggregated NET structures into the joint, changes in the macrophage differentiation (or recruitment of pro-inflammatory monocytes/macrophages), or changes in the composition of proteins coating the crystals. The observation that following engagement with TLR2, free fatty acids such as stearic acid (C18:0) act with MSU crystals to induce caspase 1 and ASC (but not NALP)-dependent IL1B release in murine macrophages and human peripheral blood mononuclear cells, suggest that a second signal is required for MSU crystal-induced IL1B release [101]. These findings may explain the clinical observation that gout flares can be triggered by a large fatty (and purine-rich) meal [102]. In contrast, stimulation of macrophages with omega-3 fatty acids including eicosapentaenoic acid and docosahexaenoic acid abolishes NLRP3 inflammasome activation and inhibits subsequent caspase 1 activation and IL1B secretion [103]. This effect of omega-3 fatty acids is mediated by G-protein-coupled receptor 120 (GPR120) and GPR40. The metabolic biosensor AMPK inhibits MSU crystal inflammation in vitro and in vivo, including NLRP3 inflammasome activation and IL1B release [104]. Tissue AMPK activity is reduced by soluble urate, fructose, alcohol, and many nutritional stressors, and in obesity and type 2 diabetes, suggesting a further link between nutritional triggers and induction of the inflammatory response to preformed crystals within the joint.

Advanced gout

Advanced gout is characterized by chronic gouty arthritis, the presence of gouty tophi and structural joint disease. Structural joint damage includes bone erosion, new bone formation, cartilage damage, and tendon deposition. Advanced gout typically occurs at least 10 years after the initial gout attack following prolonged untreated hyperuricaemia [105]. However, patients can occasionally present with tophaceous disease as the first presentation of symptomatic gout.

The gouty tophus

The tophus represents an organized chronic foreign body granulomatous inflammatory response to MSU crystals [106]. The tophus consists of three main zones; the central crystalline core with variable concentrations of MSU crystals, the surrounding cellular corona zone, and the outer fibrovascular zone [107] (Figure 39.5). Cells of the innate and adaptive immune system are present within the tophus [108]. Numerous CD68+ mono- and multinucleated macrophages are present within the coronal zone. Fewer mononucleated macrophages and no multinucleated macrophages are present in the fibrovascular zone. Macrophages are continuously recruited into the tophus, with cells closer to the crystal core expressing markers of a mature, non-migrating phenotype, and macrophages in the outer regions of the tophus expressing markers for immature freshly migrated cells [109]. Mast cells are found in similar densities in both the coronal and fibrovascular zones at relatively low densities. Neutrophils are observed infrequently in the corona zone and are absent in the fibrovascular zone. Adaptive immune cells identified within the tophus include T cells, B cells, and plasma cells [108]. CD4+ and CD8+ T cells are found scattered throughout the coronal and fibrovascular zones at relatively low densities. CD8+ T cells predominate over CD4+ T cells. B-cell aggregates are frequently identified in the fibrovascular zone. In addition, differentiated plasma cells are present in high numbers within the tophus, especially within the corona zone. Protein components within the tophus include immunoglobulins (mainly IgG and IgM), complement, myeloid-related proteins 8 and 14, and pro-inflammatory cytokines including IL1B, IL6, and TNFA [108–111]. TGFβ1 is also expressed in the coronal zone of the tophus, mostly by mononucleated cells [108].

Although tophi can become acutely inflamed, most of these lesions present as painless, uninflamed subcutaneous nodules. This presentation is perhaps surprising, given the presence of pro-inflammatory mediators expressed within the tophus. A key explanation may be the role of aggregated NETosis in inducing tophus formation by aggregating MSU crystals in a non-inflammatory state and leading to development of the crystalline core of the tophus [95]. These aggregated NETs may then inhibit the inflammatory response through proteolytic degradation of pro-inflammatory cytokines. The presence of cells expressing TGFβ1 within the tophus may further contribute to the lack of inflammatory response to the MSU crystals, and also play a role in tissue remodelling, angiogenesis, and fibrosis in granulomatous disease [112]. Ultimately, the organized architecture of the established tophus (particularly the fibrovascular zone) may allow physical containment which limits its clinically apparent MSU crystal-induced inflammation.

Structural joint damage

Bone erosion is a frequent structural manifestation of advanced gout. Gouty erosions have a typical radiographic appearance, with sclerotic rim and overhanging edge [113]. Advanced imaging studies have strongly implicated the presence of MSU crystals and tophus in the development of bone erosion in advanced gout, with the majority of large erosions having evidence of MSU crystals

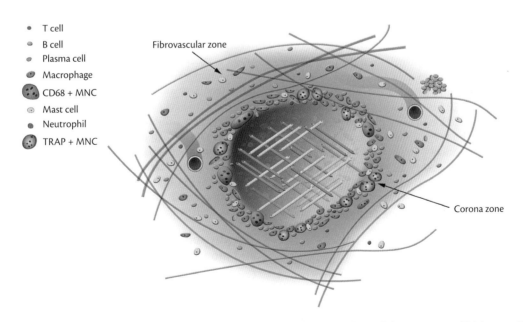

Figure 39.5 A cellular model of the gouty tophus. The central crystalline core (marked as *) is surrounded by a cellular corona zone, which is encased by a fibrovascular zone.

Dalbeth N, Pool B, Gamble GD, et al. Cellular characterization of the gouty tophus: a quantitative analysis. *Arthritis Rheum* 2010; 62:1549–56.

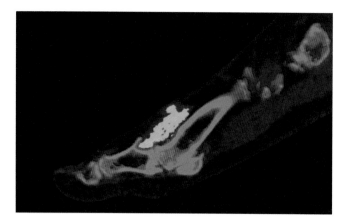

Figure 39.6 Dual-energy CT scan from a patient with tophaceous gout, demonstrating MSU crystals (green) present within a bone erosion at the first metatarsophalangeal joint.

and tophus present within the erosion on computed tomography (CT) imaging [114,115] (Figure 39.6). Bone remodelling is a balance between bone-resorbing osteoclasts and bone-forming osteoblasts. Erosive gout has been associated with abnormalities in both osteoclast and osteoblast function. Patients with erosive gout have higher circulating osteoclast precursors [116]. Osteoclast precursors are also abundant within inflamed gouty synovial fluid, and numerous osteoclasts are present at the interface between the tophus and bone erosion [116]. Although MSU crystals do not directly promote formation of osteoclast-like cells from osteoclast precursors (osteoclastogenesis) *in vitro*, stromal cells cultured with MSU crystals indirectly promote osteoclastogenesis [116]. This stromal cell effect may be due to alteration of the balance between receptor activator of nuclear factor kappa B ligand (RANKL) and its decoy receptor osteoprotegerin (OPG) [116]. RANKL is also expressed within T cells in the tophus and this expression may further account for the enhanced osteoclastogenesis observed in erosive gout [117]. Other factors that promote alternative or inflammatory pathways of osteoclastogenesis such as IL1 and TNFA are also expressed within the tophus and these cytokines may have a further influence on osteoclast formation [108,109]. In contrast to the large number of osteoclasts at the tophus–bone interface, osteoblast numbers are severely diminished or absent at these sites. MSU crystals inhibit osteoblast viability, differentiation, and function *in vitro* [118,119]. Together, the changes in both osteoclast and osteoblast function may lead to imbalance in bone remodelling with ultimate bone resorption and erosion formation at sites of MSU crystal deposition.

New bone formation is also a characteristic feature of structure damage in gout. Specific features include as spur formation, periosteal new bone formation, and sclerosis [120]. Osteophytes are also frequently observed. There is a strong relationship between the presence of bone erosion, tophus, and new bone formation in advanced gout, suggesting a connection between these lesions during the process of joint remodelling in gout [120]. The mechanisms of new bone formation in gout are currently poorly understood. However, it seems unlikely that MSU crystals directly promote new bone formation, given their inhibitory effects on osteoblasts. The processes that promote formation of the fibrovascular zone within the tophus may also contribute to the development of some forms of new bone formation.

Although ultrasound studies frequently detect the double contour sign, representing MSU crystals overlying articular cartilage [97], cartilage damage is a late feature of disease. Cartilage damage in gout is typically focal and is associated with the presence of bone erosion, synovitis, and tophus formation [121]. Analysis of mechanisms of cartilage damage can be difficult in gout, due to the frequent co-occurrence of osteoarthritis [122]. *In vitro* studies have shown that MSU crystals interact with chondrocytes to reduce cell viability and function [123]. Gene expression of cartilage matrix proteins such as aggrecan and versican is downregulated, and collagen protein secretion is reduced following culture with MSU crystals. Furthermore, chondrocytes exposed to MSU crystals up-regulate the expression of catabolic inflammatory mediators and matrix degrading enzymes such as nitric oxide, matrix metalloproteinases (MMPs) and a disintegrin and metalloproteinase with thrombospondin motifs (ADAMTS) aggrecanases [123, 124]. TLR2 signalling may play an important role in these responses [125]. Chondrocyte death can be observed adjacent to MSU crystals in histological studies of affected joints [123].

Interactions with inflamed synovial membrane may also contribute to bone and cartilage damage in gout. Histologically, tophi are frequently present within the synovium in chronic gouty arthritis [55]. Other microscopic features of chronic gouty arthritis include villous formation, chronic synovitis with granulomatous inflammation, plasma cell infiltration and synovial fibroblast proliferation [106,126]. Interactions between MSU crystals and synovial fibroblasts induce production of degradative enzymes such as MMPs which promote bone resorption and cartilage degradation [127]. Additionally, the production of pro-inflammatory cytokines such as IL1B and TNFA by macrophages within inflamed synovium may contribute to structural damage.

Although not always clinically apparent, both ultrasound and dual-energy CT studies have demonstrated the frequent involvement of tendons in advanced gout [42,128]. Within the feet, MSU crystal deposition occurs as frequently in the Achilles tendon as in the first MTP joint [128]. On imaging and histology, MSU crystals can be observed at both the enthesis and the body of the tendon [128,129]. The structural and functional impact of tendon deposition is currently unclear. However, tendon rupture is an occasional complication of advanced gout [126]. Similar to the effects on osteoblasts and chondrocytes, MSU crystals interact with tenocytes (the cells of the tendon) to reduce cell viability [129]. These crystals inhibit gene expression of collagens and tendon matrix proteins such as biglycan and tenascin C by tenocytes. In contrast to the effects on other stromal cells, MSU crystals inhibit the expression of catabolic enzymes such as MMP2, -3 and -13, and ADAMTS4 in tenocytes [129]. These enzymes are important for tendon repair and may limit the ability of the tendon to repair itself once damaged.

The physiological role of relative hyperuricaemia and monosodium urate crystal formation

Compared to most other species, serum urate concentrations are elevated in humans and other higher order primates due to evolutionary loss of the uricase gene during the Miocene period [130]. Various evolutionary advantages for relative hyperuricaemia have been postulated. These include beneficial effects of urate on water conservation, maintenance of blood pressure, locomotor activity and reaction time, fat deposition during times of starvation, and as an antioxidant (reviewed in [131]). Perhaps most compelling is the observation that MSU crystals play an important role in immune surveillance and transition from innate to adaptive immunity as an endogenous adjuvant or 'danger signal' released from dying cells [132]. MSU crystals contribute much of the endogenous activity involved in priming CD8 T-cell responses to dying cells [133]. This effect occurs through direct interactions with lipid components of the dendritic cell membrane, activation of Syk-kinase dependent signalling pathways, and increased expression of costimulatory molecules on dendritic cells [134]. MSU crystals can stimulate humoral immunity [135] and promote adjuvant responses to tumour cells and allografts [133,136]. These responses may have been particularly important in development of immunity to infectious agents [137]. Together, these observations suggest an evolutionary advantage to hyperuricaemia and formation of MSU crystals in immune surveillance and generation of adaptive immunity.

References

1. Choi HK, Mount DB, Reginato AM. Pathogenesis of gout. *Ann Intern Med* 2005; 143:499–516.
2. Campion EW, Glynn RJ, DeLabry LO. Asymptomatic hyperuricemia. Risks and consequences in the Normative Aging Study. *Am J Med* 1987; 82:421–6.
3. Rieselbach RE, Sorensen LB, Shelp WD, Steele TH. Diminished renal urate secretion per nephron as a basis for primary gout. *Ann Intern Med* 1970; 73:359–66.
4. Wyngaarden JB Kelley WN. *Gout and Hyperuricemia*. New York: Grune and Stratton; 1976.
5. Dalbeth N, Merriman TR. Hyperuricaemia and gout. In Valle-D (ed) *The Online Metabolic and Molecular Bases of Inherited Disease*: McGraw-Hill; 2013: Chapter 106.
6. Becker MA RK, Seegmiller JE Synthesis of phosphoribosylpyrophosphate in mammalian cells. *Adv Enzymol Relat Areas Mol Biol* 1979; 49:281–306.
7. Yen RC, Adams WB, Lazar C, Becker MA. Evidence for X-linkage of human phosphoribosylpyrophosphate synthetase. *Proc Natl Acad Sci U S A* 1978; 75:482–5.
8. Lesch M, Nyhan WL. A familial disorder of uric acid metabolism and central nervous system function. *Am J Med* 1964; 36:561–70.
9. Kelley WN, Rosenbloom FM, Henderson JF, Seegmiller JE. A specific enzyme defect in gout associated with overproduction of uric acid. *Proc Natl Acad Sci U S A* 1967; 57:1735–9.
10. Krenitsky TA, Elion GB, Henderson AM, Hitchings GH. Inhibition of human purine nucleoside phosphorylase. Studies with intact erythrocytes and the purified enzyme. *J Biol Chem* 1968; 243:2876–81.
11. Nishino T, Okamoto K, Eger BT, Pai EF, Nishino T. Mammalian xanthine oxidoreductase—mechanism of transition from xanthine dehydrogenase to xanthine oxidase. *FEBS J* 2008; 275:3278–89.
12. Okamoto K, Eger BT, Nishino T, Pai EF, Nishino T. Mechanism of inhibition of xanthine oxidoreductase by allopurinol: crystal structure of reduced bovine milk xanthine oxidoreductase bound with oxipurinol. *Nucleosides Nucleotides Nucleic Acids* 2008; 27:888–93.
13. Okamoto K, Eger BT, Nishino T, et al. An extremely potent inhibitor of xanthine oxidoreductase. Crystal structure of the enzyme-inhibitor complex and mechanism of inhibition. *J Biol Chem* 2003; 278:1848–55.
14. Kottgen A, Albrecht E, Teumer A, et al. Genome-wide association analyses identify 18 new loci associated with serum urate concentrations. *Nat Genet* 2013; 45:145–54.
15. Choi HK, Atkinson K, Karlson EW, Willett W, Curhan G. Alcohol intake and risk of incident gout in men: a prospective study. *Lancet* 2004; 363:1277–81.
16. Choi HK, Atkinson K, Karlson EW, Willett W, Curhan G. Purine-rich foods, dairy and protein intake, and the risk of gout in men. *N Engl J Med* 2004; 350:1093–103.
17. Choi HK, Curhan G. Soft drinks, fructose consumption, and the risk of gout in men: prospective cohort study. *BMJ* 2008; 336:309–12.
18. Faller J, Fox IH. Ethanol-induced hyperuricemia: evidence for increased urate production by activation of adenine nucleotide turnover. *N Engl J Med* 1982; 307:1598–602.
19. Raivio KO, Becker A, Meyer LJ, Greene ML, Nuki G, Seegmiller JE. Stimulation of human purine synthesis de novo by fructose infusion. *Metabolism* 1975; 24:861–9.
20. Kovarsky J, Holmes EW, Kelley WN. Absence of significant urate binding to human serum proteins. *J Lab Clin Med* 1979; 93:85–91.
21. Mandal A, Mount DB. The molecular physiology of uric acid homeostasis. Annu Rev Physiol 2015; 77:323–45.
22. Kolz M, Johnson T, Sanna S, et al. Meta-analysis of 28,141 individuals identifies common variants within five new loci that influence uric acid concentrations. *PLoS Genet* 2009; 5:e1000504.
23. Krishnan E. Chronic kidney disease and the risk of incident gout among middle-aged men: a seven-year prospective observational study. *Arthritis Rheum* 2013; 65:3271–8.
24. Enomoto A, Kimura H, Chairoungdua A, et al. Molecular identification of a renal urate anion exchanger that regulates blood urate levels. *Nature* 2002; 417:447–52.
25. Bahn A, Hagos Y, Reuter S, et al. Identification of a new urate and high affinity nicotinate transporter, hOAT10 (SLC22A13). *J Biol Chem* 2008; 283:16332–41.
26. Ekaratanawong S, Anzai N, Jutabha P, et al. Human organic anion transporter 4 is a renal apical organic anion/dicarboxylate exchanger in the proximal tubules. *J Pharmacol Sci* 2004; 94:297–304.
27. Hagos Y, Stein D, Ugele B, Burckhardt G, Bahn A. Human renal organic anion transporter 4 operates as an asymmetric urate transporter. *J Am Soc Nephrol* 2007; 18:430–9.
28. Kang DH, Han L, Ouyang X, et al. Uric acid causes vascular smooth muscle cell proliferation by entering cells via a functional urate transporter. *Am J Nephrol* 2005; 25:425–33.
29. Vitart V, Rudan I, Hayward C, et al. SLC2A9 is a newly identified urate transporter influencing serum urate concentration, urate excretion and gout. *Nat Genet* 2008; 40:437–42.
30. Caulfield MJ, Munroe PB, O'Neill D, et al. SLC2A9 is a high-capacity urate transporter in humans. *PLoS Med* 2008; 5:e197.
31. Matsuo H, Chiba T, Nagamori S, et al. Mutations in glucose transporter 9 gene SLC2A9 cause renal hypouricemia. *Am J Hum Genet* 2008; 83:744–51.
32. Bakhiya A, Bahn A, Burckhardt G, Wolff N. Human organic anion transporter 3 (hOAT3) can operate as an exchanger and mediate secretory urate flux. *Cell Physiol Biochem* 2003; 13:249–56.
33. Sato M, Mamada H, Anzai N, et al. Renal secretion of uric acid by organic anion transporter 2 (OAT2/SLC22A7) in human. *Biol Pharm Bull* 2010; 33:498–503.
34. Van Aubel RA, Smeets PH, van den Heuvel JJ, Russel FG. Human organic anion transporter MRP4 (ABCC4) is an efflux pump for the purine end metabolite urate with multiple allosteric substrate binding sites. *Am J Physiol Renal Physiol* 2005; 288:F327–33.
35. Chiba T, Matsuo H, Kawamura Y, et al. NPT1/SLC17A1 Is a renal urate exporter in humans and its common gain-of-function variant decreases the risk of renal underexcretion gout. *Arthritis Rheumatol* 2015; 67:281–7.
36. Jutabha P, Anzai N, Wempe MF, et al. Apical voltage-driven urate efflux transporter NPT4 in renal proximal tubule. *Nucleosides Nucleotides Nucleic Acids* 2011; 30:1302–11.
37. Woodward OM, Kottgen A, Coresh J, et al. Identification of a urate transporter, ABCG2, with a common functional polymorphism causing gout. *Proc Natl Acad Sci U S A* 2009; 106:10338–42.
38. Ichida K, Matsuo H, Takada T, et al. Decreased extra-renal urate excretion is a common cause of hyperuricemia. *Nat Commun* 2012; 3:764.

39. Howard RG, Pillinger MH, Gyftopoulos S, et al. Reproducibility of musculoskeletal ultrasound for determining monosodium urate deposition: concordance between readers. *Arthritis Care Res (Hoboken)* 2011; 63:1456–62.

40. Pascual E, Batlle-Gualda E, Martinez A, Rosas J, Vela P. Synovial fluid analysis for diagnosis of intercritical gout. *Ann Intern Med* 1999; 131:756–9.

41. Pascual E, Ordonez S. Orderly arrayed deposit of urate crystals in gout suggest epitaxial formation. *Ann Rheum Dis* 1998; 57:255.

42. Naredo E, Uson J, Jimenez-Palop M, et al. Ultrasound-detected musculoskeletal urate crystal deposition: which joints and what findings should be assessed for diagnosing gout? *Ann Rheum Dis* 2014; 73:1522–8.

43. Mandel NS, Mandel GS. Monosodium urate monohydrate, the gout culprit. *J Am Chem Soc* 1976; 98:2319–23.

44. Martillo MA, Nazzal L, Crittenden DB. The crystallization of monosodium urate. *Curr Rheumatol Rep* 2014; 16:400.

45. Loeb JN. The influence of temperature on the solubility of monosodium urate. *Arthritis Rheum* 1972; 15:189–92.

46. Perrin CM, Dobish MA, van Keuren E, Swift JA. Monosodium urate monohydrate crystallization. *CrystEngComm* 2011; 13:1111–7.

47. Wilcox WR, Khalaf AA. Nucleation of monosodium urate crystals. *Ann Rheum Dis* 1975; 34:332–9.

48. Burt HM, Dutt YC. Growth of monosodium urate monohydrate crystals: effect of cartilage and synovial fluid components on in vitro growth rates. *Ann Rheum Dis* 1986; 45:858–64.

49. Laurent TC. Solubility of sodium urate in the presence of chondroitin-4-sulphate. *Nature* 1964; 202:1334.

50. Katz WA, Schubert M. The interaction of monosodium urate with connective tissue components. *J Clin Invest* 1970; 49:1783–9.

51. Kam M, Perl-Treves D, Caspi D, Addadi L. Antibodies against crystals. *FASEB J* 1992; 6:2608–13.

52. Kanevets U, Sharma K, Dresser K, Shi Y. A role of IgM antibodies in monosodium urate crystal formation and associated adjuvanticity. *J Immunol* 2009; 182:1912–8.

53. Perl-Treves D, Addadi L. A structural approach to pathological crystallizations. Gout: the possible role of albumin in sodium urate crystallization. *Proc R Soc Lond B Biol Sci* 1988; 235:145–59.

54. Pascual E, Martinez A, Ordonez S. Gout: the mechanism of urate crystal nucleation and growth. A hypothesis based in facts. *Joint Bone Spine* 2013; 80:1–4.

55. Schumacher HR. Pathology of the synovial membrane in gout. Light and electron microscopic studies. Interpretation of crystals in electron micrographs. *Arthritis Rheum* 1975; 18:771–82.

56. Bellamy N, Downie WW, Buchanan WW. Observations on spontaneous improvement in patients with podagra: implications for therapeutic trials of non-steroidal anti-inflammatory drugs. *Br J Clin Pharmacol* 1987; 24:33–6.

57. Martin WJ, Harper JL. Innate inflammation and resolution in acute gout. *Immunol Cell Biol* 2010; 88:15–9.

58. Martin WJ, Walton M, Harper J. Resident macrophages initiating and driving inflammation in a monosodium urate monohydrate crystal-induced murine peritoneal model of acute gout. *Arthritis Rheum* 2009; 60:281–9.

59. Martinon F, Petrilli V, Mayor A, Tardivel A, Tschopp J. Gout-associated uric acid crystals activate the NALP3 inflammasome. *Nature* 2006; 440:237–41.

60. Amaral FA, Costa VV, Tavares LD, et al. NLRP3 inflammasome-mediated neutrophil recruitment and hypernociception depend on leukotriene B(4) in a murine model of gout. *Arthritis Rheum* 2012; 64:474–84.

61. Liu-Bryan R, Scott P, Sydlaske A, Rose DM, Terkeltaub R. Innate immunity conferred by Toll-like receptors 2 and 4 and myeloid differentiation factor 88 expression is pivotal to monosodium urate monohydrate crystal-induced inflammation. *Arthritis Rheum* 2005; 52:2936–46.

62. Netea MG, van de Veerdonk FL, van der Meer JW, Dinarello CA, Joosten LA. Inflammasome-independent regulation of IL-1-family cytokines. *Annu Rev Immunol* 2015; 33:49–77.

63. Schlesinger N, Alten RE, Bardin T, et al. Canakinumab for acute gouty arthritis in patients with limited treatment options: results from two randomised, multicentre, active-controlled, double-blind trials and their initial extensions. *Ann Rheum Dis* 2012; 71:1839–48.

64. Schlesinger N, Mysler E, Lin HY, et al. Canakinumab reduces the risk of acute gouty arthritis flares during initiation of allopurinol treatment: results of a double-blind, randomised study. *Ann Rheum Dis* 2011; 70:1264–71.

65. Chapman PT, Yarwood H, Harrison AA, et al. Endothelial activation in monosodium urate monohydrate crystal-induced inflammation: in vitro and in vivo studies on the roles of tumor necrosis factor alpha and interleukin-1. *Arthritis Rheum* 1997; 40:955–65.

66. Russell IJ, Mansen C, Kolb LM, Kolb WP. Activation of the fifth component of human complement (C5) induced by monosodium urate crystals: C5 convertase assembly on the crystal surface. *Clin Immunol Immunopathol* 1982; 24:239–50.

67. Ryckman C, McColl SR, Vandal K, et al. Role of S100A8 and S100A9 in neutrophil recruitment in response to monosodium urate monohydrate crystals in the air-pouch model of acute gouty arthritis. *Arthritis Rheum* 2003; 48:2310–20.

68. Terkeltaub R, Baird S, Sears P, Santiago R, Boisvert W. The murine homolog of the interleukin-8 receptor CXCR-2 is essential for the occurrence of neutrophilic inflammation in the air pouch model of acute urate crystal-induced gouty synovitis. *Arthritis Rheum* 1998; 41:900–9.

69. Hasselbacher P. Binding of IgG and complement protein by monosodium urate monohydrate and other crystals. *J Lab Clin Med* 1979; 94:532–41.

70. Naccache PH, Grimard M, Roberge CJ, et al. Crystal-induced neutrophil activation. I. Initiation and modulation of calcium mobilization and superoxide production by microcrystals. *Arthritis Rheum* 1991; 34:333–42.

71. Gilbert C, Poubelle PE, Borgeat P, Pouliot M, Naccache PH. Crystal-induced neutrophil activation: VIII. Immediate production of prostaglandin E2 mediated by constitutive cyclooxygenase 2 in human neutrophils stimulated by urate crystals. *Arthritis Rheum* 2003; 48:1137–48.

72. Ginsberg MH, Kozin F, Chow D, May J, Skosey JL. Adsorption of polymorphonuclear leukocyte lysosomal enzymes to monosodium urate crystals. *Arthritis Rheum* 1977; 20:1538–42.

73. Hachicha M, Naccache PH, McColl SR. Inflammatory microcrystals differentially regulate the secretion of macrophage inflammatory protein 1 and interleukin 8 by human neutrophils: a possible mechanism of neutrophil recruitment to sites of inflammation in synovitis. *J Exp Med* 1995; 182:2019–25.

74. Ryckman C, Gilbert C, de Medicis R, et al. Monosodium urate monohydrate crystals induce the release of the proinflammatory protein S100A8/A9 from neutrophils. *J Leukoc Biol* 2004; 76:433–40.

75. Martin WJ, Shaw O, Liu X, Steiger S, Harper JL. Monosodium urate monohydrate crystal-recruited noninflammatory monocytes differentiate into M1-like proinflammatory macrophages in a peritoneal murine model of gout. *Arthritis Rheum* 2011; 63:1322–32.

76. Pouliot M, James MJ, McColl SR, Naccache PH, Cleland LG. Monosodium urate microcrystals induce cyclooxygenase-2 in human monocytes. *Blood* 1998; 91:1769–76.

77. Schiltz C, Liote F, Prudhommeaux F, et al. Monosodium urate monohydrate crystal-induced inflammation in vivo: quantitative histomorphometric analysis of cellular events. *Arthritis Rheum* 2002; 46:1643–50.

78. Reber LL, Marichal T, Sokolove J, et al. Contribution of mast cell-derived interleukin-1beta to uric acid crystal-induced acute arthritis in mice. *Arthritis Rheumatol* 2014; 66:2881–91.

79. McMillan RM, Vater CA, Hasselbacher P, Hahn J, Harris ED, Jr. Induction of collagenase and prostaglandin synthesis in synovial fibroblasts treated with monosodium urate crystals. *J Pharm Pharmacol* 1981; 33:382–3.

80. Pekin TJ, Jr., Zvaifler NJ. Hemolytic complement in synovial fluid. *J Clin Invest* 1964; 43:1372–82.

81. Tramontini N, Huber C, Liu-Bryan R, Terkeltaub RA, Kilgore KS. Central role of complement membrane attack complex in monosodium urate crystal-induced neutrophilic rabbit knee synovitis. *Arthritis Rheum* 2004; 50:2633–9.

82. An LL, Mehta P, Xu L, et al. Complement C5a potentiates uric acid crystal-induced IL-1beta production. *Eur J Immunol* 2014; 44:3669–79.

83. Lunam CA, Gentle MJ. Substance P immunoreactive nerve fibres in the domestic chick ankle joint before and after acute urate arthritis. *Neurosci Lett* 2004; 354:87–90.

84. Steiger S, Harper JL. Mechanisms of spontaneous resolution of acute gouty inflammation. *Curr Rheumatol Rep* 2014; 16:392.

85. Steiger S, Harper JL. Neutrophil cannibalism triggers transforming growth factor beta1 production and self regulation of neutrophil inflammatory function in monosodium urate monohydrate crystal-induced inflammation in mice. *Arthritis Rheum* 2013; 65:815–23.

86. Savill JS, Wyllie AH, Henson JE, et al. Macrophage phagocytosis of aging neutrophils in inflammation. Programmed cell death in the neutrophil leads to its recognition by macrophages. *J Clin Invest* 1989; 83:865–75.

87. Scanu A, Oliviero F, Ramonda R, et al. Cytokine levels in human synovial fluid during the different stages of acute gout: role of transforming growth factor beta1 in the resolution phase. *Ann Rheum Dis* 2012; 71:621–4.

88. Yagnik DR, Evans BJ, Florey O, et al. Macrophage release of transforming growth factor beta1 during resolution of monosodium urate monohydrate crystal-induced inflammation. *Arthritis Rheum* 2004; 50:2273–80.

89. Chen YH, Hsieh SC, Chen WY, et al. Spontaneous resolution of acute gouty arthritis is associated with rapid induction of the anti-inflammatory factors TGFbeta1, IL-10 and soluble TNF receptors and the intracellular cytokine negative regulators CIS and SOCS3. *Ann Rheum Dis* 2011; 70:1655–63.

90. Akahoshi T, Namai R, Murakami Y, et al. Rapid induction of peroxisome proliferator-activated receptor gamma expression in human monocytes by monosodium urate monohydrate crystals. *Arthritis Rheum* 2003; 48:231–9.

91. Getting SJ, Christian HC, Flower RJ, Perretti M. Activation of melanocortin type 3 receptor as a molecular mechanism for adrenocorticotropic hormone efficacy in gouty arthritis. *Arthritis Rheum* 2002; 46:2765–75.

92. Capsoni F, Ongari AM, Reali E, Catania A. Melanocortin peptides inhibit urate crystal-induced activation of phagocytic cells. *Arthritis Res Ther* 2009; 11:R151.

93. Brinkmann V, Reichard U, Goosmann C, et al. Neutrophil extracellular traps kill bacteria. *Science* 2004; 303:1532–5.

94. Schorn C, Janko C, Latzko M, et al. Monosodium urate crystals induce extracellular DNA traps in neutrophils, eosinophils, and basophils but not in mononuclear cells. *Front Immunol* 2012; 3:277.

95. Schauer C, Janko C, Munoz LE, et al. Aggregated neutrophil extracellular traps limit inflammation by degrading cytokines and chemokines. *Nat Med* 2014; 20:511–7.

96. Pascual E, Jovani V. A quantitative study of the phagocytosis of urate crystals in the synovial fluid of asymptomatic joints of patients with gout. *Br J Rheumatol* 1995; 34:724–6.

97. Grassi W, Meenagh G, Pascual E, Filippucci E. 'Crystal clear'-sonographic assessment of gout and calcium pyrophosphate deposition disease. *Semin Arthritis Rheum* 2006; 36:197–202.

98. Rosen MS, Baker DG, Schumacher HR, Jr, Cherian PV. Products of polymorphonuclear cell injury inhibit IgG enhancement of monosodium urate-induced superoxide production. *Arthritis Rheum* 1986; 29:1473–9.

99. Terkeltaub RA, Dyer CA, Martin J, Curtiss LK. Apolipoprotein (apo) E inhibits the capacity of monosodium urate crystals to stimulate neutrophils. Characterization of intraarticular apo E and demonstration of apo E binding to urate crystals in vivo. *J Clin Invest* 1991; 87:20–6.

100. Terkeltaub R, Martin J, Curtiss LK, Ginsberg MH. Apolipoprotein B mediates the capacity of low density lipoprotein to suppress neutrophil stimulation by particulates. *J Biol Chem* 1986; 261:15662–7.

101. Joosten LA, Netea MG, Mylona E, et al. Engagement of fatty acids with Toll-like receptor 2 drives interleukin-1beta production via the ASC/caspase 1 pathway in monosodium urate monohydrate crystal-induced gouty arthritis. *Arthritis Rheum* 2010; 62:3237–48.

102. Richette P, Bardin T. Purine-rich foods: an innocent bystander of gout attacks? *Ann Rheum Dis* 2012; 71:1435–6.

103. Yan Y, Jiang W, Spinetti T, et al. Omega-3 fatty acids prevent inflammation and metabolic disorder through inhibition of NLRP3 inflammasome activation. *Immunity* 2013; 38:1154–63.

104. Wang Y, Viollet B, Terkeltaub R, Liu-Bryan R. AMP-activated protein kinase suppresses urate crystal-induced inflammation and transduces colchicine effects in macrophages. *Ann Rheum Dis* 2016; 75(1):286–94.

105. Hench PS. The diagnosis of gout and gouty arthritis. *J Lab Clin Med* 1936; 22:48–55.

106. Sokoloff L. Pathology of gout. *Arthritis Rheum* 1965; 8:707–13.

107. Palmer DG, Highton J, Hessian PA. Development of the gout tophus. An hypothesis. *Am J Clin Pathol* 1989; 91:190–5.

108. Dalbeth N, Pool B, Gamble GD, et al. Cellular characterization of the gouty tophus: a quantitative analysis. *Arthritis Rheum* 2010; 62:1549–56.

109. Schweyer S, Hemmerlein B, Radzun HJ, Fayyazi A. Continuous recruitment, co-expression of tumour necrosis factor-alpha and matrix metalloproteinases, and apoptosis of macrophages in gout tophi. *Virchows Arch* 2000; 437:534–9.

110. Kaneko K, Iwamoto H, Yasuda M, et al. Proteomic analysis to examine the role of matrix proteins in a gouty tophus from a patient with recurrent gout. *Nucleosides Nucleotides Nucleic Acids* 2014; 33:199–207.

111. Holzinger D, Nippe N, Vogl T, et al. Myeloid-related proteins 8 and 14 contribute to monosodium urate monohydrate crystal-induced inflammation in gout. *Arthritis Rheumatol* 2014; 66:1327–39.

112. Roberts AB, Sporn MB, Assoian RK, et al. Transforming growth factor type beta: rapid induction of fibrosis and angiogenesis in vivo and stimulation of collagen formation in vitro. *Proc Natl Acad Sci U S A* 1986; 83:4167–71.

113. Brailsford JF. The radiology of gout. *Br J Radiol* 1959; 32:472–8.

114. Dalbeth N, Clark B, Gregory K, et al. Mechanisms of bone erosion in gout: a quantitative analysis using plain radiography and computed tomography. *Ann Rheum* Dis 2009; 68:1290–5.

115. Dalbeth N, Aati O, Kalluru R, et al. Relationship between structural joint damage and urate deposition in gout: a plain radiography and dual-energy CT study. *Ann Rheum Dis* 2015; 74(6):1030–6.

116. Dalbeth N, Smith T, Nicolson B, et al. Enhanced osteoclastogenesis in patients with tophaceous gout: urate crystals promote osteoclast development through interactions with stromal cells. *Arthritis Rheum* 2008; 58:1854–65.

117. Lee SJ, Nam KI, Jin HM, et al. Bone destruction by receptor activator of nuclear factor kappaB ligand-expressing T cells in chronic gouty arthritis. *Arthritis Res Ther* 2011; 13:R164.

118. Chhana A, Callon KE, Pool B, et al. Monosodium urate monohydrate crystals inhibit osteoblast viability and function: implications for development of bone erosion in gout. *Ann Rheum Dis* 2011; 70:1684–91.

119. Bouchard L, de Medicis R, Lussier A, Naccache PH, Poubelle PE. Inflammatory microcrystals alter the functional phenotype of human osteoblast-like cells in vitro: synergism with IL-1 to overexpress cyclooxygenase-2. *J Immunol* 2002; 168:5310–7.

120. Dalbeth N, Milligan A, Doyle AJ, Clark B, McQueen FM. Characterization of new bone formation in gout: a quantitative site-by-site analysis using plain radiography and computed tomography. *Arthritis Res Ther* 2012; 14:R165.

121. Popovich I, Dalbeth N, Doyle A, Reeves Q, McQueen FM. Exploring cartilage damage in gout using 3-T MRI: distribution and associations

with joint inflammation and tophus deposition. *Skeletal Radiol* 2014; 43:917–24.

122. Roddy E, Zhang W, Doherty M. Are joints affected by gout also affected by osteoarthritis? *Ann Rheum Dis* 2007; 66:1374–7.

123. Chhana A, Callon KE, Pool B, et al. The effects of monosodium urate monohydrate crystals on chondrocyte viability and function: implications for development of cartilage damage in gout. *J Rheumatol* 2013; 40:2067–74.

124. Liu R, Liote F, Rose DM, Merz D, Terkeltaub R. Proline-rich tyrosine kinase 2 and Src kinase signaling transduce monosodium urate crystal-induced nitric oxide production and matrix metalloproteinase 3 expression in chondrocytes. *Arthritis Rheum* 2004; 50:247–58.

125. Liu-Bryan R, Pritzker K, Firestein GS, Terkeltaub R. TLR2 signaling in chondrocytes drives calcium pyrophosphate dihydrate and monosodium urate crystal-induced nitric oxide generation. *J Immunol* 2005; 174:5016–23.

126. Levy M, Seelenfreund M, Maor P, Fried A, Lurie M. Bilateral spontaneous and simultaneous rupture of the quadriceps tendons in gout. *J Bone Joint Surg Br* 1971; 53:510–3.

127. Hasselbacher P, McMillan RM, Vater CA, Hahn J, Harris ED, Jr. Stimulation of secretion of collagenase and prostaglandin E2 by synovial fibroblasts in response to crystals of monosodium urate monohydrate: a model for joint destruction in gout. *Trans Assoc Am Physicians* 1981; 94:243–52.

128. Dalbeth N, Kalluru R, Aati O, et al. Tendon involvement in the feet of patients with gout: a dual-energy CT study. *Ann Rheum Dis* 2013; 72:1545–8.

129. Chhana A, Callon KE, Dray M, et al. Interactions between tenocytes and monosodium urate monohydrate crystals: implications for tendon involvement in gout. *Ann Rheum Dis* 2014; 73:1737–41.

130. Wu XW, Muzny DM, Lee CC, Caskey CT. Two independent mutational events in the loss of urate oxidase during hominoid evolution. *J Mol Evol* 1992; 34:78–84.

131. Johnson RJ, Lanaspa MA, Gaucher EA. Uric acid: a danger signal from the RNA world that may have a role in the epidemic of obesity, metabolic syndrome, and cardiorenal disease: evolutionary considerations. *Semin Nephrol* 2011; 31:394–9.

132. Shi Y, Evans JE, Rock KL. Molecular identification of a danger signal that alerts the immune system to dying cells. *Nature* 2003; 425:516–21.

133. Shi Y, Galusha SA, Rock KL. Cutting edge: elimination of an endogenous adjuvant reduces the activation of CD8 T lymphocytes to transplanted cells and in an autoimmune diabetes model. *J Immunol* 2006; 176:3905–8.

134. Ng G, Sharma K, Ward SM, et al. Receptor-independent, direct membrane binding leads to cell-surface lipid sorting and Syk kinase activation in dendritic cells. *Immunity* 2008; 29:807–18.

135. Behrens MD, Wagner WM, Krco CJ, et al. The endogenous danger signal, crystalline uric acid, signals for enhanced antibody immunity. *Blood* 2008; 111:1472–9.

136. Hu DE, Moore AM, Thomsen LL, Brindle KM. Uric acid promotes tumor immune rejection. *Cancer Res* 2004; 64:5059–62.

137. van de Hoef DL, Coppens I, Holowka T, et al. Plasmodium falciparum-derived uric acid precipitates induce maturation of dendritic cells. *PLoS One* 2013; 8:e55584.

138. Dalbeth N, Stamp L. Hyperuricaemia and gout: time for a new staging system? *Ann Rheum Dis* 2014; 73:1598–600.

139. Dalbeth N. The pathological basis of hyperuricemia and gout. In Dalbeth N, Perez Ruiz F, Schlesinger N (eds) *Gout*. London: Future Medicine; 2013:24–37.

140. Dalbeth N, Merriman T. Crystal ball gazing: new therapeutic targets for hyperuricaemia and gout. *Rheumatology (Oxford)* 2009; 48:222–6.

141. Dalbeth N, Lauterio TJ, Wolfe HR. Mechanism of action of colchicine in the treatment of gout. *Clin Ther* 2014; 36:1465–79.

CHAPTER 40

The genetic basis of gout

Tony R. Merriman

Introduction

The sequencing of the human genome and identification of common inter-individual variation (polymorphism) is revealing the complexity of our genetic make-up. Genome-wide association studies (GWAS) demonstrate that some of this variation plays a role in the pathogenesis of common human disease. Typically the genetic contributions are very weak, with the additive effect of hundreds of predisposing alleles contributing to a given phenotype within a population. The existence of common disease-causing genetic variants is consistent with the idea that ancestral variations evolved in combination with an environment that provided a selective advantage to carriers of today's common causal variants. However, the presence of these variants in the modern gene pool can result in less advantageous phenotypes. Largely because of the increased lifespan allowed by our modern environment and new environmental exposures (e.g. within diet), previously advantageous phenotypes can now be disadvantageous. This chapter will review the recent advances in knowledge of the contribution of common genetic variation to gout, drawing on findings from GWAS. The genetic causes of familial hyperuricaemia and gout, caused by rare mutations, are reviewed elsewhere [1].

Heritability is defined as the proportion of variance in phenotype within a population that can be explained by inherited genetic variants. It is determined by comparing the concordance in phenotype between monozygotic (same inherited genome) and dizygotic (share half the inherited genome) twin pairs. In gout, renal uric acid handling and hyperuricaemia have a large heritable component (87% for fractional excretion of uric acid [2], 60% for serum urate [3]), although heritability estimates for gout per se are yet to be robustly determined [3,4].

Genetic associations reveal modifiable checkpoints

In a GWAS, single nucleotide polymorphisms (SNPs), that are specific points where different bases or alleles (e.g. cytosine (C) or adenine (A) in the case of SNP rs2231142 within the ABCG2 gene) are observed within a population, are typically used as markers to scan for regions of the genome associated with a defined phenotype. Association is revealed when there is a statistically significant difference in the frequency of SNP alleles between cases and controls in the case of a binary disease phenotype such as gout, or when particular alleles correlate with a continuous phenotype such as serum concentration of urate. Because of inter-SNP correlation (linkage disequilibrium) multiple SNPs are generally associated, that 'mark' the existence of a genetic variant directly responsible (aetiological)

for the phenotype (Figure 40.1). This aetiological variant could be one of the genotyped variants or it could be an ungenotyped variant that is not necessarily a SNP (e.g. an insertion/deletion of DNA). Whatever the case, it is fundamental that the aetiological variant, inherited at conception, influences the expression and function of a protein that plays a role in pathogenesis. Thus the genetic variant pinpoints a pathogenic checkpoint that has the potential to be similarly influenced by drug and/or environmental intervention to prevent or ameliorate disease.

The aetiopathogenesis of gout is dictated by several key checkpoints (Figure 40.2) [5] (see also Chapter 39). It is initiated by urate overproduction and uric acid underexcretion leading to hyperuricaemia with renal underexcretion of uric acid well established as a key cause [1]. Following that there is formation of monosodium urate (MSU) crystals in joints with gout caused by an inflammatory response to these crystals. It is reasonable to assume that progression through these checkpoints is governed by inherited genetic variants, lifetime environmental exposures, and their interaction. In order to identify genetic variants associated with gout, an obvious approach would be to compare allele frequencies between people with and without gout by GWAS. Genetic associations would mark genes involved at any one or more of the gout checkpoints. To date, however, this approach has not proven successful, largely because of the lack of availability of clinically ascertained gout sample sets of the size required (many thousands) for a GWAS in gout. However the GWAS approach has proven very successful using urate concentration as phenotype. Not only are urate levels straightforward to measure, extremely large cohorts are available for GWAS.

Genome-wide association studies in serum urate levels

Köttgen et al. reported, in a GWAS of over 140 000 European individuals using 2.8 million SNPs, statistically significant associations of 28 separate genetic loci with serum urate levels [6]. Because of the number of genetic variants studied, the p-value required for statistical significance is very low ($<5 \times 10^{-8}$), therefore a study of this size was required to provide the power to detect association with loci that have a weak effect on phenotype. The Kottgen et al. study confirmed the association with urate levels of ten loci discovered in earlier and smaller GWAS [7–11] (Tables 40.1 and 40.2). These loci are dominated by those containing genes that were either known (SLC22A11/OAT4, SLC22A12/URAT1, SLC17A1/NPT, and PDKZ1) or novel (SLC2A9/GLUT9, and ABCG2) renal and gut transporters of uric acid (see Chapter 39). The GCKR (glucokinase regulatory protein) locus implicates production of urate

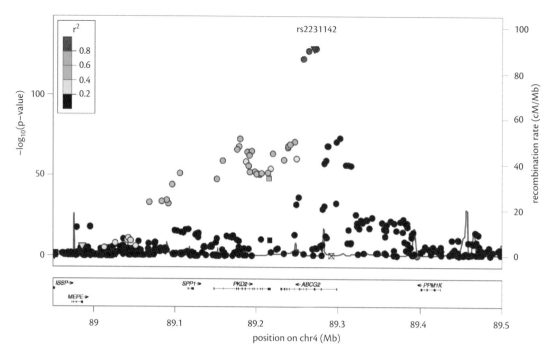

Figure 40.1 Association of the *ABCG2* locus with serum urate. Each point on the graph represents a specific single nucleotide polymorphism (SNP). The left y-axis indicates the strength of association of the SNPs and the right axis the recombination rate within the locus (indicated on the graph by the vertical peaks where excess recombination is observed). The most associated SNP is *rs2231142* (encoding Q141K; the likely aetiological variant) with other SNPs also associated with urate because of linkage disequilibrium with *rs2231142* coloured light blue, red, and green. Of note a second group of SNPs (coloured purple) are also associated with urate. That they are not in linkage disequilibrium with *rs2231142* suggests a second independent common effect at this locus.

Reprinted with permission of Macmillan Publishers Ltd. *Nat Genet*, Kottgen A, Albrecht E, Teumer A, et al., 45, copyright (2013).

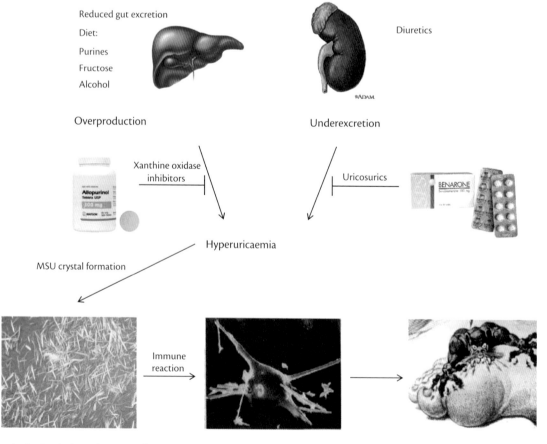

Figure 40.2 Key checkpoints in the pathogenesis of gout.

Table 40.1 GWAS meta-analyses of loci associated with serum urate and gout

	Kolz et al. (2009) [8]	Yang et al. (2010) [9]	Tin et al. (2011) [10]	Okada et al. (2012) [11]	Kottgen et al. (2013) [6]
Sample size	28 141	28 283	14 706	71 149	>140 000 (primary data)
Populations	European	European	African American	East Asian	European (primary data), African American, Indian, Japanese
Loci associated with serum urate with genome-wide significance	9 loci: *SLC2A9, ABCG2, SLC17A1, SLC22A11, SLC22A12, SLC16A9, GCKR, LRRC16A, PDZK1*	8 loci: *SLC2A9, ABCG2, SLC17A1, SLC22A11, GCKR, R3HDM2-INHBC* region, *RREB1, PDZK1*	3 loci: *SLC2A9, SLC22A12, SGK1-SLC2A12* region	4 loci: *SLC2A9, ABCG2, SLC22A12, MAF*	28 loci: 10 previously described: *SLC2A9, ABCG2, SLC17A3, SLC16A9, SLC22A11, SLC22A12, GCKR, INHBC, RREB1, PDZK1* 18 new loci: *TRIM46, INHBB, SFMBT1, TMEM171, VEGFA, BAZ1B, PRKAG2, STC1, HNF4G, A1CF, ATXN2, UBE2Q2, IGF1R, NFAT5, MAF, HLF, ACVR1B-ACVRL1, B3GNT4*
Association with gout	Not reported	The genetic urate risk score was strongly and linearly associated with gout. Except *RREB1* and *PDZK1*, all loci were associated with gout (p < 0.05)	Directionally consistent effects on serum urate and gout were observed (p-binomial <0.0001)	Not reported	Correlation between the effect on urate and the odds of gout for the replicated loci (Pearson's correlation = 0.93); 17 of the replicated serum urate associated SNPs reached statistical significance with gout (p < 0.05)

Updated and reprinted from *Rheum Dis Clin North Am*, 40/2, Merriman TR, Choi, H.K., Dalbeth, N, The genetic basis of gout, 279–90, Copyright (2014) with permission from Elsevier.

by glycolysis, with the functional relevance of the remaining loci (*SLC16A9/MCT9, INHBC*, and *RREB1*) unclear, although *MCT9* may be a renal sodium transporter and has been linked to urate via carnitine metabolism [8]. Predictably most, but not all, of these ten loci consistently associate with gout in multiple ancestral groups [6,12,13].

There is one very important caveat in interpreting the GWAS findings—the causal gene at each locus is, in the majority of instances, not obvious (Table 40.2). Extensive linkage disequilibrium (intermarker correlation) results in association signals extending for some distance across many loci. This means that multiple candidate genes can exist (see examples in Figure 40.3). In the Kottgen et al. study [6], candidate genes at each locus were identified using GRAIL [14]—a bioinformatic approach that looks for commonalities between associated SNPs, the literature, and published GWAS. To confirm the causal gene at each locus requires further genetic research, beginning with resequencing of candidate genes in each locus, with the causal gene predicted to have a larger burden of rare functional variants in extreme hyperuricaemia. This approach can be complemented by trans-ancestral mapping with the most likely common causal variant (i.e. the effect identified by Köttgen et al.) predicted to be most strongly associated with urate levels (and gout) between diverse ancestral groups. Alongside this approach identification of ancient recombinant haplotypes that differ between ancestral groups can aid in fine-mapping. A third approach is underpinned by the hypothesis that the causal variant is an 'eSNP' (expression SNP) that influences the expression of the causal gene at the locus. This is a strong hypothesis given that approximately 70% of genetic variants for common phenotypes identified by GWAS map to regulatory regions of the genome [15]. Often these regulatory regions can be outside the regulated gene—for example, the genetic variant that maps within an intron of the *FTO* gene and causes weight gain mediates its effect by regulation of expression of the neighbouring *IRX3* gene [16].

The lead associated genetic variants at *SLC2A9* and *ABCG2* collectively explain, depending on sex, 3–4% of the variance in urate levels. In the context of genetic variants associated with complex phenotypes these effects are very strong—for example, the locus most strongly associated with weight (*FTO/IRX3*) explains less than 0.5% of variance. On average, the urate-raising allele at *SLC2A9* increases serum urate by 0.373 mg/dL (0.022 mmol/L) and the urate-raising allele at *ABCG2* by 0.217 mg/dL (0.013 mmol/L) [6]. *SLC2A9* and *ABCG2* have equivalent effects in men, with *SLC2A9* a stronger effect in women than men and vice versa for *ABCG2* [6]. The collective effect of the other confirmed 26 loci identified by Kottgen et al. [6] is similar to that of *SLC2A9* and *ABCG2* combined. The importance of *SLC2A9* in urate control is emphasized by the abolition of renal reabsorption of uric acid in hypouricaemic patients with homozygous inactivating mutations [17]. Thus there is considerable research interest in understanding the molecular basis of urate control by *SLC2A9* and *ABCG2*, and their clinical significance.

SLC2A9: genetic complexity

Genetic association at the *SLC2A9* locus is extensive, encompassing hundreds of SNPs and a region larger than 500 kb [6] (Figure 40.4). Fortunately for gene mappers, only two genes are situated within this region, *SLC2A9* and *WDR1*. *WDR1* encodes a protein involved in disassembly of actin fibres that has been implicated in carditis—not an obvious urate-influencing gene. In contrast, *SLC2A9* encodes the GLUT9 protein, that is expressed in the proximal

Table 40.2 Summary of the 28 genome-wide significant urate loci detected by Köttgen et al.

	GRAIL gene	Effect size (male/female[1]) (mg/dL)	FEUA (Y/N)[2]	Association signal	Probable causal gene[3]	Strongest candidate(s)[4,5]
Old loci						
Rs1471633	PDZK1	0.059	N	Within PDZK1	PDZK1	–
Rs1260326	GCKR	0.074 (0.091/0.063)	Y	Spans >20 genes	–	GCKR
Rs12498742	SLC2A9	0.373 (0.269/0.460)	Y	Spans 4 genes	SLC2A9	–
Rs2231142	ABCG2	0.217 (0.280/0.181)	Y	Spans 4 genes	ABCG2	–
Rs675209	RREB1	0.061	Y	Upstream and within RREB1	–	RREB1
Rs1165151	SLC17A3	0.091	N	Spans 20 genes	–	SLC17A1-A4
Rs1171614	SLC16A9	0.079	N	Spans 2 genes	–	–
Rs2078267	SLC22A11	0.073	Y	Within SLC22A11	SLC22A11	–
Rs478607	SLC22A12	0.047	Y	Spans 6 genes	–	SLC22A12
Rs3741414	INHBC	0.072 (0.091/0.057)	N	Spans 7 genes	–	–
New loci						
Rs11264341	PKLR	0.050	N	Spans 2 genes	–	–
Rs17050272	INHBB	0.035	N	Intergenic	INHBB	–
Rs2307384	ACVR2A	0.029	N	Spans 3 genes	–	–
Rs6770152	MUSTN1	0.044	N	Spans 3 genes	–	–
Rs17632159	TMEM171	0.039	N	Intergenic	–	–
Rs729761	VEGFA	0.047	N	Intergenic	–	–
Rs1178977	MLXIPL	0.047	N	Spans 5 genes	–	MLXIPL
Rs10480300	PRKAG2	0.035	N	Within PRKAG2	–	PRKAG2
Rs17786744	STC1	0.029	N	Intergenic	–	–
Rs2941484	HNF4G	0.044	N	Within HNF4G		HNF4G
Rs10821905	ASAH2	0.057	N	Within A1CF		A1CF
Rs642803	LTBP3	0.036	N	Spans 6 genes	–	–
Rs653178	PTPN116	0.035	N	Spans 3 genes	–	–
Rs1394125	NRG4	0.043 (0.061/0.032)	Y	Spans 4 genes		–
Rs6598541	IGF1R	0.043	Y	Within IGFR1	–	IGFR1
Rs7193778	NFAT5	0.046	Y	Intergenic	–	–
Rs7188445	MAF	0.032	N	Intergenic	–	–
Rs7224610	HLF	0.042	Y	Within HLF	–	HLF
Rs2079742	C17ORF82	0.043	N	Downstream and within BCAS3	–	–
Rs164009	PRPSAP1	0.028	N	Within QRICH2	–	–

[1]Male and female effect sizes are given for loci where there was a significant sex-specific difference.

[2]Fractional excretion of uric acid (FEUA) was tested by Köttgen et al. [6] on a considerably smaller subset (n = 6799), meaning that inadequate power may contribute to lack of association seen at loci of weaker effect.

[3]A probable causal gene either has very strong functional evidence (SLC2A9, ABCG2) or has strong functional evidence combined with association signal restricted to the gene (PDZK1, SLC22A11) or has very strong eSNP evidence (INHBB).

[4]A 'strongest candidate' is listed when the locus contains a candidate with strong functional evidence (GCKR, SLC17A1–A4, SLC22A12) or has the association signal tightly restricted to the named gene or has strong eSNP evidence (MLXIPL).

[5]RREB1 = ras responsive element (zinc-finger) binding protein, has been genetically implicated in type 2 diabetes associated end-stage kidney disease [57]; PRKAG2 = protein kinase, AMP-activated, gamma 2 non-catalytic subunit, has been genetically implicated in blood pressure control [58]; HNF4G = hepatocyte nuclear factor 4G, has been genetically implicated in obesity [59]; A1CF = APOBEC1 (APOB mRNA editing enzyme) complementation factor; IGFR1 = insulin-like growth factor 1 receptor; HLF = hepatic leukaemia factor; MLXIPL = carbohydrate element-responsive binding protein, this locus has been identified as a pleiotropic gene for metabolic syndrome and inflammation [60].

[6]PTPN11 is ~1 Mb downstream of the association signal and does not harbour any association signal.

Reprinted from Merriman TR. An update on the genetic architecture of hyperuricemia and gout. *Arthritis Res Ther* 2015; 17:98.

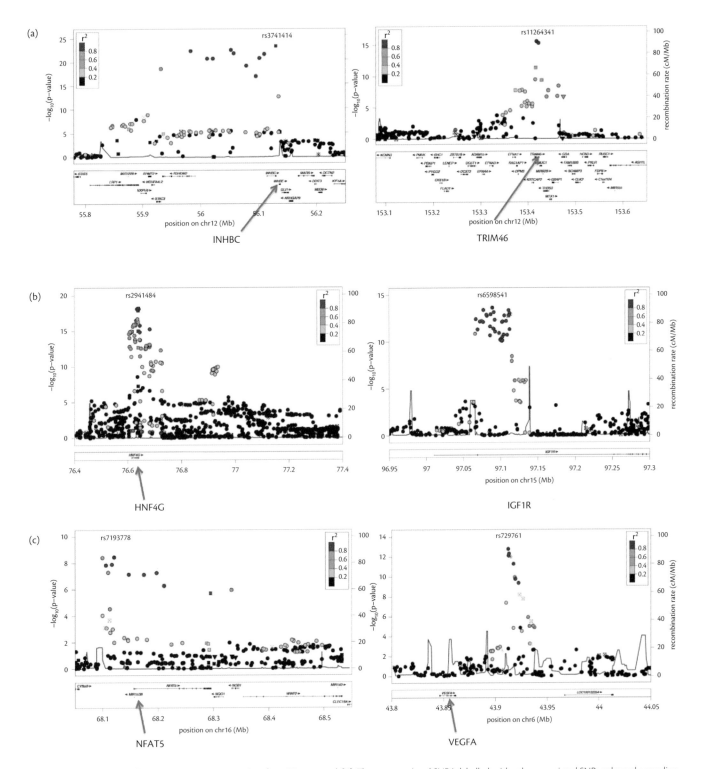

Figure 40.3 Plots of regional association in Europeans taken from Köttgen et al. [6]. The top associated SNP is labelled, with other associated SNPs coloured according to strength of linkage disequilibrium (red = high through to purple = very low). −log$_{10}$P is on the left-hand y-axis. (a) Illustrating multiple genes underlying a serum urate association signal at the INHBC and TRIM46 loci. (b) Examples of association signals that define a single causal gene of high prior probability. (The *IGF1R* gene spans the entire window.) (c) Examples of intergenic association signals.

Reprinted with permission of Macmillan Publishers Ltd. *Nat Genet*, Kottgen A, Albrecht E, Teumer A, et al., 45, copyright (2013).

renal tubule and responsible for reabsorption of filtered uric acid (reviewed in [18]). The balance of evidence very strongly supports *SLC2A9* as the gene causal of hyperuricaemia and gout at this locus. However, in contrast to the *ABCG2* locus (see next section), the precise genetic variant(s) responsible for the association at *SLC2A9* has not been identified. However, genotype-specific expression data are consistent with the possibility that the major causal serum urate-raising variant in Europeans (marked by SNP *rs12498742*) increases the expression levels of an SLC2A9 isoform (SLC2A9-S) that has a 28 residue portion missing from the N-terminus [19].

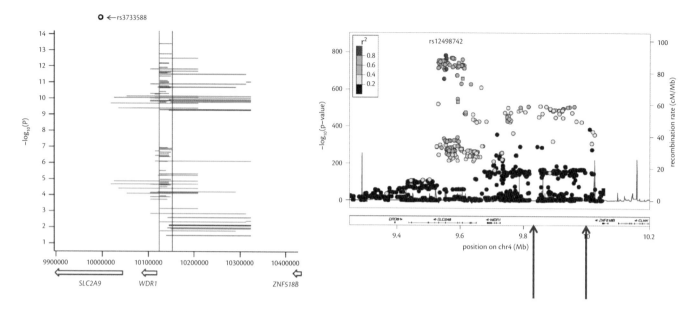

Figure 40.4 The left panel, taken from Wei et al. [26] illustrates the epistatic SNP-SNP interactions present at the *SLC2A9* locus, that concentrate on the indicated 30 kb region. The right panel, taken from Köttgen et al. [6], demonstrates the extent of extremely strong association at the *SLC2A9* locus. The approximate positions of the urate-associated copy number variants identified by Scharpf et al. [23] are arrowed. The genomic co-ordinates differ between each study because Wei et al. used Human Genome Project NCBI build 37.3 and Scharpf et al. NCBI build 36.
Kottgen A, Albrecht E, Teumer A, et al. Genome-wide association analyses identify 18 new loci associated with serum urate concentrations. *Nat Genet* 2013;45:145–54. Wei W-H, Guo Y, Kindt AS, et al. Abundant local interactions in the 4p16. 1 region suggest functional mechanisms underlying SLC2A9 associations with human serum uric acid. *Hum Mol Genet* 2014;23:5061–8.

This isoform is expressed on the apical (urine) side of the collecting duct where it presumably increases reuptake of secreted uric acid, whereas the full-length version (SLC2A9-L) is expressed on the basolateral side [20].

There is evidence that there are multiple causal variants at the *SLC2A9* locus. First, GWAS of serum urate levels in East Asians and African Americans. The East Asian GWAS [11] detected associations at *SLC2A9*, *ABCG2*, *URAT1*, and *MAF* (all common with the Kottgen et al. [6] loci identified in Europeans) and the considerably smaller African American GWAS detected association only at *SLC2A9* [21]. In both the East Asian and African American GWAS the strongest association at *SLC2A9* was with a different SNP (*rs3775948*), genetically un-correlated to the strongest SNP in Europeans (*rs12498742*). The European SNP was not associated in the East Asian GWAS probably because of the rarity of the minor allele with a prevalence of about 1%. Negating the genetic effect of *rs12498752* by a statistical genetic technique called conditional analysis demonstrates that *rs3775948* also confers an independent genetic effect in Europeans [22]. The *rs12498752* and *rs3775948* SNPs therefore each mark separate genetic effects. Second, a GWAS tested for association of common copy number variation with serum urate in Europeans [23]. This type of variation occurs when chromosomal segments over 1 kb in length deviate from the diploid state, and is a genetic and evolutionary mechanism that can generate significant changes in gene expression from a single mutation event. Examples are the immune *CCL3L1* and *FCGR3B* genes that vary from zero to copy number greater than four in the human genome. Copy number of these genes is a risk factor for autoimmune disease [24,25]. The only copy number variations associated with urate in the Scharpf et al. [23] GWAS at a genome-wide level of significance were two separate segments at the *SLC2A9* locus. These variants are 200 kb and 350 kb upstream

of *SLC2A9* (Figure 40.4) and deletion of 12 kb and 7.5 kb segments, respectively, at each copy number variant associates with, respectively, decreased and increased urate levels of approximately 5% in women and approximately 1% in men [23]. Importantly, by conditional analysis, the association of these copy number variants was genetically independent of the previously reported SNP effects at *SLC2A9* [6,11,21]. Finally a study that detected interaction between SNPs at *SLC2A9* [26] is consistent with the above-mentioned studies in providing evidence for multiple independent genetic effects at the *SLC2A9* locus—using conditional analysis they found direct evidence for five further independent genetic effects.

ABCG2

The genetic contribution of *ABCG2* to aetiology of urate control is considerably simpler than that at *SLC2A9*, with the association signal reported as being driven solely by the causal rs2231142 (Q141K) variant [27,28]. The urate-increasing and gout risk allele (141K) encodes a transporter with approximately half the uric acid transport rate of the 141Q allele [27]. However, as at *SLC2A9*, there is more recent evidence for additional independent causal genetic variants at *ABCG2* (Figure 40.1) [22]. The ABCG2 protein (also known as breast cancer resistance protein) is a multidrug transport protein transporting a wide range of molecules, including chemotherapeutic agents. It is a secretory uric acid transporter operating predominantly in the gut [27,29]. Interestingly the urate-increasing allele at rs2231142 (141K) is associated with *increased* urinary uric acid output [29,30]. In mice, an *Abcg2*-knockout also showed increased renal but decreased gut uric acid excretion [29]. This allele was also associated with a reduced increase in serum urate and glucose in response to a fructose load [30]. Collectively these results show that the urate-increasing allele at *ABCG2* does not act directly via direct effects on renal uric acid transport, rather through increased gut excretion, with the increased renal uric acid excretion associated with the urate-raising allele caused by the ABCG2-mediated 'block' in gut excretion. This has led to the proposal that *ABCG2* defines one of three pathways contributing to hyperuricaemia, namely extra-renal uric acid underexcretion, with the other two being genuine urate over-production and renal uric acid underexcretion [29].

Histone deacetylase inhibitors are able to correct the ABCG2 141K urate-increasing 'defect' [28]. The 141K variant results in reduced uric acid transport ability likely because of reduced protein expression owing to increased susceptibility to proteasomal degradation via the ubiquitin pathway [31]. Both the Q141K variation and the common cystic fibrosis-causing mutation (deletion of 508F) in the cystic fibrosis transmembrane conductance receptor (CFTR) are located in a mutational hotspot common to ABC (*ATP binding cassette*) genes involved in disease pathology (within the ATP-binding domain). Based on this and similarities between the functional effects of the Q141K and del508F variations on the respective proteins, Woodward et al. [28] demonstrated that similar small molecules that correct mutant CFTR function in cystic fibrosis can also correct the ABCG2 141K dysfunction. These molecules are histone deacetylase (HDAC) inhibitors such as the Food and Drug Administration (FDA)-approved sodium 4-phenylbutyrate [32]. Clinical trials of FDA-approved HDACs in urate-lowering in the management of gout may yield new therapy options relatively quickly. That a GWAS study first identified a role for *ABCG2* in urate control [7], illustrates the potential of genetics to directly contribute to drug discovery.

GWAS initially identify genetic variant(s) in linkage disequilibrium with a common variant that controls risk. Identification of the causal variant not only provides an opportunity for furthering understanding of pathogenesis but further analysis of the causal gene reveals other (rarer) variants causal of disease and that can also contribute to understanding of the precise molecular basis of disease [33]. At ABCG2 the Q126X variant (encoded by SNP rs72552713) is essentially unique to the Japanese population with 126X resulting in a non-functional protein, with individuals homozygous for 126X at a considerably increased risk for developing gout (prevalence of 0.9% in normouricaemic individuals and 10.1% of Japanese gout patients) [34]. Systematic resequencing of urate-associated loci in hyperuricaemic individuals drawn from other populations may identify similar variants of strong effect that may have direct clinical utility, both at *ABCG2* and other urate-associated loci.

Other uric acid transporters: SLC22A12 (URAT1), SLC22A11 (OAT4), SLC17A1 (NPT1), and PDZK1

Collectively the common genetic variants associated with serum urate levels in these four transporters explain about 1% of variance in urate levels in Europeans [9], considerably less than that explained by *SLC2A9* and *ABCG2*. This figure should not be used to underestimate the importance of these transporters in urate handling, in particular the canonical URAT1 [35]. Rather, the GWAS data indicate the presence of genetic variants in the transporters that can differentiate risk of hyperuricaemia and gout. The importance

of *URAT1* in urate control relative to *SLC2A9* is illustrated by the fact that both of the genes are the only known to harbour inactivating mutations that cause renal hypouricaemia [17,35,36].

The *SLC22A11* and *SLC22A12* genes (encoding organic anion transporter 4 (OAT4) and urate transporter 1 (URAT1), respectively) are located together on chromosome 11. Given the lack of genetic correlation between the separate variants associated with urate levels within each of the genes, the associations with urate represent independent genetic effects, with the causal variants and the molecular basis of their control of urate currently unknown. Nested within the 110 347 individuals in the serum urate GWAS of Köttgen et al. [6] were 3151 gout cases (2115 prevalent cases ascertained through self-report or medication use and 1036 incident cases ascertained by self-report of American Rheumatology Association criteria)—surprisingly given the very large number of cases there was no evidence for association of *SLC22A12* with gout (odds ratio (OR) = 1.03, p = 0.41). At *SLC22A11*, however, Köttgen et al. [6] reported association with gout (OR = 1.14, p = 2.3×10^{-5}). Conversely, in an independent European data set of 648 clinically ascertained cases there was no evidence for association with *SLC22A11* yet evidence for association at *SLC22A12* [12]. A more detailed analysis of the extended *SLC22A11–SLC22A12* locus [37] has highlighted the existence of independent common genetic effects additional to the lead effects identified by GWAS [6] and, by analysis of a Polynesian sample set, ancestral-specific effects [37]. It is likely that this general scenario will also prove to be the case at other serum urate loci—it will be important to conduct detailed genetic analyses of loci in sample sets drawn from multiple ancestral groups.

At the sodium phosphate transporter-1 (*NPT1*/*SLC17A1*) locus the causal variant is likely to be T269I (*rs1165196*), which is amongst the common variants at the locus most strongly associated with urate [6]. The presence of the urate-raising allele (269I) results in a transporter with a reduced (~30%) ability to secrete uric acid [38]. In contrast to the *SLC22A11* and *SLC22A12* genes, *SLC17A1* has been consistently associated with gout in multiple ancestral groups [39,40]. The *SLC17A3* gene (which encodes NPT4) also maps to the same locus as *SLC17A1* on chromosome 6 and contains common genetic variants strongly associated with serum urate levels [6]. Unlike NPT1, however, coding variants that affect the uric acid transport activity of NPT4 [41] are yet to be reported as genetically associated with urate levels.

Despite a clear effect of variants within *PDZK1* (which encodes a molecule known to anchor renal transport molecules to the tubule cytoskeleton) on serum urate levels, the same variants had no effect on the risk of gout in the aforementioned 3151 cases analysed in the Kottgen et al. urate GWAS (OR = 1.03, p = 0.41) [6]. However the urate-raising allele of *PDZK1* was associated with gout in a smaller study of clinically ascertained cases (OR = 1.12, p = 0.016) [12]. Why there was inconsistent association with gout is unclear, however it is notable that the same allele of the variant in *PDZK1* that is associated with increased serum urate also associates with decreased blood pressure [42]. Thus the ability to detect association with gout at *PDZK1* could depend on the proportion of analysed cases with hypertension.

Glycolytic genes

The glucokinase regulatory protein gene (*GCKR*) highlights a serum urate-controlling pathway probably distinct from renal (and gut) excretion of uric acid. It is strongly associated with serum urate in European [6] and has been consistently associated with gout in European, Chinese, and Polynesian populations [12,43]. Genetic variation in *GCKR* has also been associated with triglyceride and fasting glucose concentrations and risk of type 2 diabetes [44], indicating an aetiological link between gout and co-morbid conditions. The association of *GCKR* with serum urate is weakened when triglyceride levels are accounted for [42] and the same *GCKR* allele associated with increased urate also associates with increased triglyceride levels. Based on this observation it has been suggested that *GCKR* affects both serum urate and triglyceride levels by a common unconfirmed mediator that could be glucose-6-phosphate [42]. GCKR controls the hepatic production of glucose-6-phosphate which is catabolized for triglyceride synthesis via glycolysis, whilst glucose-6-phosphate is also a precursor for *de novo* purine (uric acid) synthesis. Other loci identified by Kottgen et al. [6] that contain glycolysis genes are *PKLR* (encodes pyruvate kinase that catalyses the final step of glycolysis, producing ATP and pyruvate), *MLXIPL* (encodes a glucose-responsive transcriptional factor that regulates *PKLR* expression), *PRKAG2* (encodes the regulatory subunit γ2 of the AMP-activated protein kinase, that senses cellular AMP:ATP ratio and activates glucose uptake and catabolism), *NFAT5* (encodes a transcription factor that can influence glucose flux and the pentose phosphate pathway) and *HNF4G* (that encodes a transcription factor responding to nutrient signals). Aside from the possible *GCKR* mechanism outlined above, it is unclear how the glycolysis genes influence serum urate levels. One proposed mechanism [6] is that they could alter the amount of lactate available physiologically—lactate influences renal uric acid excretion likely through a role as a co-transport molecule for uric acid transporters [45]. The observation that the *GCKR* and *NFAT5* loci also associate with fractional excretion of uric acid [6] supports this possibility.

Inconsistent association of urate loci with gout

It is important to demonstrate association of urate loci with gout. Elevated serum urate is the critical risk factor for development of gout. Therefore, it can be argued that genetic variants with a stronger effect on serum urate should have a greater effect on the risk of gout. While this is clearly the case for *SLC2A9* and *ABCG2*, both of which have a very strong effect on serum urate and on risk of gout, there is a clear lack of correlation within the next tier of loci of more moderate effect. The risk alleles of *GCKR*, *SLC16A9*, *SLC22A11*, and *INHBC* are associated with an average increase in serum urate of 0.004 mmol/L [6]). Of these loci the effect size in gout of *GCKR* is consistently higher with OR = 1.3–1.5 in sample sets where gout is clinically ascertained [12,43]. *INHBC* is also consistently associated in European and Polynesian with OR being approximately 1.15, although with a lower effect size than *GCKR* [6,12]. In contrast, as mentioned above, *SLC22A11* is not consistently associated with gout. The still weaker evidence for association of *SLC16A9* with gout in Köttgen et al. [6] (OR = 1.10, p = 0.017) was not replicated in a separate study [12]. Thus there are clearly inconsistent effects on association with gout between these four loci that have very similar effects on serum urate. It is also notable that the effect of *ABCG2* on gout is consistently larger than *SLC2A9* in European, Japanese, and Polynesian sample sets [6,12,13], despite *SLC2A9* having a 72% greater effect on serum

urate levels. These observations may result from a lack of independence between molecular pathways of serum urate control and clinical presentation of gout in the presence of hyperuricaemia (i.e. pleiotropic effects of the urate-associated loci) and/or confounding of serum urate and risk of gout effect sizes by unmeasured or unaccounted for environmental exposures such as alcohol and sugar-sweetened beverage consumption. Supporting the latter hypothesis is evidence for non-additive interaction of *SLC2A9* with a prevalent environmental exposure (sugar-sweetened beverages) in regulation of urate levels and risk of gout [46], and for interaction of *SLC2A9* and *SLC22A11* with diuretic use in determining the risk of gout [47]. Consequently, it will be important to continue to test urate-associated loci with gout in clinically well-phenotyped sample sets. If the inconsistent pattern of association with gout at loci such as *SLC16A9* and *SLC22A11* is evident in such data sets, it should be investigated why this is the case in clinical studies and epidemiological studies testing for non-additive interaction with environmental exposures.

Loci associated with monosodium urate crystal deposition and inflammation in gout

Only a minority of individuals with hyperuricaemia developed gout in a 5-year period [48] consistent with the hypothesis that genetic and environmental factors influence the risk of a hyperuricaemic individual developing gout. However, in contrast to the understanding of the genetic control of urate very little is known about genetic variants involved in the progression from hyperuricaemia to gout. A very small number of studies associating variants in candidate genes involved in activation of the NLRP3 inflammasome and downstream inflammatory effectors with gout have been published (e.g. [49,50]); however, they remain unreplicated. The strongest evidence for a role of an innate immune system gene in the aetiology of gout comes from a single study associating with gout the toll-like receptor 4 (*TLR4*) gene in a Chinese case–control sample set [51] which was replicated in a European sample set [52]. The TLR4 protein interacts with endogenous ligands such as MSU crystals to activate the interleukin 1 beta-generating inflammasome. The variant associated with gout (*rs2149356*) had previously been associated with other auto-inflammatory conditions. It maps to intron 4 of *TLR4* but is in strong linkage disequilibrium with two other genetic variants in the promoter of *TLR4* predicted to influence transcription binding sites and expression [53]. Interestingly, in participants with gout, the same genotype that conferred risk of gout was also associated with reduced low-density lipoprotein cholesterol and increased high-density lipoprotein cholesterol [51]. These relationships were not seen in hyper- or normouricaemia, suggesting a causal relationship between the TLR4-signaling pathway and lipoprotein metabolism in acute gout. This is consistent with an observational study that has implicated very low-density lipoprotein in the progression from hyperuricaemia to gout [54].

Concluding remarks

The genome-wide association approach has provided numerous insights into the molecular control of urate, identifying new opportunities for urate-lowering in gout. However there is a pressing need for GWAS in very large sample sets of properly phenotyped (clinically ascertained) gout cases in order to identify immune and other genetic risk factors controlling the progression from hyperuricaemia to gout. International collaborative efforts are currently underway to address this deficit [55].

References

1. Dalbeth N, Merriman TR. Hyperuricemia and gout. In Valle-D (ed) *The Online Metabolic and Molecular Bases of Inherited Disease*: McGraw-Hill, New York; 2013: Chapter 106.
2. Emmerson BT, Nagel SL, Duffy DL, Martin NG. Genetic control of the renal clearance of urate: a study of twins. *Ann Rheum Dis* 1992; 51:375–7.
3. Krishnan E, Lessov-Schlaggar CN, Krasnow RE, Swan GE. Nature versus nurture in gout: a twin study. *Am J Med* 2012; 125:499–504.
4. Kuo C-F, Grainge MJ, See L-C, et al. Familial aggregation of gout and relative genetic and environmental contributions: a nationwide population study in Taiwan. *Ann Rheum Dis* 2015; 74:369–74.
5. Merriman TR, Dalbeth N. The genetic basis of hyperuricaemia and gout. *Joint Bone Spine* 2011; 78:35–40.
6. Kottgen A, Albrecht E, Teumer A, et al. Genome-wide association analyses identify 18 new loci associated with serum urate concentrations. *Nat Genet* 2013; 45:145–54.
7. Dehghan A, Kottgen A, Yang Q, et al. Association of three genetic loci with uric acid concentration and risk of gout: a genome-wide association study. *Lancet* 2008; 372:1953–61.
8. Kolz M JT, Sanna S, Teumer A, et al. Meta-analysis of 28,141 individuals identifies common variants within five new loci that influence uric acid concentrations. *PLoS Genet* 2009; 5:e1000504.
9. Yang Q KA, Dehghan A, Smith AV, et al. Multiple genetic loci influence serum urate levels and their relationship with gout and cardiovascular disease risk factors. *Circ Cardiovasc Genet* 2010; 3:523–30.
10. Tin A, Woodward OM, Kao WH, et al. Genome-wide association study for serum urate concentrations and gout among African Americans identifies genomic risk loci and a novel URAT1 loss-of-function allele. *Hum Mol Genet* 2011; 20:4056–68.
11. Okada Y, Sim X, Go MJ, et al. Meta-analysis identifies multiple loci associated with kidney function-related traits in east Asian populations. *Nat Genet* 2012; 44:904–9.
12. Phipps-Green A, Merriman M, Topless R, et al. Twenty-eight loci that influence serum urate levels: analysis of association with gout. *Ann Rheum Dis* 2016; 75(1):124–30.
13. Urano W, Taniguchi A, Inoue E, et al. Effect of genetic polymorphisms on development of gout. *J Rheumatol* 2013; 40:1374–8.
14. Raychaudhuri S, Plenge RM, Rossin EJ, et al. Identifying relationships among genomic disease regions: predicting genes at pathogenic SNP associations and rare deletions. *PLoS Genet* 2009; 5:e1000534.
15. Maurano MT, Humbert R, Rynes E, et al. Systematic localization of common disease-associated variation in regulatory DNA. *Science* 2012; 337:1190–5.
16. Smemo S, Tena JJ, Kim K-H, et al. Obesity-associated variants within FTO form long-range functional connections with IRX3. *Nature* 2014; 507:371–5.
17. Dinour D, Gray NK, Campbell S, et al. Homozygous SLC2A9 mutations cause severe renal hypouricemia. *J Am Soc Nephrol* 2010; 21:64–72.
18. Mandal A, Mount DB. The molecular physiology of uric acid homeostasis. *Ann Rev Physiol* 2015; 77:323–45.
19. Doring A, Gieger C, Mehta D, et al. SLC2A9 influences uric acid concentrations with pronounced sex-specific effects. *Nat Genet* 2008; 40:430–6.
20. Kimura T, Takahashi M, Yan K, Sakurai H. Expression of SLC2A9 isoforms in the kidney and their localization in polarized epithelial cells. *PLoS One* 2014; 9:e84996.
21. Charles BA, Shriner D, Doumatey A, et al. A genome-wide association study of serum uric acid in African Americans. *BMC Med Genomics* 2011; 4:17.
22. Stahl E Choi H, Cadzow M, et al. Conditional analysis of 30 serum urate loci identifies 25 additional independent effects. *Arthritis Rheumatol* 2014; 66:S1294.
23. Scharpf RB, Mireles L, Yang Q, et al. Copy number polymorphisms near SLC2A9 are associated with serum uric acid concentrations. *BMC Genet* 2014; 15:81.
24. McKinney C, Merriman ME, Chapman PT, et al. Evidence for an influence of chemokine ligand 3-like 1 (CCL3L1) gene copy number on susceptibility to rheumatoid arthritis. *Ann Rheum Dis* 2008; 67:409–13.
25. McKinney C, Merriman TR. Meta-analysis confirms a role for deletion in FCGR3B in autoimmune phenotypes. *Hum Mol Genet* 2012; 21:2370–6.
26. Wei W-H, Guo Y, Kindt AS, et al. Abundant local interactions in the 4p16.1 region suggest functional mechanisms underlying SLC2A9 associations with human serum uric acid. *Hum Mol Genet* 2014; 23:5061–8.
27. Woodward OM, Kottgen A, Coresh J, et al. Identification of a urate transporter, ABCG2, with a common functional polymorphism causing gout. *Proc Natl Acad Sci U S A* 2009; 106:10338–42.
28. Woodward OM, Tuyake D, Cui J, et al. Gout-causing Q141K mutation in ABCG2 leads to instability of the nucleotide-binding domain and can be corrected with small molecules. *Proc Natl Acad Sci U S A* 2013; 110(5223–8).
29. Ichida K, Matsuo H, Takada T, et al. Decreased extra-renal urate excretion is a common cause of hyperuricemia. *Nat Commun* 2012; 3:764.
30. Dalbeth N, House ME, Gamble GD, et al. Influence of the ABCG2 gout risk 141 K allele on urate metabolism during a fructose challenge. *Arthritis Res Ther* 2014; 16:R34.
31. Furukawa T, Wakabayashi K, Tamura A, et al. Major SNP (Q141K) variant of human ABC transporter ABCG2 undergoes lysosomal and proteasomal degradations. *Pharmaceut Res* 2009; 26:469–79.
32. Rubenstein RC, Egan ME, Zeitlin PL. In vitro pharmacologic restoration of CFTR-mediated chloride transport with sodium 4-phenylbutyrate in cystic fibrosis epithelial cells containing delta F508-CFTR. *J Clin Invest* 1997; 100:2457–65.
33. Nejentsev S, Walker N, Riches D, Egholm M, Todd JA. Rare variants of IFIH1, a gene implicated in antiviral responses, protect against type 1 diabetes. *Science* 2009; 324:387–9.
34. Matsuo H, Takada T, Ichida K, et al. Common defects of ABCG2, a high-capacity urate exporter, cause gout: a function-based genetic analysis in a Japanese population. *Sci Transl Med* 2009; 1:5ra11.
35. Enomoto A, Kimura H, Chairoungdua A, et al. Molecular identification of a renal urate anion exchanger that regulates blood urate levels. *Nature* 2002; 417:447–52.
36. Shen H, Feng C, Jin X, et al. Recurrent exercise-induced acute kidney injury by idiopathic renal hypouricemia with a novel mutation in the SLC2A9 gene and literature review. *BMC Pediatr* 2014; 14:73.
37. Flynn TJ, Phipps-Green A, Hollis-Moffatt JE, et al. Association analysis of the SLC22A11 (organic anion transporter 4) and SLC22A12 (urate transporter 1) urate transporter locus with gout in New Zealand case-control sample sets reveals multiple ancestral-specific effects. *Arthritis Res Ther* 2013; 15:R220.
38. Iharada M, Miyaji T, Fujimoto T, et al. Type 1 sodium-dependent phosphate transporter (SLC17A1 protein) is a Cl⁻-dependent urate exporter. *J Biol Chem* 2010; 285:26107–13.
39. Chiba T, Matsuo H, Kawamura Y, et al. NPT1/SLC17A1 Is a renal urate exporter in humans and its common gain-of-function variant decreases the risk of renal underexcretion gout. *Arthritis Rheumatol* 2015; 67:281–7.
40. Hollis-Moffatt JE, Phipps-Green AJ, Chapman B, et al. The renal urate transporter SLC17A1 locus: confirmation of association with gout. *Arthritis Res Ther* 2012; 14:R92.
41. Jutabha P, Anzai N, Kimura T, et al. Functional analysis of human sodium-phosphate transporter 4 (NPT4/SLC17A3) polymorphisms. *J Pharmacol Sci* 2011; 115:249–53.
42. van der Harst P, Bakker SJ, de Boer RA, et al. Replication of the 5 novel loci for uric acid concentrations and potential mediating mechanisms. *Hum Mol Genet* 2010; 19:387–95.
43. Wang J, Liu S, Wang B, et al. Association between gout and polymorphisms in GCKR in male Han Chinese. *Hum Genet* 2012; 131:1261–5.

44. Vaxillaire M, Cavalcanti-Proenca C, Dechaume A, et al. The common P446L polymorphism in GCKR inversely modulates fasting glucose and triglyceride levels and reduces type 2 diabetes risk in the DESIR prospective general French population. *Diabetes* 2008; 57:2253–7.

45. Taniguchi A, Kamatani N. Control of renal uric acid excretion and gout. *Curr Opin Rheumatol* 2008; 20:192–7.

46. Batt C, Phipps-Green AJ, Black MA, et al. Sugar-sweetened beverage consumption: a risk factor for prevalent gout with SLC2A9 genotype-specific effects on serum urate and risk of gout. *Ann Rheum Dis* 2014; 73:2101–6.

47. McAdams-DeMarco MA, Maynard JW, Baer AN, et al. A urate gene-by-diuretic interaction and gout risk in participants with hypertension: results from the ARIC study. *Ann Rheum Dis* 2013; 72:701–6.

48. Campion EW, Glynn RJ, DeLabry LO. Asymptomatic hyperuricemia. Risks and consequences in the Normative Aging Study. *Am J Med* 1987; 82:421–6.

49. Chang S-J, Tsai P-C, Chen C-J, Lai H-M, Ko Y-C. The polymorphism-863C/A in tumour necrosis factor-α gene contributes an independent association to gout. *Rheumatology* 2007; 46:1662–6.

50. Liu S, Yin C, Chu N, Han L, Li C. IL-8-251T/A and IL-12B 1188A/C polymorphisms are associated with gout in a Chinese male population. *Scand J Rheumatol* 2013; 42:150–8.

51. Qing YF, Zhou JG, Zhang QB, et al. Association of TLR4 gene rs2149356 polymorphism with primary gouty arthritis in a case-control study. *PLoS One* 2013; 8:e64845.

52. Rasheed H, McKinney C, Stamp LK, et al. The toll-like receptor (TR4) variants rs2149356 and risk of gout in European and Polynesian sample sets. *PLoS One* 2016; 11:e0147939.

53. Ragnarsdóttir B, Jónsson K, Urbano A, et al. Toll-like receptor 4 promoter polymorphisms: common TLR4 variants may protect against severe urinary tract infection. *PLoS One* 2010; 5:e10734.

54. Rasheed H, Hsu A, Dalbeth N, et al. The relationship of apolipoprotein B and very low density lipoprotein triglyceride with hyperuricemia and gout. *Arthritis Res Ther* 2014; 16:495.

55. Liote F, Merriman T, Nasi S, So A. 4th European Crystal Network meeting, Paris 8-9th March 2013. *Arthritis Res Ther* 2013; 15:304.

56. Merriman TR, Choi HK, Dalbeth N. The genetic basis of gout. *Rheum Dis Clin North Am* 2014; 40:279–90.

57. Bonomo JA, Guan M, Ng MC, et al. The ras responsive transcription factor RREB1 is a novel candidate gene for type 2 diabetes associated end-stage kidney disease. *Hum Mol Genet* 2014; 23:6441–7.

58. Tragante V, Barnes MR, Ganesh SK, et al. Gene-centric meta-analysis in 87,736 individuals of European ancestry identifies multiple blood-pressure-related loci. *Am J Hum Genet* 2014; 94:349–60.

59. Berndt SI, Gustafsson S, Mägi R, et al. Genome-wide meta-analysis identifies 11 new loci for anthropometric traits and provides insights into genetic architecture. *Nat Genet* 2013; 45:501–12.

60. Kraja AT, Chasman DI, North KE, et al. Pleiotropic genes for metabolic syndrome and inflammation. *Mol Genet Metab* 2014; 112:317–38.

CHAPTER 41

Clinical presentation of gout

Tim L. Jansen

Clinical features of gout

Gout is the most common form of inflammatory arthritis. In this era, the prevalence of gout is increasing primarily due to ageing of our populations and increased occurrence of obesity [1–6]. Gout typically affects men more frequently than women, initially presenting as a peripheral joint monoarthritis. In women, gout presents more commonly after menopause and in the context of aspirin and/or diuretic use, with similar joint distribution as in men but with a more polyarticular, osteoarthritic pattern [7,8].

Pathobiologically, gout is a chronic disease of monosodium urate (MSU) crystal deposition (see Chapter 39). Hyperuricaemia is often not associated with clinical sequelae [6,8,9]. Asymptomatic hyperuricaemia may be associated with silent formation of MSU crystals in the tissue and in or around peripheral joints, tendons, or bursae, probably enhanced in the presence of a certain (collagen) matrix [10–14]. Ongoing crystal deposition may or may not result in symptoms and clinical sequelae. Stereochemical and conformational crystalline factors may influence the ability of crystals to evoke an autoinflammatory response *in vivo* [15]. Thus, not all patients experience severe acute inflammatory episodes (flares) and some will become tophaceous while having had no severe attacks at all.

Usually, though not exclusively, the first presentation is an acute, self-limiting 'flare' of extremely painful peripheral synovitis or tendonitis. This most frequently affects the first metatarsophalangeal joint (podagra) (Figure 41.1), midfoot, and/or ankle. If hyperuricaemia persists, patients develop more frequent, polyarticular flares, which may also affect joints of the upper limbs [7]. Eventually, in the situation of ongoing hyperuricaemia, tophaceous gout develops in males frequently at the ear and/or hands/olecranon/etc., and in females less at the ear but more at the fingertips; this accumulation occurs with subclinical crystal-induced chronic inflammation in response to these densely packed crystals (tophi; Figures 41.2 and 41.3), joint damage, and chronic gouty synovitis [13,15,16].

The typical presentation of gout is an acute episode of severe inflammatory arthritis with associated hyperuricaemia in middle-aged, overweight males. Some patients may report triggers for gout flares including purine-rich foods and beverages or physical exercise. The following clinical characteristics are often seen:

♦ First metatarsophalangeal joint (MTPJ1) involvement (podagra)

♦ Redness/erythema over affected joint

♦ Rapid mode of onset (within several hours)

♦ Onset during night rest

♦ Severe pain (unbearable to touch/to have bedclothes on joint/to sleep/to walk)

♦ Complete resolution between attacks (at least after the first attacks).

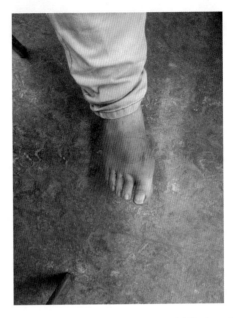

Figure 41.1 Tophaceous gout podagra, that is, severe debilitating arthritis of MTPJ1 in a 60-year-old male presenting with his first attack.

In an international study of 983 patients with a swollen joint or subcutaneous nodule, a number of features were associated with microscopically proven gout. These features are summarized in Table 41.1 [17].

This study also demonstrated frequent involvement of the MTPJ1 and ankle/midfoot regions (Table 41.2) [17].

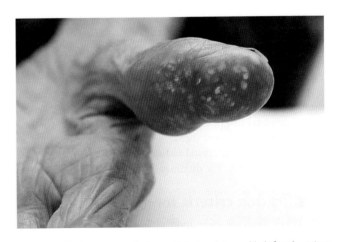

Figure 41.2 Tophaceous gout in tissue of left thumb in an elderly female patient without previous severe attacks.

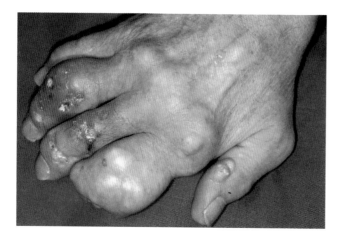

Figure 41.3 Tophaceous gout of right hand showing massive tophi with fistula through the skin in an elderly 60-plus male with severe attacks.

Patients with gout frequently have comorbid conditions such as obesity, chronic kidney disease, hypertension, and dyslipidaemia. These comorbid conditions are observed more frequently in people with gout compared with other rheumatic diseases such as rheumatoid arthritis, connective tissue disease, or polymyalgia [18].

Gout diagnosis

Wherever possible, the diagnosis of gout should be confirmed by microscopic confirmation of MSU crystals (see Chapter 42) [19]. However, joint aspiration may not always be doable or practicable, particularly in the context of anticoagulation or small joint involvement. Generally, a confident clinical diagnosis can be made in a patient with typical acute attacks of gout (e.g. recurrent episodes of podagra) [19–21]. Imaging methods such as ultrasonography and dual-energy computed tomography (DECT) scanning may also assist in identification of MSU crystals (see Chapter 43). Possibly in the future, additional cell-based tests may be an aid to clinicians in the diagnostic phase.

A diagnostic rule, available as an online gout calculator [22], is applicable in cases presenting with monoarthritis (Box 41.1).

Using this diagnostic rule, clinicians may well be able to categorize patients into three subgroups with very low, low, and high probability of having gout. This rule may assist in gout diagnosis in individuals with a monoarticular presentation even without obtaining joint aspiration and synovial fluid examination under polarized light microscopy. As no clear-cut microscopic proof is obtained, clearly false positives and false negatives may occur. False-positives may occur even at scores of 8 or higher on the diagnostic rule; in 20% of these cases an alternative diagnosis should be considered [22,23]. The midrange score leaves a high degree of uncertainty about the gout diagnosis, as the midrange gout was confirmed in only 30% of cases [22,23].

The differential diagnosis in a patient presenting with monoarthritis in a peripheral joint includes the following: septic arthritis, calcium pyrophosphate crystal arthritis, psoriatic arthritis or other forms of spondyloarthritis, rheumatoid arthritis, and osteoarthritis.

Classification criteria for gout

Aside from diagnosis of individual patients, criteria have been developed for classification purposes. Classification criteria are

Table 41.1 Features of microscopically proven gout

Feature	Frequency/level
1. Male sex preponderance	In 86% of cases
2. MTPJ1 involvement ever	In 74% of cases
MTPJ1 in isolation involved ever	In 71% of cases
MTPJ1 first ever	In 57% of cases
3. Rapid mode of onset: <4 hours	In 22% of cases
Rapid mode of onset: <12 hours	In 61% of cases
Rapid mode of onset: <24 hours	In 75% of cases
4. Pain level ever: 7 or higher	In 78% of cases
Pain level current: 7 or higher	In 81% of cases
Cannot touch	In 95% of cases
Cannot sleep	In 91% of cases
Cannot walk	In 97% of cases
5. Complete resolution after attack	In 85% of cases
6. Redness over affected joint	In 87% of cases
7. Serum urate:	
Mean (SD) highest ever SUA	0.56 (0.13) mmol/L
Mean (SD) current SUA	0.46 (0.13) mmol/L
Current SUA > 0.36 mmol/L (6 mg/dL)	In 77% of cases
Highest SUA > 0. 36 mmol/L off ULT	In 94% of cases
8. MSU crystal accumulation:	
Double contour sign at US	In 58% of cases
Snow storm effusion at US	In 31% of cases
Tophaceous accumulation at US	In 45% of cases
Macroscopic tophus/tophi	In 34% of cases
9. Other comorbidities	
Hypertension/cardiovascular disease	In 68% of cases
Renal stone disease	In 15% of cases

MTPJ1, first metatarsophalangeal joint; SD, standard deviation; SUA, serum urate; ULT, urate lowering therapy; US, ultrasound.

Taylor WJ, Fransen J, Jansen TL, Dalbeth N, Schumacher HR, Brown M, Louthrenoo W, Vazques-Mellado J, Eliseev M, McCarthy G, Stamp LK, Perez-Ruiz F, Sivera F, Ea H-K, Gerritsen M, Scire C, Cavagna L, Lin C, Chou Y-Y, Tausche A-K, Da Rocha Castelar-Pinheiro, Janssen M, Chen J-C, Slot O, Cimmino M, Uhlig T, Neogi T., Study for updated gout classification criteria (SugaR): identification of features to classify gout. *ACR Arthritis Care and Research* 2015, 2015, Wiley.

designed for research purposes to ensure relative homogeneity of study participants. Six sets of classification criteria for gout have been developed in the past but the most widely used is the 1977 American Rheumatism Association preliminary set of criteria for acute arthritis of primary gout. Most criteria sets have focused on advanced disease, or have not been developed in reference with a control group [24]. In early disease, gout may be more challenging to accurately classify since characteristic features may take years to evolve. In a recent, large, international case–control study, where studied cases were confined to those with microscopically proven gout, sensitivity across these criteria sets was better in established

Table 41.2 Affected joints in people with microscopically proven gout

Joint	Cumulative frequency (%)
Big toe/first metatarsophalangeal joint	~75
Ankle/midfoot	~50
Knee	~30
Finger	~25
Elbow	~10
Wrist	~10
Other joint	~4
Bursitis	~3
>1 site simultaneously	~10

Taylor WJ, Fransen J, Jansen TL, Dalbeth N, Schumacher HR, Brown M, Louthrenoo W, Vazques-Mellado J, Eliseev M, McCarthy G, Stamp LK, Perez-Ruiz F, Sivera F, Ea H-K, Gerritsen M, Scire C, Cavagna L, Lin C, Chou Y-Y, Tausche A-K, Da Rocha Castelar-Pinheiro, Janssen M, Chen J-C, Slot O, Cimmino M, Uhlig T, Neogi T, Study for updated gout classification criteria (SugaR): identification of features to classify gout. *ACR Arthritis Care and Research* 2015, 2015, Wiley.

disease (95% for disease duration ≤ 2 years vs 84% for disease duration > 2 years, p < 0.001) and specificity was better in early disease (80% for disease duration vs 53% for disease duration > 2 years, p < 0.001).

Updated criteria are needed because of the low specificity in both early and later disease [24]. In 2015, the American College of Rheumatology and European League Against Rheumatism (ACR-EULAR) updated these criteria [17]. The new clinical classification

---

Box 41.1 Diagnostic rule for gout: an aid for the general practitioner by providing a clinical scoring system

Patients with *monoarthritis* can be given points based on the presence of predefined variables:

◆ Male: gets 2 points

◆ Increased serum urate level: 3.5 points added, and

◆ MTPJ1 involvement: another 2.5 points adds up to 8 points.

Interpretation:

◆ Score 8 or higher: gout is the diagnosis (80% indeed is gout)

◆ Score >4 to <8: uncertain diagnosis (only 30% is gout)

◆ Score <4: no arguments for gout (<3% is gout).

Predefined specific variables 1 to 7

	Clinical scoring points
1. Male sex	2.0
2. Serum urate > 0.36mM/L	3.5
3. Patient-reported previous attacks	2.0
4. MTPJ1 involvement	2.5
5. Hypertension/cardiovascular disease	1.5
6. Onset within 1 day	0.5
7. Joint redness/rubor	1.0

https://www.radboudumc.nl/Research/Organisationofresearch/Departments/eerstelijnsgeneeskunde/Pages/Jichtcalculator.aspx

---

domains includes clinical (pattern of joint/bursa involvement, characteristics and time-course of symptomatic episodes), laboratory (serum urate, synovial fluid aspirate), and imaging (ultrasound or DECT, and plain radiography) criteria.

Conclusion

There is a wide variety of gout presentations, but the most frequent is an acute painful arthritis affecting the big toe, midfoot, ankle, or knee. If hyperuricaemia persists, gout may progress to a polyarticular, even tophaceous disease. Early diagnosis is important, and only possible if the most elementary clinical features are recognized. For diagnostic purposes, in which lifelong pharmacotherapy is considered, microscopic confirmation is ideal, sometimes even obligatory prior to prescription of a more expensive long-lasting pharmacotherapy. The diagnostic rule calculator and/or advanced imaging techniques may enhance clinical diagnosis in the absence of microscopic examination of synovial fluid. For gout classification, the older criteria sets are insufficiently specific, and the newly updated ACR-EULAR criteria are anticipated to be a major improvement.

References

1. Mikuls TR, Farrar JT, Bilker WB, et al. Gout epidemiology: results from the UK general practice research database, 1990–1999. *Ann Rheum Dis* 2005; 64:267–72.
2. Mikuls TR, Saag KG. New insights into gout epidemiology. *Curr Opin Rheumatol* 2006; 18:199–203.
3. Annemans L, Spaepen E, Gaskin M, et al. Gout in the UK and Germany: prevalence, comorbidities and management in general practice 2000–2005. *Ann Rheum Dis* 2008; 67:960–6.
4. Zhu Y, Pandya BJ, Choi HK. Prevalence of gout and hyperuricemia in the US general population: the National Health and Nutrition Examination Survey 2007–2008. *Arthritis Rheum* 2011; 63:3136–41.
5. Lawrence RC, Felson DT, Helmick CG, et al. Estimates of the prevalence of arthritis and other rheumatic conditions in the United States. Part II. *Arthritis Rheum* 2008; 58:26–35.
6. Roddy E, Doherty M. Epidemiology of gout. *Arthritis Res Ther* 2010; 12:223.
7. Ter Borg EJ, Rasker JJ. Gout in the elderly, a separate entity? *Ann Rheum Dis* 1987; 46:72–6.
8. Doherty M, Jansen TL, Nuki G, et al. Gout: why is this curable disease so seldom cured? *Ann Rheum Dis* 2012; 71(11):1765–70.
9. Zhang W, Doherty M, Bardin T, *et al.* EULAR evidence based recommendations for gout. Part II: management. Report of a task force of the EULAR Standing Committee for International Clinical Studies Including Therapeutics (ESCISIT). *Ann Rheum Dis* 2006; 65:1312–24.
10. Hershfield MS. Reassessing serum urate targets in the management of refractory gout: can you go too low? *Curr Opin Rheumatol* 2009; 21:138–42.
11. Tak HK, Cooper SM, Wilcox WR. Studies on the nucleation of monosodium urate at 37 degrees c. *Arthritis Rheum* 1980; 23:574–80.
12. Puig JG, de Miguel E, Castillo MC, et al. Asymptomatic hyperuricemia: impact of ultrasonography. *Nucleosides Nucleotides Nucleic Acids* 2008; 27:592–5.
13. Pineda C, Amezcua-Guerra LM, Solano C, et al. Joint and tendon subclinical involvement suggestive of gouty arthritis in asymptomatic hyperuricemia: an ultrasound controlled study. *Arthritis Res Ther* 2011; 13:R4.
14. Richette P, Bardin T. Gout. *Lancet* 2010; 375:318–28.
15. Jansen TL, Berendsen D, Crisan TO, et al. New gout test: enhanced ex-vivo cytokine production from PBMCs in common gout patients and a gout patient with Kearns-Sayre syndrome. *Clin Rheumatol* 2014; 33(9):1341–6.

16. Terkeltaub R. Gout. Novel therapies for treatment of gout and hyper-uricemia. *Arthritis Res Ther* 2009; 11:236.

17. Taylor WJ, Fransen J, Jansen TL, et al. Study for updated gout classification criteria (SugaR): identification of features to classify gout. *Arthritis Care Res* 2015; 67(9):1304–15.

18. Meek IL, Vonkeman HE, Van de Laar MA. Cardiovascular case fatality rate in RA is decreasing: first prospective analysis of a current low disease activity rheumatoid arthritis cohort and review of literature. *BMC Musculoskelet Disorders* 2014; 15:142.

19. Berendsen D, Jansen TL, Taylor W et al. A critical appraisal of the competence of crystal identification by rheumatologists. *Ann Rheum Dis* 2013; 72(S3):981–2.

20. Jordan KM, Cameron JS, Snaith M, et al. British Society for Rheumatology and British Health Professionals in Rheumatology guideline for the management of gout. *Rheumatology* 2007; 46:1372–4.

21. Zhang W, Doherty M, Pascual E, et al. EULAR evidence based recommendations for gout. Part I: diagnosis. Report of a task force of the Standing Committee for International Clinical Studies Including Therapeutics (ESCISIT). *Ann Rheum Dis* 2006; 65:1301–11.

22. Radboudumc. *Gout Calculator*. 2010. https://www.radboudumc.nl/Research/Organisationofresearch/Departments/eerstelijnsgeneeskunde/Pages/Jichtcalculator.aspx

23. Janssens HJEM, Fransen J, Van de Lisdonk EH, et al. A diagnostic rule for acute gouty arthritis in primary care without joint fluid analysis. *Arch Intern Med* 2010; 170:1120–6.

24. Taylor WJ, Fransen J, Dalbeth N, et al. Performance of classification criteria for gout in early and established disease. *Ann Rheum Dis* 2016; 75(1):178–82.

CHAPTER 42

Laboratory investigations in gout

Eliseo Pascual and Francisca Sivera

Serum urate

High serum urate (SUA) is a hallmark of gout and should be measured in all patients with gout before initiating urate-lowering therapy (ULT). It should also be measured serially to monitor the efficacy of ULT. SUA levels are determined by the equilibrium resulting from urate formation and its elimination. Urate is the end product of purine catabolism. Purines can be synthesized *de novo* from non-purine precursors or can be salvaged from dietary or endogenous sources. Irrespective of the way in which the purines are formed, the common steps of purine degradation include the catabolism of hypoxanthine to xanthine and xanthine to urate by the enzyme xanthine oxidase. Humans and higher primates have lost (through a mutation) the activity of the enzyme uricase, which facilitates the further transformation of urate into allantoin, more soluble and easily excreted through the kidney [1]. As a result, urate accumulates and SUA levels in humans are increased compared to most other mammals. Most of the SUA excretion is performed via the kidney, with the remaining SUA being excreted through the gut [2]. Information on the molecular determinants of renal excretion pathways has increased dramatically in the past decade [3]. It is generally believed that most hyperuricaemia in subjects with normal glomerular filtration rates (GFRs), results from a significant inefficacy of the kidneys to clear urate due to impaired tubular secretion, increased tubular resorption, or a combination of both (see Chapter 39).

Most routine assays for SUA utilize some variant of the Trinder reaction with uricase [4]. The assay is generally reliable with between-laboratory and between-method coefficients of variation less than 5%. However, there is no current consensus on the threshold that defines hyperuricaemia. Typically, and given the accepted pathophysiology of gout, hyperuricaemia is defined as above the saturation levels (7 mg/dL). However, this is inferred from the solubility limit of sodium urate in a test tube at 37°C and does not take into account local conditions such as promoters of crystallization. Given that women, especially pre-menopausal women, tend to have lower population SUA levels, different cut-off points for men and women (>7.0–7.7 mg/dL in men and >5.7–6.0 mg/dL in women) have been occasionally proposed [5,6]. While these different thresholds are based on epidemiological data, they do not reflect pathogenic differences between men and women. Given the recent findings of monosodium urate (MSU) crystal deposits in patients with asymptomatic hyperuricaemia [7,8] and the growing evidence that SUA might play a role in the pathogenesis of cardiovascular and renal disorders, several authors have suggested lowering the threshold of hyperuricaemia to 6 mg/dL [5,6], thereby equating hyperuricaemia with the currently recommended ULT target.

Even though hyperuricaemia is essential for the development of gout, a single determination of SUA during an acute gout flare can be misleading. SUA has been shown to drop during acute gout flares at the expense of an increase of renal excretion. Investigations in groups of patients undergoing gout flares have described frequencies of normouricaemia between 14% and 49% [9–12]. It is therefore advisable in the case of a suspected gout flare with normouricaemia to review previous blood tests or repeat the blood test a few weeks after flare resolution. Other inflammatory insults such as surgery might decrease SUA in a manner similar to acute gout flares [13,14].

Uric acid renal excretion

Although overproduction of urate can contribute to hyperuricaemia, in most patients—such as those with metabolic syndrome—the largest determinant of SUA concentration is renal excretion. Patients with gout have commonly been classified into over-producers or under-excretors, on the basis of the renal output of uric acid. There is no universally accepted single method of evaluating renal uric acid excretion and the evidence supporting each of them is scarce. A basic understanding of renal uric acid handling is therefore necessary in order to interpret them. Uric acid, as creatinine and most small molecules, is freely filtered in the glomeruli. Once in the tubules, uric acid undergoes a net resorption resulting in the recuperation of most of the filtered uric acid. Hyperuricaemia can result from low filtered uric acid (i.e. the hyperuricaemia in patients with severely impaired renal function) or, most commonly, from a tubular dysfunction resulting in increased net resorption [15].

Investigating uric acid renal excretion in patients with gout has two distinct aims: (1) to identify that small proportion of over-producers who might benefit from further aetiological workup, and (2) to provide information relevant to ULT choice (i.e. urico-surics vs xanthine oxidase inhibitors). Over-production of serum uric acid is an uncommon cause of gout (<10%) which can associate with a purine-rich diet, but also with acquired proliferative disorders (such as polycythemia or leukaemias), diseases with a high cell turnover (e.g. psoriasis), or very infrequent genetic disorders. Identifying over-producers amongst patients with gout might allow recognition of a severe disease or identification of a—at least partially—reversible cause. On the other hand, if uricosuric drugs are available, the renal findings might condition the choice of ULT. Uricosuric drugs are especially useful when the patients shows an impaired renal uric acid handling but increase the risk of nephrolithiasis in patients with a high uric acid renal output.

Classically, patients with gout have been considered under-excretors if the amount of uric acid on a 24-hour urine (uricosuria) sample was less than 700 mg/day [16]. However, as late as the 1990s, recommendations for performing this measurement included repeated 24-hour urine collections under a restrictive low-purine diet [17]. This approach became untenable for an unselected population and its use is currently anecdotal. A single 24-hour urine collection while on unrestricted diet is preferred. It is unknown how well the single measurement correlates with repeated measurements under restricted conditions. Uricosuria is dependent on the SUA levels (as higher SUA levels will lead to an increased total amount of uric acid in the urine) and has been shown to be a mediocre predictor of renal stone formation [18]. The 24-hour uricosuria provides data on the overall output of uric acid, but not on its tubular renal handling. With a 24-hour urine sample, the uric acid clearance can also be calculated. This measures the volume of blood cleared from uric acid for a given time (usually 1 minute).

Given that 24-hour urine sample collections have been shown to be prone to errors [19], approaches using spot urine have been developed. A high urinary uric acid to creatinine ratio (ratio > 0.63) has shown a high specificity (though low sensitivity) to diagnose over-excretors [20]. An index that provides information on the tubular handling of uric acid is the fractional excretion of uric acid (FEUA). This is the proportion of uric acid clearance to creatinine clearance and is defined by the following formula (after simplification):

$$FEUA = (UA \text{ in urine} \times \text{creatinine in blood})/(\text{Creatinine in urine} \times UA \text{ in blood}) \times 100$$

where UA = uric acid.

Given that creatinine clearance is an approximation of the glomerular filtration, it can be interpreted as the proportion of uric acid filtrated by the glomeruli that is finally excreted in the urine. It therefore estimates the net amount of uric acid reabsorbed by the tubules. Cut-off points are still unclear; in one study FEUA less than 4% in men suggest an inadequate renal handling in the presence of hyperuricaemia [21], though the threshold seems quite low. Although the renal clearance of uric acid decreases with decreasing creatinine clearance, FEUA remains quite stable in patients with moderate renal impairment. However, when the estimated creatinine clearance is below 30 mL/min, the FEUA increases disproportionately [22]. Hence, FEUA is especially useful in patients with a 'reasonable' renal function (estimated creatinine clearance > 30 mL/min). FEUA has been shown to remain stable under allopurinol therapy [23] but increases under uricosuric therapy informing of their action [23].

Another index that can be measured in spot urine is the excretion of uric acid per volume of glomerular filtration (EurGF), also known as the Simkin index. It expresses the mg of excreted uric acid per decilitre of glomerular filtration [24]:

$$EurGF = (UA \text{ in urine} \times \text{creatinine in blood})/\text{Creatinine in urine}$$

As this test is normalized for the GFR, it incorporates a meaningful correction for differences in body size. However, it does not take into account SUA levels and therefore tends to be higher with increasing hyperuricaemia [16]. EurGF also seems to work best in patients without significant renal impairment.

Even though none of the prior measurements are free from problems, it is advisable to estimate renal uric acid handling before initiating therapy.

Inflammatory markers

Serum levels of inflammatory markers such as C-reactive protein and erythrocyte sedimentation rate are elevated during acute gout flares [11] and are associated with the intensity and extension of the inflammation. These increases are non-specific for most inflammatory insults and factors such as the use of glucocorticoids can dampen the inflammatory marker increase during acute gout flares. Associated inflammatory cytokines such as interleukin 6 have also been found elevated during acute gout flares. Very severe polyarticular flares may also produce leucocytosis and neutrophilia, and if accompanied by fever may simulate a septic process.

Synovial fluid cell count and macroscopic appearance

The synovial fluid (SF) cell count reflects the degree of inflammation present in a joint. Manual counting using a haematocytometric chamber is an established standard procedure, but automatic counters can give accurate results [25]. It should be performed as soon as possible after aspiration, although even 24 hours later similar results can be obtained if the SF is preserved with EDTA and refrigerated [25] except for highly inflammatory SF, which may form a visible loose clot, trapping the cells.

Most SFs samples obtained during an acute flare of gout or calcium pyrophosphate (CPP) arthritis are in the inflammatory range—with a cloudy appearance and a high cell count, but most often below 50 000 cells/μL, which has been considered the cut-off between inflammatory and septic arthritis. However, gout or CPP arthritis may also produce effusions with counts well above 50 000 [26,27], especially when smaller joints are affected—as cellularity tends to be higher in smaller joints with clinically similar inflammation [28]. At the other side of the scale, usually in less inflamed or even uninflamed joints showing an effusion, cell counts can be quite low or in the non-inflammatory range although a search for crystals can result in identification. Cell count in SF from normal knees is lower than 100 cells/μL [29]; most SF samples obtained from uninflamed joints in patients with crystal arthritis show higher cell counts that may go up to 1000 cells/μL [30] and reflect subclinical inflammation. Especially in patients with long-standing gout—and usually not very inflamed joints—a 'milky' white SF composed exclusively of urate crystals can be seen [31]. Floating in a SF sample little white spots are occasionally seen; these are composed by large clumps of MSU crystals.

Crystal analysis

The relevant crystal arthritides are gout and CPP crystal arthropathy. Other common crystals with pathogenic importance include apatite—that cannot be identified by optical microscopy due to its submicroscopic size—and cholesterol crystals that can be seen in effusions of long duration. Other crystals occasionally reported have anecdotal importance. Therefore this discussion will be centred on the detection and identification of MSU and CPP crystals, a common cause of arthritis and from which gout must be distinguished [32].

Gout is an MSU crystal deposit disease. The crystals are responsible for all its manifestations and their deposit precedes gout clinical presentation [33,34]. MSU crystals are not found in other circumstances, so gout is best defined by their presence. Fortunately the crystals are large enough as to be easily seen and identified by optical microscopy and are regularly seen in SF of inflamed joints [35], and in previously inflamed joints of patients not treated with ULT [30,36]. Crystals can also be seen in SF samples from joints of properly treated patients before the crystals disappear [37]. Needling a tophus brings a white material composed of pure MSU crystals where they can be easily identified. In pathological preparations, MSU crystals are absent since they are dissolved by formalin during the necessary fixation process [38]. Alcohol fixation has been recommended; the authors also have good experience with frozen sections. Fortunately, crystal deposit is reversible by reducing uricaemia to its normal values. As a consequence of ULT, crystals will disappear from previously inflamed joints of properly treated patients [30,35,39,40]. According to the European League Against Rheumatism (EULAR) recommendations, MSU crystal identification is the gold standard for the diagnosis of gout [41]. EULAR also recommend a search for crystals in any SF sample obtained from any arthritis of uncertain origin, as this provides the definitive diagnosis of gout and calcium pyrophosphate deposition (CPPD) disease. Aside from their most characteristic clinical presentations [31,42], features can be quite varied and consistent with other joint diseases of less certain diagnosis. Interestingly, in the workup for the diagnosis of rheumatoid arthritis, the *Primer on the Rheumatic Diseases* recommends SF analysis to avoid mistaking polyarticular gout or CPP crystal arthritis for rheumatoid arthritis [43].

CPP crystals are regularly found in SF samples obtained from inflamed joints in its related arthropathy; chondrocalcinosis is found in a significant percentage of elderly patients and the finding of occasional crystals in SF samples of osteoarthritic joints has an uncertain clinical significance. Identification of CPP crystals in SF is considered the gold standard for CPPD disease diagnosis [44].

SF analysis is a simple and reproducible technique that can be learned after a short training period [45]. Crystal identification in SF is included in the core curriculum in rheumatology, both by the American College of Rheumatology [46] and by the European Union of Medical Specialists [47]; despite this, the procedure has been relegated and only a minority of rheumatologists routinely base the diagnosis of crystal arthritis on crystal identification [48].

The technique of crystal analysis by means of the compensated polarized microscope (an ordinary microscope fitted with proper filters) allows their differentiation by the type of birefringence (positive or negative) was initially introduced by Daniel McCarty [49]; not much has been published about the technique since. However, this can be a difficult tool for beginners who should bear in mind that both crystals are well seen with an ordinary light microscope (allowing identification by morphology) and with a simple polarized microscope (allowing differentiation by the intensity of their birefringence). After a short training, the results of crystal analysis have been found to be consistent [45].

Preparation of the sample

No fixation or staining is needed to prepare the SF sample. Fresh samples are recommended—especially for CPP—to avoid decay of the cells that may make crystal analysis difficult. Samples can be kept at 4°C and in general, examination after 24–48 hours is adequate [50]. If examination is not immediate, clotting of highly inflammatory samples can be avoided adding a drop of heparin. The glass slide and cover slid should be carefully cleaned to minimize

artefacts, the main confounder for beginners. Also the microscope lenses should be kept clean (SF may dry on the lenses rendering them quite opaque and making focusing impossible or observation less clear). A small drop of fluid directly from the syringe is placed on a glass slide and covered with a cover slid (larger drops result in thicker less appropriate preparations). The preparation is then ready for observation.

The microscope

Most modern regular microscopes used for bright field microscopy can be fitted with appropriate filters allowing simple polarized and compensated polarized microscopy; most popular microscope brands offer along with their simple laboratory microscopes an appropriate set of filters for crystal analysis (two polarized filters—polarizer and analyser—and a first-order red compensator). When asked about a polarized microscope, manufacturers may offer a geological polarized microscope, a more expensive tool with a graded rotating stage used to determine the angles of extinction (position where the crystal loses its birefringence) of different crystals. This is an unnecessary tool for rheumatology settings, where essentially we have to distinguish between two types of crystals. A 200× to 400× lens is ideal for MSU crystal detection and identification; a 600× lens is better for CPP, whose identification often relies on shape and many of the crystals are minute (Figure 42.1); this is—for this purpose—the preferred lens of the authors. A 100× and 1000× lenses are helpful in some circumstances. Starting by the simplest tool, and building up in complexity, crystal analysis can be approached as follows:

Bright field microscopy

Bright field microscopy shows the morphology of the crystals well allowing reasonable detection (if there are crystals, they are seen) and identification of MSU and CPP crystals by their shape [51]. The best observation conditions are determined by placing a preparation at the microscope stage and adapting the height of the condenser and the aperture of the diaphragm to find the best light and contrast combination at which cell details and crystals are best seen; this may vary between examiners.

All MSU crystals are needle shaped (Figures 42.2, 42.4a, and 42.5a) though their size can vary; crystals obtained by needling a tophus tend to be larger than those obtained in a SF sample likely because the different setting where they formed [52]. Crystals are seen both inside and outside the cells, and although it has been considered that only intracellular crystals result in joint inflammation, these are common in SF sample obtained from asymptomatic gouty and CPPD disease joints [53,54] (indicating a low grade of subclinical inflammation [34]). Under bright field microscopy, CPP crystal shape varies from easily recognizable rhombi and parallelepipeds to rod-looking very long rectangles and even thin needles (Figures 42.1, 42.3, 42.7, 42.8a, and 42.9a,) that can be with this microscope setting, indistinguishable from MSU crystals. When these needles are the first finding in the analysis, the search must continue until identifying characteristic CPP crystals—in which case all are most likely CPP—or it becomes clear that all crystals are needle shaped, thus suggesting MSU. The bright field is not a proper tool for distinguishing CPP from MSU in the rare SF samples that contain both—see discussion later in the chapter. Often CPP crystals show a less regular shape, on occasions because of their orientation in the microscope field; in fresh preparations cells

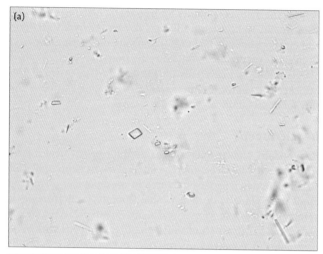

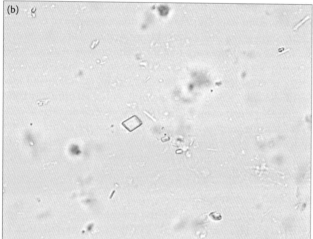

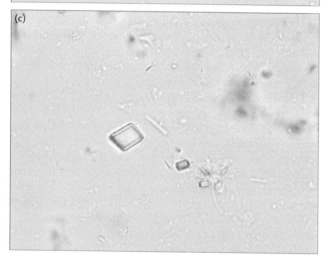

Figure 42.1 CPP crystals as seen with the ordinary bright field microscope at (a) 400×, (b) 600×, and (c) 1000×. 400× is the usual for routine analysis; 600× is a good choice for better detail, especially of small CCP crystals. 1000× is useful during the learning process to become acquainted with the different shapes and appearances of the crystals.

frequently move, and as they move, CPP crystals contained in them change shape often from the characteristic shape to more irregular ones, and observing this change of shape is a useful learning experience. Very small intracellular MSU crystals are common and are always seen as tiny needles. CPP crystals are frequently found

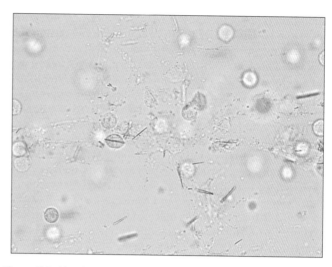

Figure 42.2 Abundant intra- and extracellular MSU crystals ordinary bright field microscope (400×). All MSU crystals are needle shaped; synovial fluid samples obtained during an attack of arthritis frequently have abundant crystals as in this figure.

inside a vacuole, but not MSU crystals. A 600× dry lens is particularly appropriate when CPP is being searched (Figures 42.1b, 42.8a, and 42.9a). As a teaching exercise, observing CPP crystals under a 1000× oil lens (Figure 42.1c) helps in becoming familiar with their shape and is worth doing. To the authors, the ordinary bright field microscope appears to best tool for CPP crystal detection (if present, it will not be missed) and the characteristic shape of CPP crystals allows definitive identification. MSU crystals are seen with ordinary light but if few, especially in very cellular or haemorrhagic fluids, they may be missed.

Uncompensated polarized microscopy

Uncompensated polarized microscopy allows detection of crystals by their birefringence. It requires the microscope to be fitted with two polarized filters, one below (polarizer) and one above (analyser) the stage. Light emitted from the source light bulb, vibrates in all

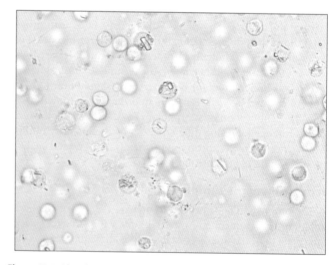

Figure 42.3 Abundant intra- and extracellular CPP crystals, ordinary bright field microscope (400×). Different shapes—characteristic rhombi and parallelepipeds—allow identification. The thinner needle-looking rods under this microscope setting, if seen isolated, could be taken for MSU crystals.

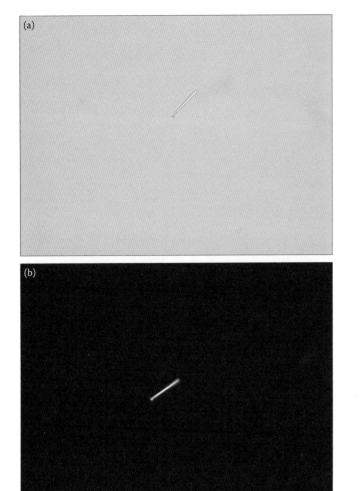

Figure 42.4 Extracellular MSU crystal 600×. (a) Ordinary bright field microscope shows the crystal by morphology. (b) Simple (uncompensated) polarized microscope shows the crystal by ITS birefringence. The blurriness of the ends of the crystal (best seen in B) result from its inclined position in the field, leaving the ends off focus (depth of field decreases as the magnification of the microscope lenses increase).

planes of space. After passing the first filter, light vibrates only in the plane that is parallel to the filter's axis; if the second filter is rotated so its axis is perpendicular to the axis of the first filter, no light will pass through. Therefore, the microscope field darkens. The SF sample is placed in between both filters. When an already polarized light passes though birefringent crystals, it decomposes into two perpendicular polarized beams of different wavelength; one of its components emerges parallel to the axis of the second filter passing through it, so crystals are seen shining in the dark microscope field. Crystals do not shine, but they allow the microscope light to be seen through the birefringent crystal. An intense microscope light helps by making the birefringent crystals appear more brilliant, facilitating crystal detection, especially that of the strongly birefringent MSU crystals (Figures 42.4b, 42.5b, and 42.6). Besides crystals, other materials—most frequently artefacts—also show birefringence and the analysts should be acquainted with them. To assure the best microscope setting for the most brilliant birefringence, a preparation with abundant MSU crystals should be placed on the microscope stage with the microscope light settled to its maximum, the diaphragm fully open (to allow for maximal light), and the height of the condenser should

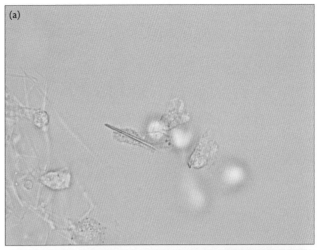
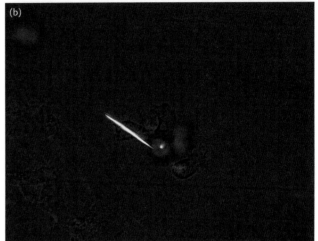
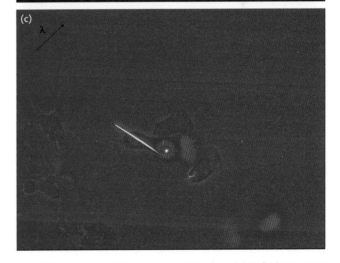

Figure 42.5 Intracellular MSU crystal 600×. (a) Ordinary bright field microscope shows the crystal by morphology. (b) Simple (uncompensated) polarized microscope shows the crystal with its strong birefringence (polarized filters slightly uncrossed to see background detail). (c) Compensated polarized microscope shows the negative sign of the birefringence (blue when perpendicular to the compensator axis marked by the arrow and λ).

be moved up and down looking for the best sight, usually close to the stage. It may be useful to slightly uncross the polarized filters to allow some background detail in order to distinguish the cell outlines and other morphological details while retaining birefringence.

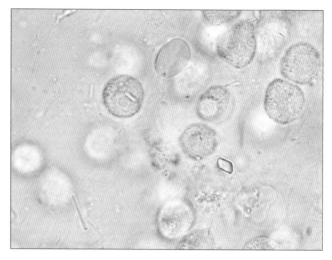

Figure 42.7 CPP crystals, ordinary microscope 1000×. A rhombus and a needle-like crystal are seen; the rhombus ascertains that these are CPP crystals, but looking for further characteristic rhombi or parallelepipeds is a good practice.

Figure 42.6 Abundant MSU crystals as seen at 100× (slightly uncrossed polarized filters to allow background detail). This microscope setting shows a large volume of synovial fluid in only one microscope field and allows easy detection of the crystals when scanty; they can be later definitively identified at a higher magnification. At this magnification the common birefringent artefacts may be taken as crystals, but large needles are usually well distinguished. (b) The same process at 200× allows a faster detection than at 400×.

Most needle-shaped MSU crystals show intense birefringence and clearly shine in the dark field. This is already noticeable at 100× and 200× (allowing examination of larger microscope fields and a faster detection when crystals are few) (Figure 42.6). Some MSU crystals show weak birefringence and an occasional crystal lacks it. This occurs if a crystal axis is positioned parallel to one of the axes of the analyser or polarizer (extinction position) and also with some small crystals. The simple polarized microscope appears as the best tool for MSU crystal detection and most often allows definitive identification based on strong birefringence and acicular shape.

On the other hand, only about a fifth of CPP crystals show any birefringence and it is fainter than that of MSU crystals [55]; only occasional CPP crystals show intense birefringence (Figures 42.8b and 42.9b). So, if searched for under simple polarized microscopy, CPP crystals are easily missed—especially if they are few and the examiner unaware of it. It is our feeling that acicular CPP crystals seldom show birefringence and, if so, it is much fainter than that

of MSU crystals. This appears an important differentiating element from MSU crystals. If CPP crystals are suspected, a search under bright light by morphology should be carried out.

Compensated polarized microscopy

Compensated polarized microscopy remains the standard for crystal identification. The technique is more complex and for those in the learning process, it appears reasonable to approach it after being well acquainted with the crystals with the ordinary and simple polarized microscopes. It adds to the previous system a first-order red compensator (retardation plate; its axis usually marked by a λ and an arrow) which helps to determine whether the long axis of the birefringent crystal is parallel to the slower or faster wavelength of the compound beam emerging from the crystal. When this ray is faster, a crystal shows yellow when parallel to the compensator axis and blue if perpendicular to it, and the crystal is said to have negative birefringence or elongation. When the vibration of the slower ray is parallel to the long dimension of the crystal, it shows blue when parallel to the compensator axis and yellow if perpendicular; it is then said to have positive birefringence or elongation [56,57]. Compensated polarized microscopy helps in the distinction of the strongly negative birefringence of MSU crystals (Figures 42.4c and 42.5c). CPP shows a weak (colours are paler than those of MSU) positive birefringence and elongated crystals (parallelepipedic crystals and some needle like) may not show it well (Figures 42.8c and 42.9c). Crystals that do not appear as birefringent under simple polarized microscope may not show colour—or appear very faint. Rhombi lack a long axis and cannot be oriented in relation to the compensator axis. Many thin rod- or needle-shaped crystals do not show clear birefringence under this system.

Although analysis with this microscope setting remains the standard tool for definitive MSU and CPP crystal distinction, the crystal nature is already evident in most occasions based on shape under ordinary microscopy and intensity of birefringence under simple polarized light. Compensated polarized microscopy is most useful in the identification of very occasional needle-like artefacts or in the rare circumstance when MSU and CPP crystals coincide in the same SF in sizable numbers.

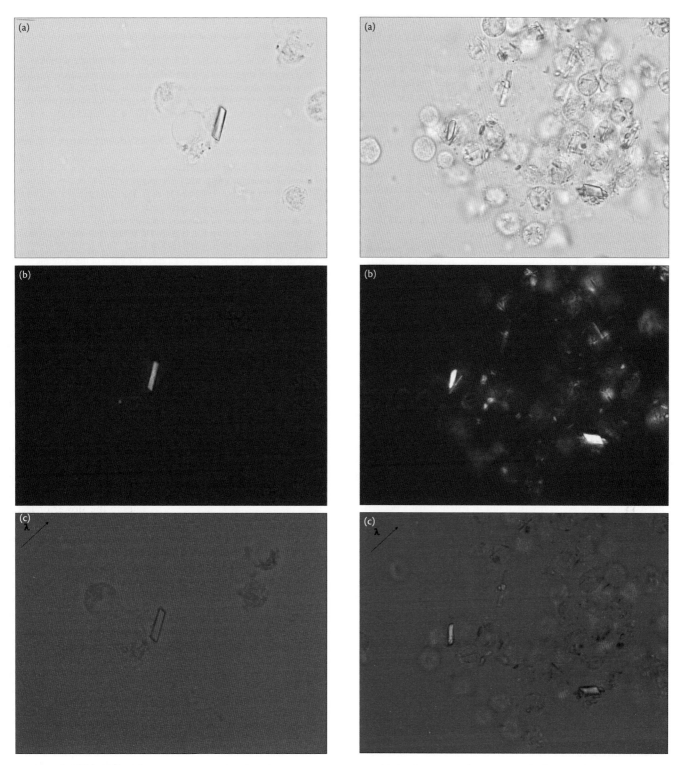

Figure 42.8 CPP crystal 600×. (a) Under ordinary bright field microscopy its parallelepipedic shape is characteristic. (b) Simple (uncompensated) polarized microscopy shows faint birefringence as many CPP crystals do. (c) Compensated polarized microscopy shows the positive sign of the birefringence (blue when parallel to the compensator axis marked by the arrow and λ).

Figure 42.9 Abundant CPP crystals; synovial fluids with so many crystals are not unusual. 600×. (a) Crystals of different shapes and sizes are seen allowing immediate identification by morphology. (b) Simple (uncompensated) polarized microscope shows that a few mostly large crystals show quite strong birefringence. A majority of the crystals—including very large ones—show faint or absent birefringence (polarized filters slightly uncrossed to see background detail). (c) Compensated polarized microscope shows the positive sign of the birefringence (blue when parallel and yellow when perpendicular to the compensator axis marked by the arrow and λ). On this occasion none of the crystals can be easily oriented in relation to the axis, a situation that it is common. Both yellow and blue are clearly less brilliant than those of MSU crystals. These three figures illustrate that the ordinary bright field microscope is the adequate tool for CPP crystal detection and identification, the other settings helping if uncertainties arise.

Some practical tips

For the beginner it is practical to approach crystal analysis in two separate steps: (1) crystal detection to ascertain whether there is any crystal—or not—in the SF sample being analysed and (2) crystal identification to properly classify detected crystals as MSU or

CPP [58,59]. It must be kept in mind that when infection occurs in a crystal-containing joint, crystals will be found in the SF. As mentioned before, the more polymorphic CPP crystals pose more difficulties than the acicular, strongly birefringent MSU crystals. Many CPP crystals (those small and not properly oriented in the microscope field and many needles, rod-shaped or less regular) may be difficult to identify until the analyst gains in experience and CPP crystals become familiar. Although to beginners the process appears to require careful analysis, experienced analysts most often recognize the crystal type at first glance. A good practice for the beginner is to observe as many SF samples as possible of inflammatory arthritides and of crystal arthritides in order to gain familiarity with the different appearances of cells and crystals. After that, the process becomes automatic on most occasions. Beginners should also become familiar with the different artefacts.

The effort needed to determine whether crystals are present or absent has received little attention. Different lengths of time of observation have been proposed, but different analysts observe at different speeds. It may be more practical to examine a number of 400× microscope fields—30 to 60—before determining that there are no crystals. This search should be made under bight light for CPP crystals and under the dark field of uncompensated polarized microscope for MSU crystals (and most samples should be examined by both means). Especially for gout, it is practical when the diagnosis appears possible and no crystals are found, to centrifuge the SF sample and examine the pellet, where crystals concentrate. MSU crystals do not occur outside of gout, so a simple crystal has to be taken as diagnostic—although a diagnosis based on such a limited finding must be taken as provisional and confirmed on another occasion or in a SF sample obtained from a different joint.

A particular problem results from the finding of an occasional CPP crystal. This occurs in osteoarthritic SFs [60], and it has been reported after meniscectomy [61] and in osteoarthritis occurring after joint dystrophies. It remains unclear how to interpret the finding of these occasional CPP crystals and how many of them or associated with which clinical features are necessary to make a sound diagnosis of CPP arthropathy.

The possibility of coincidence of MSU and CPP crystals in the same SF often is a cause of concern. This occurrence appears sporadic and no report on its clinical consequences has been published; with careful observation very occasional CPP crystals may be seen in SF samples from gouty SF containing MSU crystals, especially if the joint had osteoarthritis [62]. In any case, only MSU crystals can be eliminated by treatment.

References

1. Kratzer JT, Lanapsa MA, Murphy MN, et al. Evolutionary history and metabolic insights of ancient mammalian uricases. *PNAS* 2014; 11(10):3763–8.
2. Hosomi A, Nakanishi T, Fujita T, Tamai I. Extra-renal elimination of uric acid via intestinal efflux transporter BRCP/ABCG2. *PLoS One* 2012; 7(2):e30456.
3. Gibson T. Hyperuricemia, gout and the kidney. *Curr Opin Rheumatol* 2012; 24(2):127–31.
4. Stamp LK, Khanna PP, Dalbeth N, et al. Serum urate in chronic gout—will it be the first validated soluble biomarker in rheumatology? *J Rheumatol* 2011; 38(7):1462–6.
5. Bardin T, Richette P. Definition of hyperuricemia and gouty conditions. *Curr Opin Rheumatol* 2014; 26(2):186–91.
6. Desideri G, Castaldo G, Lombardi A, et al. Is it time to revise the normal range of serum uric acid levels? *Eur Rev Med Pharmacol Sci* 2014; 18:1295–306.
7. Pineda C, Amezcua-Guerra LM, Solano C, et al. Joint and tendon involvement suggestive of gouty arthritis in asymtpomatic hyperuricemia; an ultrasound controlled study. *Arthritis Res Ther* 2011; 13:R4.
8. de Miguel E, Puig JG, Castillo C, et al. Diagnosis of gout in patients with asymptomatic hyperuricaemia: a pilot ultrasound study. *Ann Rheum Dis* 2012; 71:157–8.
9. Logan JA, Morrison E, McGill PE. Serum uric acid in acute gout. *Ann Rheum Dis* 1997; 56:696–700.
10. Schlesinger N, Baker DG, Schumacher HRJr. Serum uric acid during bouts of acute gouty arthritis. *J Rheumatol* 1997; 24:2265–6.
11. Urano W, Yamakana H, Tsutani H, et al. The inflammatory process in the mechanism of decreased serum uric acid concentrations during acute gouty arthritis. *J Rheumatol* 2002; 29:1950–3.
12. Schlesinger N, Norquist JM, Watson DJ. Serum urate during acute gout. *J Rheumatol* 2009; 36(6):1287–9.
13. Waldron JL, Ashby HL, Razavi C, et al. The effect of the systemic inflammatory response as provoked by elective orthopaedic surgery on serum uric acid in patients without gout: a prospective study. *Rheumatology* 2013; 52:676–8.
14. Sivera F, Andres M, Pascual E. Serum uric acid drops during acute inflammatory episodes. *Ann Rheum Dis* 2010; 69(Suppl 3):122.
15. Gibson T. Hyperuricemia, gout and the kidney. *Curr Opin Rheumatol* 2012; 24:127–31.
16. Perez-Ruiz F, Calabozo M, Garcia Erauskin G, Ruibal A, Herrero-Beites AM. Renal underexcretion of uric acid is present in patients with apparent high urinary uric acid output. *Arthritis Rheum* 2002; 47(6):610–3.
17. Emmerson BT. The management of gout. *N Engl J Med* 1996; 334:445–51.
18. Yu TF, Gutman AB. Uric acid nephrolithiasis in gout: predisposing factors. *Ann Intern Med* 1967; 67:1133–48.
19. Turner WJ, Merlis S. Vicissitudes in research: the twenty-four hour urine collection. *Clin Pharmacol Ther* 1971; 12:163–6.
20. Moriwaki Y, Yamamoto T, Takahashi S, et al. Spot urine uric acid to creatinine ratio used in the estimation of uric acid excretion in primary gout. *J Rheumatol* 2001; 28:1306–10.
21. Simkin PA New standards for uric acid excretion and evidence for an inducible transporter. *Arthritis Rheum* 2003; 49(5):735–6.
22. Kannangara DRW, Ramasamy SN, Indraratna PL, et al. Fractional clearance of urate: validation of measurement in spot-urine samples in healthy subjects and gouty patients. *Arthritis Res Ther* 2012; 14:R189.
23. Fleischmann R, Kerr B, Yeh, LT, et al. Pharmacodynamic, pharmacokinetic and tolerability evaluation of concomitant administration of lesinurad and febuxostat in gout patients with hyperuricemia. *Rheumatology* 2014; 53:2167–74.
24. Simkin PA. Test of urinary excretion of uric acid. *Ann Intern Med* 1979; 91:926–7.
25. Salinas M, Rosas J, Iborra J, Manero H, Pascual E. Comparison of manual and automated cell counts in EDTA preserved synovial fluids. Storage has little influence on the results. *Ann Rheum Dis* 1997; 56:622–6.
26. Perez-Ruiz F, Testillano M, Gastaca MA, Herrero-Beites AM. 'Pseudoseptic' pseudogout associated with hypomagnesemia in liver transplant patients. *Transplantation* 2001; 71(5):696–8.
27. Frischnecht J, Steigerwald JC. High synovial fluid white in pseudogout; possible confusion with septic arthritis. *Arch Intern Med* 1975; 135:298–9.
28. Pascual Gomez E. Joint size influences on the leukocyte count of inflammatory synovial fluids. *Br J Rheumatol* 1989; 28:28–30.
29. Pascual E. Analysis of synovial fluid from healthy knees. Comparison with fluid from asymptomatic knees in RA, SLE and gout. *Br J Rheumatol* 1992; 31(Suppl 2):219.

30. Pascual E. Persistence of monosodium urate crystals and low-grade inflammation in the synovial fluid of patients with untreated gout. *Arthritis Rheum* 1991; 34:141–5.
31. Fam AG, Reis MD, Szalai JP. Acute gouty synovitis associated with 'urate milk'. *J Rheumatol* 1997; 24:2389–93.
32. Malik A, Schumacher HR, Dinnella JE, Clayburne GM. Clinical diagnostic criteria for gout: comparison with the gold standard of synovial fluid crystal analysis. *J Clin Rheumatol* 2009; 15:22–4.
33. De Miguel E, Puig JG, Castillo C, et al. Diagnosis of gout in patients with asymptomatic hyperuricaemia: a pilot ultrasound study. *Ann Rheum Dis* 2012; 71(1):157–8.
34. Pineda C, Amezcua-Guerra LM, Solano C, et al. Joint and tendon subclinical involvement suggestive of gouty arthritis in asymptomatic hyperuricemia: an ultrasound controlled study. *Arthritis Res Ther* 2011; 13(1):R4.
35. McCarty DJ, Hollander JL. Identification of urate crystals in gouty synovial fluid. *Ann Intern Med* 1961; 54:452–60.
36. Pascual E, Batlle-Gualda E, Martínez A, Rosas J, Vela P. Synovial fluid analysis for diagnosis of intercritical gout. *Ann Intern Med* 1999; 131:756–9.
37. Pascual E, Sivera F. The time required for disappearance of urate crystals from synovial fluid after successful hypouricemic treatment relates to the duration of gout. *Ann Rheum Dis* 2007; 66:1056–8.
38. Simkin PA, Bassett JE, Lee QP. Not water, but formalin, dissolves urate crystals in tophaceous tissue samples. *J Rheumatol* 1994; 21:2320–1.
39. Li-Yu J, Clayburne G, Sieck M, et al. Treatment of chronic gout. Can we determine when urate stores are depleted enough to prevent attacks of gout? *J Rheumatol* 2001; 28(3):577–80.
40. Perez-Ruiz F, Liote F. Lowering serum uric acid levels: what is the optimal target for improving clinical outcomes in gout? *Arthritis Rheum* 2007; 57:1324–8.
41. Zhang W, Doherty M, Pascual E, et al. EULAR evidence based recommendations for gout. Part I: Diagnosis. *Ann Rheum Dis* 2006; 65:1301–11.
42. Sivera F, Aragón R, Pascual E. First metatarsophalangeal joint aspiration using a 29-Gauge needle. *Ann Rheum Dis* 2008; 67:273–5.
43. Tehlirian CV, Bathon JM. Rheumatoid arthritis: A. Clinical and laboratory manifestations. In Klippel JH, Stone JH, Crofford LJ, White PH (eds) *Primer on the Rheumatic Diseases*, 13th ed. New York: Springer Science + Business Media, LCC; 2008:114–21.
44. Zhang W, Doherty M, Bardin T, et al. European League Against Rheumatism recommendations for calcium pyrophosphate deposition. Part I: terminology and diagnosis. *Ann Rheum Dis* 2011; 70:563–70.
45. Lumbreras B, Pascual E, Frasquet J, et al. Analysis for crystals in synovial fluid: training of the analysts results in high consistency. *Ann Rheum Dis* 2005; 64(4):612–5.
46. American College of Rheumatology. *Core Curriculum Outline for Rheumatology Fellowship Programs: a Competency-Based Guide to Curriculum Development*. American College of Rheumatology; 2006. http://www.rheumatology.org/educ/training/cco.doc
47. UEMS, Section of Rheumatology. *Core Curriculum for Specialist Training*. http://www.uems.eu/
48. Amer H, Swan A, Dieppe P. The utilization of synovial fluid analysis in the UK. *Rheumatology (Oxford)* 2001; 40:1060–3.
49. McCarty DJ, Hollander JL. Identification of urate crystals in gouty synovial fluid. *Ann Intern Med* 1961; 54:452–60.
50. Galvez J, Saiz E, Linares LF, et al. Delayed examination of synovial fluid by ordinary and polarized light microscopy to detect and identify crystals. *Ann Rheum Dis* 2002; 61:444–7.
51. Pascual E, Tovar J, Ruiz MT. The ordinary light microscope: an appropriate tool for the detection and identification of crystals in synovial fluid. *Ann Rheum Dis* 1989; 48:983–5.
52. Pascual E, Martínez A, Ordóñez S. Gout: the mechanism of urate crystal nucleation and growth. A hypothesis based in facts. *Joint Bone Spine* 2013; 80(1):1–4.
53. Pascual E, Jovaní V. A quantitative study of the phagocytosis of urate crystals in the synovial fluid of asymptomatic joints of patients with gout. *Br J Rheumatol* 1995; 34:724–6.
54. Martinez-Sanchis A, Pascual E. Intracellular and extracellular CPPD crystals are a regular feature in synovial fluid from uninflamed joints of patients with CPPD related arthropathy. *Ann Rheum Dis* 2005; 64:1769–72.
55. Ivorra J, Rosas J, Pascual E. Most calcium pyrophosphate crystals appear as non-birefringent. *Ann Rheum Dis* 1999; 58:582–4.
56. Nikon Microscopy. *The Source for Microscopy Education*. http://www.microscopyu.com/articles/polarized/index.html
57. Phelps P, Steele AD, McCarty DJ Jr. Compensated polarized light microscopy. Identification of crystals in synovial fluids from gout and pseudogout. *JAMA* 1968; 203:508–12.
58. Pascual E, Jovani V. Synovial fluid analysis. *Best Pract Res Clin Rheumatol* 2005; 19:371–86.
59. Courtney P, Doherty M. Joint aspiration and injection and synovial fluid analysis. *Best Pract Res Clin Rheumatol* 2009; 23:161–92.
60. Nalbant S, Martinez JA, Kitumnuaypong T, et al. Synovial fluid features and their relations to osteoarthritis severity: new findings from sequential studies. *Osteoarthritis Cartilage* 2003; 11:50–4.
61. Doherty M, Watt I, Dieppe PA. Localised chondrocalcinosis in post-meniscectomy knees. *Lancet* 1982; 29:1207–10.
62. Robier C, Neubauer M, Quehenberger F, Rainer F. Coincidence of calcium pyrophosphate and monosodium urate crystals in the synovial fluid of patients with gout determined by the cytocentrifugation technique. *Ann Rheum Dis Ann Rheum Dis* 2011; 70:1163–4.

CHAPTER 43

Imaging of gout

Robert T. Keenan, Sneha Pai, and Naomi Schlesinger

Widely used imaging in gout

Plain X-rays

The assessment of bone damage in gout traditionally relied on plain X-rays in which bone erosions serve as a marker of joint damage. However, plain X-rays are not useful early in the disease and are frequently normal. Only 45% of patients with clinically apparent gout manifest bone changes on plain X-rays, and only 6–10 years after the initial attack [1,2].

Early radiological findings in gout are limited to the soft tissues and involve asymmetric swelling in the affected joints [3]. Oedema of the soft tissues around the joints may be observed as well. Later in the disease, gout may cause subtle changes in the bony structures on plain X-rays. In the periphery of affected joints, small punched-out erosions arise. The erosions are better visualized with two views. These lesions can progress and become sclerotic as they increase in size.

Typical well-defined, 'punched out', periarticular erosions with overhanging edges are not seen on plain X-rays usually until 6–10 years after the initial acute attack [4]. Erosions are often located next to a tophus [5]. The overhanging edges are caused by a gradually expanding tophus eroding at the bone cortex with concomitant new periosteal bone formation trying to contain the tophus (Figure 43.1).

Tophi around joints can be juxta-articular, intra-articular, and subchondral and usually do not demonstrate symmetric joint involvement. The tophus, the hallmark of chronic gout, is a granulomatous immune reaction to monosodium urate (MSU) crystals [6,7].

Thus, the plain X-ray findings suggestive of gout are normal mineralization, joint space preservation, sharply marginated erosions with sclerotic borders and overhanging edges, and asymmetric polyarticular distribution. These X-ray findings indicate the chronicity of the disease process. However, plain X-rays may underestimate the size and extent of soft tissue and osseous involvement by gout.

Newer imaging modalities used in gout

Ultrasound

Over the last two decades, significant advances in ultrasound (US) have allowed the clinician new opportunities for point of care (POC) diagnosis and management of crystal arthropathies. US has contributed to the understanding of the pathology of crystalline diseases such as gout by revealing crystal deposition in and around joints at various patterns and stages [8] adding to the armamentarium of imaging modalities useful for the diagnosis and

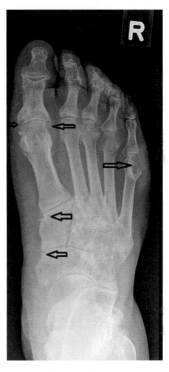

Figure 43.1 Plain radiograph of the right foot in a patient with tophaceous gout. Note the multiple erosions with overhanging edges in association with soft tissue masses (tophi) in the metatarsophalangeal (MTP) joints, especially the first and fifth MTPs, and the cuneiform and navicular bones (arrows).
Image courtesy of Professor Nicola Dalbeth, University of Auckland, Auckland, New Zealand.

management of gout (see also Chapter 17). US has proven to be more sensitive than plain X-rays in detecting early bone erosions, while also being able to reveal the structural damage to tendons and entheses [9–11]. In one study, conventional radiography was found to have a sensitivity of 31% and a specificity of 93% in showing features of gout, versus US that had a sensitivity of 96% (98/102) and a specificity of 73% in showing features of gout [12].

US imaging in gout has enabled the clinician to detect in real time synovitis and tenosynovitis by revealing synovial thickening using grey-scale US and further detect increased blood flow to the affected area using power Doppler US [13]. US's emerging role in gout doesn't stop at just detecting joint inflammation that may or may not be appreciated on clinical exam, it can also be used to facilitate joint aspiration for the confirmation of the presence of MSU crystals and also help make a diagnosis based on US-specific imaging features [12].

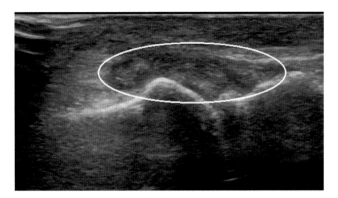

Figure 43.2 Ultrasound image of the first metatarsophalangeal joint demonstrating the hyperechoic cloudy areas or 'cottony images'.

In contrast to magnetic resonance imaging (MRI), for example, US has the ability to detect tophi smaller than 1 cm [14]. Typical features of tophi on US include ovoid shape, hypoechoic border, stippled centre, and absence of vascularity. In many gout cases, where clinically evident tophi are not appreciated, US can reveal floating hyperechoic foci (<1 mm) within synovial fluid. Likely representing microtophi surrounded by a hypoechoic area, the presence of multiple foci or microtophi, result in a snowstorm appearance and hyperechoic cloudy areas or 'cottony images' of aggregates smaller than 1 cm that can be well or poorly defined homogenous areas with a posterior acoustic shadow [15] (Figure 43.2). A study using US-guided aspiration of intra- and juxta-articular hyperechoic aggregates from joints and tendons from 49 gout patients and 8 controls showed that 78% of the gout patients' aspirated material was positive for MSU crystals and negative for 20%, while 1 patient was found to have calcium pyrophosphate crystals [9].

The double-contour (icing) sign is another gout-specific sign that was described by Thiele and Schlesinger in 2007 [16]. The double-contour sign is illustrated by two hyperechoic lines with an anechoic area between. One hyperechoic line is due to a US signal bouncing off cortical bone, for example, at the tibial plateau, while a second outer line is thought to represent the deposition of MSU crystals in a fine layer over hyaline cartilage, forming a new hyperechoic barrier with the anechoic articular hyaline cartilage in between (Figure 43.3). Consistent with these US findings, a cadaveric study

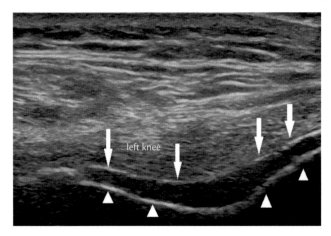

Figure 43.3 Ultrasound image of the flexed left knee showing the double-contour sign. Arrowheads demonstrate the tibial plateau, while the arrows point to the hyperechoic signal representing the deposition of the MSU crystals overlying the superficial layer of the hyaline cartilage.

from the 1950s described cartilage surfaces of gout patients as being 'diffusely dusted with white crystal deposits' [17,18].

This double-contour sign has been described in both symptomatic and asymptomatic joints, and even in asymptomatic hyperuricaemia [16,19,20]. Ottaviani and colleagues found that MSU crystal-positive gout patients with serum urate (SUA) levels greater than 10 mg/dL (600 mM) had a double-contour sign in at least one assessed joint. The investigators felt the pitfalls of the double-contour sign included varying MSU burdens amongst patient along with interpreter variability, while the sensitivity and specificity of the double-contour sign have been estimated to be 44% and 99%, respectively [21]. Although the double-contour sign is consistent with gout, the presence of the sign alone as a reliable diagnostic feature cannot yet be recommended as a replacement for the gold standard, joint aspiration and MSU crystal identification [22].

Given the ability of US to detect crystal deposition, it may prove to be useful in monitoring response to treatment. It has been shown that a target lesion in gout, as viewed by US, disappears after sustained normouricaemia is achieved. Changes can occur within half a year of achieving a SUA level of less than 6 mg/dL using urate lowering drugs [23]. Large prospective studies in crystal-proven gout patients are needed to follow US's utility in evaluating response of gout patients to treatment with urate lowering drugs [14].

It should be noted that not all sites of possible tophus deposition are accessible to US, such as intraosseous areas, and tarsus and carpus regions. Additional pitfalls with US have traditionally included low inter- and intra-observer correlation, but as improvements in technology occur, such as high-resolution US, variability has decreased and reproducibility improved [19].

When compared to plain X-ray, dual-energy computed tomography (DECT), and MRI US has a definitive advantage in POC imaging, radiation exposure, and cost (Table 43.1).

Magnetic resonance imaging

Since the first imaging of a human subject in 1977, MRI has revolutionized medical diagnosis and treatment. It has been extensively used in musculoskeletal imaging, although not as widely studied in gout as other imaging modalities discussed in this chapter [24]. Like US, MRI can reveal joint inflammation and damage, but has advantages over US regarding greater accessibility for certain joint regions and less operator dependence [25]. MRI is an excellent imaging modality to image soft tissue, synovium, cartilage, tendon, and bone with excellent contrast and resolution while lacking radiation unlike CT.

In gout, as in other inflammatory arthropathies, MRI can demonstrate features such as synovial thickening, effusions, bone erosions, and bone marrow oedema (BME) [26,27]. MRI is better than US and plain X-ray in detecting erosions [28] and can demonstrate subclinical inflammation in asymptomatic joints [28], but discrimination between other causes of joint inflammation can be subtle. Poh and colleagues described a 10-year retrospective study of patients with gout [29], observing frequent synovitis and bone erosions on MRI. In contrast to the inflammatory arthritis findings associated with rheumatoid arthritis (RA) on MRI, BME associated with gout was usually mild [29,30]. Importantly, when significant BME was observed, concomitant osteomyelitis was found. The findings not only provide impetus for strongly considering infection when extensive BME on MRI is observed in a gout patient, it also suggests the unique osteopathology of gout compared to other

Table 43.1 Comparison of imaging modalities used in gout

Imaging modality	Advantages/good visualization of:	Disadvantages	Signal measured	Cost	Radiation
Plain X-rays	Joint space narrowing		X-rays	Low	Low exposure
US	Dynamic testing/effusion, tophus/tendon pathology	Unable to evaluate deep structures; Dependent on examiner skills	Sound	Low	No radiation
MRI	Effusion, synovial proliferation, joint space narrowing, tendon pathology tophus, bone marrow oedema	High cost, availability	Alterations in magnetic fields	High	No radiation
CT	Bone/erosions/joint space narrowing/erosions	High cost; Doesn't visualize soft tissue well	X-rays	High	High exposure
DECT	Bone/erosions/joint space narrowing/erosions		X-rays	High	Feet/hands: low exposure

arthropathies such as RA [25]. A subsequent prospective study of 40 gout patients evaluating BME, erosions, tophi, and synovitis found on MRI confirmed the aforementioned study's findings of little BME in gout [31]. The study found only mild synovitis associated with gout and erosions being strongly associated with the presence of tophi. MRI has been shown to be more sensitive than US in detecting erosions, appearing as breaks in hyperechoic cortical bone, better detected in two perpendicular planes [32].

On MRI, tophi are visible as discrete masses or nodules with low signal on T1-weighted images, low to high signal intensity on T2-weighted signal, and variable contrast enhancement due to varying vascularity [33] (Figure 43.4). Using MRI as the gold standard, Perez-Ruiz and colleagues found a good correlation between US and MRI in tophus detection but only moderate agreement for measurement of tophus dimensions [34].

Limited studies comparing MRI with DECT have found that MRI has a high specificity and moderate sensitivity for detecting tophi [35,36]. One study evaluating the wrist found a good correlation between the two modalities, with MRI having a specificity of 0.98 and a sensitivity of 0.63 for detecting tophi, using DECT as a gold standard [37]. In contrast, there have been reports of tophi being mistaken for neoplasms, especially those involving bone and

tendon as some features on MRI overlap with benign conditions such as giant cell tumour of the tendon sheath, synovial sarcoma, and even metastatic cancer involving the bone [38–41].

Some authors suggest that MRI may be useful for longitudinal use in clinical trials for measuring tophus volume. Obstacles for such use are significant given the cost and the time-consuming procedure that are involved for computation of the tophus volume [25]. The clinical application of MRI in gout has limitations in addition to cost, including overlap features that may mimic neoplasms and to a lesser extent, infection. Despite some limitations, MRI may have a place in assisting diagnosis.

Computed tomography and dual-energy computed tomography scans

Computed tomography

Although CT scans allow for visualization of tophi and erosions in patients with gout, few studies have evaluated the utility of CT scans in gout. Gerster et al. [42] studied prospectively CT scans of the knees of 16 patients with MSU crystal-proven gout. One-third of patients had intra-articular opacities suspected to be tophi. The authors concluded that CT scans may be beneficial in gout patients. Dalbeth et al. [43] demonstrated that hand CT scans can estimate

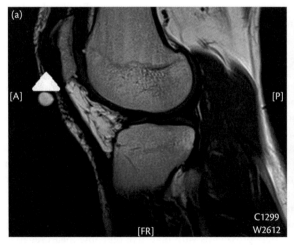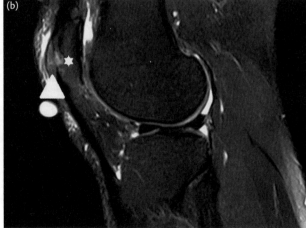

Figure 43.4 (a) Sagittal MRI of the right knee showing a low T1-weighted signal of a prepatellar tophus (arrowhead). (b) Sagittal image showing the same tophus (arrowhead) on a fat suppressed T2-weighted fast spin-echo sequence. Note the bone marrow oedema of the patella (star).

subcutaneous tophus volume reliably with excellent reproducibility. However, given the correlation between tophi identified by physical and CT assessment (r = 0.91, p < 0.0001); the authors concluded that physical measurement was equivalent to CT assessment of tophus burden. In addition, they demonstrated a close relationship between bone erosions and the presence and size of tophi [43].

Dual-energy computed tomography

Although the gold standard for diagnosing gout is visualization of MSU crystals in affected tissue, this is an invasive procedure which cannot always be performed, especially in small joints [44]. DECT identifies MSU crystals by analysing the chemical composition of the scanned tissues [44].

Historically, DECT was first utilized to detect and differentiate uric acid stones from non-uric acid stones [45]. DECT utilization in gout was first reported in 2007 [46]. Since then, many studies have confirmed the applicability of this non-invasive imaging modality in gout [47–51].

In DECT, two X-ray tubes with different voltages (80 and 140 peak kilovoltage (kVp)) are used to simultaneously acquire two sets of images of an anatomical region [52]. The settings of 80 and 140 kVp are commonly used because they provide the maximum difference and the least overlap between the spectra with standard tubes. The two settings have differences in X-ray attenuation at different photon energies. These material-specific differences of attenuation enable colour coding of the chemical composition of the scanned materials, including detection of the elemental composition of the scanned materials, including the detection of the elemental chemical composition of urate. This helps differentiate MSU crystals from other types of crystals. Post-processing of DECT data yields colour-coded (MSU deposits appear green) and three-dimensional surface rendered models which not only convey to physicians and patients the location of MSU deposits but also provide an estimate of tophus burden [53] (Figure 43.5).

The first study evaluating the utility of DECT in tophaceous gout was a case–control study by Choi et al. [47]. All 20 patients showed colour-coded MSU crystal deposits while none of the controls (n = 10) showed deposits. Since then, the sensitivity and specificity of DECT in diagnosis of acute gout has been studied by several researchers. Wu et al. [54] performed DECT in 191 patients (143 with acute gout and 48 patients with other arthritides) [54]. MSU crystals were detected in 140 of 143 (97.9%) of gout patients and 6 of 48 (12.5%) of patients with other arthritides. The sensitivity and specificity of DECT in the diagnosis of acute gout was calculated to be 97.9% and 87.5% respectively. Other studies have determined the sensitivity and specificity of DECT as 100% for both [48] and 93% and 84% respectively [51] in patients on urate-lowering therapy.

Researchers have compared utility of DECT to other imaging modalities. Gruber et al. [55] compared the sensitivity of DECT with that of US in the detection of gout in patients with clinical suspicion of gout in 37 joints. They compared these results with synovial fluid aspiration when possible. DECT detected MSU crystal deposits in 25 of 37 joints and US detected deposits in 24 of 37 joints; while 12 of 14 aspirated joints showed MSU crystals. There was a correlation between DECT and US among 32 of 37 joints (86.5%; p <0.001). The correlation between CT and synovial fluid in 12 of 14 joints (85.7%; p = 0.0119) while US findings and cytology correlated in 14 of 14 joints (100%; p < 0.001). However, this study had a number of limitations: firstly, the statistical power was limited due to the small number of patients (n = 21); secondly, there was likely a selection bias with regard to the type of patients referred by rheumatologists and only one sonographer examined all the joints.

DECT not only helps determine MSU crystal deposit volume but also gives visualization of bone and soft tissues. DECT provides better image quality with colour coding of MSU crystals and three-dimensional visualization using the same dose of radiation as regular CT scans [56]. Of the imaging techniques available today, DECT data seems to be the most reproducible between observers with a very high sensitivity (0.93) and specificity (0.78) [48,57].

However, DECT has several disadvantages: it is not widely available and is more expensive than conventional imaging [44]. Its diagnostic accuracy has not been established in early disease—reduced sensitivity in patients with acute, recent-onset gout (<6 weeks) has been reported [57]. In addition, calculating urate burden can be labour intensive [49]. Although low dose (0.5 mSv dose per region scanned) [47], exposure to ionizing radiation must also be kept in mind while ordering DECT.

DECT is an emerging modality whose utility as a monitoring tool remains to be determined. Further studies are needed to establish its use in gout diagnosis, evaluation of tophus burden, and its importance in the management of gout.

Summary

Plain X-rays remain the most widely used form of imaging in gout; however, over the last two decades there have been significant advances in gout imaging. Advanced imaging modalities such as US, MRI, CT, and DECT can reveal joint damage and tophi much earlier than a plain X-ray.

The newer imaging modalities are advancing our understanding of gout pathology, allowing us to better assess the uric acid burden, and aid us in the diagnosis of gout. The diagnosis of gout, in the future, may rely on advanced imaging without the need to aspirate joints, bursae, and tophi. In addition, advanced imaging may provide us with objective outcome measures to monitor responses to gout treatment: anti-inflammatory drugs as well as urate-lowering drugs.

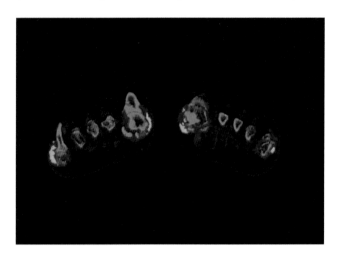

Figure 43.5 Two-dimensional dual energy computed tomography image of both feet showing urate deposition (green) at the first and fifth metatarsophalangeal joints bilaterally.

Image courtesy of Professor Nicola Dalbeth, University of Auckland, Auckland, New Zealand.

References

1. Brower AC. Gout. In Brower AC, Flemming DJ (eds) *Arthritis in Black and White*, 2nd ed. Philadelphia, PA: WB Saunders; 1997:325–41.
2. Barthelemy CR, Nakayama DA, Carrera GF, Lightfoot RW Jr, Wortmann RL. Gouty arthritis: a prospective radiographic evaluation of sixty patients. *Skeletal Radiol* 1984; 11(1):1–8.
3. Perez-Ruiz F, Dalbeth N, Urresola A, de Miguel E, Schlesinger N. Gout. Imaging of gout: findings and utility. *Arthritis Res Ther* 2009; 11(3):232.
4. Peh WCG. Tophaceous gout. Imaging consultation. *Am J Orthop* 2001; 30:665.
5. Schlesinger N, Thiele RG. The pathogenesis of bone erosions in gouty arthritis. *Ann Rheum Dis* 2010; 69(11):1907–12.
6. Palmer DG, Highton J, Hessian PA. Development of the gout tophus. An hypothesis. *Am J Clin Pathol* 1989; 91:190–5.
7. Dalbeth N, Clark B, Gregory K, et al. Mechanisms of bone erosion in gout: a quantitative analysis using plain radiography and computed tomography. *Ann Rheum Dis* 2009; 68:1290–5.
8. Delle Sedie A, Riente L, Iagnocco A, et al. Ultrasound imaging for the rheumatologist X. Ultrasound imaging in crystal-related arthropathies. *Clin Exp Rheumatol* 2007; 25(4):513–7.
9. Naredo E, Uson J, Jimenez-Palop M, et al. Ultrasound-detected musculoskeletal urate crystal deposition: which joints and what findings should be assessed for diagnosing gout? *Ann Rheum Dis* 2014; 73(8):1522–8.
10. Schueller-Weidekamm C, Schueller G, Aringer M, Weber M, Kainberger F. Impact of sonography in gouty arthritis: comparison with conventional radiography, clinical examination, and laboratory findings. *Eur J Radiol* 2007; 62(3):437–43.
11. Gerster JC, Landry M, Rappoport G, et al. Enthesopathy and tendinopathy in gout: computed tomographic assessment. *Ann Rheum Dis* 1996; 55(12):921–3.
12. Rettenbacher T, Ennemoser S, Weirich H, et al. Diagnostic imaging of gout: comparison of high-resolution US versus conventional X-ray. *Eur Radiol* 2008; 18(3):621–30.
13. Joshua F. Ultrasound applications for the practicing rheumatologist. *Best Prac Res Clin Rheumatol* 2012; 26(6):853–67.
14. Villaverde V, Rosario MP, Loza E, Perez F. Systematic review of the value of ultrasound and magnetic resonance musculoskeletal imaging in the evaluation of response to treatment of gout. *Reumatol Clin* 2014; 10(3):160–3.
15. Filippucci E, Di Geso L, Grassi W. Tips and tricks to recognize microcrystalline arthritis. *Rheumatology* 2012; 51(7):18–21.
16. Thiele RG, Schlesinger N. Diagnosis of gout by ultrasound. *Rheumatology* 2007; 46(7):1116–21.
17. Levin MH, Lichtenstein L, Scott HW. Pathologic changes in gout; survey of eleven necropsied cases. *Am J Pathol* 1956; 32(5):871–95.
18. McQueen FM, Doyle A, Dalbeth N. Imaging in the crystal arthropathies. *Rheum Dis Clin North Am* 2014; 40(2):231–49.
19. Howard RG, Pillinger MH, Gyftopoulos S, Thiele RG, Swearingen CJ, Samuels J. Reproducibility of musculoskeletal ultrasound for determining monosodium urate deposition: concordance between readers. *Arthritis Care Res* 2011; 63(10):1456–62.
20. De Miguel E, Puig JG, Castillo C, et al. Diagnosis of gout in patients with asymptomatic hyperuricaemia: a pilot ultrasound study. *Ann Rheum Dis* 2012; 71(1):157–8.
21. Filippucci E, Riveros MG, Georgescu D, Salaffi F, Grassi W. Hyaline cartilage involvement in patients with gout and calcium pyrophosphate deposition disease. An ultrasound study. *Osteoarthritis Cartilage* 2009; 17(2):178–81.
22. Ogdie A, Taylor WJ, Weatherall M, et al. Imaging modalities for the classification of gout: systematic literature review and meta-analysis. *Ann Rheum Dis* 2015; 74(10):1868–74.
23. Thiele RG, Schlesinger N. Ultrasonography shows disappearance of monosodium urate crystal deposition on hyaline cartilage after sustained normouricemia is achieved. *Rheumatol Int* 2010; 30(4):495–503.
24. McQueen FM, Doyle A, Dalbeth N. Imaging in gout—what can we learn from MRI, CT, DECT and US? *Arthritis Res Ther* 2011; 13(6):246.
25. McQueen FM, Doyle A, Dalbeth N. Imaging in the crystal arthropathies. *Rheum Dis Clin North Am* 2014; 40(2):231–49.
26. Popp JD, Bidgood WD, Jr, Edwards NL. Magnetic resonance imaging of tophaceous gout in the hands and wrists. *Semin Arthritis Rheum* 1996, 25(4):282–9.
27. Cimmino MA, Zampogna G, Parodi M, et al. MRI synovitis and bone lesions are common in acute gouty arthritis of the wrist even during the first attack. *Ann Rheum Dis* 2011; 70(12):2238–9.
28. Carter JD, Kedar RP, Anderson SR, et al. An analysis of MRI and ultrasound imaging in patients with gout who have normal plain radiographs. *Rheumatology* 2009; 48(11):1442–6.
29. Poh YJ, Dalbeth N, Doyle A, McQueen FM. Magnetic resonance imaging bone edema is not a major feature of gout unless there is concomitant osteomyelitis: 10-year findings from a high-prevalence population. *J Rheumatol* 2011; 38(11):2475–81.
30. McQueen FM, Gao A, Ostergaard M, et al. High-grade MRI bone oedema is common within the surgical field in rheumatoid arthritis patients undergoing joint replacement and is associated with osteitis in subchondral bone. *Ann Rheum Dis* 2007, 66(12):1581–7.
31. McQueen FM, Doyle A, Reeves Q, et al. Bone erosions in patients with chronic gouty arthropathy are associated with tophi but not bone oedema or synovitis: new insights from a 3 T MRI study. *Rheumatology* 2014, 53(1):95–103.
32. Carter JD, Kedar RP, Anderson SR, et al. An analysis of MRI and ultrasound imaging in patients with gout who have normal plain radiographs. *Rheumatology* 2009; 48(11):1442–6.
33. Gentili A. The advanced imaging of gouty tophi. *Curr Rheumatol Rep* 2006, 8(3):231–5.
34. Perez-Ruiz F, Martin I, Canteli B. Ultrasonographic measurement of tophi as an outcome measure for chronic gout. *J Rheumatol* 2007, 34(9):1888–93.
35. Schumacher HR, Jr, Becker MA, Edwards NL, et al. Magnetic resonance imaging in the quantitative assessment of gouty tophi. *Int J Clin Pract* 2006; 60(4):408–14.
36. Chowalloor PV, Siew TK, Keen HI. Imaging in gout: a review of the recent developments. *Ther Adv Musculoskelet Dis* 2014, 6(4):131–43.
37. McQueen FM, Doyle AJ, Reeves Q, Gamble GD, Dalbeth N. DECT urate deposits: now you see them, now you don't. *Ann Rheum Dis* 2013; 72(3):458–59.
38. Murphey MD, Gibson MS, Jennings BT, et al. From the archives of the AFIP: imaging of synovial sarcoma with radiologic-pathologic correlation. *Radiographics* 2006; 26(5):1543–65.
39. Yu JS, Chung C, Recht M, Dailiana T, Jurdi R. MR imaging of tophaceous gout. *AJR Am J Roentgenol* 1997; 168(2):523–7.
40. Girish G, Glazebrook KN, Jacobson JA. Advanced imaging in gout. *AJR Am J Roentgenol* 2013; 201(3):515–25.
41. Samuels J, Keenan RT, Yu R, Pillinger MH, Bescke T. Erosive spinal tophus in a patient with gout and back pain. *Bull NYU Hosp Jt Dis* 2010; 68(2):147–8.
42. Gerster JC, Landry M, Duvoisin B, Rappoport G. Computed tomography of the knee joint as an indicator of intraarticular tophi in gout. *Arthritis Rheum* 1996; 39(8):1406–9.
43. Dalbeth N, Clark B, Gregory K, et al. Computed tomography measurement of tophus volume: comparison with physical measurement. *Arthritis Rheum* 2007; 57(3):461–5.
44. Dalbeth N, Choi HK. Dual-energy computed tomography for gout diagnosis and management. *Curr Rheumatol Rep* 2013; 15(1):301.
45. Primak AN, Fletcher JG, Vrtiska TJ, et al. Noninvasive differentiation of uric acid versus non-uric acid kidney stones using dual-energy CT. *Acad Radiol* 2007; 14(12):1441–7.
46. Johnson TR, Weckbach S, Kellner H, Reiser MF, Becker CR. Clinical image: dual-energy computed tomographic molecular imaging of gout. *Arthritis Rheum* 2007; 56(8):2809.
47. Choi HK, Al-Arfaj AM, Eftekhari A, et al. Dual energy computed tomography in tophaceous gout. *Ann Rheum Dis* 2009; 68(10):1609–12.
48. Choi HK, Burns LC, Shojania K, et al. Dual energy CT in gout: a prospective validation study. *Ann Rheum Dis* 2012; 71(9):1466–71.

49. Dalbeth N, Aati O, Gao A, et al. Assessment of tophus size: a comparison between physical measurement methods and dual-energy computed tomography scanning. *J Clin Rheumatol* 2012; 18(1):23–7.

50. Manger B, Lell M, Wacker J, Schett G, Rech J. Detection of periarticular urate deposits with dual energy CT in patients with acute gouty arthritis. *Ann Rheum Dis* 2012; 71(3):470–2.

51. Glazebrook KN, Guimaraes LS, Murthy NS, et al. Identification of intraarticular and periarticular uric acid crystals with dual-energy CT: initial evaluation. *Radiology* 2011; 261(2):516–24.

52. Karcaaltincaba M, Aktas A. Dual-energy CT revisited with multidetector CT: review of principles and clinical applications. *Diagn Interv Radiol* 2011; 17(3):181–94.

53. Desai MA, Peterson JJ, Garner HW, Kransdorf MJ. Clinical utility of dual-energy CT for evaluation of tophaceous gout. *Radiographics* 2011; 31(5):1365–75.

54. Wu H, Xue J, Ye L, et al. The application of dual-energy computed tomography in the diagnosis of acute gouty arthritis. *Clin Rheumatol* 2014; 33(7):975–9.

55. Gruber M, Bodner G, Rath E, et al. Dual-energy computed tomography compared with ultrasound in the diagnosis of gout. *Rheumatology* 2014; 53(1):173–9.

56. Halliburton SS, Sola S, Kuzmiak SA, et al. Effect of dual-source cardiac computed tomography on patient radiation dose in a clinical setting: comparison to single-source imaging. *J Cardiovasc Comput Tomogr* 2008; 2(6):392–400.

57. Bongartz T, Glazebrook KN, Kavros SJ, et al. Dual-energy CT for the diagnosis of gout: an accuracy and diagnostic yield study. *Ann Rheum Dis* 2015; 74(6):1072–7.

CHAPTER 44

Principles of gout management

Pascal Richette

Introduction

Gout is a common arthritis due to the deposition of monosodium urate (MSU) crystals within joints, following chronic hyperuricaemia. It causes sudden acute arthritis which is mainly interleukin-1 (IL1) driven, and can lead to a severe arthropathy with major disability.

Apart from these musculoskeletal features, there are pieces of evidence to support that chronic hyperuricaemia is also associated with an increased risk of developing a myriad of comorbidities, including major cardiovascular events, some components of the metabolic syndrome, and kidney impairment [1,2].

Therefore, treatment of gout comprises both the treatment of acute flares and urate-lowering therapy (ULT) which is currently indicated in the vast majority of patients, in order to dissolve and eliminate definitively the MSU crystals.

Every physician must keep in mind that gout is a curable condition [3], and that if not properly treated, patients are exposed to an increased risk of mortality [4].

Treatment of acute attacks

In addition to rest and icing of the affected joint, several oral medications can be used for the treatment of acute flares. Whatever the medication used, the time of treatment initiation is likely of great importance: the earlier medication is introduced, the more rapidly a complete response should be obtained.

The standard oral pharmacological management of acute gout involves colchicine, non-steroidal anti-inflammatory drugs (NSAIDs), or corticosteroids, either systemic or intra-articular [5–7]. Apart from these drugs, the emerging class of IL1 blockers could become an interesting option for patients with gout and intolerance or contraindication to colchicine, NSAIDs, or corticosteroids.

Colchicine

Colchicine is an effective drug to treat flares but its frequent side effects and its complex pharmacokinetics hamper its use in all patients with gout [8]. The most important recent finding with colchicine is that low-dose (1.8 mg) is as effective as and better tolerated than high-dose colchicine (4.8 mg) when given within the first 12 hours after an attack [9]. According to the last American College of Rheumatology (ACR) guidelines for the management of gout [6], colchicine should be given to patients with recent flares with a loading dose of 1.2 mg followed by 0.6 mg 1 hour later, and then followed, as needed, after 12 hours, by continued colchicine (0.6 mg once or twice daily) until pain is relieved.

The most prevalent adverse effect of colchicine is a dose-related gastrointestinal intolerance. Toxicity of colchicine is also increased by renal, hepatic failure or by co-prescription with drugs such as ciclosporin, clarithromycin and azithromycin, diltiazem and verapamil, ketoconazole, and ritonavir. These drugs interfere with colchicine metabolism by inhibiting cytochrome P450 3A4 or P-glycoprotein [10]. Life-threatening and fatal colchicine toxicity has been reported in these patients with colchicine taken even at therapeutic doses [11]. Other potentially significant drug interactions have been reported with statins and fibrates, resulting in some cases in myopathy and rhabdomyolysis [11].

NSAIDs and corticosteroids

Alternatives to colchicine include traditional NSAIDs, coxibs, or corticosteroids. NSAIDs are widely used as first-line therapy for acute flares [6]. They should be given at maximal doses in cases of no contraindications for 1–2 weeks [5]. However, their widespread utility is limited by their gastrointestinal tolerability and cardiovascular toxicity. NSAIDs may impair renal function and should be avoided in patients with prior peptic ulcer disease, heart failure or coronary heart disease, and renal impairment.

Oral prednisolone given at a dosage of 35 mg/day for 5 days can also be used for acute flares because it is as effective as NSAIDs [12,13]. Importantly, intra-articular corticosteroids are also highly effective for acute attacks and should be the treatment of choice for an acute monoarthritis involving a joint easily punctionable [5].

Finally, for an acute attack with polyarticular arthritis, a combination therapy can be given, for instance, colchicine plus NSAIDs or oral corticosteroids plus colchicine, or intraarticular steroids with all other modalities [6].

Interleukin-1 blockers

Among the three IL1 blockers currently available for clinical use, canakinumab is the only one which has been approved by the European Medicines Agency for the symptomatic treatment of frequent acute flares. It is indicated in patients in whom NSAIDs and colchicine are contraindicated, are not tolerated, or do not provide an adequate response, and in whom repeated courses of corticosteroids are not appropriate. It is a high-affinity human anti-IL1 beta monoclonal antibody that neutralizes the bioactivity of the pro-inflammatory cytokine [14]. This activity inhibits the urate crystal-induced IL1 signalling pathway that occurs via activation of the NALP3 inflammasome [15]. Canakinumab is administered as a single 150 mg dose subcutaneously for gouty arthritis. It has been shown to be more effective than a single 40 mg dose of intramuscular injection of triamcinolone acetonide for pain relief [16].

Adverse events reported with canakinumab included infections, neutropenia, and thrombopenia [17].

Urate-lowering therapy

General principle

The goal of ULT in patients with gout is to reduce, and maintain over the long term, serum urate (SUA) levels below the saturation point for urate which is about 6.8 mg/dL (408 μmol). This therapy allows for dissolving crystal deposits and curing gout, as long as it is maintained. It reduces the size and number of tophi, and subsequently allows for their disappearance. In addition, it reduces the frequency of gout flares, and once all crystals have been dissolved, avoids their reoccurrence.

The SUA target is 6 mg/dL (360 μmol/L), but a lower level, below 5 mg/dL (300 μmol/L), to facilitate faster dissolution of crystals is recommended for patients with severe gout (tophi, chronic arthropathy, frequents attacks) until total crystal dissolution and resolution of gout has occurred [6,7].

Given the potential cardiovascular and renal toxicity of hyperuricaemia [2], recent European League Against Rheumatism (EULAR) guidelines underline the importance to not delay the initiation of ULT, but rather to consider it in every patient with a definite diagnosis of gout from the first presentation, in particular in young patients with a very high SUA (above 8.0 mg/dL; 480 μmol/L) and/or comorbidities (renal impairment, hypertension, ischaemic heart disease, heart failure) [7].

Dispersion of MSU crystals during the initial phase of deposit dissolution with ULT exposes the patient to an increased rate of flares that could contribute to poor treatment adherence. Slow titration of ULT might decrease the incidence of flares [18] and therefore, is a core aspect of the management of ULT. Prevention of flares is advised during the first 6 months of ULT and can be achieved by use of low-dose colchicine, 0.5–1 mg/day, or small doses of NSAIDs. This preventive therapy should be pursued longer for patients with tophaceous gout. Of note, if a flare occurs while on ULT, it should be treated without interrupting the ULT. Recently, reports from several trials described the efficacy of two IL1 inhibitors for the prevention of flares during the initiation of ULT. However, these agents—canakinumab, and rilonacept—are not approved for prophylaxis of flares [19].

Finally, it is preferable to start an ULT at a distance from acute attacks, because of the increased risk of flares at initiation. However, this is a matter of debate and the ACR guidelines recommend that ULT be started during an attack, if anti-inflammatory treatment has been introduced beforehand [6].

There are three ways to decrease SUA levels: (1) decreasing urate production, mainly by inhibiting the enzyme xanthine oxidase (XO), which converts hypoxanthine to xanthine and then xanthine to urate; (2) increasing the renal excretion of uric acid with uricosuric agents; and (3) degrading urate into the more soluble component allantoin with a uricase (Figure 44.1) (also see Chapter 46).

Allopurinol

Allopurinol lowers SUA levels by inhibiting XO. Allopurinol is an analogue of hypoxanthine and is converted by XO to its active metabolite, oxypurinol, an analogue of xanthine. Allopurinol inhibits XO by two mechanisms, first, as a substrate for XO, and second, oxypurinol can bind strongly to the reduced form of XO

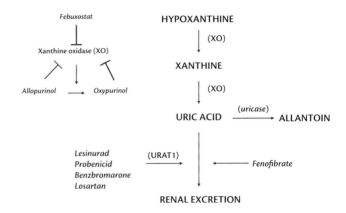

Figure 44.1 Final part of purine metabolism pathway and site of drug action.

and inhibit it (Figure 44.1). Allopurinol is rapidly metabolized (half-life approximately 1 hour) to oxypurinol, which has by far a longer elimination half-life (approximately 23 hours). Oxypurinol is eliminated almost entirely unchanged in urine, and therefore, the renal clearance of oxypurinol is the most important aspect of the pharmacokinetics of allopurinol. Indeed, the excretion of the active metabolite oxypurinol is significantly reduced in patients with impaired renal function [20].

Allopurinol should be initiated at a low dose (100 mg/day), and this dosage should be increased progressively by 100 mg increments every 2–4 weeks to reach the SUA target. In patients with normal renal function, increasing the daily dose to greater than 300 mg/day, up to 800 mg/day, is permitted although seldom practised.

Dose reduction of allopurinol in patients with renal impairment is a matter of debate. It is recommended by some national agencies, the British Society for Rheumatology, the EULAR, and others [5,7,21] but not the ACR [22]. This recommendation is based on a reported relationship between the dose of allopurinol in patients with renal impairment and the development of allopurinol hypersensitivity [20]. By contrast, some authors proposed that an initial dose of 1.5 mg allopurinol per unit estimated glomerular filtration rate followed by a slow increase in dose to reach the urate target may reduce the risk of severe allergic reaction [23,24].

Severe allopurinol-induced hypersensitivity is rare but can be life-threatening, with a mortality rate of approximately 20% [25]. The underlying mechanism of this reaction is not well known but has been attributed in part to cell-mediated immunity to allopurinol and oxypurinol, with renal clearance reduced in patients with substantial renal impairment [26]. Allopurinol-induced hypersensitivity develops early and appears to be favoured by renal failure [20], high allopurinol doses at initiation [23], co-prescription of diuretics [27], reintroduction of the drug after skin intolerance [28], and the HLA-B*5801 genotype, which is particularly frequent in some Asian subpopulations [29]. If the SUA target cannot be reached by an appropriate dose of allopurinol, allopurinol should be switched to febuxostat or a uricosuric, or combined with a uricosuric.

Febuxostat

Unlike allopurinol, febuxostat is a potent, non-purine, selective inhibitor of XO. The primary method of clearance is hepatic and only 1–6% of the drug is excreted unchanged in urine [30] (Table 44.1). Renal function has no impact on the pharmacokinetics of febuxostat. Therefore, no dose adjustment is necessary

Table 44.1 Febuxostat and allopurinol pharmacokinetics

	Febuxostat	Allopurinol (oxypurinol)
Structure	Non-purine	Purine
Inhibitor constant Ki (nM)	0.9	0.5
Enzyme selectivity	Selective inhibitor of xanthine oxidase	Non-selective inhibitor of xanthine oxidase
Clearance	Extensively metabolized in the liver and excreted by urine and faeces	Mainly excreted by urine
Half-life (hours)	5–8	14–26

for patients with mild–moderate chronic kidney disease. The two European Medicines Agency (EMA)-approved dosages, 80 mg and 120 mg/day, are more effective than allopurinol, 300 mg/day [31]. Side effects include elevated liver enzyme activity, and a not significant increased rate of serious cardiovascular events, which had led to not recommending the drug for patients with ischaemic or congestive heart failure. Finally, as for allopurinol, febuxostat impairs the XO-dependent metabolism of azathioprine, and therefore, their concurrent use must be avoided.

Uricosurics

Uricosuric agents enhance the renal excretion of uric acid, mainly through inhibition of a renal transporter (URAT1) (Figure 44.1). These agents should not be prescribed in patients with a high level of uric acid excretion, due to the risk of uric acid stone. Moreover, fluid intake should be increased in patients treated with uricosurics and urine pH maintained above 6, to prevent the development of uric acid stones [22].

Benzbromarone is a powerful uricosuric drug at a dosage of 100 mg to 200 mg/day that can be used in patients with moderate to severe renal impairment. It is more active than allopurinol taken at standard dosages [32]. Its use was restricted after reports of hepatotoxicity, but the drug can still be prescribed on a named patient basis in several European countries. Probenecid is another uricosuric which is less powerful than benzbromarone. It can be used at a dosage of 250–1000 mg twice a day. It is less effective in patients with severe renal impairment [33]. Both uricosurics are generally used in patients who are contraindicated or who failed to respond to XO inhibitors. They can be used as monotherapy or in combination with an XO inhibitor.

Lesinurad (RDEA 594) is a novel uricosuric which is currently under development. It inhibits mainly URAT1. Phase I and phase II studies have shown that lesinurad, in combination with allopurinol or febuxostat, can dose-dependently and robustly decrease the urate levels in gouty patients. It might become an interesting therapeutic option in patients not adequately controlled by available ULTs [34,35].

Pegloticase

Pegloticase is a recombinant mammalian uricase produced in *Escherichia coli* and is a tetrameric enzyme. Each subunit is conjugated with several strands of a 10-kDa monomethoxypoly (ethylene glycol) (mPEG) [36]. Uricase metabolizes urate to the more soluble allantoin that is excreted readily in the urine. It has been approved by the Food and Drug Administration in the United States and the EMA for severe tophaceous gout refractory to the previous ULT, but is no longer available in Europe. It is given as an infusion (8 mg) every 2 weeks. Pegloticase is probably the most powerful drug to debulk the urate load in patients with severe gout. However, its use is hampered by the occurrence of PEG antibodies in some patients, which results in increased drug clearance, loss of efficacy, and increased risk of subsequent infusion reactions [37].

Non-pharmacological treatments of hyperuricaemia

Epidemiological data emphasize the importance of dietary factors in the pathogenesis of gout, which has led to recommendations about weight reduction for overweight patients and the avoidance of beer, spirits, fructose-containing sodas, and consumption of red meat and seafood [5,7,22,38]. However, the impact of diet and lifestyle intervention on SUA levels is modest, leading in some studies to a 10% decrease in SUA levels [22]. Thus, these dietary modifications alone are rarely sufficient to reach the urate target in the vast majority of patients with established gout [39]. Rather, these recommendations mainly aim to promote ideal health and prevention and optimal management of life-threatening comorbidities in gout patients [22].

Patient education and management of comorbidities

Management of gout is frequently inappropriate [3]. Patient information appears to be an outstanding issue in the management of gout because educational intervention has proven to be successful [18]. Therefore, every patient should be informed about the disease, its curable nature, the targets and practicalities of drug therapy, how to prevent and handle flares, and the importance of lifestyle and dietary factors [7].

Management of comorbidities is also of outmost importance to improve cardiovascular prognosis. Therefore, all patients with gout should be systematically screened for associated comorbidities and cardiovascular risk factors, which should be addressed as an integral part of the management of gout. Of note, some therapies for these comorbidities can lower SUA levels and therefore, their use should be favoured in patients with gout. Indeed, losartan, calcium channel blockers, fenofibrate, and statins are mildly uricosuric and can slightly decrease the urate levels. By contrast, diuretics, beta-blockers, angiotensin-converting enzyme inhibitors, and non-losartan angiotensin II receptor blockers are associated with an increased risk of gout [40]. If feasible, discontinuing these drugs, in particular diuretics [41], can help to reach the urate target.

References

1. Kuo CF, Grainge MJ, Mallen C, Zhang W, Doherty M. Comorbidities in patients with gout prior to and following diagnosis: case-control study. *Ann Rheum Dis* 2016; 75(1):210–7.
2. Richette P, Perez-Ruiz F, Doherty M, et al. Improving cardiovascular and renal outcomes in gout: what should we target? *Nat Rev Rheumatol* 2014; 10(11):654–61.
3. Doherty M, Jansen TL, Nuki G, et al. Gout: why is this curable disease so seldom cured? *Ann Rheum Dis* 2012; 71(11):1765–70.

4. Perez-Ruiz F, Martinez-Indart L, Carmona L, et al. Tophaceous gout and high level of hyperuricaemia are both associated with increased risk of mortality in patients with gout. *Ann Rheum Dis* 2014; 73(1):177–82.

5. Jordan KM, Cameron JS, Snaith M, et al. British Society for Rheumatology and British Health Professionals in Rheumatology guideline for the management of gout. *Rheumatology (Oxford)* 2007; 46(8):1372–4.

6. Khanna D, Khanna PP, Fitzgerald JD, et al. 2012 American College of Rheumatology guidelines for management of gout. Part 2: therapy and antiinflammatory prophylaxis of acute gouty arthritis. *Arthritis Care Res (Hoboken)* 2012; 64(10):1447–61.

7. Richette P, Doherty M, Pascual E, et al. Updated Eular Evidence-Based Recommendations for the Management of Gout. *Ann Rheum Dis* 2014; 73(Suppl 2):783–3.

8. Richette P, Frazier A, Bardin T. Pharmacokinetics considerations for gout treatments. *Expert Opin Drug Metab Toxicol* 2014; 10(7):949–57.

9. Terkeltaub R, Furst DE, Bennet K, Kook K, Davis M. Low dose (1.8 mg) vs high dose (4.8 mg) oral colchicine regimens in patients with acute gout flare in a large, multicenter, randomized, double-blind, placebo-controlled, parallel group study. *Arthritis Rheum* 2008; 58(9, Suppl):S879.

10. Terkeltaub RA, Furst DE, Digiacinto JL, Kook KA, Davis MW. Novel evidence-based colchicine dose-reduction algorithm to predict and prevent colchicine toxicity in the presence of cytochrome P450 3A4/P-glycoprotein inhibitors. *Arthritis Rheum* 2011; 63(8):2226–37.

11. Richette P, Bardin T. Colchicine for the treatment of gout. *Expert Opin Pharmacother* 2010; 11(17):2933–8.

12. Janssens HJ, Janssen M, van de Lisdonk EH, van Riel PL, van Weel C. Use of oral prednisolone or naproxen for the treatment of gout arthritis: a double-blind, randomised equivalence trial. *Lancet* 2008; 371(9627):1854–60.

13. Man CY, Cheung IT, Cameron PA, Rainer TH. Comparison of oral prednisolone/paracetamol and oral indomethacin/paracetamol combination therapy in the treatment of acute goutlike arthritis: a double-blind, randomized, controlled trial. *Ann Emerg Med* 2007; 49(5):670–7.

14. Schlesinger N. Anti-interleukin-1 therapy in the management of gout. *Curr Rheumatol Rep* 2014; 16(2):398.

15. Martinon F, Petrilli V, Mayor A, Tardivel A, Tschopp J. Gout-associated uric acid crystals activate the NALP3 inflammasome. *Nature* 2006; 440(7081):237–41.

16. Sivera F, Wechalekar MD, Andres M, Buchbinder R, Carmona L. Interleukin-1 inhibitors for acute gout. *Cochrane Database Syst Rev* 2014; 9:CD009993.

17. Schlesinger N, Alten RE, Bardin T, Schumacher HR, Bloch M, Gimona A, et al. Canakinumab for acute gouty arthritis in patients with limited treatment options: results from two randomised, multicentre, active-controlled, double-blind trials and their initial extensions. *Ann Rheum Dis* 2012; 71(11):1839–48.

18. Rees F, Jenkins W, Doherty M. Patients with gout adhere to curative treatment if informed appropriately: proof-of-concept observational study. *Ann Rheum Dis* 2013; 72(6):826–30.

19. Latourte A, Bardin T, Richette P. Prophylaxis for acute gout flares after initiation of urate-lowering therapy. *Rheumatology (Oxford)* 2014; 53(11):1920–6.

20. Chung WH, Chang WC, Stocker SL, et al. Insights into the poor prognosis of allopurinol-induced severe cutaneous adverse reactions: the impact of renal insufficiency, high plasma levels of oxypurinol and granulysin. *Ann Rheum Dis* 2015; 74(12):2157–64.

21. Sivera F, Andres M, Carmona L, et al. Multinational evidence-based recommendations for the diagnosis and management of gout: integrating systematic literature review and expert opinion of a broad panel of rheumatologists in the 3e initiative. *Ann Rheum Dis* 2014; 73(2):328–35.

22. Khanna D, Fitzgerald JD, Khanna PP, et al. 2012 American College of Rheumatology guidelines for management of gout. Part 1: systematic nonpharmacologic and pharmacologic therapeutic approaches to hyperuricemia. *Arthritis Care Res (Hoboken)* 2012; 64(10):1431–46.

23. Stamp LK, Taylor WJ, Jones PB, et al. Starting dose is a risk factor for allopurinol hypersensitivity syndrome: a proposed safe starting dose of allopurinol. *Arthritis Rheum* 2012; 64(8):2529–36.

24. Stamp LK, O'Donnell JL, Zhang M, et al. Using allopurinol above the dose based on creatinine clearance is effective and safe in patients with chronic gout, including those with renal impairment. *Arthritis Rheum* 2011; 63(2):412–21.

25. Ramasamy SN, Korb-Wells CS, Kannangara DR, et al. Allopurinol hypersensitivity: a systematic review of all published cases, 1950–2012. *Drug Saf* 2013; 36(10):953–80.

26. Yun J, Mattsson J, Schnyder K, et al. Allopurinol hypersensitivity is primarily mediated by dose-dependent oxypurinol-specific T cell response. *Clin Exp Allergy* 2013; 43(11):1246–55.

27. Chao J, Terkeltaub R. A critical reappraisal of allopurinol dosing, safety, and efficacy for hyperuricemia in gout. *Curr Rheumatol Rep* 2009; 11(2):135–40.

28. Terkeltaub RA. Clinical practice. Gout. *N Engl J Med* 2003; 349(17):1647–55.

29. Hung SI, Chung WH, Liou LB, et al. HLA-B*5801 allele as a genetic marker for severe cutaneous adverse reactions caused by allopurinol. *Proc Natl Acad Sci U S A* 2005; 102(11):4134–9.

30. Love BL, Barrons R, Veverka A, Snider KM. Urate-lowering therapy for gout: focus on febuxostat. *Pharmacotherapy* 2010; 30(6):594–608.

31. Becker MA, Schumacher HR, Jr., Wortmann RL, et al. Febuxostat compared with allopurinol in patients with hyperuricemia and gout. *N Engl J Med* 2005; 353(23):2450–61.

32. Robinson PC, Dalbeth N. Advances in pharmacotherapy for the treatment of gout. *Expert Opin Pharmacother* 2015; 16(4):533–46.

33. Pui K, Gow PJ, Dalbeth N. Efficacy and tolerability of probenecid as urate-lowering therapy in gout; clinical experience in high-prevalence population. *J Rheumatol* 2013; 40(6):872–6.

34. Diaz-Torne C, Perez-Herrero N, Perez-Ruiz F. New medications in development for the treatment of hyperuricemia of gout. *Curr Opin Rheumatol* 2015; 27(2):164–9.

35. Fleischmann R, Kerr B, Yeh LT, et al. Pharmacodynamic, pharmacokinetic and tolerability evaluation of concomitant administration of lesinurad and febuxostat in gout patients with hyperuricaemia. *Rheumatology (Oxford)* 2014; 53(12):2167–74.

36. Ea H, Richette P. Critical appraisal of the role of pegloticase in the management of gout. *Open Access Rheumatol Res Rev* 2012; 4:63–70.

37. Sundy JS, Baraf HS, Yood RA, et al. Efficacy and tolerability of pegloticase for the treatment of chronic gout in patients refractory to conventional treatment: two randomized controlled trials. *JAMA* 2011; 306(7):711–20.

38. Zhang W, Doherty M, Bardin T, et al. EULAR evidence based recommendations for gout. Part II: Management. Report of a task force of the EULAR Standing Committee for International Clinical Studies Including Therapeutics (ESCISIT). *Ann Rheum Dis* 2006; 65(10):1312–24.

39. Bardin T. Current management of gout in patients unresponsive or allergic to allopurinol. *Joint Bone Spine* 2004; 71(6):481–5.

40. Choi HK, Soriano LC, Zhang Y, Rodríguez LA. Antihypertensive drugs and risk of incident gout among patients with hypertension: population based case-control study. *BMJ* 2012; 344:d8190.

41. Bruderer S, Bodmer M, Jick SS, Meier CR. Use of diuretics and risk of incident gout: a population-based case-control study. *Arthritis Rheumatol* 2014; 66: 185–96.

CHAPTER 45

Treatment of acute gout

Puja Khanna

Introduction

Acute gout is considered the most painful arthritis experienced by patients among various rheumatological conditions and is a common inflammatory arthritis in the adult population [1,2]. Epidemiological evidence suggests that the prevalence of gout is steadily on the rise due to longevity, coexisting comorbidities, and iatrogenic causes contributing to hyperuricaemia such as diuretic use and transplant drugs [3]. Acute gout usually presents as a self-limiting flare of synovitis that occurs due to deposition of monosodium urate (MSU) crystals [1]. Flares are characterized by the rapid onset of severe pain, swelling, warmth, erythema, and decreased range of motion in the affected joint [1,4,5]. Untreated flares can last from hours to weeks, resulting in missed work, and become chronic, which further lead to joint destruction and disability [6,7]. The frequency of flares generally increases over time in patients who continue to have hyperuricaemia and their risk factors for acute gout attacks have not been adequately addressed [1,2]. Effective treatment of acute gouty arthritis is primary focused on pain which is the primary symptom but must target both the pain and underlying inflammation. Acute gout is frequently treated with non-steroidal anti-inflammatory drugs (NSAIDs), colchicine, and corticosteroids [1,4,8]. In this chapter we will review the available therapies for management of acute gout and ones that have shown promising results.

Types of therapies

Non-pharmacological therapy for acute gout include topical ice applications and in a randomized control trial, patients who were treated with ice as an adjunct to pharmacological anti-inflammatory therapy reported a greater reduction in pain (p = 0.021) compared to the control group [9]. Joint rest and immobilization can also provide resolution of symptoms sooner [10]. Lifestyle interventions in acute gout have not been studied in a randomized controlled trial (RCT); however, weight loss is recommended as a general preventive measure [11,12]. Pharmacological options utilized in current practice entail use of monotherapy with one of the following choices: colchicine, NSAIDs, or corticosteroids. Combination therapies where NSAIDs have been used with either oral or intra-articular corticosteroids or with colchicine have been described according to recent surveys [13–16]. Current guidelines recommend caution when using colchicine and NSAIDs given their potential to cause hepatotoxicity and gastro-renal impairment respectively.

Monotherapy

Non-steroidal anti-inflammatory drugs

NSAIDs are the most commonly prescribed and self-reported class of drugs used worldwide, with more than 50 different preparation that are structurally diverse despite their similar mode of action [17]. They exert their anti-inflammatory action by inhibiting cyclooxygenase (COX), an enzyme that transforms arachidonic acid into prostaglandins. NSAIDs may be selective, inhibiting only COX1 (such as aspirin), or COX2 (such as celecoxib); or non-selective that inhibits both COX1 and COX2 (such as indomethacin or naproxen). Twenty-three studies (77%) (19 double-blind RCTs, 2 single-blind RCT, and 2 blinding not reported) have assessed the use of NSAIDs for the treatment of acute gout, all which were active comparator studies, none were placebo controlled. Fifteen studies evaluated the efficacy of indomethacin compared to other active agents. Of the indomethacin studies, four studies were compared to other active NSAID treatments [18–21], four studies to COX2 selective inhibitors [22–25], three to corticosteroids [26–28], one each to adrenocorticotropic hormone (ACTH) [29], interleukin 1 (IL1) inhibitor [30], and two to Chinese herbs (Danggui-Nian-Tong-Tang and the Simiao pill) [31,32]. There were no placebo-controlled trials, and all the 15 studies showed an improvement in pain in the indomethacin-treated subjects compared to baseline. Three studies have compared naproxen to other active medications. Two explored the efficacy of naproxen compared to etodolac [33,34] and found that there was no statistical difference between them, and that both had a statistical improvement in pain compared to baseline. One compared naproxen to prednisolone [27] and showed a similar decrease in pain with both treatments. Five studies [4,22–25] have assessed the efficacy of COX2 selective inhibitors for the treatment of acute gouty arthritis. Of these, four used indomethacin as a comparator all showing similar efficacy to indomethacin except low-dose celecoxib was statistically less effective than indomethacin [22–25]. Schumacher et al. [23] compared the efficacy of high-dose celecoxib versus low-dose celecoxib compared to indomethacin in the treatment of moderate to severe pain and inflammation associated with an acute gouty arthritis attack. This double-blind, double-dummy, active control, randomized trial randomized subjects to receive celecoxib 50 mg twice a day, celecoxib 400 mg (followed by 200 mg later on day 1 and 200 mg twice a day for 7 days), celecoxib 800 mg (followed by 400 mg later on day 1 and then 400 mg twice a day for 7 days), or indomethacin 50 mg three times a day. Subjects in the high-dose celecoxib groups

(800 mg and 400 mg) had a greater reduction in pain intensity on day 2 compared to low-dose celecoxib. However, the reduction in pain intensity on day 2 was similar between high-dose celecoxib and indomethacin three times a day. Of the five studies, four of the studies assessed COX2 inhibitors that are not available in the United States, and two studies assessed COX2 inhibitors that are no longer on the market (rofecoxib) and lumiracoxib, which is available in Mexico, Ecuador, and Dominican Republic.

Corticosteroids

The immunomodulatory actions of corticosteroids include direct inhibition of (a) transcription factor activity by transrepression, (b) expression of several proinflammatory cytokines, such as IL1, IL6, IL8 and tumour necrosis factor alpha (TNFA), and (c) interfere with phospholipase A2 and eicosanoid production. Seven studies have assessed the use of corticosteroids for the treatment of acute gout. Two compared oral corticosteroids to NSAIDs [27,28] and five compared intramuscular triamcinolone to an active comparator [5,26,29,35,36]. All seven studies showed efficacy for the use of corticosteroids in the treatment of acute gout when compared to NSAIDs, IL1 inhibition, and ACTH.

Adrenocorticotropic hormone

ACTH is a hormone secreted by the pituitary gland that stimulates the production of cortisol, corticosterone, and androgens by the pituitary gland. Although the exact mechanism of action is not well understood, ACTH is believed to exert its beneficial effect by adrenal corticosteroid release and potential activation of the melanocortin type 3 receptor. Two studies (one single-blind RCT and one RCT where blinding was not described) have assessed the use of intramuscular ACTH injection to an active comparator [29,36] and suggest a quicker resolution of pain when compared to indomethacin (p = 0.0001) and similar when compared to intramuscular triamcinolone acetonide (p = 0.89). Another retrospective cohort study supports the safety and efficacy of ACTH for the treatment of acute gout [37].

Colchicine

Colchicine is an old drug which has recently revealed new sophisticated mechanisms of action: by blocking microtubule assembly it is able to reduce neutrophil activity and migration, phagocytosis and transport of MSU crystals, and reducing adhesions molecules on endothelial cells in response to IL1 or TNFA [38-40]. Recently it has been shown that colchicine reduces NLRP3 inflammasome-driven caspase 1 activation by microtubule inhibition which decreases MSU crystal delivery [41]. Colchicine also inhibits pore formation induced by activation of P2X receptors [42]. Two studies have assessed the efficacy of colchicine, both using a placebo-controlled group, both showing a statistical decrease in pain at 24 or 48 hours [43,44] that showed oral colchicine as an effective treatment for an acute attack and had greater efficacy in treating pain compared to placebo when administered within first 12 hours of an acute attack. Although low-dose (1.2 mg, followed by 0.6 mg 1 hour later) and high-dose colchicine (4.8 mg total over 6 hours) have comparable efficacy, low-dose colchicine dosing has a significantly and markedly greater tolerability profile in the AGREE trial. In this study, 77% of subjects on high-dose colchicine developed diarrhoea compared to 23% in the low-dose group versus 14% in placebo group (p-value statistically significant in high-dose vs low-dose colchicine and placebo, but no statistical significance between low-dose

colchicine and placebo) [44]. The duration of treatment with oral colchicine for an acute gout attack was not assessed in these RCTs.

Concomitant use of P-gp and strong cytochrome P450 (CYP) 3A4 inhibitors (such as ciclosporin, clarithromycin, erythromycin, verapamil, diltiazem, ketoconazole, itraconazole, and HIV protease inhibitors) may cause severe drug interactions with colchicine, including death. A colchicine dosing regimen has been recommended if P-gp and strong CYP3A4 inhibitors are co-prescribed [45]. This combination of medications is contraindicated in patients with either renal or hepatic impairment. Myopathy including rhabdomyolysis has been described in patients receiving colchicine have been reported with concomitant use of statins and fibrates (http://www.fda.gov/Drugs/DrugSafety/PostmarketDrugSafetyInformationforPatientsandProviders/DrugSafetyInformationforHeathcareProfessionals/ucm174315.htm).

Interleukin-1 inhibitors

IL1B plays an important role in experimental and clinical gouty inflammation as MSU crystals stimulate its release by phagocytes mediated by the cryopyrin (NLRP3) inflammasome, an intracellular multiprotein complex. Cryopyrin regulates the protease caspase 1 and controls the activation of IL1B. Once caspase 1 becomes active, it cleaves IL1B to release the mature p17 form of IL1B resulting in active, secreted IL1B [46,47]. Four RCTs have assessed the efficacy of IL1 inhibitors in the treatment of an acute gout attack compared to an active comparator [5,9,30,35]. Three studies evaluating canakinumab found that it was efficacious in the treatment of acute gout when compared to intramuscular triamcinolone acetate. The fourth study looked at rilonacept compared to indomethacin and suggested that rilonacept alone or in combination with indomethacin did not provide any additional pain relief at 72 hours as compared to indomethacin alone.

Topical ice

One study has evaluated local ice as a complementary modality and showed statistical improvement in pain on a visual analogue scale (VAS) (p = 0.021) when ice treatment was added to the corticosteroid and colchicine regimen [9].

Chinese herbs

One RCT has evaluated a traditional Chinese herb used to decrease joint inflammation, the Simiao pill [32] and showed that it was more efficacious than indomethacin at day 7. Another study has compared Danggui-Nian-Tong-Tang (DGNTT) to indomethacin and found that DGNTT was not effective in treating acute gout [31].

Combination therapy

No RCT data are available for combination of two pharmacological therapies for treatment of acute gout. Two studies have used combination of pharmacological and non-pharmacological therapies. The first with oral steroid taper and colchicine compared to oral steroid taper, colchicine, and ice combination, which had a significant decrease in pain on a VAS with the addition of ice [9]. The second study compared acetaminophen/prednisone to acetaminophen/indomethacin and showed a statistical difference in the mean decrease in pain in the acetaminophen/prednisone group as compared to the acetaminophen/indomethacin group during the follow-up phase, but no significant difference during the emergency department phase [22].

Outcomes and effectiveness of the treatment choices

Oftentimes the question posed by clinicians is whether one drug is safer than the other or are NSAIDs associated with better outcomes than COX inhibitors, glucocorticoids, IL1 inhibitors, or placebo in the treatment of acute gout. NSAIDs are not significantly associated with a difference in pain reduction compared with COX inhibitors and glucocorticoids for treating acute gout. However, NSAIDs are associated with higher rates of adverse events and higher rates of withdrawal due to adverse events compared with COX inhibitors [48]. Systematic reviews on the efficacy and safety of treatments in acute gout evaluating intraarticular glucocorticoids, colchicine, NSAIDs, and IL1 inhibitors, revealed that all effectively treat acute gout but there was insufficient data to rank them; however, glucocorticoids appeared safer than NSAIDs and low-dose colchicine was safer than high-dose colchicine [49,50].

Strength of evidence from studies of acute gout therapy

Several publications have recently looked at the safety and efficacy of NSAIDs [48,49,51]. Although there was a paucity of high-quality evidence, they showed that no NSAID was superior to another and was equally efficacious as colchicine or corticosteroids or IL1

inhibitors. Glucocorticoids had a slightly better safety profile than NSAIDs. Low-dose colchicine also had a better safety profile compare to high dose. COX2 inhibitors were safer from a gastrointestinal perspective. There are 30 studies looking at various therapies in acute gout, 28 were active comparator trials, while the remaining 2 studies had a placebo-controlled group. All 30 were randomized controlled trials, of which 21 were double blind, 5 were single blind, and 3 where blinding was not described, and 1 non-blinded. The pooled mean age in years for all trials was 54.14 (SD = 11.94), and 89.7% were male. The studies had a broad range for time after onset of an acute attack until initiation of therapy. Almost one-third (30%) of studies treated subjects within 48 hours, 17% within 24 hours, one study within 12 hours, and the remaining studies ranged from 3 to 10 days of symptoms prior to initiation of therapy; 23% did not report the duration of symptoms prior to initiation of therapy. Within the various types of medications, such as NSAIDs, corticosteroids, and colchicine, there was great variability (hours to 10 days) in the duration of symptoms before initiation of therapy. For the 30 studies, the median Jadad score was 4.0 suggesting a good quality for the study design [52]. Studies that assessed efficacy of IL1 inhibitors (nm = 4, median score = 5) and corticosteroids (n = 7, median score = 5) had a higher Jadad score compared to studies of NSAIDs (n = 20, median score = 4). Studies of colchicine (n = 2) had Jadad scores of 4.0 [44] and 2.0 [43] and topical ice (n = 1) had a Jadad score of 2.0 [9]. Table 45.1 summarized the various studies and describes the strength of evidence from each study.

Table 45.1 Summary of the trials and strength of evidence for currently available therapies

Agents	No. of trials[a]	Strength of evidence	Jadad score (median)	Comparator (No. of studies if >1)	Primary endpoint	Time at evaluation of endpoint	Urate-lowering therapy (ULT) allowed
NSAIDs							
Indomethacin	14	A	3.5	NSAIDs (4), ACTH, COX2 (2), oral steroids, IM TA, rilonacept, DGNTT, Simiao Pill$^\alpha$	Variable endpoints— see comparators	Variable	NR (8), stable ULT (5), excluded ULT (1)
Naproxen	3	A	3	Etodolac (2), prednisolone	1. % decrease in pain compared to baseline (1–5 scale) (2 trials) 2. Decreased pain after 90 hours on VAS	1. Day 7 2. 90 hours	Stable ULT(2), NR (1)
Etodolac	2	A	3	Naproxen (2)	% decrease in pain compared to baseline (1-–5 scale) (2 trials)	Day 7	Stable ULT (1), NR (1)
Diclofenac	1	B	4	Rofecoxib	Pt pain score	12 hours	NR
Fenoprofen	1	B	5	Phenylbutazone	% reduction of total daily score	Days 1–4	Stable ULT
Feprazone	1	B	4	Phenylbutazone	Mean time to end of attack		NR
Flufenamic acid	1	B	4	Phenylbutazone	Number of days until pain relief		Stable ULT
Flurbiprofen	1	B	4	Phenylbutazone	Time to resolution of symptoms		NR

(continued)

Table 45.1 Continued

Agents	No. of trials[a]	Strength of evidence	Jadad score (median)	Comparator (No. of studies if >1)	Primary endpoint	Time at evaluation of endpoint	Urate-lowering therapy (ULT) allowed
Ketoprofen	1	B	3	Indomethacin	Relative rate of pain reduction compared to baseline (0–3 scale)	Day 8	NR
Ketorolac	1	B	5	Indomethacin	Mean decrease in pain (0–5 Wong–Baker scale)	2 hours	NR
Meloxicam	1	B	4	Rofecoxib	Patient pain score (5-point verbal score)	12 hours	NR
Meclofenamate Sodium	1	B	3	Indomethacin	% pain improvement (0–3 scale)	Day 7	NR
Tenoxicam	1	B	1	Indomethacin	Speed of improvement of pain	Day 6	NR
COX2 inhibitors							
Celecoxib	1	B	5	Indomethacin	Pain on VAS (0–10)	Day 2	Stable ULT
Etoricoxib	2	A	4.5	Indomethacin (2)	Likert scale of pain assessment (0–4)	Days 2–5	Stable ULT
Corticosteroids/ACTH							
Oral steroids	2	A	5	Naproxen, Indomethacin	1. Pain on VAS 2. Mean rate of decrease in pain on VAS (0–10)	1. 90 hours 2. Variable	Stable ULT (1), NR (1)
Intramuscular triamcinolone acetate (IM TA)	5	A	3	ACTH, Indomethacin, Canakinumab (3)	1. Mean time to resolution of symptoms (2 trials) 2. Mean interval to relief of pain 3. % change in pain intensity	1. Variable 2. Variable 3. 72 hours	Stable ULT (5)
IM ACTH	2	A	2	Indomethacin, IM TA	Mean interval to pain relief Mean time to resolution	Variable	Stable ULT (1), excluded ULT (1)
Oral colchicine	2	A	2.5	Placebo (2)	50% improvement on VAS (2 trials)	1. 48 hours 2. 24 hours	Stable ULT (1), NR (1)
IL1 inhibitors							
Canakinumab	3	A	5	IM TA (3)	Difference in reducing VAS pain score	72 hours	Stable ULT (3)
Rilonacept	1	B	5	Indomethacin	Reduction of pain on Likert scale (5 point)	Day 3	Stable ULT
	1	B	2	Colchicine and steroids	Relative rate of pain reduction on VAS	Day 7	Stable ULT
Simiao pill	1	B	2	Indomethacin	Clinical efficacy	Day 7	NR
DGNTT	1	B	1	Indomethacin	Pain score	Day 2–3	NR
ICE	1	B	2	Colchicine and steroids	Relative rate of pain reduction on VAS	Day 7	Stable ULT

[a]Three studies not included in table, no longer on the market. NR, not reported.

Adapted from *Seminars in Arthritis & Rheumatism* 2014. Trials reported in the Table included more than 30 subjects; all trials except colchicine were active comparator studies.

Guidelines on management of acute gouty arthritis

Timing of therapy

All major guidelines [53–58] have recommended that it is crucial to initiate acute gout therapy immediately after onset of flare and preferably as close to or within 24 hours in order for the medication to exert its optimal effects and abate the flare.

Recommendations for acute treatment

For treatment of acute gout, three guidelines, the American College of Rheumatology (ACR) [54], British Society of Rheumatology (BSR) [53], and 3e initiative [56], recommend NSAIDs, corticosteroids, or oral colchicine to be similarly effective (Table 45.2). However, the European League Against Rheumatism (EULAR) [58] recommended oral colchicine and/or NSAID as first-line agents over corticosteroids for the treatment of acute attacks. When selecting colchicine, all guidelines recommend using low-dose colchicine (1.8–2.0 mg country-specific loading dose). The ACR recommended topical ice application to be an appropriate adjunctive measure to one or more pharmacological therapies for acute gouty arthritis.

For patients with severe disease (defined as ≥7 out of 10 pain on a 0–10 VAS and/or acute polyarticular gout attack, or an attack involving at least one to two large joints), the ACR guidelines recommend initiating combination pharmacological therapy and use of IL1 inhibition [3,49,59] in subjects with refractory attacks of acute gout or contraindications to all three agents above. The BSR, EULAR and ACR all recommend combining pharmacological and non-pharmacological treatments such as rest or ice as add-on to single-drug treatment (monotherapy) for acute gouty episodes.

A recent systematic literature review for acute gout provides additional evidence to support statements of the above-mentioned guidelines [60]. Oral colchicine was demonstrated to be effective, with low-dose colchicine demonstrating a comparable tolerability profile as placebo and a significantly lower side effect profile to high-dose colchicine. The head-to-head trials between NSAIDs and COX2 inhibitors showed equivalent efficacy at regulatory-approved doses (with the exception that celecoxib that required higher doses). In this review, summary of several trials supported use of canakinumab [5,61–63] and to lesser extent anakinra [59] for patients with contraindications to standard therapies.

Prevention of acute flares when starting urate-lowering agents in chronic gout

Concurrent prophylaxis against acute gout attacks on initiation of urate-lowering therapy (ULT) also utilizes the same drugs used in management of acute flares; the exception being the dosing and duration. The 2002 Dutch guidelines recommended against chronic

Table 45.2 Summary of recommendations on management of acute gout

	2006 EULAR	2007 BSR	2012 ACR gout guidelines	3e initiative
When to start treatment	Immediately after initiation of acute attack	Not addressed	Within 24 h of initiation of attack	Not addressed
Monotherapy	NSAIDs are the drugs of choice followed by colchicine	First-line oral low-dose colchicine or NSAIDs	No preference and can be colchicine, NSAIDs, or corticosteroids	No preference and can be colchicine, NSAIDs, or corticosteroids
Oral colchicine	0.5 mg 2–4 times daily	0.5 mg 3 times a day	1.8 mg first day followed by 0.6 mg once or twice daily until end of attack	Low-dose colchicine (up to 2 mg daily)
NSAIDS and coxibs	Fast-acting NSAIDs at maximum dose are the drugs of choice; duration of therapy not addressed	Different NSAIDs are similarly effective; duration of therapy not addressed	NSAIDs or COX2 is effective at FDA/EMA-approved doses; duration for 1 week	NSAIDs or COX2 is effective; duration of therapy not addressed
Intra-articular steroids	IA steroids for acute monoarticular gouty arthritis	Effective and safe for acute gout	Recommends for acute gout in 1–2 large joints with acute gout	Effective for acute gout
Oral steroids	Effective if unable to tolerate NSAIDs or refractory gout; duration of therapy not addressed	Not addressed	Recommends oral steroids at 0.5 mg/kg for 5–10 days, or 2–5 days of full dose tapered over 7–10 days	Effective for acute gout; duration of therapy not addressed
IM steroids	Effective if unable to tolerate NSAIDs or refractory gout	Not addressed	Triamcinolone acetonide 60 mg once followed by oral prednisone. In patients who are nil by mouth, initial methylprednisolone is 0.5–2 mg/kg and repeated, as needed	Effective for acute gout
Combination therapy: with 2 pharmacological agents	Not addressed	Not addressed	When the acute attack was characterized by severe pain; acute polyarticular gout attack or an attack involving 1–2 large joints	Not addressed
Non-pharmacological	Recommends lifestyle modifications as well as ice in combination with pharmacological therapy	Should be used in combination with pharmacological therapy (i.e. ice)	Supplement first-line therapy with topical ice as needed	Not addressed

Adapted from *Seminars in Arthritis & Rheumatism* 2014. 3e, Multinational Evidence, Exchange and Expertise group; ACR, American College of Rheumatology; BSR, British Society of Rheumatology; EULAR, European League against Rheumatism; IA, intra-articular; IM, intramuscular; NSAIDs, non-steroidal anti-inflammatory; PO, oral.

colchicine. Beginning with EULAR, colchicine or NSAIDs were recommended for the first months. The British guidelines extended colchicine for 6 months (limiting low-dose NSAIDs to 6 weeks). The ACR guidelines increased duration regardless of agent (colchicine, low-dose NSAID, or low-dose steroid) to 6 months or at least 3 months beyond achieving serum uric acid for non-tophaceous patients. The 3e supported prophylaxis but was unresolved about duration. The updated EULAR guidelines recommended 6 months. Two randomized controlled trials have shown that colchicine prophylaxis for at least 6 months, when starting a ULT, reduces the risk of acute attacks [64,65]. Canakinumab has been shown to provide prophylaxis superior to colchicine when starting a ULT, although currently it is only licensed in Europe for treatment of acute gout, and is not licensed in the US for use in gout [66].

Potential targets of therapy

Among new therapies, biological anticytokine agents have been explored with the goal of targeting specific elements in the pathogenesis of acute gouty inflammation [67,68]. In this context due to the central role of IL1 in the inflammasome and toll-like receptor-dependent mechanisms associated with MSU crystal inflammation, its inhibition has been increasingly considered to prevent acute flares. IL1 inhibition has been studied in several trials [5,30,35] and seem quite efficacious for both treatment and prevention of acute gout attacks with few adverse events; costs, however, limit their use [69].

Summary

The current options for treatment of acute gout are NSAIDs, colchicine, systemic and intraarticular corticosteroids, ACTH, and anakinra. There are several new guidelines that provide case-based guidance on the use of these agents and clear evidence is available from well-done randomized studies. Drug practices, however, are dictated by the adverse events, presence of comorbidities, physicians' and patients' preferences, along with costs. It is quintessential to initiate acute therapy upon onset of symptoms to achieve optimal control of the pain and inflammation. Based on the available therapeutic options and promising new agents, efficacious treatment of acute gout can be accomplished promptly and safely.

Key points

◆ NSAIDs, COX2 inhibitors, corticosteroids, colchicine, and canakinumab (an IL1 inhibitor) have strong evidence to suggest efficacy in the treatment of acute gout.

◆ An acute gouty arthritis attack should be treated with pharmacological therapy, initiated within 24 hours of onset.

◆ NSAIDs are effective and should be individualized based on severity of the acute attack, drug interactions, and comorbidities of the patient.

◆ Oral colchicine is most effective when given promptly in the first 24 hours of acute onset of symptoms.

◆ Choice of corticosteroids in combination with colchicine can be used for refractory acute flares with polyarticular joint involvement.

◆ Established pharmacological ULT should be continued in patients without interruption during an acute attack of gout.

References

1. Neogi T. Clinical practice. Gout. *N Engl J Med* 2011; 364(5):443–52.
2. Zhu Y, Pandya BJ, Choi HK. Prevalence of gout and hyperuricemia in the US general population: the National Health and Nutrition Examination Survey 2007–2008. *Arthritis Rheum* 2011; 63(10):3136–41.
3. So A, De Smedt T, Revaz S, Tschopp J. A pilot study of IL-1 inhibition by anakinra in acute gout. *Arthritis Res Ther* 2007; 9(2):R28.
4. Cheng TT, Lai HM, Chiu CK, Chem YC. A single-blind, randomized, controlled trial to assess the efficacy and tolerability of rofecoxib, diclofenac sodium, and meloxicam in patients with acute gouty arthritis. *Clin Ther* 2004; 26(3):399–406.
5. So A, De Meulemeester M, Pikhlak A, et al. Canakinumab for the treatment of acute flares in difficult-to-treat gouty arthritis: results of a multicenter, phase II, dose-ranging study. *Arthritis Rheum* 2010; 62(10):3064–76.
6. Khanna PP, Nuki G, Bardin T, et al. Tophi and frequent gout flares are associated with impairments to quality of life, productivity, and increased healthcare resource use: Results from a cross-sectional survey. *Health Qual Life Outcomes* 2012; 10:117.
7. Sarawate CA, Patel PA, Schumacher HR, et al. Serum urate levels and gout flares: analysis from managed care data. *J Clin Rheumatol* 2006; 12(2):61–5.
8. Terkeltaub RA. Clinical practice. Gout. *N Engl J Med* 2003; 349(17):1647–55.
9. Schlesinger N, Detry MA, Holland BK. Local ice therapy during bouts of acute gouty arthritis. *J Rheumatol* 2002; 29(2):331–4.
10. Schumacher HR. Crystal-induced arthritis: an overview. *Am J Med* 1996; 100(2A):46S–52S.
11. Dessein PH, Shipton EA, Stanwix AE, Joffe BI, Ramokgadi J. Beneficial effects of weight loss associated with moderate calorie/carbohydrate restriction, and increased proportional intake of protein and unsaturated fat on serum urate and lipoprotein levels in gout: a pilot study. *Ann Rheum Dis* 2000; 59(7):539–43.
12. Moi JH, Sriranganathan MK, Edwards CJ, Buchbinder R. Lifestyle interventions for acute gout. *Cochrane Database Syst Rev* 2013; 11:CD010519.
13. Gnanenthiran SR, Hassett GM, Gibson KA, McNeil HP. Acute gout management during hospitalization: a need for a protocol. *Intern Med J* 2011; 41(8):610–7.
14. Petersel D, Schlesinger N. Treatment of acute gout in hospitalized patients. *J Rheumatol* 2007; 34(7):1566–8.
15. Schlesinger N. Management of acute and chronic gouty arthritis: present state-of-the-art. *Drugs* 2004; 64(21):2399–416.
16. Schlesinger N, Moore DF, Sun JD, Schumacher HR Jr. A survey of current evaluation and treatment of gout. *J Rheumatol* 2006; 33(10):2050–2.
17. Vonkeman HE, van de Laar MA. Nonsteroidal anti-inflammatory drugs: adverse effects and their prevention. *Semin Arthritis Rheum* 2010; 39(4):294–312.
18. Altman RD, Honig S, Levin JM, Lightfoot RW. Ketoprofen versus indomethacin in patients with acute gouty arthritis: a multicenter, double blind comparative study. *J Rheumatol* 1988; 15(9):1422–6.
19. Eberl R, Dunky A. Meclofenamate sodium in the treatment of acute gout. Results of a double-blind study. *Arzneimittelforschung* 1983; 33(4A):641–3.
20. Ruotsi A, Vainio U. Treatment of acute gouty arthritis with proquazone and indomethacin. A comparative, double-blind trial. *Scand J Rheumatol Suppl* 1978; 21:15–7.
21. Shrestha M, Morgan DL, Moreden JM, et al. Randomized double-blind comparison of the analgesic efficacy of intramuscular ketorolac and oral indomethacin in the treatment of acute gouty arthritis. *Ann Emerg Med* 1995; 26(6):682–6.
22. Rubin BR, Burton R, Navarra S, et al. Efficacy and safety profile of treatment with etoricoxib 120 mg once daily compared with indomethacin 50 mg three times daily in acute gout: a randomized controlled trial. *Arthritis Rheum* 2004; 50(2):598–606.

23. Schumacher HR, Berger MF, Li-Yu J, et al. Efficacy and tolerability of celecoxib in the treatment of acute gouty arthritis: a randomized controlled trial. *J Rheumatol* 2012; 39(9):1859–66.

24. Schumacher HR, Jr, Boice JA, Daikh DI, et al. Randomised double blind trial of etoricoxib and indometacin in treatment of acute gouty arthritis. *BMJ* 2002; 324(7352):1488–92.

25. Willburger RE, Mysler E, Derbot J, et al. Lumiracoxib 400 mg once daily is comparable to indomethacin 50 mg three times daily for the treatment of acute flares of gout. *Rheumatology (Oxford)* 2007; 46(7):1126–32.

26. Alloway JA, Moriarty MJ, Hoogland YT, Nashel DJ. Comparison of triamcinolone acetonide with indomethacin in the treatment of acute gouty arthritis. *J Rheumatol* 1993; 20(1):111–3.

27. Janssens HJ, Janssen M, van de Lisdonk EH, van Riel PL, van Weel C. Use of oral prednisolone or naproxen for the treatment of gout arthritis: a double-blind, randomised equivalence trial. *Lancet* 2008; 371(9627):1854–60.

28. Man CY, Cheung IT, Cameron PA, Rainer TH. Comparison of oral prednisolone/paracetamol and oral indomethacin/paracetamol combination therapy in the treatment of acute goutlike arthritis: a double-blind, randomized, controlled trial. *Ann Emerg Med* 2007; 49(5):670–7.

29. Axelrod D, Preston S. Comparison of parenteral adrenocorticotropic hormone with oral indomethacin in the treatment of acute gout. *Arthritis Rheum* 1988; 31(6):803–5.

30. Terkeltaub RA, Schumacher HR, Carter JD, et al. Rilonacept in the treatment of acute gouty arthritis: a randomized, controlled clinical trial using indomethacin as the active comparator. *Arthritis Res Ther* 2013; 15(1):R25.

31. Chou CT, Kuo SC. The anti-inflammatory and anti-hyperuricemic effects of Chinese herbal formula danggui-nian-tong-tang on acute gouty arthritis: a comparative study with indomethacin and allopurinol. *Am J Chin Med* 1995; 23(3–4):261–71.

32. Shi XD, Li GC, Qian ZX, Jin ZQ, Song Y. Randomized and controlled clinical study of modified prescriptions of Simiao Pill in the treatment of acute gouty arthritis. *Chin J Integr Med* 2008; 14(1):17–22.

33. Maccagno A, Di Giorgio E, Romanowicz A. Effectiveness of etodolac ('Lodine') compared with naproxen in patients with acute gout. *Curr Med Res Opin* 1991; 12(7):423–9.

34. Mizraji M. Clinical response to etodolac in the management of pain. *Eur J Rheumatol Inflamm* 1990; 10(1):35–43.

35. Schlesinger N, Alten RE, Bardin T, et al. Canakinumab for acute gouty arthritis in patients with limited treatment options: results from two randomised, multicentre, active-controlled, double-blind trials and their initial extensions. *Ann Rheum Dis* 2012; 71(11):1839–48.

36. Siegel LB, Alloway JA, Nashel DJ. Comparison of adrenocorticotropic hormone and triamcinolone acetonide in the treatment of acute gouty arthritis. *J Rheumatol* 1994; 21(7):1325–7.

37. Daoussis D, Antonopoulos I, Yiannopoulos G, Andonopoulos AP. ACTH as first line treatment for acute gout in 181 hospitalized patients. *Joint Bone Spine* 2013; 80(3):291–4.

38. Bhat A, Naguwa SM, Cheema GS, Gershwin ME. Colchicine revisited. *Ann N Y Acad Sci* 2009; 1173:766–73.

39. Cronstein BN, Molad Y, Reibman J, et al. Colchicine alters the quantitative and qualitative display of selectins on endothelial cells and neutrophils. *J Clin Invest* 1995; 96(2):994–1002.

40. Scott P, Ma H, Viriyakosol S, Terkeltaub R, Liu-Bryan R. Engagement of CD14 mediates the inflammatory potential of monosodium urate crystals. *J Immunol* 2006; 177(9):6370–8.

41. Pope RM, Tschopp J. The role of interleukin-1 and the inflammasome in gout: implications for therapy. *Arthritis Rheum* 2007; 56(10):3183–8.

42. Marques-da-Silva C, Chaves MM, Castro NG, Coutinho-Silva R, Guimaraes MZ. Colchicine inhibits cationic dye uptake induced by ATP in P2X2 and P2X7 receptor-expressing cells: implications for its therapeutic action. *Br J Pharmacol* 2011; 163(5):912–26.

43. Ahern MJ, Reid C, Gordon TP, et al. Does colchicine work? The results of the first controlled study in acute gout. *Aust N Z J Med* 1987; 17(3):301–4.

44. Terkeltaub RA, Furst DE, Bennett K, et al. High versus low dosing of oral colchicine for early acute gout flare: twenty-four-hour outcome of the first multicenter, randomized, double-blind, placebo-controlled, parallel-group, dose-comparison colchicine study. *Arthritis Rheum* 2010; 62(4):1060–8.

45. Terkeltaub RA, Furst DE, Digiacinto JL, Kook KA, Davis MW. Novel evidence-based colchicine dose-reduction algorithm to predict and prevent colchicine toxicity in the presence of cytochrome P450 3A4/P-glycoprotein inhibitors. *Arthritis Rheum* 2011; 63(8):2226–37.

46. Cronstein BN, Terkeltaub R. The inflammatory process of gout and its treatment. *Arthritis Res Ther* 2006; 8(Suppl 1):S3.

47. Martinon F, Pétrilli V, Mayor A, Tardivel A, Tschopp J. Gout-associated uric acid crystals activate the NALP3 inflammasome. *Nature* 2006; 440(7081):237–41.

48. van Durme CM, Wechalekar MD, Landewe RB. Nonsteroidal anti-inflammatory drugs for treatment of acute gout. *JAMA* 2015; 313(22):2276–7.

49. Wechalekar MD, Vinik O, Moi JH, et al. The efficacy and safety of treatments for acute gout: results from a series of systematic literature reviews including Cochrane reviews on intraarticular glucocorticoids, colchicine, nonsteroidal antiinflammatory drugs, and interleukin-1 inhibitors. *J Rheumatol Suppl* 2014; 92:15–25.

50. van Echteld I, Wechalekar MD, Schlesinger N, Buchbinder R, Aletaha D. Colchicine for acute gout. *Cochrane Database Syst Rev* 2014; 8:CD006190.

51. Zhang S, Zhang Y, Liu P, Zhang W, Ma JL, Wang J. Efficacy and safety of etoricoxib compared with NSAIDs in acute gout: a systematic review and a meta-analysis. *Clin Rheumatol* 2015; 35(1):151–8.

52. Jadad AR, Moore RA, Carroll D, et al. Assessing the quality of reports of randomized clinical trials: is blinding necessary? *Control Clin Trials* 1996; 17(1):1–12.

53. Jordan KM, Cameron JS, Snaith M, et al. British Society for Rheumatology and British Health Professionals in Rheumatology guideline for the management of gout. *Rheumatology (Oxford)* 2007; 46(8):1372–4.

54. Khanna D, Khanna PP, Fitzgerald JD, et al. 2012 American College of Rheumatology guidelines for management of gout. Part 2: therapy and antiinflammatory prophylaxis of acute gouty arthritis. *Arthritis Care Res (Hoboken)* 2012; 64(10):1447–61.

55. Romeijnders AC, Gorter KJ. [Summary of the Dutch College of General Practitioners' 'Gout' Standard]. *Ned Tijdschr Geneeskd* 2002; 146(7):309–13.

56. Sivera F, Andrés M, Carmona L, et al. Multinational evidence-based recommendations for the diagnosis and management of gout: integrating systematic literature review and expert opinion of a broad panel of rheumatologists in the 3e initiative. *Ann Rheum Dis* 2014; 73(2):328–35.

57. Yamanaka H. Japanese guideline for the management of hyperuricemia and gout: second edition. *Nucleosides Nucleotides Nucleic Acids* 2011; 30(12):1018–29.

58. Zhang W, Doherty M, Bardin T, et al. EULAR evidence based recommendations for gout. Part II: Management. Report of a task force of the EULAR Standing Committee for International Clinical Studies Including Therapeutics (ESCISIT). *Ann Rheum Dis* 2006; 65(10):1312–24.

59. Sivera F, Wechalekar MD, Andrés M, Buchbinder R, Carmona L. Interleukin-1 inhibitors for acute gout. *Cochrane Database Syst Rev* 2014; 9:CD009993.

60. Khanna PP, Gladue HS, Singh MK, et al. Treatment of acute gout: a systematic review. *Semin Arthritis Rheum* 2014; 44(1):31–8.

61. Onuora S. Crystal arthritis: canakinumab relieves gout flares when treatment options are limited. *Nat Rev Rheumatol* 2012; 8(7):369.

62. Perez-Ruiz F, Chinchilla SP, Herrero-Beites AM. Canakinumab for gout: a specific, patient-profiled indication. *Expert Rev Clin Immunol* 2014; 10(3):339–47.

63. Schlesinger N. Canakinumab in gout. *Expert Opin Biol Ther* 2012; 12(9):1265–75.

64. Borstad GC, Bryant LR, Abel MP, et al. Colchicine for prophylaxis of acute flares when initiating allopurinol for chronic gouty arthritis. *J Rheumatol* 2004; 31(12):2429–32.

65. Paulus HE, Schlosstein LH, Godfrey RG, Klinenberg JR, Bluestone R. Prophylactic colchicine therapy of intercritical gout. A placebo-controlled study of probenecid-treated patients. *Arthritis Rheum* 1974; 17(5):609–14.

66. Schlesinger N, Mysler E, Lin HY, et al. Canakinumab reduces the risk of acute gouty arthritis flares during initiation of allopurinol treatment: results of a double-blind, randomised study. *Ann Rheum Dis* 2011; 70(7):1264–71.

67. Punzi L, Scanu A, Ramonda R, Oliviero F. Gout as autoinflammatory disease: new mechanisms for more appropriated treatment targets. *Autoimmun Rev* 2012; 12(1):66–71.

68. Robinson PC, Dalbeth N. Advances in pharmacotherapy for the treatment of gout. *Expert Opin Pharmacother* 2015; 16(4):533–46.

69. Dumusc A, So A. Interleukin-1 as a therapeutic target in gout. *Curr Opin Rheumatol* 2015; 27(2):156–63.

CHAPTER 46

Long-term management of gout

Fernando Perez-Ruiz, Irati Urionagüena,
and Sandra P. Chinchilla

Introduction

Gout is the most prevalent arthritis in adults. Although well known for centuries, both academic and clinical interest seem to have diminished, and long-term management of gout is still nowadays suboptimal if not neglected in average clinical practice [1]. 'Crystal clear' conceptual issues will be addressed in this chapter concerning objectives, targets, interventions including pharmacological approaches to hyperuricaemia, and outcomes.

Gout is a chronic disease from the very first clinical manifestation and will lead, if unattended in the long term, to permanent structural damage of affected musculoskeletal structures, loss of perceived quality of life, and unrecoverable loss of function [2].

Objectives of gout management

From a clinical point of view, the milestone for the treatment of gout is long-term control of hyperuricaemia to target serum urate (SUA) levels.

Short-term objectives

At initiation of urate-lowering treatment, there is a limited-in-time risk of recurrence of the episodes of acute inflammation (EAIs), especially when a sharp decrease of SUA levels is achieved [3]. To minimize this risk, prophylaxis should be seriously considered, patients should be comprehensively informed, and rescue medication for intercurrent EAIs, tailored considering concomitant comorbid conditions, prescribed according to approved labels, and discussed with the patients to afford self-management as much as possible.

Long-term objective

The long-term objective of gout treatment is to reverse the pathophysiological mechanism that leads to monosodium urate (MSU) crystal nucleation, growth, and aggregation in tissues, namely hyperuricaemia. Achieving subsaturating SUA levels will lead to a progressive dissolution and final clearance of MSU crystals from tissues thus reducing clinical manifestations and preventing further inflammation and structural damage [4].

Serum urate targets

Adequate control of SUA levels to target during the treatment of hyperuricaemia in gout has been considered to be of the utmost importance to 'cure' gout [1,5]. Different targets could be considered during consecutive stages of the treatment of hyperuricaemia: first, a therapeutic, crystal-depleting target to ensure the complete dissolution of present MSU crystals in tissues; then, once the dissolution of the burden of deposition of MSU crystals has been achieved, a preventive target could be sequentially considered, in order to avoid new crystal formation [6].

Although it is well recognized that the target for SUA should be set to be at least less than 6 mg/dL (360 μmol/L), patients with tophi should be considered for a lower SUA target, at least less than 5 mg/dL (300 μmol/L) to promote rapid dissolution (Figure 46.1) of MSU crystals [7,8]. Lifelong control of SUA levels below the saturation threshold is strongly recommended to avoid recurrence of gout [7,8]; nonetheless, SUA targets useful for dissolving MSU crystals may not be needed in the very long term once complete depletion of deposits has been achieved, and presumably just keeping SUA levels close to 6 mg/dL (360 μmol/L) may be enough [6].

Interventions for long-term treatment

Several interventions should be considered when approaching the long-term management of gout.

Information and education

Providing information and education to the patient may well be the first intervention to be considered for the success of the treatment of gout [9]. The clinician should inform about the causes, treatment, and risk of EAIs while initiating long-term therapy, and also educate on targets, outcomes, and the importance of long-term compliance with medications and follow-up; a high rate of success has been obtained when these measures have been implemented [9], and when neglected, low rate of treatment maintenance is to be expected [10].

Urate-lowering therapy

Urate-lowering therapy (ULT) comprises any intervention, pharmacological and non-pharmacological, to achieve stable, long-term control of SUA levels to established targets. Patients with gout and hyperuricaemia are subject to be prescribed ULT, although not necessarily urate-lowering drugs (ULDs).

Lifestyle modifications and concomitant medications

Lifestyle modifications, when applicable, should include weight loss, exercise, and dietary restriction of food and beverages known to have an impact on hyperuricaemia [11]. The impact of such interventions may be limited regarding the impact on the achievement of

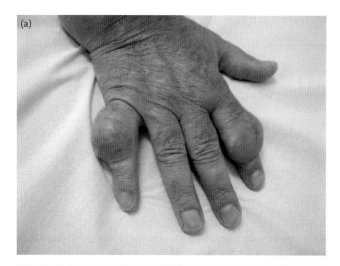

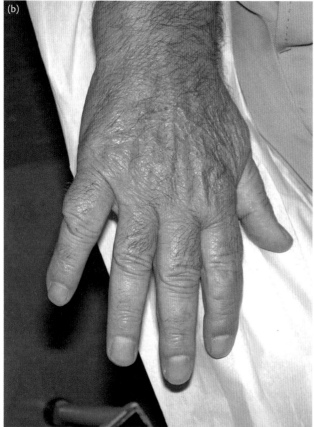

Figure 46.1 Change in tophaceous deposition in a patient with severe gout. (a) Prior to ULT; (b) after 3-year intensive urate-lowering therapy, average SUA < 4 mg/dL (240 µmol/L).
© F. Perez-Ruiz, with permission.

target SUA as in the Multiple Risk Factor Intervention Trial, where patients achieving weight reduction over 10 kg achieved an average reduction in SUA levels of 0.62 mg/dL (37 µmol/L). Nevertheless, it is beyond any discussion that such modifications will have health effects beyond their influence on gout, and especially on cardiovascular events.

Withdrawal of medications with known effect on SUA levels, such as diuretics, or prescription of medications with mild uricosuric

effect if applicable, such as losartan, atorvastatin, and fenofibrate may also be considered [12].

Urate-lowering medications

We include as ULDs those labelled for the reduction of hyperuricaemia in patients with gout, although a series of drugs are in development [13]. Not all such medications are approved worldwide and national or even local labels may also vary. Therefore, individual practice should always comply with national and local regulations.

Indications

There is no worldwide accepted consensus as when to prescribe ULDs, only that patients with recurrent episodes of acute inflammation, tophi on physical exam, or structural damage ('gouty arthropathy') are to be prescribed ULDs if needed to reach target SUA levels [7,8]. According to the 2014-updated European League Against Rheumatism (EULAR) recommendations [14], ULDs should considered and prescribed if agreed by the patient from the start of clinical manifestations in certain gout or to be prescribed in patients with more than one episode of acute inflammation a year, or just one episode in patients with chronic kidney disease (CKD), as in the American College of Rheumatology (ACR) guidelines [8]. Overall, in recent years there has been a tendency to recommend an early approach to interventions on hyperuricaemia in patients with gout, whereas the cumulative prevalence of allopurinol treatment has been shown to range from less than one-third in the first year after gout diagnosis to less than half by the ninth year in a cohort in the United Kingdom Health Improvement Network (THIN) database [15].

General considerations: efficacy, effectiveness, and safety

Urate-lowering efficacy may be defined as the percentage of reduction in SUA from baseline SUA achieved with a fixed dose of a ULD; it will depend on pharmacodynamics (PD) and pharmacokinetics (PK). Conversely, effectiveness is the percentage of patients who reach target SUA with a fixed dose of a ULD; it will be dependent on efficacy, the dose prescribed, but also on baseline SUA levels, as the higher the baseline, the harder to reach the target [16,17].

Safety will depend mainly on PD and PK of the individual ULDs; it should always be taken into account, and especially in patients with associated comorbid conditions also regarding interactions with concomitant medications. A step-up approach to effective dosing is recommended for all ULDs.

Xanthine oxidase inhibitors: allopurinol, febuxostat, and topiroxostat

Xanthine oxidase inhibitors (XOIs) include allopurinol, febuxostat, and topiroxostat. Even though the ACR guidelines make no difference between *febuxostat* and *allopurinol* as first-line ULDs, uricosurics are to be added if target SUA level is not reached, and pegloticase considered for refractory gout [8]. The 2014-updated EULAR recommendations suggest that allopurinol is to be considered as first-line treatment for patients with no renal function impairment [14], with a similar further approach afterwards. A third XOI, *topiroxostat*, is only labelled, to date, in Japan.

Allopurinol is a purine-related pro-drug available worldwide for the last five decades. Administered orally its bioavailability is close to 80% and it is afterwards metabolized into its main active metabolite, oxypurinol, which is not a selective inhibitor of XOI. Approved maximal doses vary widely, ranging from 300 to 900 mg/day, and it is recommended to start at low doses (100 mg/day) and increase dose as needed and if tolerated to reach target SUA level. Its half-life is close to 24 hours in subjects with normal renal function; accordingly, it is prescribed once daily, although a twice-daily administration may be considered for doses over 300 mg/day or in patients with poor tolerability.

Oxypurinol is almost completely cleared by the kidney as an active metabolite [18] through renal tubular urate transporters. The PK of allopurinol may change—increasing half-life and serum levels—in patients with reduced glomerular filtration and in those on drugs which enhance tubular reabsorption, such as diuretics [19].

The efficacy of allopurinol in patients with normal renal function is close to 1 mg/dL (60 μmol/L) per 100 mg/day dose [7,20], the effectiveness being dependent on the final dose prescribed. Doses are recommended to be adjusted to glomerular filtration rate (GFR) in patients with CKD: initial doses lower than 1.5 mg/day per mL of GFR have been shown to be associated with lower risk of adverse events [21], and progressive increase of doses may help achieve effectiveness [22]; step-up dosing to 4–6 mg/day per mL of GFR have also been shown to be associated with low risk of adverse events [23].

Allopurinol is generally well tolerated, not differing from other ULDs, but only doses up to 300 mg/day or lower if adjusted for GFR were considered [24,25]. The most common, but infrequent, adverse events reported are increased liver function tests and skin rash. Severe, but rare, adverse events include drug-related eosinophilia with systemic symptoms (DRESS [26], which includes what was previously known as 'allopurinol hypersensitivity syndrome') and severe cutaneous adverse reactions (SCAR [27], which includes Stevens–Johnson syndrome and toxic epidermal necrolysis). These severe and potentially fatal adverse reactions (especially DRESS when multiorgan failure develops), appear early after the initiation of allopurinol and have been associated with full, non-adjusted doses in patients with CKD and the human leucocyte antigen (HLA) allele B*5801 [27,28], through drug-specific T cells that are activated by oxypurinol bound to HLA-B*5801 [29].

Febuxostat is a new non-purine-related, selective, potent inhibitor of both isoforms (oxidized and reduced) of xanthine oxidase [30]. It is widely available, approved doses ranging from 10 mg/day for asymptomatic hyperuricaemia in Japan, to 120 mg/day for gout in the European Union (EU). Its bioavailability after oral intake is over 80%, its PK being linear with doses ranging from 10 to 120 mg/day, with an average half-life of 12 hours and is therefore to be prescribed once daily. Febuxostat is metabolized in the liver to mostly inactive metabolites that are excreted through the urine. Its PK is not significantly modified by the presence of mild to moderate renal function impairment, mild liver dysfunction, non-steroidal anti-inflammatory drugs or colchicine intake [31–33]. The efficacy of febuxostat is close to fivefold that of allopurinol milligram to milligram of dose; in clinical trials, no difference was observed between febuxostat 40 mg/day and allopurinol 300 mg/day; for 80 mg/day the reduction was 4.4 mg/dL (44.7% from baseline of 9.8 mg/dL) and 5.1 mg/dL (51.5% from a baseline of 9.9 mg/dL) for patients on febuxostat 120 mg/day [17]. As its PK is not significantly modified by mild to moderate GFR descent [34], and shows a sharp reduction of SUA levels at approved doses [35], it is an alternative to allopurinol as first-line ULD [8], especially in patients with the highest baseline SUA, with mild to moderate

renal function impairment, and on diuretics [36]. Limited experience is available in patients with renal transplant [37] and severe CKD [38].

The safety of labelled doses of febuxostat is similar to that of allopurinol at 300 mg/day or lower [24,25,35]. The most commonly observed adverse events are increase of liver function tests and thyroid-stimulating hormone levels. Severe hypersensitivity reactions are uncommon, even in patients with previous adverse events to allopurinol [39]. Cardiovascular safety from pivotal clinical trials raised some concerns, with some labels recommending not prescribing febuxostat to patients with ischaemic heart disease or chronic heart failure. To address this issue, research on high-risk population for cardiovascular events is ongoing [40].

Inhibitors of renal reabsorption of urate: uricosuric medications

Uricosurics are medications which target urate tubular transporters, mostly hURAT-1, inhibiting the reabsorption of uric acid and enhancing its leakage in the urine. Therefore, uricosurics are to be used mainly in patients with inefficient renal excretion of uric acid [41], or in combination with XOIs, as prescription in patients with efficient excretion may increase the risk of renal lithiasis [42]. A previous history of renal stones and CKD are limitations to uricosurics. Uricosurics are currently considered as second-line ULDs in monotherapy or in addition to XOIs [8,14].

Probenecid and benzbromarone are not available worldwide, or their prescription is limited, and sulfinpyrazone has been withdrawn in most countries [43]. Probenecid and sulfinpyrazone are not potent uricosurics, and therefore not effective in patients with moderate decrease in GFR. They have to be prescribed several times daily, and their tolerability at the highest doses (that are needed to be effective) is poor. Benzbromarone is a potent uricosuric drug, labelled at doses ranging from 50 to 200 mg/day in a single oral dose. It is not approved in the United States, and is restricted, if available, in most countries of the EU. It is excreted mainly through the bile, its PK is therefore not mostly dependent on renal function, and it is effective in patients with moderate renal function impairment. Benzbromarone is generally well tolerated, but infrequent cases of severe, acute liver toxicity have been reported [43].

Lesinurad has been recently approved by the Food and Drug Administration and the European Medicines Agency at doses of 200 mg once a day in combination with a XOI when target SUA is not achieved with a XOI in monotherapy. It is advised to evaluate at baseline and monitor renal function during follow-up regularly [44].

Pegloticase

Pegloticase was developed as a recombinant porcine uricase containing several residues from the baboon sequence, conjugated with nine strands of polyethylene glycol [45]. It has been labelled at doses of 8 mg administered intravenously every 2 weeks for the treatment of severe gout refractory to other ULDs available. Response (80% of the time between months 3 and 6) was observed overall in 42% of the patients in two pivotal studies [46]. The main safety concern is the development of infusion reactions, and facilities to manage these reactions must be available at the infusion centre. Lack or loss of response is associated to SUA levels over 6 mg/dL (360 μmol/L) prior to the infusion while on treatment and with the presence of anti-pegloticase antibodies, preceded infusion reactions in 79% of the patients in the phase III clinical trials.

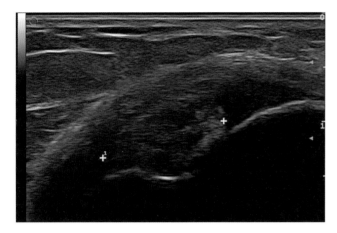

Figure 46.2 Ultrasonography of the lateral aspect of the knee showing a tophus; it can be measured for follow-up.
© F. Perez-Ruiz, with permission.

Therefore, if the pre-infusion SUA level is above target, withdrawal of treatment is recommended.

Outcomes of long-term treatment

Long-term adequate treatment of gout is associated with a reduction in the number of episodes of inflammation, which in turn is associated with improvement in patient-reported quality of life [47]. Nevertheless, the evaluation of the change of MSU crystal deposits may be especially interesting not only for clinical trials, but also for clinical practice in selected patients (Figure 46.2), in order to optimize targets for ULT [48] in patients with severe disease.

Clinical evaluation

SUA levels should be monitored during follow-up, first to assess effectiveness, second to ensure that adequate target SUA levels are sustained in the long term. Measurement of subcutaneous tophi is a reliable, easy, and inexpensive way to evaluate deposits during follow-up. Although several methods [49], including tape measures and photographs have been used, the measurement of tophi using calipers is the most reliable to date (Figure 46.3). Measurement of bursal tophi is not advised, due to the frequent presence of varying amount of fluid that may bias evaluation.

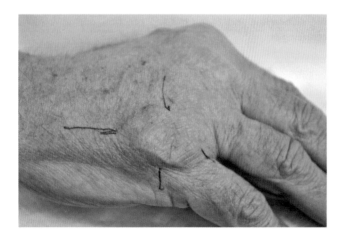

Figure 46.3 Measuring subcutaneous tophi: borders are marked using a pen.
© F. Perez-Ruiz, with permission.

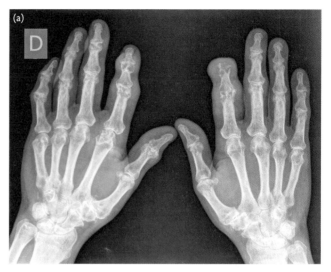

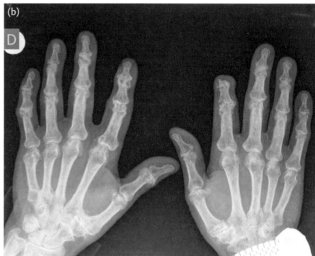

Figure 46.4 Improvement in X-ray erosion after intensive ULT: (a) baseline, (b) follow-up; nevertheless, structural cartilage damage (joint space narrowing) remains unchanged.
© F. Perez-Ruiz, with permission.

Imaging evaluation

Simple radiography (X-ray), ultrasonography (US), magnetic resonance imaging (MRI), computed tomography (CT), and dual-energy CT (DECT) has been used to date to evaluate MSU deposition and the effect of ULT, focused mostly in aggregates or tophi (Figure 46.4). Until now, only US has fulfilled most of the criteria as a valid outcome measure, but investigation is still in progress [49]. US allows the evaluation of deposits, superficial structural damage (erosions), and associated inflammation (power Doppler signal), whereas CT and DECT evaluate deposits and structural damage, but not inflammation. MRI is not specific for deposits, but may be useful to evaluate structural damage and inflammation (gadolinium-enhanced MRI).

References

1. Doherty M, Jansen TL, Nuki G, et al. Gout: why is this curable disease so seldom cured? *Ann Rheum Dis* 2012; 71(11):1765–70.
2. Perez Ruiz F, Herrero-Beites AM. Evaluation and treatment of gout as a chronic disease. *Adv Ther* 2012; 29(11):935–46.

3. Wortmann RL, MacDonald PA, Hunt B, Jackson RL. Effect of prophylaxis on gout flares after the initiation of urate-lowering therapy: analysis of data from three phase III trials. *Clin Ther* 2011; 32(14):2386–97.

4. Perez-Ruiz F, Lioté F. Lowering serum uric acid levels: what is the optimal target for improving clinical outcomes in gout? *Arthritis Rheum* 2007; 57(7):1324–8.

5. Perez-Ruiz F. Treating to target: a strategy to cure gout. *Rheumatology* 2009; 49:ii9–12.

6. Perez-Ruiz F, Herrero-Beites AM, Carmona L. A two-stage approach to the treatment of hyperuricemia in gout: the 'Dirty Dish' hypothesis. *Arthritis Rheum* 2011; 63(12):4002–6.

7. Zhang W, Doherty M, Pascual E, et al. EULAR evidence based recommendations for gout Part II. Management. Report of a Task Force of the EULAR Standing Committee for international clinical studies including therapeutics (ESCISIT). *Ann Rheum Dis* 2006; 65:1312–24.

8. Khanna D, Fitzgerald JD, Khanna PP, et al. 2012 American College of Rheumatology guidelines for management of gout. Part 1: Systematic nonpharmacologic and pharmacologic therapeutic approaches to hyperuricemia. *Arthritis Care Res (Hoboken)* 2012; 64(10):1431–46.

9. Rees F, Jenkins W, Doherty M. Patients with gout adhere to curative treatment if informed appropriately: proof-of-concept observational study. *Ann Rheum Dis* 2013; 72(6):826–30.

10. Annemans L, Spaepen E, Gaskin M, et al. Gout in the UK and Germany: prevalence, comorbidities and management in general practice 2000-2005. *Ann Rheum Dis* 2007; 67:960–6.

11. Choi HK, Curhan G. Gout: epidemiology and lifestyle choices. *Curr Opin Rheumatol* 2005; 17(3):341–5.

12. Perez-Ruiz F. New treatments for gout. *Bone Joint Spine* 2007; 74(4):313–5.

13. Diaz-Torne C, Perez-Herrero N, Perez-Ruiz F. New medications in development for the treatment of hyperuricemia of gout. *Curr Opin Rheumatol* 2015; 27(2):164–9.

14. Richette P, Doherty M, Pascual E, et al. Updated EULAR evidence-based recommendations for the management of gout. *Ann Rheum Dis* 2014; 73(Suppl 2):783.

15. Cea Soriano L, Rothenbacher D, Choi HK, Garcia Rodriguez LA. Contemporary epidemiology of gout in the UK general population. *Arthritis Res Ther* 2011; 13:R39.

16. Perez-Ruiz F, Calabozo M, Fernandez-Lopez MJ, et al. Treatment of chronic gout in patients with renal function impairment. An open, randomized, actively controlled. *J Clin Rheumatol* 1999; 5:49–55.

17. Becker MA, Schumacher HR Jr, Wortmann RL, et al. Febuxostat compared with allopurinol in patients with hyperuricemia and gout. *N Engl J Med* 2005; 353(23):2450–61.

18. Day RO, Graham GG, Hicks M, et al. Clinical pharmacokinetics and pharmacodynamics of allopurinol and oxypurinol. *Clin Pharmacokinet* 2007; 46(8):623–44.

19. Stamp LK, Barclay ML, O'Donnell JL, et al. Furosemide increases plasma oxypurinol without lowering serum urate—a complex drug interaction: implications for clinical practice. *Rheumatology (Oxford)* 2012; 51(1670):1676.

20. Jansen TL, Richette P, Perez-Ruiz F, et al. International position paper on febuxostat. *Clin Rheumatol* 2010; 29:835–40.

21. Stamp LK, Taylor WJ, Jones PB, et al. Starting dose is a risk factor for allopurinol hypersensitivity syndrome: a proposed safe starting dose of allopurinol. *Arthritis Rheum* 2012; 64(8):2529–36.

22. Jennings CG, Mackenzie IS, Flynn R, et al. Up-titration of allopurinol in patients with gout. *Semin Arthritis Rheum* 2014; 44(1):25–30.

23. Perez-Ruiz F, Hernando I, Villar I, Nolla JM. Correction of allopurinol dosing should be based on clearance of creatinine, but not plasma creatinine levels. Another insight to allopurinol-related toxicity. *J Clin Rheumatol* 2005; 11:129–33.

24. Seth R, Kydd AS, Buchbinder R, Bombardier C, Edwards CJ. Allopurinol for chronic gout. *Cochrane Database Syst Rev* 2014; 10:CD006077.

25. Castrejon I, Toledano E, Rosario MP, et al. Safety of allopurinol compared with other urate-lowering drugs in patients with gout: a systematic review and meta-analysis. *Rheumatol Int* 2015; 35(7):1127–37.

26. Markel A. Allopurinol-induced DRESS syndrome. *IMAJ* 2005; 7:656–60.

27. Mockenhaupt M, Viboud C, Dunant A, et al. Stevens-Johnson syndrome and toxic epidermal necrolysis: assessment of medication risks with emphasis on recently marketed drugs. The EuroSCAR-Study. *J Invest Dermatol* 2007.

28. Lonjou C, Borot N, Sekula P, et al. A European study of HLA-B in Stevens-Johnson syndrome and toxic epidermal necrolysis related to five high-risk drugs. *Pharmacogenet Genomics* 2008; 18(2):99–107.

29. Yun J, Marcaida MJ, Eriksson KK, et al. Oxypurinol directly and immediately activates the drug-specific T cells via the preferential use of HLA-B*58:01. *J Immunol* 2014; 192(7):2984–93.

30. Okamoto K, Eger BT, Nishino T, et al. An extremely potent inhibitor of xanthine oxidoreductase. Crystal structure of the enzyme-inhibitor complex and mechanism of inhibition. *J Biol Chem* 2003; 278(3):1848–55.

31. Khosravan R, Grabowski BA, Mayer MD, et al. The effect of mild and moderate hepatic impairment on pharmacokinetics, pharmacodynamics, and safety of febuxostat, a novel nonpurine selective inhibitor of xanthine oxidase. *J Clin Pharmacol* 2006; 46:88–102.

32. Khosravan R, Wu JT, Joseph-Ridge N, Vernillet L. Pharmacokinetic interactions of concomitant administration of febuxostat and NSAIDs. *J Clin Pharmacol* 2006; 46(8):855–66.

33. Khosravan R, Kukulka MJ, Wu JT, Joseph-Ridge N, Vernillet L. The effect of age and gender on pharmacokinetics, pharmacodynamics, and safety of febuxostat, a novel nonpurine selective inhibitor of xanthine oxidase. *J Clin Pharmacol* 2008; 48(9):1014–24.

34. Mayer MD, Khosravan R, Vernillet L, et al. Pharmacokinetics and pharmacodynamics of febuxostat, a new non-purine selective inhibitor of xanthine oxidase in subjects with renal impairment. *Am J Ther* 2005; 12(1):22–34.

35. Tayar JH, Lopez-Olivo MA, Suarez-Almazor ME. Febuxostat for treating chronic gout. *Cochrane Database Syst Rev* 2012; 11:CD008653.

36. Perez-Ruiz F, Dalbeth N, Schlesinger N. Febuxostat, a novel drug for the treatment of hyperuricemia of gout. *Future Rheumatol* 2008; 3(5):421–7.

37. Tojimbara T, Nakajima I, Yashima J, Fuchinoue S, Teraoka S. Efficacy and safety of febuxostat, a novel nonpurine selective inhibitor of xanthine oxidase for the treatment of hyperuricemia in kidney transplant recipients. *Transplant Proc* 2014; 46(2):511–3.

38. Shibagaki Y, Ohno I, Hosoya T, Kimura K. Safety, efficacy and renal effect of febuxostat in patients with moderate-to-severe kidney dysfunction. *Hypertens Res* 2014; 37(10):919–25.

39. Stamp LK. Safety profile of anti-gout agents: an update. *Curr Opin Rheumatol* 2014; 26(2):162–8.

40. MacDonald TM, Ford I, Nuki G, et al. Protocol of the Febuxostat versus Allopurinol Streamlined Trial (FAST): a large prospective, randomised, open, blinded endpoint study comparing the cardiovascular safety of allopurinol and febuxostat in the management of symptomatic hyperuricaemia. *BMJ Open* 2014; 4(7):e005354.

41. Perez-Ruiz F, Calabozo M, Garcia-Erauskin G, Ruibal A, Herrero-Beites AM. Renal underexcretion of uric acid is present in patients with apparent high urinary uric acid output. *Arthritis Rheum* 2002; 47(6):610–3.

42. Perez-Ruiz F, Hernandez-Baldizon S, Herrero-Beites AM, Gonzalez-Gay MA. Risk factors associated with renal lithiasis during uricosuric treatment of hyperuricemia in patients with gout. *Arthritis Care Res (Hoboken)* 2010; 62(9):1299–305.

43. Perez-Ruiz F, Herrero-Beites AM, Atxotegi J. Uricosuric therapy of hyperuricemia in gout. In Terkeltaub RA (ed) *Gout & Other Crystal Arthropathies*. Philadelphia, PA: Elsevier; 2011:148–53.

44. Perez-Ruiz F, Sundy JS, Miner JN, et al. Lesinurad in combination with allopurinol: results of a phase 2, randomized, double-blind study in patients with gout with an inadequate response

to allopurinol. *Ann Rheum Dis* 2016. [Epub ahead of print]. DOI: 10.1136/annrheumdis-2015-207919.

45. Sherman MR, Saifer MGP, Perez-Ruiz F. PEG-uricase in the management of treatment-resistant gout and hyperuricemia. *Adv Drug Deliv Rev* 2008; 60(1):59–68.

46. Sundy JS, Baraf HSB, Yood RA, et al. Efficacy and tolerability of pegloticase for the treatment of chronic gout in patients refractory to conventional treatment. Two randomized controlled trials. *JAMA* 2011; 306(7):711–20.

47. Khanna PP, Perez-Ruiz F, Maranian P, Khanna D. Long-term therapy for chronic gout results in clinically important improvements in the health-related quality of life: short form-36 is responsive to change in chronic gout. *Rheumatology (Oxford)* 2011; 50(4):740–5.

48. Perez-Ruiz F, Schlesinger N, Dalbeth N, Urresola A, De Miguel E. Imaging of gout: findings and utility. *Arthritis Res Ther* 2009; 11(3):232.

49. Dalbeth N, Schauer C, MacDonald P, et al. Methods of tophus assessment in clinical trials of chronic gout: a systematic literature review and pictorial reference guide. *Ann Rheum Dis* 2011; 70(4):597–604.

CHAPTER 47

Asymptomatic hyperuricaemia: to treat or not to treat?

Thomas Bardin

Introduction

Asymptomatic hyperuricaemia is a frequent finding, which has been variously interpreted across time. Its association with hypertension, the metabolic syndrome, and cardiovascular diseases has long been recognized (reviewed in [1]). Following the lack of independent association between asymptomatic hyperuricaemia and cardiovascular death in the Framingham Heart Study [2], it has been recommended not to treat asymptomatic hyperuricaemia but to focus on the associated comorbidities which were believed to explain the increased cardiovascular risk associated with hyperuricaemia in non-adjusted analysis. Hyperuricaemia indeed associates with various comorbidities in a dose-dependent fashion [3,4]. Even if the issue is still disputed, the dogma not to treat asymptomatic hyperuricaemia has been recently challenged by a large number of results from animal and human studies that supported the view that hyperuricaemia was an independent cardiovascular risk factor and might predict the development of other well-established risk factors for cardiovascular disease [5].

Definition of hyperuricaemia

The definition of hyperuricaemia varies across studies, and can be different for men and women. For gout we proposed a serum urate (SUA) threshold of 360 µmol/L (6 mg/dL) in men and women as it seemed that the lifelong risk of urate deposition started at this value in both sexes [6]. For cardiovascular diseases, the potential risk appears to similarly increase continuously with SUA; few studies aimed at determining the SUA at which cardiovascular risk started to increase. The SUA threshold might depend on the age and sex and could be lower than 360 µmol/L (6 mg/dL), especially in women. For hypertension, Gaffo et al. [7] found that, in the cohort of young adults they examined, the risk of developing hypertension during follow-up started at 345 µmol/L in men and 214 µmol/L in women. In the Framingham cohorts [8], SUAs higher than 300 µmol/L (5 mg/dL) were associated with an increased risk of type 2 diabetes. In the Pressiori Arteriose E Loro Assessioni (PAMELA) study [9], receiver operator characteristic analysis of data identified a cutoff value of 324 µmol/L (5.4 mg/dL) and 285 µmol/L (4.9 mg/dL) for the best prediction of cardiovascular and all-cause mortality respectively.

Epidemiological aspects

Serum urate varies with age, sex, ethnicity, and time in the normal populations [10]. Women have lower SUA than men until menopause [11], when SUA increases due to the loss of uricosuric oestrogen secretion. Hyperuricaemia is a frequent condition, especially in men. Prevalence estimates have depended on the retained definition of hyperuricaemia, the time of the study, and the population studied. Highest prevalences have been reported in Taiwan aboriginals [12,13] and New Zealand Māori [14]. In the US National Health and Nutrition Survey (NHANES) 2007–2008, the prevalence of hyperuricaemia, defined as greater than 420 µmol/L (7 mg/dL) was estimated at 23% and was higher in black people (25.7% versus 22.1% in non-black people) [3]. In Italy, prevalence of hyperuricaemia (defined as >360 µmol/L (6 mg/L) was estimated in 2009 at 11.9% [15]. Both studies showed the prevalence to increase with time, making even more important the question of treating or not treating asymptomatic hyperuricaemia.

Asymptomatic hyperuricaemia and the risk of gout and nephrolithiasis

Hyperuricaemia is the main, if not the only, risk factor for gout. However, not every hyperuricaemic individual will develop gout and it is commonly estimated that only about 15% of hyperuricaemic individuals suffer from gout. The risk of gout increases with the level of hyperuricaemia, as nicely shown 30 years ago by the elegant Normative Aging Study [16]. It also increases with the duration of hyperuricaemia as monosodium urate (MSU) crystal formation is a slow process. However, the risk of gout is not considered as an indication to treat asymptomatic hyperuricaemia by urate-lowering drugs (ULDs), as the risk/benefit ratio of these drugs is probably unfavourable in such a situation, if one takes apart the potential cardiovascular risk. Ultrasound scans can detect asymptomatic MSU deposits in approximately 30% of asymptomatic hyperuricaemia patients [17]. It is likely that these asymptomatic deposits increase the risk of developing clinical gout, but no study has yet investigated this question. Asymptomatic hyperuricaemia can be associated with increased concentration of uric acid in the urine, a known risk factor for uric acid nephrolithiasis and a debated factor for calcium oxalate stones (18), but no ULD has been approved to prevent this risk when no lithiasis has developed.

Animal studies of the cardiovascular risk associated with hyperuricaemia

Animal studies support a pathological role for hyperuricaemia in the development of hypertension, renal disease, and the metabolic syndrome. Mild and chronic hyperuricaemia in rats was first obtained by the group of Richard Johnson by enriching the diet with oxonic acid, an inhibitor of urate oxidase which normally keeps SUA low in these animals. They observed that hyperuricaemic rats developed hypertension, which could be reversed by ULDs, provided these were given early [19]. Kidney changes included mild tubular atrophy and a primary preglomerular arteriolopathy, which was still observed when blood pressure was maintained as normal by diuretics, but was prevented by enalapril and losartan, suggesting that it was mediated by activation of the renin–angiotensin system. Urate was shown to stimulate smooth muscle vascular cells proliferation *in vitro* and this was similarly mediated by the renin–angiotensin system [20]. Importantly, after an early phase when hyperuricaemia-induced hypertension could be corrected by ULDs, came a second phase, with irreversible salt-sensitive hypertension which could not be improved anymore by ULDs [21]. If one translates these animal findings to humans, ULDs should be beneficial only at the onset of hyperuricaemia, and this could be a major limitation of their therapeutic use. Renal lesions in these hyperuricaemic animals included overtime glomerulosclerosis and interstitial disease. Hyperuricaemia was also shown to worsen renal function in the 5/6 nephrectomy model [22], ciclosporin-induced renal disease [23] in diabetic nephropathy [24] in mice, whereas lowering urate could improve these kidney diseases [25]. The Johnson group later produced hyperuricaemia in rats by feeding them with a fructose-enriched diet [26]. Fructose-fed rats again developed renal hypertension that could be alleviated by allopurinol. Additional features of the metabolic syndrome were observed, such as hypertriglyceridaemia and hyperinsulinaemia, the latter being corrected by ULDs. Hyperuricaemic animals gained weight and this was reduced by allopurinol.

Another group recently produced a third animal model of hyperuricaemia, by selectively deleting the intestine Glut9 transporter in mice, therefore decreasing the intestinal secretion of acid uric and increasing SUA, despite increased uricuria [27]. This lead to a full metabolic syndrome including gain weight, hypertension, hypertriglyceridaemia and hypercholesterolaemia, liver steatosis, increased fasting glycaemia, and hyperinsulinaemia. Allopurinol was shown to prevent gain weight, hypertension, hypercholesterolaemia, and liver steatosis.

Taken together, these various animal models strongly suggest that hyperuricaemia may induce the main features of the metabolic syndrome and kidney disease, and that ULDs may prevent most of these features. Box 47.1 shows the main cellular mechanisms implicated in the deleterious effects of urate [28,29]. Schematically these mechanisms seem to be related to increased intracellular concentrations, whereas extracellular urate has long been known to exhibit beneficial antioxidant properties.

Human studies

Hyperuricaemia and mortality

Several studies of large prospectively followed cohorts aimed to determine if baseline hyperuricaemia was associated with increased

---

Box 47.1 Potential cellular mechanisms of urate toxicity

- Inhibition of NO synthetase, reduction of endothelial NO production [30]
- Stimulation of NADPH oxidase [31]
- Release of alarmins from the endothelial cell [22,32]
- Stimulation of the renin–angiotensin system [22]
- Stimulation of the proliferation of vascular smooth muscle cells [20,22]
- Stimulation of MCP1 production in vascular smooth muscle cells [33]
- Increased COX2 endothelial expression and thromboxane stimulation [22]
- Activation of circulating platelets [34]
- Increase in the production of proinflammatory cytokines [35]
- Induction of renal inflammation via activation of tubular NF kappa B signalling pathway [36]
- Induction of an epithelial-mesenchymal transition [37]
- Induction of insulin resistance through impairment of insulin-mediated release of NO leading to decrease of glucose uptake by skeletal muscle and peripheral tissues
- Induction of oxidative stress and inflammation in the adipocytes [38].

---

mortality, in particular cardiovascular mortality, after adjustment for accepted cardiovascular risk factors [2,9,39–44]. The cut-off value to define hyperuricaemia and the adjustment variables varied across studies. Most but not all of these studies were positive. A meta-analysis of 11 studies available in April 2013 concluded that an elevated SUA increased the risks of all-cause mortality (relative risk (RR) 1.24, 95% confidence interval (CI) 1.08–1.42) and cardiovascular mortality (RR 1.37, 95% CI 1.19–1.57). The increase in all-cause mortality was observed among men but not in women; the risk of cardiovascular mortality was found to be more pronounced in women [45]. In addition to studies in the general population, SUA has also been shown to be a significant independent predictor of all-cause and/or cardiovascular mortality for patients with gout [43,46], chronic kidney disease (CKD) [47], coronary heart disease [48], hypertension [49], patients at high risk of cardiovascular disease [50], and overweight/obese individuals (51). A few studies suggested that very low SUAs were also predictive of increased mortality [40,49,52,53], including in renal failure patients [54]. This finding—which appears to require confirmation—might be explained by the antioxidant effect of circulating urate or by the fact that low SUA may be linked to malnutrition and poor general health.

Hyperuricaemia and hypertension

In cross-sectional studies, hyperuricaemia significantly associates with hypertension [4,55]. In longitudinal studies, hyperuricaemia predicts hypertension. Numerous studies of large prospective cohorts have now shown that baseline SUA antedated the development of hypertension. Two recently published meta-analyses confirmed the incidence of hypertension to continuously increase with baseline hyperuricaemia [56,57]. In these two meta-analyses, the adjusted RR of hypertension for a 60 µmol/L (1 mg/dL) SUA increase was 1.13 (95% CI 1.06–1.20) and 1.15 (95% CI 1.06–1.26) respectively. The effect was consistent across diverse populations, although it seemed higher in black individuals and lower in US-based studies [56]. The risk appeared more pronounced in younger individuals and women. The question of the time frame during which hypertension develops following hyperuricaemia remains little addressed. In the Framingham cohort, the adjusted risk was significant at a 4-year follow-up, when an SD increment in SUA was comparable with a 5-year age increment [58]. It became non-significant in the multivariate analysis made at the 12-year follow-up period, possibly due a larger effect at a young age and a higher background of incident hypertension not linked to SUA after 12 years, but the lower number of individuals analysed at this longer follow-up might also have made the analysis underpowered.

In children, the association of hyperuricaemia with primary hypertension appears even stronger. In a prospective evaluation of children referred for hypertension with no renal failure, Feig et al. reported that 89% of 63 children with primary hypertension had SUA higher than 330 µmol/L (5.5 mg/dL). This contrasted with the 40 young patients with secondary hypertension, of whom only 30% were hyperuricaemic, suggesting that hyperuricaemia was not secondary to hypertension itself but was more likely to play a role in the pathophysiology of primary hypertension [59]. In primary hypertension and control groups, but not in secondary hypertension, SUA correlated with systolic and diastolic blood pressures. Childhood hyperuricaemia has been shown to predict adult hypertension [60].

Together with the animal study results, these data have prompted intervention trials to evaluate the effect of urate-lowering therapy on blood pressure. In 2013, Agarwal et al. published the results of their meta-analysis of ten clinical studies (nine randomized, one prospective) with a total of 738 participants, that investigated the effect of allopurinol on blood pressure [61]. The daily dose of allopurinol varied widely across studies, from 100 mg to 900 mg, and so did the ages of the included patients from 15 to 78 years, the study durations, from 1 to 24 months, and the number of comorbidities of included patients. From these very heterogeneous studies, the authors concluded that allopurinol was associated with a small but significant reduction of systolic (in the range of 3 mmHg) and diastolic (about 1.3 mmHg) blood pressures. The beneficial effect of allopurinol was also recently observed in a study of the GPRD database that compared 365 individuals, aged over 65 years, who were started on allopurinol, to 6678 propensity matched controls. In this study, allopurinol associated with a dose-dependent decrease in diastolic and systolic blood pressures [62]. However, the most convincing data came from two randomized placebo-controlled studies performed in adolescents, in whom hyperuricaemia was likely to be of recent onset, which may have favoured an effect of SUA on blood pressure at a time when blood pressure increase was still reversible. In a short-term (4 weeks) crossover study of 30 adolescents with newly diagnosed essential hypertension and SUA of at least 360 µmol/L (6 mg/dL), allopurinol 400 mg/day decreased the renin levels and normalized blood pressure in 20 patients [63]. A second study enrolled 60 obese, prehypertensive adolescents who were randomized to placebo, allopurinol 200 mg twice daily, or probenecid 500 mg twice daily for 7 weeks [64]. Subjects treated with both types of urate-lowering

drugs experienced a highly significant reduction of blood pressure and of systemic vascular resistance. These results favour the idea that hyperuricaemia (and not xanthine oxidase activity) can cause hypertension. Interestingly whereas patients treated with placebo continued to gain weight, those on ULDs did not, a finding consistent with the observation that hyperuricaemia predicted gain weight and hypertension in one human study [65] and in the fructose-fed rats [26]. However, the hypothesis that hyperuricaemia might induce weight gain has recently been very much challenged by the Mendelian randomization analysis of two Danish cohorts, which demonstrated that weight gain increased SUA and did not support the reverse mechanism [66].

Hyperuricaemia and kidney function

Recent studies [67,68] have confirmed that hyperuricaemia and gout frequencies increased in parallel with decline in the estimated glomerular filtration rate (eGFR). Hyperuricaemia similarly increased with proteinuria. A recent meta-analysis of 17 studies estimated the prevalence of CKD stage higher than 3 in gout patients at 24% (95% CI 19–28%) [69]. An explanation for this association has been to consider hyperuricaemia as a marker rather than a pathological factor of CKD. Urate indeed is excreted through the kidneys and SUA usually rises when renal function deteriorates, despite increased elimination by the intestine. The classical gouty nephropathy has been denied for years, as MSU crystals in the medulla did not correlate with renal function decline, and renal changes could be explained by the frequently associated hypertension. However, the finding of similar lesions, apart from MSU crystals, in hyperuricaemic rats has revived the hypothesis that soluble urate may be toxic to the kidney. In line with this hypothesis, most longitudinal studies of normal baseline renal function cohorts have shown that hyperuricaemia was an independent predictor for the development of incident kidney disease [29]. This observation, when made in healthy, normotensive individuals, appears not to be mediated by hypertension or hyperuricaemic drugs (70). In addition some, but not all, studies found that hyperuricaemia was predictive of renal function deterioration in various nephropathies, in particular immunoglobulin A [71,72], diabetic [73–75], and chronic allograft nephropathies [76,77].

Pilot studies have been performed to test the ability of ULDs to improve renal function in CKD. After intensive screening (most Korean CKD patients were already treated by allopurinol), Siu et al. were able to randomize 51 hyperuricaemic patients with mild to moderate CKD into allopurinol (100–300 mg/day) or placebo. At 1 year, the allopurinol-treated patients had less renal disease progression [78]. A larger study was subsequently published by Goicoechea et al. [79], which included 113 hyperuricaemic CKD patients, who, in addition to standard treatment, were randomly assigned to either allopurinol (100 mg/day) or no additional treatment. After 2 years, eGFR increased in the allopurinol group by 1.3 ± 1.3 mL/min whereas it decreased in the non-treated group by 3.3 ± 1.2 mL/min. Wang et al. [80] recently published a meta-analysis of 11 RCTs, among which 6 were written in Chinese. Studies enrolled a total of 753 patients; allopurinol (100 to 300 mg/day) was tested in 11 studies and rasburicase and benzbromarone in one each. The meta-analysis confirmed that urate lowering was associated with a protection of renal function. Interestingly, in a Chinese report, benzbromarone was said to have a good effect so that protection might not be explained by xanthine oxidase inhibition. However there was great heterogeneity, in particular in their duration (1 month to 2 years), of the analysed trials, which enrolled overall few patients. Although the presently available data can be considered as encouraging, further studies, including large RCTs, are obviously needed to correctly assess the effect of ULDs on renal failure.

Hyperuricaemia, the metabolic syndrome, and diabetes

Cross-sectional studies show a strong association of hyperuricaemia with the metabolic syndrome, both in gouty [81] and asymptomatic patients [82,83]. The association is stronger in women, increases with the level of hyperuricaemia, involves all the individual components of the syndrome, and has also been observed in children [84]. Diseases commonly associated with the metabolic syndrome such as non-alcoholic fatty liver disease [83,85] and obstructive sleep apnoea [86] have an increased prevalence in hyperuricaemic subjects, even after adjustment for various variables including weight. Longitudinal studies have shown hyperuricaemia to be a risk marker for the metabolic syndrome, which persists after adjustments for body mass index [87–90]. Whereas type 1 diabetes negatively associates with gout [91]—a finding that could be explained by the increased urinary urate excretion caused by polyuria—the risk of hyperinsulinaemia and type 2 diabetes is increased in hyperuricaemic patients, as shown by several prospective studies [8,90,92]. An explanation for the association between hyperuricaemia, hyperinsulinaemia, and type 2 diabetes could rely on the promoting effect of insulinaemia on renal tubular reabsorption of urate, but the sequence of events and the results of animal studies (see above) support the hypothesis that hyperuricaemia is not a consequence of but a risk factor for type 2 diabetes.

A short-term and small randomized placebo-controlled study found that allopurinol was able to reduce the incidence of metabolic syndrome following a high fructose diet in humans, with, however, no effect on blood fasting glucose [93].

Hyperuricaemia and the heart

Coronary artery disease

Several epidemiological studies have investigated the association of coronary artery disease (CAD) with hyperuricaemia [94–99]. A majority supported an independent association of CAD with hyperuricaemia. The association appeared as weaker than with gout and was stronger in women, in younger patients, and in those with fewer cardiovascular risk factors. A cross-sectional study of acute coronary syndrome patients disclosed more coronary artery calcification in hyperuricaemic patients with asymptomatic MSU deposition than in those with no crystal deposition [100]. A recent pathological study found negatively birefringent crystals in coronary arteries in 6 of 55 hearts explanted during transplantation, suggesting that MSU crystal deposition might play a role in the CAD risk associated with hyperuricaemia [101], in addition to the proatherotic effect of excessive soluble urate [5].

Hyperuricaemia appears as predictive of a poor outcome in patients with CAD. In a prospective study of 8149 patients with stable CAD after percutaneous coronary intervention, followed-up for 1 year, the adjusted hazard ratio for mortality was 1.71 (95% CI 1.22–2.39) for patients in the highest quartile of SUA (>450 μmol/L (7.5 mg/dL) as compared to the others, and was evaluated at 1.10

(95% CI 1.01–1.20) for each 60 μmol/L (1 mg/dL) increase in SUA level [102]. The same group observed, in an even larger cohort of CHD patients, that the relationship between mortality and SUA followed a J-shaped curve with lowest risk of death in patients with uric acid levels between 310μmol/L (5.17 mg/dL) and 406 μmol/L (6.76 mg/dL) [103]. Hyperuricaemia was also associated with an increased mortality rate in another large study of recent myocardial infarction (MI) patients [104]. A study of patients undergoing primary coronary intervention observed increased hospitalization and mid-term (2-year) mortality rates in patients with hyperuricaemia [105].

A majority of studies that investigated the benefits of ULDs in hyperuricaemic coronary heart disease (CHD) patients concluded that the effect of allopurinol was beneficial. Allopurinol has been shown to improve endothelium function in hyperuricaemic patients [106,107], including in patients with stable CAD [108,109]. Case–control studies suggested that allopurinol use could protect from MI [110,111]: de Abajo et al. observed a sharp (~50%) reduction of non-fatal MI in patients exposed to greater than 300 mg allopurinol daily, for more than 180 days [111]. RCTs support the same conclusions. In CKD patients, Goicoechea et al. observed that major cardiovascular events, including MI, were significantly decreased in the allopurinol group as compared to placebo [79]. A placebo-controlled crossover trial in 65 patients with well-characterized stable CHD, concluded that allopurinol, 600 mg/day, increased total exercise time but also the time to ST-segment depression and the time to symptoms, with effect sizes similar to those associated with traditional antianginal drugs [112]. The same group showed, in another small placebo-controlled trial, that allopurinol 600 mg/day given for 9 months also regressed left ventricular (LV) hypertrophy, LV end-systolic volume, and improved endothelial function in CAD patients with LV hypertrophy [113]. Finally, very early (<12 hours) xanthine oxidase inhibition by allopurinol appeared to improve the short-term prognosis of hyperuricaemic patients with acute MI undergoing primary percutaneous coronary intervention in a small randomized, placebo-controlled trial [114].

Heart failure

A recent meta-analysis concluded that elevated SUA above 420 μmol/L (7 mg/dL) in men and 360 μmol/L (6 mg/dL) in women was associated with a significantly increased risk of heart failure (HF) and that hyperuricaemia was a marker of poor prognosis in patients with HF [115]. Tamariz et al. found that the risk of increased all-cause mortality in hyperuricaemic HF patients became significant from 420 μmol/L (7 mg/dL) to 480 μmol/L (8 mg/dL) [116]. A study of 6224 subjects with HF followed-up for a mean of 498 days found that treatment with allopurinol was independently associated with improved survival [117]. Two very small RCTs also found a positive effect of allopurinol (118, 119). However, more recent, larger studies failed to show that allopurinol improved survival in hyperuricaemic HF patients [120,121]. Overall, the presently available data therefore do not support the idea that decreasing an over-expressed xanthine oxidase activity in HF might be beneficial by inhibiting free radical production by the enzyme [122]. A small study showed no benefit of benzbromarone [123].

Atrial fibrillation

Hyperuricaemia has been shown to be associated with an increased risk of atrial fibrillation [124]. A recent meta-analysis confirmed the association of high SUA with atrial fibrillation in both longitudinal and cross-sectional studies [125]; hyperuricaemia might also increase the risk of left atrial thrombosis and ischaemic stroke associated with atrial fibrillation [126]. No data are available on the effect of ULDs.

Hyperuricaemia and stroke

Prospective studies have shown that hyperuricaemia was associated with an increase in both stroke incidence and mortality [127]. The increased incidence was found to start at SUAs lower in men than in women: between 360 μmol/L (6 mg/dL) and 420 μmol/L (7 mg/dL) in men, and between 300 μmol/L (5 mg/dL) and 360 μmol/L (6 mg/dL) in women [128].

Hyperuricaemia and peripheral artery disease

Gout [129] and hyperuricaemia [130,131] have been found to be associated with peripheral arterial disease.

Mendelian randomization approach of the link between SUA and cardiovascular diseases

In Mendelian randomization studies, a genotype associated with the risk factor of interest is used as an instrumental variable to account for potential confounders and reverse causality. This appears as a very promising tool in the field, given the complexity of the adjustments made in traditional analysis, which may be incomplete. In addition, the fact that hyperuricaemia may play a role in the genesis of traditional risk factors such as hypertension and CKD further complicates multivariable analysis interpretation. Reverse causality cannot be totally excluded in the longitudinal studies that showed association between hyperuricaemia and cardiovascular/renal risk, as preclinical atherosclerosis or kidney involvement could lead to higher urate levels, and favour, independently of urate, the incidence of clinical disease. Numerous genes have been reported to play a part in regulation of SUA levels via genome-wide association studies [132]. However, each of these genes has a minimal impact in SUA variance so that negative results of Mendelian randomization studies must be taken with some caution, as studies may be underpowered unless extremely large cohorts are examined. A study by Palmer et al. in two Danish cohorts did find a weak association of SUA with ischaemic heart disease or blood pressure level. However, no association was seen between these outcomes and a single nucleotide polymorphism (SNP) in the *SLC2A9* gene, which accounted for only 2% of the SUA variance of the studied population [66]. Another study disclosed no association between a different SNP in the *SLC2A9* gene and carotid intima–media thickness [133]. In contrast, a different SNP in the *SLC2A9* gene leading to higher SUA was found to be associated with higher systolic blood pressure [134], and a careful analysis of an Amish cohort found an association of a variant of the same *SLC2A9* gene with hypertension [135]. The later study included only 516 adults, who were put on a standardized diet before obtaining blood pressure measurements. The use of a genetic risk score for high urate might strengthen the power of Mendelian randomization studies, as combining the effects of several genes increases the SUA related changes. In a study including eight gene variants, the score was related with cardiovascular death [136]. However, in a study by Hughes et al., a urate genetic risk score was associated with improved, and not decreased, renal function [137]. In another genetic risk score study, Sedaghat

et al. found 30 gene variants that were associated with increased SUA but with lower blood pressure [138]. In the later study, the results were sensitive to diuretic therapy, and there was no relationship between a *SLC2A9* SNP and blood pressure in patients not treated with diuretics, further highlighting the complexity of the relationship between urate and cardiovascular disease and the persisting possibility of confounders in this type of analysis. These results, together with the lack of agreement between the presently available Mendelian randomization studies, highlight the need for additional studies which, in addition to exploring very large numbers of subjects, should be designed to investigate the effect of urate in defined groups, with attention to concurrent treatments and salt intake.

Hyperuricaemia and cancer

Gout has been associated with various cancers and particularly prostate cancer in a National Health Insurance database of Taiwan [139]. Interestingly, MSU crystals have been observed in prostatic cancer tissues [101]. Other studies have found that hyperuricaemia was associated with a lower incidence of lung cancer [140] and improved survival of colon and pancreas cancer [141,142] so that no clear picture of a potential role of urate in carcinogenesis can be presently pictured.

Serum urate and degenerative diseases of the central nervous system

A number of studies suggested that patients with neurodegenerative disorders had lower SUA than controls, leading to the hypothesis that urate might have a beneficial effect on the central nervous system. A meta-analysis of studies comparing SUA in patients with Alzheimer's disease and matched controls concluded that Alzheimer's disease was associated with lower urate blood concentrations [143]. Similarly, gout negatively associates with Alzheimer's disease [144]. Parkinson's disease also appears to be associated with lower SUA levels [145–147] and gout has been associated with a lower risk of Parkinson's disease [148]. Low serum and cerebral spinal fluid urate concentrations correlated with a greater decline of Parkinson's disease patients [149]. Although a causality link seems far from established, these data may support avoidance of extreme urate lowering (e.g. below 180 μmol/L or 3 ml/dL) when treating hyperuricaemia in the long run.

Should we treat or not treat asymptomatic hyperuricaemia?

Given the amount of data that now suggest that asymptomatic hyperuricaemia might be deleterious for the kidney, the heart, and arteries, it appears reasonable to seriously consider the treatment of hyperuricaemic subjects. This can be achieved, to some extent, by diet and lifestyle changes, and the risk/benefit ratio of dietary advices and exercise appears as, in any case, highly favourable. In particular, weight loss is indicated in the overweight, because of the risk or coexistence of metabolic syndrome. Similarly, hyperuricaemia should prompt a search for and treatment of other cardiovascular risk factors. Drug-induced hyperuricaemia is mainly related to diuretic intake, and despite the hyperuricaemia they induce, diuretics remain largely indicated as the first-line drugs for the management of hypertension because of their good patient acceptability and efficacy. In many countries, including France, nephrologists monitor SUA in their kidney transplant patients and manage hyperuricaemia either by avoiding calcineurin inhibitors which can be substituted by the non-hyperuricaemic mycophenolate mofetil, or by substituting azathioprine to be able to use xanthine oxidase inhibitors [150].

The awareness of the links of gout with cardiovascular diseases has led the European League Against Rheumatism (EULAR) recommendation task force to broaden the indications of ULDs in gout management and to recommend considering the indication of ULDs from the first definite gout flare [151]. The Japanese Society of Gout and Nucleic Acid Metabolism has recommended the treatment of asymptomatic hyperuricaemia above 540 µmol/L (9 mg/dL) in patients with no cardiovascular risk factor and above 480 µmol/L (6.8 mg/dL) in patients with at least one risk factors [152]. Management of asymptomatic hyperuricaemia was not in the scope of the American College of Rheumatology [153] and EULAR [151] recommendations. In contrast, the third initiative specifically did not recommend pharmacological treatment of asymptomatic hyperuricaemia to prevent gouty arthritis, renal disease, or cardiovascular events [154]. In Europe and America, no ULD has been approved for the management of asymptomatic hyperuricaemia, even if the European labelling of febuxostat allows treatment of asymptomatic MSU deposits. The lack of approval is explained by the persistence of debates about the toxicity of soluble urate, and to the impossibility of clearly defining the benefit of ULDs, facing the lack of large RCTs investigating their effect on cardiovascular and renal hard clinical outcomes. Such studies are clearly needed, which should also settle the issues of the level of SUA to be targeted and the type of drugs to be used for cardiovascular benefits. If preliminary data suggest that urate lowering either by a xanthine oxidase inhibitor or a uricosuric drug could be used to target hypertension [64], xanthine oxidase inhibition could be a better tool in other vascular diseases such as CAD, in which the effects of uricosurics have not yet been investigated.

References

1. Feig DI, Kang DH, Johnson RJ. Uric acid and cardiovascular risk. *N Engl J Med* 2008; 359(17):1811–21.
2. Culleton BF, Larson MG, Kannel WB, Levy D. Serum uric acid and risk for cardiovascular disease and death: the Framingham Heart Study. *Ann Intern Med* 1999; 131(1):7–13.
3. Zhu Y, Pandya BJ, Choi HK. Prevalence of gout and hyperuricemia in the US general population: the National Health and Nutrition Examination Survey 2007–2008. *Arthritis Rheum* 2011; 63(10):3136–41.
4. Juraschek SP, Kovell LC, Miller ER, Gelber AC. Dose-response association of uncontrolled blood pressure and cardiovascular disease risk factors with hyperuricemia and gout. *PLoS One* 2013; 8(2):e56546.
5. Richette P, Perez-Ruiz F, Doherty M, et al. Improving cardiovascular and renal outcomes in gout: what should we target? *Nat Rev Rheumatol* 2014; 10(11):654–61.
6. Bardin T. Hyperuricemia starts at 360 micromoles (6mg/dL). *Joint Bone Spine* 2015; 82(3):141–3.
7. Gaffo AL, Jacobs DR, Jr, Sijtsma F, et al. Serum urate association with hypertension in young adults: analysis from the Coronary Artery Risk Development in Young Adults cohort. *Ann Rheum Dis* 2013; 72(8):1321–7.
8. Bhole V, Choi JW, Kim SW, de Vera M, Choi H. Serum uric acid levels and the risk of type 2 diabetes: a prospective study. *Am J Med* 2010; 123(10):957–61.
9. Bombelli M, Ronchi I, Volpe M, et al. Prognostic value of serum uric acid: new-onset in and out-of-office hypertension and long-term mortality. *J Hypertens* 2014; 32(6):1237–44.
10. Bardin T, Richette P. Definition of hyperuricemia and gouty conditions. *Curr Opin Rheumatol* 2014; 26(2):186–91.
11. Hall AP, Barry PE, Dawber TR, McNamara PM. Epidemiology of gout and hyperuricemia. A long-term population study. *Am J Med* 1967; 42(1):27–37.
12. Ko YC, Wang TN, Tsai LY, Chang FT, Chang SJ. High prevalence of hyperuricemia in adolescent Taiwan aborigines. *J Rheumatol* 2002; 29(4):837–42.
13. Chou CT, Lai JS. The epidemiology of hyperuricaemia and gout in Taiwan aborigines. *Br J Rheumatol* 1998; 37(3):258–62.
14. Brauer GW, Prior IA. A prospective study of gout in New Zealand Maoris. *Ann Rheum Dis* 1978; 37(5):466–72.
15. Trifiro G, Morabito P, Cavagna L, et al. Epidemiology of gout and hyperuricaemia in Italy during the years 2005-2009: a nationwide population-based study. *Ann Rheum Dis* 2013; 72(5):694–700.
16. Campion EW, Glynn RJ, DeLabry LO. Asymptomatic hyperuricemia. Risks and consequences in the Normative Aging Study. *Am J Med* 1987; 82(3):421–6.
17. Chowalloor PV, Keen HI. A systematic review of ultrasonography in gout and asymptomatic hyperuricaemia. *Ann Rheum Dis* 2013; 72(5):638–45.
18. Curhan GC, Taylor EN. 24-h uric acid excretion and the risk of kidney stones. *Kidney Int* 2008; 73(4):489–96.
19. Mazzali M, Hughes J, Kim YG, et al. Elevated uric acid increases blood pressure in the rat by a novel crystal-independent mechanism. *Hypertension* 2001; 38(5):1101–6.
20. Mazzali M, Kanellis J, Han L, et al. Hyperuricemia induces a primary renal arteriolopathy in rats by a blood pressure-independent mechanism. *Am J Physiol Renal Physiol* 2002; 282(6):F991–7.
21. Watanabe S, Kang DH, Feng L, et al. Uric acid, hominoid evolution, and the pathogenesis of salt-sensitivity. *Hypertension* 2002; 40(3):355–60.
22. Kang DH, Nakagawa T, Feng L, et al. A role for uric acid in the progression of renal disease. *J Am Soc Nephrol* 2002; 13(12):2888–97.
23. Mazzali M, Kim YG, Suga S, et al. Hyperuricemia exacerbates chronic cyclosporine nephropathy. *Transplantation* 2001; 71(7):900–5.
24. Kosugi T, Nakayama T, Heinig M, et al. Effect of lowering uric acid on renal disease in the type 2 diabetic db/db mice. *Am J Physiol Renal Physiol* 2009; 297(2):F481–8.
25. Mazali FC, Johnson RJ, Mazzali M. Use of uric acid-lowering agents limits experimental cyclosporine nephropathy. *Nephron Exp Nephrol* 2012; 120(1):e12–9.
26. Nakagawa T, Hu H, Zharikov S, et al. A causal role for uric acid in fructose-induced metabolic syndrome. *Am J Physiol Renal Physiol* 2006; 290(3):F625–31.
27. DeBosch BJ, Kluth O, Fujiwara H, Schurmann A, Moley K. Early-onset metabolic syndrome in mice lacking the intestinal uric acid transporter SLC2A9. *Nat Commun* 2014; 5:4642.
28. Johnson RJ, Perez-Pozo SE, Sautin YY, et al. Hypothesis: could excessive fructose intake and uric acid cause type 2 diabetes? *Endocr Rev* 2009; 30(1):96–116.
29. Johnson RJ, Nakagawa T, Jalal D, et al. Uric acid and chronic kidney disease: which is chasing which? *Nephrol Dial Transplant* 2013; 28(9):2221–8.
30. Khosla UM, Zharikov S, Finch JL, et al. Hyperuricemia induces endothelial dysfunction. *Kidney Int* 2005; 67(5):1739–42.
31. Sanchez-Lozada LG, Lanaspa MA, Cristobal-Garcia M, et al. Uric acid-induced endothelial dysfunction is associated with mitochondrial alterations and decreased intracellular ATP concentrations. *Nephron Exp Nephrol* 2012; 121(3–4):e71–8.
32. Rabadi MM, Kuo MC, Ghaly T, et al. Interaction between uric acid and HMGB1 translocation and release from endothelial cells. *Am J Physiol Renal Physiol* 2012; 302(6):F730–41.
33. Kanellis J, Watanabe S, Li JH, et al. Uric acid stimulates monocyte chemoattractant protein-1 production in vascular smooth muscle cells via

mitogen-activated protein kinase and cyclooxygenase-2. *Hypertension* 2003; 41(6):1287–93.

34. Mustard JF, Murphy EA, Ogryzlo MA, Smythe HA. Blood coagulation and platelet economy in subjects with primary gout. *Can Med Assoc J* 1963; 89:1207–11.

35. Netea MG, Kullberg BJ, Blok WL, Netea RT, van der Meer JW. The role of hyperuricemia in the increased cytokine production after lipopoly-saccharide challenge in neutropenic mice. *Blood* 1997; 89(2):577–82.

36. Zhou Y, Fang L, Jiang L, et al. Uric acid induces renal inflammation via activating tubular NF-kappaB signaling pathway. *PLoS One* 2012; 7(6):e39738.

37. Ryu ES, Kim MJ, Shin HS, et al. Uric acid-induced phenotypic transition of renal tubular cells as a novel mechanism of chronic kidney disease. *Am J Physiol Renal Physiol* 2013; 304(5):F471–80.

38. Sautin YY, Nakagawa T, Zharikov S, Johnson RJ. Adverse effects of the classic antioxidant uric acid in adipocytes: NADPH oxidase-mediated oxidative/nitrosative stress. *Am J Physiol Cell Physiol* 2007; 293(2):C584–96.

39. Fang J, Alderman MH. Serum uric acid and cardiovascular mortality the NHANES I epidemiologic follow-up study, 1971–1992. National Health and Nutrition Examination Survey. *JAMA* 2000; 283(18):2404–10.

40. Tomita M, Mizuno S, Yamanaka H, et al. Does hyperuricemia affect mortality? A prospective cohort study of Japanese male workers. *J Epidemiol* 2000; 10(6):403–9.

41. Meisinger C, Koenig W, Baumert J, Doring A. Uric acid levels are associated with all-cause and cardiovascular disease mortality independent of systemic inflammation in men from the general population: the MONICA/KORA cohort study. *Arterioscler Thromb Vasc Biol* 2008; 28(6):1186–92.

42. Chen JH, Chuang SY, Chen HJ, Yeh WT, Pan WH. Serum uric acid level as an independent risk factor for all-cause, cardiovascular, and ischemic stroke mortality: a Chinese cohort study. *Arthritis Rheum* 2009; 61(2):225–32.

43. Stack AG, Hanley A, Casserly LF, et al. Independent and conjoint associations of gout and hyperuricaemia with total and cardiovascular mortality. *QJM* 2013; 106(7):647–58.

44. Odden MC, Amadu AR, Smit E, Lo L, Peralta CA. Uric acid levels, kidney function, and cardiovascular mortality in US adults: National Health and Nutrition Examination Survey (NHANES) 1988-1994 and 1999-2002. *Am J Kidney Dis* 2014; 64(4):550–7.

45. Zhao G, Huang L, Song M, Song Y. Baseline serum uric acid level as a predictor of cardiovascular disease related mortality and all-cause mortality: a meta-analysis of prospective studies. *Atherosclerosis* 2013; 231(1):61–8.

46. Perez-Ruiz F, Martinez-Indart L, Carmona L, et al. Tophaceous gout and high level of hyperuricaemia are both associated with increased risk of mortality in patients with gout. *Ann Rheum Dis* 2014; 73(1):177–82.

47. Heras M, Fernandez-Reyes MJ, Sanchez R, et al. Serum uric acid as a marker of all-cause mortality in an elderly patient cohort. *Nefrologia* 2012; 32(1):67–72.

48. Lin GM, Li YH, Zheng NC, et al. Serum uric acid as an independent predictor of mortality in high-risk patients with obstructive coronary artery disease: a prospective observational cohort study from the ET-CHD registry, 1997-2003. *J Cardiol* 2013; 61(2):122–7.

49. Verdecchia P, Schillaci G, Reboldi G, et al. Relation between serum uric acid and risk of cardiovascular disease in essential hypertension. The PIUMA study. *Hypertension* 2000; 36(6):1072–8.

50. Ioachimescu AG, Brennan DM, Hoar BM, Hazen SL, Hoogwerf BJ. Serum uric acid is an independent predictor of all-cause mortality in patients at high risk of cardiovascular disease: a preventive cardiology information system (PreCIS) database cohort study. *Arthritis Rheum* 2008; 58(2):623–30.

51. Skak-Nielsen H, Torp-Pedersen C, Finer N, et al. Uric acid as a risk factor for cardiovascular disease and mortality in overweight/obese individuals. *PLoS One* 2013; 8(3):e59121.

52. Kuo CF, See LC, Yu KH, et al. Significance of serum uric acid levels on the risk of all-cause and cardiovascular mortality. *Rheumatology (Oxford)* 2013; 52(1):127–34.

53. Gerber Y, Tanne D, Medalie JH, Goldbourt U. Serum uric acid and long-term mortality from stroke, coronary heart disease and all causes. *Eur J Cardiovasc Prev Rehabil* 2006; 13(2):193–8.

54. Suliman ME, Johnson RJ, Garcia-Lopez E, et al. J-shaped mortality relationship for uric acid in CKD. *Am J Kidney Dis* 2006; 48(5):761–71.

55. Krishnan E. Interaction of inflammation, hyperuricemia, and the prevalence of hypertension among adults free of metabolic syndrome: NHANES 2009–2010. *J Am Heart Assoc* 2014; 3(2):e000157.

56. Grayson PC, Kim SY, LaValley M, Choi HK. Hyperuricemia and incident hypertension: a systematic review and meta-analysis. *Arthritis Care Res (Hoboken)* 2011; 63(1):102–10.

57. Wang J, Qin T, Chen J, et al. Hyperuricemia and risk of incident hypertension: a systematic review and meta-analysis of observational studies. *PLoS One* 2014; 9(12):e114259.

58. Sundstrom J, Sullivan L, D'Agostino RB, et al. Relations of serum uric acid to longitudinal blood pressure tracking and hypertension incidence. *Hypertension* 2005; 45(1):28–33.

59. Feig DI, Johnson RJ. Hyperuricemia in childhood primary hypertension. *Hypertension* 2003; 42(3):247–52.

60. Alper AB, Jr, Chen W, Yau L, et al. Childhood uric acid predicts adult blood pressure: the Bogalusa Heart Study. *Hypertension* 2005; 45(1):34–8.

61. Agarwal V, Hans N, Messerli FH. Effect of allopurinol on blood pressure: a systematic review and meta-analysis. *J Clin Hypertens (Greenwich)* 2013; 15(6):435–42.

62. Beattie CJ, Fulton RL, Higgins P, et al. Allopurinol initiation and change in blood pressure in older adults with hypertension. *Hypertension* 2014; 64(5):1102–7.

63. Feig DI, Soletsky B, Johnson RJ. Effect of allopurinol on blood pressure of adolescents with newly diagnosed essential hypertension: a randomized trial. *JAMA* 2008; 300(8):924–32.

64. Soletsky B, Feig DI. Uric acid reduction rectifies prehypertension in obese adolescents. *Hypertension* 2012; 60(5):1148–56.

65. Masuo K, Kawaguchi H, Mikami H, Ogihara T, Tuck ML. Serum uric acid and plasma norepinephrine concentrations predict subsequent weight gain and blood pressure elevation. *Hypertension* 2003; 42(4):474–80.

66. Palmer TM, Nordestgaard BG, Benn M, et al. Association of plasma uric acid with ischaemic heart disease and blood pressure: mendelian randomisation analysis of two large cohorts. *BMJ* 2013; 347:f4262.

67. Juraschek SP, Kovell LC, Miller ER, 3rd, Gelber AC. Association of kidney disease with prevalent gout in the United States in 1988–1994 and 2007–2010. *Semin Arthritis Rheum* 2013; 42(6):551–61.

68. Jing J, Kielstein JT, Schultheiss UT, et al. Prevalence and correlates of gout in a large cohort of patients with chronic kidney disease: the German Chronic Kidney Disease (GCKD) study. *Nephrol Dial Transplant* 2015; 30(4):613–21.

69. Roughley MJ, Belcher J, Mallen CD, Roddy E. Gout and risk of chronic kidney disease and nephrolithiasis: meta-analysis of observational studies. *Arthritis Res Ther* 2015; 17(1):90.

70. Bellomo G, Venanzi S, Verdura C, et al. Association of uric acid with change in kidney function in healthy normotensive individuals. *Am J Kidney Dis* 2010; 56(2):264–72.

71. Syrjanen J, Mustonen J, Pasternack A. Hypertriglyceridaemia and hyperuricaemia are risk factors for progression of IgA nephropathy. *Nephrol Dial Transplant* 2000; 15(1):34–42.

72. Shi Y, Chen W, Jalal D, et al. Clinical outcome of hyperuricemia in IgA nephropathy: a retrospective cohort study and randomized controlled trial. *Kidney Blood Press Res* 2012; 35(3):153–60.

73. Hovind P, Rossing P, Tarnow L, Johnson RJ, Parving HH. Serum uric acid as a predictor for development of diabetic nephropathy in type 1 diabetes: an inception cohort study. *Diabetes* 2009; 58(7):1668–71.

74. Jalal DI, Rivard CJ, Johnson RJ, et al. Serum uric acid levels predict the development of albuminuria over 6 years in patients with type 1 diabetes: findings from the Coronary Artery Calcification in Type 1 Diabetes study. *Nephrol Dial Transplant* 2010; 25(6):1865–9.

75. Zoppini G, Targher G, Chonchol M, et al. Serum uric acid levels and incident chronic kidney disease in patients with type 2 diabetes and preserved kidney function. *Diabetes Care* 2012; 35(1):99–104.

76. Akalin E, Ganeshan SV, Winston J, Muntner P. Hyperuricemia is associated with the development of the composite outcomes of new cardiovascular events and chronic allograft nephropathy. *Transplantation* 2008; 86(5):652–8.

77. Haririan A, Metireddy M, Cangro C, et al. Association of serum uric acid with graft survival after kidney transplantation: a time-varying analysis. *Am J Transplant* 2011; 11(9):1943–50.

78. Siu YP, Leung KT, Tong MK, Kwan TH. Use of allopurinol in slowing the progression of renal disease through its ability to lower serum uric acid level. *Am J Kidney Dis* 2006; 47(1):51–9.

79. Goicoechea M, de Vinuesa SG, Verdalles U, et al. Effect of allopurinol in chronic kidney disease progression and cardiovascular risk. *Clin J Am Soc Nephrol* 2010; 5(8):1388–93.

80. Wang H, Wei Y, Kong X, Xu D. Effects of urate-lowering therapy in hyperuricemia on slowing the progression of renal function: a meta-analysis. *J Ren Nutr* 2013; 23(5):389–96.

81. Choi HK, Ford ES, Li C, Curhan G. Prevalence of the metabolic syndrome in patients with gout: the Third National Health and Nutrition Examination Survey. *Arthritis Rheum* 2007; 57(1):109–15.

82. Choi HK, Ford ES. Prevalence of the metabolic syndrome in individuals with hyperuricemia. *Am J Med* 2007; 120(5):442–7.

83. Li Y, Xu C, Yu C, Xu L, Miao M. Association of serum uric acid level with non-alcoholic fatty liver disease: a cross-sectional study. *J Hepatol* 2009; 50(5):1029–34.

84. Sun D, Li S, Zhang X, Fernandez C, et al. Uric acid is associated with metabolic syndrome in children and adults in a community: the Bogalusa Heart Study. *PLoS One* 2014; 9(10):e89696.

85. Keenan T, Blaha MJ, Nasir K, et al. Relation of uric acid to serum levels of high-sensitivity C-reactive protein, triglycerides, and high-density lipoprotein cholesterol and to hepatic steatosis. *Am J Cardiol* 2012; 110(12):1787–92.

86. Hirotsu C, Tufik S, Guindalini C, et al. Association between uric acid levels and obstructive sleep apnea syndrome in a large epidemiological sample. *PLoS One* 2013; 8(6):e66891.

87. Ryu S, Song J, Choi BY, et al. Incidence and risk factors for metabolic syndrome in Korean male workers, ages 30 to 39. *Ann Epidemiol* 2007; 17(4):245–52.

88. Wang JY, Chen YL, Hsu CH, et al. Predictive value of serum uric acid levels for the diagnosis of metabolic syndrome in adolescents. *J Pediatr* 2012; 161(4):753–6 e2.

89. Sui X, Church TS, Meriwether RA, Lobelo F, Blair SN. Uric acid and the development of metabolic syndrome in women and men. *Metabolism* 2008; 57(6):845–52.

90. Carnethon MR, Fortmann SP, Palaniappan L, et al. Risk factors for progression to incident hyperinsulinemia: the Atherosclerosis Risk in Communities Study, 1987-1998. *Am J Epidemiol* 2003; 158(11):1058–67.

91. Rodriguez G, Soriano LC, Choi HK. Impact of diabetes against the future risk of developing gout. *Ann Rheum Dis* 2010; 69(12):2090–4.

92. Dehghan A, van Hoek M, Sijbrands EJ, Hofman A, Witteman JC. High serum uric acid as a novel risk factor for type 2 diabetes. *Diabetes Care* 2008; 31(2):361–2.

93. Perez-Pozo SE, Schold J, Nakagawa T, et al. Excessive fructose intake induces the features of metabolic syndrome in healthy adult men: role of uric acid in the hypertensive response. *Int J Obes (Lond)* 2010; 34(3):454–61.

94. Wheeler JG, Juzwishin KD, Eiriksdottir G, Gudnason V, Danesh J. Serum uric acid and coronary heart disease in 9,458 incident cases and 155,084 controls: prospective study and meta-analysis. *PLoS Med* 2005; 2(3):e76.

95. Krishnan E, Baker JF, Furst DE, Schumacher HR. Gout and the risk of acute myocardial infarction. *Arthritis Rheum* 2006; 54(8):2688–96.

96. Choi HK, Curhan G. Independent impact of gout on mortality and risk for coronary heart disease. *Circulation* 2007; 116(8):894–900.

97. Bos MJ, Koudstaal PJ, Hofman A, Witteman JC, Breteler MM. Uric acid is a risk factor for myocardial infarction and stroke: the Rotterdam study. *Stroke* 2006; 37(6):1503–7.

98. Holme I, Aastveit AH, Hammar N, Jungner I, Walldius G. Uric acid and risk of myocardial infarction, stroke and congestive heart failure in 417,734 men and women in the Apolipoprotein MOrtality RISk study (AMORIS). *J Intern Med* 2009; 266(6):558–70.

99. Kuo CF, See LC, Luo SF, et al. Gout: an independent risk factor for all-cause and cardiovascular mortality. *Rheumatology (Oxford)* 2010; 49(1):141–6.

100. Andres M, Quintanilla MA, Severa F, Vela P, Ruiz-Nodar JM. Asymptomatic deposit of monosodium urate crystals associates to a more severe coronary calcification in hyperuricemic patients with acute coronary syndrome (abstract). *Arthritis Rheum* 2014; 66:S365.

101. Park JJ, Roudier MP, Soman D, Mokadam NA, Simkin PA. Prevalence of birefringent crystals in cardiac and prostatic tissues, an observational study. *BMJ Open* 2014; 4(7):e005308.

102. Ndrepepa G, Braun S, King L, et al. Association of uric acid with mortality in patients with stable coronary artery disease. *Metabolism* 2012; 61(12):1780–6.

103. Ndrepepa G, Braun S, King L, et al. Uric acid and prognosis in angiography-proven coronary artery disease. *Eur J Clin Invest* 2013; 43(3):256–66.

104. Levantesi G, Marfisi RM, Franzosi MG, et al. Uric acid: a cardiovascular risk factor in patients with recent myocardial infarction. *Int J Cardiol* 2013; 167(1):262–9.

105. Kaya MG, Uyarel H, Akpek M, et al. Prognostic value of uric acid in patients with ST-elevated myocardial infarction undergoing primary coronary intervention. *Am J Cardiol* 2012; 109(4):486–91.

106. Mercuro G, Vitale C, Cerquetani E, et al. Effect of hyperuricemia upon endothelial function in patients at increased cardiovascular risk. *Am J Cardiol* 2004; 94(7):932–5.

107. Kanbay M, Huddam B, Azak A, et al. A randomized study of allopurinol on endothelial function and estimated glomerular filtration rate in asymptomatic hyperuricemic subjects with normal renal function. *Clin J Am Soc Nephrol* 2011; 6(8):1887–94.

108. Higgins P, Dawson J, Lees KR, et al. Xanthine oxidase inhibition for the treatment of cardiovascular disease: a systematic review and meta-analysis. *Cardiovasc Ther* 2012; 30(4):217–26.

109. Rajendra NS, Ireland S, George J, et al. Mechanistic insights into the therapeutic use of high-dose allopurinol in angina pectoris. *J Am Coll Cardiol* 2011; 58(8):820–8.

110. Grimaldi-Bensouda L, Alperovitch A, Aubrun E, et al. Impact of allopurinol on risk of myocardial infarction. *Ann Rheum Dis* 2015; 74(5):836–42.

111. de Abajo FJ, Gil MJ, Rodriguez A, et al. Allopurinol use and risk of non-fatal acute myocardial infarction. *Heart* 2015; 101(9):679–85.

112. Noman A, Ang DS, Ogston S, Lang CC, Struthers AD. Effect of high-dose allopurinol on exercise in patients with chronic stable angina: a randomised, placebo controlled crossover trial. *Lancet* 2010; 375(9732):2161–7.

113. Rekhraj S, Gandy SJ, Szwejkowski BR, et al. High-dose allopurinol reduces left ventricular mass in patients with ischemic heart disease. *J Am Coll Cardiol* 2013; 61(9):926–32.

114. Rentoukas E, Tsarouhas K, Tsitsimpikou C, et al. The prognostic impact of allopurinol in patients with acute myocardial infarction undergoing primary percutaneous coronary intervention. *Int J Cardiol* 2010; 145(2):257–8.

115. Huang H, Huang B, Li Y, et al. Uric acid and risk of heart failure: a systematic review and meta-analysis. *Eur J Heart Fail* 2014; 16(1):15–24.

116. Tamariz L, Harzand A, Palacio A, et al. Uric acid as a predictor of all-cause mortality in heart failure: a meta-analysis. *Congest Heart Fail* 2011; 17(1):25–30.

117. Gotsman I, Keren A, Lotan C, Zwas DR. Changes in uric acid levels and allopurinol use in chronic heart failure: association with improved survival. *J Card Fail* 2012; 18(9):694–701.

118. Doehner W, Schoene N, Rauchhaus M, et al. Effects of xanthine oxidase inhibition with allopurinol on endothelial function and peripheral blood flow in hyperuricemic patients with chronic heart failure: results from 2 placebo-controlled studies. *Circulation* 2002; 105(22):2619–24.

119. Farquharson CA, Butler R, Hill A, Belch JJ, Struthers AD. Allopurinol improves endothelial dysfunction in chronic heart failure. *Circulation* 2002; 106(2):221–6.

120. Hare JM, Mangal B, Brown J, et al. Impact of oxypurinol in patients with symptomatic heart failure. Results of the OPT-CHF study. *J Am Coll Cardiol* 2008; 51(24):2301–9.

121. Givertz MM, Anstrom KJ, Redfield M, et al. Effect of xanthine oxidase inhibition in hyperuricemic heart failure patients: the EXACT-HF study. *Circulation* 2015; 131(20):1763–71.

122. Tamariz L Hare JM. Xanthine oxidase inhibitors in heart failure. *Circulation* 2015; 131(20):1741–4.

123. Ogino K, Kato M, Furuse Y, et al. Uric acid-lowering treatment with benzbromarone in patients with heart failure: a double-blind placebo-controlled crossover preliminary study. *Circ Heart Fail* 2010; 3(1):73–81.

124. Nyrnes A, Toft I, Njolstad I, et al. Uric acid is associated with future atrial fibrillation: an 11-year follow-up of 6308 men and women—the Tromso Study. *Europace* 2014; 16(3):320–6.

125. Tamariz L, Hernandez F, Bush A, Palacio A, Hare JM. Association between serum uric acid and atrial fibrillation: a systematic review and meta-analysis. *Heart Rhythm* 2014; 11(7):1102–8.

126. Chao TF, Liu CJ, Chen SJ, et al. Hyperuricemia and the risk of ischemic stroke in patients with atrial fibrillation—could it refine clinical risk stratification in AF? *Int J Cardiol* 2014; 170(3):344–9.

127. Kim SY, Guevara JP, Kim KM, et al. Hyperuricemia and risk of stroke: a systematic review and meta-analysis. *Arthritis Rheum* 2009; 61(7):885–92.

128. Huang J, Hu D, Wang Y, Zhang D, Qu Y. Dose-response relationship of serum uric acid levels with risk of stroke mortality. *Atherosclerosis* 2014; 23 4(1):1–3.

129. Baker JF, Schumacher HR, Krishnan E. Serum uric acid level and risk for peripheral arterial disease: analysis of data from the multiple risk factor intervention trial. *Angiology* 2007; 58(4):450–7.

130. Tseng CH. Independent association of uric acid levels with peripheral arterial disease in Taiwanese patients with type 2 diabetes. *Diabet Med* 2004; 21(7):724–9.

131. Yang X, Sun K, Zhang W, et al. Prevalence of and risk factors for peripheral arterial disease in the patients with hypertension among Han Chinese. *J Vasc Surg* 2007; 46(2):296–302.

132. Kottgen A, Albrecht E, Teumer A, et al. Genome-wide association analyses identify 18 new loci associated with serum urate concentrations. *Nat Genet* 2013; 45(2):145–54.

133. Oikonen M, Wendelin-Saarenhovi M, Lyytikainen LP, et al. Associations between serum uric acid and markers of subclinical atherosclerosis in young adults. The cardiovascular risk in Young Finns study. *Atherosclerosis* 2012; 223(2):497–503.

134. Mallamaci F, Testa A, Leonardis D, et al. A polymorphism in the major gene regulating serum uric acid associates with clinic SBP and the white-coat effect in a family-based study. *J Hypertens* 2014; 32(8):1621–8.

135. Parsa A, Brown E, Weir MR, et al. Genotype-based changes in serum uric acid affect blood pressure. *Kidney Int* 2012; 81(5):502–7.

136. Kleber ME, Delgado G, Grammer TB, et al. Uric acid and cardiovascular events: a Mendelian randomization study. *J Am Soc Nephrol* 2015; 26(11):2831–8.

137. Hughes K, Flynn T, de Zoysa J, Dalbeth N, Merriman TR. Mendelian randomization analysis associates increased serum urate, due to genetic variation in uric acid transporters, with improved renal function. *Kidney Int* 2014; 85(2):344–51.

138. Sedaghat S, Pazoki R, Uitterlinden AG, et al. Association of uric acid genetic risk score with blood pressure: the Rotterdam study. *Hypertension* 2014; 64(5):1061–6.

139. Kuo CF, Luo SF, See LC, et al. Increased risk of cancer among gout patients: a nationwide population study. *Joint Bone Spine* 2012; 79(4):375–8.

140. Horsfall LJ, Nazareth I, Petersen I. Serum uric acid and the risk of respiratory disease: a population-based cohort study. *Thorax* 2014; 69(11):1021–6.

141. Dziaman T, Banaszkiewicz Z, Roszkowski K, et al. 8-Oxo-7,8-dihydroguanine and uric acid as efficient predictors of survival in colon cancer patients. *Int J Cancer* 2014; 134(2):376–83.

142. Stotz M, Szkandera J, Seidel J, et al. Evaluation of uric acid as a prognostic blood-based marker in a large cohort of pancreatic cancer patients. *PLoS One* 2014; 9(8):e104730.

143. Schrag M, Mueller C, Zabel M, et al. Oxidative stress in blood in Alzheimer's disease and mild cognitive impairment: a meta-analysis. *Neurobiol Dis* 2013; 59:100–10.

144. Lu N, Dubreuil M, Zhang Y, et al. Gout and the risk of Alzheimer's disease: a population-based, BMI-matched cohort study. *Ann Rheum Dis* 201; 75(3):547–51.

145. de Lau LM, Koudstaal PJ, Hofman A, Breteler MM. Serum uric acid levels and the risk of Parkinson disease. *Ann Neurol* 2005; 58(5):797–800.

146. Jesus S, Perez I, Caceres-Redondo MT, et al. Low serum uric acid concentration in Parkinson's disease in southern Spain. *Eur J Neurol* 2013; 20(1):208–10.

147. Schlesinger I, Schlesinger N. Uric acid in Parkinson's disease. *Mov Disord* 2008; 23(12):1653–7.

148. Alonso A, Rodriguez LA, Logroscino G, Hernan MA. Gout and risk of Parkinson disease: a prospective study. *Neurology* 2007; 69(17):1696–700.

149. Ascherio A, LeWitt PA, Xu K, et al. Urate as a predictor of the rate of clinical decline in Parkinson disease. *Arch Neurol* 2009; 66(12):1460–8.

150. Jacobs F, Mamzer-Bruneel MF, Skhiri H, et al. Safety of the mycophenolate mofetil-allopurinol combination in kidney transplant recipients with gout. *Transplantation* 1997; 64(7):1087–8.

151. Richette P, Doherty M, Pascual E, et al. *The 2014 EULAR Recommendations on the Management of Gout.* 2014 EULAR Annual Congress, Paris, France, June 2014.

152. Yamanaka H. Japanese guideline for the management of hyperuricemia and gout: second edition. *Nucleosides Nucleotides Nucleic Acids* 2011; 30(12):1018–29.

153. Khanna D, Fitzgerald JD, Khanna PP, et al. 2012 American College of Rheumatology guidelines for management of gout. Part 1: systematic nonpharmacologic and pharmacologic therapeutic approaches to hyperuricemia. *Arthritis Care Res (Hoboken)* 2012; 64(10):1431–46.

154. Sivera F, Andres M, Carmona L, et al. Multinational evidence-based recommendations for the diagnosis and management of gout: integrating systematic literature review and expert opinion of a broad panel of rheumatologists in the 3e initiative. *Ann Rheum Dis* 2014; 73(2):328–35.

SECTION 14

Calcium pyrophosphate crystal deposition

CHAPTER 48

Epidemiology and risk factors for calcium pyrophosphate deposition

Abhishek Abhishek and Michael Doherty

Introduction

Calcium pyrophosphate (CPP) crystal deposition (CPPD) is the commonest cause of articular cartilage calcification—chondrocalcinosis (CC). CPPD is recognized to occur mainly in the elderly, although young-onset CPPD (<55–60 years old) may occur at sites of prior joint injury and osteoarthritis (OA) (usually mono- or oligo-articular) or be due to genetic or metabolic disorders (usually polyarticular). CPPD is frequently asymptomatic, being noticed as an incidental finding of CC on imaging studies, but can also cause acute CPP crystal synovitis and associate with chronic symptomatic arthropathy with structural features of OA.

The sensitivity to detect CPPD *in vivo* varies according to the method used. Most epidemiological studies of CPPD have used standard musculoskeletal radiographs to detect CC because these are relatively inexpensive and widely available. However, plain radiographs are relatively insensitive in detecting CC and although alternative radiographic methods (e.g. use of mammography films) may increase sensitivity these are rarely undertaken. Ultrasonography appears more sensitive than plain X-rays (Chapter 51) but is less convenient in terms of population studies. Definitive diagnosis by demonstration of CPP crystals, for example, in aspirated synovial fluid, again is unfeasible in epidemiological studies. For these reasons, the epidemiology of CPPD is not well defined, and epidemiological studies often use radiographic CC as a surrogate for CPPD. In this chapter, we describe the epidemiology of CPPD within these limitations.

History

The first description of articular cartilage calcification is attributed to Robert Adams, a Dublin surgeon (*c*.1854). The advent of radiography led to articular cartilage calcification being observed more frequently, and in 1960, Zitnan and Sitaj suggested that it was the cardinal manifestation of a distinct disease entity '*chondrocalcinosis articularis*' [1]. In 1962, McCarty et al. demonstrated CPP crystals in joints of patients with apparently acute 'gouty' arthritis many of whom had radiographic CC [2]. Subsequently, basic calcium phosphate (BCP) crystals, predominantly carbonated hydroxyapatite, were identified in synovial fluid and articular cartilage showing that CC is not exclusively due to CPPD. Furthermore mixed CPP and BCP deposition is common, especially in the context of marked structural OA [3].

Classification

The classification of arthropathy associated with CPPD has evolved from a complex system based on similarity to other conditions (e.g. pseudogout, pseudo-osteoarthritis, etc.) [4] to a simpler system recommended by the European League Against Rheumatism which emphasizes the main presentations of CPPD [5] (Box 48.1). This change was necessary as the previous system was potentially confusing. For example, patients frequently change from one phenotype to the other or have different phenotypes at different joints; terms such as 'pseudogout' make patients think that they have something to do with gout; the term 'pseudo-' implies that CPP crystals are only of secondary importance to urate crystals; and the multiple terms were used inconsistently in the literature. In this recent classification, the crystals are termed CPP (the 'dihydrate' is omitted), and the umbrella term CPPD (previously used as the abbreviation for CPP dihydrate crystals) is used for all instances in which CPP crystals occur [5].

Box 48.1 Classification of CPPD

- *Asymptomatic CPPD*: CPPD with no apparent clinical consequence.

- *OA with CPPD*: CPPD in a joint that also shows structural changes of OA, on imaging or histological examination (previously 'pseudo-OA'). As with OA without CPPD, this can be symptomatic or asymptomatic.

- *Acute CPP crystal arthritis*: acute onset, self-limiting painful synovitis with CPPD (previously 'pseudogout').

- *Chronic CPP crystal inflammatory arthritis*: chronic inflammatory arthritis associated with CPPD (previously 'pseudo-rheumatoid arthritis').

Joints affected by calcium pyrophosphate crystal deposition

CPPD can occur in any synovial or fibrocartilaginous joint, however, in descending order of frequency it most commonly occurs in the knees, wrists, symphysis pubis, and hips [6–9]. While previous studies reported that it is rare to get radiographic CC in the absence of any knee involvement, a recent plain radiograph study suggested that up to 40% of people with radiographic CC at any joint do not have knee involvement [10]. However, this may not hold true if more sensitive imaging techniques are used. For example, in a recent joint ultrasound examination study of 42 patients with CPPD, almost all had knee CC [11].

Incidence

The incidence of CPPD in the general population has not been examined formally. However, in hospital-based imaging or synovial fluid studies of middle-aged or older adults with knee OA, the annual incidence of radiographic knee CC has been estimated as 0.8–2.1% and that of CPPD within the knee (either synovial fluid CPP crystals or radiographic CC) as 2.7–5.5% [12]. However, such studies suffer from selection bias in that most participants studied were symptomatic hospital-referred patients with knee OA and this is likely to lead to gross over-estimation of incidence.

Prevalence

A limited number of studies have assessed the population prevalence of radiographic CC (Table 48.1). Results vary according to the age range of the population sample, and the joint(s) being assessed. In studies of middle-aged and older people from Europe and the United States, the prevalence of CC at the knee, knee or hand/wrist, and knee or hips/symphysis pubis are reported as 7.0–8.1%, 10.0%, and 10.4% respectively [7–9]. As expected, radiographs underestimate the true prevalence of CPPD, and between one-quarter to one-half of OA knees with CPP crystals do not have radiographic CC [12].

In comparative terms, in an Italian study CPPD appeared to be the fourth most prevalent condition after OA, gout, and rheumatoid arthritis in community-dwelling adults, with a prevalence of 0.42% [13]. However, studies restricted to older people or hospital-based studies report a significantly higher prevalence of CPPD. CPPD is reported in all ethnicities but seems to be more common in Caucasians than in Chinese [14] and those from the Middle-East.

Risk factors

Age, sex, and body mass index

It is clear in all studies that CPPD shows a strong positive association with increasing age (Box 48.2). In a community-based study from Nottingham, United Kingdom, the prevalence of knee CC increased from 3.7% at age 55–59 years to 17.5% at age 80–84 years [9]. Similarly, in the Framingham study, there was more than a doubling in the prevalence of knee CC with each 10-year increase in age after the age of 60 years (relative risk (95% confidence interval (CI)) 2.40 (1.97–2.91)) [8].

Although some small studies and a large study from China reported a higher prevalence of CC in women [14], a recent meta-analysis and results from large community-based studies from Nottingham (United Kingdom), and Framingham (United States) suggest that sex does not associate with CPPD [5]. Similarly, body mass index (BMI) does not associate with CPPD [5].

Heredity

CPPD is rarely inherited as a monogenic autosomal dominant disease. Many instances of such hereditary transmission occur due to mutations in the *ANKH* (ankylosis human) gene [15]. Familial CPPD can also occur as part of a severe dysplastic OA phenotype associated with mutations in the procollagen type 2 gene, *CCAL1*, and osteoprotegerin genes. Although one sibling study did not suggest a genetic contribution to the risk of apparently sporadic CC [16], polymorphisms in the *ANKH* gene also associate with sporadic CPPD. Two independent studies from Oxford and Nottingham in the United Kingdom show that the −4 base pair G to A polymorphism in the 5′-UTR of *ANKH* associates with radiographic CC [17,18], and that this is independent of age, sex, BMI, and OA [18].

Osteoarthritis

OA associates with CPPD, and this association is independent of age [8,9]. While OA at knees, wrists, scaphotrapezoid joint, and metacarpophalangeal joints associates with CC [19–22], hip OA does not associate with hip CC or with CC at other joints [7,23] suggesting that the association between CPPD and OA may be joint specific. Although CPPD may rarely occur in rapidly progressive destructive large joint OA [24], prospective studies show that CC either protects against or does not associate with risk of progression of knee OA [25,26]. Furthermore, knee CC does not associate with incident knee OA suggesting that CPPD is not a cause of OA [27].

Table 48.1 Prevalence of chondrocalcinosis

Region	Age (range)	Joints examined	CC crude prevalence
Marche, Italy [13]	18–91	Symptomatic joints	0.42%
Nottingham, UK [9]	40–86	Knee	7.0%
Framingham, US [8]	63–93	Knee	8.1%
Veneto Region, Italy [7]	>65	Knee, pelvis	10.4%
Osona, Spain [6]	60–88	Wrist, hand, knee	10.0%

Box 48.2 Risk factors for CPPD

- Increasing age
- Osteoarthritis[a]
- Meniscectomy
- Metabolic diseases: hyperparathyroidism, haemochromatosis,[b] hypomagnesaemia, hypophosphatasia, CKD 5[c]
- Hereditary—mutations in *ANKH* gene (common), part of severe dysplastic OA phenotype.

[a]Except for hip OA.
[b]Causes structural arthropathy in addition to CPPD.
[c]Risk factor for acute CPP crystal arthritis.

Metabolic diseases

Haemochromatosis, hyperparathyroidism, hypomagnesaemia, and hypophosphatasia are the main metabolic diseases that have been shown to predispose to CC due to CPPD. These all increase extracellular levels of inorganic pyrophosphate (see Chapter 49) and their presence should be screened for in young (<55 years) people with CPPD, especially those with polyarticular CC [28,29]. As hyperparathyroidism gets more prevalent with increasing age, it should be screened for in older patients with CPPD. Other diseases which are common and age associated, such as diabetes and hypothyroidism, have been linked to CPPD but once adjusted appropriately no association is apparent [28,30].

Haemochromatosis

Haemochromatosis is the only metabolic disease associated with CPPD that results in structural arthropathy in addition to CC, and this commonly affects the knees, wrists, hips, metacarpophalangeal joints, and ankles [31]. Population-based studies suggest that homozygosity for H63D—which carries a smaller risk of iron overload—and not for C282Y associates with CPPD [32]. This finding is counterintuitive, and may be due to variable penetrance of *HFE* mutations, channelling bias, or the possibility that factors unrelated to iron overload predispose to CPPD.

Hyperparathyroidism

Hyperparathyroidism associates with CPPD (pooled odds ratio (OR) (95% CI) 3.03 (1.15–8.02) [5]. Patients with hyperparathyroidism develop CPPD at a younger age [33,34]. However, as expected, the association between CC and hyperparathyroidism is not independent of age since hyperparathyroid patients with CC tend to be older than hyperparathyroid patients without CC. The recently reported association between CC and low cortical bone mineral density (BMD) but not low cancellous BMD may also be mediated by parathyroid hormone [23].

Hypomagnesaemia

Hypomagnesaemia, due either to chronic persistent renal loss, for example, the Gitelman variant of Bartter syndrome [35] or from gastrointestinal losses due to intestinal failure, associates with CPPD. In a cross sectional study, CC associated with intestinal failure (OR (95% CI) 7.0 (1.45–66.1)), and this association was significantly higher in patients with lower serum magnesium levels (OR (95% CI) 13.5 (2.76–127.3)) [36]. Similarly, acute hypomagnesaemia can also associate with acute CPP crystal arthritis, presumably due to partial dissolution of pre-existing CPP crystals that then more easily 'shed' from cartilage into the joint space. Finally, the reported association between chronic diuretic use and knee CC is believed to be mediated by diuretic-induced hypomagnesaemia [9].

Hypophosphatasia

The association between hypophosphatasia and CC is based on several case reports of young-onset florid polyarticular CC [28]. Similarly, the suggested associations between rare diseases such as Wilson disease, ochronosis, and CPPD are also based on isolated case reports [28].

Other joint disorders

CC is reported to associate with gout [37] but not with hyperuricaemia [38]. This raises the possibility that the association between CC and gout is either due to a shared predisposition to crystal formation or to epitaxy—the nucleation of one crystal type on another. A recent meta-analysis suggests that there is a negative association between CPPD and rheumatoid arthritis (pooled OR (95% CI) 0.18 (0.08–0.41)) (5), which is supported mechanistically by the subnormal levels of inorganic pyrophosphate that occur in rheumatoid synovial fluid [39].

Local joint insults such as meniscectomy appear to increase the risk of CC, as well as OA. For example, knees which underwent meniscectomy are fivefold more likely to develop CC than the unoperated knee [40]. Similarly, self-reported varus knee alignment in the third decade associates with subsequent knee CC, and this is independent of age, sex, BMI in the 20s, and knee OA [15]. However, current knee alignment does not associate with knee CC supporting a causal association between early-life knee malalignment and CC.

Risk factors for acute calcium pyrophosphate crystal arthritis

An age-sex matched study using the UK Clinical Practice Research Datalink reported that hyperparathyroidism, OA, and loop diuretic use independently associates with acute CPP crystal arthritis (adjusted ORs 1.35–4.87) [41]. It also reported that renal failure (CKD 5) is also associated with acute CPP crystal arthritis [41].

Conclusion

CPPD is uncommon under the age of 55 years and becomes increasingly common, particularly at the knee. The main attributable risk factors recognized are ageing and OA. Rarely, CPPD can be inherited or result from predisposing metabolic diseases that elevate extracellular pyrophosphate levels. However, further studies using non-invasive sensitive imaging modalities such as ultrasound are required to better determine the population prevalence and incidence of CPPD and to obtain estimates of these for each clinical phenotype.

References

1. Zitnan D, Sitaj S. [Chondrocalcinosis polyarticularis (familiaris): roentgenological and clinical analysis.]. *Cesk Rentgenol* 1960; 14:27–34.
2. McCarty DJ, Kohn NH, Faires JS. The significance of calcium phosphate crystals in the synovial fluid of arthritic patients: the "pseudogout syndrome": I. Clinical aspects. *Ann Intern Med* 1962; 56(5):711–37.
3. Fuerst M, Bertrand J, Lammers L, et al. Calcification of articular cartilage in human osteoarthritis. *Arthritis Rheum* 2009; 60(9):2694–703.
4. McCarty DJ. Calcium pyrophosphate dihydrate crystal deposition disease: nomenclature and diagnostic criteria. *Ann Intern Med* 1977; 87(2):241–2.
5. Zhang W, Doherty M, Bardin T, et al. European League Against Rheumatism recommendations for calcium pyrophosphate deposition. Part I: terminology and diagnosis. *Ann Rheum Dis* 2011; 70(4):563–70.
6. Sanmarti R, Panella D, Brancos MA, et al. Prevalence of articular chondrocalcinosis in elderly subjects in a rural area of Catalonia. *Ann Rheum Dis* 1993; 52(6):418–22.
7. Ramonda R, Musacchio E, Perissinotto E, et al. Prevalence of chondrocalcinosis in Italian subjects from northeastern Italy. The Pro.V.A. (PROgetto Veneto Anziani) study. *Clin Exp Rheumatol* 2009; 27(6):981–4.
8. Felson DT, Anderson JJ, Naimark A, Kannel W, Meenan RF. The prevalence of chondrocalcinosis in the elderly and its association with knee osteoarthritis: the Framingham Study. *J Rheumatol* 1989; 16(9):1241–5.

9. Neame RL, Carr AJ, Muir K, Doherty M. UK community prevalence of knee chondrocalcinosis: evidence that correlation with osteoarthritis is through a shared association with osteophyte. *Ann Rheum Dis* 2003; 62(6):513–8.

10. Abhishek A, Doherty S, Maciewicz R, et al. Chondrocalcinosis is common in the absence of knee involvement. *Arthritis Res Ther* 2012; 14(5):R205.

11. Filippou G, Filippucci E, Tardella M, et al. Extent and distribution of CPP deposits in patients affected by calcium pyrophosphate dihydrate deposition disease: an ultrasonographic study. *Ann Rheum Dis* 2013; 72(11):1836–9.

12. Abhishek A, Doherty M. Epidemiology of calcium pyrophosphate crystal arthritis and basic calcium phosphate crystal arthropathy. *Rheum Dis Clin North Am* 2014; 40(2):177–91.

13. Salaffi F, De Angelis R, Grassi W. Prevalence of musculoskeletal conditions in an Italian population sample: results of a regional community-based study. I. The MAPPING study. *Clin Exp Rheumatol* 2005; 23(6):819–28.

14. Zhang Y, Terkeltaub R, Nevitt M, et al. Lower prevalence of chondrocalcinosis in Chinese subjects in Beijing than in white subjects in the United States: the Beijing Osteoarthritis Study. *Arthritis Rheum* 2006; 54(11):3508–12.

15. Abhishek A, Doherty M. Pathophysiology of articular chondrocalcinosis—role of ANKH. *Nat Rev Rheumatol* 2011; 7(2):96–104.

16. Zhang W, Neame R, Doherty S, Doherty M. Relative risk of knee chondrocalcinosis in siblings of index cases with pyrophosphate arthropathy. *Ann Rheum Dis* 2004; 63(8):969–73.

17. Zhang Y, Johnson K, Russell RG, et al. Association of sporadic chondrocalcinosis with a -4-basepair G-to-A transition in the 5'-untranslated region of ANKH that promotes enhanced expression of ANKH protein and excess generation of extracellular inorganic pyrophosphate. *Arthritis Rheum* 2005; 52(4):1110–7.

18. Abhishek A, Doherty S, Maciewicz R, et al. The association between ANKH promoter polymorphism and chondrocalcinosis is independent of age and osteoarthritis: results of a case-control study. *Arthritis Res Ther* 2014; 16(1):R25.

19. Sanmarti R, Kanterewicz E, Pladevall M, et al. Analysis of the association between chondrocalcinosis and osteoarthritis: a community based study. *Ann Rheum Dis* 1996; 55(1):30–3.

20. Al-Arfaj AS. The relationship between chondrocalcinosis and osteoarthritis in Saudi Arabia. *Clin Rheumatol* 2002; 21(6):493–6.

21. Bourqui M, Vischer TL, Stasse P, Docquier C, Fallet GH. Pyrophosphate arthropathy in the carpal and metacarpophalangeal joints. *Ann Rheum Dis* 1983; 42(6):626–30.

22. Peter A, Simmen BR, Bruhlmann P, Michel BA, Stucki G. Osteoarthritis of the scaphoidtrapezium joint: an early sign of calcium pyrophosphate dihydrate disease. *Clin Rheumatol* 2001; 20(1):20–4.

23. Abhishek A, Doherty S, Maciewicz R, et al. Association between low cortical bone mineral density, soft-tissue calcification, vascular calcification and chondrocalcinosis: a case-control study. *Ann Rheum Dis* 2014; 73(11):1997–2002.

24. Gerster JC, Vischer TL, Boussina I, Fallet GH. Joint destruction and chondrocalcinosis in patients with generalised osteoarthrosis. *Br Med J* 1975; 4(5998):684.

25. Neogi T, Nevitt M, Niu J, et al. Lack of association between chondrocalcinosis and increased risk of cartilage loss in knees with osteoarthritis: results of two prospective longitudinal magnetic resonance imaging studies. *Arthritis Rheum* 2006; 54(6):1822–8.

26. Ledingham J, Regan M, Jones A, Doherty M. Factors affecting radiographic progression of knee osteoarthritis. *Ann Rheum Dis* 1995; 54(1):53–8.

27. Felson DT, Zhang Y, Hannan MT, et al. Risk factors for incident radiographic knee osteoarthritis in the elderly: the Framingham Study. *Arthritis Rheum* 1997; 40(4):728–33.

28. Jones AC, Chuck AJ, Arie EA, Green DJ, Doherty M. Diseases associated with calcium pyrophosphate deposition disease. *Semin Arthritis Rheum* 1992; 22(3):188–202.

29. Richette P, Bardin T, Doherty M. An update on the epidemiology of calcium pyrophosphate dihydrate crystal deposition disease. *Rheumatology (Oxford)* 2009; 48(7):711–5.

30. Chaisson CE, McAlindon TE, Felson DT, et al. Lack of association between thyroid status and chondrocalcinosis or osteoarthritis: the Framingham Osteoarthritis Study. *J Rheumatol* 1996; 23(4):711–5.

31. Sahinbegovic E, Dallos T, Aigner E, et al. Musculoskeletal disease burden of hereditary hemochromatosis. *Arthritis Rheum* 2010; 62(12):3792–8.

32. Alizadeh BZ, Njajou OT, Hazes JM, et al. The H63D variant in the HFE gene predisposes to arthralgia, chondrocalcinosis and osteoarthritis. *Ann Rheum Dis* 2007; 66(11):1436–42.

33. Pritchard MH, Jessop JD. Chondrocalcinosis in primary hyperparathyroidism. Influence of age, metabolic bone disease, and parathyroidectomy. *Ann Rheum Dis* 1977; 36(2):146–51.

34. Yashiro T, Okamoto T, Tanaka R, et al. Prevalence of chondrocalcinosis in patients with primary hyperparathyroidism in Japan. *Endocrinol Jpn* 1991; 38(5):457–64.

35. Gitelman HJ, Graham JB, Welt LG. A new familial disorder characterized by hypokalemia and hypomagnesemia. *Trans Assoc Am Physicians* 1966; 79:221–35.

36. Richette PA, Lahalle G, Vicaut S, et al. Hypomagnesemia associated with chondrocalcinosis: a cross-sectional study. *Arthritis Rheum* 2007; 57(8):1496–501.

37. Stockman A, Darlington LG, Scott JT. Frequency of chondrocalcinosis of the knees and avascular necrosis of the femoral heads in gout: a controlled study. *Ann Rheum Dis* 1980; 39(1):7–11.

38. Hollingworth P, Williams PL, Scott JT. Frequency of chondrocalcinosis of the knees in asymptomatic hyperuricaemia and rheumatoid arthritis: a controlled study. *Ann Rheum Dis* 1982; 41(4):344–6.

39. Pattrick M, Hamilton E, Hornby J, Doherty M. Synovial fluid pyrophosphate and nucleoside triphosphate pyrophosphatase: comparison between normal and diseased and between inflamed and non-inflamed joints. *Ann Rheum Dis* 1991; 50(4):214–8.

40. Doherty M, Watt I, Dieppe PA. Localised chondrocalcinosis in post-meniscectomy knees. *Lancet* 1982; 1(8283):1207–10.

41. Rho YH, Zhu Y, Zhang Y, Reginato AM, Choi HK. Risk factors for pseudogout in the general population. *Rheumatology (Oxford)* 2012; 51(11):2070–4.

CHAPTER 49

Pathophysiology of calcium pyrophosphate deposition

Abhishek Abhishek and Michael Doherty

Introduction

Calcium pyrophosphate (CPP) dihydrate crystal formation requires a sufficient extracellular ionic product of inorganic pyrophosphate (PPi) and calcium, as well as a cartilage matrix environment that facilitates crystal nucleation and growth. CPP crystals are formed extracellularly *in vivo* and are deposited predominantly in the middle layer of fibrocartilage and articular hyaline cartilage. Consequently, they frequently cause no symptoms for extended periods of time. However, they are extremely phlogistic (less so than monosodium urate (MSU) on a weight basis) and when shed into joints cause an acute inflammatory response. They may also exert mechanical effects on the cartilage in which they form. In this chapter we describe the biochemical changes that result in CPP crystal formation, and review the mechanisms by which they cause inflammation.

Inorganic pyrophosphate and calcium pyrophosphate crystal formation

Despite a high turnover (approximately several kilograms/day), both intracellular and extracellular PPi concentrations are maintained at a low level by several ubiquitous pyrophosphatase enzymes that rapidly metabolize PPi complexed with magnesium to orthophosphate (Pi). PPi largely derives from breakdown of nucleoside triphosphates (NTPs) and is a by-product of many biosynthetic reactions in the body. As for uric acid and MSU crystals, having sufficiently elevated PPi is a prerequisite for CPP crystal formation [1]. In a chicken embryo growth plate matrix vesicle (MV) model, CPP crystals formed exclusively when the Pi/PPi ratio was less than 6, and their formation was inhibited when the Pi/PPi ratio was greater than 28.4. In contrast, optimal formation of apatite crystals occurred when the Pi/PPi ratio was greater than 140 and their formation was completely inhibited when this ratio was less than 70 [2]. PPi is also required for the initial nucleation of apatite from amorphous calcium phosphate and for subsequent crystal growth; however, higher levels of PPi inhibit this by preventing crystal nucleation and retarding crystal growth [2]. By the same mechanism, PPi also inhibits abnormal calcification in the vasculature, saliva, and the urinary tract, and is used commercially as an industrial water softener. PPi is therefore a key regulator of apatite formation, modest levels of PPi stimulating but high levels of PPi inhibiting apatite crystal formation and growth.

Patients with calcium pyrophosphate crystal deposition (CPPD) have high synovial fluid PPi levels, and the plasma and urinary

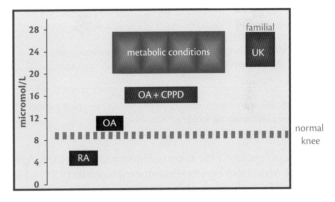

Figure 49.1 Synovial fluid pyrophosphate (PPi) levels in healthy and diseased joints. Note subnormal levels of synovial fluid PPi in rheumatoid arthritis (RA), and high levels in joints with osteoarthritis (OA) +/− calcium pyrophosphate crystal deposition (CPPD), metabolic diseases associated with CPPD, and in familial CPPD.

concentrations are normal, which strongly supports local production of PPi as the main contributor to a high ionic product [1,3]. Compared to normal knees, elevated synovial fluid PPi concentrations are reported both in OA with CPPD and in OA without apparent CPPD, with less impressive elevations in acute CPP crystal arthritis [1]. Conversely the synovial fluid PPi levels are lower than normal in rheumatoid arthritis (RA), reflecting increased clearance or inhibitory effects of inflammatory cytokines on PPi synthesis [1]. Synovial fluid PPi is also elevated in metabolic diseases like hyperparathyroidism, hypomagnesaemia, and haemochromatosis, and in familial CPPD (Figure 49.1) [4–6].

Source of extracellular inorganic pyrophosphate

All PPi in the body is made endogenously with none coming from the diet. PPi cannot cross cell membranes passively due to its size. Extracellular PPi (ePPi) is derived either from local extracellular production or by transmembrane transport of PPi produced within cells. The multi-pass transmembrane ankylosis protein (ANK in mice, ANKH in human) is the key PPi transporter [7–9]. Loss-of-function mutations in *ANK* result in high intracellular PPi (iPPi) and low ePPi (Figure 49.1), causing abnormal mineralization due to loss of the normal inhibitory effect of ePPi on apatite formation—the ankylosis mouse phenotype [7] (Figure 49.2). Conversely, gain-of-function polymorphisms and mutations in *ANKH* result in greatly elevated ePPi and subsequent CPPD and have been identified as

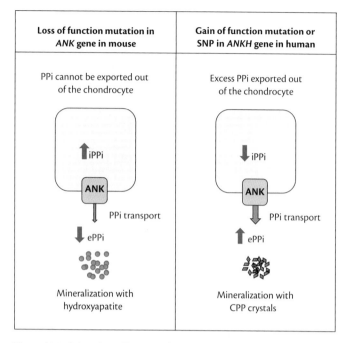

Figure 49.2 Gain or loss of function of ANK(H) decides the type of calcium crystal formed. SNP, single nucleotide polymorphism.

the cause of familial CPPD in several human kindreds [8,9]. Apart from PPi, *ANKH* also exports adenosine triphosphate (ATP) which can be broken down extracellularly to release PPi [10].

Phosphodiesterase nucleotide pyrophosphatase (PDNP) enzymes which include ectonucleotide pyrophosphatase/phosphodiesterase 1 (ENPP1, also known as plasma cell membrane glycoprotein 1, located on the membranes of cells and MVs), autotaxin (secreted from cells), and PDNP3 (intracellular) hydrolyse the phosphodiester 1 bond of NTP to produce PPi [11] (Figure 49.3). Of these, ENPP1 is the most significant contributor to extracellular

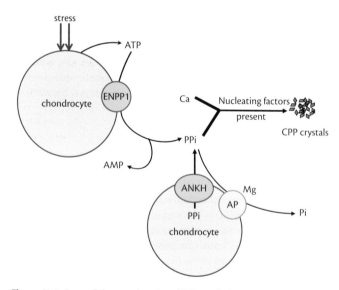

Figure 49.3 Extracellular pyrophosphate (PPi) metabolism. AMP, adenosine monophosphate; ANKH, ankylosis human protein; AP, alkaline phosphatase; ATP, adenosine triphosphate; Ca, calcium; ENPP1, ectonucleotide pyrophosphatase/phosphodiesterase 1; Mg, magnesium; Pi, phosphate; PPi, pyrophosphate.

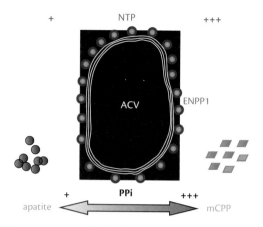

Figure 49.4 Pyrophosphate (PPi) level determines the calcium crystal formed. High PPi level—CPP crystal formed, low PPi level hydroxyapatite crystal formed. ACV, articular cartilage vesicle; NTP, nucleotide triphosphate; PPi, pyrophosphate; mCPP, monoclinic CPP crystal; ENPP1, ectonucleotide pyrophosphatase/phosphodiesterase 1.

NTP breakdown, and knockout mouse models suggest that ENPP1 and not ANKH produces most of the ePPi [12]. ENPP1 activity is upregulated in OA and with ageing. As with loss of function mutations in *ANKH*, loss of function mutations in the *ENPP1* gene cause low ePPi levels and are recognized to cause the extremely rare and fatal generalized arterial calcification of infancy, again due to uninhibited apatite formation. The release of ATP, the principal extracellular substrate of ENPP1 from chondrocytes, is potentiated by mechanical loading, increased cell activity, cell division, and injury [1,13]. Extracellular ATP concentration largely determines the ePPi levels and the type of calcium crystal formed [1,14]. For example, the addition of plentiful ATP to cultured articular chondrocyte vesicles results in high ePPi levels which encourage CPP crystal formation, while restricted ATP results in lower ePPi levels which stimulate formation of BCP crystals [2,14,15] (Figure 49.4). As with intracellular PPi, the ePPi level is tightly regulated. ePPi complexed with magnesium is normally rapidly hydrolysed by the cell-membrane bound alkaline phosphatases (TNAP) to Pi, which can readily cross cell membranes. The mechanism of predisposition to CPPD in metabolic diseases includes:

◆ increased PPi (due to increased adenylate cyclase activity) +/− increased calcium levels in hyperparathyroidism

◆ reduced breakdown of PPi by alkaline phosphatase in hypomagnesaemia and hypophosphatasia

◆ inhibition of alkaline phosphatase and promotion of CPP crystal nucleation by iron in haemochromatosis

◆ increased PPi levels, generally believed to be due to increased ANKH activity in familal CPPD.

Effect of cytokines and growth factors on inorganic pyrophosphate levels

Known regulators of ePPi include transforming growth factor beta (TGFβ), interleukin 1 beta (IL1B), and insulin-like growth factor 1 (IGF1). TGFβ, an important growth factor in OA and osteophyte formation, promotes ENPP1, ANKH, cartilage intermediate layer protein (CILP), and transglutaminase activity and down-regulates

Table 49.1 Regulators of pyrophosphate metabolism

Substrate	Substrate expression	
	Factors increasing	Factors reducing
ENPP1	TGFβ[a], ageing, thyroid hormone, retinoic acid[b]	IL1B, IGF1[c]
TNAP	IL1B, thyroid hormone	TGFβ[d]
ANKH	TGFβ	IGF1, TNF
Transglutaminase	TGFβ, ageing	IGF1
CILP	TGFβ, ageing	IGF1

[a]Effect of TGFβ on ENPP1 is antagonized by IL1B and IGF1.

[b]Effect of retinoic acid on ENPP1 is mediated in part by activation of latent TGFβ.

[c]Effect of IGF1 on ENPP1 is antagonized by CILP-1.

[d]Effect of TGFβ on TNAP is antagonized by IL1B.

TNAP activity which increases ePPi levels [9] (Table 49.1). IGF1 has the opposite effect to TGFβ, and reduces ePPi levels. Inflammatory cytokines such as IL1B down-regulate ENPP1 and ANKH activity and promote TNAP activity resulting in lower ePPi levels, which may explain the negative association between RA and CPPD.

Pi and PPi levels are inter-related by several biofeedback mechanisms. For instance, a TGFβ-induced increase in ANKH expression is mediated by the influx of Pi through PIT1, and PIT2, and by the influx of calcium by L- or T-type voltage dependent calcium channels [16,17]. A gain in ANKH activity increases the expression of PIT1 resulting in high intracellular Pi levels which then stimulates TNAP activity thereby lowering ePPi concentration [18]. Apart from this, elevated extracellular Pi increases the effect of TGFβ on ANKH, ENPP1, and PIT1 mRNA and protein expression thereby increasing ePPi [19].

Type 2 transglutaminase and factor XIIIa also promote CPP crystal formation [20]. This may be due to transglutaminase-mediated activation and incorporation of latent TGFβ in the extracellular matrix, post-translational modification of extracellular matrix favouring crystal formation, stimulation of phospholipase A$_2$ with resulting cartilage degradation, and inhibition of TNAP [21–23]. Osteopontin, a calcium-binding matricellular protein present in the pericellular location, also increases CPPD by activating transglutaminases [24].

Calcium pyrophosphate crystal formation

The formation of CPP crystal in vivo appears restricted principally to fibro- and hyaline articular cartilage (less commonly seen in capsule, tendon, or ligaments). However, they also form in the areas of chondroid metaplasia in the synovium [25]. Of the 12 known crystallographic forms of CPP crystals, only the rod-like monoclinic (M-) or squat triclinic (T-) forms are deposited in vivo. Formation of M-CPP and T-CPP is slow, occurring via intermediate crystal species, with T-CPP being the final, most stable form in post-mortem menisci, and in in vitro gel and aqueous models.

Unlike MSU crystals which form readily in supersaturated solutions, CPP crystals require exacting physicochemical conditions or prolonged incubation [26]. In addition, CPPD only occurs in larger animals such as primates and dogs. Thus, to date, an animal model of CPPD has not been developed, and most knowledge is derived from models employing gels (non-biological, gelatin, or native collagen gels).

From these experimental studies the following generalities are implied. In addition to the ionic product (Ca^{2+} × PPi), local magnesium concentration influences CPPD by inhibiting crystal nucleation and growth and by enhancing crystal dissolution. Pi, chondroitin sulphate, and large proteoglycans are also inhibitory to crystal nucleation and growth. With proteoglycan this effect depends on the spatial arrangement of carboxylate ligands, which may operate via calcium binding or spatial regulation of Mg^{2+}, phosphate, or unidentified small-molecular-weight promoters and inhibitors. Conversely, nucleating and growth-promoting factors include iron (Fe^{3+} > Fe^{2+}) and seeded MSU crystals. Interestingly, seeded apatite has little epitaxial effect but efficiently traps PPi, leading to more stable CPP growth. A possible promoting role for collagen and acidic phospholipid has been suggested.

Histological studies suggest that CPP crystals always form extracellularly, initially in pericellular locations usually in the collagenous matrix in the midzone of fibro- and hyaline articular cartilage [27]. A very close association is reported with hypertrophic or metaplastic chondrocyte phenotypes containing Sudan-positive lipid granules. In addition, Sudan-positive lipid may occur around CPP crystals, the involved matrix often being proteoglycan deplete and degenerate [27]. Such findings support the importance of tissue ('soil') factors, implying that reduction of inhibitors (e.g. proteoglycan) and an increase in promoters (e.g. lipid) combine to promote CPP crystal formation. The relative importance of soil and seed (e.g. ePPi) factors may vary in different clinical settings.

Calcium pyrophosphate crystal-induced inflammation

CPP crystals induce inflammation predominantly by their effects on the innate immune system. As with acute gout, activation of the NALP3 inflammasome which results in production of IL1B seems to be central to acute inflammation induced by CPP crystals [26]. IL1B then orchestrates the release of other cytokines such as TNFA. This is because CPP crystal-induced TNFA release lags behind IL1B secretion, and is blocked by both IL1B maturation blocker, and IL1 receptor antagonists [26]. The inflammatory infiltrate in acute CPP crystal arthritis is predominantly neutrophilic and there is a paucity of mononuclear cells. This may be as CPP crystals preferentially induce IL8 (chemotactic to neutrophils) and not macrophage inflammatory protein 1 alpha (MIP1A, chemotactic to macrophages) production [28]. Additionally, while the IL8 secretion induced by TNFA and granulocyte-macrophage colony-stimulating factor is further potentiated by CPP crystals, the MIP1A secretion induced by TNFA is inhibited by CPP crystals [28]. Apart from recruiting neutrophils preferentially, CPP crystals also inhibit neutrophil apoptosis by inhibiting pro-apoptotic cysteine protease caspase 3 and activating ERK1/2, p38, and Akt [29]. This may explain the prolonged neutrophilic inflammatory response in acute CPP crystal arthritis.

Neutrophils that phagocytose CPP crystals respond with increased metabolic activity, and the release of myeloperoxidase, IL1B, IL8, and neutrophil extracellular trap (NET) [30]. NETs are neutrophil fragments composed of chromatin and myeloperoxidase and can damage bystander cells [30]. Apart from this, CPP crystals also induce superoxide production and the release of lysosomal enzymes and lipoxygenase-derived products of arachidonic acid, such as leukotriene B4, following phagocytosis. Additionally, CPP crystals also increase the release of IL6 [31], and activate toll-like receptor 2 which leads to several downstream changes (e.g. NO production) that may adversely affect the chondrocyte and the cartilage matrix [32].

CPP crystals activate complement via effects on both classic and alternative pathways. Hageman factor is also activated *in vitro*, leading to the generation of kallikrein, bradykinin, plasmin, and other soluble mediators. Many of these effects result from direct crystal contact, though some (e.g. classic pathway complement activation) may be enhanced or mediated via immunoglobulin G (IgG) adsorbed on to the crystal surface [33]. In biological systems, the CPP crystals avidly attract both anionic and cationic proteins, with some preferential selection for immunoglobulin, especially IgG. Although the altered stereochemical configuration of adsorbed IgG may be pro-inflammatory, other protein binding may be inhibitory. Of most interest in this respect are apolipoprotein B-containing low-density and high-density lipoproteins, binding with which, for example, inhibits CPP-induced inflammation [34–36].

Certain physical characteristics of CPP crystals affect their inflammatory potential [33]. In general, smaller, protein-coated, and M-CPP crystals are more inflammatory. This may result from mechanical effects (e.g. greater ease of phagocytosis) or merely reflect the greater surface area/volume presented for protein or membrane interactions [33]. 'Roughness' and net negative surface charge are also important [33]. Crystal surfaces of inflammatory membranolytic crystals are irregular and possess a high density of charged groups that give a high negative zeta potential, whereas surfaces of non-inflammatory crystals (e.g. diamond) are smooth, with low or zero zeta potential. Basic brushite and apatite are intermediate in these respects and result in modest inflammatory effects.

Less is known of chronic CPP-induced tissue damage, though postulated mechanisms include matrix metalloproteinase expression, NO release, persistent synovial inflammation, altered cell metabolism, prostaglandin E2 release, and altered osteoblast activity [32]. There are limited data on the possible mechanical effects of intra-articular crystal deposits. Deposits that are harder or softer than the surrounding cartilage, especially loosely packed crystal deposits associate with abnormal shear stress, while very densely packed and tightly bound spherical aggregates will themselves carry a certain amount of load [37,38]. Crystals that reach the cartilage surface and synovial fluid potentially could act as wear particles to encourage fibrillation.

Crystal shedding

The preferred mechanism to explain the occurrence of CPP crystals within synovial fluid is shedding from preformed deposits within cartilage [39]. This could be accomplished by a reduction in crystal size, fissuring of cartilage, or alteration in cartilage matrix that allows crystals to escape. Although not directly visualized, circumstantial evidence in support includes the provocation of acute CPP crystal arthritis by joint lavage with crystal solubilizing agents, parathyroidectomy associated with reduced ionized calcium (reduced crystal size), trauma (micro-fissuring, 'shaking loose'), thyroxine replacement (change in interstitial matrix), and co-occurrence of acute CPP crystal arthritis and sepsis ('enzymatic strip mining'). Direct evidence for this comes from the reduction in radiographic

chondrocalcinosis documented during acute CPP crystal arthritis [39,40].

Shedding might expose previously protected crystals to soluble mediators and cells and thus trigger the acute attack. The CPP crystals are subsequently taken up and processed by neutrophils and synoviocytes. However, such 'trafficking' through the joint is slow and CPP crystals are still identifiable in synovial fluid as the attack settles and even long after it has resolved. What 'turns off' the attack remains unexplained. Nevertheless, coating by inhibitory proteins appears a plausible explanation.

Pathological changes

CPP crystals are virtually confined to locomotor structures. They form close to hypertrophic chondrocytes in a cartilage matrix that is rich in electron-dense amorphous material including proteoglycans (e.g. dermatan sulphate), collagen fibres (e.g. type 1 collagen), lipids, cellular debris, and S-100 protein [27,41,42]. Of these, both dermatan sulphate and S-100 protein have calcium binding properties and such extracellular materials may act as CPP crystal nucleating and growth promoting factors. Furthermore, metabolically active hypertrophic chondrocytes are rich in iPPi and readily release ATP [42].

Microscopy usually shows rounded, sharply demarcated crystal deposits within a granular matrix in the midzone of the cartilage [27,41]. The cartilage morphology may appear macroscopically fairly normal or show the spectrum of changes observed in OA. CPP crystals are deposited in the plane of the collagen fibres with collagen fibres being observed in early deposits [42]. However, identifiable collagen fibres may be absent in the fully formed tightly packed deposits [42]. The earliest CPPD is perilacunar, but with widespread chondrocalcinosis superficial cartilage may be involved, with tophus-like deposits predominating in the midzone. Surrounding cartilage may appear normal or show loss of metachromasia, chondrocyte cloning, or fibrillation and occurrence of associated lipid-laden hypertrophic metaplastic chondrocytes has been described [27]. In synovium, CPP crystals usually occur superficially in the interstitial space and synoviocyte vacuoles, often surrounded by fibrocytes and connective tissue. Neutrophil and lymphocyte infiltrates may be present but the prominent response is lining cell hyperplasia. Tophus-like deposits, surrounding giant cell reactions and osteochondral bodies, are occasional findings. In advanced disease, masses of CPP crystals may virtually replace ischaemic-appearing villi.

Summary and conclusion

Factors promoting CPP crystal formation and the mechanisms by which they cause inflammation are becoming better understood. However, the inability to dissolve CPP crystals *in vivo* and to potentially provide a cure for CPPD significantly reduces the volume of basic research in this common condition.

References

1. Rachow JW, Ryan LM. Adenosine triphosphate pyrophosphohydrolase and neutral inorganic pyrophosphatase in pathologic joint fluids. Elevated pyrophosphohydrolase in calcium pyrophosphate dihydrate crystal deposition disease. *Arthritis Rheum* 1985; 28(11):1283–8.
2. Thouverey C, Bechkoff G, Pikula S, Buchet R. Inorganic pyrophosphate as a regulator of hydroxyapatite or calcium pyrophosphate dihydrate

mineral deposition by matrix vesicles. *Osteoarthritis Cartilage* 2009; 17(1):64–72.

3. Micheli A, Po J, Fallet GH. Measurement of soluble pyrophosphate in plasma and synovial fluid of patients with various rheumatic diseases. *Scand J Rheumatol* 1981; 10(3):237–40.

4. Pattrick M, Hamilton E, Hornby J, Doherty M. Synovial fluid pyrophosphate and nucleoside triphosphate pyrophosphatase: comparison between normal and diseased and between inflamed and non-inflamed joints. *Ann Rheum Dis* 1991; 50(4):214–8.

5. Doherty M, Hamilton E, Henderson J, Misra H, Dixey J. Familial chondrocalcinosis due to calcium pyrophosphate dihydrate crystal deposition in English families. *Br J Rheumatol* 1991; 30(1):10–5.

6. Doherty M, Chuck A, Hosking D, Hamilton E. Inorganic pyrophosphate in metabolic diseases predisposing to calcium pyrophosphate dihydrate crystal deposition. *Arthritis Rheum* 1991; 34(10):1297–303.

7. Ho AM, Johnson MD, Kingsley DM. Role of the mouse ank gene in control of tissue calcification and arthritis. *Science* 2000; 289(5477):265–70.

8. Zhang Y, Johnson K, Russell RG, et al. Association of sporadic chondrocalcinosis with a -4-basepair G-to-A transition in the 5'-untranslated region of ANKH that promotes enhanced expression of ANKH protein and excess generation of extracellular inorganic pyrophosphate. *Arthritis Rheum* 2005; 52(4):1110–7.

9. Abhishek A, Doherty M. Pathophysiology of articular chondrocalcinosis—role of ANKH. *Nat Rev Rheumatol* 2011; 7(2):96–104.

10. Costello JC, Rosenthal AK, Kurup IV, et al. Parallel regulation of extracellular ATP and inorganic pyrophosphate: roles of growth factors, transduction modulators, and ANK. *Connect Tissue Res* 2011; 52(2):139–46.

11. Johnson KH, Hashimoto S, Lotz S, et al. Up-regulated expression of the phosphodiesterase nucleotide pyrophosphatase family member PC-1 is a marker and pathogenic factor for knee meniscal cartilage matrix calcification. *Arthritis Rheum* 2001; 44(5):1071–81.

12. Harmey D, Hessle L, Narisawa S, et al. Concerted regulation of inorganic pyrophosphate and osteopontin by akp2, enpp1, and ank: an integrated model of the pathogenesis of mineralization disorders. *Am J Pathol* 2004; 164(4):1199–209.

13. Graff RD, Lazarowski ER, Banes AJ, Lee GM. ATP release by mechanically loaded porcine chondrons in pellet culture. *Arthritis Rheum* 2000; 43(7):1571–9.

14. Ryan LM, Kurup IV, Derfus BA, Kushnaryov VM. ATP-induced chondrocalcinosis. *Arthritis Rheum* 1992; 35(12):1520–5.

15. Derfus BA, Rachow JW, Mandel NS, et al. Articular cartilage vesicles generate calcium pyrophosphate dihydrate-like crystals in vitro. *Arthritis Rheum* 1992; 35(2):231–40.

16. Oca P, Zaka R, Dion AS, Freeman TA, Williams CJ. Phosphate and calcium are required for TGFbeta-mediated stimulation of ANK expression and function during chondrogenesis. *J Cell Physiol* 2010; 224(2):540–8.

17. Cailotto F, Reboul P, Sebillaud S, et al. Calcium input potentiates the transforming growth factor (TGF)-beta1-dependent signaling to promote the export of inorganic pyrophosphate by articular chondrocyte. *J Biol Chem* 2011; 286(22):19215–28.

18. Wang W, Xu J, Du B, Kirsch T. Role of the progressive ankylosis gene (ank) in cartilage mineralization. *Mol Cell Biol* 2005; 25(1):312–23.

19. Hamade T, Bianchi A, Sebillaud S, et al. Inorganic phosphate (Pi) modulates the expression of key regulatory proteins of the inorganic pyrophosphate (PPi) metabolism in TGF-beta1-stimulated chondrocytes. *Biomed Mater Eng* 2010; 20(3):209–15.

20. Rosenthal AK, Masuda I, Gohr CM, Derfus BA, Le M. The transglutaminase, factor XIIIA, is present in articular chondrocytes. *Osteoarthritis Cartilage* 2001; 9(6):578–81.

21. Rosenthal AK GC, Henry LA, Le M. Participation of transglutaminase in the activation of latent transforming growth factor beta1 in aging articular cartilage. *Arthritis Rheum* 2000; 43(8):1729–33.

22. Rosenthal AK, Derfus BA, Henry LA. Transglutaminase activity in aging articular chondrocytes and articular cartilage vesicles. *Arthritis Rheum* 1997; 40(5):966–70.

23. Heinkel D, Gohr CM, Uzuki M, Rosenthal AK. Transglutaminase contributes to CPPD crystal formation in osteoarthritis. *Front Biosci* 2004; 9:3257–61.

24. Rosenthal AK, Gohr CM, Uzuki M, Masuda I. Osteopontin promotes pathologic mineralization in articular cartilage. *Matrix Biol* 2007; 26(2):96–105.

25. Beutler A, Rothfuss S, Clayburne G, Sieck M, Schumacher HR, Jr. Calcium pyrophosphate dihydrate crystal deposition in synovium. Relationship to collagen fibers and chondrometaplasia. *Arthritis Rheum* 1993; 36(5):704–15.

26. Martinon F, Petrilli V, Mayor A, Tardivel A, Tschopp J. Gout-associated uric acid crystals activate the NALP3 inflammasome. *Nature* 2006; 440(7081):237–41.

27. Ishikawa K, Masuda I, Ohira T, Yokoyama M. A histological study of calcium pyrophosphate dihydrate crystal-deposition disease. *J Bone Joint Surg Am* 1989; 71(6):875–86.

28. Hachicha M, Naccache PH, McColl SR. Inflammatory microcrystals differentially regulate the secretion of macrophage inflammatory protein 1 and interleukin 8 by human neutrophils: a possible mechanism of neutrophil recruitment to sites of inflammation in synovitis. *J Exp Med* 1995; 182(6):2019–25.

29. Liu-Bryan R, Liote F. Monosodium urate and calcium pyrophosphate dihydrate (CPPD) crystals, inflammation, and cellular signaling. *Joint Bone Spine* 2005; 72(4):295–302.

30. Pang L, Hayes CP, Buac K, Yoo DG, Rada B. Pseudogout-associated inflammatory calcium pyrophosphate dihydrate microcrystals induce formation of neutrophil extracellular traps. *J Immunol* 2013; 190(12):6488–500.

31. Guerne PA, Terkeltaub R, Zuraw B, Lotz M. Inflammatory microcrystals stimulate interleukin-6 production and secretion by human monocytes and synoviocytes. *Arthritis Rheum* 1989; 32(11):1443–52.

32. Liu-Bryan R, Pritzker K, Firestein GS, Terkeltaub R. TLR2 signaling in chondrocytes drives calcium pyrophosphate dihydrate and monosodium urate crystal-induced nitric oxide generation. *J Immunol* 2005; 174(8):5016–23.

33. Swan A, Heywood B, Chapman B, Seward H, Dieppe P. Evidence for a causal relationship between the structure, size, and load of calcium pyrophosphate dihydrate crystals, and attacks of pseudogout. *Ann Rheum Dis* 1995; 54(10):825–30.

34. Burt HM, Jackson JK, Rowell J. Calcium pyrophosphate and monosodium urate crystal interactions with neutrophils: effect of crystal size and lipoprotein binding to crystals. *J Rheumatol* 1989; 16(6):809–17.

35. Ohnuma S. [A role for lipoproteins in the recovery from CPPD crystal-induced arthritis]. *Nihon Seikeigeka Gakkai zasshi* 1994; 68(11):953–60.

36. Kumagai Y, Watanabe W, Kobayashi A, et al. Inhibitory effect of low density lipoprotein on the inflammation-inducing activity of calcium pyrophosphate dihydrate crystals. *J Rheumatol* 2001; 28(12):2674–80.

37. Clift SE, Hayes A, Miles AW, Harris B, Dieppe PA. Load concentrations around crystal aggregates in articular cartilage under short-term loading. *Proc Inst Mech Eng H* 1993; 207(1):35–40.

38. Hayes A, Harris B, Dieppe PA, Clift SE. Wear of articular cartilage: the effect of crystals. *Proc Inst Mech Eng H* 1993; 207(1):41–58.

39. Doherty M, Dieppe PA. Acute pseudogout: 'crystal shedding' or acute crystallization? *Arthritis Rheum* 1981; 24(7):954–7.

40. Dieppe PA, Alexander GJ, Jones HE, et al. Pyrophosphate arthropathy: a clinical and radiological study of 105 cases. *Ann Rheum Dis* 1982; 41(4):371–6.

41. Ohira T, Ishikawa K, Masuda I, Yokoyama M, Honda I. Histologic localization of lipid in the articular tissues in calcium pyrophosphate dihydrate crystal deposition disease. *Arthritis Rheum* 1988; 31(8):1057–62.

42. Masuda I, Ishikawa K, Usuku G. A histologic and immunohistochemical study of calcium pyrophosphate dihydrate crystal deposition disease. *Clin Orthop Rel Res* 1991(263):272–87.

CHAPTER 50

Clinical features of calcium pyrophosphate crystal deposition

Abhishek Abhishek and Michael Doherty

Introduction

Calcium pyrophosphate deposition (CPPD) is generally asymptomatic. It may be detected incidentally on radiographs performed for another purpose. However, it can cause both acute arthritis and chronic musculoskeletal symptoms, most commonly in the elderly [1–4]. In this chapter we will describe both the common and the rare clinical manifestations of CPPD using the European League Against Rheumatism (EULAR) classification of clinical presentations of CPPD [5].

Acute calcium pyrophosphate deposition crystal arthritis

This is a common cause of acute arthritis in older people, and acute attacks may be the only manifestation of otherwise asymptomatic CPPD. The typical attack of acute calcium pyrophosphate (CPP) crystal arthritis develops rapidly (over a few hours), with pain, stiffness, and swelling, and is usually maximal within 6–24 hours of onset (Figure 50.1). As in gout, the pain may be described as the 'worst ever' and the patient may be unable to tolerate even light pressure from clothes or bedding. The patient is unable to fully move the joint and holds it in a position that minimizes the intra-articular pressure (i.e. the 'loose-pack position', such as fixed-flexion at the knee or elbow, and internally rotated,

and adducted at the shoulder). Overlying erythema is common and the joint swelling may be more widespread than expected, especially in those with acute CPP crystal arthritis of the wrist, ankle, or metacarpophalangeal joints. Examination reveals a swollen, often erythematous joint which is warm to touch, and tender to palpate. There may be a large or tense effusion. Marked joint line tenderness is usual and there is universal stress pain (pain progressively worse as the joint is moved into its tight-pack positions) and a restricted range of movement. Pitting periarticular oedema is common especially in those with wrist, ankle, and mid-foot involvement. Fever may be present and can be marked. Confusion may be present in an elderly patient with florid or polyarticular acute CPP crystal synovitis. Acute attacks are self-limiting and usually resolve within 1–3 weeks. Some patients have problematic recurrent haemarthrosis, particularly of the shoulder and knee. Synovial fluid leakage may occur with extensive swelling and bruising of the adjacent tissues (Figure 50.2). Although any joint can be affected, acute attacks most frequently occur in knees (commonest), wrists, shoulders, elbows, and ankles (Figures 50.3 and 50.4). Rarely the first metatarsophalangeal joint may be affected ('pseudo-podagra'), simulating acute gout. Concurrent attacks in more than one joint is unusual (<10% of cases) and polyarticular attacks are rare. In patients with osteoarthritis (OA), the attacks may superimpose on chronic symptomatic arthropathy.

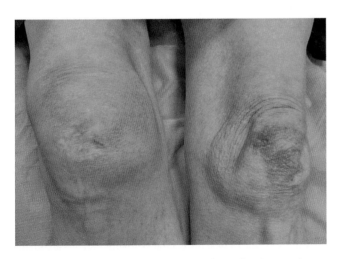

Figure 50.1 Swollen right knee with overlying erythema; there is a tense knee effusion with obvious distention of the suprapatellar pouch.

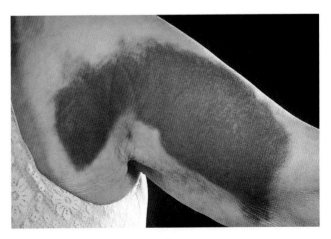

Figure 50.2 Joints with a large tense effusion may leak synovial fluid into the soft tissues. Note subcutaneous haemorrhage in the upper arm of an elderly lady with acute CPP crystal arthritis. This can also occur at the knees.

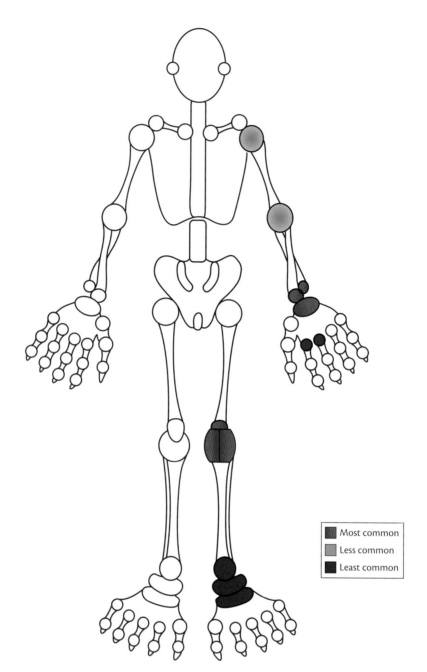

Figure 50.3 Joints commonly affected by acute CPP crystal arthritis, and by CPPD with OA.

Most episodes of acute CPP crystal arthritis develop spontaneously, but several provoking factors may precipitate the attack (Box 50.1). The commonest precipitating factor is intercurrent illness (e.g. chest or urinary tract infection). The frequency of attacks of acute CPP crystal arthritis varies from person to person. While some people get relatively infrequent episodes, others may have frequent acute attacks. The reason for this is not entirely clear.

CPP crystal-associated bursitis, tenosynovitis, and tendonitis may also occur but appear to be rare. For example, olecranon, prepatellar and retrocalcaneal bursitis have been reported in patients with CPPD. Acute inflammatory episodes in the triceps, flexor digitorum, and Achilles tendons, and tenosynovitis of the wrist flexors and extensor tendons have also been reported [6]. Flexor tendon involvement may associate with carpal tunnel syndrome, and may cause combined median and ulnar nerve entrapment at the wrist, the entrapment appearing to relate more to soft tissue swelling than structural arthropathy. Tendon rupture (e.g. hand extensors, Achilles) is a rare complication.

Chronic arthropathy

Chronic arthropathy most commonly presents as OA with CPPD, and far less commonly as chronic CPP crystal inflammatory arthritis. The two manifestations may coexist in different joints in the same patient, and a single joint may evolve from one phenotype to another. Additionally, patients with either condition may develop superimposed attacks of acute crystal synovitis. Patients are mainly elderly, and large and medium-sized joints are targeted, with the knees being the most commonly and severely affected joint,

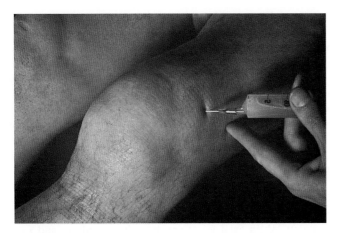

Figure 50.4 Acute CPP crystal arthritis: there may be a large effusion, and the aspirated fluid may be turbid.

followed by wrists, shoulders, elbows, hips, and mid-tarsal joints. Symptoms are often restricted to just a few joints, though involvement of multiple joints can also occur.

Osteoarthritis with CPPD

Symptomatic OA with CPPD presents the same symptoms and signs as OA without CPPD. Pain is predominantly usage related but may be accompanied by some night pain, especially in large joints, and morning and inactivity stiffness are not marked. Examination reveals varying degrees of joint-line tenderness, restriction of movement, bony swelling, coarse crepitus, and malalignment and deformity. Clinical signs of inflammation (stress pain, effusion, synovial thickening, and increased warmth) are usually absent or only mild to modest, and mainly identified clinically as mild to modest effusions at the knee. Although predominantly anecdotal, clinical experience suggests that OA with CPPD associates with more inflammatory symptoms and signs (e.g. more stiffness and effusion) and an atypical distribution of structural arthropathy (e.g. more pronounced involvement of the MCP, radiocarpal, midcarpal, glenohumeral, ankle, and midfoot joints)

Box 50.1 Triggers of acute CPP crystal arthritis

Joint injury:

- Intercurrent illnesses (e.g. chest infection, urinary tract infection, myocardial infarction)
- Surgery (especially parathyroidectomy)
- Blood transfusion, parenteral fluid administration
- Joint lavage.

Possible:

- Intra-articular hyaluronan injection
- Bisphosphonate use—initiation of oral weekly alendronate, and intravenous neridronate or pamidronate; also reported after cyclical etidronate therapy
- Thyroxine replacement therapy.

Note: most cases of acute CPP crystal synovitis develop spontaneously.

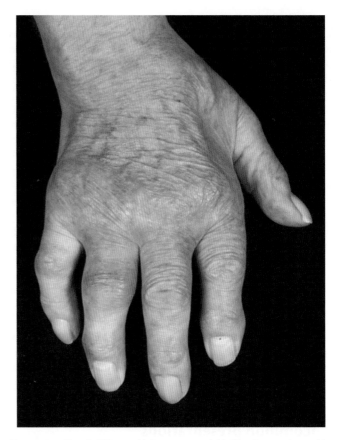

Figure 50.5 Chronic CPP crystal inflammatory arthritis. Note increased synovial thickening in the metacarpophalangeal joints.

when compared with OA alone [5]. Examination often reveals more widespread asymptomatic OA changes and presence of generalized nodal OA with Heberden and Bouchard nodes is common. Though less well documented, it is likely that asymptomatic OA with CPPD is also common in the eighth and ninth decades of life, as is asymptomatic OA.

Chronic CPP crystal inflammatory arthritis

Some patients present with chronic oligoarthritis or polyarthritis with more overt inflammatory symptoms and signs and occasional systemic upset (with elevation of C-reactive protein and erythrocyte sedimentation rate (ESR)). There may be additional episodes of superimposed acute crystal synovitis. Therefore, this condition should be considered in the differential diagnosis of rheumatoid arthritis (RA) and other chronic inflammatory joint diseases in older adults [7]. On examination there may be signs of OA but also signs of synovitis, for example, warmth, joint line and/or capsular tenderness, stress pain, joint effusion, and marked synovial thickening (Figure 50.5). It is usually most evident clinically at knees, wrists, and metacarpophalangeal and glenohumeral joints.

Outcome of chronic arthropathy associated with CPPD

The natural history of chronic CPPD-associated arthropathy is not well documented. Previously in Europe it was often termed 'chronic pyrophosphate arthropathy' without any distinction between 'non-inflammatory' (OA with CPPD) and 'inflammatory' (chronic CPP crystal inflammatory arthritis) arthropathy. Thus, previous long-term outcome studies are difficult to interpret in the context of the new EULAR nomenclature. While some studies suggested that chondrocalcinosis (CC) does not lead to progressive joint space narrowing in knees with OA over a 2.5- to 3-year period [8], other studies raise the possibility that CC and CPPD may associate with worsening joint space narrowing. For example, rapidly progressive arthropathy has been associated with CPPD, both in anecdotal case reports, and in a small case–control study in which CC at distant joints associated with rapidly progressive hip OA [2]. Similarly, in another hospital-based prospective study of 350 OA knees, the presence of synovial fluid CPP crystals or radiographic articular CC associated with radiographic progression, especially bone attrition (odds ratio 3.44, 95% confidence interval 1.97–6.02) and clinical deterioration, suggesting that CPPD may be a marker for poor prognosis in knee OA [9]. Rapidly progressive large joint arthropathy has also been associated with CPPD ('pseudo-neuropathic' arthritis) [4]. However, as with OA it seems likely that OA plus CPPD shows a spectrum of severity, ranging from asymptomatic and stable through to more symptomatic and progressive, and that there are no true discrete subsets within this clinical spectrum. Further research is required to determine whether the presence of CPPD is a true risk factor for clinical and structural outcomes and whether chronic inflammatory CPP crystal arthritis is a discrete subset of CPPD.

Uncommon presentations

Familial CPPD

A hereditary form of CC was first reported by Zitnan and Sitaj in seven Czechoslovakian kindreds in 1963. Subsequently, there have been several case reports of familial CPPD from all over the world. In some families, CPPD may be part of a hereditary premature dysplastic OA phenotype, while in others, it may be the only manifestation presenting with recurrent episodes of acute CPP crystal arthritis [10,11].

The pattern of inheritance in familial CPPD varies, though autosomal dominance is usual. Two familial phenotypes have been emphasized:

- Early-onset (third to fourth decade) florid polyarticular CC, and variable severity of arthropathy ranging from mild to destructive [12]
- Late-onset (sixth to seventh decade) oligoarticular CC mainly confined to the knees, and arthritis resembling sporadic OA with CPPD [13].

The latter phenotype may be more common than recognized. The late onset of disease expression and geographic dispersal of families pose difficulty in this respect. Some families may also have early-onset diffuse idiopathic skeletal hyperostosis with inflammatory back pain, peripheral and axial enthesophytes, and spinal ankylosis [14]. Premature CPPD due to a mutation in the *ANKH* gene also associates with childhood febrile seizures in one kindred in the United Kingdom [15].

Axial CPPD

Some people develop spinal CPPD. Although mostly asymptomatic when present in the disc material [16], it can associate with the crowned dens syndrome, or with acute localized meningism and/or myeloradiculopathy. Crowned dens syndrome (so-called because there is a crown of calcification in the cruciate, transverse, alar, and apical ligaments around the dens) presents with acute cervico-occipital pain, fever, and neck stiffness accompanied by an acute inflammatory reaction [17]. The symptoms last for a few days to a few weeks, and the severity of pain may range from mild to severe. This syndrome can be misdiagnosed as meningitis, epidural abscess, polymyalgia rheumatica, giant cell arteritis, or as cervical spondylitis, and its diagnosis requires a high index of suspicion as in some patients it may be the first presentation of CPPD [18].

Severe spinal stiffness, particularly in Czech, Chilean, and other familial forms, may present as 'pseudo-ankylosing spondylitis' and indeed, spinal ankylosis may occur in the Chilean families [19]. Acute attacks in axial joints are difficult to confirm, and some self-limiting spinal syndromes, described in relation to the periodontoid, cervical, and lumbar regions, may reflect acute CPP crystal arthritis, especially in the elderly. Other uncommon and atypical spinal manifestations of CPPD include neurological syndromes related to axial compression, foramen magnum syndrome, cervical radiculomyelopathy, thoracic cord compression, cauda equina syndrome, lumbar radiculopathy, and lumbar canal stenosis.

Tophaceous CPPD

Tophaceous ('tumoural') CPPD is rare. This usually presents as slow-growing painless lumps. However, they may rarely cause bone erosion and destruction. Lesions are solitary and usually develop in areas of chondroid metaplasia without predisposing metabolic abnormality or CPPD elsewhere. They can be intra- or periarticular in location. Tophaceous CPPD most commonly occurs at the temporomandibular joint [20]. Other less common locations include hands, cervical spine, feet, hips, acromioclavicular joints, knees, and elbows. Malignancy is often suspected and the diagnosis usually follows examination of excised material.

Differential diagnosis

Acute CPP crystal arthritis

In typical cases, when pain and synovitis are marked and at their worst within 24 hours, the principal differential diagnosis is another crystal-induced arthritis. This is usually gout and differentiation primarily rests on synovial fluid analysis or on the demonstration of the characteristic double-contour sign on ultrasound. Rarely, calcium oxalate crystals can cause acute synovitis, sometimes with intra-articular calcification evident on radiographs, in people with end-stage renal disease who are on dialysis, and in those with primary hyperoxaluria. Acute synovitis within a few hours of an intra-articular steroid injection suggests an acute inflammatory reaction to corticosteroid crystals, which usually settles without further progression over several days.

The presence of acute synovitis in one or a few joints with overlying erythema, fever, constitutional upset, and cloudy and/or purulent joint fluid, particularly in the setting of preceding surgery, trauma, or infective illness, should always lead to the consideration and exclusion of septic arthritis. As septic arthritis may rarely coexist with crystal synovitis, Gram stain and culture of joint fluid (with culture of blood and possibly urine, sputum, or other body fluids as appropriate) should be undertaken in an unwell patient, when the attack has been triggered by intercurrent illness or surgery, or when the attack is less typical (e.g. possibly progressive for more than 24 hours) even if CPP crystals are identified and/or radiographic CC is demonstrated.

Occasionally uniform blood-staining of joint fluid may lead to consideration of other causes of haemarthrosis, especially bleeding disorder (low vitamin C levels in the elderly may encourage haemarthrosis) or subchondral fracture (particularly with preceding trauma). However, if CPP crystals are identified, there is no bleeding diathesis, no radiographic fracture, and no evidence of lipid droplets in the aspirated synovial fluid, the diagnosis of acute CPP crystal arthritis alone can be accepted. If localized pain and tenderness persist following resolution of synovitis, repeat radiographs (± subsequent bone scan) may be justified to detect a missed fracture.

Chronic arthropathy

In most cases the characteristic distribution, radiographic features, and synovial fluid analysis permits easy diagnosis. In older patients, however, a marked inflammatory component, polyarthritis with metacarpophalangeal joint involvement, and modest elevation of ESR may lead to consideration of RA. Nevertheless, the following usually permit distinction: infrequency of metatarsophalangeal arthropathy; infrequency of tenosynovitis; absence of extra-articular features; lack of juxta-articular osteopenia and marginal erosions; lack of seropositivity for rheumatoid factor and anti-CCP antibodies; and presence of synovial fluid CPP crystals and/or CC.

Patients with marked proximal shoulder and hip girdle stiffness and elevated ESR due to chronic glenohumeral and hip involvement are differentiated from those with polymyalgia rheumatica mainly by careful locomotor examination and by positive joint fluid and radiographic findings. Oral corticosteroids often improve symptoms in such patients but rarely give the rapid 'cure' of polymyalgia: response to local intra-articular corticosteroid may be more impressive.

Differentiation from uncomplicated OA is often by the different pattern of distribution between and within articulations (e.g. greater involvement of lateral tibiofemoral joint, wrist joint, and trapezioscaphoid arthropathy without involvement of the first metacarpophalangeal joint); a more florid inflammatory component; presence of superimposed acute attacks; radiographic findings of CC; and demonstration of synovial fluid CPP crystals. Although rapidly progressive and destructive CPPD arthropathy may resemble a neuropathic joint radiographically, such joints arise in the absence of overt neurological or serological abnormality. Finally, tophaceous CPPD should be considered with malignancy and tophaceous gout in the differential diagnosis of periarticular swellings. Biopsy and histopathological examination is required for the correct diagnosis.

References

1. Dieppe PA, Alexander GJ, Jones HE, et al. Pyrophosphate arthropathy: a clinical and radiological study of 105 cases. *Ann Rheum Dis* 1982; 41:371–6.

2. Doherty M, Dieppe P. Clinical aspects of calcium pyrophosphate dihydrate crystal deposition. *Rheum Dis Clin North Am* 1988; 14:395–414.

3. Kohn NN, Hughes RE, McCarty DJ Jr, Faires JS. The significance of calcium phosphate crystals in the synovial fluid of arthritic patients: the 'pseudogout syndrome': I. Clinical aspects. *Ann Intern Med* 1962; 56:711–37.

4. McCarty DJ. Calcium pyrophosphate dihydrate crystal deposition disease—1975. *Arthritis Rheum* 1976; 19(Suppl 3):275–85.

5. Zhang W, Doherty M, Bardin T, et al. European League Against Rheumatism recommendations for calcium pyrophosphate deposition. Part I: terminology and diagnosis. *Ann Rheum Dis* 2011; 70:563–70.

6. Gerster JC, Lagier R. Upper limb pyrophosphate tenosynovitis outside the carpal tunnel. *Ann Rheum Dis* 1989; 48:689–91.

7. McCarty DJ, Solomon SD, Warnock ML, Paloyan E. Inorganic pyrophosphate concentrations in the synovial fluid of arthritic patients. *J Lab Clin Med* 1971; 78:216–29.

8. Neogi T, Nevitt M, Niu J, et al. Lack of association between chondrocalcinosis and increased risk of cartilage loss in knees with osteoarthritis: results of two prospective longitudinal magnetic resonance imaging studies. *Arthritis Rheum* 2006; 54:1822–8.

9. Ledingham J, Regan M, Jones A, Doherty M. Factors affecting radiographic progression of knee osteoarthritis. *Ann Rheum Dis* 1995; 54:53–8.

10. Abhishek A, Doherty M. Pathophysiology of articular chondrocalcinosis—role of ANKH. *Nat Rev Rheumatol* 2011; 7:96–104.

11. Baldwin CT, Farrer LA, Adair R, et al. Linkage of early-onset osteoarthritis and chondrocalcinosis to human chromosome 8q. *Am J Hum Genet* 1995; 56:692–7.

12. Gruber BL, Couto AR, Armas JB, et al. Novel ANKH amino terminus mutation (Pro5Ser) associated with early-onset calcium pyrophosphate disease with associated phosphaturia. *J Clin Rheumatol* 2012; 18:192–5.

13. Rodriguez-Valverde V, Tinture T, Zuniga M, Pena J, Gonzalez A. Familial chondrocalcinosis. Prevalence in Northern Spain and clinical features in five pedigrees. *Arthritis Rheum* 1980; 23:471–8.

14. Bruges-Armas J, Couto AR, Timms A, et al. Ectopic calcification among families in the Azores: clinical and radiologic manifestations in families with diffuse idiopathic skeletal hyperostosis and chondrocalcinosis. *Arthritis Rheum* 2006; 54:1340–9.

15. McKee S, Pendleton A, Dixey J, Doherty M, Hughes A. Autosomal dominant early childhood seizures associated with chondrocalcinosis and a mutation in the ANKH gene. *Epilepsia* 2004; 45:1258–60.

16. Berlemann U, Gries NC, Moore RJ, Fraser RD, Vernon-Roberts B. Calcium pyrophosphate dihydrate deposition in degenerate lumbar discs. *Eur Spine J* 1998; 7:45–9.

17. Bouvet JP, le Parc JM, Michalski B, Benlahrache C, Auquier L. Acute neck pain due to calcifications surrounding the odontoid process: the crowned dens syndrome. *Arthritis Rheum* 1985; 28:1417–20.

18. Salaffi F, Carotti M, Guglielmi G, Passarini G, Grassi W. The crowned dens syndrome as a cause of neck pain: clinical and computed tomography study in patients with calcium pyrophosphate dihydrate deposition disease. *Clin Exp Rheumatol* 2008; 26:1040–6.

19. Reginato AJ. Articular chondrocalcinosis in the Chiloe Islanders. *Arthritis Rheum* 1976; 19(Suppl 3):395–404.

20. Zweifel D, Ettlin D, Schuknecht B, Obwegeser J. Tophaceous calcium pyrophosphate dihydrate deposition disease of the temporomandibular joint: the preferential site? *J Oral Maxillofac Surg* 2012; 70:60–7.

CHAPTER 51

Investigations of calcium pyrophosphate deposition

Abhishek Abhishek and Michael Doherty

Introduction

The definite diagnosis of calcium pyrophosphate crystal deposition (CPPD) requires synovial fluid examination and identification of calcium pyrophosphate (CPP) crystals [1]. If synovial fluid examination is not feasible, radiological investigations can be carried out to support the diagnosis of CPPD as suggested by the European League Against Rheumatism (EULAR) recommendations [1]. Once the presence of CPP crystals is confirmed or radiographic articular chondrocalcinosis (CC) demonstrated, consideration should be given to the need for further investigations to determine if an underlying metabolic predisposition is present. However, every patient with CPPD does not require extensive testing for underlying metabolic abnormality, and the need for such testing depends on the patient's age, presence of osteoarthritis (OA), and the number of joints with CPPD. Additional ancillary haematological, biochemical, and serological investigations may be required for the differential diagnosis of suspected acute CPP crystal arthritis, OA with CPPD, or chronic CPP crystal inflammatory arthritis. In this chapter we will describe the investigations that are helpful in demonstrating the presence of CPP crystals, identifying any underlying metabolic predisposition, and in the differential diagnosis of clinical presentations of CPPD.

Blood tests

Patients with acute CPP crystal arthritis often demonstrate a marked acute phase response with leucocytosis (predominantly neutrophilia) and increased platelet count. Elevated C-reactive protein (CRP) levels, high erythrocyte sedimentation rate (ESR) and increased plasma viscosity are often present. These changes normalize when the acute attack subsides. As acute CPP crystal arthritis may be provoked by infection, targeted questioning for symptoms suggestive of chest or urinary tract infection should form a part of the initial clinical assessment, and further investigations, for example, chest X-ray, blood culture, urine dipstick, and urine culture may be performed if required. As expected, CPPD with OA or asymptomatic CC does not associate with raised inflammatory markers. However, chronic CPP crystal inflammatory arthritis may present with raised inflammatory markers (CRP and/or ESR), but typically is negative for rheumatoid factor and anti-CCP antibodies.

Metabolic disease predisposition to CPPD is rare, and routine screening of all patients with CPPD is unrewarding. Nevertheless, CPPD/CC and arthritis may be the initial features of hyperparathyroidism, haemochromatosis, hypomagnesaemia, and adult-onset hypophosphatasia, and screening tests are warranted in those with early-onset CPPD (younger than 55 years), florid polyarticular CC, clinical presentation with recurrent acute attacks, or additional clinical or radiographic clues that suggest an underlying metabolic abnormality [2]. Screening tests include calcium, alkaline phosphatase, magnesium, ferritin and transferrin saturation, and liver function tests. Parathyroid hormone levels should also be checked as some patients with hyperparathyroidism may have normal serum calcium. After the age of 55 years the presence of hyperparathyroidism should be looked for in all patients with CPPD because both conditions are more common in this age group [2,3]. Testing for iron overload (e.g. serum ferritin, transferrin saturation) should be carried out first if haemochromatosis is suspected. Genotyping for C282Y and H63D polymorphisms in the *HFE* (high ferritin) gene should not be used to screen for haemochromatosis as these polymorphisms have variable penetrance and haemochromatosis can also result from other rarer mutations [4]. Testing for iron overload is especially relevant in those with CC and an atypical distribution of early-onset OA affecting metacarpophalangeal joints, ankle, and hips.

Tests for rarer diseases associated with CPPD are only warranted if there are clinical features suggestive of these conditions or in those with polyarticular CPPD at a very young age. Depending on other manifestations, these tests include serum copper and caeruloplasmin (low in Wilson's disease); plasma homogentisic acid (elevated in alkaptonuria); 24-hour urinary calcium (low 24-hour excretion in the presence of high serum calcium and normal or slightly elevated parathyroid hormone level suggests familial hypocalciuric hypercalcaemia); serum insulin-like growth factor 1 (elevated in acromegaly) and serum phosphate (low serum phosphate in presence of high urinary phosphate excretion, normal serum calcium, 25-OH vitamin D, 1,25 $(OH)_2$ vitamin D, and parathyroid hormone suggests X-linked hypophosphataemic rickets). Genotyping for mutations and polymorphisms, especially in the *ANKH* gene, may be carried out in those with a family history of premature CPPD if there is no evidence of an associated metabolic predisposing condition. However, such genetic testing is often not available in most clinical centres.

Synovial fluid examination

The aspirated synovial fluid in acute CPP crystal arthritis is often turbid, and can be blood stained. Synovial fluid viscosity is reduced with elevated cell counts (usually >90% neutrophils). In a large case series, the mean synovial fluid white cell count in acute CPP crystal arthritis was over 19 000/mm^3 with over 76% being polymorphonuclear cells [5]. The synovial fluid white cell count may also be mildly elevated in the intercritical period (mean: 301 cells/μL; 95% confidence interval (CI) 217–386), with the majority of white cells (mean 83%; 95% CI: 80–86%) being mononuclear rather than polymorphonuclear [6]. The gross appearance, viscosity, and cell count in OA + CPPD is variable and ranges from inflammatory to bland. However, the white blood cell count and percentage of polymorphonuclear cells is significantly higher in OA synovial fluid positive for CPP crystals compared to those without CPP crystals [5].

Although CPP crystals are robust, examination of fresh synovial fluid is ideal and avoids the problems of cell disruption (most CPP crystals are intracellular) and post-aspiration artefact. Centrifugation of the sample at a low speed (which prevents the accumulation of debris) and examination of the aspirate from the base of the tube can increase the diagnostic yield [5]. However, if examination of fresh synovial fluid is not possible, the synovial fluid may be stored at 4°C or at a stable room temperature of 20°C for up to 3 days without any significant reduction in the semi-quantitative crystal counts [7].

The identification of synovial fluid CPP crystals remains the gold standard for the diagnosis of CPPD. The initial search for these crystals should be carried out under light microscopy (400× or 1000×) since most CPP crystals (80%) are not birefringent and may not be visualized under non-compensated polarized light microscopy [8]. However, once a CPP crystal is identified by its morphology it should be examined under polarized light. Phase contrast microscopy is additionally useful in showing intracellular CPP crystals. CPP crystals are generally rhomboid or rod shaped, occasionally acicular, and approximately 2–10 μm long (Figure 51.1). A minority show weak positive birefringence and inclined extinction (15–20°) under compensated polarized microscopy. 'Twinning' of crystals, with a chip left at one corner, is seen occasionally. CPP crystals can be present intracellularly in both actively inflamed and intercritical joints [6]. CPP crystals are less readily identified and often less numerous than monosodium urate (MSU) crystals, and they can often be missed [9]. A careful search in areas of cellular debris,

and examination of a centrifuged deposit, may increase detection. Lack of consistency between different observers in identifying CPP crystals is a potential problem; however, training in crystal identification improves the levels of inter-observer agreement [10]. CPP crystal may occasionally coexist with MSU crystals depending on the joint aspirated. A retrospective study of over 2300 synovial fluid samples suggested that they coexist in 0.7% of crystal positive samples [5].

Several methods like the Diff Quik stain and dried cytospin preparation allow long-term storage of synovial fluid slides [11,12]. Neutral buffers should be used to avoid dissolution in histological samples as CPP crystals may be lost during decalcification. Identification of CPP crystals by more definitive analytic means such as infrared spectrophotometry, electron microscopy, and X-ray diffraction is ideal, but these methods are not used in routine clinical practice as they often require a high crystal load for analysis, are expensive, rarely available, and time-consuming.

Synovial fluid Gram stain and culture should be performed when septic arthritis is a possible differential diagnosis, especially in cases of acute CPP crystal arthritis triggered by inter-current illness. Acute CPP crystal arthritis and septic arthritis can rarely coexist, and the mere identification of CPP crystals and a negative initial Gram stain is not sufficient in excluding septic arthritis in the clinical scenario where septic arthritis is a possibility [13]. In a retrospective study from a tertiary hospital, four of the 265 synovial fluid samples had CPP crystals and coexistent infection [13]. Of these, CPP crystals were present in three samples, while MSU crystal was present in one [13]. However, it is important to bear in mind that all four patients had significant co-morbidities (e.g. diabetes, AIDS), and one had concomitant femoral popliteal bypass infection [13]. Coexistence of both MSU and CPP crystal types and infection has also been reported [14]. If sepsis develops in a joint with CPPD the inflammation created by the infection may encourage release of crystals from cartilage, a process referred to as crystal shedding through 'strip mining' [15].

Rarely, histological examination is used to detect CPPD, for example, in meniscectomy or arthroplasty samples. Such specimens should be preserved un-decalcified, for example, in phosphate buffered neutral 10% formalin, as the CPP crystals are dissolved during the decalcification process.

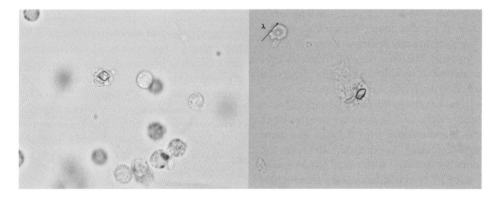

Figure 51.1 The left-hand image is a synovial fluid CPP crystal viewed under phase contrast microscopy (×400). Note the straight borders and distinct angles that confirm it as a crystal and the rhomboid shape that is consistent with CPP. As with most CPP crystals it is intracellular and on polarized light microscopy it was non-birefringent. The right-hand picture shows another synovial fluid sample viewed under compensated polarized light microscopy (×400). Again a definite intracellular rhomboid crystal is apparent but this one demonstrates weak positive birefringence.

Images courtesy of Professor Eliseo Pascual, Hospital General Universitario de Alicante, Spain.

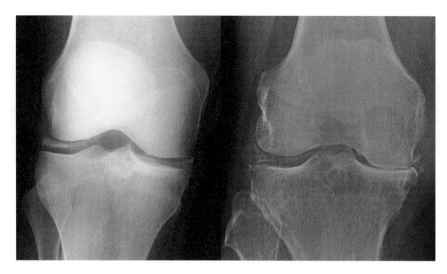

Figure 51.2 The left-hand image shows meniscal calcification (chondrocalcinosis). Note lateral meniscus is more heavily calcified than the medial meniscus, and there are no radiographic changes of osteoarthritis. The right-hand image shows chondrocalcinosis—wedge-shaped calcification of the lateral meniscus—with radiographic changes of osteoarthritis. Note there is sclerosis, joint space narrowing, and osteophytosis in the medial tibiofemoral compartment.

Imaging

Imaging features of CPPD include articular cartilage calcification and radiographic changes of structural arthropathy. Plain radiography, ultrasonography (US), and computed tomography (CT) can be used to identify CPPD. Of these, plain radiography and US scanning are commonly used in clinical practice. CT scans are used rarely due to the amount of radiation exposure. However, CT may be particularly useful in demonstrating axial CPPD, for example, peri-odontoid calcification in the crowned dens syndrome. Magnetic resonance imaging is rarely used as it has very low sensitivity for detecting CPPD [16]; however, it may be useful in the evaluation of patients with neurological symptoms due to axial CPPD syndromes.

Imaging features of CPPD include articular cartilage calcification, and radiographic changes of structural arthropathy. On plain radiographs CPPD is often visualized as linear calcification or as irregular spotty calcification arranged in a linear fashion (Figure 51.2). Linear calcification, parallel to the underlying cortex most commonly occurs in hyaline articular cartilage, whereas shaggy irregular spots arranged in a linear pattern are more common in the fibrocartilage, and may be observed in the meniscus of the knee, triangular cartilage of the wrist, and hip labrum (Figures 51.2–51.4). Cloudy synovial calcification is less common, but may occur, especially in metacarpophalangeal joints. Linear calcification can also be observed in capsules. Bursae and tendons often have more irregular deposits. Tophaceous CPPD is rare and presents irregular calcified deposits predominantly in periarticular

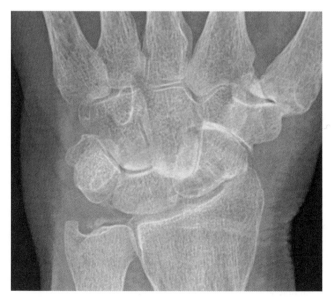

Figure 51.3 The wrist radiograph shows irregular, and shaggy triangular cartilage calcification. Note sclerosis of the mid-carpal joints, especially the trapezioscaphoid and the scaphotrapezoid joint.

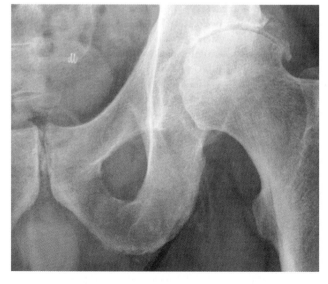

Figure 51.4 The pelvis radiograph shows hyaline cartilage calcification (linear and parallel to the cortex of the underlying femoral head) and diffuse labral calcification in the left hip. Changes of osteoarthritis are also present. There is irregular, linear calcification in the symphysis pubis.

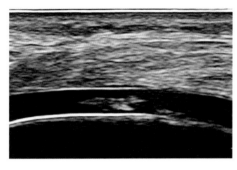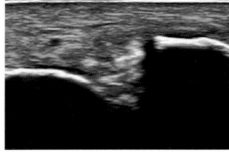

Figure 51.5 Knee ultrasound scan. Left panel shows irregular, shaggy calcification in the middle layer of the hyaline articular cartilage, and right panel shows calcification in the meniscal fibrocartilage.

Images courtesy of Dr Georgios Filippou PhD MD, Rheumatologist, University of Siena, Siena, Italy.

locations. As expected, plain radiographs are not sensitive in detecting small deposits of CPPD which are better visualized on a US scan. US is even more sensitive than CT scanning in detecting CPPD. In one study comparing the diagnostic utility of plain radiography, US scanning, and CT scanning, US imaging detected CPP crystals in 100%, CT scanning in 72%, and radiographs in 52% patients with crystal-proven CPPD [17].

US has excellent sensitivity and specificity for detecting articular and soft tissue calcification (see also Chapter 17). On US, CPPD appears as hyperechoic deposits in one of the following patterns (Figure 51.5) [18]:

* Thin hyperechoic bands, parallel to the surface of the hyaline cartilage (frequently observed in the knee)

* 'Punctate' pattern, composed of several thin hyperechoic spots, more common in fibrous cartilage and in tendons

* Homogeneous hyperechoic nodular or oval deposits localized in bursae and articular recesses (frequently mobile).

Calcification due to CPPD is reported to have a sparkling appearance. CPP deposits tend to create posterior shadowing only when their size exceeds 10 mm [18]. In contrast, calcifications that present a hypoechoic appearance with posterior shadowing even at an early stage (2–3 mm in diameter) are considered typical of basic calcium phosphate crystal deposition [18].

US examinations are more sensitive than plain radiography in detecting CPPD [18–20]. US has excellent specificity (96.4%) and good sensitivity (86.7%) with a positive predictive value of 92% and a negative predictive value of 93% for detecting CPPD compared to synovial fluid examination in patients with symptomatic arthritis [19]. However, US may not be as good as joint aspiration and synovial fluid examination in patients with acute CPP crystal arthritis. In a study of 54 Dutch patients presenting to the hospital with acute mono- or oligoarthritis, there were six cases with crystal-proven acute CPP crystal arthritis. US of the index joint, contralateral joint, and four other joints did not demonstrate any intra-articular cartilage calcification that is regarded as typical of CPPD [21]. Thus, further studies are required to explore the diagnostic utility of US in the setting of acute CPP crystal arthritis.

US, however, can be used to distinguish between MSU and CPP crystal deposition, with involvement of the chondrosynovial margin occurring in gout, and intracartilaginous hyperechoic spots occurring in joints with CPPD [22].

CPPD associates with OA, and is reported to modify the distribution of OA with greater involvement of lateral tibiofemoral joints, metacarpophalangeal joints, and trapezioscaphoid joints [23,24]. Whether the radiographic phenotype of structural arthropathy associated with CPPD (i.e. OA with CPPD) differs from that of OA without CPPD is not well established. Conflicting results have been reported with some studies reporting an association with osteophytosis (Figure 51.3) while other studies suggest that CPPD does not modify the phenotype of OA [23,25,26]. A systematic review and meta-analysis by the EULAR Task Force failed to identify any such difference, although these findings are limited by a lack of good quality studies [1]. Thus, further research is required to identify the structural radiographic changes that can be attributed to CPPD.

References

1. Zhang W, Doherty M, Bardin T, et al. European League Against Rheumatism recommendations for calcium pyrophosphate deposition. Part I: terminology and diagnosis. *Ann Rheum Dis* 2011; 70(4):563–70.
2. Richette P, Bardin T, Doherty M. An update on the epidemiology of calcium pyrophosphate dihydrate crystal deposition disease. *Rheumatology* 2009; 48(7):711–15.
3. Jones AC, Chuck AJ, Arie EA, Green DJ, Doherty M. Diseases associated with calcium pyrophosphate deposition disease. *Semin Arthritis Rheum* 1992; 22(3):188–202.
4. Hanson EH, Imperatore G, Burke W. HFE gene and hereditary hemochromatosis: a HuGE review. *Am J Epidemiol* 2001; 154(3):193–206.
5. Oliviero F, Scanu A, Galozzi P, et al. Prevalence of calcium pyrophosphate and monosodium urate crystals in synovial fluid of patients with previously diagnosed joint diseases. *Joint Bone Spine* 2013; 80(3):287–90.
6. Martinez Sanchis A, Pascual E. Intracellular and extracellular CPPD crystals are a regular feature in synovial fluid from uninflamed joints of patients with CPPD related arthropathy. *Ann Rheum Dis* 2005; 64(12):1769–72.
7. Tausche AK, Gehrisch S, Panzner I, et al. A 3-day delay in synovial fluid crystal identification did not hinder the reliable detection of monosodium urate and calcium pyrophosphate crystals. *J Clin Rheumatol* 2013; 19(5):241–5.
8. Ivorra J, Rosas J, Pascual E. Most calcium pyrophosphate crystals appear as non-birefringent. *Ann Rheum Dis* 1999; 58(9):582–4.
9. Swan A, Amer H, Dieppe P. The value of synovial fluid assays in the diagnosis of joint disease: a literature survey. *Ann Rheum Dis* 2002; 61(6):493–8.
10. Lumbreras B, Pascual E, Frasquet J, et al. Analysis for crystals in synovial fluid: training of the analysts results in high consistency. *Ann Rheum Dis* 2005; 64(4):612–15.

11. Selvi E, Manganelli S, Catenaccio M, et al. Diff Quik staining method for detection and identification of monosodium urate and calcium pyrophosphate crystals in synovial fluids. *Ann Rheum Dis* 2001; 60(3):194–8.

12. Graf SW, Buchbinder R, Zochling J, Whittle SL. The accuracy of methods for urate crystal detection in synovial fluid and the effect of sample handling: a systematic review. *Clin Rheumatol* 2013; 32(2):225–32.

13. Shah K, Spear J, Nathanson LA, McCauley J, Edlow JA. Does the presence of crystal arthritis rule out septic arthritis? *J Emerg Med* 2007; 32(1):23–6.

14. Jarrett MP, Grayzel AI. Simultaneous gout, pseudogout, and septic arthritis. *Arthritis Rheum* 1980; 23(1):128–9.

15. Gordon TP, Reid C, Rozenbilds MA, Ahern M. Crystal shedding in septic arthritis: case reports and in vivo evidence in an animal model. *Aust N Z J Med* 1986; 16(3):336–40.

16. Abreu M, Johnson K, Chung CB, et al. Calcification in calcium pyrophosphate dihydrate (CPPD) crystalline deposits in the knee: anatomic, radiographic, MR imaging, and histologic study in cadavers. *Skeletal Radiol* 2004; 33(7):392–8.

17. Barskova VG, Kudaeva FM, Bozhieva LA, et al. Comparison of three imaging techniques in diagnosis of chondrocalcinosis of the knees in calcium pyrophosphate deposition disease. *Rheumatology* 2013; 52(6):1090–4.

18. Frediani B, Filippou G, Falsetti P, et al. Diagnosis of calcium pyrophosphate dihydrate crystal deposition disease: ultrasonographic criteria proposed. *Ann Rheum Dis* 2005; 64(4):638–40.

19. Filippou G, Frediani B, Gallo A, et al. A 'new' technique for the diagnosis of chondrocalcinosis of the knee: sensitivity and specificity of high-frequency ultrasonography. *Ann Rheum Dis* 2007; 66(8):1126–8.

20. Gutierrez M, Di Geso L, Salaffi F, et al. Ultrasound detection of cartilage calcification at knee level in calcium pyrophosphate deposition disease. *Arthritis Care Res* 2014; 66(1):69–73.

21. Lamers-Karnebeek FB, Van Riel PL, Jansen TL. Additive value for ultrasonographic signal in a screening algorithm for patients presenting with acute mono-/oligoarthritis in whom gout is suspected. *Clin Rheumatol* 2014; 33(4):555–9.

22. Filippucci E, Riveros MG, Georgescu D, Salaffi F, Grassi W. Hyaline cartilage involvement in patients with gout and calcium pyrophosphate deposition disease. An ultrasound study. *Osteoarthritis Cartilage* 2009; 17(2):178–81.

23. Riestra JL, Sanchez A, Rodriques-Valverde V, Castillo E, Calderon J. Roentgenographic features of the arthropathy associated with CPPD crystal deposition disease. A comparative study with primary osteoarthritis. *J Rheumatol* 1985; 12(6):1154–8.

24. Sanmarti R, Kanterewicz E, Pladevall M, et al. Analysis of the association between chondrocalcinosis and osteoarthritis: a community based study. *Ann Rheum Dis* 1996; 55(1):30–3.

25. Hansen SE, Herning M. A comparative study of radiographic changes in knee joints in chondrocalcinosis, osteoarthrosis and rheumatoid arthritis. *Scand J Rheumatol* 1984; 13(1):85–92.

26. Neame RL, Carr AJ, Muir K, Doherty M. UK community prevalence of knee chondrocalcinosis: evidence that correlation with osteoarthritis is through a shared association with osteophyte. *Ann Rheum Dis* 2003; 62(6):513–8.

CHAPTER 52

Treatment of calcium pyrophosphate deposition

Abhishek Abhishek and Michael Doherty

Introduction

The treatment of calcium pyrophosphate crystal deposition (CPPD) depends on its clinical manifestations. Asymptomatic CPPD (chondrocalcinosis) does not require any treatment, although screening for underlying metabolic predispositions may be warranted (see Chapter 51). Other manifestations of CPPD, specifically acute CPP crystal arthritis, symptomatic osteoarthritis (OA) with CPPD, or chronic CPP crystal inflammatory arthritis should be managed to provide optimum symptom control. Unlike urate crystal deposition there is no definitive treatment to prevent or remove CPP crystals so the management of CPPD is predominantly symptomatic. There is a paucity of trial data specific to CPPD and most treatment recommendations are empirical and largely extrapolated from trial evidence relating to gout or OA. The European League Against Rheumatism (EULAR) has recently developed consensus driven evidence based recommendations for the management of CPPD [1] and this review largely reflects those guidelines.

Acute calcium pyrophosphate crystal arthritis

The aims of treatment of acute CPP crystal arthritis are a prompt reduction in symptoms, and rapid mobilization once symptoms improve. Rapid mobilization is important because many patients are elderly and prone to complications due to prolonged immobility. As acute CPP crystal arthritis frequently affects only one or a few joints (e.g. knee, wrist, or elbow), local treatment is preferred over systemic therapy. Any triggering illnesses should be identified and treated. See Box 52.1.

Aspiration and injection

In most cases, joint aspiration, as much as possible to dryness, rapidly relieves symptoms by reducing intra-articular hypertension and capsular distension. This may be the only treatment required. However, if undertaken early within 12–24 hours of onset, re-accumulation is usual so combined aspiration and intra-articular injection of corticosteroid to suppress the acute synovitis is usually preferred. As usual, arthrocentesis requires sterile equipment and a sensible aseptic approach with the patient relaxed on a couch [2].

Intra-articular injection of slow-release, intermediate-acting corticosteroids (e.g. triamcinolone acetonide or methylprednisolone) may be carried out either at the time of initial joint aspiration or as a second procedure once the diagnosis is confirmed. There are no

---

Box 52.1 Treatment of acute CPP crystal arthritis

- Patient education
- Rest, ice packs
- Joint aspiration +/− corticosteroid injection
- Colchicine/oral corticosteroids/NSAIDs*
- Anti-IL1 agents (e.g. anakinra) in refractory cases.

*Avoid in the elderly.

---

clear guidelines on the dose of corticosteroid that is most effective for this indication in individual joints. However, commonly used doses are 40 mg triamcinolone acetonide or 40–80 mg of methylprednisolone for larger joints (e.g. knee, shoulder); 20 mg triamcinolone or methylprednisolone for intermediate joints such as wrists and elbows; and smaller doses of methylprednisolone (5–10 mg) for small joints such as metacarpophalangeal joints (fluorinated triamcinolone should be avoided for small superficial joints because of the risk of subcutaneous fat atrophy and depigmentation from back-flow along the needle track) [2]. Many physicians also inject 1–2 mL 2% lignocaine in addition to the corticosteroid for faster pain relief (NB if mixed from two vials this can cause some flocculation of methylprednisolone). Although some doctors prefer the reassurance of a negative Gram stain and/or culture before injecting, this obviously delays optimum control of symptoms, so with typical presentations, combined initial aspiration and injection is optimal. However, since septic arthritis and acute CPP crystal arthritis rarely may coexist, where the index of suspicion for septic arthritis is high (i.e. in patients in whom intravenous antibiotics would be initiated pending the culture results), corticosteroid injection should only be carried out after a negative culture report is obtained.

Joint lavage (normal saline, room temperature) can help settle acute attacks but is usually reserved for troublesome relapsing or prolonged episodes poorly responsive to corticosteroid injection.

Other treatments

Ice packs may be applied locally for symptomatic relief. Temporary rest when the joint is acutely inflamed also provides symptomatic relief. Simple analgesics and non-steroidal anti-inflammatory drugs (NSAIDs) may have additional benefits. If an NSAID, including a selective COX2 inhibitor (coxib), is used, co-prescription of a proton pump inhibitor is required as suggested by the NICE guideline (http://www.nice.org.uk/guidance/CG177). However, NSAIDs are often contraindicated in older patients, especially those with comorbidity, and their use should be discouraged given the high risk of gastrointestinal and renal side effects in this population. Oral colchicine may be effective but is rarely warranted. If used it should be given at a low dose (e.g. 0.5 or 0.6 mg, two or three times daily) to reduce the incidence of gastrointestinal side effects, especially in older or frail patients or in those with renal impairment. One small study in patients with recurrent acute CPP crystal arthritis (n = 10) suggested that colchicine also may be effective in the prophylaxis of acute CPP crystal arthritis [3]. As for gout, colchicine, a microtubule assembly inhibitor, may work by inhibiting CPP crystal endocytosis or its presentation to the inflammasome [4].

In the older patient with acute CPP crystal arthritis, a short course of systemic corticosteroid may be preferable to an NSAID or colchicine (once infection has been excluded as a trigger) and produces a more rapid relief compared to these other agents [5]. Again, there is a lack of guidance on the doses of corticosteroids that are effective for this purpose. However, common practice would be intramuscular injection of slow-release, intermediate-acting corticosteroid (e.g. 120 mg methylprednisolone), or oral prednisolone at a dose of 15–30 mg/day (depending on age, frailty, and comorbidity), tapered rapidly over a period of 2 weeks. This approach is particularly suitable for patients with severe polyarticular attacks or in whom aspiration and injection is impractical (e.g. in primary care). Adrenocorticotrophic hormone (ACTH) may be an effective alternative in controlling acute CPP crystal arthritis. A recent retrospective case series reported a dramatic response, with attenuation of signs of inflammation within 24 hours, in 13 of 14 patients with monoarticular acute CPP crystal arthritis who were given a single intramuscular injection of 1 mg (100 units) of synthetic depot ACTH as sole therapy after, with just one patient requiring a second injection the next day [6].

Anakinra (interleukin 1 (IL1) receptor antagonist) has been used both in the treatment and prophylaxis of polyarticular acute CPP crystal arthritis unresponsive to oral corticosteroids [7]. However, the usefulness of this agent for prophylaxis was not confirmed in a recent case series of three patients with chronic CPP crystal arthritis (two due to haemochromatosis), and anakinra may be less effective in the presence of structural arthropathy or in those with chronic joint inflammation [8]. A larger case-series of 16 patients, most with polyarticular acute CPP crystal arthritis refractory to corticosteroids or NSAIDs and/or colchicine (mean (standard deviation) swollen joint count, disease duration, C-reactive protein (CRP), and prednisolone dose: 5.9 (2.1), 10.7 (6.6) days, 97.2 (57.4) mg/L and 22.8 (7.5) mg/day respectively), reported a good or partial improvement in 14/16 on day four after receiving anakinra injections (100 mg/day for 3 days) [9]. There was a significant reduction in the swollen joint count, CRP, and prednisolone dose by day four. Some patients were on anakinra for a longer duration (8 days to 6 months). However, over a third of patients had a relapse when anakinra was stopped (given its short-term immunosuppressive effect) and other treatments (e.g. methotrexate, colchicine, or corticosteroid injections) were required. Thus there are data to support consideration of anakinra in the treatment of acute CPP crystal arthritis if other conventional treatment options fail to be effective, though randomized controlled trials are required

to demonstrate its efficacy before wider use can be recommended. Similarly, other longer-acting biological agents that inhibit IL1 such as canakinumab and rilonacept that are effective in treating or preventing acute attacks of gout may be effective in the treatment and/or prophylaxis of acute CPP crystal arthritis.

Osteoarthritis with calcium pyrophosphate crystal deposition

The overall aim of management of OA with CPPD is the same as that for OA. A variety of strategies are employed, and evidence supporting their use is extrapolated from OA trials (Box 52.2). Whether CPPD affects treatment outcomes in those with OA remains unknown.

An individualized package of care needs to be devised with full involvement of the patient in decision-making. The following core non-pharmacological treatments should be considered for every person with OA (see Chapter 21):

- Education regarding the nature of their arthritis and its treatment

- Advice regarding regular local muscle strengthening and general aerobic/fitness exercises

- Interventions aimed to minimize adverse mechanical factors, for example, pacing of activities, weight loss if overweight or obese, footwear modification, walking aids, environmental adaptations etc. and adjunctive analgesics should also be considered, with oral paracetamol and/or topical NSAID gel or cream (especially for knees and wrists) the first to consider.

Despite the presence of structural abnormality, intra-articular corticosteroid injection often improves symptoms. Though often temporary, lasting for a few months at a time, this may improve the patient's confidence, encourage adherence with other aspects of treatment (e.g. weight loss), and provide a useful relatively pain-free interval for effective physiotherapy or enjoyment of an important life event (e.g., holiday).

One small, double-blind, placebo-controlled study of 6 months' duration reported reduction in knee pain in patients with knee OA plus CPPD from daily oral magnesium carbonate supplements (equivalent to 30 mEq magnesium daily) regardless of whether hypomagnesaemia was present [10]. However, there was no reduction in radiographic chondrocalcinosis. A double-blind controlled study of intra-articular radiocolloid (yttrium-90) injection for CPPD with OA of the knee showed efficacy even in cases with gross structural change [11]. The number needed to treat (NNT) for

---

Box 52.2 Treatment of OA + CPPD

- Patient education

- Core treatment for OA—exercises, physiotherapy, weight loss (if appropriate), simple analgesics

- Treatment of any superimposed acute CPP crystal arthritis attacks

- Radiosynovectomy

- Total joint replacement.*

*Same indications as for OA alone.

greater than 33.3% improvement in knee pain and 50% improvement in global knee symptoms was 2. Radiosynovectomy is also useful for the treatment of recurrent haemarthrosis, often a problem in the shoulder, presumably by inducing synovial fibrosis.

Chronic calcium pyrophosphate crystal inflammatory arthritis

Oral NSAIDs (with gastro-protection) and/or colchicine, low-dose corticosteroids, hydroxychloroquine, and methotrexate all have been suggested as pharmacological options for treatment of chronic CPP crystal arthritis [1]. The recommendation regarding the use of NSAIDs and low-dose corticosteroids is supported solely by expert opinion and clinical experience. The use of colchicine is based on the findings of a study on patients with knee OA and persistent inflammation due to CPP crystals, in whom colchicine (0.5 mg twice daily regularly for 8 weeks and then taken as necessary) resulted in a greater than 30% improvement in pain (NNT = 2 at 4 months, and 4 at 5 months) [12]. A small (n = 36), double-blind, placebo-controlled study reported rapid clinical benefit from oral hydroxychloroquine over a 6-month period (NNT = 2 for 30% reduction in swollen and tender joint counts) [13]. However, the findings of this study have not been replicated in a larger trial. See Box 52.3.

Two small retrospective case series have reported beneficial effects of methotrexate in chronic CPP inflammatory arthritis. In a retrospective review of patients with this condition, methotrexate (median dose 12.5 mg/week) reduced symptoms, clinically assessed joint inflammation, ESR, and CRP with a mean time to improvement of 7–8 weeks [14]. Similar findings were reported from a retrospective case series from Spain [15]. However, another retrospective case series was negative in this respect [16], and a prospective, double-blind, randomized, placebo-controlled cross-over trial did not report any statistically significant improvement with methotrexate [17]. In the prospective trial, 26 patients with recurrent mono- or oligoarthritis (at least three flares/6 months) or persistent polyarthritis secondary to CPP crystals, who had an unsatisfactory response or were contraindicated to oral NSAID or low-dose glucocorticoids, were randomized to subcutaneous injections of methotrexate (7.5 mg/week increased to 15 mg/week) or placebo for 3 months with a 2-month washout period in between [17]. There were no differences in the 44-joint Disease Activity Score, swollen joint count, tender joint count, CRP, number of flares, and severity of pain between the two periods [17]. Therefore

overall there is no convincing evidence to recommend methotrexate in the treatment of recurrent acute or chronic CPP crystal inflammatory arthritis.

Some patients with persistent mono- or oligoarthritis or recurrent monoarthritis may benefit from radiosynovectomy. Rilonacept (IL1 Trap) which is beneficial in the treatment of patients with chronic gouty arthritis may also be effective in patients with refractory CPP crystal-related arthritis, though this has not been studied formally.

Other treatment

Stronger analgesics, for example, NSAIDs (including selective COX2 inhibitors) or opioids may improve symptoms but carry an appreciable risk of side effects and drug interactions. Such drugs should be used with caution in the elderly. If prescribed, the patient should be clearly informed regarding optimal usage, the requirement for drugs should be regularly reviewed, and 'repeat' prescribing avoided.

Surgery

Patients with progressive or destructive large joint arthropathy who require joint replacement appear to derive benefits equal to those with uncomplicated OA, without any increase in the risk of prosthetic failure [18]. In a retrospective case series of 1500 primary total knee arthroplasties for OA, the presence of chondrocalcinosis at the time of surgery was not associated with differences in postoperative range of motion or knee society score [18]. Similarly, a retrospective case series (n = 206 patients, 234 knees) reported that radiographic knee chondrocalcinosis did not influence outcomes after unicompartmental knee arthroplasty in terms of 15-year cumulative survival rates, use of NSAIDs, radiographic progression of OA in the adjacent tibiofemoral compartment, failure of the anterior cruciate ligament, or aseptic loosening of the prosthesis [19].

Treatment of underlying metabolic abnormality

Treatment of underlying metabolic diseases that predispose to CPPD is appropriate. However, other than possibly for correction of hypomagnesaemia, such treatment does not appear to influence the outcome of CPP crystal-associated disease [20]. For example, surgical treatment of hyperparathyroidism does not result in resolution of CPPD or improvement in its symptoms [21]. Parathyroidectomy may even precipitate acute CPP crystal arthritis (attributed to a sudden reduction in serum calcium), but normalization of biochemical abnormalities does not result in resolution of chondrocalcinosis, or improvement in joint symptoms over the next decade or so [21]. Similarly, iron chelation therapy does not reverse the structural arthropathy of haemochromatosis [20].

Strategies for crystal dissolution

Although there is interest in the possibility of modifying CPP crystal formation and dissolution, a strategy to safely dissolve CPP crystals *in vivo* has not been developed to date. Joint lavage with calcium-chelating agents such as magnesium sulphate provokes acute CPP crystal arthritis, perhaps through partial dissolution that then encourages crystal shedding [22]. Phosphocitrate inhibits the deposition and growth of CPP crystals *in vitro* [23] and

---

Box 52.3 Treatment of chronic CPP crystal inflammatory arthritis

- Patient education
- Periodic joint aspiration and corticosteroid injections
- Low-dose colchicine (1 mg/day) or oral corticosteroids (prednisolone 7.5 mg/day)
- Hydroxychloroquine
- Anti-IL1 agents (e.g. anakinra) in refractory cases
- Radiosynovectomy—persistent mono- or oligoarticular disease.

polyphosphates such as sodium metaphosphate and pentasodium triplyphosphate dissolve synthetic CPP crystals and CPP crystals from human menisci without cell damage [24], but these have not been tested in animals or humans. Clearly such potential treatment strategies are likely to require local intra-articular rather than systemic administration.

In conclusion, the objectives of management of CPPD are to relieve symptoms and to prevent acute attacks without the option of influencing CPP crystal deposition [1]. It is evident that the research evidence to support management recommendations for symptomatic CPPD is sparse and further clinical trials in CPPD are needed [1].

References

1. Zhang W, Doherty M, Pascual E, et al. EULAR recommendations for calcium pyrophosphate deposition. Part II: management. *Ann Rheum Dis* 2011; 70(4):571–5.
2. Courtney P, Doherty M. Joint aspiration and injection and synovial fluid analysis. *Best Pract Res Clin Rheumatol* 2013; 27(2):137–69.
3. Alvarellos A, Spilberg I. Colchicine prophylaxis in pseudogout. *J Rheumatol* 1986; 13(4):804–5.
4. Martinon F, Petrilli V, Mayor A, Tardivel A, Tschopp J. Gout-associated uric acid crystals activate the NALP3 inflammasome. *Nature* 2006; 440(7081):237–41.
5. Werlen D, Gabay C, Vischer TL. Corticosteroid therapy for the treatment of acute attacks of crystal-induced arthritis: an effective alternative to nonsteroidal antiinflammatory drugs. *Rev Rhum Engl Ed* 1996; 63(4):248–54.
6. Daoussis D, Antonopoulos I, Yiannopoulos G, Andonopoulos AP. ACTH as first line treatment for acute calcium pyrophosphate crystal arthritis in 14 hospitalized patients. *Joint Bone Spine* 2014; 81(1):98–100.
7. McGonagle D, Tan AL, Madden J, Emery P, McDermott MF. Successful treatment of resistant pseudogout with anakinra. *Arthritis Rheum* 2008; 58(2):631–3.
8. Couderc M, Mathieu S, Glace B, Soubrier M. Efficacy of anakinra in articular chondrocalcinosis: Report of three cases. *Joint Bone Spine* 2012; 79(3):330–1.
9. Ottaviani S, Brunier L, Sibilia J, et al. Efficacy of anakinra in calcium pyrophosphate crystal-induced arthritis: a report of 16 cases and review of the literature. *Joint Bone Spine* 2013; 80(2):178–82.
10. Doherty M, Dieppe PA. Double blind, placebo controlled trial of magnesium carbonate in chronic pyrophosphate arthropathy *Ann Rheum Dis* 1983; 42(S):106–7.
11. Doherty M, Dieppe PA. Effect of intra-articular yttrium-90 on chronic pyrophosphate arthropathy of the knee. *Lancet* 1981; 2(8258):1243–6.
12. Das SK, Mishra K, Ramakrishnan S, et al. A randomized controlled trial to evaluate the slow-acting symptom modifying effects of a regimen containing colchicine in a subset of patients with osteoarthritis of the knee. *Osteoarthritis Cartilage* 2002; 10(4):247–52.
13. Rothschild B, Yakubov LE. Prospective 6-month, double-blind trial of hydroxychloroquine treatment of CPDD. *Compr Ther* 1997; 23(5):327–31.
14. Chollet-Janin A, Finckh A, Dudler J, Guerne PA. Methotrexate as an alternative therapy for chronic calcium pyrophosphate deposition disease: an exploratory analysis. *Arthritis Rheum* 2007; 56(2):688–92.
15. Andres M, Sivera F, Pascual E. Methotrexate is an option for patients with refractory calcium pyrophosphate crystal arthritis. *J Clin Rheumatol* 2012; 18(5):234–6.
16. Doan TH, Chevalier X, Leparc JM, et al. Premature enthusiasm for the use of methotrexate for refractory chondrocalcinosis: comment on the article by Chollet-Janin et al. *Arthritis Rheum* 2008; 58(7):2210–11.
17. Finckh A, Mc Carthy GM, Madigan A, et al. Methotrexate in chronic-recurrent calcium pyrophosphate deposition disease: no significant effect in a randomized crossover trial. *Arthritis Res Ther* 2014; 16(5):458.
18. Lee GC, Lotke PA. Does chondrocalcinosis affect Knee Society scores and range of motion after TKA? *Clin Orthop Relat Res* 2014; 472(5):1512–7.
19. Hernigou P, Pascale W, Pascale V, Homma Y, Poignard A. Does primary or secondary chondrocalcinosis influence long-term survivorship of unicompartmental arthroplasty? *Clin Orthop Relat Res* 2012; 470(7):1973–9.
20. Jones AC, Chuck AJ, Arie EA, Green DJ, Doherty M. Diseases associated with calcium pyrophosphate deposition disease. *Semin Arthritis Rheum* 1992; 22(3):188–202.
21. Glass JS, Grahame R. Chondrocalcinosis after parathyroidectomy. *Ann Rheum Dis* 1976; 35(6):521–5.
22. Bennett RM, Lehr JR, McCarty DJ. Crystal shedding and acute pseudogout. An hypothesis based on a therapeutic failure. *Arthritis Rheum* 1976; 19(1):93–7.
23. Cheung HS, Kurup IV, Sallis JD, Ryan LM. Inhibition of calcium pyrophosphate dihydrate crystal formation in articular cartilage vesicles and cartilage by phosphocitrate. *J Biol Chem* 1996; 271(45):28082–5.
24. Cini R, Chindamo D, Catenaccio M, Lorenzini S, Selvi E, Nerucci F, et al. Dissolution of calcium pyrophosphate crystals by polyphosphates: an in vitro and ex vivo study. *Ann Rheum Dis* 2001; 60(10):962–7.

SECTION 15

Basic calcium phosphate crystal deposition

CHAPTER 53

Basic calcium phosphate crystal deposition

Nicola Dalbeth

What are basic calcium phosphate crystals?

Basic calcium phosphate (BCP) crystals are a heterogeneous group of ultramicroscopic calcium-containing crystals associated with periarticular and articular disorders (reviewed in [1,2]). Individual crystals measure 20–100 nm in diameter. The crystals typically clump in synovial fluid (clumps measure 5–20 μm) and are not usually visible using standard light microscopy or polarizing light microscopy methods. The most recognized forms of BCP crystals are hydroxyapatite ($Ca_{10}(PO_4)_6(OH)_2$), carbonate apatite ($Ca_{10-w-y/2}(PO_4)_{6-x}(CO_3)_y(OH)_{2-y}(CO_3)_{y/2} \cdot nH_2O$), octacalcium phosphate ($Ca_8H_2(PO_4)_6 \cdot 5H_2O$), and tricalcium phosphate ($Ca_3(PO_4)_2$). Other BCP crystals include dicalcium phosphate dihydrate, calcium phosphate dihydrate, and magnesium-substituted apatite (whitlockite) crystals. These crystals deposit in tendons, ligaments, synovium, and cartilage, and can also be observed in non-articular tissues such as skin, breast, and arteries.

How do BCP crystals form?

Under normal physiological conditions, tissue mineralization is a tightly regulated process that is initiated by chondrocyte- and osteoblast-derived matrix vesicles (MVs) that contain calcium and inorganic phosphate ions (Pi) [3]. Within the joint, articular cartilage MVs are the primary source of calcium-containing crystals (BCP and calcium pyrophosphate (CPP)). The preferential formation of BCP or CPP calcium-containing crystals is dependent on the concentrations of extracellular inorganic phosphate (ePi) and extracellular inorganic pyrophosphate (ePPi). High ePi and low ePPi favours formation of BCP crystals (see also Chapter 49). PPi antagonizes the ability of Pi to crystallize with calcium to form BCP and also suppresses BCP crystal propagation. The extracellular concentrations of Pi and PPi are regulated by the activity of a series of proteins including ankylosis human (ANKH), ectonucleotide pyrophosphatase/phosphodiesterase 1 (ENPP1, also known as plasma cell membrane glycoprotein 1), and tissue non-specific alkaline phosphatase (TNAP) (Figure 53.1) [4–6]. ANKH transports intracellular PPi across the cell membrane, promoting high ePPi concentrations and CPP crystal formation. TNAP promotes catabolism of ePPi to ePi, promoting BCP crystal formation. ENPP1 converts nucleotide triphosphate into ePPi and adenosine monophosphate (AMP). Additional molecules that also influence PPi and Pi concentrations are PiT1 (plasma cell membrane glycoprotein 1) which transports ePi into the cell, and CD73

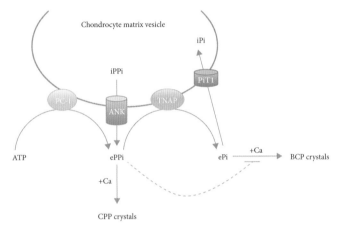

Figure 53.1 Regulation of pyrophosphate (PPi) and phosphate (Pi) balance. Calcium (Ca) complexes with PPi to form CPP crystals or with Pi to form BCP crystals. High extracellular PPi (ePPi) levels occur with increased ANK or PC-1 (ENPP-1) activity. High ePPi inhibits BCP crystal formation. Increased TNAP activity or low ANK or PC-1 activity increases Pi levels, promoting BCP crystal formation. iPPi, intracellular PPi; iPi, intracellular phosphate; PC-1, plasma cell membrane glycoprotein 1 (also known as ectonucleoside triphosphate pyrophosphatase phosphodiesterase, ENPP1); PiT1, plasma cell membrane glycoprotein 1; TNAP, tissue non-specific alkaline phosphatase.

(ecto-5′-nucleotidase) that converts AMP to ePi and adenosine, which in turn inhibits TNAP [7–9]. Animal models associated with BCP crystal deposition in articular cartilage, synovitis, osteoarthritis (OA), and extracellular PPi deficiency include the murine progressive ankylosis (*ank/ank*) mice and the ENPP1-deficient tip-toe walking (*ttw/ttw*) mice [10,11]. In humans, clinical syndromes associated with gain-of-function ANKH mutations lead to excessive CPP crystal formation [12], and loss of function ENPP1 or CD73 mutations lead to extensive periarticular and vascular BCP crystal deposition [7,13].

Tissue responses to BCP crystals

BCP crystals interact with many cells within the joint to promote both inflammatory and degradative pathways. These cells include macrophages, synovial fibroblasts, and chondrocytes. Following injection of BCP crystals *in vivo*, an inflammatory response is rapidly induced, with recruitment of neutrophils and mononuclear cells into the inflamed area. This cellular response is self-resolving [14].

Various types of BCP crystals have different capacity to induce the acute inflammatory response, with octacalcium phosphate generally considered the most proinflammatory [15]. Furthermore, the shape of hydroxyapatite crystals also influences the inflammatory response, with needle-shaped or irregular clump and rod forms having greater proinflammatory effects in macrophages [16]. The macrophage inflammatory response to BCP crystals is also inversely related to particle and pore size, with crystals of 1–2 micron diameter and pore size of 10–50 Å the most bioactive [17].

Macrophages respond to BCP crystals by internalization into vacuoles and secretion of soluble proinflammatory cytokines including TNFA, IL1B, and IL8 [17]. The PKC, ERK1/2, and JNK intracellular signalling pathways play an important role in the BCP crystal-induced macrophage secretion of TNFA, with activation of ERK1/2 being dependent on upstream activation of PKC [17]. Exposure of macrophages to BCP crystals also leads to activation of Syk and PI3 kinase, and macrophage production of proinflammatory cytokines in response to BCP crystals can be suppressed with Syk and PI3 kinase inhibitors [18]. Similar to the macrophage response to monosodium urate and calcium pyrophosphate crystals [19], BCP crystals induce mature IL1B release through activation of the NLRP3 inflammasome in macrophages [15,16]. This activation is dependent on potassium efflux, reactive oxygen species (ROS) generation, phagocytosis, and lysosomal protease release [16]. In various in vivo models, acute inflammation induced by BCP crystals is attenuated in mice lacking NLRP3, ASC, and caspase 1, confirming the central role of NLRP3 activation in BCP crystal-induced tissue inflammation in vivo [15,16,18]. Activation of the Syk and PI3 kinase pathway within macrophages also leads to production of S100A8, a known TLR4 ligand, which can act as Signal 1 for NLRP3 inflammasome activation to induce gene expression of pro-IL1B [18]. The role of NLRP3 activation in joint damage associated with BCP crystals is less clear. In in vivo models that induce cartilage damage through intra-articular injection of BCP crystals, synovial inflammation and cartilage damage is not altered in mice deficient for components of the NLRP3 inflammasome, IL1A or IL1B [20]. In contrast, in an ANK-deficient model of arthritis (characterized by extensive BCP crystal deposition and joint damage), decreased joint damage was observed in mice deficient for caspase 1 or NLRP3 [16].

BCP crystals induce fibroblast mitogenesis, which may contribute to synovial lining proliferation in vivo [21]. BCP crystals induce fibroblast production of degradative enzymes including matrix metalloproteinases (MMP)-1, -3, -8, -9, and -13 [22–26]. BCP crystals induce both cyclooxygenase 1 and cyclooxygenase 2, with increased PGE2 production [27,28]. Endocytosis is required to induce MMP expression, and mitogenesis is accompanied by collagenase induction and secretion [29]. Activation of protein kinase C plays a key role in BCP crystal-induced mitogenesis in fibroblasts. BCP crystals also activate the transcription factors nuclear factor kappa B and activator protein 1 in human fibroblasts [30].

BCP crystals are also internalized by chondrocytes; internalization leads to activation of catabolic pathways with release of PGE2, nitric oxide (NO), and degradative enzymes including MMP1 and MMP13 [31–33]. BCP crystal induction of NO production and inducible NO synthase gene expression in chondrocytes is mediated through the p38 and JNK–MAPK signalling pathways [33]. BCP crystals also induce chondrocyte apoptosis through mechanisms that are dependent on cell-crystal contact and intra-lysosomal crystal dissolution [34]. Culture of chondrocytes with BCP crystals leads to increased intracellular calcium (iCa) content; variation in iCa content is associated with BCP crystal-induced cartilage matrix degradation, in a manner that is independent of MMPs or ADAMTS [35]. BCP crystals also induce IL6 production in chondrocytes (through involving Syk and PI3 kinases, Jak2 and Stat3 pathways) [36]. IL6 production leads to further pathways that promote BCP crystal formation, leading to a positive amplification loop of BCP crystal formation [36].

In summary, BCP crystals induce proinflammatory and catabolic pathways in joint tissues that collectively promote development of synovitis and joint damage. Although it is assumed that the degradative enzymes produced in response to BCP crystals induce bone loss, the mechanisms of bone resorption in BCP crystal-associated disease are unknown. It is also unclear why calcification occurs within tendons in asymptomatic individuals, and how acute inflammatory episodes are triggered in those with previously asymptomatic BCP crystal deposition.

Clinical syndromes associated with BCP crystal deposition

BCP crystals are associated with inflammatory and destructive joint syndromes. These crystals may also be present in the absence of symptoms, for example, identified as an incidental finding on plain radiography or computed tomography. Radiographic shoulder calcific tendinitis was first described in 1907 [37] with basic calcium crystals within calcific tendon deposits reported in 1966 [38]. The role of BCP crystals causing a specific form of inflammatory arthropathy was initially reported in 1976 [14], with description of a destructive arthritis associated with BCP crystals and collagenase activity in synovial fluid (Milwaukee shoulder syndrome) published in 1981 [39].

Periarticular BCP crystal deposition

Periarticular BCP crystal deposition may be detected as an incidental finding in an asymptomatic individual (typically on plain radiography or computed tomography), as acute calcific periarthritis/tendinitis, or as chronic periarticular pain. Some authors have described that calcium apatite is the dominant form of BCP crystals in calcific periarthritis [40]. A large longitudinal radiographic study demonstrated calcific deposits in the shoulders of 2.7% of adults, most of whom were asymptomatic at the time of assessment [41]. Symptomatic disease developed subsequently in 10.9% of these individuals with tendon calcification. These findings suggest that BCP crystal deposition precedes development of the inflammatory response to these crystals.

Calcific periarthritis

Acute calcific periarthritis is a well-recognized presentation of BCP crystal deposition. Calcific tendinitis may occur due to tendon degeneration causing secondary calcification [42]. The tendon response to injury or degeneration leads to transformation of tendon tissue to fibrocartilaginous material containing chondrocyte-like cells that are capable of BCP crystal deposition from extracellular MVs [43,44]. Three phases of disease are thought to occur; the formative precalcific phase characterized by a fibrocartilaginous metaplasia, the calcific phase (which is usually asymptomatic), and the resorptive phase, presenting as an acute inflammatory episode that is triggered by rupture or resorption of the calcific deposit [45].

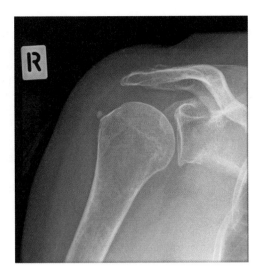

Figure 53.2 Calcific tendinitis of the supraspinatus tendon. Note the calcific deposit close to the insertion of the supraspinatus tendon.
Image courtesy of Dr Anthony Doyle.

The most widely recognized presentation of calcific periarthritis is acute calcific tendinitis affecting the rotator cuff tendons of the shoulder, most frequently the supraspinatus tendon (Figure 53.2). In acute calcific tendinitis of the shoulder, patients typically present with an acutely inflamed shoulder, with associated pain, swelling, erythema, warmth, and restricted movement. The onset is typically spontaneous, although a history of minor trauma or over-use may be reported. An acute phase response with raised inflammatory markers (C-reactive protein and erythrocyte sedimentation rate) may be present. Plain radiographs during the acute inflammatory episode typically show poorly defined calcification [46], which is usually more easily viewed by computed tomography [47]. The acute inflammatory episode typically resolves over a number of weeks. Resolution of symptoms is often associated with disappearance of the periarticular calcification. Persistent calcification may be associated with chronic shoulder pain, tendon rupture, or frozen shoulder syndrome.

Less frequently, other large joints such as the hip (most often affecting the gluteus medius tendon), knee, wrist, and ankle may be affected by acute calcific periarthritis. Acute calcific retropharyngeal tendinitis is a rare presentation affecting the superior fibres of the longus colli muscle tendons. Other periarticular structures such as ligaments and bursae may also be affected. Bone erosion may also be present. More than one site may be involved, with an oligo- or polyarticular presentation. Rarely, smaller joints, including the first metatarsophalangeal joint (hydroxyapatite pseudopodagra) may be affected. Acute neck pain due to BCP crystal deposition around the odontoid process may present as a 'crowned dens' syndrome, similar to that observed in CPP crystal deposition.

Initial treatment of acute calcific periarthritis includes medical therapy with non-steroidal anti-inflammatory drugs (NSAIDs) and colchicine. Local corticosteroid injection may be useful, although there is a potential concern that this may increase the likelihood of further calcification. In a small case series of patients with acute calcific tendinitis and persistent symptoms despite high-dose NSAIDs, a 3-day treatment with the interleukin 1 receptor antagonist anakinra led to rapid resolution of pain, normalization of shoulder function, and improvement in inflammatory markers [48].

For patients with calcific tendinitis of the shoulder who have persistent calcification and symptoms despite NSAIDs, needle aspiration, irrigation, and local corticosteroid injection is frequently undertaken. A randomized controlled trial of ultrasound (US)-guided needling and lavage plus subacromial corticosteroids versus subacromial corticosteroids alone for calcific tendinitis of the shoulder demonstrated improved 1-year outcomes in shoulder function and calcification size in the needling group compared to the group having subacromial corticosteroids alone [49]. A further clinical trial has demonstrated benefit of disodium EDTA in calcific tendinitis of the shoulder, administered through single needle mesotherapy and 15 minutes of pulsed-mode 1 MHz US, with improved pain and function at 1 year [50]. In this study, calcifications disappeared completely in 62.5% of participants in the disodium EDTA group and none in the control group after 1 year. In a recent systematic literature review of extracorporeal shock wave therapy (ESWT) for the treatment of chronic calcific tendonitis of the rotator cuff, 20 randomized controlled trials compared ESWT energy levels and placebo were identified [51]. These studies consistently showed that high-energy ESWT was significantly better than placebo in decreasing pain and improving function and resorption of calcifications in calcific tendinitis. If non-surgical treatments fail in calcific tendinitis of the shoulder, surgical debridement with or without subacromial decompression may be of benefit but partial tendon tears may occur following surgery and clinical symptoms may not be entirely restored [52].

Intra-articular BCP crystal deposition

As with periarticular BCP crystal deposition, intra-articular BCP crystal deposition may be asymptomatic and identified as an incidental finding. The most widely recognized clinical presentation of intra-articular deposition is a destructive arthropathy (most frequently as Milwaukee shoulder syndrome) [14,39]. BCP crystal deposition within the joint may also be associated with an acute synovitis or severe OA [53,54]. The relationship between OA and BCP crystals is discussed in detail later in this chapter.

BCP crystal-associated destructive arthritis

Milwaukee shoulder syndrome is the prototypical BCP crystal-associated destructive arthritis, typically affecting elderly women with rotator cuff rupture [39]. The condition is frequently bilateral, with the dominant side most severely affected. Affected patients typically present with chronic shoulder pain, swelling, and restricted shoulder movement and function (Figure 53.3). Plain radiographs show evidence of an effusion and superior subluxation of the humoral head (consistent with a rotator cuff tear). Marked cartilage and subchondral bone destruction may occur (Figure 53.4). An effusion is usually easily visible on joint examination, and examination of synovial fluid shows a relatively non-inflammatory pattern, with a low white cell count and predominantly mononuclear cells. A haemorrhagic effusion may be present. The synovial fluid is characterized by high collagenase activity and the presence of BCP crystals using various techniques including alizarin red S staining (Figure 53.5). Synovial histology shows non-specific changes of vascular congestion, synovial cell hyperplasia with villi and fibrin deposition without a pronounced inflammatory response [55,56]. There have been no randomized controlled trials of treatments for Milwaukee shoulder syndrome. Management is usually symptomatic and conservative, including analgesics, NSAIDs if tolerated,

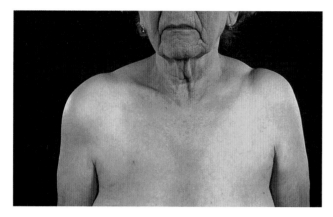

Figure 53.3 Milwaukee shoulder syndrome. Note the large effusion in the right shoulder.

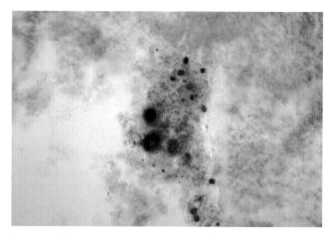

Figure 53.5 Alizarin red S staining (at acidic pH) of synovial fluid showing aggregates of positively staining BCP crystals.
Image courtesy of Dr Michael Doherty.

arthrocentesis or tidal irrigation with intra-articular corticosteroids [57], and arthroplasty if there is sufficient bone stock remaining.

Occasionally other large joints such as the hips, knees, and mid-tarsal joints may be affected in a similar manner to Milwaukee shoulder syndrome [14,53]. Patients present with a rapidly progressive, destructive arthropathy, with large cool effusions and instability of the joint due to joint destruction. More than one joint may be affected. Plain radiographs show marked and progressive destructive changes and deformity, with cartilage and atrophic bone loss (Figure 53.6). Articular or periarticular calcification may be evident. As with Milwaukee shoulder syndrome, aspirated synovial fluid shows a non-inflammatory pattern with alizarin red S staining confirming the presence of numerous clumps of BCP crystals. The principles of management at other joints are similar to that described for Milwaukee shoulder syndrome.

Acute synovitis associated with intra-articular BCP crystals

In addition to the chronic forms of arthritis associated with BCP crystal deposition, an acute arthritis may occasionally present [53]. This arthritis affects younger individuals, most often in the knee,

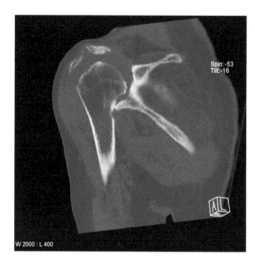

Figure 53.4 Computed tomography scan of a patient with Milwaukee shoulder syndrome. Note the joint effusion, superior subluxation of the humeral head, loss of cartilage, and bone damage.
Image courtesy of Dr Anthony Doyle.

and is typically self-resolving. Calcification of articular or periarticular structures may not be present, and the diagnosis is made through identification of BCP crystals in synovial fluid. The true incidence of acute synovitis associated with BCP crystal deposition is unknown.

Non-articular BCP crystal deposition

BCP crystals may also deposit in non-articular locations. These locations include arteries (e.g. calcium hydroxyapatite crystals causing vascular calcification), breast tissue (e.g. microcalcifications containing calcium hydroxyapatite crystals associated with malignant human breast lesions), subcutaneous tissues (e.g. calciphylaxis), and throughout cutaneous and subcutaneous tissue in systemic sclerosis, dermatomyositis, and tumoural calcinosis.

Both joint-associated and non-articular BCP crystal deposition are more common in patients with conditions leading to high serum calcium, including primary hyperparathyroidism and chronic kidney disease with associated parathyroid disease. Such deposition may be asymptomatic, but may also cause restricted joint movement and recurrent episodes of focal acute inflammatory episodes.

Identification of BCP crystals

A key barrier to diagnosis and research in BCP crystal arthropathy is the lack of a reliable and feasible test to accurately identify BCP crystal deposition. In contrast to MSU and CPP crystals, which can be readily identified using polarizing light microscopy in clinical practice, BCP crystals are not birefringent and are not easily visualized using standard microscopic techniques. Imaging methods may assist with BCP crystal identification, and new spectroscopic and chemical methods have been described.

Imaging techniques for identification of BCP crystals and diagnosis of BCP crystal arthropathy

Plain radiography is often sufficient for diagnosis of acute calcific periarthritis/tendinitis, with calcific deposits visible at characteristic locations, for example, near the insertion of the supraspinatus tendon (Figure 53.2) [46]. Plain radiography may also be sufficient

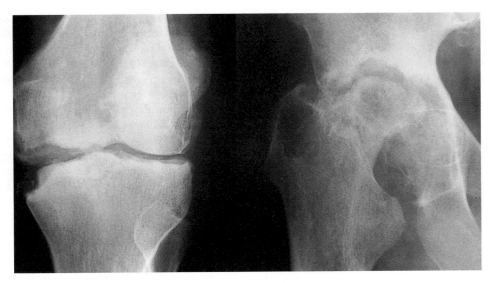

Figure 53.6 BCP crystal-associated destructive arthritis. Marked bone atrophy at the hip and knee in a patient with apatite-associated arthropathy.

to document BCP crystal-associated destructive arthritis particularly if capsular or periarticular calcification is present in addition to the destructive bone and cartilage changes [58].

Advanced imaging methods may assist with detection of BCP crystals and also allow assessment of disease complications. Computed tomography has higher resolution and may allow detection of smaller areas of calcification and calcific deposits at atypical sites that are not easily visible on plain radiography [59,60]. On magnetic resonance imaging (MRI), calcific deposits are of low signal on T1- and T2-weighted images (Figure 53.7). Synovitis, tenosynovitis, joint effusion, cartilage damage, and bone disease (erosion and bone marrow oedema) are well visualized on MRI (although these features are not specific for BCP crystal-associated arthritis) [61]. US allows identification of calcific deposits and also features of bursitis or tendinitis associated with calcific tendinitis

[62]. On US, calcific deposits can appear arc shaped (most commonly), fragmented, or punctate, and less frequently nodular or cystic [63]. US-guided aspiration of calcific deposits can provide good symptomatic relief in patients with chronic shoulder pain associated with calcific deposits [49].

Microscopy and other methods of BCP crystal identification

Due to their small size and lack of birefringence, BCP crystals are not typically visible using widely used microscopic techniques. Large clumps of BCP crystals may be visible on light microscopy, but these may be mistaken for artefact. Alizarin red S staining of synovial fluid improves sensitivity for BCP crystal clumps (Figure 53.5) [64]. This staining method detects both BCP and CPP

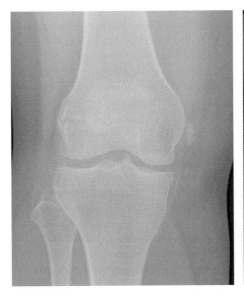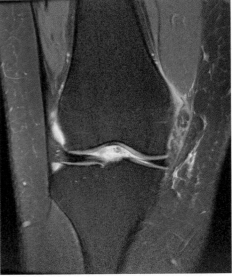

Figure 53.7 Plain radiographic and magnetic resonance imaging (MRI) appearance of calcific tendinitis. Paired radiographs (left panel) and T2-weighted coronal MRI image (right panel) of the right knee showing calcific deposit in the medial collateral ligament.
Images courtesy of Dr Anthony Doyle.

crystals, and differentiation of BCP crystals using this technique requires careful assessment of crystal morphology. False-positive results are common [65]. Other microscopic staining methods such fluorescent dyes and tetracycline-binding methods may improve sensitivity and accuracy, but these assays are not in widespread clinical use [66,67].

Many other methods have been studied and reported to improve detection of BCP crystals (reviewed in [2]). Scanning electron microscopy, transmission electron microscopy, and atomic force microscopy provide improved resolution and sensitivity but are not feasible techniques for routine clinical detection of BCP crystals [53,68,69]. Spectroscopic techniques that have been used to identify BCP crystals in research settings including Raman spectroscopy and Fourier-transform infrared spectroscopy (with or without enhancement using a synchrotron system) [70–72]. These technologies are expensive, and require highly specialized equipment that is not widely available. Calcium/phosphate analysis of synovial fluid samples using colorimetric or spectrophotometric methods may be compromised by interference and artefact [73,74]. X-ray diffraction and radioassays have been developed for research purposes but require complex protocols that are, again, not feasible for routine clinical testing [75,76]. Methods in development include isolation of crystals using bisphosphonate-coated magnetic beads [77].

Principles of treatment of BCP crystal deposition

As described for specific conditions associated with BCP crystals, treatment of acute inflammatory episodes includes NSAIDs and corticosteroids. Although there are no randomized controlled trials, colchicine or IL1 inhibitors may also be of benefit [48].

Removal of crystals is a useful treatment goal. For persistent calcific tendinitis, various strategies for removing focal crystal deposits have clinical efficacy, with clinical trial data supporting the role of US-guided aspiration of calcific deposits [49], ESWT [51], and disodium EDTA-based mesotherapy [50]. However, for syndromes associated with intra-articular BCP crystal deposition, there are no available systemic therapies to promote dissolution of BCP crystals. Phosphocitrate is a naturally occurring compound that inhibits hydroxyapatite crystal formation, and also attenuates many of the cellular responses to BCP crystals *in vitro* [78–81]. In guinea pig model of meniscal calcification, intraperitoneal administration of a formulation of phosphocitrate (CaNaPC) inhibited meniscal calcification and progression of OA [82]. Phosphocitrate can also inhibit disease progression in the *ank/ank* mouse [83]. There are no data to support the use of this compound in humans with BCP crystal associated arthropathies.

The role of BCP crystals in the pathogenesis of osteoarthritis

BCP crystals are frequently identified in joints affected by OA, and are infrequently observed in joints affected by rheumatoid arthritis [84]. Although many different methods have been used to identify these crystals, most studies have reported that calcium-containing crystals are present within synovial fluid of 30–60% of patients with OA [84,85]. BCP crystals are observed more frequently in synovial fluid from joints with more severe OA [86]. In a longitudinal study of sequential synovial fluid examination in patients with OA over a mean duration of 3.6 years, BCP crystals were observed in 23% of synovial fluid samples at first aspiration, and 58% at the final aspiration [86]. In a study of joints with severe OA requiring joint replacement, all cartilage specimens had evidence of mineralization, with the prominent mineral composed of BCP rather than CPP [54]. In these joints, the severity of articular damage closely correlates with the extent of cartilage mineralization. The widespread deposition of BCP crystals in human knee cartilage affected by OA has been confirmed by other groups; with deposition present in all compartments and in both superficial and deep cartilage layers [87]. BCP crystals are also observed in the synovial membranes of patients with OA, including in low-grade disease [20,88]. Although some commentators consider BCP crystals an 'innocent bystander' or epiphenomenon in the pathogenesis of OA [89], others argue that they play an important role in the development and progression of OA [90].

In vitro, BCP crystals induce many processes implicated in OA pathogenesis that collectively promote cartilage catabolism and joint inflammation. As described, these crystals can induce expression of catabolic enzymes such as MMP1 and MMP13 in chondrocytes and fibroblasts [24,25,31,32]. Furthermore, gene expression of tissue inhibitors of metalloproteinases (TIMP1 and TIMP2) is also inhibited in fibroblasts following exposure to BCP crystals [91]. These effects are inhibited by addition of phosphocitrate to cell cultures [91]. In fibroblasts cultured with BCP crystals, induction of cyclooxygenase 1 and 2 is followed by PGE2 production [27,28]. Mature IL1B, an important cytokine in OA pathogenesis, is released by macrophages in response to BCP crystals, following NLRP3 activation [15,16]. Macrophage expression of catabolic enzymes including ADAMTS4, MMP3, and MMP9 is also induced by BCP crystals [20]. BCP crystals also induce proteoglycan loss in human cartilage explants [36].

Animal model data provide some support for the role of BCP crystals in OA pathogenesis. Intra-articular injection of BCP crystals leads to synovial inflammation, cartilage degradation, and chondrocyte apoptosis, in a manner that is independent of IL1 [20]. In meniscectomized mice, increasing deposits of BCP crystals are observed around the joint, and the presence of these crystals is associated with cartilage degradation and IL6 expression [36]. In the *ank/ank* mouse, low extracellular levels of PPi lead to widespread BCP crystal deposition. In this mouse, joint calcification and degeneration are observed [10]. However, these mice also have a number of other phenotypic abnormalities including spontaneous ankyloses of peripheral and axial joints. Similarly, mice with spontaneous ENPP1 mutations have marked hypermineralization abnormalities and OA, but also ossification of the posterior longitudinal ligament of the spine [11].

Many observations support the hypothesis that cartilage injury or damage leads to a positive cycle of chondrocyte MV formation, and induction of genes that promote tissue mineralization [92,93]. Interaction of BCP crystals with joint tissue leads to pro-catabolic and inflammatory pathways that may lead to further tissue damage within the joint, leading to further cycles of BCP crystal formation and joint damage [36]. Induction of chondrocyte hypertrophy leads to increased mineral formation by chondrocytes [54]. Similarly, chondrocytes from osteoarthritic joints express genes that promote mineralization [93]. In joints with severe OA, the ability of chondrocytes to produce BCP crystals closely correlates with the extent of cartilage mineralization [54]. Phosphocitrate, the inhibitor of

BCP crystal formation, can reduce meniscal calcium deposits and arrest OA disease progression in a guinea pig OA model with associated meniscal calcification [82], suggesting that BCP crystal formation may be a useful therapeutic target in OA.

References

1. Ea HK, Liote F. Diagnosis and clinical manifestations of calcium pyrophosphate and basic calcium phosphate crystal deposition diseases. *Rheum Dis Clin North Am* 2014; 40:207–29.
2. MacMullan P, McMahon G, McCarthy G. Detection of basic calcium phosphate crystals in osteoarthritis. *Joint Bone Spine* 2011; 78:358–63.
3. Hsu HH, Anderson HC. The deposition of calcium pyrophosphate and phosphate by matrix vesicles isolated from fetal bovine epiphyseal cartilage. *Calcif Tissue Int* 1984; 36:615–21.
4. Ho AM, Johnson MD, Kingsley DM. Role of the mouse ank gene in control of tissue calcification and arthritis. *Science* 2000; 289:265–70.
5. Siegel SA, Hummel CF, Carty RP. The role of nucleoside triphosphate pyrophosphohydrolase in in vitro nucleoside triphosphate-dependent matrix vesicle calcification. *J Biol Chem* 1983; 258:8601–7.
6. Hessle L, Johnson KA, Anderson HC, et al. Tissue-nonspecific alkaline phosphatase and plasma cell membrane glycoprotein-1 are central antagonistic regulators of bone mineralization. *Proc Natl Acad Sci U S A* 2002; 99:9445–9.
7. St Hilaire C, Ziegler SG, Markello TC, et al. NT5E mutations and arterial calcifications. *N Engl J Med* 2011; 364:432–42.
8. Montessuit C, Caverzasio J, Bonjour JP. Characterization of a Pi transport system in cartilage matrix vesicles. Potential role in the calcification process. *J Biol Chem* 1991; 266:17791–7.
9. Solomon DH, Wilkins RJ, Meredith D, Browning JA. Characterisation of inorganic phosphate transport in bovine articular chondrocytes. *Cell Physiol Biochem* 2007; 20:99–108.
10. Hakim FT, Cranley R, Brown KS, et al. Hereditary joint disorder in progressive ankylosis (ank/ank) mice. I. Association of calcium hydroxyapatite deposition with inflammatory arthropathy. *Arthritis Rheum* 1984; 27:1411–20.
11. Sakamoto M, Hosoda Y, Kojimahara K, Yamazaki T, Yoshimura Y. Arthritis and ankylosis in twy mice with hereditary multiple osteochondral lesions: with special reference to calcium deposition. *Pathol Int* 1994; 44:420–7.
12. Pendleton A, Johnson MD, Hughes A, et al. Mutations in ANKH cause chondrocalcinosis. *Am J Hum Genet* 2002; 71:933–40.
13. Rutsch F, Vaingankar S, Johnson K, et al. PC-1 nucleoside triphosphate pyrophosphohydrolase deficiency in idiopathic infantile arterial calcification. *Am J Pathol* 2001; 158:543–54.
14. Dieppe PA, Crocker P, Huskisson EC, Willoughby DA. Apatite deposition disease. A new arthropathy. *Lancet* 1976; 1:266–9.
15. Pazar B, Ea HK, Narayan S, et al. Basic calcium phosphate crystals induce monocyte/macrophage IL-1beta secretion through the NLRP3 inflammasome in vitro. *J Immunol* 2011; 186:2495–502.
16. Jin C, Frayssinet P, Pelker R, et al. NLRP3 inflammasome plays a critical role in the pathogenesis of hydroxyapatite-associated arthropathy. *Proc Natl Acad Sci U S A* 2011; 108:14867–72.
17. Nadra I, Mason JC, Philippidis P, et al. Proinflammatory activation of macrophages by basic calcium phosphate crystals via protein kinase C and MAP kinase pathways: a vicious cycle of inflammation and arterial calcification? *Circ Res* 2005; 96:1248–56.
18. Cunningham CC, Mills E, Mielke LA, et al. Osteoarthritis-associated basic calcium phosphate crystals induce pro-inflammatory cytokines and damage-associated molecules via activation of Syk and PI3 kinase. *Clin Immunol* 2012; 144:228–36.
19. Martinon F, Petrilli V, Mayor A, Tardivel A, Tschopp J. Gout-associated uric acid crystals activate the NALP3 inflammasome. *Nature* 2006; 440:237–41.
20. Ea HK, Chobaz V, Nguyen C, et al. Pathogenic role of basic calcium phosphate crystals in destructive arthropathies. *PLoS One* 2013; 8:e57352.
21. Cheung HS, Story MT, McCarty DJ. Mitogenic effects of hydroxyapatite and calcium pyrophosphate dihydrate crystals on cultured mammalian cells. *Arthritis Rheum* 1984; 27:668–74.
22. McCarthy GM, Cheung HS, Abel SM, Ryan LM. Basic calcium phosphate crystal-induced collagenase production: role of intracellular crystal dissolution. *Osteoarthritis Cartilage* 1998; 6:205–13.
23. McCarthy GM, Macius AM, Christopherson PA, Ryan LM, Pourmotabbed T. Basic calcium phosphate crystals induce synthesis and secretion of 92 kDa gelatinase (gelatinase B/matrix metalloprotease 9) in human fibroblasts. *Ann Rheum Dis* 1998; 57:56–60.
24. Molloy ES, Morgan MP, Doherty GA, et al. Mechanism of basic calcium phosphate crystal-stimulated matrix metalloproteinase-13 expression by osteoarthritic synovial fibroblasts: inhibition by prostaglandin E2. *Ann Rheum Dis* 2008; 67:1773–9.
25. Cheung HS, Halverson PB, McCarty DJ. Release of collagenase, neutral protease, and prostaglandins from cultured mammalian synovial cells by hydroxyapatite and calcium pyrophosphate dihydrate crystals. *Arthritis Rheum* 1981; 24:1338–44.
26. Reuben PM, Wenger L, Cruz M, Cheung HS. Induction of matrix metalloproteinase-8 in human fibroblasts by basic calcium phosphate and calcium pyrophosphate dihydrate crystals: effect of phosphocitrate. *Connect Tissue Res* 2001; 42:1–12.
27. McCarty DJ, Cheung HS. Prostaglandin (PG) E2 generation by cultured canine synovial fibroblasts exposed to microcrystals containing calcium. *Ann Rheum Dis* 1985; 44:316–20.
28. Molloy ES, Morgan MP, Doherty GA, et al. Mechanism of basic calcium phosphate crystal-stimulated cyclo-oxygenase-1 up-regulation in osteoarthritic synovial fibroblasts. *Rheumatology (Oxford)* 2008; 47:965–71.
29. Cheung HS, Devine TR, Hubbard W. Calcium phosphate particle induction of metalloproteinase and mitogenesis: effect of particle sizes. *Osteoarthritis Cartilage* 1997; 5:145–51.
30. McCarthy GM, Augustine JA, Baldwin AS, et al. Molecular mechanism of basic calcium phosphate crystal-induced activation of human fibroblasts. Role of nuclear factor kappab, activator protein 1, and protein kinase c. *J Biol Chem* 1998; 273:35161–9.
31. Cheung HS, Halverson PB, McCarty DJ. Phagocytosis of hydroxyapatite or calcium pyrophosphate dihydrate crystals by rabbit articular chondrocytes stimulates release of collagenase, neutral protease, and prostaglandins E2 and F2 alpha. *Proc Soc Exp Biol Med* 1983; 173:181–9.
32. McCarthy GM, Westfall PR, Masuda I, Christopherson PA, Cheung HS, Mitchell PG. Basic calcium phosphate crystals activate human osteoarthritic synovial fibroblasts and induce matrix metalloproteinase-13 (collagenase-3) in adult porcine articular chondrocytes. *Ann Rheum Dis* 2001; 60:399–406.
33. Ea HK, Uzan B, Rey C, Liote F. Octacalcium phosphate crystals directly stimulate expression of inducible nitric oxide synthase through p38 and JNK mitogen-activated protein kinases in articular chondrocytes. *Arthritis Res Ther* 2005; 7:R915–26.
34. Ea HK, Monceau V, Camors E, et al. Annexin 5 overexpression increased articular chondrocyte apoptosis induced by basic calcium phosphate crystals. *Ann Rheum Dis* 2008; 67:1617–25.
35. Nguyen C, Lieberherr M, Bordat C, et al. Intracellular calcium oscillations in articular chondrocytes induced by basic calcium phosphate crystals lead to cartilage degradation. *Osteoarthritis Cartilage* 2012; 20:1399–408.
36. Nasi S, So A, Combes C, Daudon M, Busso N. Interleukin-6 and chondrocyte mineralisation act in tandem to promote experimental osteoarthritis. *Ann Rheum Dis* 2015.
37. Painter CF. Subdeltoid bursitis. *Boston Med Surg J* 1907; 156:345–9.
38. McCarty DJ, Jr., Gatter RA. Recurrent acute inflammation associated with focal apatite crystal deposition. *Arthritis Rheum* 1966; 9:804–19.
39. McCarty DJ, Halverson PB, Carrera GF, Brewer BJ, Kozin F. 'Milwaukee shoulder'—association of microspheroids containing hydroxyapatite crystals, active collagenase, and neutral protease with rotator cuff defects. I. Clinical aspects. *Arthritis Rheum* 1981; 24:464–73.

40. Hamada J, Ono W, Tamai K, Saotome K, Hoshino T. Analysis of calcium deposits in calcific periarthritis. *J Rheumatol* 2001; 28:809–13.

41. Bosworth BM. Calcium deposits in the shoulder and subacromial bursitis: a survey of 12,122 shoulders. *JAMA* 1941; 116:2477–82.

42. Refior HJ, Krodel A, Melzer C. Examinations of the pathology of the rotator cuff. *Arch Orthop Trauma Surg* 1987; 106:301–8.

43. Sarkar K, Uhthoff HK. Ultrastructural localization of calcium in calcifying tendinitis. *Arch Pathol Lab Med* 1978; 102:266–9.

44. Gohr CM, Fahey M, Rosenthal AK. Calcific tendonitis: a model. *Connect Tissue Res* 2007; 48:286–91.

45. Uhthoff HK, Loehr JW. Calcific tendinopathy of the rotator cuff: pathogenesis, diagnosis, and management. *J Am Acad Orthop Surg* 1997; 5:183–91.

46. McKendry RJ, Uhthoff HK, Sarkar K, Hyslop PS. Calcifying tendinitis of the shoulder: prognostic value of clinical, histologic, and radiologic features in 57 surgically treated cases. *J Rheumatol* 1982; 9:75–80.

47. Farin PU. Consistency of rotator-cuff calcifications. Observations on plain radiography, sonography, computed tomography, and at needle treatment. *Invest Radiol* 1996; 31:300–4.

48. Zufferey P, So A. A pilot study of IL-1 inhibition in acute calcific periarthritis of the shoulder. *Ann Rheum Dis* 2013; 72:465–7.

49. de Witte PB, Selten JW, Navas A, et al. Calcific tendinitis of the rotator cuff: a randomized controlled trial of ultrasound-guided needling and lavage versus subacromial corticosteroids. *Am J Sports Med* 2013; 41:1665–73.

50. Cacchio A, De Blasis E, Desiati P, et al. Effectiveness of treatment of calcific tendinitis of the shoulder by disodium EDTA. *Arthritis Rheum* 2009; 61:84–91.

51. Bannuru RR, Flavin NE, Vaysbrot E, Harvey W, McAlindon T. High-energy extracorporeal shock-wave therapy for treating chronic calcific tendinitis of the shoulder: a systematic review. *Ann Intern Med* 2014; 160:542–9.

52. Balke M, Bielefeld R, Schmidt C, Dedy N, Liem D. Calcifying tendinitis of the shoulder: midterm results after arthroscopic treatment. *Am J Sports Med* 2012; 40:657–61.

53. Schumacher HR, Smolyo AP, Tse RL, Maurer K. Arthritis associated with apatite crystals. *Ann Intern Med* 1977; 87:411–6.

54. Fuerst M, Bertrand J, Lammers L, et al. Calcification of articular cartilage in human osteoarthritis. *Arthritis Rheum* 2009; 60:2694–703.

55. Halverson PB, Garancis JC, McCarty DJ. Histopathological and ultrastructural studies of synovium in Milwaukee shoulder syndrome—a basic calcium phosphate crystal arthropathy. *Ann Rheum Dis* 1984; 43:734–41.

56. Garancis JC, Cheung HS, Halverson PB, McCarty DJ. 'Milwaukee shoulder'—association of microspheroids containing hydroxyapatite crystals, active collagenase, ad neutral protease with rotator cuff defects. III. Morphologic and biochemical studies of an excised synovium showing chondromatosis. *Arthritis Rheum* 1981; 24:484–91.

57. Epis O, Caporali R, Scire CA, et al. Efficacy of tidal irrigation in Milwaukee shoulder syndrome. *J Rheumatol* 2007; 34:1545–50.

58. Watt I. Radiology of the crystal-associated arthritides. *Ann Rheum Dis* 1983; 42(Suppl 1):73–80.

59. Hall FM, Docken WP, Curtis HW. Calcific tendinitis of the longus coli: diagnosis by CT. *AJR Am J Roentgenol* 1986; 147:742–3.

60. Kraemer EJ, El-Khoury GY. Atypical calcific tendinitis with cortical erosions. *Skeletal Radiol* 2000; 29:690–6.

61. Flemming DJ, Murphey MD, Shekitka KM, et al. Osseous involvement in calcific tendinitis: a retrospective review of 50 cases. *AJR Am J Roentgenol* 2003; 181:965–72.

62. O'Connor PJ, Rankine J, Gibbon WW, et al. Interobserver variation in sonography of the painful shoulder. *J Clin Ultrasound* 2005; 33:53–6.

63. Chiou HJ, Chou YH, Wu JJ, et al. Evaluation of calcific tendonitis of the rotator cuff: role of color Doppler ultrasonography. *J Ultrasound Med* 2002; 21:289–95.

64. Paul H, Reginato AJ, Schumacher HR. Alizarin red S staining as a screening test to detect calcium compounds in synovial fluid. *Arthritis Rheum* 1983; 26:191–200.

65. Gordon C, Swan A, Dieppe P. Detection of crystals in synovial fluids by light microscopy: sensitivity and reliability. *Ann Rheum Dis* 1989; 48:737–42.

66. Hernandez-Santana A, Yavorskyy A, Loughran ST, McCarthy GM, McMahon GP. New approaches in the detection of calcium-containing microcrystals in synovial fluid. *Bioanalysis* 2011; 3:1085–91.

67. Rosenthal AK, Fahey M, Gohr C, et al. Feasibility of a tetracycline-binding method for detecting synovial fluid basic calcium phosphate crystals. *Arthritis Rheum* 2008; 58:3270–4.

68. Cunningham T, Uebelhart D, Very JM, Fallet GH, Vischer TL. Synovial fluid hydroxyapatite crystals: detection thresholds of two methods. *Ann Rheum Dis* 1989; 48:829–31.

69. Blair JM, Sorensen LB, Arnsdorf MF, Lal R. The application of atomic force microscopy for the detection of microcrystals in synovial fluid from patients with recurrent synovitis. *Semin Arthritis Rheum* 1995; 24:359–69.

70. Hornez JC, Chai F, Monchau F, et al. Biological and physico-chemical assessment of hydroxyapatite (HA) with different porosity. *Biomol Eng* 2007; 24:505–9.

71. Muehleman C, Li J, Aigner T, et al. Association between crystals and cartilage degeneration in the ankle. *J Rheumatol* 2008; 35:1108–17.

72. Rosenthal AK, Mattson E, Gohr CM, Hirschmugl CJ. Characterization of articular calcium-containing crystals by synchrotron FTIR. *Osteoarthritis Cartilage* 2008; 16:1395–402.

73. Yavorskyy A, Hernandez-Santana A, Shortt B, McCarthy G, McMahon G. Determination of calcium in synovial fluid samples as an aid to diagnosing osteoarthritis. *Bioanalysis* 2010; 2:189–95.

74. Yavorskyy A, Hernandez-Santana A, McCarthy G, McMahon G. Detection of calcium phosphate crystals in the joint fluid of patients with osteoarthritis—analytical approaches and challenges. *Analyst* 2008; 133:302–18.

75. Calafiori AR, Di Marco G, Martino G, Marotta M. Preparation and characterization of calcium phosphate biomaterials. *J Mater Sci Mater Med* 2007; 18:2331–8.

76. Halverson PB, McCarty DJ. Identification of hydroxyapatite crystals in synovial fluid. *Arthritis Rheum* 1979; 22:389–95.

77. Hernandez-Santana A, Yavorskyy A, Olinyole A, McCarthy GM, McMahon GP. Isolation of calcium phosphate crystals from complex biological fluids using bisphosphonate-modified superparamagnetic beads. *Chem Commun (Camb)* 2008:2686–8.

78. Williams G, Sallis JD. Structure—activity relationship of inhibitors of hydroxyapatite formation. *Biochem J* 1979; 184:181–4.

79. Cheung HS, Sallis JD, Mitchell PG, Struve JA. Inhibition of basic calcium phosphate crystal-induced mitogenesis by phosphocitrate. *Biochem Biophys Res Commun* 1990; 171:20–5.

80. Cheung HS, Sallis JD, Struve JA. Specific inhibition of basic calcium phosphate and calcium pyrophosphate crystal-induction of metalloproteinase synthesis by phosphocitrate. *Biochim Biophys Acta* 1996; 1315:105–11.

81. Morgan MP, Whelan LC, Sallis JD, et al. Basic calcium phosphate crystal-induced prostaglandin E2 production in human fibroblasts: role of cyclooxygenase 1, cyclooxygenase 2, and interleukin-1beta. *Arthritis Rheum* 2004; 50:1642–9.

82. Cheung HS, Sallis JD, Demadis KD, Wierzbicki A. Phosphocitrate blocks calcification-induced articular joint degeneration in a guinea pig model. *Arthritis Rheum* 2006; 54:2452–61.

83. Krug HE, Mahowald ML, Halverson PB, Sallis JD, Cheung HS. Phosphocitrate prevents disease progression in murine progressive ankylosis. *Arthritis Rheum* 1993; 36:1603–11.

84. Swan A, Chapman B, Heap P, Seward H, Dieppe P. Submicroscopic crystals in osteoarthritic synovial fluids. *Ann Rheum Dis* 1994; 53:467–70.

85. Gibilisco PA, Schumacher HR, Jr, Hollander JL, Soper KA. Synovial fluid crystals in osteoarthritis. *Arthritis Rheum* 1985; 28:511–5.

86. Nalbant S, Martinez JA, Kitumnuaypong T, Clayburne G, Sieck M, Schumacher HR, Jr. Synovial fluid features and their relations

to osteoarthritis severity: new findings from sequential studies. *Osteoarthritis Cartilage* 2003; 11:50–4.

87. Nguyen C, Ea HK, Bazin D, Daudon M, Liote F. Osteoarthritis, a basic calcium phosphate crystal-associated arthropathy? Comment on the article by Fuerst et al. *Arthritis Rheum* 2010; 62:2829–30.

88. van Linthoudt D, Beutler A, Clayburne G, Sieck M, Fernandes L, Schumacher HR, Jr. Morphometric studies on synovium in advanced osteoarthritis: is there an association between apatite-like material and collagen deposits? *Clin Exp Rheumatol* 1997; 15:493–7.

89. Pritzker KP. Counterpoint: Hydroxyapatite crystal deposition is not intimately involved in the pathogenesis and progression of human osteoarthritis. *Curr Rheumatol Rep* 2009; 11:148–53.

90. McCarthy GM, Cheung HS. Point: Hydroxyapatite crystal deposition is intimately involved in the pathogenesis and progression of human osteoarthritis. *Curr Rheumatol Rep* 2009; 11:141–7.

91. Bai G, Howell DS, Howard GA, Roos BA, Cheung HS. Basic calcium phosphate crystals up-regulate metalloproteinases but down-regulate tissue inhibitor of metalloproteinase-1 and -2 in human fibroblasts. *Osteoarthritis Cartilage* 2001; 9:416–22.

92. Jubeck B, Gohr C, Fahey M, et al. Promotion of articular cartilage matrix vesicle mineralization by type I collagen. *Arthritis Rheum* 2008; 58:2809–17.

93. Nguyen C, Bazin D, Daudon M, et al. Revisiting spatial distribution and biochemical composition of calcium-containing crystals in human osteoarthritic articular cartilage. *Arthritis Res Ther* 2013; 15:R103.

Index

Tables, figures, and boxes are indicated by an italic *t*, *f*, and *b* following the page number.